World Health Systems

World Health Systems

XIAOMING SUN

WILEY

Published by John Wiley & Sons, Inc., Hoboken, New Jersey.
Published simultaneously in Canada.

For general information on our other products and services or for technical support, please contact our Customer Care Department within the United States at (800) 762-2974, outside the United States at (317) 572-3993, or fax (317) 572-4002.

Wiley publishes in a variety of print and electronic formats and by print-on-demand. Some material included with standard print versions of this book may not be included in e-books or in print-on-demand. If this book refers to media such as a CD or DVD that is not included in the version you purchased, you may download this material at http://booksupport.wiley.com. For more information about Wiley products, visit www.wiley.com.

Library of Congress Cataloging-in-Publication Data is Available:

ISBN 978-1-119-50887-8 (hardback)
ISBN 978-1-119-50890-8 (ePDF)
ISBN 978-1-119-50892-2 (ePub)

Cover Design: Wiley
Cover Image: © Creative-Touch/iStock.com

Printed in the United States of America

V10015190_102919

Contents

PART IV: CHARACTERISTICS OF HEALTH SYSTEMS IN DEVELOPING COUNTRIES

PART V: HEALTH SYSTEMS IN DEVELOPING COUNTRIES

Chapter 18: Health Systems in Seven Asian Countries　765

Foreword

With the advent of the third healthcare revolution and its gradual inclusion in government agendas, the *World Health Report 2013* proposed a key issue of our time, namely, universal health coverage (UHC). The goal of UHC is to provide all people with access to necessary and affordable health services. UHC aims to reduce the inequalities in health coverage within an entire country or area and is a key component in sustainable development and poverty reduction.

As a basic socioeconomic system, a health system is intricately linked with the social, political, and economic development and policies of a specific period in time. It is clear that China is currently in a crucial transitional period of refining a socialist market economy that is operating within the context of rapid industrialization and urbanization. Hence, healthcare reforms in China still face three challenges when resolving the issues of limited access and high costs: First, there is a gap between the high demand for healthcare by the public and the limited capacity of the state. Second, there is a discrepancy between the public's medical needs and the supply of health services. Third, there is a conflict between the satisfaction of medical staff and the satisfaction of the public. A new solution for effectively resolving these differences is to strengthen governance at the source and enhance system construction. By changing the models of healthcare services and health-seeking behaviors, a health system can place greater emphasis on disease prevention and truly shift from a disease-centered model to a health-centered model. This shift, in turn, will enable the health system to achieve the original goal and ultimate target of providing higher-quality healthcare to the population.

There are inherent logical relationships between the healthcare and social security systems of a country and its political system, economic level, traditional history and culture, and other "native" factors. Nevertheless, the global issues encountered by China in healthcare reforms may have also occurred at some stage in certain developed countries or may currently exist in different forms or to different extents in certain developing countries that are also in transition. For example, these issues may involve the relationship between economic development and investment in healthcare, the balanced distribution of health resources, or the establishment of an orderly hierarchical medical system. Tackling these issues will require us to study and understand the recurring patterns in the development of medical and health services and social security systems from a global perspective. We should also draw extensively from the positive experiences of countries at different levels of development and incorporate these experiences within the real-life conditions of China and Shanghai.

This book starts from a multidisciplinary standpoint and provides a comprehensive explanation of the structures of health systems and the determinants of health. This book also summarizes the basic models and selection of world health systems and systematically compares the characteristics of health system models, development processes, reform measures, and performance evaluations of 12 representative developed countries and 18 representative developing countries. In addition, the book summarizes the common characteristics, experiences, insights, and developmental trends of health system reforms in countries with different levels of development in order to reflect on how these countries have overcome the universal challenges that all countries face. Clearly, this discussion is extremely insightful for our current journey as we explore the improvement of new healthcare reforms in China.

Here, three specific questions at different levels, which readers can discuss and explore, may be raised.

The first question is at the macro level: How can effective institutional arrangements between the government and the market be achieved in the field of healthcare? The world does not currently have an answer to this question. This issue is especially sensitive for China, which is now in a key period of transformation, so the slightest mistake in this regard may affect the progress of socioeconomic transition across the entire country. Among developed countries, the National Health Service in the UK emphasizes planned interventions, whereas the US has implemented a commercial health insurance system that focuses on market regulation. Among the BRICS countries (Brazil, Russia, India, China, and South Africa), the systems in China and Brazil are mainly based on the state's macroeconomic control, which is subject to moderate market regulation; India and South Africa primarily rely on the spontaneous regulation of the market; and Russia depends on the joint forces of market incentives and state regulation. However, there are substantial differences in the improvement of health performance among the BRICS countries, and these differences are not significantly associated with national income levels. On the surface, no two countries share the same health system. However, further investigation reveals that it is still possible to classify these systems and to identify the patterns resulting from their institutional development. The formation of these systems is generally closely related to two factors. The first is the country's level of economic development, and the second is the country's choice of political system. Does the country prioritize market competition to improve the efficiency of healthcare services, or does it prioritize balanced planning to improve the equality of healthcare services? Each country has to choose the emphasis on and extent of these two priorities. If we take the level of economic development as the vertical axis and the degree of marketization and planning in the health system as the horizontal axis, each country will find its own position within this coordinate system. This book aims to classify and explain these patterns by comparing the different health systems of different countries.

Are China's healthcare reforms currently experiencing over- or undermarketization? I believe that both aspects are present. Overmarketization is manifested in the imperfect compensation mechanisms of public hospitals, operational chaos in drug production, and artificially high drug prices, which have led to issues of fairness. Undermarketization is manifested in the inability to reflect the value of labor and technology, barriers to institutional approval, and staff turnover, which may result in lower service efficiency.

With regard to basic medical and health services guaranteed by the new healthcare reforms, government leadership should continue to be strengthened for public and quasi-public goods, with simultaneous efforts to resolve internal market failures and inadequacies. For the development of the health service industry, such as private healthcare institutions and high-end medical services, commercial health insurance, biomedicine, and information technology, China should rely more heavily on interventions by the invisible hand of the market to meet public demand for these diversified health services.

The second question is at the meso level: What direction should be taken in the development of administrative systems for health services and health security? In the early twenty-first century, the social and health insurance systems of Japan, Germany, and other countries combined the functions of healthcare and social security, which facilitated the centralization and coordination of health service provision, health insurance, and supervision by the government. Among developing BRICS countries, India has established an integrated health administrative system based on its national conditions (i.e., the Ministry of Health and Family Welfare), and Brazil has also established an administrative system that brings together healthcare, health insurance, and pharmaceuticals under the Ministry of Health. China's health management and health security are currently in a fragmented state. For instance, health insurance is scattered among a number of departments, including the National Health and Family Planning Commission, the People's Insurance Company of China, the Food and Drug Administration, and the Ministry of Civil Affairs, and this fragmentation can easily lead to divided policies and the waste of resources. The relevant departments are more inclined to promote isolated reforms from the perspective of localized interests. Hence, they may fail to integrate effectively into a continuous and coordinated system that is centered on patients' health, which is not beneficial to the efficiency and quality of the overall health system. If China can take advantage of this tide of comprehensive and deepened reforms, discard the obstacles of entrenched interests, and achieve breakthroughs in the organization of the medical and healthcare management systems, then, within the context of a large-department system, will China be able to reap more benefits in the promotion of synergistic and joint reforms in the fields of healthcare, health insurance, and medicine?

The third question is at the micro level: Can the more mature family physician and hierarchical medical system of developed countries be applied to developing countries, and can it be embedded within China's system of health and medical services? Although the family physician system originated in Europe, the US, and other developed countries, it is not exclusive to developed countries. For example, in Latin America, the Cuban government began implementing the family physician system in urban and rural areas in 1984 and promoted the system nationwide in the 1990s. In the face of China's aging population, the continuous increase in health needs, and the rise of medical costs, it is necessary to strategically shift forward the allocation of health resources, encourage high-quality medical resources to trickle down, strengthen the construction of the primary health care system, and enhance the public's health awareness and competency.

These measures will gradually realize the transformation from disease insurance to health insurance discussed in this book, which will ensure that health services will be more efficient, thereby reducing the economic burden of healthcare on China's residents. China's policy actions in the new healthcare reforms are to "safeguard basic health needs, strengthen primary health care, and build a sound mechanism" in order to establish an orderly and effective system of medical and health services. The community general practitioner (GP) system may be a path for China's future healthcare reforms. Since the new healthcare reforms, Shanghai has been at the forefront of the country in its implementation of the GP system, and it has achieved a certain level of progress. However, many obstacles and doubts still remain. For example, there is the issue of introducing effective policies to ensure that becoming a community GP is the preferred career choice for an excellent doctor. In that case, the public will feel confident seeking medical treatments from these GPs, and only critically ill patients or difficult cases will be referred by the GPs to specialists in large hospitals.

Another issue is ensuring that the health insurance payment mechanism for GP services can be transformed from a fee-for-service system to the more advanced capitation system in order to implement a healthcare system that involves designated healthcare institutions, community first-contact care, and hierarchical referral systems. Finally, there is the issue of constructing the internal interest-oriented mechanisms of regional medical consortiums.

Can strong evidence or reasonable solutions to address these questions be found in this book? Should China rely on the experiences and initiatives of developed countries, or are the practices and patterns of developing countries more applicable? Where can we find more scientific and more rigorous evidence to support the government's determination to promote the reform ideas mentioned above? Readers who are interested in these questions can refer to the 2005 first edition and 2012 second edition of *Medical Service and Insurance System in Developed Countries and Areas*, which can be read in conjunction with this book. Different readers may have different reactions. This book is based on the admirable international vision upheld by Dr. XIAOMING SUN, his keen long-term observations on the reforms and developmental trends in international health systems, and his reflections on these observations, with a special emphasis on his focused research on developing countries in recent years. It systematically introduces much of the latest objective data, reform content, and empirical analysis, which further enables the book to be more comprehensive, rich, and detailed. Regardless of whether the readers are policymakers, scholars, or even members of the public, this book may provide each and every one of its readers with a valuable basis for the implementation of new healthcare reforms. Therefore, I am very glad to have been given the opportunity to write this Foreword. I also urge all readers to share with the author any ideas or opinions you may have after reading this book, which will allow us to contemplate and design more rational and scientific models together. Doing so will help us to promote new healthcare reforms in Shanghai, or even in China, and will encourage the active offering of advice and suggestions to the relevant decision-making departments of the government, thus enabling us to contribute to China's early establishment of a complete, scientific, and rational health system.

Professor YONGHAO GUI
Vice President of Fudan University
Dean of Shanghai Medical College
May 2019

Preface

China's national conditions have caused the vast majority of high-ranking health management positions to be held by medical experts. Each one of these experts had to face certain inner struggles when they were transferred from a clinical position to a management position, because being a physician is a skilled and dignified profession that is noble and highly respected. Thus, at the start of their appointments, such experts believe that health management is an experience that depends merely on prestige and power or that the work involved is more procedural and routine, with a low level of technical content. I was no exception. In the late 1980s, I faced these struggles as well when I transitioned from a role as a physician to a health management position.

When I was first introduced to the field of health management, my attitude was fundamentally changed. I began to like this discipline and gradually became hooked on it, even to the point of losing control. In early 1990, I was fortunate enough to receive the Sino-British Friendship Scholarship, which allowed me to systematically focus on this subject in the UK. Through this study, I discovered an inexhaustible system of scientific knowledge, and I came to realize that the research, innovation, and practice of health and insurance systems in the world were as diverse, variable, and progressive as art. This field had a "soul" that was filled with endless appeal.

After many years of study and accumulation, I wrote and published *Medical Service and Insurance System in Developed Countries and Areas* in 2005 and completed the revised edition, which included more novel and comprehensive content, in 2012. The book received a warm response and encouragement from academic peers, authorities related to healthcare reforms, and its readers. During the preparation work for the revised edition, I was inspired by Professor Liang Hong from Fudan University, which led to the following notion: Can further research be conducted on the health services and social security systems of developing countries? Under the constraints of economic development, have the vast number of developing countries also accumulated relevant experiences? Based on the considerations of the following aspects, I believe that the answer is affirmative.

First, the twenty-first century is the century of life and health sciences. On a micro level, this topic is reflected in the rapid development of gene technology. On a meso level, it is manifested as the dramatic improvements in new diagnostic and treatment methods, such as the rapid breakthroughs and popularization of organ transplants, catheterization, and minimally invasive techniques as well as the rapid progress of enhanced prevention and control in public health. On a macro level, the focus is on the design, practice, and continuous reform and improvement of health services and health insurance systems. Among the 191 sovereign nations in the world, no two countries have completely identical medical and health systems. The establishment and development of a system is determined by the core values of a country and its citizens. This is also the case for the reformation of health and social security systems. The goal is to pursue fairness and efficiency. However, both cannot be achieved simultaneously, and a compromise has to be reached between the two. If this were not the case, there would not be so many systems in the world, and there would not be such extensive debates that make healthcare reform a global challenge. The US system, which emphasizes market efficiency, and the UK system, which emphasizes equitable planning, are the two most typical extremes of the numerous systems that exist in the world. The general directions of their current reforms are to learn from each other's strengths but to also abide by the bottom lines of their value orientations in order to take small steps toward a middle ground. The systems of other developed countries and areas are somewhere in between these two extreme systems. Of these systems, the most representative are the German and Canadian systems, and the others differ only in the extent of their tendencies in either direction. Over the past decade, the general orientation of global healthcare reforms has been to emphasize equitable planning and the responsibilities of the government due to the belief that people's right to health is part of their right to life. Hence, a certain level of efficiency can be sacrificed to ensure that each person's right to life is treated equally.

Since the 1990s, the economies of developing countries have generally shown continuous and rapid development, and their strengths have significantly increased. For example, in the past 10 years, the economic growth of Asian countries, such as China and India, has far outstripped the average levels of OECD countries. These countries are greatly influencing and promoting the reshuffling of global interests. Some studies have predicted that, by 2050, BRICS countries (Brazil, Russia, India, China, and South Africa) will be ranked as the world's strongest economies. Hence, there is reason to believe that the socioeconomic development of and the progress of civilization in developing countries will receive increasing international attention and concern. Within this overarching context, I believe that it will be consistent with the development needs of the future era if researchers are able to comprehensively and systematically present and analyze the models and reforms of health systems in developing countries at a higher level.

Second, from a practical standpoint, the new round of healthcare reforms in China has entered the "deep-water zone" and the "conflict-of-interest zone." Based on the country's national conditions, we need to absorb the concepts or practices of healthcare reforms that have been implemented internationally and have shown good results and that can also be reproduced and promoted in China. Although the numerous developing countries have different national conditions, all of them have undeveloped socioeconomic conditions, and, hence, all are faced with similar issues, such as economic transformation, a widening wealth gap, a large population with high mobility, an urban–rural dual structure, and so on. Each country is striving to try different solutions. Here, perhaps, lie the experiences and patterns in healthcare reforms that are suitable for us to learn from! For example, this book mentions that the healthcare institutions in South Africa and Egypt are implementing the separation of medical services and drug sales and the rigorous development of commercial health insurance; some developing countries in Eastern Europe and Latin America are developing the family physician system and have exerted good control over the increase in medical costs. These practical journeys in reform have immense research value in helping us to construct a medical and health system with both Chinese and contemporary characteristics.

Just as the models of developed countries should not be imitated, the paths taken by developing countries should also be modified. By analyzing both of these models in parallel and making mutual references, we can begin from a higher standpoint and can also adopt more rational thinking. By taking a wider perspective in research, we can present a more objective picture. After analyzing developing countries to a certain extent, this thought prompted me to extract the results from research on both types of countries and integrate them in this one book, *World Health Systems*. The value orientations contained within these systems are inextricably linked with the theories of political science and economics and are rooted within their respective socioeconomic development levels. Therefore, the point of departure for this book is still economic theory supplemented by political science, with the aim of conducting an in-depth exploration of health systems and reform measures that can balance both fairness and efficiency.

It should be noted that in the 30 years since the 1980s, reformation of the health and social security systems in developed countries and areas was relatively active. Various theories and reform practices were fully manifested during this period, and, hence, they comprise the foundation of the evolution and formation of current models. Therefore, 600 articles of the greatest significance have been carefully selected for this book from among the few thousand articles that have been published worldwide in the past 30 years. Referencing, collation, and analyses were then conducted by combining these articles with my own observations, experiences, and research during my 10 years of studies abroad in more than a dozen countries, including the UK, the US, Canada, and Australia. Furthermore, I have also focused on collecting and compiling official global socioeconomic development and health statistics released by the WHO, UNICEF, the World Bank, and other organizations, as well as health survey reports and policy options for specific areas or individual countries published by third-party nongovernmental organizations.

In contrast, due to economic and system changes, culture, language, and a variety of factors, data related to the status and reformation of health systems in developing countries are significantly sparser than data in developed countries are. In particular, it is difficult to find international reports related to countries with less developed economies, which has brought about significant difficulties when writing this book. Therefore, in the selection of typical developing countries, the BRICS countries were regarded as the iconic, leading countries in order to combine the principles of representativeness and regional balance.

This book is divided into five parts and includes a total of 21 chapters.

Part I focuses on analyzing the theoretical basis for the establishment of world health systems, introducing the world's socioeconomic development and health status on a macro level, and comprehensively elaborating the institutional structures of health systems and the determinants of health. In addition, Part I summarizes the basic models and selection of world health systems, policies for social medical aid systems, and the common characteristics of and trends in the health system reforms of countries with different levels of development. Parts II and III discuss the health systems of developed countries and areas. A systematic summary is presented on the role played by the governments of developed countries in the health service market, the basic policies of drug administration, and the models of healthcare cost containment. Then, using a storyboard format, we focus on each representative developed country and area and perform an in-depth analysis on the characteristics of its health system model. The analysis includes the mode of operation and development of the health policy systems and the reform measures and performance evaluations at different stages. The aim is to present readers with a detailed description of each school of thought in order to extract the differences and features of different developed countries and areas. Parts IV and V discuss the health systems of developing countries, with a focus on the comparative study of the health service systems and their reform outcomes in BRICS countries. An overview is presented on the insights from the reform experiences of the health services and social security systems of developing countries. In addition, we explore the main structures, features, and value orientations of future reforms in the health systems of 18 representative developing countries.

Today, health economics and health management have become scientific disciplines with strict definitions and formal requirements in their quantitative methods and their systematic discussions. An increasing number of fields are involved in these sciences, and more esoteric methods are being used. This book focuses on introducing the ways of asking questions and the methods of solving problems that are employed by health and health insurance authorities in countries and areas with different levels of development. The ultimate aim of this book is to include a wide range of different perspectives and to be easily accessible to a wide audience. A detailed reference index has also been included at the end of the book, and interested readers may refer to the original literature.

I would like to express my gratitude to my alma maters, the Keele University Center of Health Planning and Management, the University of Leeds Nuffield Institute of Health Sciences, and the Harvard School of Public Health. Not only have the outstanding experts and professors in these institutions nurtured my academic talent, scientific thinking, and practical abilities, but they have also provided a large number of valuable references and data. During the process of writing this book, I have received the support of several leaders, experts, and scholars in China and abroad, especially that of the vice president of Fudan University, Professor Gui Yong-Hao, who also penned the Foreword. Professor Gui Yong-Hao has been a collaborator of mine for many years and has provided many valuable suggestions. In addition, I am grateful for the unwavering support of my colleagues at the Pudong Institute for Health Development, including Lou Ji-Quan, the executive vice president; Zhang Yi-Min; Li Yan-Ting; Liu Shan-Shan; Jing Li-Mei; Shu Zhi-Qun; Bai Jie; Ding Ye; and Qiao Yun. Dr. Zhang Yi-Min, in particular, assisted me by revising the logical framework of the entire book and undertaking manuscript compilation. In addition, I would like to thank Lei Peng, Zou Tao, Wang Xi, Chen Xi, Zhang Fen, Geng Huai-Zong, Lu Wei, Huang Jiao-Ling, and Liu Rong, who were involved in the data collection, data processing, and proofreading of some chapters. Furthermore, I am grateful for my colleagues at the original Shanghai Municipal Health Bureau, who provided their assistance in the writing of the first two editions of the monograph on developed countries and areas. I hereby express my sincerest gratitude for your hard work and selfless help.

Due to the wide range of areas, abundant statistics, and numerous references covered in this book, as well as the author's limited awareness and knowledge, it is inevitable that many mistakes will be made. I invite all experts, peers, and general readers to correct any mistakes they encounter.

XIAOMING SUN
May 2019

About the Book

This book is divided into five parts – Overview, Characteristics of Health Systems in Developed Countries and Areas, Health Systems in Developed Countries and Areas, Characteristics of Health Systems in Developing Countries, and Health Systems in Developing Countries – which are divided into a total of 21 chapters.

Part I is the book's overview and includes six chapters. In this part, we explore the theoretical basis for the establishment of world health systems from a multidisciplinary perspective, introduce the world's socioeconomic development and health status on a macro level, and comprehensively elaborate the institutional structures of health systems and determinants of health. In addition, Part I also summarizes the basic models and selection of world health systems, the policies for social medical aid systems, and the common characteristics of and trends in health system reforms in countries with different levels of development.

Parts II and III include eight chapters and mainly focus on the health systems of developed countries and areas. First, we present a systematic summary of the role played by the governments of developed countries in the health service market, basic policies of drug administration, and models of healthcare cost containment. Based on the classification of health systems into five categories (national health service, social health insurance, commercial health insurance, savings health insurance, and other improved models), we use a storyboard format to focus on each representative developed country and area (the UK, Canada, Australia, Sweden, Germany, France, Japan, Poland, the US, Singapore, Hong Kong, and Taiwan) in order to perform an in-depth analysis of the characteristics of each country's health system model. The analysis includes the mode of operation and development of the health policy systems and the reform measures and performance evaluations at different stages. The aim is to present readers with a detailed description of each school of thought in order to extract the differences and features of different developed countries and areas.

Parts IV and V include seven chapters and mainly focus on describing the health systems of developing countries. We provide definitions of the social formations and structures of developing countries and focus on the comparative study of the health service systems and their reform outcomes in the BRICS countries (Brazil, Russia, India, China, and South Africa). An overview of insights from the reform experiences of the health services and social security systems of developing countries will also be presented. In addition, we perform detailed and in-depth explorations of the main structures, features, and value orientations of future reforms in the health systems of 18 representative developing countries. Like the iconic BRICS countries, these countries are grouped into four regions – namely, Asia (China, India, Thailand, Vietnam, the Philippines, Armenia, and Kyrgyzstan), Africa (South Africa, Egypt, and Morocco), Europe (Russia, Hungary, the Czech Republic, and Bulgaria), and America (Brazil, Cuba, Chile, and Mexico).

About the Author

XIAOMING SUN is Shanghainese. He graduated from Shanghai Medical University in the 1980s with a Bachelor of Medicine. He furthered his studies in the UK between 1990 and 1997. In 1993, he received a Master's in General Practice (M.Sc.) from the University of Leeds. In 1996, he was awarded a PhD in Health Planning and Management from Keele University and remained at the university as a Research Fellow. During his time in the UK, he joined the Royal Society of Medicine, where he began attending international academic conferences and publishing academic papers. From 2007–2008, he was a Takemi Fellow at the Harvard School of Public Health, where he conducted research and practice for one year. In 1997, he was employed by the Shanghai Municipal People's Government and undertook management in the health administration department. He was promoted to chief physician in 2000. In 2005, he became a professor at Fudan University and a doctoral supervisor at the School of Public Health, as well as a professor and chief physician at Zhongshan Hospital, which is affiliated with Fudan University. In 2013, he was a doctoral supervisor for the Department of General Practice at Fudan University. In addition, he has also served as the vice president of the Shanghai Medical Association, the vice president of the Shanghai Medical Doctor Association, the vice chairman and committee member of the Chinese Medical Association General Practice Branch, the president of the Shanghai Community Health Association, and in other roles.

PART ONE

Overview

HEALTH SYSTEMS ARE CLOSELY related to human survival, development, and the quality of life. Not only is the healthy development of humans the primary condition for the development of social productivity, it is also the ultimate goal of all social production activities performed by humans.

At the turn of the twenty-first century, the development and reform of health systems in all countries worldwide became a topic of great concern. Healthcare reform in the US was one of the three issues raised by President Obama during his presidential election, and it was passed by Congress in March 2010. These healthcare reforms ultimately achieved the dream of universal health insurance. The specific schemes that were implemented included establishing health insurance exchanges, reforming commercial health insurance, improving the quality of medical and health services, placing greater emphasis on disease prevention, and encouraging rehabilitation in the community or at home. The draft bill proposed the establishment of public health insurance and regulated the transfer from private to public health insurance. It imposes a health insurance mandate on US residents that does not permit insurance companies to deny coverage or increase premiums for individuals with preexisting conditions. The entire reform process was convoluted and fraught with difficulties. Hillary Clinton, who was responsible for healthcare and insurance reforms during the Clinton presidency, wrote in her memoirs, "The problem of reform was like Mount Everest in the field of human social policy." The healthcare reforms advocated by Obama have also been constantly hampered by the Republicans. The election of Donald J. Trump – who promised during his campaign to dismantle "Obamacare" – posed the stiffest challenge yet for the landmark bill. And the future of Obamacare remains unclear. Thus, it can be said that the reform of the US healthcare system has been extremely challenging.

The goals and principles of healthcare reform are the same in all countries. On the one hand, when the government leads and promotes reforms, the health system needs to continue meeting the health needs of the people in a fair, accessible, and efficient manner,

1

thereby improving health levels and promoting the progress of medical science and technology. On the other hand, the government must ensure that the costs are not too high; maintain a fiscal balance; regulate the burdens borne by the government, businesses, and individuals; guarantee the balance of payments of social insurance funds; and maintain social stability. Reform is precisely this balance of interests and has to be implemented with great care. With China's recent socioeconomic development, its total GDP is now the second largest in the world, and, hence, this steady development should tend to increase the government's financial investment to improve the level of health security and reduce the healthcare burden on individuals, especially those with serious illnesses. At the same time, China should also emphasize the development of community health and general medicine, ensure that health resources and patient treatment trickle down, and reform the payment methods for health insurance, thereby achieving the containment of total healthcare costs.

China is also at a crucial juncture in healthcare and health insurance system reforms and is faced with a global problem, the conflict between continuously meeting the public's health needs and effectively containing the rapid growth in healthcare costs. The Shanghai Municipal Health Bureau often proudly states, "We are using the economic capacity of a developing country to maintain the health levels of developed countries and areas." However, there are many contradictions and crises hidden behind these words. The medical and health industries need to flourish, but there is a relative lack of investment and compensation. The health needs of the public need to be met, but the corresponding health insurance is still insufficient in terms of breadth and depth. The government's positive investment in and compensation of healthcare institutions is still not a smooth process, whereas the fierce competition in the healthcare market and the demands of modernization have forced healthcare institutions to seek compensation from society and the people. These various challenges have gradually increased, leading to conflicts between the healthcare and health insurance systems and the needs and capacity of society. Increasing attention has been given to the limited accessibility to and high costs of healthcare, and the calls for reform have grown louder and, thus, have finally placed healthcare reforms on the government's agenda. This increasing attention necessitates the reexamination of our current conflicts and conundrums from a theoretical level while also drawing from the experiences and lessons of reform practices in developed countries and areas. In reality, a number of similar contradictions and problems have already arisen during the development of the healthcare services and health insurance industries in developed countries and areas. Moreover, different types of reforms have been proposed, intensely debated, and implemented. Other developing countries, especially the BRICS countries (Brazil, Russia, India, China, and South Africa), are now also facing similar issues. These experiences and lessons will benefit the theoretical research and reform practices in China's health industry.

The US, European nations, and other developed countries have employed the theories and principles of economics, sociology, and public policy to conduct analysis and research on the health and insurance systems. This discipline has developed rapidly over the past 30 years. Many well-known universities have established corresponding institutes and academic groups that have conducted extensive research and practice, leading to the publication of numerous academic papers and study results. Thus, a relatively complete discipline has been formed. As health services and insurance systems usually fall within the domain of the public sector, developed countries and areas have paid more attention to macro-level policy research. Hence, more studies have focused on analyzing and solving problems from the perspectives of resource utilization efficiency and fair and accessible services.

CHAPTER ONE

Theoretical Foundations for the Establishment of World Health Systems

SECTION I. THEORIES OF ECONOMIC DEVELOPMENT

Since the 1930s, five major schools of economics have deeply influenced and dominated the establishment and transformation of the healthcare and insurance systems in developed countries and areas. These schools of economics have become the main theoretical basis for the analysis and evaluation of each country's healthcare and insurance system. The theories of economic development since the 1990s, in particular, have had an even more profound impact.

"Economic development" refers to the modernization process of a country's economic and social structure that is based on economic growth. In other words, it is the balanced, sustainable, and coordinated development of a country's economic, political, sociocultural, environmental, and structural changes. Indicators for measuring economic development include not only indicators of economic growth but also indicators of social development, such as the total population size and net population growth, the domestic development index, the urbanization level, the tertiary industrial structure, residents' living conditions, the number of doctors per 1,000 people, the average population life expectancy, the government integrity index, and so on; indicators of educational development, such as total expenditure on public education as a percentage of GDP, national average years of schooling, the percentage of current college students in the college-age population, and so on; indicators of social equality and stability, such as the Gini coefficient, Engel's coefficient, gross national happiness, the index of sustainable economic welfare, the income gap warning line, income hierarchy standards, the poverty incidence, social security coverage, and so on; and environmental indicators, such as natural resource and energy efficiency, the environmental pollution composite index, and so on.

The main theoretical bases for economic development include Marx's theory of human needs and all-round development, the theory of balanced growth, the theory of the share economy (Weitzman et al.), theories of innovation (e.g., institutional innovation theory by

3

North et al. and technological innovation theory by Schumpeter et al.), theories of sustainable development (e.g., coordinated development of population, resources, and environment; cost-of-growth theory; return-to-nature theory; the theory of sustainable improvement in the human quality of life; and ecological development theory), and so on.

The theory of economic development, in a narrow sense, is development economics. This theory studies the industrialization process of less economically developed countries, which involves replacing an agricultural economy, which is based on individual manual production, with an industrial economy, which is based on machine production. From a historical perspective, developed countries have generally undergone three important stages of economic development, which have also formed three different modes of economic development.

The first mode of economic development involves models driven by the input of production factors and capital investment. The time period of this mode of development lasted approximately from the Industrial Revolution in the late eighteenth century until the beginning of the Second Industrial Revolution in the late nineteenth century. The historical background for this mode of economic development was the rise of the Industrial Revolution, which ushered in the replacement of workshop craft production with large machine production. Economic development in this stage required extensive machine manufacturing and the support of other heavy industries. The main driving force of economic development was manifested as high investment-driven growth.

The second mode of economic development involves models driven by technological innovation. The time period of this mode of development began around the late nineteenth century and ended in the mid-twentieth century. During this stage, limitations in the factors of production meant that economic growth based on the input of resources became unsustainable. Hence, the driving force of economic development became technological improvements and increased production efficiency.

The third mode of economic development involves models driven by information technology. The time period for this mode of development began around the 1950s and continues to the present. The main representatives of this stage of development are early-industrialized developed countries. These countries achieved industrialization at an earlier stage and have gradually entered the information age, which is characterized by the knowledge economy. The driving force of economic growth during this period is mostly based on information technology centered on the Internet and the application of high-end technology.

In a broader sense, the theory of economic development is the theory of the modernization process of a country's economic and social structure, which is based on economic growth.

1. Classical Political Economics

As the economic study of the transition from workshop craft production to large-scale mechanized production, the classical political economics of the UK are the predecessor to modern theories of economic development. The core of economic development theory in classical political economics is the idea that economic growth arises from the interaction between capital accumulation and the division of labor. That is, capital accumulation drives the specialization of production and the division of labor. The division of labor, in turn, enables society to generate greater capital accumulation by increasing total output and allows capital to flow towards production areas with the highest efficiency, thereby forming a positive cycle of economic development. In his discourse on how to increase national wealth, Adam Smith stated that there are two primary means by which to increase wealth. The first is to improve labor productivity through the division of labor, and the second is to increase the number of people engaged in productive labor. The theory of economic development in classical political economics encompasses three major features: (1) Its methods of analysis do not merely involve the analysis of socioeconomic development from an economic perspective but also include the comprehensive examination of various factors influencing economic development, including society, political systems, and ethics. (2) Classical political economics holds that economic development is a process that involves the integration of internal factors, such as labor, capital, and land, and external factors, such as technological changes and socioeconomic systems. Economic development always involves the confrontations of power and conflicts of interest among different economic agents. Hence, the process of economic development is fraught with contradictions and conflicts. Thus, a reasonable system should be established to legally regulate the power relations among different economic agents in order to ensure the normal operation of economic activities and to effectively achieve economic development. (3) Classical political economics holds that economic activities and economic development are the processes resulting from human rationality. To the "economic man," who seeks to maximize his own interests, rationality is the intrinsic motivation for and fundamental guarantee of economic activity and economic development. The economic man is an abstraction of the average person in economic life who can perform calculations, is rational, and pursues his self-interests or maximizes his utility. The economic activity of the economic man is rational behavior. The pursuit of self-interest is the fundamental and universal motivation that drives the economic behavior of humans. Economic agents who engage in production and exchange are all rational individuals pursuing their self-interest, and each economic man will attempt to obtain the maximum benefit at minimal cost. Given the premise of a natural order (e.g., market mechanisms and good legal and social systems), the free actions of economic man in pursuit of maximizing his self-interests will drive economic development and maximize social benefits. Therefore, economic development should necessarily be a spontaneous and harmonious process.

Classical political economics propose that private property rights and free competition systems are the most suitable social systems for the self-serving nature and profit-oriented rationality of humans. Therefore, this school of thought advocates for the establishment and protection of private property rights and free competition systems, the reduction of government intervention in the economy, and the freedom of the "invisible hand" to guide economic growth, thereby consolidating and developing the capitalist mode of production. In general terms, the theory of economic development in classical political economics holds that rationality determines the system, and the system achieves rationality. Its theoretical paradigm of economic development is the integrated paradigm that combines rationalism and institutionalism – that is, an institutionalism paradigm based on rationality. This basic feature of economic development theory in classical political economics later became the historical origin of two major paradigms in economic development – the institutionalism paradigm and the rationalism paradigm.

Since the mid-1980s, a number of development economists have used institutional structure as a research methodology to study the issues of economic development in different countries. They believe that a key reason that developing countries are less developed is the lack of efficient political and economic systems, such as a property rights system. If departments providing public goods are too uniform, the mechanisms of competition will be lacking. If power is too concentrated, any mistake in decision-making will have an overall impact, resulting in great losses. Imperfect and unsound market systems and market institutions distort price signals and hinder fair competition. Development economists propose that in the economic development of developing countries, increases in the rate of capital accumulation must also be accompanied by corresponding and extremely important changes to systems and institutions. In fact, in some sense, institutional reform plays an even more important role in economic development than does capital accumulation.

Neo-institutionalism states that institutions have three main functions in economic development. First, institutions can provide legal protection for physical and intellectual property, encourage innovation, and form the driving force of development. Second, institutions can influence the market through laws, rules, and ethical norms, thereby increasing the efficiency of resource allocation. Third, institutions can increase information transparency using rules, such that all individuals are able to make more accurate judgments about the behavioral responses of others and of society in general. The analytical paradigm of neo-institutionalism emphasizes the endogenous effects of institutional and temporal factors and believes that institutions are important. Not only do institutions determine the inter-relations among people, but they also form the incentive structure for political, economic, and social transactions. Therefore, neo-institutionalism focuses on factors that determine economic performance, such as institutional incentives and information.

2. Welfare Economics

(1) Welfare Economics and Its Advocacy of Social Security Policy

The publication of *The Economics of Welfare* by Pigou in 1920 was the hallmark of welfare economics. Pigou defined the subject of welfare economics as the study of enhancing the economic welfare of the world or of a country. Based on the theory of cardinal marginal utility, Pigou proposed two fundamental theorems of welfare. The first is that the higher the total national income, the greater the social and economic welfare, and the second is that the more equalized the distribution of national income, the greater the social and economic welfare. He believed that economic welfare is determined to a large extent by the amount of national income and the distribution of national income among the members of society. Therefore, in order to increase economic welfare, production should increase total national income, and inequalities in the distribution of national income must be eliminated.

Pigou proposed that during the process of income redistribution, the increase in utility received by the poor is greater than the loss of utility experienced by the wealthy, so the total utility of society increases. Hence, social security policy that involves income redistribution will expand a country's economic welfare. In view of this notion, he advocated the following ideas with regard to social security: (1) increasing the necessary monetary subsidies to improve the labor conditions of workers, such that workers receive the appropriate material assistance and social services for illness, disability, unemployment, and pension; (2) imposing a progressive income tax on wealthy individuals with high incomes and increasing unemployment benefits and social relief for low-income workers or individuals who have lost the ability to work, so as to achieve the equalization of income and, hence, increase general welfare; (3) implementing a universal social security system, or a system of universal subsidy based on a minimum income, thereby achieving social equity through effective income transfer payments.

Pigou's welfare economics can be regarded as the most important theoretical foundation for the social security systems of developed countries and areas. These ideas have had a profound impact on the establishment and development of social security in all countries.

Following the economic crisis of the Western world from 1929 to 1933, economists from the UK, the US, and other countries made extensive modifications and additions to welfare economics within this new historical context. It is generally accepted that the notion of welfare economics established by Kaldor, Hicks, Lerner, and Scitovsky on the basis of the Pareto principle is known as new welfare economics.

Over the past 20 years, Western economists have focused their discourse on the theory of external economies, the theory of the second best, the theory of relative welfare, the theory of the equity-efficiency trade-off, the theory of macro welfare, and other topics in welfare economics. In their view, the state can achieve the rational allocation of resources through government interventions in price and output adjustments. Although this allocation system may seem unreasonable from certain perspectives, any further changes may lead to even more unreasonable conditions.

Despite the substantial differences between the theories of new and old welfare economics, their starting points in welfarism, that is, the realization of equality, efficiency, and social welfare, are interlinked.

In summary, the value orientations of social security theory in welfarism are as follows:

1. **Equality.** The most prominent feature of Western social security theory is the predominant position occupied by the relationship between equality and efficiency in economic research. In particular, the economic theory of social security uses equality as its starting point, while welfare economics also uses social equality as its starting point to argue for the maximization of social welfare. This field considers social security to function as a mechanism for security and stability in order to meet the goal of social equality in order to compensate for the defects of market allocation. Therefore, social security must be considered a basic right and obligation of citizens that must be safeguarded in the law and enforced. Welfare economics advocates for the principle of a progressive income tax and a system of interpersonal income transfer payments, which forms a unique ideology of "robbing the rich and giving to the poor." This ideology is still the theoretical foundation for the social security systems of many countries to this day.

2. **Universality.** Welfarism emphasizes the universality of social welfare and the concepts of humanitarianism and human rights. Its service recipients are all members of society. The universality of social security is manifested in two ways. First, social security is a basic human right. Hence, it should be freely available to all, and no group should be excluded due to differences in race, gender, occupation, age, and so on. Second, the threshold of the social security system should be low, and the system should be easily accessible to members of society. It should be freely available to all in theoretical terms but is difficult to access in reality.

3. **Welfare.** The implementation of the welfare state is the best interpretation of the theories of welfare social security. Welfarism asserts that the goal of social security is to safeguard the security of every citizen from birth to death for all aspects of life and possible risks, including illnesses, disasters, old age, childbirth, death, widowhood, loneliness, disability, and so on. The welfare of social security is manifested in three ways. The first is that individuals do not pay or pay low levels of social security fees; welfare expenses are essentially borne by enterprises and the government. The second is the comprehensiveness of the social security program, and programs with high standards generally include "cradle-to-grave" coverage. The third is that the aim of social security is not purely to prevent and eliminate poverty but also to maintain the quality of life of the population at a certain standard and to enhance individuals' senses of security. Thus, the aim is not only to meet the people's social security needs but also to satisfy their social welfare needs.

The equality, universality, and welfare advocated by welfarism are, in essence, unified by equality, which serves as its cornerstone. Universality and welfare are the rational extensions of equality. To this day, equality remains the core foundation for the social security systems of most countries in the world. This fact is precisely the reason why social welfare ideology has been regarded as the origin and mainstream thought of social security theory.

(2) Beveridge's Main Theory of the Welfare State

The term "welfare state" was coined in 1941 by the British Archbishop of Canterbury William Temple in his book *Citizen and Churchman*. The welfare state refers to the concept whereby material goods are produced by enterprises, whereas the government provides an increasing number of social services and infrastructure improvements that are indispensable to raising the standards of civilization and culture, including social security, public health care, housing, cultural education, and so on. The aim of establishing a welfare state is to consciously utilize the strength of political power, organization, and management to rectify the shortcomings of allocations by market mechanisms for powerless workers, thereby providing particular members of society with material assistance. It is generally accepted that the majority of developed countries began moving towards the welfare state after World War II.

In 1941, the UK government commissioned Professor Beveridge, who was the former Director of the Labor Exchanges and Director of the London School of Economics, to formulate a plan for post-war social security. At the end of 1942, he published a report entitled "Social Insurance and Allied Services," which is also known as the Beveridge Report. Its central concept is that "social security should aim at guaranteeing the minimum income needed for subsistence"; "social security means security of income up to a minimum standard"; and "social insurance and national assistance organized by the State are designed to guarantee . . . a basic income for subsistence." The report recommended that UK social policy should aim to abolish the five Giant Evils: want, disease, squalor, ignorance, and idleness. It advocated a national security system that provides every citizen with seven aspects of social security: children's allowances, a pension, disability benefits, unemployment benefits, funeral grants, assistance for the loss of a subsistence source, and women's welfare. The basic methods by which these welfare aims are achieved include social insurance, national assistance, and voluntary insurance. The Beveridge Report proposed the three guiding principles of social security.

1. *Principle of universality.* The scope of social security should not be restricted to the poorest sections of society but should include all citizens, and insurance contributions should be paid at a flat rate regardless of income level.
2. *Principle of unified government management.* The organization and implementation of various social security measures should be carried out by the government through the redistribution of national income. The state is responsible for preventing poverty and misfortune; social welfare is a government responsibility.
3. *Principle of comprehensive security or citizen needs.* By being fully and gainfully employed, each citizen has the right to receive assistance from society to ensure that his standard of living reaches the national minimum. Beveridge not only established the main content, basic functions, and principles of social security in theoretical terms but also explained the mechanisms of social security in practice. Beveridge's theory of social security laid the foundation for the development of modern theories of social security and is a milestone in the development history of social security theory.

(3) Influence of Welfare Economics on the Construction of Healthcare Services and Social Security Systems

In 1948, the UK announced that it had established the world's first welfare state. Thereafter, economically developed countries, including Northern European countries such as Sweden, Denmark, and Norway, and other Western European countries such as France, the Germany Federal Republic, Austria, Belgium, the Netherlands, Switzerland, and Italy, all began following the example set by the UK in the implementation of social welfare policy and established their own welfare states. Subsequently, the US, Australia, New Zealand, and Japan also established their own social security systems according to the welfare state approach. The main contents of these social security systems were the universal provision of high-quality health services and health security systems. With the establishment and development of health services and health security systems, welfarism and welfare states have made an immense impact on the development of human society. The ideas of welfarism still have a profound impact on the future construction of health services and health security systems in all countries throughout the world.

3. Keynesian Economics

(1) Origins of the Theory of Keynesian Economics

In 1936, Keynes published *The General Theory of Employment, Interest, and Money*, which aimed to identify the causes and rescue measures of capitalist recessions. In Keynesian economics, social security theory is established based on demand management. Keynes asserted that a country's production and employment status are mainly dependent on effective demand. However, due to the effects of three major psychological laws, there will often be inadequate effective demand, which will result in economic crises and unemployment. Therefore, the state must intervene in the free-market economy and apply fiscal policies in order to guide the tendencies of consumer demand through purposeful and conscious fiscal expenditure and revenues. The guiding principle for government intervention is that the state should utilize changes in the taxation system, restrictions of interest rates, and other measures in order to provide relief to the unemployed and the poor through interpersonal fiscal transfer payments, thereby stimulating consumer demand.

His theoretical system and analytical methods have opened up a whole new perspective: the equalizing effect of social security on market economics. According to Keynesian thought, economic depression and widespread unemployment stem from inadequacies in effective demand, which in turn is due to low consumption levels. As the poor tend to consume more than the rich do, taxes should be increased on the rich and then redistributed via transfer payments to the poor in order to reduce savings and increase expenditure on consumption, thereby achieving macroeconomic equilibrium. Based on this idea, Keynes' successors argued for the long-term equalizing effect of social security on macroeconomics. Keynesian theory triggered a protracted "Keynesian Revolution" involving government intervention in the economy.

Keynesian economics transformed the blueprint of Western economics and shaped the fundamental economic systems of Western countries. After Keynes, laissez-faire liberalism had all but disappeared from the markets, and Western mainstream economic theories were marked with the stamp of Keynesian economics (i.e., the emphasis on effective government intervention in markets). Typical theories included the idea of a "social market economy" by Alfred Müller-Armack and Ludwig Erhad and its practical implementation in

Germany. The concept of a social market economy was first proposed by Professor Müller-Armack – specifically, that a social market economy is not a laissez-faire market economy but rather a market economy that is consciously controlled from the perspective of social policy. Müller-Armack once stated that a social market economy is based on the laws of a market economy but is supplemented by the economic system of social security. Its significance lies in combining the principle of market freedom with that of social equality.

By the 1980s, a new school emerged that advocated government intervention: New Keynesian economics. These economists proposed that government initiatives should abide by the principle of maximizing public welfare or generally assumed that the government has good intentions, and, hence, the policies formulated by the government should, in theory, focus on maximizing social welfare. They strongly advocated that government interventions should play the following roles in market failure: maintaining competition and restricting monopolies, directly conducting economic affairs and providing typical public goods, utilizing monetary and fiscal policies to regulate the related economic variables so as to achieve the stability of the macroeconomic environment, actively regulating income redistribution to abolish poverty and inequality, and defining and protecting property rights to encourage the internalization of economic externalities.

The greatest contribution of Keynesian economics to social security theory is the introduction of the concept of an equalizer in social security, that is, to regard social security as an important means for state intervention in the economy and also as an equalizer or stabilizer for adjusting economic operations.

(2) Influence of Keynesian Economics on the Establishment of Social Security Systems

Keynes deduced the necessity of state intervention in the macroeconomy by analyzing the shortcomings of the capitalist economy, and he justified the stabilizing effect of social security on economic fluctuations based on measures of state intervention. Therefore, Keynesian theory fundamentally demonstrates the rationality of and necessity for the existence of a social security system. This theory resulted in the birth of the modern social security system in the US. Since then, all countries in the world, especially developed countries, have applied Keynesian theory when establishing social security systems but have also strengthened government intervention in public utilities, including health services and social security systems. Keynesian theory was also used as the foundation of practice and played a crucial role in driving the establishment of health services and health security systems.

4. Liberal Economics

(1) Economic Theories of Liberalism

The economic theories of liberalism are deeply rooted in western economics and can be said to be the traditional school of western economics. However, with regards to the field of social security theory, liberal economic theories did not have the opportunity to rival the reigning welfare economics before World War II. Then, in the 20–30 years after World War II, the domination of Keynesian economics did not leave any room for the development of liberal economic theories. It was not until after the 1970s, with the crisis of Keynesian economics in the theoretical domain and that of Western social security in the practical domain, that liberal theories underwent a resurgence, the most representative of which was neoliberalism. Neoliberalism launched fierce attacks against Keynesian state intervention, the "mixed economy," and social welfare systems, claiming that these concepts had violated the principles of the free-market economy. Since the 1980s, and especially in the 1990s, the ideology of Western liberalism and its policies have once again influenced all spheres of socioeconomic life from a different angle. Liberalization and privatization have become important threads that run through Western socioeconomic development. In the field of social security, the sudden rise of corporate and commercial insurance plans has constituted a key component in the privatization of social insurance and has played an even more important role in subsequent development.

Neoliberalism, represented by Milton Friedman, criticized state-owned enterprises and the social welfare system on the grounds of upholding a free-market economy, opposing state intervention in the economy, and alleviating the state's spending burden. In the view of neoliberalists, strengthening the role of the government is a curse on economic interests and individual freedoms. They claim that excessive macroeconomic management and social security will lead to bureaucracy and, thus, result in inefficiency. The only solution is to reduce social welfare and accept high levels of unemployment in the short term. The central tenet of neoliberalism is the restoration of a free-market economy and the stimulation of strong individualism. Neoliberal policies played a primary role in effectively stimulating the redevelopment of the Western economy throughout the 1980s.

Representatives of neoliberalism, including modern monetarism, social market economy, and public choice, all believe that social security undermines the functions of market mechanisms and seriously affects the market order of free competition. Therefore, neoliberalism opposes the welfare state and advocates for the marketization, privatization, and diversification of social security.

According to the views of neoliberalism, not only should businesses be privatized and marketized, but welfare and social security, including health services and health security, should also be privatized, marketized, and commercialized, such that the welfare received by each individual is determined by that individual's ability to pay. Doing so inevitably leads to a widening gap in the social security treatment received by different social classes, which will exacerbate social inequality. However, neoliberalism claims that this process will address the drawbacks of the capitalist social welfare system, as it will stimulate the labor motivation of workers and the investment motivation of capitalists, which will benefit economic development. Friedman pointed out that in order to ensure the effective operation of the free market, we should not strive for equality as advocated by the welfare state but instead should maintain inequality. He stated, "A society that puts equality above freedom will get neither." The US health insurance system is a typical example, in that it overemphasizes the public's freedom of choice, leading to uneven healthcare coverage and insufficient equality. Although the US spends 16% of its GDP on healthcare, it has achieved poor outcomes, and up to 15% of the population does not have health insurance (approximately 40 million). Within three months of the financial crisis in September 2008, the number of people without health insurance increased by a further 6 million. In comparison, France spends 11% of its GDP on healthcare, and all residents of France are covered by health insurance.

(2) Influence of Neoliberalism on the Health Security System

In response to the failures of Keynesian economic theories and the crises experienced by welfare-type social security systems, monetarism and supply-side economics used the principle of economic interest as their starting point to put forward policy suggestions on reducing social security expenditures. These policies have been widely adopted and implemented in the reforms of social security systems in different countries. The efficiency of health services is mainly reflected in the effective control of healthcare costs and the improvement of healthcare services. In the past 20 years, Western developed countries have identified effective methods for managing the rise in healthcare costs, and key issues include the organization and financing of health services. The most effective methods include diversified insurance plans that are financed by the national budget or under a global budget and healthcare cost-sharing systems. The current problems not only include controlling costs but also include providing a variety of cost-effective health services while ensuring that patients and the public are reasonably satisfied.

The US health security system is a typical case of a social security system that is influenced by neoliberalism. The US health security system is essentially based on the principles of neoliberalism. It is operated by the market; the government only assumes limited responsibility, such as providing healthcare and assistance to the elderly and the poor. In other words, the government only intervenes in issues that cannot be solved by the market.

The influence of neoliberalism on health services and health security systems can be seen from the fact that an increasing number of countries worldwide have begun to adopt multilevel health services and health security systems. The diversification of health services and social security systems is manifested in the simultaneous adoption of administrative means and market-based instruments, the close cooperation between governmental and nongovernmental organizations and between for-profit and nonprofit organizations, and cost-sharing among individuals and families, businesses, communities, and the government. Diversified health service and social security systems consist of two parts. The first is the government's promise to satisfy basic healthcare and basic social security, and the second is provided by multiple agents, including specialized health services, supplementary health insurance cooperatives with voluntary participation, and the government's medical aid system.

5. Information and Institutional Economics

(1) Analysis of Health Services and Health Security Systems based on Information Economics

In 1961, George J. Stigler published "The Economics of Information" in the *Journal of Political Economy*. In the same year, William Vickrey published "Counterspeculation, Auctions, and Competitive Sealed Tenders" in the *Journal of Finance*. The publication of these two articles marked the birth of information economics. Many key topics in information economics are based on game theory, such as, for example, signaling and adverse selection, mechanism design, contracts and moral hazard, auctions, reputation, and so on. Most of these issues involve information asymmetry. In essence, information economics is the application of information asymmetry to game theory in economics. In the literature on information science, players in a game who possess private information are known as "agents," and those who do not possess private information are known as "principals." Thus, all analyses in information economics can be conducted within the framework of principal–agent problems.

1. Information Asymmetry and Adverse Selection   When individuals conduct transactions, the quality of the product is an important feature. In many cases, only the seller truly knows the quality of the product, whereas the buyer does not. Different sellers (manufacturers) provide goods of different quality, and sellers of poor quality goods (defective goods or "lemons") will hide the information on product quality to protect their own interests. At this point, all sellers claim that they have high-quality goods. Since the buyers are unable to distinguish between sellers who are telling the truth and those who are telling lies, they can only decide on the quantity to be purchased and the price to be paid based on their estimation of the overall market. When high-quality goods and lemons are treated in the same way by the customers, the lemons have an advantage in terms of cost, and, hence, may gain the upper hand in sales. When customers find that the purchased goods are not of the quality that they expected, they will lower their expectations of product quality even further and the price that they are willing to pay decreases. At this point, high-quality goods with higher costs may be eliminated from the market, leaving behind the lemons. This outcome, in which high-quality goods fail in competition and defective goods remain, goes against the selection rule of survival of the fittest in market competition.

In 1970, Akerlof analyzed the used car market (lemon market) and proposed the theory of adverse selection. Adverse selection explains the damaging effect of fake and defective goods on the market. Such goods may push high-quality goods out of the market and will eventually destroy consumers' trust in the market, which will cause the market to shrink. This occurrence is common in the market and has currently arisen in the local vicious competition found in the service market of private medical institutions.

However, in such situations, it is the buyers rather than the sellers who are able to withhold information, as in the case of the health insurance market. In health insurance, individuals who know that they have poor health and may need to be hospitalized at any time will take the most initiative in purchasing insurance, whereas those with good health will have a far lower willingness to purchase insurance. Under these circumstances, an insurance company will increase insurance prices (reduce the amount of compensation), which may run the risk of driving away healthy customers from the insurance market, leaving behind customers who are at risk of illnesses at any time or who need compensation. This example illustrates the problem of adverse selection.

During the transaction process, the price mostly relates to the quantity. However, when quality information is unclear in a transaction, the traditional price competition model loses its explanatory power for economic phenomena. Hence, information on quality becomes crucial for the existence of the market. Evidently, this type of problem is not limited merely to the used car and insurance markets. In practice, it is an extremely widespread problem that is prevalent in an economic society. We can see that if these problems are not properly dealt with in an economic society (i.e., distinguishing between high and low quality), then the market may not exist. This principle implies that the issue of distinguishing between goods of different quality and different features is an important component in the non-price system of an economic society.

Information screening and methods of product differentiation can be established by those who do not have private information, that is, the agents (i.e., used car buyers and insurance companies) can formulate a set of strategies or contracts for the car sellers or insured parties to choose from. For example, in the health insurance market, insurance companies can formulate contracts for insured parties with different features. Naturally, when products of different quality are mixed together such that consumers or customers are not able to differentiate between them, businesses will also actively reveal their own characteristics to show that their goods are of better quality so that customers can differentiate them from poorer quality goods. One of the key functions of economic systems is to ensure that participants in the economic society can display their true signals through the economic system. When agents with private information attempt to use signal transmission activities to differentiate their own features from those of other members of society, an economic system that shares the common trust of society plays an important role.

The problem of adverse selection shows that screening the authenticity of information is extremely important to the market economy. The principal can screen the characteristics of agents who possess private information through the use of contract diversification. However, it is also very important to screen the authenticity of information transmitted by the agents. At this point, the government and legal departments play an important role in signal management. An economic system established on this basis should become a basic tool or means for the effective transmission of authentic information.

2. Moral Hazard   After both parties to a transaction have signed a contract, if the interests of the principal are also dependent on the actions of the agent, then the principal may face a "moral hazard" when achieving his interests. This is because the principal cannot confirm whether the agent is willing to or is actively trying to achieve the principal's interests. In economics, moral hazard mainly involves an agent's action selection that cannot be clearly defined in the contract. The agent has private information, which is hidden from the principal, regarding this action selection, and the principal is unable to observe these actions. Hence, the agent's action selection affects the interests of the principal. For example, when a patient seeks medical treatment from a hospital, he has already paid the treatment fees. Thus, according to the contract, the patient should receive the corresponding treatment. However, what standard of physician will the hospital provide for the patient's treatment, and will the physician be conscientious and responsible? The selection of these actions depends on the hospital, and the average patient does not know if he has received the best or most appropriate treatment that the hospital can provide.

3. Incentive Measures   The key to avoiding the occurrence of moral hazard is to provide others with the incentive to perform actions that will benefit oneself. It should be said that a promise is itself an incentive, and the price system is also intended to motivate others to engage in certain actions. However, when there is information asymmetry, this method is inadequate. Mechanism design theory illustrates the basic idea of determining the final price to be paid (e.g., a manager's or employee's salary) based on the ex-post outcome. An alternative is to partially (or completely) transform the principal's ex-post risk caused by moral hazard into the agent's own risk within the contract. For instance, the fixed quota system is one such mechanism. Without a contract, the risk is borne by the principal, but after a contract is in place, the risk is borne by the agent. Individual rational decision-makers will allow others to face moral hazard but will not perform actions that will hurt their own interests. However, this scenario further involves more complicated issues, including choosing the specific forms that these incentives should take and identifying methods that are more rational under different circumstances. For example, individuals can formally resolve the issue of mutual incentives through contractual agreements, which can specify the interests of both parties in more detail under all possible circumstances. Such contractual solutions to the problem must be legally binding.

In addition, individuals can also resolve this issue through the notion of "reputation." It is not possible for any individual to maintain stable, long-term relationships with different societies. Thus, reputation becomes important capital for profit-making. If reputation is used to solve the problem of moral hazard, then the need for professional ethics arises in the economic society. The economic society will form requirements and evaluation standards for the professional ethics of different occupations. Individuals who do not conduct their professional activities according to these standards may lose their professional qualifications, and this threat will cause members of society to restrain themselves from undertaking unethical behaviors. Thus, the formation of social professional ethics and the punishment of unethical behavior are important measures by which to resolve moral hazard.

In the practice of health insurance, mechanism design is especially important to health insurance management and healthcare institutions due to the presence of third-party payments. The various approaches in the settlement of healthcare costs are intended to induce healthcare institutions to adopt behaviors that will benefit health insurance institutions. However, the theories of information economics tell us that urging healthcare institutions to establish good professional ethics is also an important approach.

4. Analysis on Adverse Selection and Moral Hazard in Health Insurance Management

(1) Uncertainties in the health insurance market   There are numerous particularities and uncertainties in the health insurance market. From the perspective of information asymmetry, the first is the presence of adverse selection, and the second is the problem of moral hazard. After comparing the health market with a standard competitive market, economists have found that the former consists of numerous particularities. The differences between a standard competitive market and the health market are shown in Table 1.1.

Due to the differences of the health insurance market from a standard competitive market, there is an extreme dearth of information. This lack of information is mainly reflected in a few ways. First, patients lack health-related information and do not possess expert knowledge. Second, consumers can only consult physicians to understand this information, but physicians are precisely the sellers of these products. Hence, it is difficult for physicians to impart this information to patients in a fair and comprehensive manner. Third, even when consumers receive some information, they may not be able to make an accurate judgment. Finally, errors in judgment are likely to result in wrong choices, and wrong choices are associated with very high costs. Compared to the case of other products, these wrong choices are often unchangeable, unrepeatable, or even irreversible. Therefore, patients are dependent on the information provided by physicians and find it difficult to make their own decisions.

(2) Excessively high transaction costs   The transaction costs of private health insurance systems are considered to be higher than those of social health insurance systems. Part of the reason is that accounting and litigation costs, which are due to the lack of information, account for a substantial portion of the transaction costs of the former type. There are two direct consequences of higher transaction costs. First, there is a lower level of medical welfare. Proponents of social health insurance have cited this reason to assert that even having no insurance is better than having private health insurance. In the absence of third-party payments, transaction costs can be avoided, which can improve the utilization efficiency of

TABLE 1.1 Differences Between a Standard Competitive Market and the Health Market

Standard Competitive Market	Health Market
Many buyers	Limited number of hospitals
Homogenous goods	Nonhomogeneous goods
Adequate information for buyers	Inadequate information for buyers
Companies aim to maximize profits	Most providers are not-for-profit
Payments made directly by consumers	Consumers pay only part of the costs

funds. Second, private health insurance causes the prices of health insurance products to increase. Insurance products have high prices due to transaction costs, and the percentage of the population who cannot afford insurance may increase each year. This possibility is another important reason cited by proponents of social health insurance. These claims are substantiated by reality. Take the US, for example, where the private health insurance system is widely prevalent. The percentage of the population without insurance in 1980 was 12.5%. By 2002, this percentage rose to 15.5%, meaning that 36.5 million people did not have any health insurance. In 2010, this number increased to 16.3%, which implies that the number of people without health insurance had risen to 49.9 million. This outcome is related to increases in the prices of health insurance products.

(3) Adverse selection   Adverse selection is one of the major reasons leading to insufficient supply in the health insurance market. Different individuals have different probabilities of contracting diseases. In theory, individuals with poor health will need to pay higher premiums to purchase health insurance. However, the result of adverse selection is that high-risk individuals will hide their true risk statuses, and the pool of consumers who actively purchase insurance may consist entirely of individuals with poor health. The eventual outcome is the continuous reduction of the population with health insurance. Individuals with below-average risk must bear the costs of having an average risk level, causing them to think that the insurance is not cost-effective, which reduces their purchase demand. Individuals with above-average risk will need to increase their insurance premiums, or they may be rejected. The continuation of this vicious cycle causes an increasing number of people to withdraw from the market. Many countries have imposed mandatory social health insurance to solve the problem of adverse selection on a fundamental level.

(4) Moral hazard   Both social health insurance and market-based private health insurance face the problem of moral hazard. In the case of third-party payments, both doctors and patients may reach an agreement due to shared interests, which leads to excessive service and consumption, thus jointly sacrificing the third-party interests of the health insurance sector. Therefore, the key challenge in health insurance lies in the health consumption process after enrollment. However, the standards of health and treatment outcomes are more difficult to define and measure compared to those of other goods. The standardization, programming, and normalization of health behaviors and processes are challenging, and, hence, the supervision of health consumption is constrained both by cost and technology. From a broader perspective, moral hazard will also be manifested beyond health consumption, as insured parties may spend less effort on avoiding risks, such as by not paying attention to their diets, smoking, or not exercising. The reduction in individuals taking health precautions will necessarily affect health insurance demand, and the result will inevitably lead to the deviation of private and social costs. The more comprehensive the social health insurance is, the less responsibility the insured party will bear with regards to their health service behaviors, and the more likely it is that they will over-consume. This outcome is also a reason why the level of health security should not be too high.

By analyzing the health services and health insurance markets using information economics, we find that the sustainable development and long-term management of health and insurance systems is far more challenging than establishing such a system is. Although information economics cannot provide targeted and immediate effects in the management of health insurance, its theories can serve as a profound analysis on the loopholes and draw-backs in the application of health services and health insurance. Therefore, these theories can be used as powerful tools to analyze and evaluate the design, policy formulation, and management operations of health services and health insurance systems.

(2) Analysis of Health Service and Health Security Systems Based on Institutional Economics

Institutional economics is a branch of economics that focuses on institutions, which orig-inated from the German historical school in the late nineteenth century. This field studies the influence of institutions on economic behaviors and economic development as well as the influence of economic development on institutions. Institutions refer to rules in inter-personal interactions and the structure and mechanisms of social organizations. John R. Commons proposed that an institution was a series of behavioral codes or rules though which collective action controls individual action. Schultz defined institutions as rules of conduct that involve social, political, and economic behaviors. North pointed out that insti-tutions are a series of man-made rules, legal norms, behavioral ethics, and ethical norms. They are the "rules of the game" of a society, which aim to restrain individual actions that maximize subjective benefits or effects. These constraints govern human interactions. Kasper and Streit stated, "Institutions are widely accepted, man-made rules which con-strain possibly arbitrary and opportunistic behavior in human interaction. Institutions are shared in a community and are always enforced by some sort of sanction." Although each of the definitions above has its own focus, all of them share a common meaning. That is, insti-tutions are rules and constraints to limit and govern individual actions. Moreover, these rules and constraints are manmade. Therefore, in the process of institutional evolution, individuals can take the initiative to change old institutions and formulate and implement new institutions.

Institutional economics places great emphasis on the role of rules. Rules are the means or measures used to constrain the members of an organization and compel them to work towards a common direction. They are the operational mechanisms of institutions. To achieve the development of institutions, it is first necessary to refine the mechanisms or rules of the institutions. At the same time, corresponding adjustments must be made to the institutions when problems are uncovered. The adjustment of institutions is essentially the control and regulation of human behavior, whereas the operation of institutions is also dependent on human actions. The relationship between humans and institutions is bidi-rectional. On the one hand, all institutions are formed, maintained, and developed through human behaviors. On the other hand, all human actions and their underlying motivations are also constrained and influenced by established institutions. Perfect and lawful rules or operational mechanisms of institutions will promote the continuous development and improvement of institutions.

The field of institutional economics also believes that the evolution of institutions is closely associated with their environmental conditions. The operation of institutions is achieved by specific organizations, whereas the existence and development of any organiza-tion cannot be separated from its environmental conditions. A given set of environmental conditions will give rise to corresponding institutions. As the environment changes, the rules of the organization, that is, the operational mechanisms of the institutions, will also need to undergo corresponding adjustments; otherwise, the institutions may disintegrate. Of course, powerful institutions may also have an impact on the environmental conditions to some extent. However, a discussion of institutions that is divorced from environmental conditions is meaningless. The current differences among the health systems of different countries exist precisely because each country has combined its national needs with its historical and cultural environment to produce a health security system that conforms to its actual circumstances.

The concepts of institutional functions, including institutional structure, institutional change, institutional efficiency, institutional allocation, institutional coupling, institutional conflicts, and institutional vacuums, are important analytical tools in institutional economics. They play a crucial role in studying institutional evolution, evaluating institutional performance, and identifying the problems that exist in institutions. North proposed that institutional change is the spontaneous process of incremental alteration to capture potential opportunities for profit during institutional disequilibria. However, in practice, the selection of the mode of institutional change is mainly constrained by the power structure among interest groups and the preference structure of society. The health security systems of all countries are also constantly undergoing transformation. The public will always include institutions in their complaints about health insurance. Hence, institutional economics can indeed provide some theoretical guidance regarding the healthcare and health security systems.

1. Path Dependence of Institutional Change   Path dependence refers to the fact that once a specific system has been chosen, the presence of certain factors, such as economics of scale, learning effects, coordination effects, and adaptive expectations, results in the self-reinforcement of the system such that the system continues to follow the established direction. Since the theory of path dependence was proposed, it has been widely used in all aspects of choice and customs. To a certain extent, all of the choices made by humans are subjected to the dreaded influence of path dependence, and all theories related to customs can be explained using path dependence.

Based on Arthur's path dependence in technological change and David's path dependence in historical change, North introduced the theory of path dependence in his analytical framework of institutional change. From this analysis, he established the path dependence theory of institutional change. This theory has become extremely important and well-known in the current new institutional economics.

North asserted that path dependence is akin to inertia in physics. Once something takes a certain path, it may produce dependence on this path because, as with the physical world, economic life also has mechanisms for increasing returns and self-reinforcement. These mechanisms imply that once a certain path has been chosen, it will receive continuous self-reinforcement in future development. By following a set path, changes in economic and political institutions may enter the trajectory of a virtuous cycle and undergo rapid optimization, or they may follow the wrong initial path and undergo a downward slide. A system that reaches lock-in will find it extremely difficult to escape. Doing so often requires the help of external effects, such as the introduction of exogenous variables or changes in political power, in order to reverse the original direction. This is due to the background considerations of interests and the costs that can be borne. After an institution has been established, organizations will form vested interest groups that have a strong demand for the existing institution. It is only by consolidating and strengthening the existing system can they guarantee their continued interests, even if a new institution would be more efficient overall. As for individuals, once they have made a choice, they will continually invest their efforts, money, and various material resources. They will not change paths easily even if they discover that the path they have selected is unsuitable because this change will render their previous substantial investments worthless. This idea is known as "sunk costs" in economics. Sunk costs are a major reason for path dependence.

2. Theoretical Perspective of Institutional Structure

Institutional structure refers to the sum of formal and informal institutional arrangements for a given object. Here, a given object can refer to a country, a society, or a specific concrete activity. Formal institutions include political rules, economic rules, and contracts as well as the hierarchical structure constructed from this series of rules. From the constitution, to statutory and common law, to specific bylaws, and finally to individual contracts and from general rules to particular specifications, institutions collectively constrain human actions. Informal institutions are formed subconsciously through long-term human interactions that have lasting vitality and constitute a part of the culture that has been passed down through generations. From a historical perspective, before the establishment of formal institutions, the relationships among individuals were maintained mainly based on informal institutions. Even in developed market economies, formal institutions are only a small part of the total set of constraints that determine choices. The majority of economic operations is still constrained by informal institutions. In North's view, informal institutions include values, ethical norms, moral codes, customs, and ideology. In informal institutions, ideology occupies a core position because it implicitly contains values, ethical norms, moral codes, and customs. It can also formally constitute an a priori model of certain formal institutional arrangements.

According to the theory of new institutional economics, a contract can simply be understood as an agreement reached by two parties on certain mutual obligations in a legal bilateral transaction (Furubotn and Richter, 1998). All transactions are carried out through some form of contract. Therefore, health insurance can also be understood as a legal contract signed between the government, healthcare institutions, and individuals concerning the transaction of health resources. Adopting the perspective of contract economics not only allows us to examine the transaction itself at the level of health insurance mechanisms, it also deepens the scope of research to the institutional level, on which the survival of health insurance mechanisms depends. As stated by the German economist W. Eucken (1951), contracts are not only the means by which to engage in transactions, but they can also be used to create economic organizations and power structures in different economic situations.

Health insurance itself has a clear contractual nature. The health insurance contract is a long-term contractual relationship that emphasizes not only specialized cooperation but also the maintenance of long-term contractual relationship. To maximize their expected returns in the resource transaction of health insurance, the government and an individual will stipulate the attributes and conditions of the transaction based on the situation at the time of establishing the health insurance system, in accordance with economic principles. Provisions that cannot be clearly stipulated at that time or costly terms are be dealt with accordingly or await reforms in due course. Therefore, health insurance contracts can be considered as typical relational contracts. With regards to the completeness of the contract, as the actions and decisions of the public and the government are constrained by limited rationality and information asymmetry, it is impossible to predict all changes in the health insurance contract, and, hence, it is also not possible to formulate complete and nonexhaustive contractual terms. The presence of transaction costs could also cause the government to artificially design an imperfect health insurance system during its establishment. Dimensions that are too costly or fundamentally cannot be defined are temporarily excluded from the health insurance system and will be dealt with by future reforms or constrained by the law, customs, and other institutions.

Due to the incompleteness of health insurance contracts, the key to preserving health insurance mechanisms lies in how the government prevents individuals and healthcare institutions from exploiting the incompleteness of the contract and using too many healthcare resources. The field of new institutional economics generally believes that implicit contractual guarantees are more suitable for the requirements of a competitive contracting process and are more effective than explicit contractual guarantees at ensuring the implementation of incomplete contracts. New institutional economics emphasizes the importance of implicit contracts, whereas the key to implicit contracts is addressing the issue of "quasi-rent." Quasi-rent in health insurance refers to the opportunism that may encroach on health resources, which mainly comes from information asymmetry among the state, healthcare institutions, and individuals, as well as to the related incomplete social security contract. Health insurance quasi-rent is mainly divided into the quasi-rents of individuals using their information advantage and the quasi-rents of healthcare institutions using their information advantage. Individual quasi-rent is similar to commercial insurance. The information advantage of individuals in the noncommercial health insurance market also leads to moral hazard and adverse selection. Due to third-party payments, the moral hazard in this case is often manifested as individual over-consumption of health resources (e.g., the use of health services, expensive drugs and advanced medical equipment, long hospital stays, etc.).

SECTION II. THEORIES OF PUBLIC GOODS

1. Concept and Characteristics of Public Goods

The theory of public goods is one of the hot topics in economic theory. Its theoretical innovations can provide guidance for the effective supply of public goods. In a narrow sense, public goods refer to nonrivalrous *and* nonexcludable goods. In a broader sense, public goods refer to nonrivalrous *or* nonexcludable goods, which include three major types: pure public goods, club goods, and common-pool resources. Samuelson, Buchanan, and Ostrom have described the typical problems faced by public goods in the broader sense. Examples include the free-rider problem, exclusion costs, the tragedy of the commons, and financing and distribution problems. These economists have also proposed corresponding theoretical models based on the different types of goods and their respective problems, such as the theory of pure public goods, club theory, and the theory of common-pool resources. There are differing criteria for the classification of goods, including the excludability and rivalry criterion, the publicness criterion, and the relative costs criterion. For example, Head and Shoup found that relative cost can be used to differentiate between public goods and private goods. This finding is also known as the economic efficiency criterion. They proposed that, regardless of how a service is being supplied, if it can be rendered at a lower cost under non-excludable conditions at a given time or place, then it is a public good. Holtermann proposed that the criteria for defining public goods should be the attributes of the goods. Different economic goods have different publicness levels corresponding to different allocations of property rights. However, Barzel believes that, due to the presence of information costs, it is impossible to fully define any individual right. Part of the value of ecological resources remains in the public domain due to the lack of any definition of its rights. Hudson and Jones also asserted that changes in property rights and technology will cause changes in the attributes of a particular good, and the only classification criterion remaining is publicness.

Public goods can be consumed or enjoyed by the vast majority of the public and are produced and provided by the government (or the public sector). Once public goods are provided, they can be enjoyed by everyone, and no effective measures can be taken to induce the beneficiaries to actively and voluntarily pay for these public goods. Due to the inability to recover costs or make profits, private individuals and businesses are unwilling to invest in public goods. Public goods generally cannot be provided by the market; they can and must only be led by the government or the public sector. As such goods are nonexcludable, everyone believes that they can enjoy the benefits of public goods regardless of whether they have paid the costs. Hence, consumers are not motivated to pay voluntarily, and they will tend to become free riders, thus causing the inability to recover investments in these goods. This free-riding phenomenon will inevitably lead to an insufficient market supply of public goods, which will result in market failure.

In theoretical terms, defining whether a good or service is a public good depends on whether it has two characteristics: nonexcludability and nonrivalrous consumption. Nonexcludability means that when one party provides a public good, it cannot effectively exclude others from consuming this good, regardless of the providing party's intentions. The inability to exclude others from enjoying the benefits of the public good may be because it is technologically infeasible or extremely difficult or because the cost of exclusion is too high, rendering exclusion impractical. Nonrivalrous consumption refers to the situation in which the marginal cost of adding one more consumer to a particular good is zero (i.e., for a given amount of a public good, the marginal cost of allocating the good to one more consumer is zero). This definition does not imply that the marginal cost of providing one more unit of public good is zero. In this case, the marginal cost of providing one more unit of public good is positive, which is similar to that of other goods, because the provision of public goods also consumes a limited amount of resources. Based on these two criteria, we can classify different goods as pure public goods, quasi-public goods, and private goods. Goods that possess both of the characteristics above are pure public goods. Goods that do not possess either of these characteristics are private goods. Goods that only possess one of these characteristics are quasi-public goods. It should be noted that in a strict sense, the definitions of the two characteristics above are not absolute but are dependent on technological conditions and specific environments. When determining whether a type of good is a public good, it is necessary to consider the number of beneficiaries and whether these beneficiaries can be excluded from using this good. If there are numerous beneficiaries and it is technologically infeasible to exclude any beneficiary, then a good can be regarded as a public good. Samuelson's classical definition of public goods is goods for which each individual's consumption does not lead to subtractions from any other individual's consumption of that good.

In the real world, true pure public goods are very rare, and most goods can be regarded as quasi-public goods in between pure public goods and private goods. Based on the differences between and relationships among public goods, quasi-public goods, and private goods, we will analyze the scope, scale, and funding sources for the government's supply of public goods. We will also explore the division of labor among the different levels of government in this process and, hence, analyze the different methods of supplying public and quasi-public goods. Finally, we will discuss the theoretical and practical significance of public goods theory for China's new healthcare reforms. By applying the theories of public goods, we can determine the scope and scale of public goods in the domain of China's health system reforms, thus allowing us to clarify the nature of public health spending, that is, the public goods financed by the government. In the field of healthcare reforms, the role of government finance should be limited to the public attributes of public and quasi-public goods, and it should gradually withdraw from the private attributes of private and quasi-public goods. In other words, government finance should withdraw from the commercial and rival domains. Analyzing existing problems from the perspective of public economics and identifying the phenomena of market failure in China's current healthcare reforms according to public goods theory will give us insights into perfecting China's health system reforms.

2. Classification Criteria of Public Goods

Based on the classification criteria, the concept of public goods is the inverse of that of private goods, which refers to indivisible, nonexcludable, and nonrivalrous goods with utility in consumption activities. Such goods are also known as collective consumption goods. Goods can be classified into four different types according to whether they are nonexcludable and nonrivalrous in the consumption process: (1) Goods that are both nonexcludable and non-rivalrous are pure public goods. (2) Goods that are both excludable and rivalrous are pure private goods. (3) Goods that are nonexcludable and rivalrous are common-pool resources. (4) Goods that are excludable and nonrivalrous are quasi-public goods or mixed goods.

3. Theoretical Analysis of Public Goods

In the term "public goods," "public" means "shared." Under given conditions, the interests of public goods do not belong to an individual's private property rights. According to the principle of market exchange, it is difficult to produce exchange behavior for such goods, and the relationship between the consumers and the supplier is interrupted. Although there is market demand, there is no market supply. At this point, the government must intervene to compensate for this market defect, leading to the birth of public goods. There are three typical characteristics that can distinguish public goods from private goods. The first is nonexcludability; if a public good is provided to a specific group, then an individual cannot prevent others from consuming that good or extremely high costs are associated with preventing others from consuming that good. The second is nonrivalry; the same unit of the public good can be consumed by multiple individuals, and the supply to one individual does not reduce the supply to other individuals. The third is indivisibility. Comparatively speaking, public goods (e.g., national defense and foreign affairs) are indivisible, and economies of scale must be considered for the majority of public goods. For example, railways, bridges, and museums cannot be divided. Public goods can be further categorized as pure public goods and quasi-public goods. A typical example of a pure public good is national defense. Quasi-public goods can be even further divided into two types. The first type is natural-monopoly public goods, which are goods related to economies of scale, such as sewer systems, water, and power supply systems. The second type is merit goods, which are public goods that should be consumed or received by everyone regardless of their income level, such as primary and secondary education, healthcare, and pension insurance. Merit goods are the opposite of demerit goods. The former generally refers to goods (or services) with high utility that can benefit individuals and society, such as primary education and seatbelts on aircrafts. In contrast, tobacco and marijuana are typical demerit goods. The difference between merit goods and public goods lies in whether there is consumer excludability. There are vast differences among public goods, quasi-public goods, and private goods, which are shown in Table 1.2.

Health service products are typical merit goods that are rivalrous. When the number of consumers increases from zero to a relatively large positive number (i.e., the point of congestion) then an increase in consumers will reduce the overall utility. The consumption process of health services and health insurance has strong characteristics of private goods. Hence, if the government offers free healthcare or charges a nominal fee, the public may overconsume this product, which will exacerbate congestion. In reality, the public will always hope that the state will provide free healthcare services. This is a typical free-riding state of mind, which is prevalent in welfare states. The nature of public goods is such that private individuals (manufacturers) are unwilling to provide such goods. Hence, it is beyond doubt that the government should be the main provider of public goods. In contrast, the nature of private

TABLE 1.2 Differences between Public Goods and Private Goods

Features	Pure Public Goods	Quasi-Public Goods	Private Goods
Divisible during consumption?	No	Partially divisible	Yes
Exclusive upon purchase?	No	Basically not	Yes
Method of purchase	Indirect payment (e.g., taxes)	Partially direct, partially indirect	Direct payment by self
Principle of distribution	Political vote	Political vote and market purchase	Market price
Individual freedom of choice?	No	Virtually none	Yes
Can it be enjoyed without purchase?	Yes	Partially	No
Can its quality be determined?	Not easily	Not very easily	Easily
Wastage during use	Not easily wasted	Relatively high waste	Relatively low waste
Examples	National defense, police	Compulsory education	Hairdresser, clothes, radio

goods includes excludability in property rights and divisibility in consumption, which implies that private manufacturers are willing to produce such goods. If no one is producing such goods, their prices will increase, which will attract a large number of producers to this sector. Conversely, too many producers flooding a market leads to overproduction, and prices fall, which once again causes many producers to withdraw automatically. Hence, for private goods, as long as a policy monopoly is avoided, production by manufacturers is much more efficient than that by the government. The interests and risks are all borne by the manufacturers, and there are no concerns about the lack of alternative choices for the consumers.

The providers of quasi-public goods are not homogeneous. It is generally accepted that it is ideal for public goods to be produced by manufacturers and subsidized by the government. Consumers need quasi-public goods. However, due to restrictions in consumption, manufacturers cannot guarantee their returns without government subsidies, which affect their production. However, if such goods are completely produced by the government, it may lead to communalism, which will reduce efficiency.

At the same time, it is not possible to absolutely reject the government's role in the production of private goods. If the government intends to fulfill the following two objectives, then it is not only possible but also necessary for the government to produce private goods. The first objective is to limit the usage of such goods to ensure the rational utilization of resources. Furthermore, the scarcity of resources implies that there is a need to limit the use of certain resources to ensure sustainable socioeconomic development. However, the private sector may plunder these scarce resources for their immediate gains, resulting in the depletion of some resources. The other objective is to disrupt monopolies and achieve social equality. If it is the government's intention to fulfill these aims, then it should produce private goods. Generally speaking, the government's production of private goods involves the resolution of the principal-agent interest mechanism and the agency cost problem. If these two problems can be resolved, then the performance of the government may be superior in the production of private goods.

The supply of public goods mainly involves two problems, namely, efficiency and price. As public goods are nonexcludable, they inevitably give rise to the free-rider problem. In general, the free-rider problem has two causes: moral behavior and natural behavior. Moral behavior is due to human self-interest, also known as egoism, whereas natural behavior is due to the nonexcludability of public goods. That is, if a consumer needs to consume this type of good and does not need to pay any fees, then these conditions imply that the consumer will not pay a meaningless price. Free-riding means that the cost of resources cannot be recovered, which affects the return on capital investment and is a manifestation of inefficiency. The production behavior under such conditions will result in a serious shortage of public goods, thereby leading to the loss of social welfare. This outcome is often the case for health services under excessive health security.

The following methods can generally be used for the pricing of the public goods supply. The first is the principle of marginal-cost pricing. The most appropriate level of general welfare corresponds to selling all goods at their marginal costs. The second is the introduction of competitive price mechanisms. These include the implementation of price hearing systems to form a mechanism of public pricing among producers, consumers, and managers; open bidding systems, which introduce competition mechanisms among manufacturers; the price regulation of the public goods supply; government pricing; and price limiting of public goods.

Health security comes under the scope of quasi-public goods, as it has the characteristics of both public and private goods. The consumption of such a good should be paid for by individuals, but its costs should also be partially supported by the government to ensure its efficient supply. There are two possible methods for doing so. The first is for public goods to be supplied by private individuals and subsidized by the government, and the second is for the government and private individuals to cooperate in the joint provision of public goods.

Under perfect market conditions, the supply and demand of health insurance goods involves individual residents raising and paying the increased healthcare costs, whereas the provision of health services is completely regulated by market demand. The health insurance products that can be accessed by individual residents are determined by their financial abilities. The total amount of individual payments determines the amount of supply; a higher amount of payments leads to a greater supply of services.

However, in reality, it is difficult to operate the health service market based on the general principles of market supply and demand because, in the health service market, there is information asymmetry between the service providers and consumers. Physicians can directly influence the patient's level of demand by changing the patient's perception of his own needs and inducing his satisfaction with the pursuit of cutting-edge medical technology. Thus, an inverse relationship cannot be formed between an increase in price and the service quantity demanded, implying that healthcare costs will remain high, ultimately leading to the failure of market rules. We can observe in real life that since consumers are lacking in professional knowledge when they utilize healthcare services, it is physicians who guide, and even dictate, the healthcare services that consumers use. Physicians also hold the power in deciding the quantity of supply. Over time, in order to seek greater economic gains, physicians (with the exception of ethical physicians with patients' best interests in mind) and healthcare institutions will inevitably exploit their excessive power in supply determination to increase healthcare consumption. However, due to the uneven distribution of wealth in society and the concentration of wealth among a privileged few, the price of healthcare services will rise more rapidly than the financial ability of the majority of the general population. That is, under a self-funded health system with a proportion of low-income residents who cannot access healthcare services, there may be an increasing number of residents who are unable to receive the healthcare services that come with socio-economic development. Therefore, we can see that health service and health security products are special goods. Although the general theories of supply and demand can be used to analyze basic trends, these theories cannot fully explain the supply and demand and price determination of health service and health security products. In particular, physicians may exploit their power to determine consumption to induce demand, and consumers may over-utilize limited health resources within the context of third-party payments in health insurance. To address these issues, we need another theory, namely, information economics, for further research and analysis.

SECTION III. THEORIES OF SOCIAL EQUALITY

The representative theories of equality in contemporary Western society posit that equality is a cyclical process that involves four aspects: equality of starting conditions, equality of opportunity, equality of process, and equality of outcomes. The association between social security and social equality is as follows: Equality is the core concept of social security. The social security system originates from the demand for equality. The design of the social security system should embody the principle of equality. Its own equality will ensure the equality of opportunity and protect the equality of process. The social security system has a function in equality, that is, to compensate for the inequality of starting conditions and reduce the inequality of outcomes, thereby increasing the overall level of equality in society.

Equality is the rational allocation of political, economic, and other interests among all members of society. It entails equal rights, rational distribution, equal opportunities, and justice. It is subject to the influence of the given social and political environment, interest structure, ideology, religious ethics, philosophical thoughts, and cultural traditions. Hence, everyone has different views of equality.

1. Concept of Equality in Classical Liberalism

Classical liberalism posits that equality refers to the equality of starting conditions, that is, the equality of rights and not the equality of welfare. The role of the government is to ensure that everyone shares the same rights and freedoms rather than directly providing happiness and well-being. Classical liberalism advocates for the principle of value neutrality and denies the positive significance of the state in society. However, modern administrative theories assert that the government is not value-neutral, as it needs to protect the right to freedom while also striving for the core value of equality. In terms of its views on equality, classical liberalism insists on the equality of starting conditions and the equality of rights but not the equality of welfare.

2. Concept of Equality in Utilitarianism

The main representatives of utilitarianism are Jeremy Bentham and John Stuart Mill. Bentham insisted on the hedonism of morality and posited that the approval or disapproval of an action is based on whether the action has augmented or diminished the happiness of all parties involved. If the party involved is an individual, then the happiness of the individual is used as a criterion. If the party involved is the government, then the happiness of society is used as a criterion, and this happiness follows the law of diminishing marginal utility.

Mill, on the other hand, insisted on the hedonism of the spirit, that is, that the quality of happiness should be considered along with its quantity. Under the principle of the "greatest happiness for the greatest number," utilitarianism holds that the main responsibility of the state and the government is to ensure survival, achieve prosperity, promote equality, and preserve safety. Utilitarianism requires people to not only not harm others but also benefit others in an attempt to maintain the "greatest happiness for the greatest number." As stated by Mill, "The utilitarian morality does recognize in human beings the power of sacrificing their own greatest good for the good of others." Any sacrifice for the good of others is praised in utilitarianism.

3. Concept of Equality in Rawlsianism

Rawls first proposed a hypothetical "original position," which he argued will guarantee the equality of the basic contract it reaches and the justice of any principle that has unanimous agreement. When individuals make choices in the original position, they insist on two principles. The first principle is the priority of rights and liberties, and the second principle is the priority of fairness and justice in efficiency and welfare. Justice has priority over the efficiency principle and the principle of greatest benefit; equal opportunity has priority over the difference principle. The difference principle is also known as the "maximin principle," which states that unless there is a distribution that improves the statuses of both individuals, if one individual receives nothing, then an equal distribution is preferred, regardless of how much improvement the other individual will experience.

4. Concept of Equality in the School of New Public Administration

Represented by Frederickson, the school of new public administration regarded equality as the third normative pillar of public administration, along with efficiency and economy. To this end, Frederickson proposed the compound theory of equity to explain a series of social equity problems, including employment, contracts, government services, public policy, and the social, economic, and political sectors. This theory mainly comprises the following types of equality: (1) simple individual equality, which refers to one-to-one single relationships of equality; (2) segmented equality, which assumes equality of individuals within the same category but inequality between the categories; (3) block equality, which calls for equality between different groups and subclasses; (4) the domains of equality, which can be defined narrowly or broadly, as domains are constantly shifting, aggregating, or breaking apart and may involve intergenerational problems of equality; (5) equalities of opportunity, which include prospect and means equalities of opportunity; and (6) the value of equality, which is the notion of a person's equality in public administration that respects the individual rather than a notion of equality that is neutral, arbitrary, and insensitive to variations in people's needs.

5. Concept of Equality in Marxism

The concept of equality in Marxism generally includes three aspects. First, permanent and absolute equality does not exist from the perspective of human social development. Equality is a historical and transient category constrained by the conditions of productivity in real life. Second, the qualitative definition of equal distribution in future society depends on the public ownership of the means of production. Third, the form taken by equal distribution in future society is not static but is ever-changing.

In theoretical terms, equality is not a single concept but a comprehensive theoretical system. At different historical stages, there have been great dissimilarities in the concept, content, and implementation of equality. The reason for these differences is the conflict between the concreteness and complexity of society in the abstraction and simplification of the concept of equality. China is currently in a stage of social transformation, which is both a period of major strategic opportunities and one with numerous potential risks. Properly addressing the issue of equality will have important significance to the harmonious and sustainable development of the whole society. Based on the theories of equality, the government should not pursue efficiency excessively while ignoring the basic values of democracy, equality, and justice. Instead, it should actively respond to the preferences of citizens and service users and determine the role of the government while also respecting the value of efficiency that is in line with its goals.

A variety of social contradictions have emerged recently in Chinese society. Under these circumstances, it is insufficient to use only one theory of social equality to consolidate the different contradictions in society. The views of Marx and Engels on equality have laid the legitimate basis and moral foundations for system reforms and an institutional framework in contemporary China. This is the mainstream view of equality in China. However, in practice, China is faced with confrontations and conflicts among different views of equality. Hence, during the process of establishing and promoting a socialist concept of equality, China should also absorb and learn from the Western concepts of equality, which will have great significance for building a harmonious society. Whether in theory or in practice, the utilitarian concept of equality, the concept of income equality in classical liberalism, and the Rawlsian concept of equality, which are found in welfare economics, will serve as valuable theoretical references as China establishes and develops its social welfare and social security systems and a distribution system for health resources.

SECTION IV. THEORIES OF UNIVERSAL HEALTH COVERAGE

1. Proposal of UHC Theory

The World Health Organization (WHO) first proposed the concept of universal health coverage (UHC) in The World Health Report 2000. According to the definition of The World Health Report 2000, "universal coverage" means the "effective health protection and spreading of financial risks for all citizens; providing basic and accessible healthcare packages to all according to their needs and preferred choices, regardless of their income, social status, or place of residence; and the high-quality delivery of essential care for everyone, rather than all possible care for the whole population."

At the 58th World Health Assembly in 2005, the WHO formally proposed to its Member States the goal of moving towards health systems with universal coverage. In this meeting, the WHO urged all Member States to commit in 2005 to establishing their own health financing systems so that all people have access to health services and do not suffer financial hardships in paying for them. This goal was defined as "universal coverage," also known as "universal health coverage."

Based on the document of this meeting, UHC was defined as "access to key promotive, preventive, curative, and rehabilitative health interventions for all at an affordable cost, thereby achieving equity in access. The principle of financial-risk protection ensures that the cost of care does not put people with serious illnesses at risk of financial catastrophe." Subsequently, in the World Health Report 2010, the WHO once again called upon all

Member States to move toward the goal of universal coverage, and the main topic of the 2010 report was "Health Systems Financing: The Path to Universal Coverage."

2. Definition and Implications of UHC Theory

The WHO report gave a detailed elaboration of how countries can modify their financing systems to move more quickly towards the goal of providing universal coverage and sustaining the results that have been achieved. The report stated that the WHO Member States have formulated their own goals for developing their own health-financing systems so that all people have access to health services and do not suffer financial hardships paying for them. This report provides a set of actions for countries at all stages of development, which are based on new research results and lessons learned from the experiences of different countries. The report also suggests ways that the international community can support low-income countries to achieve universal coverage and improve their health statuses. Achieving UHC and ensuring that every citizen can receive fair, accessible, high-quality, and reliable health services and security will have an important and positive effect on political stability, building a social safety net, and promoting social equality. China has always attached great importance to improving the health of its citizens. Since 2009, the various measures to deepen healthcare reform have laid a solid foundation for achieving UHC.

The World Health Report 2013, entitled "Research for Universal Health Coverage," emphasized that research plays a vital role in the process of promoting UHC and that research should be used to provide everyone with high-quality health services. UHC refers to a system that ensures that everyone has access to the health services they need without the risk of financial ruin or impoverishment. The WHO 132nd Session of the Executive Committee in January 2013 and the 66th World Health Assembly in May 2013 comprehensively summarized the latest progress made towards the Millennium Development Goals set in 2000. In particular, substantial improvements have been made in decreasing child and maternal mortality rates and in controlling major diseases. In addition, the post-2015 global development agenda was confirmed, and one of its most important goals was to achieve UHC. This goal is the foundation and premise for achieving the WHO's fundamental mission, which is the "attainment by all peoples of the highest possible level of health."

In recent years, during a systematic discussion by the United Nations agencies (including the WHO) on the Post-2015 Development Agenda, it was once again emphasized that a major post-2015 challenge that the world must face is the formulation of a universally accepted and feasible goal for UHC. Currently, the consensus reached by the international community on the concept of UHC includes equitable access to health resources, equitable access to health services, and equitable access to social security systems. This conceptual framework is aligned with the target model of health systems advocated by the World Bank (Availability, Accessibility, Affordability; the 3As), and is in line with the basic policy framework of China's deepening healthcare reforms. Correspondingly, the policy priorities for attaining UHC and deepening healthcare reform must also focus on the following three aspects:

1. Ensuring the accessibility and availability of health resources implies that there must be sufficient resource input in the field of healthcare, including human resources, financial resources, and facilities for health.
2. The affordability of healthcare costs and protection against the risk of diseases refer to the level of health security. This domain can be divided into three dimensions. The first dimension is the coverage population. If the health security system aims to achieve

equitable coverage, then priority should be given to ensuring that the poor enroll in insurance; it should also ensure that the rich subsidize the poor and the healthy subsidize the sick. The second is the content of insurance. Not only should hospitalization costs be reimbursed, outpatient costs should also be reimbursed, which can be extended to health promotion, disease prevention, health rehabilitation for key populations, long-term elderly care, and palliative care. This is a necessary trend in the development of health insurance systems in modern society. The third is the level of insurance (i.e., the ratio of reimbursement), which should avoid the impoverishment of patients caused by the self-funding of healthcare costs. The specific policy is that the pay line should not affect a patient's medical-seeking behavior, whereas the cap line should not be the upper limit to prevent overdrafts of the health insurance funds but should ensure that the enrolled families can avoid impoverishment or disruptions in daily living due to disease. This dimension is one of the essential differences between a social health security system and commercial health insurance.

3. All citizens should be guaranteed access to safe, high-quality, and effective health services that they need – that is, healthcare services should be provided based on need rather than an individual's ability to pay. UHC ensures that every individual can access good quality health services without suffering financial hardships in paying for them. This coverage, in turn, requires a strong, efficient, and well-functioning health system that can provide basic drugs and technology as well as an adequate number of motivated and proactive healthcare workers. The challenge faced by most countries is the expansion of health services and the use of limited resources to meet growing demand. Therefore, it is very important to actively perform research on UHC.

The World Health Report 2013 urged the following: (1) increased international and national investment and support for research, especially targeting the improvement of health service coverage between and within countries; (2) closer collaboration between researchers and policy-makers, that is, a movement of research activities away from academic institutions and into public health planning, which is closer to health service supply and demand; (3) well-trained and motivated teams of researchers in all countries to build up countries' research capacities; (4) a comprehensive code of conduct for good research in each country; and (5) the use of global and national research networks to promote collaborations and information exchange in coordinated research activities.

Along with rapid economic development, changes in the spectrum of disease, and growing demand for disease risk protection, the calls for reforms of the healthcare system are becoming louder. At present, China is undergoing five key healthcare reforms. Together, the Urban Employee Basic Medical Insurance, Urban Residents Basic Medical Insurance, and the New Rural Co-operative Medical Care Scheme (NRCMS) have covered 95% of urban and rural residents. The achievements attained by this reform measure are even more remarkable in rural areas. Through economic incentives and administrative interventions, the NRCMS has covered more than 800 million rural residents. From an economic perspective, since the NRCMS is generally coordinated and managed at the county level, the central and province-level governments have increased their efforts in transfer payments to provide the NRCMS with adequate subsidies. These subsidies will help to incorporate more rural families into the health insurance system. From an administrative perspective, the NRCMS incorporates the target responsibility system for the management of local officials, which has helped to reduce personal out-of-pocket expenses and to provide medical aid to poor rural residents. In summary, the NRCMS is currently operating smoothly and is maintaining good momentum in terms of financing and enrollment. It is also closely integrated with economic adjustments.

Recently, the WHO and the World Bank jointly held a meeting to discuss how countries can achieve UHC. The meeting concluded that countries continue to face many challenges in attaining UCH, including a shortage of human resources and uneven distributions of health resources between urban and rural areas and between rich and poor areas. Furthermore, all countries are faced with the serious issue of reaching a balance between ensuring the accessibility of health services and setting a level of healthcare expenditure that the government can afford. Addressing these issues will require the political commitments of policy-makers at the highest level to UHC as well as improvements in information systems and more accountability of the government and healthcare providers for health outcomes. In addition, the progress of UHC should be monitored while also incorporating the key roles of researchers, civil society groups, and international institutions. In response to the demands of all countries, the WHO and the World Bank have already begun formulating a monitoring framework to help countries track their progress towards UHC. Over the past decade, China has continuously deepened its health system reforms and has made remarkable strides in the establishment of a basic health security system and moving toward UHC. After five years of implementing the new round of healthcare reforms, it is especially important for China to further clarify the concept of UHC, continuously improve the relevant policies, and formulate strategies and plans for achieving UHC.

SECTION V. THEORY OF PERFORMANCE EVALUATION FOR WORLD HEALTH SYSTEMS

1. Definition of Concepts Related to Performance Evaluation

The concept of "performance" originated from business management, which includes two levels: business results and employee productivity. As the problems of low service quality and low productivity are also present in the field of healthcare, the theory and practice of performance evaluation have gradually been extended to include health systems. The WHO defines a health system as all activities with the primary purpose of promoting, restoring, and maintaining health. The basic goals of a health system include contributing to the improvement of residents' health, good responsiveness, and equitable sharing of healthcare costs. The performance of a health system refers to the execution ability of the overall health system and its affiliated institutions in achieving its health goals. Attaining a good level of health system performance requires a country to set development goals for its health system as a yardstick and to make timely modifications of its development direction so as to achieve the ultimate goal of providing high-performance health services to the public. In practice, countries around the world have already established different performance evaluation frameworks to monitor, evaluate, and manage their own health systems.

Performance evaluation is an effective method for monitoring a health system and improve the quality of health services. Hence, governments around the globe have been paying great attention to performance evaluation. The performance of a health system has a direct impact on the accessibility of health services and the equity of health, which ultimately determines the health level of the population. The World Health Report 2000 introduced the theme "Health Systems: Improving Performance," which was a turning point for governments across the world to transform their health development strategies. A consensus was reached by all countries that the contribution of health services to improving the population's health has not reached its fullest potential. The reason for this is not merely due to the limitations of health technology; the true obstacle is the low resource integration and utilization of the overall health system (i.e., low performance levels).

2. Model of Performance Evaluation for Health Systems

As the public's health expectation increases, its health level is determined by the performance of the health system. Even among countries with the same level of income, there is significant variation in the performance of healthcare work. Hence, it is necessary for decision-makers in health policy to understand the opportunities and challenges faced by health systems in order to improve their performance and, hence, improve the health of the population. The WHO defines a health system as all organizations, institutions, and resources associated with health actions. Any action performed by individual healthcare services, public health services, and nonhealth sectors that are related to improving the population's health can be referred to as a "health action." Therefore, based on the broader definition, the scope of health systems needs to be expanded, and all actions with a view to improving health should come under the scope of a health system. The World Health Report 2000 presented a new framework for the analysis of national health systems. It proposed that a health system should have three main goals:

1. *Access to good health.* Not only does this goal imply increasing health levels, raising healthy life expectancy, and reducing the burden of disease, but it also includes improving the status of the population distribution and alleviating the inequitable distribution of health status, with a particular emphasis on improving the health status of the poor.
2. *Strengthening the responsiveness to the population's expectations.* This goal refers to the design of relationships between institutions. It is based on the universal, reasonable demands of the population and the outcome (nonhealth outcome) of responding to these demands appropriately. This concept touches on two aspects. The first is respecting the dignity of the individual, the autonomy and privacy of individuals and families for their own health and treatment, and basic human rights. The second is the responsiveness to health service users (recipients), which includes service satisfaction, whether prompt attention is paid to a patient's needs, the utilization of social support networks, the infrastructure and environment of healthcare institutions, and the possibility of choice for health service users.
3. *Ensuring the fairness of health-financing.* This goal includes two aspects. The first is the fairness of financing. Financing is considered fair when each family contributes the same level to the health system. The second is protection against serious illnesses such that no individual faces financial risk due to paying for healthcare costs. The financing system is unfair if a family's disposable funds are needed to cover the high costs of serious illnesses. Fair and reasonable financing involves spreading the risk of paying for healthcare costs across all families according to their ability to pay. A fair health system should be able to protect everyone in society, including the poor, and should not allow the impoverishment of some families due to medical costs.

In the World Health Report 2000, the WHO ranked health systems based on the evaluation outcomes of these three basic goals. It also suggested that the performance in achieving these goals is determined by four health service functions: service provision, financing, resource generation, and stewardship. See Figure 1.1.

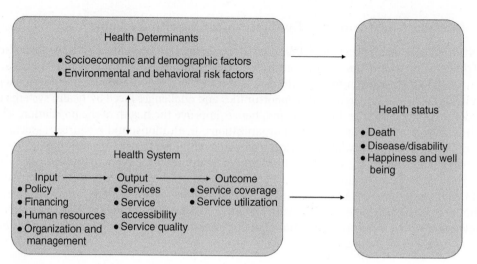

FIGURE 1.1   Model of framework for the performance evaluation of health systems.

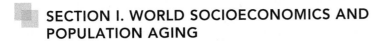

CHAPTER TWO

World Socioeconomic Development and Health Status

SECTION I. WORLD SOCIOECONOMICS AND POPULATION AGING

1. Economic Crisis and Transformational Development

In 2008, the global financial crisis triggered by the subprime mortgage crisis in the US caused a deep economic recession in many countries, which resulted in a high unemployment rate, a rapid increase in poverty, and the intensification of social conflicts. Given the double blow of the financial crisis and the sovereign debt crisis, many countries were mired in difficulties. At present, both developed countries (e.g., Greece and Ireland) and developing countries (e.g., Portugal and Brazil) are faced with problems such as budget deficits and current account deficits. In 2003, Greece's total debt-to-GDP ratio was 97.4%, and that of Portugal was 59.4%. By 2012, this indicator soared to 156.9% and 123.6%, respectively for these two countries. Within this context, economic recovery became the top priority of the governments and central banks of all countries. The increasing need to stretch fiscal funds meant that governments were forced to make spending cuts, including in healthcare, which further worsened the difficult conditions faced by the poor and unemployed.

As the central focus of government expenditures, public health and medical care inevitably became key areas of spending cuts in all countries. A series of policies on public health and medical care were introduced to ease the financial risks, some of which focused on lowering the spending on public health and the health sector more broadly. These policies involved substantial reductions of workers' wages in the public health care system, planned batch layoffs of public healthcare workers, hiring freezes of new workers, reduced spending on various public healthcare programs, and controlling the price and use of patented drugs. In contrast, some countries increased their spending on public healthcare

33

programs. These countries increased the ratio of social insurance taxes, raised the fees for users of public health resources, and increased taxes on tobacco, alcohol, and drugs. Some countries focused on improving the efficiency of public health and the health sector. These countries improved their health information systems and established electronic health records. To summarize these policies, the policies adopted by the majority of countries can be categorized into three groups. The first group comprises policies related to achieving a balanced budget in the public health system to ensure that it does not become a burden to the national budget. The second group deals with guaranteeing the equality and accessibility of public health in the face of economic downturn and public spending cuts. The third group involves actively using the financial crisis to improve the operational efficiency of the public health system through policies. Among these three categories of policies, the first is the most immediate and the most common way to control a financial crisis. In order to achieve a balanced budget in its public health system, Greece reduced its national public health expenditure as a ratio of GDP by 0.5%, which represented a reduction of €1.4 billion (€560,000 in spending cuts came from workers' salaries and welfare and €840,000 came from reducing the operating costs of public hospitals) in 2011. Since 2010, Estonia no longer fully funds the cost of nursing care during hospitalization, and the copayment rate is fixed at 15%. Due to the impact of the financial crisis, governments have reduced their investments in healthcare and social security to varying degrees. As a result, the health and well-being of many countries have also deteriorated. On the one hand, certain communicable diseases that had essentially been eradicated have begun to come back. For example, malaria, which was considered to be eradicated on the European continent, has once again reappeared in Greece. It is difficult to claim that this situation is unrelated to Greece's health spending cuts. Other countries have also experienced sharp rises in the incidence of cardiac diseases, depression, and suicide due to financial problems. On the other hand, the economic crisis has also curtailed the treatment of healthcare workers, which has influenced the quality of healthcare. In a few developing countries hit by the economic crisis, numerous healthcare workers became unemployed, whereas others did not receive their wages for many months. Some public hospital suppliers even stopped delivering goods to the hospitals.

In the vast majority of countries, the global financial crisis has widened the wealth gap even further. Currently, the income gaps of non-OECD countries are generally higher than those of OECD countries. For example, the income gaps of India, China, and Russia are much higher than those of OECD countries. Although the levels of economic growth in developing countries, such as India, China, and Vietnam, have been higher than the average levels of OECD countries over the past 10 years, the economic development of these countries will inevitably widen the wealth gap. This situation is therefore a test of each country's wisdom in making the best of limited social security funds to reduce the poverty gap.

It is precisely the many economic and financial challenges, as well as the various global trends and specific factors of the current era, that have prompted most countries to embark on the active transformations of their health systems. As early as the 1990s, countries had already begun to carry out transformational development. However, the macroeconomic policies that were implemented were mainly aimed at raising the economic growth point and very rarely involved the problem of social equality. As a result, the health and social security systems also underwent haphazard changes and did not receive sufficient attention. With the advent of a new century and the impact from a new round of financial crises, countries gradually began to realize that their past pursuits, which focused solely on economic development and neglected social equality, were biased.

2. Current Status and Trends of World Population Aging

Population aging refers to the phenomenon involving the continuous increase in the proportion of the elderly population in a country or a region over a period of time. Internationally, an aging country, city, or region is generally defined as one in which those over the age of 60 account for more than 10% of the population or those over the age of 65 account for more than 7% of the population. In 1992, the 47th United Nations (UN) General Assembly adopted the "Proclamation on Aging" and decided to observe the year 1999 as the International Year of Older Persons. In 2002, the "Madrid International Plan of Action on Aging" was adopted at the Second World Assembly on Aging in response to the opportunities and challenges posed by population aging in the 21st century. Figure 2.1 shows the trends and forecasts of global population aging provided by the Population Division of the UN Department of Economic and Social Affairs in 2000. It is estimated that by 2050, elderly persons will exceed 30% of the total population in developed countries.

In the final few weeks of the twentieth century, the global population exceeded the 6 billion mark. UN experts have predicted that the global population will rise sharply by 3 billion from its current levels and reach the alarming figure of 9 billion by 2050. However, due to the drastic reduction in human fertility and mortality in the twenty-first century, the issue of the declining workforce due to population aging has temporarily displaced the worries over the population explosion and has become the greatest challenge facing humans in the twenty-first century. According to figures released by the United Nations Population Fund (UNPFA), the global average fertility rate has decreased from five births per woman in 1960 to the current level of 2.7 births per woman. At the same time, the global average life

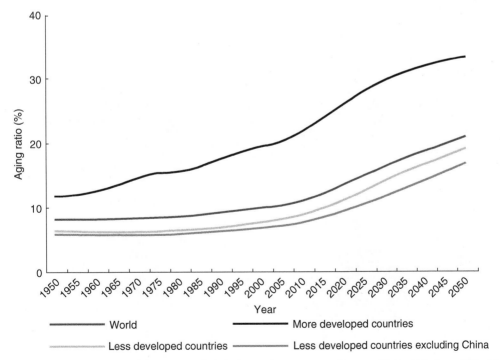

FIGURE 2.1   Trends and forecasts of global population aging *Source*: United Nations "World Population Prospects," 2011 revision.

expectancy has increased from 46 years to 68 years in the past half-century. In 1950, an estimated 200 million people worldwide were aged 60 years or over, and this figure reached 300 million by 1970. According to a UN report, in 2002, the worldwide population aged 60 years or over had risen to 630 million. The global population age-sex pyramids published in the latest 2011 revision of the UN's "World Population Prospects" can be found in Figure 2.2.

According to UN statistics, the population aged 60 years or over outnumbers the population aged 15 years or under for the first time in advanced countries and regions, such as Europe, the US, and Japan. Europe was the earliest to enter an aging society and is known as the oldest region in the world. The three countries that have been most affected by population aging are Spain, Italy, and Japan. It is projected that by 2050 the proportion of the elderly in Spain will rise from the current level of 22% to 44%, that of Italy will increase to 42%, and that of Japan will increase to 60%. In addition, Russia, Sweden, Switzerland, Germany, and Belgium are also experiencing serious population aging. In 1996, the average percentage of the population aged 65 years or over in Europe was 14%, followed by North America (13%) and Oceania (10%), and the youngest region was Africa (3%). By the end of the twentieth century, the percentage of people aged 65 years or over in Italy was 18%, followed by Greece (17.2%), Belgium (16.8%), Spain (16.7%), France (15.9%), Germany (15.8%), the UK (15.8%), Austria (15.5%), Portugal (15.3%), Denmark and Finland (14.8%), Luxembourg (14.3%), the Netherlands (13.6%), and Ireland (11.2%).

In 2000, the global population of individuals aged 60 years or over was approximately 600 million, which accounted for 9.8% of the total population. By 2005, this figure had risen to 820 million, accounting for 13.8% of the total population, and it has been increasing at a rate of 2.4%–3.0% each year. It is forecasted that by 2025, this figure could reach 2 billion

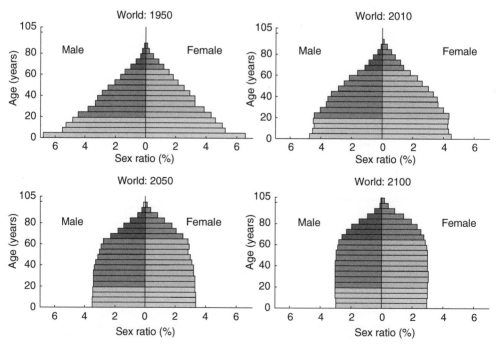

FIGURE 2.2 Global population age-sex pyramids. *Source*: United Nations "World Population Prospects," 2011 revision.

and account for 21.3% of the total population. At this point, the proportion of the population aged 60 years or over will exceed that of children aged 15 years or younger for the first time, and the entire global population will become an aging society. Europe is the region with the fastest rate of aging in the world. By 2050, an average of one in every three people will be aged 65 years or over. The percentage of people aged 80 years or over will exceed 10% in 13 countries, and Italy will be the leading country at 14%. The number of people aged 100 years or over will increase drastically by 16-fold to 2.2 million, indicating that an average of 1 in 5,000 people will be a centenarian. At this point, the elderly population in Asia alone will be 1 billion, which implies that the elderly population will no longer be a minority in all countries. UN experts have stressed that in the next 50 years, parts of Europe and Asia will face the increasingly serious problem of population aging due to the continual decline in birth rates and the prolonged life expectancy of humans. This situation is of particular concern in Japan. Fifty years from now, individuals aged 60 years and over will account for 32.9% of the population in Japan. In Europe, the US, Russia, and China, the percentage of the population aged 60 years and over will account for 31.7%, 24.6%, 22.4%, and 20.3% of the respective populations.

Based on these figures, it has been projected that there will be major structural changes in the global population by the mid-twenty-first century. With the slower growth rate of the productive population and newborns, the social costs due to a sharp rise in the elderly population will fall to an ever-shrinking productive population. The first countries to experience an increasing dependency ratio will be European countries and Japan. Nonetheless, this shift will be gradual, and if the actual retirement age can be raised to 65 years, the existing system will be able to maintain the feasibility of its insurance statistics. In quantitative terms, the shrinking productive population will need to bear the health security costs for a growing elderly population, which may result in an intolerable situation. The aging population and declining birth rate will trigger a global crisis in social and economic tensions, potentially bringing several challenges. First, an increase in the cost-of-living index will accompany a decrease in the actual living standards of residents. Second, the mass withdrawal of elderly people from the labor market and the resulting shortage of labor will lead to economic stagnation or recession. In Canada, for example, population aging has made it necessary for both spouses in most families to work in order to maintain their daily expenses. If one spouse retires or is unemployed, the other needs to work 65–80 hours per week to meet the annual living expenses of the family. For Canadian airlines, the cabin crew mostly consists of women aged 40 or 50 years and above, which demonstrates the aging workforce of the labor market. Finally, an overburdened health and social insurance system will imply that the corresponding quality of service cannot be guaranteed.

It has been forecasted that in the next 25 years, 75% of the elderly population in the world will be concentrated in developing countries, which will be a heavy burden for these countries' development. According to the UNPFA, the global total fertility rate (which is the sum of all age-specific fertility rates and represents the total number of children to be born per woman until the age of 49 years) has decreased by half, from 4.9 in the 1960s to 2.6 in the 2010s. This decline has been even greater in developing countries. Since 1960, the average fertility of these countries has already decreased by more than half (implying that the average woman in a developing country will have more than three fewer children in her lifetime than the average such woman would have had in 1960). It was originally believed that low fertility was a phenomenon that was peculiar to well-educated and highly modernized developed countries. However, the population of developed countries only accounts for less than one-fifth of the global population. Hence, we can speculate that the current low global fertility rate is also driven by low fertility rates in developing countries. According to the US Census Bureau, nearly all East Asian countries are characterized by low fertility rates, which is also the case in most Southeast Asian countries (e.g., Vietnam and Thailand), most Caribbean countries, and an increasing number of Latin American countries (Chile, Brazil, Costa Rica, Suriname, and Uruguay). Low fertility rates have also spread to countries in the part of the Islamic world that spans from North Africa through the Middle East to Asia, such as Algeria, Tunisia, Lebanon, Azerbaijan, Uzbekistan, and Brunei. Compared with other Western countries, many developing countries lack retirement pension plans and social welfare policies with universal coverage and are experiencing population aging before the completion of industrialization. Moreover, they face serious shortages of capital, technical, and infrastructure reserves to cope with the problems of population aging. Hence, the hardships they face when dealing with population aging are compounded, and they are under more severe pressure than developed countries are. Therefore, all developing countries, including China, must quickly learn from the experiences and lessons of developed countries and areas and begin to examine the solutions to the problems caused by the drastic increase in the elderly population, including issues in health services and health security systems.

3. Impact of Population Aging on Healthcare Costs

The extension of human life expectancy worldwide is one of the major achievements of social development and public health. However, it has also led to hidden worries in human society, one of which is the rapid rise of healthcare costs. According to OECD projections, half of the growth in age-related social spending between 2000 and 2050 will be due to healthcare and long-term care. Age-related social spending as a share of GDP will increase from less than 19% in 2000 to 26% in 2050, of which healthcare, long-term care, and pension spending will account for half. Within the past 10 years in Shanghai, the costs of the Shanghai Municipality Urban Employee Basic Medical Insurance grew 2.5-fold, with an average growth of 15.3% per year.

In the next 10 years, the health insurance spending of insured persons aged 60 years or over will increase from the current level of around RMB19 billion to RMB29.043 billion.

Due to the decline of physiological function and reduced physical resistance, the elderly population has a far higher incidence of diseases relative to other age groups. The elderly are especially susceptible to hypertension, diabetes, stroke, cancer, dementia, and other chronic diseases, which are direct causes of disability and mortality. Long-term chronic diseases have led to a rapid increase in the burden of disease. According to the 2008 National Health Services Survey in China, the two-week prevalence (i.e., the ratio of the number of patients to the total number of respondents in two weeks) of the population aged 60 years and over was 2.2 times higher than that of the total population (43.2% vs. 18.9%), and the chronic disease prevalence of the population aged 60 years and over was also 2.2 times higher than that of the total population (43.8% vs. 20%), with an average of two to three diseases per capita. Compared to the first survey conducted in 1993, there were significant increases in the two-week and chronic disease prevalences of the elderly population, especially for cancer, cardiovascular diseases, diabetes, and geriatric mental disorders. According to a UN report, only 10% of the global population aged 75 years or over have successfully maintained their physical health, whereas the rest are suffering from various diseases and disabilities, which imposes a heavy burden on society. It is extremely rare for individuals to continue maintaining their physical health once they have entered old age, and many of them begin to enjoy their golden years when they are 50–60 years old. A survey conducted by the Singapore Geriatric Research Institute in 2002 indicated that the elderly population of Singapore had a higher risk of developing diabetes, heart disease, stroke, and arthritis than they did 15 years prior. Only 13% of the elderly suffered from heart disease 15 years prior, but this percentage increased to 36.5% in 2001. Currently, in Taiwan, every eight productive individuals have to bear the cost of one elderly person, and up to 56% of the elderly population suffer from various geriatric chronic diseases. Each elderly person seeks medical assistance five times every three months, on average. One-tenth of the elderly population requires special care, one-third has cardiovascular diseases, and more than 90,000 elderly individuals are unable to live independently. According to the 2008 Chinese National Health Services Survey, in terms of disability, 4% of the elderly population are long-term bed-ridden, 7.3% have hearing problems, and 7% do not have self-care abilities (of which 3% are completely unable to participate in self-care). Population aging has also led to the sharp increase in the prevalence and burden of psychiatric disorders. For example, there are four million patients with Alzheimer's disease (dementia) in the US. The direct and indirect costs of treatment for dementia amount to US$300 billion each year. US experts have estimated that in the absence of effective prevention and treatment, 1 in 10 people in the US may suffer from Alzheimer's disease by the mid-twenty-first century, resulting in massive spending that will pose a serious threat to the US national economy.

Elderly patients suffer from many difficult and complicated diseases. Compared to other patients, they are more likely to be high risk and have higher surgery ratios, longer lengths of hospital stay, and greater examination and treatment costs. Studies have shown that the healthcare expenditures across a person's lifetime are mainly concentrated in old age. Furthermore, geriatric diseases share a few common characteristics: long durations, frequent recurrences, and high degrees of difficulty to cure. Hence, the healthcare expenditures of elderly persons aged 65 years or over are much higher than those of younger individuals (generally equivalent to a 3:1 ratio). In the UK, half of healthcare costs are incurred by people aged 60 years or over, and in the US, one-third of healthcare costs are incurred by people aged 65 years or over. In Australia, the healthcare expenditure per capita of people aged 60 years or over is six times that of children aged 15 years or under; in Hungary, it is 10 times higher. In Japan, the healthcare costs of the elderly are five times those of the rest of the population, which are approximately 50% of total healthcare costs.

According to the *World Development Report 1993* by the World Bank, a large-scale sample survey of developed and developing countries and areas found that the proportion of the population that is elderly can explain 92% of healthcare costs and public fund spending. In other words, the rapid growth of healthcare costs and pensions is mainly due to population aging.

4. Strategies for Actively Coping with Population Aging

There is a growing contradiction between the increasing healthcare expenditures due to population aging and the limited health resources available to society, which poses a major challenge to health insurance in all countries. In response, countries worldwide, especially developed countries and areas with serious population aging issues, have proactively explored the expansion of their health insurance financing, the establishment of specialized health insurance and healthcare systems for the elderly, and the reinforcement of community health services.

(1) Multichannel Increase in Health Insurance Financing

As a result of population aging, the working-age population in the majority of countries will decrease, which will reduce the number of health insurance contributors and cause a corresponding drop in the sources of health insurance funds. For instance, in the case of Germany's statutory health insurance, the current average level of contributions at 14% is based on 70% paying employees and 30% nonpaying retirees and unemployed persons. In the next 30 to 40 years, the proportion of contributors will drop to 60%, whereas that of nonpaying retirees and unemployed persons will increase to 40%, which represents a substantial gap in the financing of the health insurance funds.

The measures adopted by all countries to expand the financing of health insurance funds are mainly based on expanding the premium base and increasing the health insurance contribution rate. For example, in France, the "Contribution sociale généralisée (General Social Contribution)" was introduced in 1991, which incorporated a variety of alternative incomes under its premium (tax) base, including pensions, unemployment benefits, inheritance income, and property income (income from shares, rental income, and bank interests). Moreover, the rate for this tax has been increasing each year. In 1991, it was 1.1%, followed by 2.4% in 1993, 3.4% in 1996, and 7.5% in 1998. The entirety of the "General Social Contribution" is spent on health insurance. Since September 1999, Japan has increased the government-managed health insurance rate from 8.2% to 8.5% of monthly salary. In Germany, the average rate of contribution to the statutory health insurance has increased from 8.2% in 1970 to 14% in 2002. Furthermore, a few countries have also subsidized health insurance funds by issuing lotteries and levying tobacco surcharges. For example, the French government has imposed a 10.7% cut on the wholesale prices of drugs and mandated pharmaceutical companies to pay 4% of their operating revenues to the government, which have become a second channel for health insurance financing.

(2) Establishment of a Separate Health Insurance System for the Elderly

Due to the high disease incidence and relatively low income of elderly persons, some countries have established a specialized health security system for the elderly, which the government directly subsidizes or provides certain preferential policies on taxation and investments, in order to solve the health security problem of the elderly population.

The US healthcare program for the elderly (Medicare) was introduced in 1965, and its recipients are mainly elderly and disabled individuals aged 65 years or over (including their dependents or surviving dependents aged 65 years or over) who have contributed to social insurance taxes for more than 10 years. This program includes two parts: hospital insurance and supplementary medical insurance. Hospital insurance includes inpatient hospital stays and related medical services, with voluntary participation in supplementary insurance. As one of the two public health insurance programs run by the US government, hospital insurance occupies an extremely important position in the overall US health security system. The number of people in the US enrolled in hospital insurance was only 19.082 million in 1966, but it rose to 33.719 million people in 1990 and further increased to 36.544 million people in 1994. The supplementary medical insurance within Medicare covers a broader scope than the hospital insurance does. It is not limited to insured persons aged 65 years or over eligible for old-age or disability insurance but is also applicable to all people aged 65 years or over who have enrolled voluntarily and pay a monthly premium. All individuals eligible for benefits under hospital insurance can also enroll in the supplementary medical insurance by paying monthly premiums. In Japan, the health insurance system for the elderly was established in 1983, and its main recipients are all persons aged 70 years or over and bedridden individuals aged over 65 years and under 70 years. Seventy percent of this system is financed by health insurance premiums from the National Health Insurance, and 30% is financed by all levels of government. Within the next few years, the proportion of the healthcare costs for the elderly borne by the government will increase to 50%.

(3) Establishment of a Long-Term Care Insurance System Suitable for the Elderly

The Obama administration's Affordable Care Act created a nationwide voluntary insurance program, the Community Living Assistance Services and Supports Act. Although this program does not come under the health insurance program, it stipulates that all employees (except for those who opt out) will be subjected to automatic deductions from their monthly wages as premiums. The premiums are age-related and will be used to finance the hiring of service staff to care for the daily living of the insured in the event of functional impairments.

Based on the high prevalence of chronic disease among the elderly and the needs of some patients for long-term care, Germany, Japan, Singapore, and other countries have also proposed long-term care insurance for the elderly. The establishment of long-term care insurance for the elderly will help to improve the quality of care services they receive, increase the use of community health service institutions, and, thus, gradually reduce the utilization of hospital services and the number of hospital beds occupied by the elderly.

Germany established independent statutory care insurance in 1995. The contribution rate of the statutory care insurance is 1.7%, borne in equal halves by the employee and employer. All persons insured by the statutory health insurance are enrolled in the care insurance. Currently, among the 1.95 million people requiring care in Germany, aside from a small number requiring accident and postnatal care, most of the other recipients are persons aged 80 years and above. Care insurance provides a care service fee of €384 per month to home care staff and €205 per month to family caregivers.

Japan established its long-term care insurance for the elderly, which was relatively completed as of April 1, 2000. The insurers are the local governments below the prefecture level (city, town, or village). The government bears 50% of the funds for long-term care insurance, of which 25% are borne by the central government, 12.5% by the prefecture government, and 12.5% by the city, town, or village government.

The individuals covered by the long-term care insurance are divided into people aged 40–64 years and people aged 65 years or over. The premiums they pay are 17% and 33%, respectively. Elderly individuals who require care services can apply for them, and a government long-term care approval board will determine the amount of benefits to be paid according to the six levels of care required: partial, mild, moderate, severe, very severe, and exceptionally severe.

Singapore's population structure is relatively young. Currently, there are only 200,000 individuals aged over 65 years, accounting for 7% of the total population. By 2030, this figure will increase to 800,000 and account for 18% of the total population. As Singapore's health insurance system will face serious challenges posed by population aging in the near future, the government established the ElderCare Fund in 2000 as a precautionary measure to reduce the tax burden of a shrinking working population. Its interest income is used to subsidize community hospitals, nursing homes, daytime rehabilitation, home health check-ups, home care, and the operating costs of nursing homes run by voluntary welfare organizations. This fund mainly targets the elderly from low- and lower-middle income households. In 2001, Singapore introduced the ElderShield insurance plan, which pays for the long-term care of elderly persons with severe disabilities, including the costs of home care. ElderShield is an actuary-based lifetime insurance with low premiums that can be paid using a health savings (Medisave) account. An insured person starts paying premiums from 40 years of age until 65 years of age. The cash payout of this insurance program is SGD 300 per month with a maximum payout period of 60 months.

(4) Strengthen Community Health Services

Community health services focus on the basic healthcare of people. These services comprise a primary healthcare system that fully utilizes community resources to provide basic healthcare, health education, health promotion, preventive healthcare, rehabilitation, and necessary social services. With regards to the utilization of health services, 90% of clinic visits involve community health services, and 10% involve hospital services. In an aging society, government or health insurance agencies can monitor and intervene in the high-risk elderly population through community health service providers to promote economic, rapid, and convenient detection methods. Doing so enables the early discovery, diagnosis, and treatment of chronic noncommunicable diseases, thus achieving the aim of saving healthcare costs. Based on the different healthcare needs of the elderly, community health providers can also prepare health records, develop family sickbeds, and provide outpatient care, home care, daytime observation, hospice care, and other services. Countries around the world are paying more attention to the role of community health services.

Obama's Affordable Care Act required USD 10 billion to be spent each year for five consecutive years, 2010–2014, to continue developing the "National Action Plan for Aging and Disability Resource Centers." This program is jointly managed by the US Senior Citizens Bureau and the federal Centers for Medicare and Medicaid Services. It aims to encourage state governments to set up community-based resource centers for disease care and rehabilitation, which will provide the elderly and disabled with timely and easy access to information on these topics.

Not only is the UK the birthplace of community health services, it is also widely recognized as having community health services with the most comprehensive organizational structures and service functions. These services are mainly provided by general practitioners (GPs). British law stipulates that nonemergency patients must first consult their own GPs for medical treatment; otherwise, they will not be able to receive free medical service. It is generally accepted that this "gatekeeper" system of British GPs is a key reason for the UK's low growth in healthcare costs.

To strengthen its community services, Germany adjusted the professional structure of physicians. The proportion of GPs was increased by modifying the ratio of specialists to GPs from 6:4 to 4:6, and the income of GPs was also increased in order to encourage more healthcare workers to engage in community health services.

(5) Reform of Health Insurance Payment Methods

Payments based on diagnosis-related groups (DRGs) involve the classification of hospital inpatients into groups based on their diagnoses, ages, and other factors. Each group is then classified into different levels based on disease severity and the presence of complications. The corresponding cost reimbursement standards are then determined for the different levels in each group. Based on this cost standard, a one-time payment can be made to a service provider for the full treatment course of a certain severity level in a particular DRG. At present, more than a dozen countries in the world, particularly in Europe, have adopted DRG-based payment systems. DRG-based payment systems enable the standardized utilization of medical resources by formulating unified reimbursement standards for DRG quotas, which ensures that the consumption of hospital resources is proportional to the number and medical needs of hospital inpatients. As the reimbursements of costs incurred by hospitals are pre-paid according to case quotas, the prepayment income received by hospitals is related to each case and its diagnosis rather than the actual cost of treatment for each case.

Hospital profitability is determined by the difference between the DRG standard costs and the actual costs incurred, which in turn encourages hospitals to proactively reduce costs to gain profit. Thus, hospitals can minimize the durations of patients' hospital stays, thereby effectively suppressing supplier-induced demand and enabling the possibility of containing the consumption of healthcare costs.

SECTION II. GLOBAL HEALTH STATUS AND CURRENT CHALLENGES

With the advancement of society, substantial achievements have been made in the improvement of human health, with remarkable progress and changes in the four major indicators of health evaluation. In 2012, the global average life expectancy was 72.7 years for women and 68.1 years for men, the infant mortality rate was 35 per 1,000 live births, the under-five mortality rate was 48 per 1,000 live births, and maternal mortality rate was 210 per 100,000 live births. In addition, with the development of the economy, the health goals of governments around the world and the public's understanding of health have both changed, resulting in new content and requirements for the concept of health.

1. Update on the Concepts of Health

Owing to the very nature of health, its importance cannot be overemphasized. In the words of the Nobel laureate Amartya Sen, "Health, like education, is among the basic capabilities that gives value to human life." According to the results of a global survey, which was commissioned by the UN Secretary-General Kofi Annan in preparation for the UN Millennium Summit, good health consistently ranked as the number one desire of all people around the world. The suffering and premature death caused by diseases have made disease control the central concern of all societies, which has also motivated the world to enshrine health as one of the basic human rights in international law. However, what is health, and how is health determined? The answers to these questions have always been in constant dispute. As society advances, there have been gradual transformations in our understanding and in medical models of diseases, which have accompanied by continuous changes and updates in the concept of health.

(1) Simple Concepts of Health

The ancient Greek physician Hippocrates believed that the human body contained four humors: blood, phlegm, yellow bile, and black bile. Thus, he considered a state of health to be when the four humors were balanced in the correct proportions; otherwise, health was lost. This is the ancient, primitive concept of health. After the application of microscopy to medicine in the seventeenth century, the ecological concept was proposed, which posits that health is a state of dynamic equilibrium among three elements: pathogenic factors, the host, and the environment. However, more emphasis was placed on the role of pathogenic factors. On this basis, sociologists proposed that a state of health could only be achieved through the coordination of individual behavioral factors, host factors, and environmental factors. As progress was made in the biological sciences, the formation of biological disciplines, such as anatomy, histology, physiology, biochemistry, and genetics, enabled humans to understand the phenomenon of life and the relationship between health and disease from a biological perspective. In particular, after the establishment of cytology in the mid-nineteenth century, the biomedical model of health – which considered health as a biological adaptation and a state of internal equilibrium in the body – gradually occupied a dominant position. The biomedical model has played a major facilitatory role in the development of medicine. In the field of basic medicine, the understanding of the human body progressed from the macroscopic level to the microscopic cellular and molecular levels, which led to the founding of gene theory. In terms of clinical medicine, antimicrobial drugs were discovered, the sterilization of surgical operations was achieved, and the problems of pain, infection, and blood loss were resolved. Thus, a number of diseases with high morbidity and mortality in the population were controlled and eliminated. With regard to public health, environmental improvements and immunization programs for children drastically reduced the incidence of deadly infectious diseases, which decreased infant mortality and increased the average life expectancy. Although the biomedical concept of health emphasizes that life activities form a unified whole in terms of structure, function, and information exchange, it neglects the fact that humans are amalgamations of biological and social characteristics.

(2) Transformations in the Concept of Health Caused by Changes in Medical Models

Due to the achievements of biomedical models, most developed countries and areas have completed their first health revolution since the 1950s, which succeeded in controlling acute communicable diseases that endanger human health. The spectrum of human diseases and causes of death underwent substantial changes, and the main diseases affecting human health and lives have gradually shifted from acute communicable diseases to chronic noncommunicable diseases. Therefore, the primary task of the second health revolution is to control chronic noncommunicable diseases. Although communicable diseases have yet to be fully controlled in developing countries, the incidence and mortality rates of cardiovascular disease and malignant cancers have also been gradually increasing each year. Hence, developing countries are currently in the transition period between the first and second health revolutions. At the same time, our understanding of human nature has transcended from that of a biological, natural man to that of a soci-economic man. Our understanding of the genesis and development of diseases has ascended from the biological level to the psychological and social level. Our concept of health has become increasingly holistic and multilevel. With the development of the economy and increases in national incomes, the public has higher expectations for healthcare. People are no longer satisfied with the absence of illness and good physical condition but are also demanding reasonable nutrition, appropriate working and living conditions, good lifestyles, balanced and healthy mental states, the ability to engage in social activities, a higher quality of life, and longer life expectancies.

Medical models have gradually been updated from biomedical models to biopsychosocial models. The field of medicine will shift from being disease-oriented to being health-oriented and from being centered on individual patients to being centered on all groups in society. The focus of medicine will shift from diagnosis and treatment to preventive healthcare. The task of medicine will gradually transform from the prevention and treatment of diseases to people-oriented, comprehensive protection and improvement of human health and the quality of life.

(3) The Concept of Health Proposed by the World Health Organization

In 1974, the World Health Organization (WHO) stated that "health is a state of complete physical, mental and social well-being, and not merely the absence of disease or infirmity."

The 27th Session of the World Health Assembly in 1974 stressed that new knowledge, new technology, and new methods should be applied in medicine to promote health and to investigate the role of psychological and social factors in disease and healthcare. To ensure that the public had a complete and accurate understanding of the concept of health, the WHO proposed 10 standards for the measurement of health:

1. Sufficient energy and ability to cope easily with daily life and work without feeling overly nervous or fatigued.
2. An optimistic and positive attitude and a willingness to take on tasks without being picky.
3. The ability to obtain adequate rest with good sleep quality.
4. Strong adaptability and ability to adjust to changes in the external environment.
5. A basic level of resistance against the common cold and infectious diseases.
6. Maintenance of an optimal body weight and symmetrical body proportions with coordinated head, shoulder, and arm positions when standing.
7. Clear vision with quick reactions and eyelids that are not prone to inflammation.
8. Clean, defect-free, and pain-free teeth and gums of normal color and without bleeding.
9. Healthy hair with no dandruff.
10. Full muscles and elastic skin.

The introduction of this new concept of health led to extensive debate. Some believed that this concept of health was too broad, such that it was beyond the scope of medical capacity and could not be achieved. However, with the shift in medical models and deeper research in social medicine, people have gradually come to realize that this definition is an active concept that reveals the essence of human health, which regards humans on a higher level as members of society. This concept unites natural man and social man and, thus closely links the body with the spirit and human health with the biological, psychological, and social. It is not only the goal pursued by human beings, but it also reveals the various levels involved in the definition of health and is of important practical significance.

The changes in modern health and medical models have led to a shift from a patient-centered approach to an approach oriented towards the overall population, which has had an immense impact on traditional health services. First, health services have expanded from treatment services to prevention services. Preventive healthcare emphasizes interactive thinking and is present throughout the process of life. It focuses on three levels of prevention: primary prevention, which involves adopting effective measures before the onset of disease to prevent its occurrence; secondary prevention, which involves early detection and timely treatment at the initial stage of the disease; and tertiary prevention, which involves disease treatment and rehabilitation to prevent disability. Second, health services have expanded from technical services to social services. Physicians are required to have both medical knowledge and knowledge of human science. In addition to treating diseases, physicians should also be able to apply social medical diagnoses to discover the health problems of residents and identify the risk factors that endanger their health. Based on their findings, they should provide health guidance and health promotion, thereby guiding individuals to adopt healthy lifestyles and behaviors. Third, health services have expanded from physiological services to psychological services. Modern medical models require health services to adopt a holistic approach. Thus, when providing physical care, psychological services should also be given to patients and the general population. Physicians should understand the psychological factors that may influence patients and should continuously enrich the contents and measures of psychological services.

(4) Universal Coverage of Health Security

Achieving the universal coverage of health security is currently a major global trend. By comprehensively surveying the features in the historical development of health security worldwide, we know that the goal has always been to improve health security coverage until universal coverage is achieved. As a crucial step in achieving universal health coverage (UHC), the universal coverage of health security can be based on the path to achieving UHC.

The realization of UHC is also a topic of significant concern worldwide. The WHO pointed out that for a community or a country to achieve UHC, the following factors are essential:

1. A robust, efficient, well-functioning health system that can meet key health needs through integrated, people-centered healthcare services (including services for HIV, tuberculosis, malaria, noncommunicable diseases, and maternal and child health). Such a system includes the provision of information encouraging the public to stay healthy and prevent diseases, early detection of health status, capacity for disease treatment, and the rehabilitation of patients.
2. Ensuring affordability by establishing a system of financing health services so that individuals do not experience financial hardships when using health services. This goal can be achieved in a number of ways.
3. Access to basic drugs and technology for diagnosis and treatment of medical problems.
4. Well-trained and enthusiastic healthcare workers with the full capacity to deliver services and meet the needs of patients based on the best available evidence.

The promotion and protection of health contributes to the enhancement of human well-being and is a facilitator of sustainable socioeconomic development. Thirty years ago, the Declaration of Alma-Ata stated that "primary health care for all people" contributes not only to a better quality of life but also to world peace and security.

There are numerous factors that can influence health. The WHO defines the Social Determinants of Health (SDH) as the factors affecting health beyond the direct causes of diseases that result from the basic structures and social conditions of social stratification within the living and working environments of the people. They are the "cause of cause" of diseases and include all of the social conditions in which people live and work, such as poverty, social exclusion, living conditions, and so on.

As we can see, the methods to promote and maintain health have exceeded the purview of the health sector. The conditions in which people grow, live, work, and age have immense impacts on their lives and deaths. By incorporating the influences of education, housing, nutrition, and employment issues on health, we can arrive at the theory of "Health in All Policies (HiAP)."

In China, the majority of functions in health security do not come under the jurisdiction of the health sector. Hence, to achieve the universal coverage of health security, it is necessary to fully implement the contents of HiAP. HiAP was first proposed by the Finnish EU Presidency in 2006 and aims to achieve common goals through intersectoral cooperation. It reiterated the importance of public health in policies and the structural factors that affect health. In 2013, the 8th Global Conference on Health Promotion was held in Helsinki, Finland, with HiAP as the theme of the conference. In her speech at the conference, WHO Director-General Margaret Chan stated that the social determinants of health are exceptionally broad and that policies in other sectors can have a profound effect on health. When addressing the problems of health, policymakers should make full use of the HiAP strategy and lend the strength of multisectoral collaboration to protect health policies from the effects of commercial interests. The conference reviewed and adopted the Helsinki Statement and "Health in All Policies: Framework for Country Action," which called on all countries to place an emphasis on the social determinants of health and to provide organizational and technical measures to support the implementation of the HiAP strategy.

(5) Four-Dimensional Concept of Health

From the biological-medical model of health proposed in modern society to the three-dimensional concept of complete physical, mental, and social well-being proposed by the WHO in the 1940s and 1950s, we can see that there have been substantial changes in our understanding and pursuit of health. This is especially true in recent decades, where the changes in the social environment and personal lifestyles brought about by rapid economic development have posed a large number of new problems with regards to human health. To this end, in the 1990s, the WHO incorporated "moral health" into the concept of health, and the new definition includes physical, mental, social, and moral health – that is, the four-dimensional concept of health.

2. Comparison of World Health Statuses

In "World Health Statistics 2014," the WHO used a comprehensive health indicator – the disability adjusted life expectancy (DALE) or the healthy life expectancy – to measure the health levels of the citizens in each country. The 191 Member States were ranked according to this indicator. We can see from Table 2.1 that the DALE basically represents the actual health level of each country. This statistic reflects the differences in the health levels among the countries presented and is consistent with the gaps found by other common health indica-tors (e.g., the infant mortality rate, the maternal mortality rate, and average life expectancy).

As of 2012, the three major health indicators had shown significant improvements for all countries, but the gap between countries with different levels of economic development was still substantial. The health levels of developed countries and areas were much higher

TABLE 2.1 Health Indicators in 2012 of Countries with >100 Million People

Country	DALE (years)	Total Population (million)	Infant Mortality Rate (per 1,000 live births)	Maternal Mortality Rate* (1/100,000)	Life Expectancy (years)
			Health Indicators		
Japan	75	127.3	2	6	84
United States	70	317.5	6	28	79
China	68	1,384.8	12	32	75
Russia	61	143.2	9	24	69
Brazil	64	198.7	13	69	74
India	57	1236.7	44	190	66
Nigeria	46	168.8	78	560	54

* Indicates data from 2013.

than those of developing countries. This distinction was especially prominent in Japan, which topped the global rankings for average life expectancy (84 years), infant mortality rate (2 per 1,000 live births), and maternal mortality rate (6/100,000).

In terms of the global average, girls born in 2012 can expect to live about 73 years and boys about 68 years, which is six years longer than the global average life expectancy of children born in 1990. The World Health Statistics 2014 reported that low-income countries showed the greatest improvement in average life expectancy, which increased by nine years from 1990 to 2012. The six countries with the highest gains in life expectancy were Liberia (a gain of 20 years, from 42 years in 1990 to 62 years in 2012), Ethiopia (from 45 years to 64 years), Maldives (from 58 years to 77 years), Cambodia (from 54 years to 72 years), Timor-Leste (from 50 years to 66 years), and Rwanda (from 48 years to 65 years). The gap between rich and poor countries was still substantial, as people in high-income countries had a higher probability of living longer than that of people in low-income countries. In high-income countries, boys born in 2012 are expected to live for 76 years, which is 16 years longer than boys born in low-income countries (60 years). The difference is even more pronounced in girls, with a gap of 19 years between high-income (82 years) and low-income (63 years) countries. Women in Japan have the highest life expectancy in the world at 87 years, followed by women in Spain, Switzerland, and Singapore. The 10 highest female life expectancies by country are all above 84 years, and the nine highest male life expectancies by country are all above 80 years. Iceland, Switzerland, and Austria have the highest male life expectancies. At the other end of the scale, the male and female life expectancies of nine sub-Saharan countries, Angola, Central African Republic, Chad, Côte d'Ivoire, Democratic Republic of Congo, Lesotho, Mozambique, Nigeria, and Sierra Leone, are still below 55 years.

Figure 2.3 shows the relationship between the average life expectancy at birth and GDP per capita in 176 countries around the world. We can see that a higher level of income per capita generally corresponds with a higher level of average life expectancy. In addition, the figure also shows that countries with similar incomes per capita may have vast differences in life expectancy at birth, especially among poorer countries. For example, the average life expectancy of Sierra Leone (GDP per capita of US$679) is 22 years shorter than that of Nepal (GDP per capita of US$694) and that of South Sudan (GDP per capita of US$1045) is 17 years shorter than that of Cambodia (GDP per capita of US$1007). The difference between life expectancies in Nigeria and Philippines is 15 years, and that between China and South Africa is 11 years. Figure 2.3 also shows that there is a relatively large gap the GDPs per capita of countries with similar life expectancies. For example, the average life expectancies of Italy and Switzerland were both 83 years, but the GDP per capita of the former was US$35,926, and that of the latter was US$84,815. There are also differences between Poland (average life expectancy: 77 years, GDP per capita: US$13,648) and Peru (average life expectancy: 77 years, GDP per capita: US$6,662) and between Kazakhstan (average life expectancy: 68 years, GDP per capita: US$13,610) and Nepal (average life expectancy: 68 years, GDP per capita: US$694). These findings indicate that the level of income per capita within a certain period of time is not, as suggested by conventional curves, an absolute limiting factor on the rate of health development.

In the World Health Report 2008, the classic Preston curve was used to characterize the definitive relationship between health and wealth, but the report also noted that the Preston curve has been shifting over the years. Figure 2.4 shows that from 1975 to 2005, the relationship between economic growth and life expectancy at birth has shown three distinct patterns. Within these 30 years, the majority of countries experienced increases in the life expectancy at birth and significant economic growth. The first pattern is that the

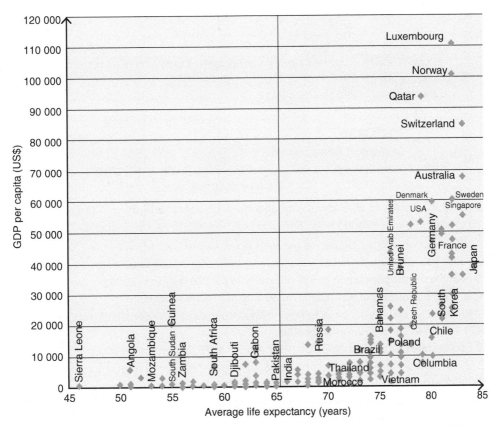

FIGURE 2.3   Relationship between life expectancy at birth and GDP per capita in 176 countries worldwide. *Source:* Average life expectancy (2012) – World Health Organization (2012); GDP per capita – World Bank (2013).

Note: Only the names of a few representative countries are labeled.

total population in many Asian (including India), Latin American, and low-income countries has increased from 1.1 billion in 1975 to 2 billion in 2005. GDP per capita in these countries has increased by 1.6-fold, and the life expectancy at birth has increased by 12 years. The second pattern is that high-income countries and countries with GDPs in the range of 3,000–10,000 international dollars (I$) in 1975 also experienced significant economic growth and increased life expectancies. The third pattern is that in other parts of the world, the growth in GDP was not accompanied by an increase in life expectancy. The newly independent states in Eastern Europe showed significant increases in GDP per capita. However, the widespread poverty accompanying the dissolution of the Soviet Union meant that the life expectancy of women has stagnated at 1980s levels, whereas that of men has plummeted, especially for those lacking education and job security. By 1980, China had increased the life expectancy of its inhabitants far beyond those of other low-income countries in the 1970s. As the Chinese economic reform progressed in the 1980s, China's GDP per capita grew at an astonishing rate. However, its access to healthcare and social security continued to deteriorate, especially in rural areas. This reduced access slowed down the pace of China's health development, which suggests that a regression in average life expectancy was only avoided due to the higher living standards associated with rapid economic growth.

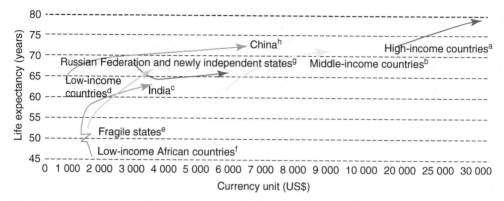

FIGURE 2.4 Trends in GDP per capita and life expectancy at birth for 133 countries from 1975 to 2005. *Source:* World Health Organization, The World Health Report 2008.

Note: The countries in the figure are grouped according to GDP in 1975.

[a] 27 countries, total population of 766 million in 1975, 953 million in 2005.

[b] 43 countries, total population of 587 million in 1975, 986 million in 2005.

[c] India, total population of 621 million in 1975, 1.103 billion in 2005.

[d] 17 low-income countries, not including African countries and fragile states, total population of 471 million in 1975, 872 million in 2005.

[e] 20 fragile states, total population of 196 million in 1975, 374 million in 2005.

[f] 13 low-income African countries, not including fragile states, total population of 71 million in 1975, 872 million in 2005.

[g] Russian Federation and 10 newly independent states, total population of 186 million in 1985 (no data for 1975), 204 million in 2005.

[h] China, total population of 928 million in 1975, 1.316 billion in 2005.

There is also a set of low-income countries defined as "fragile states" according to the low-income countries under stress (LICUS) criteria for 2003–2006. These countries account for about 10% of the global population, and 66% of this population is in Africa. These countries had the lowest life expectancy at birth in 1975, and both their GDPs and their life expectancies have stagnated. Extended internal conflicts and poor governance are common in these countries, and they face similar difficulties: fragile social orders, disintegration of social relations, corruption, breakdown in the rule of law, and a lack of mechanisms to generate legitimate power and authority.

Furthermore, certain low-income African countries share similar characteristics and circumstances as these fragile states. In fact, many of them have experienced sustained internal and external conflicts over the past 30 years. If the LICUS classification had existed at that time, they would have been classified as fragile states as well. Economic development in these countries has been extremely limited, as has been the increase in average life expectancy. However, these countries' average life expectancies were not the lowest, as many countries in southern Africa were impacted by the AIDS pandemic. The latter countries have experienced some economic growth since 1975 but have also seen a significant reversal in life expectancy.

3. Key Issues in Human Health

In many parts of the world, reducing the risk of communicable diseases and controlling communicable, parasitic, and nutrient-deficiency diseases remains a daunting task. Furthermore, certain communicable diseases that were previously under control, such as tuberculosis and malaria, have now started to reappear due to the emergence of drug-resistant bacteria. Moreover, new communicable diseases, including AIDS, are showing clear global trends of spreading. Noncommunicable diseases that are related to human socioeconomics, urbanization, population aging, behaviors, and lifestyle have also become the main causes of death in many developed and developing countries and areas.

New problems have begun to emerge even before the old issues have been resolved. Society now faces the following challenges in health.

(1) Extreme Imbalance in Social Health Conditions

With socioeconomic development and technological advancement, there have been improvements in people's living and working conditions. However, there are still significant disparities among different regions and countries, between rural and urban areas, and among different social classes within the same country.

Malnutrition is a worldwide social health problem despite the multiple ways it manifests in different regions and countries. According to the estimates of the UN Food and Agriculture Organization and the World Bank, between 500 million and 1 billion people in the world (mostly in developing countries) are undernourished. Among the 1.1 billion inhabitants of high-income countries (countries in Europe, North America, Japan, and Oceania), the rate of population growth is very low (0.7%), whereas the level of food production is high, resulting in malnutrition due to overeating (e.g., obesity). Among the 800 million inhabitants of middle-income countries in Asia and Africa (except China), although population growth is high (2.8%), the rate of economic development is also rapid, and food production is greatly increasing. Thus, a considerable proportion of the population in these countries (high-income class) suffers from overnutrition. Among the poorer countries in Asia and Africa (1.2 billion inhabitants, GDP per capita below US$200), an estimated one-third to one-half of the population is severely undernourished, especially among children.

The impact of global warming and environmental pollution on health should not be underestimated. In China and other Asian countries with planned economies, the GNP per capita is below average, but significant malnutrition is uncommon. A similar situation is observed for environmental sanitation. In overall terms, the living conditions of human beings have improved, but there are imbalances among different regions. In developing countries, the main problems are the lack of basic sanitation facilities and environmental pollution caused by energy-intensive and highly polluting industries. In more developed countries, the prominent problems are environmental hazards related to industrialization and urbanization, industrial pollution, traffic problems, noise, and the degradation of air and water quality. Rural areas have poorer basic sanitation facilities than urban areas have. According to a WHO survey in 1995, 83% of urban residents had access to running water and 79% had reasonable sanitation facilities, whereas in rural areas, only 22% of residents had an adequate water supply and 15% had satisfactory sanitation services. In the early 1970s, a survey on living conditions found that 75% of urban households had electric equipment, in contrast to only 25% of rural households (5% for some countries). With increasing industrialization, urbanization, and utilization of chemical substances, the extent of environmental pollution (including air, water, soil, and food) is gradually becoming worse, and the living environment of human beings is further deteriorating.

(2) Widespread Inequalities in Health Status

First, there are health inequities among countries. The global average life expectancy in 2009 was 71 years, but that of developed countries was 80 years, that of developing countries was 71 years, and that of the least developed countries was 57 years. With regard to the infant mortality rate, that of developed countries was 4 per 1,000 live births, that of developed countries was 11 per 1,000 live births, and that of the least developed countries was 36 per 1,000 live births. As for the proportion of deaths from communicable diseases, that of poor countries was 60 per 1,000 live births, whereas that of rich countries was only 8–10%. Looking at the distribution of mortality, more than half of the deaths in poor countries occurred under the age of 15 years, whereas in rich countries, only 4% of deaths occurred under the age of 15 years.

Second, there are health inequities within each country. In both rich and poor countries, there is a clear difference in health status among different social classes. For example, a study in the UK showed that the mortality rate of individuals with lower socioeconomic status was significantly different from that of those with higher status, and this difference had a graded association with health. In underdeveloped and developing countries, this disparity is mainly determined by socioeconomic status and equality of access to healthcare services.

(3) Key Changes in the Spectrum of Disease and Causes of Death

Noncommunicable diseases are one of the main challenges of health and development in the twenty-first century. These diseases bring about suffering in patients and endanger countries' socioeconomic statuses, especially among low- and middle-income countries. No government can afford to ignore the increasing burden of noncommunicable diseases. Without evidence-based actions, the human, social, and economic costs of noncommunicable diseases will continue to increase and will far exceed the capacity of any country to deal with this issue.

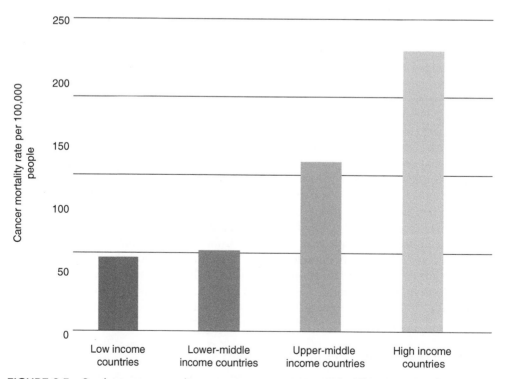

FIGURE 2.5   Crude cancer mortality rates among countries with different income levels in 2012. *Source:* World Health Organization, *Global Status Report on Noncommunicable Diseases 2014.*

In 2012, the total number of deaths worldwide was 56 million, of which 38 million (68%) were due to noncommunicable diseases. The WHO Global Status Report on Noncommunicable Diseases 2014 also showed that there were differences in the crude cancer mortality rates among countries with different income levels in 2012 (see Figure 2.5). Three-quarters (28 million) of deaths from noncommunicable diseases and most premature deaths (82%) occurred in low- and middle-income countries. However, the majority of premature deaths caused by noncommunicable diseases are preventable. China's premature deaths from noncommunicable diseases are not especially severe when compared to those of similar countries (upper-middle-income level), but its situation is very serious from a global perspective.

The data indicates that of the premature deaths in China, 19% were due to the four groups of diseases mentioned earlier. In our survey, we found that the average for nine countries, including Australia, Sweden, and Japan, was only 9%. Therefore, China should adopt measures and policies to reduce this figure.

Based on the current development of low- and middle-income countries, it is estimated that the economic losses caused by noncommunicable diseases from 2011 to 2025 will reach US$7 trillion. Thus, the enormous cost of inaction far exceeds that of implementing a comprehensive set of influential measures to reduce the burden of noncommunicable diseases (US$11.2 billion per year). In recognition of the destructive impact that noncommunicable diseases have on society, the economy, and public health, the leaders of the world adopted a political declaration in September 2011 that included a strong commitment to addressing the global burden of noncommunicable diseases and called for the WHO to take action to support all national efforts. One of the tasks was to develop a 2013–2020 Action Plan for the Global Strategy for the Prevention and Control of Noncommunicable Diseases, which included nine voluntary global targets and a global monitoring framework. In 2013, the WHO approved this Global Action Plan and its voluntary global targets.

The main causes of death have gradually transitioned from acute communicable diseases, parasitic diseases, and malnutrition in the past to cardiovascular diseases, cancers, and accidental injuries. The burden of disease analyzed using the disability-adjusted life year (DALY) indicated that from 1990 to 1999, the contribution of mortality from communicable, parasitic, and nutrient-deficiency diseases to total DALYs decreased from 45.8% to 42.8%, whereas that of chronic noncommunicable diseases increased from 42.2% to 43.2% and that of accidental injuries increased from 12.0% to 13.2%. In developed countries and areas, the proportion of deaths from cardiovascular diseases has decreased slightly but still accounts for nearly half of deaths. In developing countries, communicable diseases are still the primary threat to health, but the risk of cardiovascular diseases and cancers is gradually increasing. Table 2.2 shows the changing trends in the composition of the leading causes of global deaths.

(4) Impact of Social Diseases on Health

Increasing emphasis has been placed on the relationship between health and social diseases, which are adverse behavioral factors related to human health, including smoking, alcohol consumption, drug use, stressful lifestyles, and unhealthy behaviors.

Smoking is a major cause of declining health and premature death. In most European countries, the smoking prevalence among adult men is above 50%, and that among adult women is between 10% and 50%. As for countries in Asia, Africa, America, and Oceania, the smoking prevalence among adult men is mostly above 40% and even reaches 70% in some countries (Japan, the Philippines, and South Africa), but that among women is very low and rarely exceeds 30%.

TABLE 2.2 Composition Changes in the Leading Causes of Global Deaths

Cause of Death	Developed Countries			Developing Countries		
	1985	1990	1997	1985	1990	1997
Communicable and parasitic diseases	5	4	1	45	44	43
Circulatory system diseases	51	48	46	16	17	24
Cancer	21	21	21	6	7	9
Respiratory system diseases	4	3	8	6	6	5
Perinatal and maternal diseases	1	1	1	10	10	9
Other diseases	18	23	23	17	16	10
Total	100	100	100	100	100	100

Although many survey studies have confirmed the effects of smoking (including passive smoking) on human health (including the health of the next generation), the cultivation, processing, and consumption of tobacco has only continued to increase. Furthermore, tobacco production in developing countries is growing at a faster rate than that of developed countries. Among the top 10 tobacco-producing countries, five are developing countries (Brazil, China, India, Indonesia, and Turkey). Understanding the relationship between smoking and health and addressing the issue of smoking control have become key topics in current preventive medicine and public health.

Excessive alcohol consumption has an impact not only on individual health but also on family and society as a whole. The amount of ethanol (alcohol) consumption is positively correlated with the prevalence of cirrhosis. However, ethanol consumption is increasing in nearly all countries. In many European countries, the pure alcohol consumed per capita per year is above 10 L (e.g., France, 16.8 L; Italy, 13.6 L; Austria, 12.4 L; Portugal, 11.7 L; Spain, 11.4 L; Switzerland, 10.8 L).

The abuse of psychotropic drugs is on the rise throughout the world. In some countries in Southeast Asia and the Western Pacific Region, opiate addiction has become a serious and long-term problem. The rate of heroin abuse among urban youths has been increasing each year, and the emergence of new drugs has brought about even more serious challenges.

More youths worldwide are engaging in sexual behaviors at an earlier age. The incidence of sexually transmitted diseases, especially gonorrhea, has risen significantly among youths, and teenage pregnancy has been gradually increasing. A survey conducted in certain Latin American countries found that among women below 20 years of age, 50% had given birth to their first child, 25% had their second child, and 10% had their third child. In developing countries, maternal complications are one of the major causes of death among women aged 15–19 years.

(5) Improvements Needed in Public Health Emergency Response Systems

In 2002–2003, atypical pneumonia caused considerable damage in both Mainland China and Hong Kong, but it was well-controlled in the US, where the losses were reduced to a reasonable extent. This outcome was due to the effective role played by the rapid public health response system in the US. Global warming has resulted in the frequent occurrence of natural disasters worldwide, which is a major threat to public health and poses new challenges to the public health emergency response systems in all countries.

On May 12, 2008, a 7.8-magnitude earthquake hit Wenchuan in Sichuan Province. On September 25, 2008, the Ministry of Civil Affairs reported that 69,227 people were confirmed dead, 374,643 were injured, and 17,923 were missing. According to official statistics, On September 25, emergency rescue workers had rescued and relocated 1,486,407 people in total. Based on the report of the Ministry of Health, On December 22, a total of 96,544 people had been hospitalized due to injuries from the earthquake (not including the number of injured people treated in the quake zone), of whom 93,518 had been discharged, 352 remained hospitalized, and 153 were injured people transferred from Sichuan to other provinces. In total, 4,273,551 injured people were rescued and treated.

On August 28, 2008, as Hurricane Katrina approached the US port city of New Orleans at a speed of 282 kilometers per hour, Mayor Ray Nagin ordered a mandatory evacuation of the city on the same day. Measures were taken to avoid all possible losses.

On March 11, 2011, a 9.0-magnitude earthquake struck off the Pacific coast of Japan to the east of the northeastern Miyagi Prefecture at a depth of 10 kilometers, followed by 168 aftershocks registering magnitudes of over 5.0. A total of 14,704 people were confirmed dead or injured, and 10,969 were missing. After a string of accidents in multiple units of the Fukushima Nuclear Power Plant, radiation levels exceeding the local standard value could be detected in many parts of Japan. The sudden threat of natural disasters to human life is beyond the realm of normalcy. Hence, a complete and sound response system is particularly important for the protection of human life and health.

SECTION III. PROPOSING THE CONCEPT OF GLOBAL HEALTH AND ITS DEVELOPMENT TRENDS

1. Definition and Evolution of Global Health

(1) Definition of Global Health

Global health, or global sanitation, has its focus on the health of populations within a global context and not just on the health of populations in individual countries. Its emphasis is on health issues that transcend national borders or have a global political or economic impact. In 2005, participants of the Global Health Summit held in Philadelphia, Pennsylvania signed the Philadelphia Accord, which cited the wording of the American Medical Association in its definition of global health. That is, global health is "health issues and major controversies that transcend national boundaries or that may be affected by the conditions and experiences of certain countries, such that joint action is the best solution to these problems."

Different scholars have different opinions regarding the attributes of "global health." Brown et al. argued that the term "international health" originated from the joint efforts between countries in the control of infectious diseases and requires two or more countries, whereas "global health" implies the common concerns of the global population over the health issues of the whole planet, which weakens the concept of individual nations. The latter concept is more consistent with the blurring of national boundaries in globalization. In their article, Bunyavanich and Walkup also raised a similar view, suggesting that the term "global" highlights the "irrelevance of geopolitics in addressing health issues" while also echoing the WHO strategy of achieving health for all. In addition, "global health" emphasizes the commonalities in healthcare knowledge, provisions, and policies shared by people of all nations that are a manifestation of globalization in health. Kickbusch proposed that "global health" refers to "health issues that transcend national boundaries and

governments and call for actions on the global forces that determine the health of people."
These forces include not only countries but also various newly emerging actors.

(2) Evolution of Global Health

The term "global health" first appeared in the 1970s and has gradually become a dominant term in the field of international public health since the 1990s. Its predecessor was "international health." In the mid-fourteenth century, the Black Death was a devastating blow to Europe. To control this epidemic, certain port cities in Italy, led by Venice, began to impose a 40-day embargo on foreign ships and established a quarantine system in 1377. This system controlled the spread of the disease to some extent, but it was not conducive to the development of the European economy, as the primary mode of trade was by sea. In order to find a balance between disease control and economic development, the first International Sanitary Conference was held in Paris in 1851. This conference was the first multinational gathering in history that brought together public health managers and researchers to address cross-border health issues. Hence, 1851 has been regarded as the starting point of international health.

In 1907, the Office of International Public Hygiene was established. It was the first international organization in the world, and its main functions involved research on infectious diseases, organizing regular international health conferences, and implementing conference resolutions. After World War I, the Allies set up a dedicated Health Organization in the League of Nations, which mainly engaged in research on disease epidemiology and technology development. It coexisted with the International Office of Public Hygiene but had different functions, and it persisted until World War II. As the main battlefield of World War II, Europe suffered major losses, and neither the International Office of Public Hygiene nor the Health Organization of the League of Nations was able to continue assuming the responsibility for international health.

In 1945, at the UN Conference in San Francisco, the delegations of Brazil and China jointly proposed the establishment of a worldwide health organization, which became the World Health Organization, founded in 1948. The International Office of Public Hygiene and the Health Organization of the League of Nations were both incorporated within this new organization. In the few decades since its establishment, the WHO has made remarkable achievements in disease control, health promotion, and strengthening primary healthcare, and, thus, an international health system centered on the WHO has gradually formed. With the globalization of the concept of the free market, the spread of capital, goods, people, ideas, thoughts, and values began to transcend national boundaries. Economic, political, and social interdependence gradually deepened, and global integration occurred at an accelerated pace. This globalization also had an impact on the health sector. Since the 1990s, the concept of global health began to emerge and gradually replaced the concept of international health.

2. Research Areas Related to Global Health

The aim of global health is to improve living conditions, reduce disease transmission, and promote global stability. It highlights the fact that global health concerns the health of human populations and is the shared responsibility of all citizens of the world. Therefore, global health not only involves the traditional domain of public health (mainly concerning the prevention and control of diseases) but also extends to many other areas. One of the more prominent aspects of global health is the integration of global health with diplomacy.

(1) Global Health and Health

A substantial proportion of the problems that need to be addressed and solved in global health are within the traditional domain of public health, specifically including disease prevention and the extension of life expectancy. Within this domain, infectious diseases are a major concern of global health. The continued progress of globalization has enabled infectious diseases to spread globally at an accelerated pace. According to the WHO's World Health Report 2007, the greater interdependence between countries, higher population mobility, and increased speed of transportation have strengthened the ability of infectious diseases to spread on a global level, thereby increasing the speed of transmission.

In 2003, severe acute respiratory syndrome (SARS), avian influenza, and the H1N1 (influenza A) virus were transmitted across all parts of the world within a very short period of time. The globalization of production processes, the expansion of trade, and the frequent movement of products have contributed to the transmission of infectious diseases. Much of the food consumed by people comes from distant parts of the world. Problems occurring at any stage of planting, breeding, processing, transportation, and sales may lead to the transmission of infectious diseases. Mad cow disease and hoof-and-mouth disease are two well-known such examples.

(2) Global Health and Diplomacy

Public health has always been a low priority in foreign policy, and its role in international relations has not been taken seriously. However, in recent years, the advancement of globalization has imbued public health with more global characteristics. People are also gradually recognizing the higher level of interactions between public health and foreign policy, which highlights the role of health in diplomacy. Furthermore, the solutions to health issues, especially global health issues that concern all countries, also require the interventions such as diplomatic negotiations and consultations. This integration of health and diplomacy not only helps sovereign nations solve their own global health issues but has also produced two major results: the Framework Convention on Tobacco Control (FCTC) and International Health Regulation (IHR). These legally binding instruments, which are the results of international negotiations and consultations, have played an important role in global health issues.

3. Challenges and Opportunities Concerning Global Health

Global health issues are global by nature. Hence, global health is of paramount importance to the moral, practical, and strategic considerations for the peace, prosperity, and welfare of all countries. However, the rapid means of travel, international trade, commercial exchanges, and convenient global communication of the modern era have also brought about new challenges and opportunities to global health. The key aspects are discussed next.

First, although breakthroughs in vaccines, antibiotics, clean water, environmental health, and other areas of science and technology have contributed to global health, globalization has also led to a sharp increase in cross-border health risks. These risks include newly emerging and reemerging infectious diseases, the global spread of diseases linked to the consumption of harmful products or unhealthy lifestyles, environmental pollution, the impact of climate change in human health, and so on. In particular, HIV infections, the increasing number of chronic diseases, and the unprecedented worldwide flow of goods and people are significant challenges in public health.

Second, a variety of factors, including poverty and disparities in health conditions, urgently need to be addressed.

Third, the social determinants of many health issues are becoming more globalized. Hence, in order to deal with these determinants, it is necessary to take joint action with the nonhealth sector and even more crucial to promote the cooperation and understanding of public health in all countries. To successfully prevent the outbreak of new diseases and promote health status, healthcare workers and the general public must adopt a global outlook and think beyond national borders. Consideration must be given to global events that may have an impact on the public as well as the impacts of the actions of one nation on that nation's neighbors across the globe.

Fourth, there is a need to formulate a timetable that will enable governments, nongovernmental organizations, religious groups and advisory bodies, publicly and privately funded health programs, integrated health and environment promotion organizations, professional health associations and societies, public education systems in all countries, and the media to undertake their respective obligations in promoting global health, thereby creating favorable circumstances for health governance.

SECTION IV. EXPLORING THE INTEGRATION OF HEALTHCARE AND PREVENTION IN HEALTH INSURANCE

The compensation of economic losses caused by diseases is the primary purpose of establishing a health security system. However, with the changes in the concept of health, especially with the influence of its modern concept, people's understanding of the function of health security has also been changing continuously.

1. Gradual Transition from Disease Insurance to Health Insurance

In the early stages of establishing a health security system, countries first prioritized sickness allowances in health security and then proceeded to include treatment costs within the scope of health security. The first items to be included in the treatment costs are the treatment costs that have a relatively large impact on people's standard of living. For example, the costs of inpatient medical services were included first, and this coverage was then expanded to general medical services. In countries with relatively complete health security systems, elderly care and preventive healthcare have also been included in the scope of health security. As the concept of health began to change, people gradually realized that including preventive healthcare in the scope of health security could facilitate the decrease in disease incidence or the early detection of diseases. This, in turn, was beneficial to the containment of healthcare costs and could also help to fundamentally improve the level of health.

In the formulation of the US Healthy People 2000 plan, clinical preventive services were listed as one of the three main objectives. Clinical preventive services encompass four main aspects: early disease screening, disease counselling and guidance, immunization, and chemoprevention. The early identification of patients, early diagnosis, early treatment, and improving the prevention and treatment of diseases could have important economic and social significance. For example, cervical cancer is the leading cause of death among female cancer patients in developing countries, resulting in approximately 150,000 deaths per year. In developed countries and areas, the use of Pap smear tests for screening is extremely common. This method mainly targets women above the age of 35 years, and screening is performed once every five to 10 years. Inexpensive outpatient treatments (e.g., cryotherapy of abnormal cells) are provided to women with serious precancerous symptoms. If this treatment is coupled with good followup services, then such preventive work is extremely cost-effective.

The US Preventive Service Task Force (USPSTF) was established in 1984. Since 1998, the Agency for Healthcare Research and Quality has been responsible for providing the USPSTF with ongoing funding and technical support. The recommendations of this task force are seen as the gold standard for clinical disease prevention. Obama's Affordable Care Act requires that any Grade A or Grade B preventive service recommended by this task force must be offered free of charge to insured persons under Medicare, Medicaid, and all commercial health insurance. In addition, it is also internationally recognized that in countries with high incidences of breast cancer, performing mammography in women over 50 years of age can significantly reduce the mortality rate of women in this age group.

In 1990, the UK National Health Service switched from a fee-for-service system for the payment of free GP services to a payment-by-results system. For example, GPs were given different remunerations depending on the coverage levels of childhood immunization and cervical cancer screening within their catchment area. This policy enabled the mobilization of GPs to actively engage in preventive work. In Germany's Statutory Health Insurance, the preventive services provided include health counseling, vaccinations, cancer screenings once a year for women aged 20 years and over and men aged 45 years and over, and physical examinations every two years for adults aged 35 years and over to check for cardiovascular diseases, diabetes, and nephropathy.

2. Strengthening Health Education and Advocating Healthy Lifestyles

Chronic noncommunicable diseases, represented by cardiovascular diseases and malignant cancers, have gradually become the leading causes of deaths in the global population.

The treatment of chronic diseases is often costly and ineffective. Modern medical research has shown that diet and lifestyle changes and minimizing other risk factors are the best ways to avoid the incidence of such diseases and to reduce unnecessary healthcare expenditures. At present, the control of chronic noncommunicable diseases mainly depends on population-based prevention. Population-based prevention is the targeted dissemination of necessary preventive knowledge to the recipients of preventive healthcare. It aims to establish effective knowledge, attitudes, and behaviors for effective health education habits combined with targeted self-management performed by individuals. It is only by ensuring that all members of society understand and possess a certain level of health knowledge that the overall health of society can effectively be improved. Doing so requires enhancing the breadth and depth of disseminating medical and health knowledge such that all members of society are able to establish a correct understanding of self-care, consciously adopt active measures to safeguard and promote health, and develop lifestyles that meet the requirements for health. These lifestyles include adequate exercise, reasonable diets and nutrition, normal social activities, abstaining from unhealthy behaviors, and so on. To achieve all these goals requires a certain level of health knowledge.

In 1989, the provisions of the German Healthcare Reform Act required all sickness funds to return "no claim bonuses," equivalent to one month's premiums, to insured persons who had not submitted claims for medical treatment within a year. In the same year, German law stipulated that the sickness funds were responsible for undertaking health promotion and that all sickness funds must educate all citizens (especially those with low incomes) on health knowledge. The Federal Joint Committee required that all funds must spend a minimum of 5 Marks per person on advocating health education.

3. Promoting the Capitation System to Enhance Preventive Healthcare

The health maintenance organization (HMO) is also widely used in the cost containment models of developed countries and is an early mode of operation for managed care.

In 1973, the US federal government enacted the Health Maintenance Organization Act, which strongly encouraged the development of HMOs. An HMO is the most complicated mode of operation in managing and controlling healthcare services and expenditures. HMOs can be categorized as open-panel and closed-panel HMOs. The independent group model HMO and the network model HMO have also been developed in recent years. In an open-panel HMO, physicians or other obligors sign a contract with the HMO as an independent entity. The open-panel model is further divided into the independent practice association and the direct contract model. In a closed-panel HMO, the contracted physicians and their clinics are limited to providing medical services to members of the HMO and not to other patients.

A common feature of HMOs is that insured persons are limited to physicians and hospitals within the service network of the HMOs. If patients seek medical services beyond the service network, the HMOs will not cover the expenses incurred or will only cover a limited amount of the medical expenses. The GP management model is adopted for outpatient care, where GPs act as gatekeepers who manage and coordinate the use of various medical services and determine referrals for specialist and inpatient care.

The capitation system involves prepaying healthcare providers a total sum of medical expenses based on the service population, service volume, or measured average costs. It is a method of settling healthcare expenditures in which healthcare providers can control the outgoing expenses, retain their savings, and cover any overexpenditures. This approach can promote healthcare institutions to form internal cost-containment mechanisms for healthcare services and consciously adopt measures to control costs, for example, by actively performing preventive care, health education, regular health checkups, and so on. Doing so can help to minimize morbidity, thereby reducing expenditures and encouraging physicians to provide better quality service at lower costs.

Survey statistics from developed countries indicate that after implementing a capitation system, the healthcare spending per capita decreased by 10–40% and the hospitalization rate decreased by 25–45%.

The statutory health insurance programs of the UK, Denmark, and the Netherlands have adopted capitation systems. Prior to 1980, Italy adopted this approach for a proportion of its insured persons. After 1980, this approach became common practice nationwide. The capitation system is widely used among HMOs in the US. Indonesia and Costa Rica have also adopted this payment method for healthcare costs. In 1989, Ireland discontinued its existing compensation system based on the number of treatments and first visits and adopted the capitation system.

The DRG-based system has also been widely implemented in the US and Taiwan, which has resulted in significant cost-containment effects. The fee-for-service system is characterized by its simplicity and ease of operation. It offers patients a greater choice of physicians and can basically meet the needs of patients. However, the income of the healthcare providers is directly proportional to the amount of services provided, which leads to the overprovision of medical services by healthcare providers and incentivizes healthcare consumption. This overconsumption ultimately results in the rapid growth of healthcare costs, causing overpayment by health insurance funds and increased patient burden. The DRG-based payment system uses the International Classification of Diseases (ICD-9) to classify diseases based on diagnosis, age, and sex into several major groups. Each group is then divided into DRGs according to disease severity, and the presence of comorbidities and complications. This is combined with evidence-based medicine to calculate the medical cost standard for each DRG based on clinical pathways, which is then prepaid to the healthcare providers.

SECTION V. PROGRESS IN MEDICAL TECHNOLOGY AND ITS IMPACT ON HEALTHCARE COSTS

1. Current Status of and Trends in the Development of Medical Technology

The dramatic changes in healthcare over the past 100 years can be attributed to the rapid advances in biomedical sciences and medical technology. In the late nineteenth and early twentieth centuries, the establishment of cytopathology, genetics, and a series of basic disciplines in biomedical sciences became a significant landmark in the development of modern medicine. The other landmark in the development of modern medical technology is the close combination of medicine with natural sciences and technologies.

The medical advancements of the twentieth century were deeply impressive due to the dizzying array of diagnostic and therapeutic instruments and devices that were available in large, modernized hospitals. These advancements range from X-ray and electrocardiography in the early twentieth century, to electron microscopy, endoscopy, tracers, and diagnostic ultrasonography in the mid-twentieth century, and then to computed tomography, positron emission tomography, and magnetic resonance imaging (MRI). These instruments have revolutionized the field of diagnostics, enabling us to achieve modern clinical diagnoses that are accurate, precise, dynamic, microquantitative, automated, and noninvasive. Furthermore, renal dialysis machines, pacemakers, organ transplants and artificial organs, minimally invasive surgery, and a new generation of drugs have also demonstrated the important role of new technologies and new materials in clinical treatment.

After the mid-twentieth century, significant progress was made in surgery, marked by cardiac surgery and transplant surgery. In 1967, when Barnard succeeded in transplanting a woman's heart into the body of a 54-year-old male, transplant surgery received the same extent of public attention as space travel. As humans gained further understanding of the immune system, the development of immunosuppressive agents solved the problem of rejection and opened up new areas in transplant surgery. Over the past 100 years, not only has rapid progress been made in surgery, but its nature has also undergone a transformation. In the early twentieth century, surgery essentially involved suturing and resection. However, it has now transformed into precise repair and seamless replacement. With the discovery of endoscopic surgery, surgery has also developed in the direction of becoming more refined and minimally invasive.

After the 1950s, the establishment of molecular biology enabled scientists to conduct more in-depth research to elucidate the structures and functions of the human body on a molecular level, thus providing theoretical guidance to solve major medical problems, such as cancer, immunity, genetics, tissue regeneration, anti-aging, and drug development.

Basic scientific research has transformed people's understanding of the body's battle against diseases. The defective genes of many genetic disorders as well as the related genes and viral pathogenic genes of other diseases have also been identified. This research further confirmed that genes are essentially the material basis for determining the birth, aging, illness, death, and all other phenomena of human life. In addition, genetic engineering has also promoted the emergence the new drugs and sequences.

In 1986, US scientists proposed the Human Genome Project (HGP), which aimed to determine the entire sequence of the human genome. This project was officially launched in 1990, and the US announced its completion in 2003. The achievements of the HGP will continue to be an inexhaustible source of knowledge for modern biology and medicine. Furthermore, immune theory and technology have also permeated and influenced the entire field of medicine. Recognizing the mutual effects of the immune system with the nervous and endocrine systems has contributed to a deeper understanding of the integrity and organic interconnections of the human body. The development of neuroscience gave new hope to the treatment of Parkinson's disease and other disorders of the central nervous system. Since the 1990s, more attention has been paid to the importance of an integrative perspective in the brain sciences, that is, to recognize the multifaceted and multilevel nature of neural activity. Therefore, we can see that the development of molecular biology, neuroscience, immunology, and endocrinology has not only deepened our understanding of the basic structure and function of the human body but has also revealed the integrity and organic interconnections of the body from different perspectives. Modern medicine has begun to focus its attention on exploring the mysteries of life based on the interrelationships and integration among different levels in the movement of life substances. This work has greatly improved the progress of clinical medicine.

Following its conquest of numerous serious diseases and the alleviation of suffering, the goal of medicine now seems unclear and confused. The principle of "technology for good" emerged alongside the rapid development of medical technology, which has solidified people's ambitious vision of medicine, that is, "whatever can be done, must be done." There was a belief that humans could eliminate all disease and suffering and that all damaged human organs could be replaced like spare parts in a machine. However, even as the development of medical technology continues to improve the level of human health, the total number of diseases has increased instead. On one hand, this process is inevitable as our understanding of the human body continues to deepen. On the other hand, it is possible that people are increasingly viewing the normal processes of human life, such as menopause and the decline of body functions with age, as diseases that need to be alleviated by drugs, Nevertheless, one thing is certain: the development of medical science and technology has led to changes in healthcare costs. Health security not only concerns the quality of healthcare but should also consider the costs of health security.

2. Impact of High-Tech Medicine on Healthcare Costs

The rise of high technology is a double-edged sword that has promoted medical advances that have improved the level of health and created greater social value but has also led to the rapid rise of healthcare costs and greatly exacerbated the burden on society.

(1) Development of High-Tech Medicine Has Exacerbated the Unequal Distribution of Health Resources

The extensive and costly treatments highlighted in clinical medicine have saved the lives of critically ill patients and delayed the process of death. However, this tendency to focus on the disease and ignore the patient while also placing a heavy economic burden on the patient and society has drawn an increasing amount of criticism. Solving the contradiction between developing sophisticated and applicable technology while also coordinating the conflict of caring for patients and treating diseases have become urgent issues in modern society. A US official responsible for health administration once calculated that the cost of one artificial heart transplant is equivalent to that of 11,900 general outpatient clinic visits. Given a fixed amount of healthcare resources, this method of funding implies that performing one artificial heart transplant is equivalent to rejecting 11,900 general patients. The reverse implies that only one cardiac patient will lose the chance of prolonging their life. If a dying patient can be given an artificial heart with the provision of expensive medical services but millions of expectant mothers cannot receive prenatal care due to a lack of funds, we must ask whether there is equality in this situation.

Many experts believe that the current sophisticated medical technologies are mostly post-treatment technologies with limited treatment scopes and efficacies. The higher the level of specialist technology is, the lower its benefits to the population are. Hence, the lower its equality is, the smaller its effect on enhancing the overall health of the population is.

(2) Misdiagnosis Caused by Overdependence on Medical Technology Has Led to Rising Healthcare Costs

Since the emergence of high-tech medicine, there has been an overdependence by physicians and an overconfidence by patients in this technology. During the healthcare process, physicians place a greater emphasis on examination reports and often ignore the effects of the patient's psychosocial factors on the disease. Moreover, what patients most expect is to receive the specific examinations they want, instead of providing the physicians with as much psychosocial and biological information as possible, which will help the physicians' analysis and diagnosis. This expectation not only dilutes the doctor–patient relationship but also easily leads to misdiagnosis and mistreatment.

Furthermore, due to the mechanization, remote control, informatization, and acceleration of certain healthcare activities, there is less contact between nurses and patients, which has reduced direct interactions and has affected patients' emotional expression and transmission. This has led to the formation of a healthcare worker–medical device–patient relationship between doctors and patients and between nurses and patients, which is known internationally as a "health hazard."

For example, mitral valve prolapse is a disease observed in 1969 based on X-ray imaging, which was replaced by M-mode ultrasound in the 1970s for its diagnosis. Several studies reported that the detection rate of mitral valve prolapse was very high among women, possibly exceeding 10%, and it was the most common heart disease. By the late 1970s, after the development of two-dimensional echocardiography, it was found that a significant proportion of the diagnoses based on M-mode ultrasonography were misdiagnoses. If physicians had performed more physical examinations in greater detail, instead of relying solely on the ultrasound results, then these misdiagnoses could have been completely avoided. Evidently, the overdependence on high-tech equipment contradicts the requirements of modern biopsychosocial medical models, which can easily lead to misdiagnosis and mistreatment. Not only does this cause significant physiological and psychological trauma to patients, it also leads to a substantial waste in health resources.

(3) Abuse of High-Tech Medicine Leading to the Waste of Healthcare Resources

It takes a certain amount of time for people to fully understand a new medical technology. There have been cases in which immature technologies have been widely promoted, consuming a large amount of health resources, but have ultimately been shown to be ineffective or even harmful. For example, the administration of thalidomide to pregnant women led to fetal deformities; oxygen therapy in premature babies led to retrolental fibroplasia; and the invention and extensive application of gastric cryosurgery was ineffective in treating ulcers and resulted in the death of patients. Therefore, this technology must be used with caution; otherwise, it may cause harm to patients and lead to a waste of healthcare resources. However, in the context of the current commodity economy, many hospitals have tried to maximize their profits by adopting various material incentives that encourage physicians to order high-tech tests and prescribe expensive drugs. When ordering tests, physicians often do not consider their suitability for disease diagnosis and the patients' financial abilities but are more inclined to consider their own economic interests. Direct consequences of this incentive structure are excessive tests and excessive prescriptions. This situation seriously affects the mutual trust and mutual communication between physicians and patients, which has had adverse effects on diagnosis and treatment. Thus, the calls for solving the problems of inaccessible and unaffordable healthcare have been growing louder.

The development of medical science and technology may lead to unnecessary healthcare needs and increased healthcare supply. Not only does this process increase the number of patients, it also results in a decline in the overall health of the population. A study in the US showed that at least 20% of clinical tests are unnecessary. Another survey of a teaching hospital found that 47% of clinical tests can be canceled without affecting the quality of healthcare. A survey of coronary artery bypass in the US showed that 25% of surgeries in that year lacked medical indications.

A few foreign health economists have suggested that the development of medical technology can be divided into three stages:

1. The first is the nontechnology stage, where hospitals and health services play an insignificant role in improving health status and treatment costs are low.
2. The second is the clinical technology stage, where the treatment of many diseases, such as organ transplants and the surgical treatment of cancer, becomes possible. The treatment costs are high in this stage.
3. The third is known as the health intervention technology stage, where there is a clearer understanding of the pathogenesis of diseases, and preventive measures can be taken to control the occurrence of disease, as, for example, through the application of immunotherapy. At the same time, measures can also be adopted to promote and improve the lifestyle, behaviors, and environment of the population. This type of high technology places a greater emphasis on social health interventions in the population. The growth of healthcare costs in this stage is relatively reasonable. It requires considerable investments from social funds into the field of preventive healthcare and produces better health outcomes. Over the past 30 years, the health sector has mainly been developing "semi-technologies" for the treatment of many diseases, and the advancement of these technologies has led the rapid rise in healthcare costs.

3

Health System Structure and Determinants of Health

 ## SECTION I. STRUCTURE OF HEALTH SYSTEMS AND THEIR RELATIONSHIPS

1. Goals and Boundaries of Health Systems

Of the approximately 191 independent countries in the world, there are no two with health systems that are identical. In fact, the structure and operating mode of health systems undergo constant changes even within the same country. However, there are several common methods available to analyze these systems in any country at any given point in time. Just like a car has engine, tires, and seats, every health system has specific components, but the characteristics of these components might differ substantially between countries.

Although systems must be comprehensively analyzed, there should be a boundary to this comprehensiveness, and the goals of a health system are defined by its boundaries. Undoubtedly, the primary goal of a health system is to promote health or recovery from disease or injury. However, health systems clearly have secondary goals as well, such as creating healthcare jobs or keeping workers healthy in order to maintain their productivity.

Is healthcare the ultimate goal, or does it serve to improve happiness, economic productivity, and military strength? This is a philosophical question. Regardless of its ultimate purpose, the primary and direct goal of healthcare is to improve and protect people's health. Moral and legal issues would inevitably arise if healthcare services served only to generate income for physicians or any other purpose unrelated to health.

There are still ambiguities to be resolved, even when using the narrow definition of health systems (i.e., a system with the primary goal of improving and protecting people's health). For example, hospital bedside care is clearly a healthcare service that falls within the scope of health systems, but what about nursing-home care for the elderly? Similarly, providing vitamins to children with rickets clearly belongs within the scope of health systems, but what about the provision of nutritious lunches to schoolchildren? These two examples – nursing homes and nutritious lunches – can significantly improve the health of their target population, but health improvement is not their primary objective. In other words, health protection is merely a byproduct, rather than the primary goal, of providing care to the elderly or lunches to schoolchildren.

In that case, what content should be included within the scope of health systems? As each country provides a range of different healthcare services, examining the complex resources and activities involved in these services will reveal a number of main categories. In early societies, where cities had not yet formed and governments were still in their rudimentary stages, the health system was centered solely on the care provided by shamans to patients. In later sections, we will discuss how highly developed health systems have evolved. Here, we only need to be aware that the structure and function of all health systems in modern society are becoming increasingly complex.

Currently, there are five major categories of interrelated activities that can be easily identified within the health systems of all countries: (1) creation or retrieval of certain resources (human and material); (2) establishment of healthcare programs on the basis of these resources (with varying forms among countries), which generally also include informal private healthcare markets; (3) multiple sources of funding used to create healthcare resources and provide healthcare services; (4) some form of management to provide better healthcare services in both public and private programs; (5) ultimately, the provision of healthcare services to both healthy individuals and patients, which will vary in form among different countries, even among different population groups within the same country. In short, the main components in the health system of any country can be generalized using the following five terms: production resources, project organization, financial support, management methods, and service provision.

Figure 3.1 shows the main interrelationships among these components. It should be noted that the health system refers only to the space within the dotted lines (i.e., the boundaries); the components beyond the boundaries are the healthcare issues and needs that must be addressed by the system (left) and the outputs of the system (right).

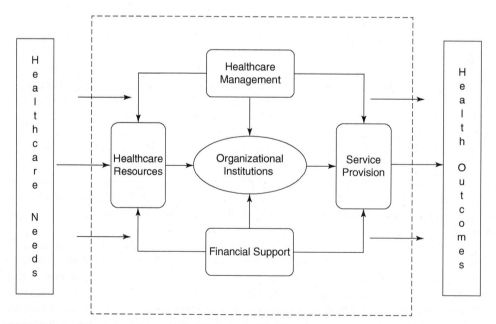

FIGURE 3.1   Schematic diagram of national health systems.

The health systems of all countries have been evolving over several centuries and have all come under the influences of various social phenomena, such as religion, science, industry, urbanization, communication technology, international trade, wars, and politics. The economic development and mainstream political ideologies of each country play decisive roles in the functioning of each component of the health system.

In order to fully demonstrate the relationships between the five major components of health systems, more lines and arrows must be added to the schematic diagram in Figure 3.1. Additionally, each component can be divided into innumerable subcomponents, some of which can be regarded as subsystems that can further be delineated into more subsystems. For instance, the main component Healthcare Resources contains the subcomponent Healthcare Workforce Development, which can be further divided into Nursing Education. Alternatively, the main component Organizational Institutions almost always contains Spontaneous Healthcare Agencies, which in turn may also contain Organizations for the Prevention and Control of Tuberculosis. Thus, it is easy to see that through in-depth studies of health systems in each country, each of these categories varies in its contents and features across different countries.

Within the greater context of our current understanding of the definition of health systems, we will examine in detail the specific contents of these five components within the health systems of different countries.

2. Medical and Health Resources

Each healthcare system includes several types of resources. For example, such systems must provide healthcare workers (healthcare workforce), healthcare facilities that enable these workers to carry out their tasks (the most basic facility being the residences of traditional practitioners), goods and supplies (mainly drugs) for patient care, and comprehensive knowledge systems for the treatment and prevention of diseases. The concrete application of these knowledge systems is often referred to as techniques.

The four types of resources already mentioned should either be producible or readily available. In general, the healthcare workforce or healthcare workers either need to be trained or recruited from other countries. Financial support (along with human and material resources) is essential to the construction of healthcare facilities. Medical supplies, such as drugs, bandages, and laboratory equipment can be manufactured, imported, and acquired from nature (e.g., herbal medicines), whereas knowledge can be obtained through research, observation, learning (the most common approach), and consolidating experiences. The generation and acquisition of healthcare resources will be elaborated upon in the following sections.

(1) Healthcare Workforce

The diversity and size of the healthcare workforce has increased exponentially with the development of the health sciences. Due to various historical reasons, physicians are often regarded as playing the most crucial role in all healthcare systems, alongside numerous other types of healthcare workers. Developed countries typically have healthcare workforces that are of relatively greater diversity than those of less-developed countries.

Despite their crucial role in the healthcare system of all countries, the definition of "physician" remains elusive. Several years ago, the member states of the World Health Organization (WHO) attempted to achieve a global consensus on and recognition of the unique qualities and functions of physicians. In 1972, such a consensus was finally achieved following a lengthy debate. According to this definition, a physician must be admitted to state-recognized medical schools in their country of residence, successfully complete the required medical courses, acquire the necessary skills to independently engage in medical practices (including prevention, diagnosis, treatment, and rehabilitation skills), and obtain a medical license according to law, before they can engage in improving community and individual health.

In other words, after undergoing training in compliance with the statutory standards of their respective countries, physicians must be equipped with the necessary skills to independently engage in the health improvement of the population. In reality, it is almost impossible to establish an internationally recognized standard because the requirements for medical education and practices vary greatly across countries.

Based on this definition, all countries have professional healthcare workers who have undergone some form of formal education and training and are regarded as experts in the diagnosis, treatment, and prevention of diseases, as well as overall health improvement. Medical colleges and institutions are affiliated with universities in most but not all countries. Medical education typically begins with the study of the basic sciences, such as chemistry, biology, physics, anatomy, physiology, and pathology. This is followed by various theoretical courses on clinical medicine, including pediatrics, surgery, obstetrics, gynecology, psychiatry, and internal medicine. Furthermore, increasing attention has been paid to the psychosocial aspects of diseases and the strategies used for health promotion and disease prevention during the training of physicians. Finally, medical students must participate in clinical training by taking examinations and treating different patients, in order to apply their theoretical knowledge into practice. The sequence, duration, and teaching methods of the aforementioned processes vary substantially across different countries, and even across different schools within the same country.

Newly graduated medical doctors are generalists in the diagnosis and treatment of diseases, and are commonly referred to as "general practitioners." With the advancement of medical knowledge, science, and technology, as well as the development of the medical profession, greater emphasis has been placed on people-oriented values and concepts. In all healthcare systems, especially those of developed and industrialized countries, physicians can also further their medical training in various specialties to become medical specialists, which can be achieved by completing several years of residency at hospitals. Specialists typically incur greater service charges than do general practitioners due to the lengthy and expensive courses involved in training a specialist. Therefore, the training and recruitment of specialists will increase a country's healthcare expenditures.

The medical specialties of physicians can be classified along the following lines: Organ- or system-based specialties, such as ophthalmology, cardiology, and neurology; technique-based specialties, such as radiology, pathology, and anesthesiology; demographic-based specialties, such as pediatrics, obstetrics, and the emerging field of geriatrics. Internal medicine can be further subdivided into cardiology, endocrinology, gastroenterology, nephrology, etc. Surgeons, who are required to perform surgery, might focus on certain organs or body parts, such as the skeletal system (orthopedic surgery) or nervous system (neurosurgery). In light of the global trend towards increasing specialization, many countries have begun to raise the status of general practitioners through the following measures: providing them with regular continuing education and training courses, raising their salaries, and providing support in the form of healthcare assistants in community centers. Several countries have implemented postgraduate programs for general or family practitioners and regard general medicine as a medical specialty.

Other independent healthcare practitioners, such as traditional practitioners or therapists (commonly referred to as "barefoot doctors" or "rural doctors" in China) are the most widely distributed categories of primary healthcare workers worldwide. They provide patients with the most direct, simple, and fundamental healthcare services. Traditional practitioners are the oldest "physicians" in history and have existed before the emergence of modern medicine. To date, they still play an important role and generally outnumber modern physicians in most developing countries, particularly in remote rural regions.

There are hundreds of different types of traditional practitioner. The theoretical foundation of their therapeutic approaches typically includes the following aspects: (1) religious or supernatural understanding of diseases; (2) experience in the use of traditional herbal medicines or other natural substances; and (3) some combination of the previous two aspects. Some of these traditional practitioners (especially in Asia) undergo short-term formal training, whereas others might only learn their skills from an "old master" as apprentices. Traditional therapists are typically classified as an independent healthcare workforce, but sometimes they are (fully or partially) included in the healthcare programs launched by the government. Conversely, they are legally prohibited from practicing in many developed countries and regions.

Traditional birth attendants, who are usually mature women with multiple childbirth experiences, form a category of healthcare workers that is closely related to traditional therapists in almost all developing countries. They usually assist or supervise the process of childbirth not only in rural areas but also in urban areas. However, traditional birth attendants should not be confused with well-trained registered midwives or nurse midwives because the former mainly rely on their experience with local customs and traditional childbirth practices. Traditional birth attendants are widely included in obstetric services in developing countries. Furthermore, the healthcare authorities in many countries have begun systematically training them in healthcare practices. They are occasionally provided with the appropriate equipment for cutting the umbilical cord and trained in appropriate disinfection practices by the government.

In many developing and developed countries, there is another type of healthcare service provider that should not be referred to as physicians or therapists. They are known as religious or cult practitioners, as they perform medical practices based on ancient religions or experiences. In reality, their therapeutic theories have only gradually emerged in the modern era. These healthcare service providers include chiropractors and homeopathic practitioners – the former claim to treat any illness via spinal adjustment while the latter employ over-diluted medications for the treatment of almost any illness. Other, similar types of cult practitioners include naturopathic practitioners and nutritional therapists, who seek to treat all types of diseases through special diets. The believers of Christian Science treat illnesses through prayer and religious dialogue. Osteopathic practitioners, who once followed similar theoretical principles as chiropractors, have gradually broadened their concepts to coincide with modern medicine (also known as allopathic therapy). The legal rights of the aforementioned medical practitioners are protected by law in many countries, which ensures that they can continue providing services to patients seeking their aid.

Other types of independent medical practitioners have a more solid scientific basis but specialize only in certain body parts. The most well known among them are dentists (who specialize in teeth and periodontal tissues) and stomatologists (who specialize in oral health). In most healthcare systems, dentists must receive a university education, which is characterized by the same learning intensity as physicians. Similar to physicians, dentists can also further specialize in different fields, including pediatric dentistry, periodontal diseases, malocclusion (orthodontics), and other dental diseases.

Some highly or moderately developed countries also have other types of independent healthcare workers specializing in other organs. Optometrists (sometimes referred to as opticians) specialize in the correction of refractive errors through eyeglasses but are not qualified to treat other ocular diseases. Podiatrists are trained in the treatment of relatively common foot disorders, such as bunions and plantar warts. However, there are still controversies in some countries regarding which symptoms require the attention of physicians or the aforementioned practitioners.

The healthcare workforce in the field of psychiatry is especially complicated: some healthcare workers can legally and independently provide services to patients, whereas others must work under the supervision of a physician. In the health systems of certain countries, psychologists (those with higher educational qualifications only) and occasionally social workers (psychiatric social workers only) are allowed to directly provide treatment to patients.

Pharmacists are healthcare professionals who specialize in pharmacy. However, their independence varies greatly across healthcare systems. Pharmacists can independently prescribe some drugs (such as aspirin) to patients in any country, but most countries legally require written prescriptions from physicians for many drugs. However, in reality, pharmacists do not fully obey such laws or regulations and may dispense controlled drugs, such as penicillin and digitalis, without a physician's prescription. Unqualified pharmacists, who are in fact drug dealers, occasionally carry out these illegal prescriptions.

Among the support workers for physicians and independent healthcare practitioners, nurses are the primary type of support workers and are arguably the most important type of healthcare worker throughout the world. Nurses can be further categorized according to their academic qualifications, training levels, and responsibilities, but all of them practice under the direct or indirect supervision of physicians, dentists, or other independent healthcare workers. The earliest nurses were Catholic nuns who cared for bedridden patients in hospitals. However, nurses are being trained for more tasks as healthcare systems become increasingly complex. They are primarily trained at hospitals but can also be trained elsewhere depending on the duration and content of the training course.

The most familiar hospital-based nurse training program requires students to train for three years in nursing schools and hospitals after completing 10–12 years of basic education. These nursing graduates must then pass an examination to become certified as "registered" nurses. In addition, in response to the increasing demands in hospitals and other healthcare facilities, the healthcare systems in most countries also employ numerous nursing associates or assistants who have completed brief training programs. For instance, nursing assistants must have received 4–8 years of basic education, followed by 1–2 years of professional nursing education. In addition, some nursing personnel, often referred to as nursing aides or care workers, primarily acquire simple professional skills through on-the-job training.

In addition to hospital nurses, there are other types of nurses who assume different roles. For instance, nurses at community health centers and other healthcare facilities mainly engage in providing outpatient services, whereas school nurses mainly provide nursing and health education to students. Factory nurses assume similar roles to school nurses. Therefore, nurses play a crucial role in public health programs because they are responsible for outpatient appointments, immunizations, home visits, and supervision of other healthcare workers. Nurses sometimes work with physicians in private clinics or provide home-based care services. However, the vast majority of them work in organized governmental or nongovernmental healthcare institutions.

As hospitals and other organizational healthcare programs employ a large number of healthcare workers, it is necessary to supervise these personnel. Undergraduate-level nursing education, as well as master's and doctorate-level education, have been established in many countries to train senior nurses who can assume supervisory or educational roles. Although nurses at all levels still work under the supervision of physicians, nurses often make autonomous decisions regarding everyday nursing care. At present, there is a world-wide trend toward assigning physicians' duties to nurses. In the health system of certain countries, specialized nurses are also trained as nurse practitioners with additional medical courses, such that they can undertake the diagnosis and treatment of common diseases.

In some countries, nurses must undergo an additional 1–2 years of training to become certified nurse midwives (i.e., obstetric nurses), such that they can assume obstetrical roles at hospitals. Furthermore, some nurses receive additional specialized training to become anesthetic nurses. In a theoretical sense, both types of specialized nurses work under the supervision of physicians, but this supervision is minimal. The same is true for specialized midwives who are not professional nurses but have received training for a similar duration to nurses at hospitals.

In addition to nurses, there are numerous other healthcare workers who engage in supporting the diagnostic and treatment duties of physicians. For instance, medical laboratory technicians or technologists trained at different professional levels are essential for the diagnostic process. They may be trained and educated at comprehensive universities, polytechnics, hospitals and other institutions to specialize in such things as blood tests, biochemical analysis, bacterial testing, histopathological slide preparation, and examination, in hospitals, outpatient centers, research institutes, and private companies.

Similarly, the development of radiology and electrocardiography (ECG) has led to the emergence of numerous types of X-ray or medical imaging technicians and ECG technicians, respectively. The invention of electroencephalography (EEG) and other diagnostic instruments, such as computed tomography (CT) and magnetic resonance imaging (MRI), has also led to the emergence of a large number of technicians.

Physicians also need other types of auxiliary health workers during the course of treating patients. Dietitians are experts in the selection, procurement, preparation, and distribution of foods for both patients and healthy individuals. They are usually female and have completed secondary education in most developing countries or university education in developed countries. From a public health perspective, dietitians specialize in population dietary habits, dietary needs, possible malnutrition, and strategies for improving community nutrition. Dietitians are usually medical specialists, but some have received only nutritional training (strictly speaking, dietitians are not considered support workers for physicians). Additionally, there are also other types of healthcare workers, such as record custodians and specially trained clerks in charge of keeping medical records.

Corresponding healthcare workers are available to assist in the rehabilitation of patients with various physical disabilities, including physiotherapists, occupational therapists, and speech therapists. Healthcare workers who test for hearing ability are referred to as audiologists. In general, medical social workers assist a wide range of physicians in helping patients and ensuring the rational use of community resources. In addition, there are assistants for all the aforementioned healthcare workers, including laboratory assistants and physiotherapist assistants, who constitute the second tier of support workers.

The advancement of science and technology has led to the emergence of an increasing number of new healthcare careers. For example, respiratory therapists specialize in the oxygenation and treatment of patients with pulmonary diseases. Hearing aid technicians, family-planning specialists (contraception), and emergency care workers have also emerged in response to new healthcare needs. The advent of advanced medical instruments such as hemodialysis machines for renal dialysis and cardiopulmonary bypass pumps for thoracic surgery has also prompted the need for other professional technicians.

Apart from physicians and psychiatrists, we have previously mentioned independent health practitioners for psychiatric disorders and mental health. In some healthcare systems, psychologists, social workers, and other healthcare workers serve as support workers for physicians and are part of the mental health team. Some countries have also introduced the position of psychiatric nurse, who receive completely different training from general registered nurses. Psychiatric hospitals might employ these specially trained psychiatric nurses to care for psychiatric patients.

Pharmacists were defined earlier as technicians who practice independently and are responsible for dispensing drugs directly to patients. However, pharmacists also assist physicians in prescribing medicines to patients. Despite their ancillary roles, pharmacists are legally responsible, to a certain extent, for ensuring the rationality and appropriate dosage of prescriptions issued by physicians. Because modern pharmaceutical companies currently manufacture most drugs, the functions of pharmacists are often limited to the maintenance of drug inventories, the appropriate storage of drugs, labeling, and providing explanations during drug dispensing (pharmacists sometimes issue alerts or recommendations to physicians regarding pharmacologically incompatible drugs for certain patients).

Regardless of whether their role is independent or ancillary, pharmacists often require the assistance of pharmacy clerks. In fact, all independent healthcare workers require assistants. For instance, opticians, optical technicians, and polishing technicians are required for the fabrication of spectacle lenses prescribed by optometrists, who then perform the basic frame adjustment.

Dentists require a variety of chairside dental assistants to perform their duties effectively. Dental technologists or dental technicians are responsible for denture construction. Oral hygienists at schools or workplaces are responsible for the dental care and teeth cleaning either under the instruction of dentists or independently. In some countries, denture technicians are qualified to replace the entire upper and lower rows of teeth in patients without the intervention and guidance of dentists, regardless of whether relevant legislation has been enacted.

Nominally supervised healthcare workers who directly provide healthcare services have been gaining more attention in modern healthcare systems. This is because the demand for direct healthcare services has significantly outgrown the existing workforce of physicians and other independent healthcare workers. There has been a worldwide consensus regarding the need for healthcare services among rural and urban poor populations, which has prompted the recruitment of community health workers (CHWs), who complete simple training courses to provide basic disease prevention and healthcare services to local residents. The course content and duration for CHWs vary widely, ranging from several years of training after high school to several weeks of training after primary school. Physicians or other systematically trained healthcare workers nominally supervise them, but CHWs work independently in most cases.

Under the influence of the WHO, CHWs and even social workers who have received only a few weeks of training are qualified to provide a very wide range of healthcare services that cover all aspects of primary healthcare. Social workers mainly rely on their experience to receive continuing education. On the other hand, some social workers only provide a single service, such as immunization, control of mosquito-borne disease, or surveillance and treatment of infectious ocular diseases. Both all-rounded and specialized social workers have become increasingly important in most developing countries. In a theoretical sense, they are required to work under supervision, but the relevant supervision is often inadequate, which can lead to many problems. This will be discussed later.

School dental nurses, also known as dental therapists, provide various dental care services to schoolchildren, occasionally under the guidance of dentists. The first school dental nurses appeared in New Zealand in 1920. Currently, over 20 countries have established this position to provide dental services to children. School dental nurses are generally females and have received two years of training after high school in almost all pediatric oral care skills, including dental filling and extraction. They also provide oral health education.

Public health workers are another crucial type of healthcare workers who work under supervision to directly provide healthcare services to the public. With the increasing maturity of healthcare systems, community-based health-related activities have been extensively established to achieve health promotion, prevention of specific diseases, and efficiency of healthcare services. At the national, provincial, municipal, and metropolitan levels, professionally trained physicians lead public healthcare workers; however, at the grassroots level, public healthcare workers work independently.

Healthcare workers with specialized knowledge and skills are required for disease prevention via environmental monitoring and control. They are broadly referred to as public health experts or environmentalists but can be further classified into various categories. For instance, health engineers are responsible for the construction and operation of tap water and waste-disposal systems, whereas health inspectors at different levels are required to monitor environmental health. Public health experts who have received many years of training typically assume management roles, whereas other personnel with less training work under their supervision. The control of disease vectors, such as insects, is another branch of environmental health. Furthermore, employees of waterworks or wastewater-treatment plants also require special training.

Health education is another type of profession that has emerged in recent years. Its target population is sometimes focused on schoolchildren; however, it is usually aimed at serving the general public. The prevalence of certain diseases has also prompted the recruitment of corresponding experts, such as sexually transmitted disease (STD) experts and malaria inspectors. The management of hospitals and other large-sized healthcare facilities requires healthcare management personnel who are specially trained in knowledge on finances, human relations, procurement, and maintenance. On the other hand, the healthcare management of certain regions requires another type of healthcare management personnel. In recent years, there has been a need for greater healthcare planning to meet future healthcare demands, which has led to the emergence of health information specialists who collect, maintain, and analyze large amounts of data.

In general, public health nurses (PHNs) receive one or more years of public health training following their professional nursing education. They generally supervise other healthcare workers in public health agencies, serve at tuberculosis, leprosy, and STD clinics, or provide primary healthcare. Occasionally, they also perform routine physical examinations for pregnant women, newborns, and children, and would only refer severe cases to physicians. Many PHNs also conduct home visits to monitor infectious diseases or newborns. Another type related to PHNs is the visiting nurse, who provides home-based bedside care to patients with chronic diseases.

In summary, we have briefly outlined all the current types of the healthcare workforce in healthcare systems across the world. The healthcare workforce can roughly be divided into four main categories, which will enable us to identify common patterns across countries with varying backgrounds: (1) physicians, (2) other independent healthcare workers who directly provide services, (3) support workers for independent healthcare workers, (4) nominally supervised healthcare workers who directly provide health services to patients. There is no clear distinction between these four types of healthcare workers, and certain types (e.g., pharmacists, PHNs, and psychologists) have vastly different definitions depending on the specific national healthcare systems. As mentioned earlier, the education, training, and roles of the different personnel also vary greatly.

The supply and utilization of the healthcare workforce within each healthcare system are constantly changing. Ancient, individual medical practices can no longer cope with current complex healthcare situations; instead, these situations require healthcare teams consisting of physicians, pharmacists, nurses, dentists, technicians, public health experts, CHWs, management personnel, etc. These teams can be rationally and meticulously organized, but can also be loosely organized. As seen above, the fluctuations in the healthcare workforce of different countries have revealed an increasing trend towards greater organization, which may help to improve the efficiency of national healthcare systems.

(2) Healthcare Facilities

The second category of resources in healthcare systems concerns the workplaces in which healthcare workers provide their services – healthcare facilities. These workplaces, with the exception of patients' homes, must be equipped with the necessary facilities and resources to ensure that healthcare work can proceed normally. There are six major categories of healthcare facilities: hospitals, general clinics, specialist clinics, long-term care facilities, environmental health protection facilities, and other specialized healthcare facilities; these can all be further divided into subcategories.

1. Hospitals   Hospitals are the oldest form of healthcare facility, and their primary purpose is to provide shelter and bedside care for critically ill patients. Hospitals mainly refer to general hospitals, which primarily serve patients with acute and chronic diseases as well as patients with severe injuries. General hospitals can vary in size and technical level. Small hospitals often have limited facilities, whereas large hospitals tend to be equipped with various advanced technical resources. Even the definition of "general" hospital also differs across countries. For example, in some countries, general hospitals do not have obstetrics and gynecology departments, and others do not include infectious diseases.

There are numerous types of specialist (i.e., nongeneral) hospitals. Institutions for psychiatric disorders have been established in almost all healthcare systems. Although some general hospitals may admit psychiatric patients, psychiatric hospitals are fully specialized in the treatment of acute and chronic psychiatric patients. Intellectually disabled patients are often housed in separate institutions, but can sometimes be admitted to psychiatric hospitals.

Specialist hospitals also refer to other types of hospitals specialized in the treatment of perinatal cases (neonatal, pregnancy, and birth), gynecological diseases, or pediatric patients. Some specialist hospitals are specialized in the treatment of infections or infectious diseases. In the past, there were numerous specialist hospitals or sanctuaries catering to tuberculosis due to the high incidence and prolonged course of this disease. However, these have now been significantly reduced. In addition, in many developing countries, there are hospitals that specialize in the treatment of patients with chronic leprosy. Many specialist hospitals are dedicated to bone and joint diseases or orthopedic surgery, as well as to the rehabilitation of physical disabilities. The number of hospitals specializing in tumors and cardiovascular diseases is increasing due to the high incidence rates of these conditions in many countries.

Some general hospitals are dedicated to serving specific groups, such as active-duty military personnel, veterans, and indigenous communities. General hospitals have been established in many large-scale factories, mines, and farms (e.g., plantations) for the employees of these institutions and their families. General hospitals have also been established in some colleges and universities to serve students. Even prisons have hospitals dedicated to serving inmates.

Other than patient-based classification, hospitals can also be classified according to ownership. In general, investors own hospitals, and they may sell the hospitals or legally change ownership. Government or public hospitals, nonprofit hospitals, and commercial or private hospitals are the most common types of ownership, each of which can be further sub-divided.

National, provincial, state, prefectural, municipal, and county governments control public hospitals. Nonprofit hospitals are donated and controlled by various religious or non-religious organizations. One or multiple physicians usually own private hospitals, but some are also owned by a group of investors.

For all three types of ownership, the hospital may be an independent institution or form part of a network of multiple institutions. The national government may control the network of military hospitals or indigenous healthcare facilities. The municipal governments of some major cities may also control a network of general hospitals. Religious organizations, especially the Catholic Church, often donate toward the building of general hospitals on a national or even international scale. In recent years, private companies in some countries now own an increasing number of large-sized general hospitals or specialist hospitals.

Hospitals ownership varies greatly across the different types of national healthcare systems. From a global perspective, there has been a steady growth in hospital supply (often measured using the number of hospital beds) and the ratio of hospital beds to the population over the last century. The percentage distribution of hospitals with different types of ownership has a significant impact on healthcare services. The type of ownership can also affect the internal organizational structure and healthcare service provision of individual hospitals.

The capabilities of hospitals are gradually increasing alongside the development of healthcare systems. Hospitals were once limited to providing bedside care for critically ill patients but are now capable of providing services to outpatients and mobile patients, conducting health education and medical research, and developing medical education and other preventive services. Sometimes, healthcare workers are also appointed to provide patients with on-site services and serve as personal healthcare service management centers in certain regions.

2. General Clinics   General clinics are healthcare facilities that serve only outpatients and have a slightly shorter history than do hospitals. As described earlier, although most hospitals have an outpatient department, general outpatient clinics specialize in the treatment of patients who do not need bed rest. There are a large number of these institutions, and they are generally referred to as healthcare centers or community health centers. Occasionally, major healthcare centers (which have a capacity of around 50,000 people) also consist of subcenters (with a capacity of about 10,000), or even simple healthcare stations with only a single healthcare worker.

The majority of healthcare centers and related units are state owned, but some belong to charitable and religious organizations. These healthcare centers play varying roles in the healthcare systems of different countries, but they can generally be found in greater numbers and play more extensive roles in developing countries. Healthcare centers and subcenters also have varying workforce allocations. In wealthy countries, this mostly includes several physicians, nurses, and other personnel, whereas, in developing countries, this may only include support workers or a single physician and a few other healthcare workers.

Healthcare centers provide both preventive and curative services, which are sometimes referred to as primary healthcare services. Healthcare centers often focus on preventive care for mothers and children, and disease treatment usually depends on the abilities of the employed healthcare workers. Some healthcare centers are equipped with small laboratories for diagnosis and pharmacies to dispense drugs for everyday ailments.

The main outpatient facilities in certain healthcare systems are referred to as general clinics because they consist of multidisciplinary physician teams. These teams are sometimes comparable to those found in large-sized general hospitals, except for the fact that general clinics do not provide beds. Conceptually, such clinics are an advanced form of healthcare centers and are commonly seen in state-controlled healthcare systems.

Both healthcare centers and general clinics reflect the global trend toward well-organized healthcare-service provision. For centuries, well-organized healthcare facilities have been considered indispensable for patients requiring bedside care. At present, there is also a growing recognition of the need for well-organized outpatient services, which have now emerged in both private and public medical institutions.

Finally, we should not overlook the facilities that serve as workplaces for physicians and other healthcare workers in general outpatient services (variously referred to as offices, surgeries, wards, private clinics, etc.) because they play a unique role in almost all healthcare systems. These facilities vary significantly in size, type, and the number of equipment. In the major cities of many countries, such facilities might contain a large number of independent physicians and healthcare workers, as well as pharmacies, laboratories, and medical equipment stores that are centralized in a single building, which are convenient for patients.

3. Specialist Clinics   Healthcare centers primarily serve the general public, but here are several types of clinics that focus on outpatient services for specific groups. Similar to specialist hospitals, such clinics may serve military personnel, workers, or prison inmates. Some specialist clinics also specifically target the treatment and prevention of certain diseases or health problems and are often referred to as centers for disease prevention and control.

These clinics can be classified according to their ownership, most of which are controlled by public healthcare agencies or the Ministry of Health. Furthermore, all countries have established official centers of prevention and control to provide medical examinations for children under five years of age, provide advice on breastfeeding, proper diet and infant care, and vaccinations, and they carry out follow-up care for infants with congenital anomalies. These centers are often referred to as infant-care centers, infant-welfare centers, maternal and child health centers, and so on. These agencies have far-reaching benefits for protecting infant and child health and reducing infant mortality. However, in most (but not all) countries, these centers offer very limited treatment for infants with congenital anomalies. Furthermore, there are relatively few agencies that offer antenatal check-ups for pregnant women.

There is a wide variety of clinics for public health diseases that are responsible for the surveillance and follow-up of patients with tuberculosis, STDs, malnutrition, leprosy, schistosomiasis, paralytic diseases (in both adults and children), cancer, eye diseases, dental diseases, skin diseases, cardiovascular disease, mental disorders, drug abuse, and so forth. Some clinics also offer contraceptive (birth control) and immunization services. Most of these clinics have been established by official healthcare agencies, but a minority of them have been established by voluntary organizations or other government agencies and are generally subsidized by the Ministry of Health.

Outpatient departments that cater to all types of patients have become an increasingly important part of hospitals, especially public hospitals. These departments may offer a range of specific specialist services, such as surgery, gynecology, pediatrics, cardiology, and plastic surgery, on a particular day of the week. In addition, most general hospitals maintain 24-hour emergency services due to a large number of patients seeking emergency medical attention due to accidental injury. Accordingly, hospital outpatient departments often bring together a diverse group of patients seeking medical treatment from internists or surgical specialists.

Clinics have also been established in factories, particularly those with hundreds of thousands of employees, to provide medical examinations, first aid, or treatment of occupational injuries for employees. In general, larger companies provide more comprehensive healthcare services, and the precise allocation of healthcare workers depends on the size of these clinics. They are also bound by law to uphold particular health standards.

School-based health centers (SBHCs) are commonly established in schools and are mostly staffed with nurses. SBHCs in primary schools are responsible for immunization and early warnings of infectious diseases, whereas SBHCs in high schools often provide treatment for sports injuries, drug abuse, STDs, and common respiratory infections. In contrast, SBHCs in universities offer more comprehensive treatment and preventive services, generally employing full-time or part-time physicians, as undergraduate students tend to live away from home.

In countries where the majority of physicians are engaged in private practice, physicians often jointly establish "cooperative clinics," which may be composed of physicians within different or the same specialties. In healthcare systems where specialists tend to work in hospitals, these clinics predominantly employ general practitioners. However, each general practitioner might target specific groups of patients, such as women, children, or the elderly.

In a small number of countries, cooperative clinics mainly serve patients covered by private health insurance. This practice was known as "mutual aid" in Cuba before 1959. A similar practice called "prepaid health plans" was also implemented in the US, but this model was later replaced by Health Maintenance Organizations (HMOs) after 1970. Countries such as Australia and Indonesia are also currently interested in this form of outpatient services for middle-class populations who can afford private insurance premiums.

Clinic facilities may also be donated by voluntary organizations, which cater to the organizations' specific fields of interest, such as mental disorders, cancer diagnosis, disabled children, and so on. In addition, governmental welfare agencies may establish specialized clinics for destitute or elderly populations, or patients with psychiatric disorders. The Ministry of Agriculture may establish clinics for rural families or specific disadvantaged groups, such as migrant workers. Furthermore, many developing countries have clinics that have been established and are currently operated by religious missionary groups for residents in remote rural areas.

4. Long-Term Care Facilities   As mentioned earlier, some hospitals primarily focus on caring for patients with chronic diseases, such as psychiatric disorders, tuberculosis, or leprosy. In many countries, there are also hospitals that specifically target patients with normal chronic diseases or those who are incapable of self-care, most of whom are elderly individuals. These facilities are particularly important in wealthy industrialized countries, as they have a higher percentage (over 10%) of elderly adults (generally defined as individuals aged 65 years and over) in the population. These institutions may exist in different forms across the healthcare systems of different countries and may come under government departments, nonprofit voluntary organizations (usually religious organizations), or private institutions.

There are different tiers of healthcare facilities catering to the elderly and patients with chronic diseases. Some general hospitals provide 24-hour active medical care only to long-term patients. Additionally, some countries have developed specialized geriatric medicine for this group of patients. General hospitals providing long-term care mainly focus on physical and mental rehabilitation, which is reflected in their allocation of personnel and facilities.

Although some chronic patients do not require active medical intervention, they are still in need of nursing care and bedside care, and hence, they require a different type of healthcare facility. In some countries, these healthcare facilities are referred to as nursing homes, professional nursing facilities, or rehabilitation hospitals. Although they mainly house sick elderly patients, these facilities are also sometimes referred to as retirement homes. Some patients might be completely bedridden, whereas others might only be able to perform minimal activities of daily living (ADLs).

A handful of geriatric institutions target patients who are physically weak but do not need clinical care – these are known as nursing homes, senior living apartments, or adult daycare centers. Users of these facilities are often treated as "clients" rather than as patients and are typically incapable of independent self-care and lack cohabiting family or friends. Such institutions are invariably found in wealthier countries due to the high level of routine maintenance costs, which are unaffordable in low-income countries.

Rehabilitation centers are another category of institutions for patients of any age group (but with a greater focus on younger patients). Despite providing similar service intensities as hospitals, these centers are more adept at physiotherapy. Patients with severe neurological disorders, such as spinal cord injury, can improve their physical abilities through long-term physiotherapy and occupational therapy; they are also taught to use various assistive devices, such as prostheses, wheelchairs, and crutches. Some patients stay full-time at the rehabilitation centers, whereas others visit the facilities regularly. The large-scale development of rehabilitation centers originated from the immense destructive power of World War II, but they have since shifted their focus from exclusively serving war-disabled patients to ordinary injured patients.

"Hospices" have also been established in some wealthy countries to accommodate terminally ill patients. The majority of patients requiring hospice care are patients with cancer and other terminal illnesses, where only pain relief can be provided. Furthermore, hospices comfort grieving family and friends and provide maximum comfort to dying patients.

Finally, the most common form of long-term care facility that should not be overlooked is home-based care. In light of the continuous increase in operating and material costs for various healthcare facilities, many countries have established service systems that allow frail or disabled patients to recuperate at home alone or under the care of family members. These systems consist of meal delivery services, which deliver daily meals to patients' doorsteps, and home-visit nurses, who regularly visit patients at home to help them take their medicine, change their wound dressings, or ensure their personal hygiene. These services may be provided either by voluntary organizations or public agencies. In certain major cities, hospitals organize home-based care programs for long-term patients and provide necessary technicians and beds to patients who need hospitalization.

5. Environmental Health Protection Facilities Although such facilities do not provide healthcare services, they could effectively protect the population from environmental hazards. The vast differences in environmental health facilities across the healthcare systems of different countries can be largely attributed to differences in economic development and urbanization.

One of the hallmarks of modern civilization is the public water supply, which provides water that is safe for drinking and for other purposes. Various health-engineering strategies have been employed to extend piping and drinking water to urban housing and other buildings. In most countries, multiple physicochemical treatments, which must be determined according to the water source, are essential to ensure the purity of the water supply. Regardless of how sophisticated the pipework systems are, regular water quality tests are necessary to ensure the continued safety of drinking water.

The majority of the world's population still resides in rural areas, which require very different facilities for the provision of safe drinking water compared to urban areas. Instead of being supplied via indoor faucets and cisterns, safe drinking water in rural areas is usually supplied through wells or storage tanks that each family must visit each day to obtain water. The water for these wells or tanks can be derived from various sources, such as rivers, precipitation, and springs. In the absence of water treatment facilities, it is often dangerous to draw water directly from rivers or lakes.

Human waste disposal facilities are crucial to all healthcare systems. In general, wastewater treatment networks have been installed in major cities but require continuous maintenance. The problem of human waste disposal in smaller towns and rural areas largely remains unsolved. In developed countries, sewage is processed through sewage treatment plants before being discharged into rivers or the sea to reduce environmental pollution. Farmers in rural areas, as well as the residents of many towns and cities in developing countries, must rely on septic tanks or dry toilets for the treatment of their excreta. The large-scale construction of such small-scale facilities must often be accomplished via organized healthcare programs.

Different healthcare systems also have various facilities that protect environmental health to varying degrees. All cities in the world must dispose of solid waste (i.e., garbage), for which a variety of methods are used, such as garbage trucks or designated sites for waste disposal. The latter may include remote location, designated landfills, garbage incinerators, waste shipment overseas, or other methods.

The discharge of industrial waste into rivers has resulted in serious issues in water pollution. However, there is increasing awareness among the public of the harmful effects of toxic industrial waste. The disposal of radioactive waste materials from nuclear power plants also represents a major challenge in some countries. Insect-borne diseases have to be controlled via the removal of sewage from swamps. A hygienic living environment implies that the residents are protected from rodent and insect infestations. Furthermore, the purification of industrial waste, exhaust gases, and other volatile substances is necessary for the prevention of air pollution.

6. Other Professional Healthcare Facilities   There are also other types of facilities that should be considered as part of the healthcare system resources in most, if not all, countries. Drugs and some medical supplies are made available in pharmacies, which are ubiquitous. Drugs can be chosen by patients or prescribed by physicians (depending on the local laws and law enforcement). Pharmacies that sell numerous nonmedical products, such as cosmetics, tobacco products, and candies, are often known as grocery stores.

In some countries, nearly all pharmacies and grocery stores are privately owned and operated, whereas in other countries, they may form part of a nationwide franchise. Typically, pharmacies and grocery stores are small, private enterprises, but in some healthcare systems they are considered public healthcare facilities like hospitals. Furthermore, in many healthcare systems, where standard healthcare services are either unavailable or unaffordable to low-income individuals, pharmacies or grocery stores are considered convenient healthcare resources that individuals can visit whenever necessary.

Medical laboratories are another basic healthcare facility where physical specimens are examined for medical diagnosis. The vast majority of medical laboratories are affiliated with hospitals or other healthcare facilities. However, independent laboratories that are privately operated by individuals or institutions are present as well. Large medical laboratories might have different departments for bacteriological specimen testing, histopathological examinations, blood tests, chemical tests, etc.

In the healthcare systems of some countries, laboratories within the same region form a network where simple medical tests are outsourced to small peripheral laboratories, whereas complex tests are sent to larger, more central laboratories. In addition, some countries also distinguish between laboratories that specialize in public health tests (e.g., water quality testing, food testing, or specimen testing for suspected cases of infectious diseases) and those testing patient specimens; however, this distinction is gradually fading.

Blood banks refer to facilities in which human blood and blood products of different blood types are stored. As with laboratories, blood banks are usually affiliated with large hospitals; occasionally, however, blood products are kept in separate institutions for disaster relief. In addition to storing blood at low temperatures, blood banks also perform the identification, testing, and transport of blood specimens to ensure their safety and effectiveness. Blood banks are also responsible for the collection of blood from healthy donors.

Some special public or private facilities may provide various types of prosthetic devices, including orthopedic devices (e.g., crutches, corset belts, hernia belts, and wheelchairs) and implanted devices (e.g., stents and prostheses). In some healthcare systems, optical stores are separated from optometrists or ophthalmologists, whereby the latter is responsible for determining the necessary corrective lenses for individuals. Additionally, some stores are dedicated to selling hearing aids.

(3) Healthcare Products

The third type of fundamental resource that can be found in all healthcare systems is the collection of physical and chemical products for the prevention and treatment of diseases. The most common form of healthcare products is drugs and biopharmaceuticals, which are used worldwide. The second category is medical supplies for disease treatment and diagnosis. The third category is precision instruments for disease diagnosis and treatment, which is currently increasing in number.

(1.). Drugs and Biopharmaceuticals   Minerals, plants, and animal products have been utilized for the treatment of diseases since ancient times. As a result of continuous advancement in human knowledge, drugs can now be manufactured via chemical synthesis. Before the dawn of modern chemistry, drugs were mostly extracted from herbs, and this practice is still widely employed in developing countries (in fact, herbal medicines are still used to a certain extent in all countries); collectively, such herbal medicines are called traditional medicines to distinguish them from modern drugs.

Traditional health practitioners, who also provide diagnosis and prescriptions to their patients, prepare most traditional medicines. In fact, traditional therapists usually provide free health counseling services and only charge for prescriptions. There is a vast body of literature on the prescriptions used to treat various symptoms (e.g., pain, fever, diarrhea, headache) in India and China (collectively known as traditional Chinese medicine or TCM in China), with less attention being paid to the disease diagnosis. Some traditional health practitioners are aware of the immense value of modern drugs (e.g., penicillin) and hence will also employ them in their practice.

Innumerable types of modern drugs are manufactured by pharmaceutical companies worldwide, but the majority of such companies are based in the US, Germany, Switzerland, the United Kingdom, and a few other countries. Drugs manufactured in pharmaceutical factories in these countries are then exported and sold worldwide. Many pharmaceutical companies have also established branches in developing countries to produce pills and oral liquids from raw materials, which are then packaged and sold in local markets (corrective measures are typically required for such drugs, as both physicians and patients are often unaware of their variety and prices; this will be discussed later).

Most industrialized countries have enacted patent protection laws, granting exclusive marketing rights (EMR) to manufacturers who first discovered and manufactured a novel drug over a certain period of time (20 years in most European countries). This right is asserted through the product name of the drug. Other pharmaceutical companies are allowed to manufacture and commercialize the same drug, but only under a different product name and they are required to pay royalties (per pill) to the patent holder. Once the patent expires, any company can produce the drug under the generic name (i.e., the chemical name) stipulated by the government, and generic drugs usually are sold at a cheaper price than the original product. Despite numerous controversies over the marketing of generic drugs, they are preferred in almost every healthcare program due to cost considerations.

Given the increasing competition in the pharmaceutical industry, almost all pharmaceutical companies invest heavily in advertising their products and mainly target physicians. These advertisements can appear in medical journals, as targeted email advertising, or on-site marketing by medical representatives. Pharmaceutical companies also often directly advertise over-the-counter drugs to the general public. Because imported drugs are more expensive, specialized institutions have emerged to manufacture generic drugs within the countries where these drugs are ultimately sold.

Drug dispensing, especially for imported drugs, has always been a complicated issue in healthcare systems throughout the world. Most countries are required to provide drugs to public hospitals, healthcare-facility networks, and countless retail pharmacies, as well as raw materials to government-owned pharmaceutical factories. This need has led to the development of pharmaceutical wholesalers. Local factories established by foreign pharmaceutical companies typically have their own sales channels. Warehouses are usually required for the storage of medicines because they are often imported in large quantities. Refrigeration is also required for effective storage and transport of biopharmaceuticals (e.g., vaccines and immunosuppressants), because the success of immunization often relies on the appropriate maintenance of a cold chain.

(2.). Medical Supplies Hospitals, healthcare centers, and other healthcare facilities require a constant supply of soaps and disinfectants for sanitation; various types of bandages for wounds and postoperative care; sutures for wound closure during surgery; splints and special plaster for the treatment of fractures and dislocations; laboratory reagents; and X-ray films.

All these supplies are either manufactured by the national healthcare system or imported from foreign countries. Even some of the simplest diagnoses and treatments are unattainable without these medical supplies. Bed sheets and insecticides are often not considered as medical supplies despite their frequent use in the daily management of hospitals. However, it is important to note that an effective procurement plan is required to ensure an adequate supply of these materials. In addition, hospitals require an adequate supply of paper and stationery for recording and storing medical information. However, the advancement of information technology, the implementation of procurement plans, information exchange, and recording have become more convenient.

(3.). Medical Equipment A vast array of medical equipment is used for the diagnosis, treatment, and prevention of diseases in modern medicine. For example, syringes are used for immunization. Thermometers, despite being a seemingly simple piece of equipment, must still be imported for most countries. The same is true of stethoscopes, sphygmomanometers, otoscopes, ophthalmoscopes, and so forth. Modern laboratories require hundreds of types of equipment, including microscopes, chromatography systems, centrifuges, incubators, refrigerators, and so on. In fact, in large-sized hospitals in highly developed countries, automated hematology analyzers that enable 12 or 24 tests per drop of blood are considered essential; however, such equipment is almost unimaginable in most developing countries.

Medical advancements have increased the number of available equipment for use in physical examinations. The stethoscope was a major invention in the early nineteenth century and can be considered a hallmark of modern medicine. Electrocardiography (ECG) has also become an indispensable instrument in modern medical examinations. Endoscopes, such as the vaginal speculum, cystoscope, proctoscope, and gastroscope, are medical tools required for observations conducted via various bodily orifices. Additionally, electroencephalography (EEG) is used to examine the brain, and electromyography is used to assess muscle function.

Modern surgery requires an even greater variety of medical equipment for such purposes as cutting, clamping blood vessels, examining organs, and sealing surgical incisions. Obstetric forceps and other instruments are needed in obstetrics. Various precision instruments are required for eye and vision testing in modern ophthalmology. The equipment for anesthetizing patients during surgery is also becoming more complicated, and cardiopulmonary bypass (CPB) and other advanced technologies are required for organ transplantation.

The instruments commonly used in the radiology departments of modern hospitals for examination are also constantly being upgraded. The simple single-irradiation X-ray generator invented by Wilhelm Conrad Röntgen has long been obsolete and has been replaced by more sophisticated radiography instruments, such as CT and MRI, which are capable of irradiation from varying projecting angles to reproduce the three-dimensional structure of human bodies. Ultrasound instruments are sometimes adopted for diagnostic purposes in order to prevent the possible harmful effects of X-ray.

High-tech therapeutic methods also employ a wide variety of medical equipment. Lasers are used to create incisions in minimally invasive procedures, and hemodialysis machines can greatly improve the life expectancy of patients with advanced kidney disease. The newly invented vascular catheterization technique is capable of dilating blocked arteries and extending the life expectancy of patients with coronary artery embolisms. Intravenous infusion and pure oxygen inhalation have become commonplace in modern hospitals. Furthermore, radiotherapy has become the standard therapy for treating cancer and other diseases.

In many developing countries, the advanced technologies mentioned earlier can only be found at top-tier central hospitals or may be completely absent in the country. However, simple equipment, medical supplies, and medicines are indispensable to healthcare systems. Most countries still rely on imports for the majority of medical supplies, with the exception of a handful of highly developed countries.

(4) Knowledge

Knowledge is the fourth type of resource for all healthcare systems and is often neglected. Innovative research is required for the acquisition of new knowledge. Most healthcare systems rely on knowledge systems where old knowledge from past generations is documented and taught to healthcare workers. New knowledge on disease prevention and treatment is typically disseminated via journals, books, and sometimes speeches in conferences.

Health science research is carried out to a certain extent in all healthcare systems to obtain new knowledge. Some of these studies may never be published, but most of them will form a part of the collective experiences to guide healthcare workers in their daily operations. Health-science research is usually conducted in more formal environments, such as universities, health ministries, specialized research institutes, hospitals, and clinics. Some results may only be published in local journals.

Highly industrialized developed countries have completed the largest number of existing medical studies and rigorous medical investigations. New findings are also rapidly published and widely disseminated, which can help improve the health status of the global population. Furthermore, the subdivision of medicine and related disciplines has given rise to hundreds of research institutes, which specialize in specific problems faced by health systems of individual countries, such as infectious diseases, malnutrition, cancer, cardiovascular diseases, blindness, occupational diseases, psychiatric disorders, or other conditions. These research institutes often fund universities and other institutions in their specific research areas.

On the other hand, the main problem faced by less advanced developing countries is the dissemination of new knowledge and information to those living in remote areas. Poor communication may lead to the inability of providing life-saving medical information to farmers living in poor and remote areas. In some healthcare systems, the Ministry of Health or other relevant departments might perform targeted measures to help disseminate important new knowledge.

Technology is a collective term for knowledge embodied within drugs and specialized equipment. Unfortunately, many new therapeutic and preventive technologies have not been adequately evaluated. As new technologies are generally very costly, more people have begun to push for detailed and meticulous analyses of the value of such technologies prior to their promotion. Such assessments and their results can be conducted and published in a number of ways.

3. Organizations and Institutions

(1) The Ministry of Health

With the expansion of healthcare services and the important role played by the government in health protection, there has been a corresponding increase in the functions fulfilled by the Ministry of Health and the development of a more complex organizational structure. No two countries have adopted the same roles and organizational structure for their Ministry of Health, because they reflect the history of these countries. In addition, different governments assign different roles to the Ministry of Health, which is a feature that differs substantially from those of other government agencies. Therefore, this book can only provide a very general description of the structures and functions of the Ministry of Health.

1. Preventive Services In general, the health ministries of most countries were initially established to combat infectious diseases through various means; hence, they are almost always responsible for disease prevention. In the organizational chart of a given Ministry of Health, the task of disease prevention may be assigned to one or several departments. However, regardless of the administrative arrangement, the control of infectious diseases remains a prominent duty of the Ministry of Health. As certain diseases have caused particularly serious problems in some countries, special administrative units have been established that are responsible for the control of these diseases, which include malaria, tuberculosis, STDs, leprosy, vector-borne infections, and so on.

In addition, the Ministry of Health is generally responsible for protecting the public from environmental pollution. Safe drinking water and proper disposal of human waste are the prerequisites for health protection in every country. In many countries, the multiple aspects of environmental health fall under the direct responsibility of other agencies, but the Ministry of Health still has a role in ensuring a long-term, ongoing monitoring of the country's compliance with environmental standards.

Other departments under the umbrella of the Ministry of Health also assume some of the roles related to disease prevention. In general, there is a dedicated department for disease prevention among infants and school-age children. Furthermore, this department, or a similar one, is also responsible for the health of pregnant women, and is often referred to as "the department of maternal health." Departments of maternal health are also in charge of family planning and contraception in many countries, which helps to promote maternal health and control population growth. Population control is highly valued in some countries, which makes the department responsible for family planning an important agency under the Ministry of Health; in some cases, this department could even be completely independent of the Ministry of Health.

Another function of the Ministry of Health is the implementation of nutrition and health education for disease prevention and health promotion. Such education is often delivered in the form of nutrition promotion programs, such as providing nutritious lunches to schoolchildren and dietary supplements for malnourished preschool children. Nutrition research institutes are also utilized to help study the nutritional status of the population and identify foods that are more suited to the local dietary structure. The primary role of health education is to compile information on the major health issues and encourage active participation of local residents in the activities launched by the Ministry of Health.

Disease-prevention activities initiated by the Ministry of Health might focus on other issues based on the local health status. For instance, a major task of health ministries in industrialized countries is the prevention of accidents on the road, at home, or in other public places, and the prevention of accidental injuries. The Ministry of Health may also need to adopt targeted measures during outbreaks of trachoma and other eye diseases. Another example of special healthcare planning handled by the Ministry of Health is the prevention of dental diseases via water fluoridation and oral healthcare services.

2. Therapeutic Services   Great importance is generally attached to departments under the Ministry of Health that provide therapeutic or curative services to patients. In some cases, these departments are responsible only for monitoring the hospitals directly under the Ministry of Health, whereas in other cases, they are also responsible for all public and private hospitals in the country. In some healthcare systems, designated large-sized tertiary research and teaching hospitals are affiliated with other institutions beyond the control of the Ministry of Health. In such systems, the Ministry of Health is responsible only for secondary healthcare institutions. The departments responsible for therapeutic care generally establish standards for healthcare institutions nationwide based on certain indicators, such as the numbers of beds, physicians, nurses, medical technicians per 100 patients or per 1,000 people within the service area.

The responsibilities of therapeutic services may sometimes include the monitoring of large-sized outpatient facilities, such as large-sized healthcare centers and general clinics. However, if such healthcare institutions provide immunization and other preventive healthcare services as well, the departments responsible for preventive services might administer them. Another function of this department is the workforce allocation and operations of medical laboratories, as the work performed by these laboratories are often closely associated with certain treatment regimens. Since curative services might also include emergency and outpatient services, they may need to collaborate with voluntary organizations, such as the Red Cross. They may also be responsible for the supervision of pharmacies.

3. Training   Many Ministries of Health have a dedicated department for training healthcare workers, because their respective countries are often devoted to developing pools of various types of healthcare workers. With the exception of a few countries (mainly socialist countries), such training typically refers to continuing education for established nurses, physicians, laboratory technicians, health inspectors, dietitians, and CHWs, rather than the medical, dentistry, and pharmacy degrees offered in universities. Training for this group of workers is generally conducted at hospitals or healthcare centers directly under the Ministry of Health but might sometimes be carried out under separate higher vocational education programs.

The departments in charge of training may also need to prepare appropriate instruction manuals and audiovisual materials for the training of healthcare workers and are sometimes involved in organizing continuing education programs to update healthcare workers on the latest scientific advances. These training departments may sometimes organize special conferences for physicians and other relevant graduate-levels professionals. Generally, they are also responsible for the registration of physicians, nurse practitioners, and other healthcare workers nationwide. However, departments or agencies other than the Ministry of Health might also undertake such licensing work.

The type, size, and distribution of the healthcare workforce must be taken into consideration when planning the healthcare system of a country. In order to meet the healthcare demands of the people, it is necessary to provide a variety of healthcare workers, who are available almost any time and at any place. This is achieved in most countries by relying on the power of the market. However, the roles played by government planning and intervention are expanding in this regard. Hence, the training programs organized by the Ministry of Health are often closely related to its planning efforts.

4. Other Primary Functions of the Ministry of Health   Almost all health ministries around the world have to fulfill the three primary functions mentioned earlier and are required to undertake clear obligations. However, they are also required to fulfill other functions and are responsible for certain major issues. Therefore, the Ministry of Health will generally have heavyweight departments responsible for environmental hygiene, even though this issue should, in theory, fall under preventive services. Drug regulation, and sometimes even drug manufacturing, may be controlled by a separate department, even though it should, in theory, be considered a therapeutic service. There are also departments responsible for psychiatric healthcare services, alcohol abuse, drug abuse, and other issues. In industrialized countries, the control of chronic noncommunicable diseases also requires special attention, particularly for cardiovascular diseases and cancer, as well as general issues and rehabilitation programs related to aging. As previously mentioned, some departments are responsible for family planning and population control.

5. Institutional Functions of the Ministry of Health   Corresponding to the functions mentioned earlier, all Ministries of Health also have departments for administering and coordinating various personnel and functions to support and promote various activities. In general, there is an administrative department in charge of finance and human resources to support the activities launched by the department of professional services. The administrative department is usually responsible for communicating with the National Treasure or Ministry of Finance. As a government agency that fulfills public functions, the administrative department must operate in compliance with governmental rules and regulations and is generally responsible for supervising the annual budget of the Ministry of Health. If a specific program requires additional funds in a given fiscal year, the administrative department has the authority to approve budget adjustments to cover these extra expenses. It may also be responsible for the procurement of medical supplies and equipment, as well as the transportation of relevant products.

Another key institutional function of most health ministries is healthcare planning. Even though most countries have a specialized planning agency (usually affiliated with the office of the prime minister or president), the concrete plans for healthcare are still formulated by the Ministry of Health. Additionally, health research and statistics (which may be referred to using other terminology) are another institutional function that is also closely associated with healthcare planning. The statistical analyses of data on births, deaths, and notifiable diseases can be considered as one of the earliest functions of the Ministry of Health.

Finally, most health ministries have a department of internal affairs or foreign affairs. In developing countries, this department might be responsible for matters related to the receipt of foreign assistance, which is an extremely important function. Moreover, all countries must cooperate with other countries and international organizations (e.g., WHO and UNICEF) with regards to various health issues. In most wealthy countries, this department might be responsible for the supervision of foreign assistance on behalf of donor countries.

Previous analyses on the functions of the Ministry of Health have mainly focused on the central government or the highest level of government. However, with the exception of a few smaller countries, almost all central governments consider it necessary to divide their countries into various administrative units. The exact means of delineating these administrative boundaries and tiers vary across different countries according to the country's demographic and historical factors. Most countries adopt a top-down, three-tier administrative system. Different terms are used to refer to these administrative divisions. Here, we refer to the three administrative levels as a province (also known as a state or a territory), city (also referred to as a county or a region), and district (also referred to as a municipality or a community). The administrative level referred to as a province in one country might also be known as a county or even a republic in other countries.

In some countries, the second administrative level (i.e., province, state, or republic) has considerable autonomy. Education and health in these federal states are often governed by these local governments. Nevertheless, delineating the administrative divisions in any country will also grant a certain degree of autonomy to these local governments. Similarly, centralization can also be observed in countries with the highest level of federalism. In other words, the power structures of countries are often very complex and cannot be simply categorized into centralized and decentralized.

In view of this complexity, health ministries often have a department devoted to ensuring smooth communication between the central government and local healthcare agencies. This department is responsible for or helps to ensure the orderly allocation of personnel and proper operation of provincial agencies. Problems in these domains should first be handled by this department, and external advice should be sought when necessary. This central department must also take the lead in communicating with local health agencies during nationwide health campaigns or amendments to health regulations.

The relationships among the different administrative levels of the Ministry of Health are often depicted as a pyramid. Undoubtedly, different countries will delegate different roles to each administrative level. However, in most cases, certain preventive services (e.g., maternal and child healthcare services) are completely delegated to lower administrative levels, whereas the management of large-sized hospitals under therapeutic services tends to remain at the central level. The general pattern is as follows: the second level of government (i.e., the provincial government) shares the same scope of public functions as the central government, whereas the lower levels of government (i.e., city and district levels) have a narrower scope of functions. It should also be noted that the scope of functions might vary across provinces and cities, especially in federal countries. However, even in highly centralized countries, the province may assume a broader scope of responsibility under the initiative taken by the provincial leaders of healthcare.

Additionally, the scope of responsibilities also depends on the personalities of the leadership of the provincial, city or district governments. For example, provincial governors with good political prestige are more willing to encourage health innovations. Furthermore, the leadership style of the Ministry of Health can affect provincial healthcare, while the leadership style of the provincial government can affect municipal healthcare. Some healthcare systems experience more effective internal communication, whereas other systems experience intermittent communication between different levels, thus leading to poor leadership and teamwork.

Evidently, it is impossible to summarize the health ministries of all countries in a single sentence. The Ministry of Health in one system might be powerful and influential, whereas in others, it might only have a weak influence, or it might be a combination of the two in a third system (i.e., influential in certain functions and completely ineffective in other functions). The influence wielded by the Ministry of Health is not related to the types of services it provides. Instead, it depends heavily on the role of other agencies within the healthcare system, especially that of the private healthcare markets. Since many countries have well-developed private healthcare institutions, the health ministries of these countries tend to focus on the impoverished sectors of the population. In such cases, the Ministry of Health only has a greater influence on the public in terms of preventive services.

However, the hierarchical structure of the Ministry of Health changes continuously in response to the emergence of new health issues or new preventive and therapeutic approaches. One good example is the worldwide epidemic of acquired immune deficiency syndrome (AIDS) in the 1980s. In addition, the health ministries of all countries made corresponding organizational adjustments following the WHO/UNICEF International Conference on Primary Health Care in 1978. Regime changes or leadership replacements often result in the adjustment of functions and departments between the Ministry of Health and other ministries. Attempts at new approaches are often made when the Ministry of Health has operated under a particular system for a prolonged period, which inevitably leads to a series of problems. Such changes can either be horizontal (i.e., on the same administrative level) or vertical (i.e., between different administrative levels) adjustments in function.

(2) Other Government Agencies

Regardless of the scope of functions fulfilled by the Ministry of Health, there will always be other government agencies in all healthcare systems that undertake some healthcare-related functions. These agencies might undertake more responsibilities if the Ministry of Health has a particularly narrow scope of functions, but even when the Ministry of Health assumes a broader scope, certain healthcare-related functions are still delegated to other government agencies.

The workforce allocation of the Ministry of Health and their subsidiary departments vary greatly across different countries. A specific public function (e.g., traffic and transportation) might be directly assigned to a minister or cabinet member in certain countries, whereas in others, a certain ministry might govern them. The term "ministry" is used in this book to refer to agencies that oversee public services on behalf of the state, irrespective of whether the ministry has an official ministerial position.

1. Social Security   About half of all countries provide basic healthcare services to all or some civilians that are funded by statutory health insurance. In the vast majority of these countries, this responsibility is assigned to government departments other than the Ministry of Health, the most common of which is the Ministry of Labor given that the concept of social security was derived from labor unions of factory workers. In other countries, however, social security services are governed by the Department of Health and Social Security, as such services are associated with public health. Social security is sometimes assigned to the same department as the social welfare scheme (not covered by statutory health insurance), an independent department, or another government agency.

In many healthcare systems, the primary role of social security is to provide financial support. However, in some healthcare systems (especially those in developing countries), social security involves the direct provision of healthcare services to the public. Either way, social security plays a pivotal role in the operation of healthcare systems. Although social insurance might only serve to provide financial support for the private healthcare market, it can have a strong effect on the market operation in all countries. The terminology used to refer to social insurance is often confusing, with different terms being used to describe the same concepts, such as sickness insurance, health insurance, compulsory health insurance, prepaid healthcare plan, and social security.

Occupational injury insurance, also known as workers' compensation, represents a special and more common type of social security scheme compared to the national healthcare schemes. Workers' compensation might form a part of the health insurance schemes in social security or a separate insurance scheme. Usually, the Ministry of Labor or sometimes a dedicated public committee, even in cases where general health insurance is overseen by other departments, governs it. As the definition of occupational injury varies substantially across different countries, workers also enjoy vastly different benefits under this form of health insurance.

For most types of health insurance, beneficiaries receive financial compensation due to a loss in their ability to work. This is often referred to as disability insurance and can be further divided into short-term disability benefits and long-term disability benefits. Disability insurance is of great importance for healthcare because individuals require funds to cover their basic needs. Similarly, there are other social security schemes, such as unemployment benefits and pension schemes, which subsidize certain groups of people living in poverty. These schemes have clear health implications; they can help those in need live a healthier lifestyle such as by providing funds for medical treatment.

2. Occupational Health and Safety Planning   The Ministry of Labor is usually responsible for the safety and sanitation of factories and other workplaces, including the organization of field inspections and implementation of technical standards at workplaces. As this does not include the provision of welfare, these responsibilities are generally not delegated to the social security department. In exceptional circumstances, these may fall under the duties of the Ministry of Health or agencies specializing in general manufacturing inspections for industrial enterprises.

These duties are mainly preventive, and their actual degree of implementation varies considerably. Workers are being exposed to more risks alongside increasing industrialization and automation. For instance, farm mechanization and the use of fertilizers and pesticides in the agricultural sector might entail certain health risks. There has been a great deal of controversy in both developed and developing countries over the pros and cons of using various equipment and chemicals from the perspective of their impact on human health.

3. The Ministry of Education   Schools at all levels are linked to healthcare systems. In general, primary school students must receive health education. Both primary and secondary schools in many wealthy countries have health teachers (typically nurses) who perform first aid and routine physical examinations for students. The Ministry of Health may assign health teachers to a school but in most cases, the schools employ health teachers directly, just like other teachers.

Universities and other higher education institutions might offer more comprehensive personal healthcare services for their students. In addition, colleges and universities often have affiliated institutions dedicated to training physicians, dentists, pharmacists, clinical psychologists, and other healthcare workers. Notably, although the Ministry of Education often controls physician training, it still requires cooperation with the Ministry of Health to meet the needs of national healthcare systems.

4. Environmental Protection Agency (EPA)   In some countries, a ministry or other public agencies address common environmental issues. Aside from the protection of wild animals and some purely aesthetic environmental projects, these agencies also focus on environmental projects that have a direct influence on health. The alleviation of water and air pollution has become an important topic following world population growth and accelerated urbanization.

The EPA might be directly responsible for waterworks, sewage treatment, and solid waste (garbage) disposal in major cities, as well as the management of industrial waste. The improper disposal of nuclear waste could lead to considerable health risks for a country's population. Following the development of civilian nuclear energy, the EPAs of some countries also required to monitor nuclear waste disposal and prevent radiation leakage accidents from nuclear power plants.

5. The Ministry of Agriculture   Food production is of great significance to health. In addition, the Ministry of Agriculture may also directly provide healthcare services. For instance, agricultural ministries in developed countries often provide training for rural families on proper health and nutrition. The Ministry of Agriculture might teach farmers residing in rural areas predominated by cash crops to grow vegetables in their own yards, and usually it has a specialized animal husbandry department responsible for improving the health of livestock. Another important public health function of this ministry is the control of the transmission of zoonotic diseases, such as bovine brucellosis and tuberculosis.

The agricultural ministries of many developing countries are also responsible for various rural development projects, such as the construction of rural healthcare centers and healthcare stations. In some countries, the Ministry of Agriculture has the statutory obligation to drill wells and ensure the safety of drinking water in rural areas, which enables the identification of water sources for irrigation and domestic use.

6. The Ministry of Public Works   Many countries have a specialized ministry responsible for major construction projects, such as roads, bridges, schools, hospitals, and healthcare centers. Indeed, such a ministry usually carries out the construction of healthcare facilities, even if these projects are initiated or funded by the Ministry of Health or Ministry of Social Security. Sometimes, the construction of healthcare centers is subcontracted to private companies, but the Ministry of Public Works still holds the ultimate responsibility. Additionally, the Ministry of Public Works might be responsible for the construction of water supply networks and sewerage networks in major cities.

7. The Ministry of the Interior   Among the many ministries of a given country, the Ministry of the Interior (also known as the Ministry of Home Affairs or Ministry of Internal Affairs) typically assumes the broadest scope of responsibilities. In some countries, where the government has yet to attach sufficient importance to health issues and the Ministry of Health is not yet an independent ministry, the duties of health protection are delegated to an agency subordinate to the Ministry of Interior. At this point, environmental health protection and the prevention of disease outbreaks are regarded as the responsibilities of the police, which in turn are supervised by the Ministry of the Interior. Even after the establishment of the Ministry of Health, the Ministry of the Interior still retains some inspection tasks related to public health.

In a few less-industrialized countries, the Ministry of Labor is unnecessary. As such, the Ministry of the Interior tends to be responsible for inspecting the sanitation of factories. The Ministry of the Interior might also have specialized departments dedicated to various social welfare services, such as ensuring the well-being of the elderly, providing shelters for the homeless, rehabilitating workers with occupational disabilities, providing drug rehabilitation services, and combating human trafficking and prostitution.

The major cities of some countries do not fall under the jurisdiction of their respective provincial or state governments. Thus, the public health issues of these cities do not fall under the control of provincial health departments or the Ministry of Health. In such cases, municipal public health issues are fully or partially administered by the Ministry of the Interior.

8. The Ministry of Commerce   Drugs and other medical products that are needed in a healthcare system must be acquired via commercial trade. Pharmacies, grocery stores, and stores trading in prostheses, hearing aids, and eyeglasses are usually registered with a country's Ministry of Commerce. Business registration is often a requirement for business management rather than health needs, but it may also be the only avenue to access information related to this type of healthcare resources.

The Ministry of Commerce, which can influence health, also manages advertising. The Ministry of Commerce implements relevant specifications to strictly regulate pharmaceutical advertising. Similarly, tobacco and alcohol advertising has been restricted (due to its harmful effects on health) by the Ministry of Commerce in many countries.

9. Social Welfare   The scope of social welfare usually includes the protection of the elderly, orphans, and refugees, which generally falls under the responsibility of the Ministry of Social Welfare, although it is sometimes incorporated under the Ministry of Health or Ministry of Labor. Either way, social welfare has a major impact on health. Healthcare services are often needed in nursing homes and orphanages. Furthermore, many countries take in millions of economic and political refugees from different countries, and healthcare services are always needed in the refugee camps. The responsibility of meeting these needs are generally borne by the Ministry of Social Welfare but may also be borne by the Ministry of Health.

Poor and disabled individuals in wealthy countries are sometimes able to live in their own homes through financial assistance from social welfare agencies, who pay for their necessary healthcare services in the mainstream private healthcare market. Additionally, social welfare agencies may also establish general hospitals that provide healthcare services to individuals living in poverty.

10. Transportation and Public Utilities The maintenance of large-sized public transport facilities, such as railways, barge fleets, and airplanes has contributed to the creation of certain special healthcare programs. In many countries, the aforementioned public facilities remain state-owned even when the majority of their economic activities have been privatized. This also applies to other public utilities, such as telephones and telegraphs, electricity, water, and gas. Almost all public utility departments provide special health insurance schemes for their employees.

A large number of engineering-related problems are encountered during the construction of these facilities in very remote areas. Hence, the provision of healthcare services is especially crucial at this stage. Special health insurance schemes continue to evolve with the economic development of a nation, as well as the development of public transport and works.

11. The Ministry of Justice All countries have a judicial system that deals with illegal and criminal behaviors, and this system inevitably involves prisons and detention camps. Prisoners in developed countries are provided with healthcare services, which are often disregarded by the public. The responsibility for providing such services is mainly delegated to the prison administrative authorities.

12. Military and Veterans Affairs With the exception of a small number of countries, most countries have a military authority known as the Ministry of Defense or Ministry of National Security. The military is generally divided into the army, navy, and air force. Soldiers are provided with comprehensive military healthcare services to maintain their health, regardless of whether the country is at war or at peace.

Almost all countries attach considerable importance to their military forces; therefore, the healthcare services offered to soldiers usually have adequate healthcare workers and are equipped with the most advanced medical equipment and supplies in the country. Although urban and rural healthcare services may have many shortcomings in developing countries, the army and navy of these countries are typically provided with adequate healthcare resources. For instance, if a country can afford to import only one piece of expensive medical equipment, that equipment is usually placed in a large-sized military hospital.

Politicians are generally eligible to receive treatment in military hospitals because of their highly advanced healthcare facilities, as are dignitaries and wealthier citizens. In most countries, military dependents are also eligible to access healthcare services in military hospitals or have their medical fees in other hospitals reimbursed by the Ministry of Defense. Military physicians are typically military officers, and auxiliary healthcare workers also tend to have some military rank. In most countries, the most important military hospitals are situated within the capital cities, whereas other military healthcare facilities are established in military garrisons.

Veterans and retired military personnel are highly respected in many countries, especially those who have served in wars. As a commendation for their services, retired soldiers tend to have continued access to military healthcare services. Whereas for most military personnel, the scope of these healthcare services is often limited to health issues caused by military service, higher-ranking military officers can access healthcare services for any health issues. Soldiers in a handful of countries can access this type of special healthcare services for the rest of their lives, regardless of whether the disease is related to military service.

13. The Ministry of Finance   Typically, the Ministry of Finance, the Treasury, or other agencies with similar functions are responsible for taxation and budget allocation. Given that state revenues are limited and official budgets often exceed existing funds, the Ministry of Finance typically has the final decision on national healthcare planning. Sometimes, the president or prime minister assumes these ministerial duties, and the decision comes from the highest level of the country. Occasionally, when state revenues cannot be transferred to the government in time, the Ministry of Finance also has the right to decide which public programs should not be funded (temporarily). In general, all ministries and national commissions, such as the Ministry of Health, will submit annual draft budgets to the Ministry of Finance for confirmation.

14. National Planning   Since World War II, nearly all countries have formulated their own national economy and social development plans. This does not imply that every country has established a specialized national planning agency. Instead, some countries may have delegated these tasks to different ministries. However, the Ministry of Finance typically has a hand in all of these tasks. Many developing countries and all socialist countries have a well-established central planning agency, which usually wields a large amount of power. For such countries, national planning typically includes the healthcare industry as part of its agenda, or the broader issue of social welfare (which includes healthcare). The central planning agency usually collaborates with the planning department of the Ministry of Health and helps to coordinate the efforts of the Ministry of Health with other ministries, such as the Ministry of Public Works and the Ministry of Education in constructing healthcare facilities or training physicians, respectively.

Although the previous sections provided an extensive overview of the healthcare functions fulfilled by other government agencies, there are doubtlessly some omissions. Some countries might have a ministry overseeing indigenous and ethnic minorities, and one of the roles of such a ministry would be the provision of healthcare services for these groups. Furthermore, some socialist countries have established a Ministry Light Industry to oversee the production of drugs. Some governments also have branches that deal exclusively with affairs related to women and the elderly, where the provision of healthcare forms an indispensable part of their duties. Ultimately, it is important to remember that healthcare functions permeate all aspects of central and local governments and far exceed the scope of responsibilities undertaken by the Ministry of Health.

(3) Voluntary Organizations

In every country, there are numerous programs launched by nongovernmental organizations (NGOs) that directly and indirectly affect the national healthcare system. These voluntary organizations are typically greater in number and have greater influence in wealthy, industrialized countries because of the larger middle-class populations, whose family members (usually women) tend to have more spare time and money for various social causes. Nevertheless, NGOs exist in all countries and their activities can have a certain impact on the healthcare system.

Voluntary organizations are founded for various reasons. They are often formed by groups of citizens to call for more action on issues that have not been given sufficient attention by the government. Most disease-specific voluntary organizations are established under these circumstances. Other voluntary organizations are founded to increase awareness and serve certain groups of people, such as the elderly. Some voluntary organizations are supported by the government and are used to tackle issues through the private sector that the government is unwilling to handle directly. Certain voluntary organizations are also founded to serve only their own benefits.

Voluntary organizations are sometimes founded for humanitarian and religious purposes. A proportion of the funds used for their activities are commonly obtained through donations, but in many countries, voluntary organizations are also subsidized by the government due to the indispensable roles they play. Currently, there are many ingenious means for these organizations to raise funds, such as through selling charitable commemorative stamps for the Christmas holidays.

1. Disease-Specific Voluntary Organizations The first large-scale, disease-specific voluntary organization in history was launched to tackle tuberculosis. Before the discovery of the tuberculosis pathogen, numerous tuberculosis-specific organizations had been founded in dozens of countries to aid patients with the disease. Before the government took similar actions, the private sector had already established several sanatoriums and specialized clinics. In general, the primary goal of these voluntary healthcare institutions was to provide care for patients with the disease. However, after the government took over their original responsibilities, they have moved on to raising funds for research and development, public health promotion, and training physicians in the treatment of tuberculosis. Since tuberculosis is now under control in some countries, these tuberculosis-specific organizations have shifted their focus to other diseases.

Voluntary organizations have also been established to address certain serious chronic diseases. Social healthcare groups have begun to focus on STDs. In some of the poorest countries, the treatment of leprosy has begun to be funded by the private sector. Poliomyelitis, also known as polio or infantile paralysis, has attracted the widespread attention of voluntary organizations. The adversities faced by cancer patients have also drawn the focus of many voluntary organizations, which help in providing care for patients with cancer and funding cancer research and development. Voluntary organizations focusing on cardiovascular diseases are now widely supported in many developed countries.

Voluntary organizations have attached particular importance to some rare but highly serious diseases, such as multiple sclerosis, epilepsy, and other neurological diseases. Some countries have established voluntary organizations for congenital diseases, such as cystic fibrosis and hemophilia. Children with intellectual disability and congenital or acquired disabilities receive a great deal of care, sympathy, and support from voluntary organizations. The parents of children with such diseases usually initiate such voluntary organizations, and one of their major goals is to draw the government's attention to the suffering of these patients.

Some voluntary organizations focus on helping patients with vision and hearing impairments by establishing schools that teach Braille to children with vision impairments, as well as speech-reading and sign language to children with hearing impairments. Other voluntary activities include organizing transportation, training guide dogs, and calling for the government to provide barrier-free facilities via legislation for visually impaired individuals who use white canes.

A number of voluntary organizations focusing on specific disorders operate like support groups. For instance, the best-known support group, Alcoholics Anonymous (AA), has successfully helped many individuals with long-term alcoholism through psychological and spiritual support in many countries. There are similar initiatives for drug dependence, but with less success. The previously mentioned hemophilia- and epilepsy-specific organizations tend to have similar functions as support groups.

2. Institutions for Specific Groups   Children, especially poor and vulnerable children, are arguably the population most in need of support worldwide. There are numerous volunteer organizations for children in nearly all countries (even in the least developed countries), and these organizations tend to be sponsored by mothers from wealthier families. The most common form of volunteering involves the provision of supplementary food, and other forms include child day care, the provision of clothes, or the organization of rural outings for urban children. Such activities have received tremendous public support. Hence, in some countries, it is even customary for the First Lady to be an honorary chairman of children's organizations.

As population aging is increasing in more industrialized countries, many active voluntary organizations have emerged that focus on improving the health and well-being of elderly individuals. The core strategy of such organizations is to improve the activity levels of the elderly, because this can prevent the early onset of muscle weakness and inability to perform self-care. Other voluntary organizations provide meals and other forms of assistance to weak or disabled elderly individuals.

Disabled veterans are another group requiring unique volunteer services, especially when there is a lack of government support. The same applies to indigenous and ethnic minorities living in poverty. Ethnic minorities, in particular, often require aid from volunteer organizations because their healthcare needs tend to be neglected by mainstream culture. In short, charity aid is crucial for those who live in poverty, regardless of their age.

3. Organizations with Specific Healthcare-Related Functions   Almost every country in the world has a Red Cross or Red Crescent Society to provide rescue services during emergencies. These societies were initially established during wartime but nowadays continue to operate even in times of peace. They typically have their own ambulances and blood banks and are prepared to provide all types of assistance in the event of natural disasters. The Red Cross also provides education on swimming safety and fire prevention, as well as other knowledge and skills. Ambulance service teams in some countries belong to another long-standing organization – the St. John Ambulance.

Another important area of volunteer activities is the dissemination of information on family planning and contraception. Most countries have recognized the importance of birth control but there are a few countries that still prohibit contraception for religious reasons. Volunteer organizations that promote family planning often receive more government subsidies than do other healthcare-related volunteer organizations because the governments often wish to control population growth via unofficial channels. Family planning services may or may not include abortion services for pregnant women.

Volunteer organizations in many countries also provide bedside nursing services for bedridden or convalescing patients at home. Major cities in many wealthy countries have Visiting Nurses Associations, which usually consist of ordinary residents. However, the government sometimes pays them to provide nursing care for disabled low-income individuals. The service provided by visiting nurses is drawing increased attention due to its lower cost compared to hospitals or nursing homes.

4. Professional Health Associations (also known as industry associations) Healthcare workers in most countries have established national or local professional associations. The main objective of such associations is to serve the interests of individual professional healthcare workers, but they also have an impact on the national healthcare system as a whole.

Among these associations, physician associations are the most well-established and have played a substantial role in the continuing education of physicians. They represent all physicians when negotiating with the government about medical fees or salaries. In addition, physician associations can serve as guardians of medical ethics by investigating allegations of medical malpractice against physicians. Furthermore, in some countries, they insure their members for medical malpractice lawsuits.

Certain countries have another type of medical association, often known as a "college" or academic association, which is responsible for monitoring compliance with medical ethics. New medical graduates are often required by law to register and maintain their memberships in physician associations in order to obtain their medical licenses and retain status as registered physicians. Physicians who have been found to violate medical ethics by their peers may have their membership canceled and thereby lose their medical license.

Similar associations have also been established for dentists, nurses, pharmacists, laboratory technicians, and other healthcare professionals. For some professions, such as optometrist and orthopedist, there is controversy over whether their healthcare services require government approval. Associations often strive for the widest definitions possible when determining at which point optometric and orthopedic treatments exceed the legally permissible boundaries, and thereby cross over into medicine. Similar controversies have arisen, igniting extensive debate, over the licensing of osteopathic, chiropractic, homeopathic, and acupuncture treatments. Associations have also been established for hospitals, rehabilitation facilities for chronic diseases, and other healthcare facilities for educational or political purposes. These professional associations negotiate with the government or NGOs on behalf of their member hospitals and often make substantial contributions to improving the management of healthcare facilities.

There is an increasing number of organizations that have been spontaneously established, which primarily serve an educational purpose. Aside from organizing meetings and publishing academic articles, these associations also strive to improve public understanding of the medical profession. The associations of some specialties, such as pediatrics, propose pediatric health standards to the government. Unfortunately, serious discrepancies may sometimes arise between these professional associations and the government on certain issues, such as the salary of healthcare workers and various legal provisions. Under these circumstances, professional associations might call for work stoppages and labor strikes. Similar incidents could occur between associations representing nurses or other healthcare workers and the hospitals that employ them.

5. Religious Organizations As mentioned previously, nearly all countries have hospitals established and funded by religious organizations. Furthermore, the religious groups of Europe and North America have long supported missionary physicians in developing countries and have funded the construction of thousands of hospitals, healthcare centers, and dispensaries in the remote areas of low-income countries. Following the independence of these African and Asian colonies, most of these healthcare institutions were integrated into the country's healthcare systems. Despite charging fees for treatment, missionary physicians were originally funded by foreign religious charities. Almost all religious groups – including Buddhism, Christianity, Hinduism, Judaism, and Islam – organize health-related activities as part of providing humanitarian aid to the poor and sick. For example, many

Buddhist temples offer rehabilitation services for patients with addiction; Christian and Jewish social welfare institutions offer healthcare services directly to low-income families; and the Salvation Army provides aid for destitute populations, especially those living in the slums of major cities. The ultimate aim of these institutions might be to seek religious conversion, but the provision of healthcare services is used as a means to achieve this aim.

6. Charitable Organizations   Philanthropists in some of the wealthiest countries might establish or donate to charitable foundations, which aim to sponsor healthcare programs. For example, the well-known Rockefeller Foundation, which was founded in the US, has contributed substantially to public health and medical education. Similar charities have also been established in the UK, European countries, and Japan.

Most charitable foundations fund a wide range of humanitarian operations, whereas some focus on specific healthcare issues, such as the Nuffield Trust Fund for Local Hospitals in England, the Sasakawa Foundation in Japan, and the Robert Wood Johnson Foundation in the US. The Mill Burbank Memorial Foundation is a smaller-scale foundation with the sole mission of improving the level of healthcare services in the US.

A charitable foundation might rely on substantial donations from individual donors. However, most community organizations in industrialized countries, such as community welfare funds, United Way Association, and charity alliances, raise funds through many small donations from the public and businessmen. These charitable organizations also support various volunteer healthcare institutions, which may not need to raise funds through other channels.

7. General Social Groups   Apart from the aforementioned volunteer activities, there are a large number of general social groups that might be involved in healthcare activities. These general social groups usually target a specific population, such as women, youth, workers, and farmers.

Women's organizations come in various forms, such as elite women's clubs in wealthy communities, large-scale women's labor organizations, or associations initiated by workers' wives. These women's organizations often offer healthcare services for pregnant women and children, along with immunization, family planning, and nutrition education. They might also provide volunteer services at hospitals, where they help to care for patients without family or the elderly. There are also parent–teacher associations (PTAs), which are established by parents (usually mothers) and schoolteachers in developed countries, aimed at promoting school-based healthcare services for students.

Labor organizations, especially trade unions, are committed to improving the working environment of factories and providing education on occupational safety. Trades unions have played an important role in expanding the coverage of social security worldwide. Furthermore, workers in developing countries often volunteer to participate in civil constructions, such as roads and buildings, in order to improve the quality of the local healthcare resources.

Rural and peasant organizations have actively promoted the quality of healthcare and drinking water among farmers and residents of rural areas. They are involved in mobilizing farmers to participate in well-digging and agricultural irrigation, constructing healthcare stations, and fundraising for basic healthcare services. Youth organizations, on the other hand, come in different forms. Boy Scouts and Girl Scouts of different age groups have been established in highly industrialized countries to provide basic training in various fields, including healthcare courses. Youth organizations in developing countries may also participate in other activities, such as environment cleaning and mobilization of family members to receive vaccination.

Political groups are organizations that are joined by people from all walks of life, usually with the intention of promoting a particular political agenda, such as supporting healthcare legislation. These political groups allow members to participate in their projects, such as the construction of healthcare centers, in order to enhance their team spirit and enthusiasm.

(4) Enterprises

Enterprises also contribute to healthcare, but to a lesser extent compared to volunteer organizations. Many major companies are either required by law or their own human resource regulations to offer healthcare schemes to their employees. However, there are certain differences between urban and rural enterprises.

1. Urban Enterprises   The vast majority of manufacturers in both developed and developing countries are small-sized enterprises. In most countries, small-sized factories are defined as those with fewer than 100 employees; these factories seldom provide employees with healthcare services. Medium-sized factories are defined as those with 100–500 employees, and large-sized factories as those with more than 500 employees.

In medium-sized factories, there are usually well-trained first aid workers on-site for the treatment of injuries or sudden illnesses. In developed countries, such first aid workers are usually nurses, but in developing countries, they might be clerks or workers trained in basic nursing skills. Some factories may be located near a designated hospital with on-call physicians in case of emergencies.

Large-sized factories or other enterprises (such as transport networks) often have designated physicians who visit the workplace at a fixed time on a daily basis to provide physical examinations for employees and pre-employment medical examinations. Ideally, these physicians should perform health risk assessments in the working environment; unfortunately, occupational physicians rarely possess these skills, except for those working in large-sized enterprises with thousands of employees in highly developed countries. Employees in urban enterprises who require more comprehensive healthcare services are usually referred to a local hospital.

2. Rural Enterprises   The most common rural enterprises include manors and plantations growing specific crops, or mining companies and oil refineries. Rural enterprises with fewer than 100 employees are less likely to provide employees with healthcare services, whereas enterprises with more than 100 employees, particularly those with more than 500 employees, tend to be equipped with healthcare facilities. An enterprise is more likely to provide healthcare facilities if employees' families are also entitled to healthcare services.

In developing countries, government healthcare facilities that are established near rural enterprises might be sufficient to meet employees' healthcare demands. However, the chance of this occurring is regarded as negligible because government healthcare facilities tend to be established elsewhere, and large-sized rural enterprises are often required to take care of their own employees. Hence, rural enterprises in remote areas are often required to establish healthcare programs for their employees and dependents. Furthermore, it is generally more affordable for rural enterprises, especially foreign-funded enterprises, to recruit physicians and nurses with high salaries due to their profitable revenues.

Large-sized rural enterprises, such as oil refineries, rubber factories, tea estates, and sugarcane estates, might have a well-established network of healthcare facilities, whereby healthcare stations and central hospitals are established near workplaces to serve employees. The degree to which occupational healthcare services are offered is largely determined by the economic development and political ideology of the country. For instance, welfare states impose relatively more stringent laws on both state-owned and private enterprises.

(5) Private Market

It is believed by some that there is no room for purely commercial healthcare programs in countries with extensive governmental and non-governmental healthcare services. However, the reality is quite different. No governmental or nongovernmental healthcare program can fully meet the preventive or therapeutic needs of all citizens in nearly all healthcare systems. For this reason, almost all countries have a certain proportion of purely commercial or for-profit healthcare services with varying market sizes. These commercial markets can be analyzed based on the following categories.

1. Traditional Therapeutic Approaches   Almost all traditional health practitioners provide services in private healthcare markets, usually at a lower cost. Sometimes, they are compensated with goods for the healthcare services they provide. Traditional health practitioners are commonly found in the rural areas of developing countries, as they are both culturally and psychologically close to the locals. Most traditional health practitioners are engaged in other full-time employment and provide traditional therapies on a part-time basis. Only a handful of skilled traditional health practitioners develop such a solid reputation that they can provide services on a full-time basis for higher treatment fees in cities. The health ministries of some countries may recruit traditional health practitioners to participate in official healthcare programs, but this number is generally very small (with the exception of China).

As previously described, traditional birth attendants (TBAs) usually serve on a part-time basis for lower fees in private markets, and they are often compensated with goods for their services. In developing countries, each village has their own local TBA, and a number of TBAs can also be found in cities. Traditional health practitioners are only occasionally recruited by the Ministry of Health to offer public healthcare services. In contrast, TBAs often receive official recognition and may even obtain formal healthcare training. All health ministries have realized that there is a large number of TBAs in their respective countries and their demand among pregnant women is high. Hence, it is wiser to provide them with proper healthcare training, rather than to ignore them.

Unlicensed drug distributors are another common healthcare-related occupation in the private healthcare markets of developing countries. In addition to distributing modern drugs, these distributors often sell preparations of traditional herbs. They are unable to diagnose diseases and usually sell medicines based on patients' requests or their own assumptions. Their quoted prices often fluctuate and are typically very expensive because most of their medicines are derived from the black market.

2. Private Clinics of Physicians and Dentists   Physicians and dentists who work full-time in the commercial market can be found in almost all countries. These professionals might have begun their private practice at the start of their careers or after retiring from public hospitals. As with any independent small business owner, physicians and dentists in private practice have substantial decision-making power in their own offices or clinics, typically having their own support staff and equipment.

In many wealthy industrialized countries, the funding sources of health insurance are social insurance or other public schemes, but their healthcare services are still provided by physicians in the private market. In countries that lack similar reimbursement policies, the patients of physicians in private practice tend to be mid- to high-income individuals. However, poorer families might also seek treatment in private practice in cases of severe medical conditions, especially for children.

In many developing countries and some developed countries, physicians and dentists work at governmental or other healthcare facilities for four to six hours per day and spend their spare time serving patients in their private practice (possibly in collaboration with other physicians). Because the salary for physicians is lower in developing countries, it would be difficult for physicians and their family to lead a decent life without the income from private practice. Hence, the Ministry of Health usually does not intervene in private practice, because this is the only way to recruit physicians to fill less attractive positions at hospitals. However, the employment of physicians in both public and private healthcare markets has given rise to various issues. For instance, they may rush to complete their tasks in public healthcare institutions in order to spend more time in private practice for a higher pay.

3. Pharmacies and Grocery Stores Apart from pharmacies in socialist countries and those in public hospitals and healthcare centers, the vast majority of pharmacies and grocery stores are privately owned, and they tend to sell both prescription and nonprescription drugs. However, in many developing countries, there is no distinction between prescription and nonprescription drugs, which gives patients access to all drugs. Medical expenses for prescription drugs might be reimbursed by a healthcare scheme or paid by the patients themselves.

Most private pharmacies keep long open hours and are open daily, allowing patients to seek help from pharmacists (or unqualified personnel employed in pharmacies) outside of physicians' working hours. However, some patients visit pharmacists during physicians' working hours to avoid paying consultation fees. This has given rise to the saying, "Pharmacists are the doctors of the poor." Likewise, stores that sell prostheses, hearing aids, and artificial eyes are primarily privately owned, profit-driven stores.

4. Private Hospitals A large proportion of private hospitals are operated by religious organizations and nonprofit organizations, but some operate like for-profit private enterprises. One or more physicians, as well as other investors might own such private hospitals. They are usually smaller in size and primarily serve wealthy patients who can afford their medical fees. Private hospitals are usually established in cities due to the higher concentration of wealth. Occasionally, these hospitals serve patients covered by third-party insurance, such as workers with occupational injuries.

Patient comfort is a primary feature of private hospitals, which often manifests as attentive nursing care, nutritious and delicious meals, single-bed rooms, individual televisions for each patient, and so on. Because these amenities and services are somewhat expensive, this will reduce the funds available for diagnostic and therapeutic equipment. Hence, the current trend among private hospitals is to provide treatments for relatively simple medical conditions, such as pregnancy, appendicitis, and other minor illnesses. Wealthy individuals usually choose to receive treatment in larger and more advanced hospitals in case of severe illnesses.

Large public and nonprofit hospitals tend to have a few VIP wards that charge extra fees, which can serve wealthy patients and individuals of prominent social status. There has been a great deal of controversy regarding the provision of such luxury private wards in public hospitals.

In recent years, a new problem has emerged in commercial hospitals. Some large-sized enterprises have established or acquired hospital franchises. This situation has mainly arisen in the US and Western Europe, where there is a large amount of capital available via the stock market. Studies have shown that such for-profit hospitals tend to provide high-quality services but at much higher costs. In other words, a large number of small-sized hospitals can give rise to scale effects, but this will generate greater profits rather than lower prices.

Here, it is also necessary to provide an overview of the commercial healthcare market. In general, the size of the commercial healthcare market is inversely proportional to the capabilities of the Ministry of Health, social security services, and other healthcare planning initiatives. Larger private markets emerge when healthcare planning is weakly organized and the needs of the people cannot be met. Conversely, if the development of social healthcare services is strong and the coverage is comprehensive, then the private healthcare market will be smaller. Nevertheless, even healthcare systems with well-organized and advanced public healthcare services retain a private market for wealthy individuals dissatisfied with public healthcare services. The private market can be considered a safety valve, because the inability to serve wealthy individuals may give rise to unnecessary political difficulties. The key point here is the relative size of the private market.

The private healthcare market is clearly different from conventional, organized healthcare services, but its features are susceptible to economic factors, such as demand and supply equilibrium, price, and competition. However, the economy is often unable to exert its full effects, especially in complicated issues such as healthcare. It is often difficult for patients to make fully rational decisions about the healthcare services they need before putting forward a "demand." In fact, physicians (suppliers) make most healthcare decisions, rather than patients (consumers). Furthermore, given the nature of the illness, patients are unable to shop around and compare the price or quality of the same treatment provided in other locations or by different physicians or dentists.

Therefore, there is an increasing trend in the majority of countries toward strengthening the organization, increasing standards, and ensuring the effective management of resources and services (with a few notable exceptions). In other words, most countries are gradually replacing their private healthcare market with healthcare programs initiated by social organizations, despite inconsistencies in the rate of social change between these countries. In the late 1980s, the political forces of several countries once encouraged the privatization of healthcare services, but this is probably an interim transition in the long-term trends of social development.

4. Economic Support

(1) General Taxes

The healthcare programs launched by the Ministry of Health and other government agencies are mostly funded by general taxes. Taxes are levied in all countries to support community-based preventive healthcare services, including environmental and individual sanitation. Therapeutic services, on the other hand, are allocated slightly less funding. Taxes have also been used to fund training courses for various types of healthcare workers and to construct healthcare facilities.

General taxes refer to the taxes levied by all levels of government (central, provincial, and municipal), such as personal income tax and corporate sales tax. Most countries have adopted a progressive tax, whereby high-income groups and enterprises are subjected to higher tax rates on their net income than is the low-income group. Developing countries tend to attach considerable importance to property and sale taxes, because it is often difficult to levy income taxes. Imported or large-sized products (e.g., cars, refrigerators, etc.) are subjected to special taxes. Alcoholic beverages, tobacco, and other luxury goods, such as hotels and restaurants, are also heavily taxed. Agricultural and mineral products are subjected to sale taxes or export duties. Other sources of government revenue include various licensing fees for businesses, occupations, driving, or public performances.

Most of the aforementioned taxes are transferred to the treasuries of either the central or the local government. The Ministry of Health must compete with other government agencies for these tax revenues, which is a process that is subjected to numerous political forces. Consequently, many health ministries prefer to rely on health-specific allocations or health-related revenues, such as income from social security.

(2) Social Security

Social insurance or social security is a special fund for medical services and other social purposes. This fund is typically collected via statutory contributions at a stipulated percentage of wages or salaries from both employers (e.g., industrial enterprises with more than 20 employees) and employees on a regular (e.g., monthly) basis. As these social security funds are typically not included as part of government finances, they are often considered a deposit rather than a tax. There may be an upper limit for the percentage of employees' wages allocated to social security (e.g., 5% of their monthly salary, no more than US$1,000 per month). The employees' monthly wages or salary may or may not have a similar upper limit. The social security law of some countries also requires the government to contribute a certain amount of funds.

The statutory contributions might be deposited in a central social security fund. However, for historical reasons, some countries require the social security contributions to be deposited into local independent insurance funds, which are restricted by numerous laws and regulations. For example, these local funds might be used to pay nationwide standardized fees to physicians for the provision of specific healthcare services. Social insurance contributions are levied independently by each province or state in some federal countries, such as Canada and the US. There might also be other differences in the specific measures adopted for social security funds.

A wide range of healthcare services is covered by social insurance funds, with varying requirements. The insured person may sometimes be required to bear the partial costs of each healthcare service or make copayments. In other cases, the insured person must pay the full medical fees to the healthcare institution before they can apply for an 80% or 90% reimbursement from the insurance fund. In some countries, physicians are paid by the funds on a monthly basis according to the number of patients they see, instead of according to the services provided. In many developing countries and some developed countries, social security institutions have their own general hospitals and hence only need to pay the salaries of physicians and other healthcare workers under their employment. Due to the differences in specific circumstances, social insurance is commonly referred to as "welfare."

(3) Voluntary Insurance

Before the implementation of statutory health insurance, many people have long been voluntarily purchasing healthcare insurance as a precaution against serious illness. In most countries, voluntary health insurance against diseases (including loss of income and medical costs) has become statutory insurance. Until the 1980s, voluntary insurance remained the primary source of medical expenses in Australia, South Africa, the US, and other countries. Voluntary insurance is largely associated with employment, whereby employers are required to pay most or part of the insurance premiums.

There are numerous carriers for voluntary insurance. Commercial insurance companies are one of the major carriers, and mainly offer life insurance, accident insurance, and accidental death and injury insurance policies. Special insurance agencies funded by physicians, hospitals, and professional organizations also participate in the insurance industry. There are also less common insurance funds offering more comprehensive coverage that are designed based on the consumer population. Some countries have already implemented social security schemes, and healthcare services are sometimes even covered by the Ministry of Finance. Hence, individuals who choose to purchase voluntary insurance are high-income earners who demand private healthcare services.

(4) Charitable Donations

The majority of the aforementioned charitable healthcare institutions are funded through charitable donations. Unlike purchasing insurance, donors are often motivated by a desire to help others rather than to receive benefits in return. Wealthy countries often donate extensively to these institutions due to their large middle-class populations, who typically have some disposable income. Charitable foundations are also funded through donations.

In many industrialized countries, fundraising has become a career due to the frequent demand for donations by various charitable organizations that serve healthcare and other humanitarian purposes. These charitable organizations may compile electronic lists of possible donors to specific causes. However, fundraising costs may take up a large proportion of the donations solicited. For this reason, charitable donations are generally not considered an important part of national healthcare systems. Although charitable donations primarily serve as the main source of income for charitable healthcare institutions, these donations are occasionally channeled to select hospitals, universities, or even government agencies.

In poorer developing countries, the source of charitable donations is mainly attributed to a handful of wealthy individuals or members of royal families. Arguably, the greatest donations in these countries are the contributions of volunteer healthcare workers who serve the communities without compensation.

Lottery. Charitable organizations and occasionally governments often organize lotteries or "lucky draw" activities to raise funds for hospitals and healthcare programs. However, the costs of creating and distributing lottery tickets and purchasing prizes can often use up a large proportion of the raised funds.

Foreign Aid. Foreign aid represents a unique type of charitable donation that most developing countries receive to help develop their healthcare systems. The earliest form of foreign aid involved the construction of hospitals and clinics by foreign missionaries. To date, such healthcare institutions are still in operation worldwide. Since World War II, two major types of healthcare assistance and guidance have been provided by developed countries to developing countries: multilateral aid and bilateral aid. Both are often provided in forms other than cash, which include technical support, medical equipment, medical supplies, and consultations, which are the key elements that contribute to a comprehensive healthcare program.

The WHO and UNICEF are considered the most important multilateral aid organizations. However, the United Nations Development Program (UNDP), World Bank, and United Nations Population Fund (UNFPA) also provide financial support to some healthcare programs. Together, these organizations represent almost every country in the world and have organized innumerable healthcare development programs. These programs are often referred to as examples of "cooperation" instead of "aid."

Bilateral aid typically consists of specific aid programs delivered by a donor country to a recipient country via either government or private organizations. Examples include the construction of a hospital by Japan in Myanmar, or the family planning program implemented by the US in Kenya. Occasionally, there are ulterior motives behind these donations, but these programs undeniably facilitate healthcare development in the recipient countries.

Privately funded programs might also be sponsored by different charitable organizations from donor countries.

(5) Individuals and Families

In all healthcare systems, individuals and families must bear a portion of the medical fees, regardless of the percentage borne by governmental or other social insurance schemes. Because diseases and accidents are unpredictable life events, some families without sufficient social support become burdened with massive medical costs.

In most countries, individuals can spend a considerable amount of money on routine healthcare, such as by purchasing nonprescription drugs, paying for health insurance out-of-pocket, or consulting private physicians. Personal healthcare expenditures are generally proportional to household income, meaning that wealthy individuals have higher healthcare expenditures. However, low-income families are more susceptible to severe illnesses. Because healthcare expenditures often account for a greater proportion of the household income among low-income families, this has made the issue of inequality more prominent.

Some countries have advocated for minimizing government-funded health coverage while maximizing personal healthcare expenditures. In these countries, even public hospitals and healthcare centers impose medical fees. In certain particularly impoverished countries, public hospitals merely provide beds and charge patients for drugs, medical tests, and X-ray examinations. Patients must rely on families for daily meals, with the exception of patients without any family.

(6) Summary

The allocation ratio of these economic resources varies across countries. Unfortunately, it is difficult to obtain concrete data in this area. If such data are available, they can accurately reflect the nature of the healthcare system and determine whether a country views the health of its citizens as its social responsibility.

Another measure of financial support is the percentage of total government expenditure allocated to healthcare. Typically, the budget allocated for healthcare declines as the government budget for military expenditures increases.

A country's emphasis on its healthcare system is also reflected in the correlation between its total health expenditure (i.e., the sum of public and private expenditure) and its financial strength or gross national product (GNP). The percentage of the total healthcare expenditure has increased throughout the 20th century in both developing and developed countries. This is due to various factors, such as advancements in the health sciences and changes in demographic or social factors. The ratio of the GNP spent on healthcare in wealthy countries has always been higher than that in poor countries. Despite notable improvements in the latter, this discrepancy still exists. In the following chapters, we will examine the characteristics of different types of countries and the reasons for these changes.

5. Health Management

Management is second only to finance in supporting healthcare resources, programs, and services. Here, the term "management" is used to refer to various management procedures, including planning, administration, regulation and supervision, and legislation.

With the exception of some socialist countries, no country has a sufficiently comprehensive and coherent healthcare system that can be fully analyzed using the four aspects mentioned earlier. In fact, most healthcare systems are collections of "programs" or subsystems, each of which has slightly different management characteristics from the others. A country's overall culture or ideology has a pervading influence on all subsystems. However, there will be differences in the specific implementation of these management procedures; for instance, the management of government departments, volunteer organizations, and private companies are different from each other.

(1) Planning

The planning of healthcare systems can be classified into multiple categories. A highly centralized management system could be established to supervise every aspect of the whole system or only be applied to the Ministry of Health. The objectives of planning might not be limited to human and material resources but might also include the specific standards for all healthcare services, including individual and environmental healthcare standards.

Adopting a highly centralized system in national planning can potentially influence all major healthcare services, which not only include programs initiated by the Ministry of Health but also independent social security healthcare planning, universities that provide training for healthcare workers, and water-supply facilities constructed by the Ministry of Internal Affairs. However, the planning department of the Ministry of Health usually carries out planning if it is applicable only to the ministry itself. In that case, healthcare workers providing services in private markets (physicians, dentists, pharmacists, etc.) are entirely excluded from the planning in terms of personnel allocation and medical practice. However, the planning of healthcare systems does sometimes include the private market to ensure a reasonable allocation of healthcare workers to all regions in the country.

Healthcare planning can be carried out using various approaches. Policymakers might estimate the objective healthcare needs of the population through surveys or other research methods. They may actively respond to perceived healthcare needs, or passively make adjustments based on the existing resources. The locations of healthcare centers or hospitals might not only be determined based on objective formulations derived from analyzing the changes in healthcare needs but also be based on the personal preferences of influential leaders alone. Although healthcare planning is generally carried out by central government agencies, nongovernmental experts might be invited to advise on certain aspects, such as physical examinations for newborn infants.

To what extent is the power to carry out healthcare planning decentralized in dominant countries? Is it necessary for the central government to issue standard requirements or guidance if local agencies are delegated with considerable responsibility for such planning? Does a local authority carry out the approval of the central government necessary for the implementation of healthcare planning? Do certain NGOs participate in the planning process? It is only by answering these questions that we can fully understand the characteristics of planning.

(2) Administration

The terms "administration" and "management" are often used interchangeably, but here, the former specifically refers to the policy decisions of project leaders, and the degree of supervision and control they have over a project to ensure its effective implementation and achieve specific goals. Different administrative policies have been adopted across different healthcare systems.

The administrative style can be divided into various types, such as autocratic, democratic, and a range of intermediates between these two extremes. An autocratic administrative style is preferred in some political contexts, whereas a democratic style is preferred in others. The autocratic style might be fully embraced by a country when facing a crisis during a particular historical period; however, in other times, management can only succeed if every policy is extensively debated. The management of both large- and small-scale healthcare programs involves at least the following eight functions.

1. *Organization:* Any project must be divided into multiple tasks, which are then completed by individuals with suitable skills. All these tasks are interlinked by temporal, physical, or spatial relationships. This function requires the deployment of personnel to certain geographic locations for certain tasks, which may only be accomplished using certain equipment. Needless to say, the purpose of organizing resources is to improve the efficiency by using the minimum amount of time, resources, and energy to achieve one's goals. In that case, how should these organizational processes be conducted?

2. *Staffing and budgeting:* The initiation of a project requires the appointment of personnel who are sufficiently competent for the task or who will receive the relevant training. Ensuring that the personnel possess the relevant skills is not the only factor that is considered when appointing staff. Other factors include ensuring that the personnel will demonstrate good performance and consistency. Reasonable staff management should also take other factors into consideration, such as salaries, working conditions, and working relationships. How should these issues be addressed?

   Once the personnel have been appointed, the expenditures for other items, including equipment, supplies, communication, and travel expenses, can then be estimated. In general, the budget needs to be approved by senior management before the project can be implemented. Another factor that needs to be considered in budgeting is whether provisions have been made for dealing with contingencies.

3. *Supervision:* Appropriate and feasible supervision is necessary following the appointment of appropriate personnel. Although some personnel are diligent and require minimal supervision, others might require close supervision. Supervision can have a positive effect and encourage the completion of tasks, but it might also lead to fear among personnel and can lower their enthusiasm. These characteristics of management should be fully comprehended when studying the healthcare system of a country.

4. *Consultation:* Providing consultation for personnel is closely associated with supervision. This is because healthcare workers will always encounter problems with a project regardless of their capabilities. Managers might resolve these problems, but sometimes, a third-party consultant is required. Healthcare workers can also advise colleagues who encounter similar problems. In addition, the persistent recurrence of a problem should serve as a reminder for managers to hold regular staff meetings.

   The involvement of local residents in the project management process is a special approach to consultation, whereby feedback on healthcare services, solicited through neighborhood committees, can benefit any project considerably. It is an opportunity to obtain suggestions for improvement from the residents. Community engagement can serve as a long-term consultation mechanism for both the project teams and residents. Does the involvement of local residents also gain their trust as beneficiaries of the project?

5. *Procurement and logistics:* Most well-organized healthcare programs rely on reliable supplies of drugs and other materials through diversified supply chains. In general, medical supplies are delivered regularly from a centralized warehouse to each medical

facility in the area. Certain special items may be supplied to facilities based on a preestablished annual procurement plan, or via a purchasing order issued by a specific unit on an as-needed basis. Developing countries rely on imports for most medical supplies, making it infeasible for them to purchase the supplies in bulk due to inadequate foreign-exchange reserves.

Some healthcare facilities purchase medical supplies directly from the local market. Despite the higher net costs, this resolves potential shipping issues and allows them to meet healthcare demands more rapidly and effectively. Medical supplies can be transported together or separately from the primary order for use in other projects, such as school or agricultural projects.

6. *Recording and reporting:* Daily records and regular reporting are essential for the project management team to understand the daily operations of their project and respond to changes in healthcare demands in a timely manner. Healthcare programs usually require the recording of patient information, diagnostic results, service contents, medications, and may sometimes even require financial information. The number of participants in certain activities, such as health education and training courses, also needs to be recorded. Has this information been recorded?

   The information recorded then forms the basis for reports that are submitted regularly to the senior management team. Aside from the quantitative data of healthcare services, these reports can also include current problems or suggestions for policy changes to improve the project. An experienced manager should be capable of extracting hidden issues from these reports.

   Rapid communication is yet another important management method. Communication tools, such as telephone, fax, and mail, should not be taken for granted, as it is difficult to guarantee that these devices or services are always available.

7. *Coordination:* One major task in the management process is the coordination of projects among different administrative functions, including the coordination among different healthcare programs, as well as the coordination between healthcare programs and projects in other fields. Sometimes, discrepancies between healthcare programs and programs in other fields can be resolved via a simple discussion; other times, discrepancies cannot be resolved at all through coordination. Ultimately, the success of interdisciplinary cooperation is dependent on the quality of the two-way communication between administrative personnel in the social fields involved.

8. *Assessment:* Finally, health programs must be assessed at different levels, including internal assessments within a specific healthcare unit or hospital, district- or province-level healthcare assessments, assessments for a particular type of project (e.g., tuberculosis and family planning), and nationwide healthcare assessments. Healthcare assessment has become increasingly important due to the worldwide increase in healthcare expenditures.

There are countless methods of healthcare assessment with varying levels of complexity. Long-term recording and monitoring of nationwide or regional mortality trends, such as infant mortality rate and life expectancy at birth, is arguably the most commonly adopted method. These data largely reflect the actual situation in a country or region, but might not be able to illustrate the value and actual operation of the healthcare system. It is well known that the effects of environmental and social factors on mortality are comparable to or greater than are those of the healthcare system. These factors include employment, housing, education, income levels, agricultural status, and so on.

Mortality rate is an outcome indicator for healthcare and many other disciplines. However, mortality rate can only be used to objectively reflect the outcomes of healthcare programs after appropriate research parameters have been established. Other important indicators include input and process indicators. For instance, the training and allocation of 1,000 nurses in a province would be considered an input indicator, as nurses provide healthcare services that are beneficial to patients.

Let us take, for example, a process indicator, which shows a childhood vaccination rate of 80% within a region. Assuming an equal level of vaccine effectiveness, this region has a higher quality healthcare program when compared to a region with a vaccination rate of 40%. If we also assume that the vaccine is effective in preventing a specific infectious disease, then the overall incidence rate of the vaccinated disease would be considered an outcome indicator of this vaccination project (given that both regions are comparable in all other respects).

Different countries are effective to varying degrees in assessing their healthcare systems. Assessments are usually carried out by a third-party unrelated to the project or activity, in order to ensure reliability. For some healthcare programs, the assessment results are incorporated directly into daily records as part of their management efforts, thus allowing the managers to receive feedback on the project's processes and outcomes. Such feedback can also be related to expenditures, which in turn enables managers to track the costs incurred in relation to their funding status.

(3) Regulation and Supervision

The establishment and implementation of standards form a part of the management of healthcare systems. In general, supervision refers to the surveillance by government agencies of commercial activities. Most cases of supervision belong to this category. In other cases, supervision might refer to surveillance by higher-level government agencies or other departments on lower-level government agencies. Here, we discuss the four main categories of supervisory targets.

1. Environmental Conditions Healthcare-related supervision can be extended to the establishment and implementation of environmental standards, such as quality standards for water purity (especially drinking water). In addition, there are numerous rules and regulations for the management of human waste, particularly in urban areas. Some laws also require the physical or chemical treatment of sewage prior to its discharge into a river or other water bodies, in order to reduce environmental pollution. Similarly, the disposal of industrial waste must comply with relevant regulations.

Many countries have issued relevant rules and regulations to reduce air pollution caused by both industrial and domestic waste. In major cities, many rules and regulations have been imposed on the automotive industry because passenger car emissions are the main contributor to air pollution. Relevant legislation have also been enacted to protect air quality, including the restrictions on open burning and outdoor bonfires.

The contamination of dairy products during the collection and processing of raw milk can have severe harmful effects on the populations of countries that consume large amounts of animal milk (mainly cow's milk, but the milk of other animals as well). Hence, many countries have enacted numerous rules and regulations concerning milk disinfection. Similarly, animal slaughter and the storage and processing of meat products must comply with the relevant standards and regulations. The inspection of food establishments is practiced in most developed countries but is usually not performed in developing countries (with the exception of major cities).

The enforcement of healthcare regulations requires a large number of law-enforcement officers with relevant skills. However, such enforcement resources are typically lacking, even in the most developed countries. Supervision is meaningless without enforcement or with weak enforcement.

2. Pharmaceuticals Pharmaceutical surveillance is an important component in the management of healthcare systems. There have been all-too-frequent tragedies resulting from the illegal commercialization of harmful or toxic pharmaceuticals by private pharmaceutical companies in pursuit of profit. Moreover, false therapeutic claims are made for many pharmaceutical drugs.

Therefore, many countries have been implementing a series of laws and regulations concerning the production and distribution of pharmaceutical drugs to ensure their safety and therapeutic efficacy. Along with the advances in pharmacology, evidence is now legally required to support claims that a drug has therapeutic benefits for specific diseases. Some countries have also imposed restrictions on the type of pharmaceutical drugs that can be imported.

The implementation of these rules and regulations requires on-site inspections of pharmaceutical manufacturers and extensive reports in the early phases of clinical trials of pharmaceutical drugs. Additionally, the laws and regulations typically impose detailed restrictions on the labels and advertising content of pharmaceutical drugs. Are there sufficient resources for such supervision?

3. Healthcare Workers and Facilities The professional certification and occupational licensing of healthcare workers are also regulated by healthcare systems. Indeed, medical licensing for physicians is required in every country. Aside from completing the required medical degree, physicians must also undergo practical training programs (such as internships or practicing in rural areas) to obtain a professional license. Physicians in some countries must join a medical ethics association in order to demonstrate their morality. Furthermore, the government departments of some countries have set up examinations for healthcare workers. Special licensing requirements are also imposed for graduates of foreign medical schools. In addition, there are regulations related to professional grades in the medical field, but these tend to be formulated by the respective professional associations rather than the government.

Comprehensive training programs are needed for nurses, pharmacists, dentists, and other healthcare workers to obtain their professional licenses. The classification and standards of licensed healthcare workers vary considerably across countries. Some auxiliary healthcare workers are only required to undergo healthcare training programs organized by the public health department. According to the regulations, they should practice in accredited medical units, but some may also be involved in illegal private medical practices.

Professional licenses and certification usually have permanent validity unless they are revoked due to criminal behavior or serious misconduct. However, a few countries require regular license renewal for certain categories of healthcare workers. Healthcare workers are also usually required to attend some degree of continuing education or must renew their certification by passing examinations.

Many countries have established standards for hospitals, which include the building structure, bed size, fire-control system, surgical theaters, and laboratories, as well as hospital practices such as environmental sanitation, safe operation in X-ray rooms, and the qualification of healthcare workers. In some countries, the same standards are applicable to all hospitals, whereas, in other countries, these standards are only applicable to public healthcare institutions. In addition to government-issued standards, NGOs also tend to formulate their own standards for hospitals. For instance, hospital associations might supplement the aspects that are not covered by the government standards, such as the maintenance of medical records, specifications for healthcare workers, and correct surgical procedures. Such certifications are issued by NGOs in order to highlight to the public that certain hospitals have relatively higher quality, whereas non-accredited hospitals may have hidden risks.

The standards issued by governmental organizations and NGOs are generally applicable to other healthcare facilities, such as rehabilitation centers that provide long-term care. Certain departments in laboratories, blood banks, and other institutions may have to comply with other standards issued by NGOs or the governmental departments.

4. Personal Healthcare Services   The licensing of healthcare workers refers to the standards formulated for their medical practice. Well-trained healthcare workers may also work according to specific principles. In addition, most healthcare systems issue codes of conduct for other types of healthcare workers, but these may be informal.

These informal regulations may have first appeared in hospitals as self-regulatory codes of conducts when physicians, nurses, and other healthcare workers worked together. In such environments, everyone pays attention to their own behaviors to earn the respect of their colleagues. However, the codes of conduct are subject to change according to the nature of the hospital leadership and the overall culture of the healthcare system. Such self-regulation may also exist in healthcare centers and general clinics.

Under the health insurance system, physicians' income can also be used to assess their level of professionalism, as it is associated with their own professional conduct. Statistical analyses have found that some physicians engage in over-prescription of laboratory tests, physical examinations, and drugs, as well as unnecessary surgeries. Although no conclusions can be drawn based on these data, they are sufficient to initiate an investigation of these physicians. Similar supervision can also be applied to dental services.

The judicial system allows for indirect supervision via medical malpractice lawsuits by patients. The legal and practical aspects of medical malpractice lawsuits vary substantially across different countries, such that these lawsuits are easily accepted by courts in some countries, but not in others.

(4) Legislation

The healthcare system is directly or indirectly supported by the legal system. Various laws overtly and subtly influence the five components of healthcare systems; hence, they form a part of the management of healthcare systems. As seen before, many aspects of supervision, as well as other aspects of healthcare systems, are based on legislation.

Broadly speaking, the healthcare system is supported by the law in the following six ways.

1. *Promotion of resource production*: The law may stipulate the funding sources for training physicians, nurses, and other healthcare workers and guarantee that there is sufficient funding. These laws may also stipulate that medical graduates must serve in rural areas in order to obtain their medical licenses. Some new types of healthcare work require legal approval, and there may be corresponding standards for the issuance of medical licenses.

As a rule, both the financial allocation and actual construction of hospitals and healthcare centers must be legally approved. The law might also specify that certain healthcare services can only be provided in healthcare facilities of a certain size and capacity within a regional network.

2. *Project approval:* The majority of the healthcare programs mentioned before must be legally approved. The Ministry of Health is generally established on a legal basis, even though the law only provides a general definition of its functions. Nonetheless, the law typically delineates a broad scope for the functions of the Ministry of Health with the aim of protecting public health. Similarly, the law may also assign the responsibility of ensuring workers' safety and health to the health department of the Ministry of Labor, which often has a broad scope.

Different countries have different laws regulating the financial affairs. In democratic countries, an annual budget must be approved according to specified legal procedures, whereas in other countries, the government directly authorizes the executive departments for the use of funds. Regardless of the approach adopted, publicly and sometimes privately funded healthcare programs require legal approval. Similarly, numerous projects, such as the control of disease transmission, environmental health, family planning, and water fluoridation for tooth decay also require legal approval.

3. *Social coordination of gealth security:* Several forms of financial support for healthcare services are either fully or partially provided by law. For instance, in social security schemes, the law clearly requires enterprises and employees to regularly contribute social insurance premiums. Even private insurance companies must comply with the law when issuing voluntary health insurance. Similarly, charitable organizations are required to operate within a legal framework.

Taxes are the main source of income for most governmental healthcare workers, and the levying of taxes is stipulated in the law. For example, the rates of personal income tax, property tax, and financial transaction tax are implemented according to legal requirements. Corresponding legislative authorization is required for taxes that are levied by governmental bodies below the level of the central government.

4. *Quality assurance*: The management of healthcare workers and hospitals mentioned earlier is generally conducted on a legal basis, and the ultimate aim is to protect the public from medical malpractice. The law is indispensable for protecting members of the public from nonbeneficial services or harmful treatments driven by the pursuit of profit. Peer reviews are also required by law to maintain a code of professional conduct.

5. *Prohibition of harmful behaviors*: Most regulations related to environmental health impose restrictions on individual or collective behaviors, such as littering or discharging toxic waste into sources of drinking water. Similarly, the laws impose speed limits for vehicles and require motorcyclists to wear a helmet.

These laws are issued to protect civilians and the society as a whole. However, their implementation might lead to controversy as they often restrict individual freedoms. For instance, the law restricts the advertising of tobacco and cigarettes because they are harmful to individuals or others around them. Based on a country's national constitution and judicial framework, courts must often determine whether or at what point the protection of public health is more important than guaranteeing these individual rights. The legitimate scope of the regulatory authority held by the government changes constantly alongside an increasing understanding of the social determinants of healthcare and disease.

6. *Protection of individual rights*: Laws have been established in many countries to protect individual rights within the healthcare system. Patients have the right to know the risks of surgery and must provide their informed consent. In addition, the law might protect the right of employees to be informed about the risk of exposure to harmful substances at the workplace.

6. Service Provision

(1) Primary Healthcare Services

Primary healthcare services refer to the majority of services involved in health promotion and disease prevention at both environmental and individual levels. The WHO considers primary healthcare to include at least the following eight types of services: (1) health education on diseases and disease prevention and control; (2) improvement of food supply and promotion of balanced nutrition; (3) ensurance of an adequate water supply and good basic public health; (4) maternal and child healthcare services, including family planning; (5) epidemic prevention of major infectious diseases; (6) prevention and control of endemic diseases; (7) Ensurance of the correct treatment for common diseases and injuries; (8) provision of basic drugs. Although these categories seem to be targeted at developing countries, in reality, they are applicable to the primary healthcare of all countries. In developed countries, the absence of adequate food and clean water is almost unimaginable, as these resources are readily available, but food supplies and water purification are still crucial to human health. The WHO hopes that all countries will provide primary healthcare services, in order to ensure equal and timely access to healthcare services for all.

1. Preventive Services   Among the eight categories of primary healthcare services listed by the WHO, the first six all involve disease prevention and healthcare. Differences exist in the specific methods by which these health services are provided to different social classes (e.g., urban workers) within the same country, not to mention the differences in specific healthcare practices across different countries (e.g., clean water supply and maternal and child care).

Some regions of developing countries still rely on well water, and women are required to carry home water in large jugs balanced on their heads. In contrast, those living in skyscrapers in cities can simply turn on their stainless-steel water taps in the kitchen to obtain clean water. In some developed countries, indoor water supply is available even in the rural areas, whereas rich urban residents may think that filling their water bottles before going to the countryside feels like a vacation. As can be seen, there are considerable differences among the different countries and social groups in this regard.

In terms of maternal and child care, different nursing methods may be used even within the same healthcare system. Low-income individuals might seek antenatal checkups from assistant midwives at worn-out or excessively busy outpatient departments in public hospitals. They may also receive antenatal check-ups at the obstetrics and gynecology clinics of local public hospitals or community health centers established by local religious organizations. The spouses of skilled workers might undergo antenatal check-ups at general clinics designated by their social insurance, which has dedicated obstetricians or at private clinics of general practitioners. On the other hand, wealthy individuals might prebook their antenatal check-ups at the offices of private obstetricians equipped with excellent facilities, where pregnant women are examined by physicians assisted by well-trained nurses on a comfortable examination chair with clean linen sheets. In all the cases mentioned, the people in charge of antenatal check-ups have different sources of incomes; some of these individuals serve on a full-time basis and are taxpayer-funded; some serve on a part-time basis and are paid by social security funds; some are paid directly by patients. Moreover, the training, equipment, and supplies available to these professionals also vary considerably even within the same healthcare system. This difference would undoubtedly be much larger across different systems.

There are also significant variations in other preventive services of primary healthcare. Dental care, health education, vaccination, malaria control, and other services have different characteristics in different social environments within the same healthcare system. Evidently, these differences would be greater across different healthcare systems. A full understanding of a national health system requires recognition of its diversity. Even though some systems may have greater internal variations, this type of diversity is commonly found. Unfortunately, many analyses of national healthcare systems tend to oversimplify this diversity and generalize the uniform and universal characteristics within the system.

2. Therapeutic Services The WHO has pointed out that the most basic primary healthcare must consist of the aforementioned eight categories of services, among which the last two are considered therapeutic services. "The correct treatment of common diseases and injuries" might sound simple but it encompasses an exceedingly broad and diverse range of content. There might be only a dozen or so common diseases in an ordinary community, but the primary healthcare for these diseases involves diverse resources, careful organization, funding, management, and so on. This has led to considerable intra- and intercountry differences in the models of healthcare service provision.

For example, therapeutic methods for the common cold vary greatly within the same healthcare system. Patients may be asked to convalesce at home (e.g., rest and drink hot tea), consult physicians at community health centers, or seek medical attention at UNICEF-supported mobile clinics (generally stocked with many drugs), or consult general practitioners in small-sized healthcare centers in the city. The patient might also consult otolaryngology specialists in private clinics, consult military physicians at military hospitals, seek medical attention from well-trained nurses at large-sized industrial clinics, consult private internists, or use any number of other therapeutic approaches. Due to the differences in therapeutic approaches even within the healthcare system of the same country, such a minor illness might result in different prescriptions issued by physicians, diagnostic medical check-ups, check-up times, waiting times, level of concern of healthcare workers, payment methods, and so on.

Based on the geographical area of the healthcare system, it is possible to identify the main model of primary healthcare service provision. This can range from private general practitioners in the cities of industrialized countries to witch doctors in the rural areas of the poorest developing countries. Most patients in developing and developed countries seek medical attention from healthcare workers in healthcare centers or general clinics. In addition, patients from all the aforementioned countries seek treatment for common diseases at the outpatient departments of general hospitals.

The provision of healthcare services during the transition from primary to secondary healthcare remains controversial. Perhaps this is because there are differences even in the definitions of primary healthcare between different countries and social groups. However, in order to facilitate the comparison between countries, we will adopt the definition provided by the WHO – i.e., primary healthcare is the provision of at least the eight categories of the services mentioned earlier. We may also add two further categories to this list: (9) simple prevention and treatment of dental diseases (which can also be regarded as common diseases but are unique in their technical aspects); and (10) prediction of possible serious physical or mental illnesses requiring secondary or tertiary healthcare services.

(2) Secondary Healthcare Services

There is no unified definition or scope for secondary healthcare. To enable the comparison of medical models of different countries, we believe that secondary healthcare should include the following four categories of services: (1) special outpatient treatment; (2) general hospitalization; (3) treatment by nonmedical experts; (4) general long-term treatment.

1. Special Outpatient Treatment   The diagnostic or therapeutic skills required to treat many diseases are beyond the capacity of primary healthcare workers, including CHWs and general practitioners. For example, the diagnosis and establishment of sophisticated treatment regimens for tuberculosis, adult diabetes, childhood epilepsy, and so forth require special diagnostic examinations beyond the capacity of primary healthcare services. In addition, special training programs are required to tailor selected drugs and dosages to individual patients.

When these diseases are detected in primary healthcare facilities, physicians will transfer these patients to secondary healthcare facilities, such as healthcare centers with adequate healthcare workers or the outpatient department of district-level general hospitals. In developing countries with hospitals where care is covered by social security, the general clinics in most urban areas typically provide secondary healthcare services. In developed countries and some major cities in developing countries, private physicians might also provide secondary healthcare services to high-income patients.

The treatment of diseases in secondary healthcare facilities may require extremely expensive drugs. For example, all the aforementioned conditions require long-term treatments that are very expensive – to the point where they are unaffordable for most families. Therefore, secondary healthcare services usually require financial support from social security programs for drugs. In addition, adjustments need to be made in the patients' diet, work, and living environment; hence, only patients who are relatively well off can afford such healthcare.

2. General Hospitalization   All forms of hospitalization, including hospitalization at small-sized healthcare facilities in small towns, are considered examples of secondary healthcare. Hospitalization aims to provide care and observe patients during their disease progression, which requires a suitable amount of healthcare workers and equipment. Some people consider childbirth assisted by TBAs as a form of primary healthcare. This is because the medical services, equipment, supplies, and medicines at hospitals are not available to TBAs who assist home deliveries. Hence, even the crudest hospitals are able to provide secondary healthcare services.

Naturally, vast differences exist in the specific conditions of hospitalizations. For instance, in many developing countries, some hospitals have only 20 or fewer beds with a single full-time physician, several nurses, one laboratory technician, a chef, and a doorman. On the other hand, some local hospitals might have 100–200 beds with 10–20 well-trained specialists, as well as laboratories, radiology departments, other outpatient departments with sophisticated instruments, and fully equipped surgical and delivery rooms. In most countries, hospitals employ only full-time physicians, but hospitals in a few developed countries have more flexible policies. In the latter case, the community specialists and general practitioners care for patients in the hospital for only a few hours per day. The level of secondary healthcare can be influenced by a number of hospital-related conditions, including the quality of nursing care, hospital records, food, drug therapies, and departmental composition.

3. Treatment by Nonmedical Experts   There are several types of healthcare workers who are not physicians but contribute equally to secondary healthcare. For instance, the services provided by optometrists, who prescribe corrective lenses appropriate for each patient, and podiatrists, who examine minor foot illnesses, are considered secondary healthcare services. Other examples include the services provided by physiotherapists, occupational therapists, and speech therapists, as well as the complicated dental implants and other dental treatments performed by dentists.

Not every country has these nonmedical experts, and where these services are available, there are considerable variations in their methods of service provision. Secondary healthcare services offered by these experts might be provided at formal medical institutions, such as the outpatient departments of general hospitals and general clinics, where the healthcare workers are generally paid a salary and work under the supervision of physicians. However, these experts may also practice independently at their own clinics, and their treatment fees may be paid by patients or by specialized institutions.

4. Long-Term Treatment   We have previously highlighted the diverse types of institutions that provide long-term therapeutic services. Although these therapeutic services do not require high levels of professional skills, they clearly exceed the scope of primary healthcare. Within the institutions that provide such long-term therapeutic services, the most important characteristic of the personnel is their attitude, rather than their skill. For example, personnel might attach more importance to the feelings of chronic patients or elderly patients when planning their treatment. This attitude is extremely necessary when providing treatment.

Patients with chronic diseases who convalesce at home may also receive home-based nursing care, meal delivery, or other organized services. Much like the living conditions of families differ according to their economic statuses, the provision of long-term healthcare services is also influenced by differences in personnel and equipment.

In some countries, long-term healthcare institutions have attracted investments from private enterprises. In industrialized countries, the aging population has led to increased demand and growing prices for long-term healthcare. Consequently, wealthy individuals are able to obtain high-quality services, whereas low- and middle-income individuals only have access to lower-quality services or home-based care.

(3) Tertiary Healthcare Services

Tertiary healthcare refers to the most complex and expensive healthcare services a country can offer. In many countries, they are available in only one or a few hospitals. Physicians, technicians, and other healthcare workers with many years of professional training provide tertiary healthcare services. The purchase and maintenance of the equipment used for tertiary healthcare are unaffordable for some developing countries. Fortunately, only a limited number of patients require tertiary healthcare.

Some tertiary healthcare services are entirely diagnostic, such as CT and MRI. Tertiary therapeutic services include hemodialysis, brain surgery, heart surgery, and organ transplantation. Inevitably, tertiary healthcare generally requires meticulous planning and teamwork. Regardless of whether they are publicly or privately funded, or whether they are affiliated with government agencies or charitable organizations, the methods for providing tertiary healthcare services are often highly organized.

High-tech healthcare services are often considered to be examples of tertiary healthcare. In addition, rehabilitation programs for individuals with severe disabilities are also considered tertiary healthcare services because they are expensive, time-consuming, and complicated. In the more affluent countries, there are specialized facilities that mainly provide rehabilitation and healthcare services for patients with quadriplegia due to spinal cord injuries. Through such rehabilitative care, painstaking effort, and high-end equipment, these patients can master a great number of skills using their remaining finger and jaw muscles. Highly experienced nurses are also indispensable in such cases.

The therapeutic services provided by well-established psychiatric hospitals are another form of tertiary healthcare service. Patients with severe psychiatric disorders require long-term and complicated healthcare, which combines psychotherapy, psychotropic medication, and community-based therapeutic services. Psychiatric treatment is relatively rare in developing countries due to the prolonged and expensive course of treatment; even in developed countries, they are often only affordable to wealthy individuals.

Based on our understanding of these three types of healthcare services, we can see that not only are the methods of service provision across different countries diverse but also different social groups within the same country receive vastly different healthcare services. In most cases, we find that a small group of people receive services for all three types of healthcare that differs from that provided to the general public.

For instance, the dependents of military personnel are covered by the military healthcare system, even after the military personnel retires. If the children of military personnel decide to join the military as well, they receive healthcare services from cradle to grave under this self-contained healthcare system. The majority of individuals living in the same country also receive different healthcare services due to a number of factors, such as their own socioeconomic status, state of illness, and region of residence. Even individuals from well-off families might experience differences in the healthcare services provided.

From a different perspective, children with severe intellectual disabilities are admitted to specialized welfare institutions. They might spend their entire lives in these institutions, which provide them with primary, secondary, and tertiary healthcare services. Their lives, whether good or bad, will certainly not be the same as those of their families or most other people.

It is inevitable that our explanations here have oversimplified primary, secondary, and tertiary healthcare services to a certain extent. In fact, the boundaries between these three categories of healthcare services are often quite vague. Nevertheless, this simplification can facilitate the establishment of effective healthcare systems, in order to maximize the use of resources. It also helps us in analyzing the actual operations of different healthcare systems.

In many healthcare systems, healthcare institutions are categorized as primary, secondary, or tertiary according to the specific healthcare services provided. This policy is commonly referred to as regionalization, and is generally adopted by healthcare systems that prioritize social coordination. The principle of regionalization can provide guidance for healthcare planning and policies and is particularly valuable in systems with limited resources.

SECTION II. KEY FACTORS INFLUENCING HEALTH SYSTEMS

Section I provided an overview of the structure of different health systems. However, these structures are seldom designed in advance. As such, we can only derive the five major components influencing these systems and their interrelations by analyzing the existing health systems. Through this analysis, we will learn that these components have been influenced by long-term historical evolution. Each of the five components exhibits its own characteristics, but collectively they determine the health system of a country.

1. Economic Factors

Economic development has a significant influence on a country's health system. This is because the economy determines the health status (i.e., type of diseases) of the country's population, which in turn has an impact on the development of the healthcare system. There are extensive differences in the health systems between poor and wealthy countries. In the former, infectious diseases are rampant and children commonly suffer from malnutrition, whereas the main issues faced by the latter are chronic diseases in the elderly population. Even if a given health system does not always meet the health needs of the population, the demand for healthcare will clearly affect its design.

The level of economic development has other effects on health systems, particularly in the supply and demand of healthcare resources, including healthcare workforce, facilities, products, and knowledge. For example, the quantity and quality of physicians are influenced by the wealth of a country due to the substantial resources required to train a physician. The conventional approach to determining a country's economic development is looking at its gross domestic product (GDP), which refers to the value of all final products and services produced by the country per year. The number of healthcare workers (percentage of total population) in a country increases with economic development, albeit at different rates. In fact, if we list the GDP per capita and the number of physicians for all countries, we will observe clear inconsistencies across different countries. This is mainly attributed to the fact that under the same level of economic development, some countries attach greater political value to the recruitment of physicians whereas others consider it too expensive to train such a large number of physicians. Similar relationships exist between the level of economic development and the availability of other healthcare resources, such as the number of hospital beds.

In most countries, the quality of healthcare resources is positively correlated with their quantity. Therefore, wealthy countries (e.g., Sweden and Greece) tend to have better quality healthcare workers, facilities, and overall hospital conditions than do poorer countries (e.g., Sudan and Colombia).

A country's economic strength not only determines the quantity and quality of healthcare resources but also affects the practices of healthcare workers. Wealthy countries have a relatively active market economy, which provides a large private market for physicians and other health practitioners. Medical fees might be paid out-of-pocket by the patients or through voluntary health insurance (e.g., the US) or social insurance (e.g., France and Japan). Most physicians participate in private practice to some degree, even in countries such as France and Japan where almost all citizens are covered by social security.

On the other hand, the vast majority of physicians in Latin American countries, such as Ecuador and Peru, cannot earn satisfactory incomes from private clinics. Therefore, they search for salaried positions, working 4–6 hours per day at social security hospitals, health ministries, military units, private enterprises, and so forth and spend their spare time serving patients in private practice. Only a small number of physicians are capable of living off their own private practice, as the medical fees are unaffordable to most patients.

In developed countries, physicians in private practice or private hospitals are subsidized by public finances, which enable economically disadvantaged residents to receive healthcare services from private institutions. In poorer countries, patients living in poverty might seek treatments at public healthcare institutions where physicians are paid a salary. The efficient use of government funds is highly valued in these countries due to limited finances. Both these approaches reflect how the delivery mode of healthcare services is determined by a country's level of economic development.

A country's wealth can be primarily attributed to its degree of industrialization, and it has a number of effects on the healthcare system. Developed countries often have higher degrees of urbanization, better transportation and communication systems, and higher education level among residents, all of which influence the demand and supply of healthcare services. For instance, cities tend to have larger hospitals, more skilled physicians, and advanced facilities. In contrast, countries with a greater rural population (e.g., India and Nigeria) not only face a shortage of drugs but also lack scientific support for the prescription of drugs. Naturally, there are many drawbacks to living in densely populated cities, but cities tend to adopt better approaches in disease prevention and treatment. The geographical allocation of healthcare resources in every country is typically based on the economic level of each region.

The country's level of economic development also determines its dependence on other countries for drugs, medical equipment, and even scientific technology. There are almost no pharmaceutical companies capable of manufacturing modern drugs in less-developed countries, which must rely on imports for these drugs at higher prices. Even if a country is able to manufacture drugs locally, raw pharmaceutical materials must often be imported. India began to develop its pharmaceutical industry (under the guidance of foreign experts) immediately after its independence. Similar actions were adopted by China and Cuba after their social revolutions in 1949 and 1959, respectively.

Scientific research not only requires high-end equipment but also substantial resources for training scientists. Hence, most scientific discoveries related to disease prevention and treatment are made in highly developed countries, such as European or North American countries. It is, however, not our intention to ignore the achievements of Ayurveda and TCM, which will be further elaborated in later chapters. Fortunately, scientific knowledge is shared internationally via scientific publications or other avenues due to internationally accepted ethical norms.

Finally, the percentage of a country's healthcare input is also influenced by its wealth. Wealthy and poor countries allocate 5–10% and 2–5% of their GNP, respectively, to the healthcare industry. Developing countries have relatively fewer resources allocated to health systems because the majority of their expenditure is allocated to daily necessities, such as food and housing. In other words, the health systems in poorer countries are only allocated a small slice of the economic pie.

2. Political Factors

In contrast to economic factors, political factors play an equally or even more important role in a country's healthcare system. Political factors play a crucial role as they can exert a joint effect with economic factors, which thereby influence economic operations. Under the guidance of different ideologies, political factors often have an effect on all aspects of the quantity and delivery method of healthcare services across different countries.

Political factors are not limited to the traits of the ruling party or the current legal form of the central government. Even long-past political events are still capable of influencing the characteristics of the current healthcare system. Even when a social revolution alters the entire structure of the society, its previously established power structure (e.g., the administrative division of province and cities) tends to remain unchanged. During the course of history, historical events have had an inevitable influence on the current policies, and past events are merely a preface to the present.

The US gained its independence in 1776 after the American Revolution against the British monarchy. One of the core elements of the American revolutionary ideology was opposition to political centralization, regardless of whether the power was centralized in the hands of a monarch in London or other nobility. The US Constitution was established during the American Revolution to minimize political centralization and to allow for greater checks and balances of power between the legislative, executive, and judicial branches of the government. The US Constitution also guarantees the sovereignty of each state (originally 13 British colonies), and most of their duties were preserved. These duties do not come under the authority of the federal government but are state affairs. One such duty is the protection of citizens' health. In the 243 years since the US gained its independence, healthcare programs, such as medical licensing, public health programs, and hospital planning are still the responsibility of state governments rather than the federal government.

Another example is the French Revolution of 1789. The French Revolution not only targeted the monarch but also his allies (feudal landlords and the Roman Curia). The Roman Curia had amassed vast fortunes, while also controlling and operating most French hospitals at the time. When the parliamentary system was first established in the French First Republic, hospital ownership was shifted to secular power. France was eventually divided into 90 provinces, each of which was responsible for managing the church hospitals contained therein. However, the Napoleonic Code that was promulgated after the Great French Revolution established a highly centralized political system whereby the central government has the right to appoint the chief minister in each province, who is then responsible for managing public properties, such as hospitals, in the province. The chief minister appoints healthcare officers, who are then responsible for the healthcare programs within the province. The healthcare officers work under the guidance of the Provincial Assembly, which is comprised of elected officials who represent each district within the province. To date, the public hospitals in France are still owned and controlled by local governments in accordance with the laws and regulations of the central government. These are the outcomes and continuation of the French Revolution.

Following the outbreak of the Crimean War in Russia (1853–1956), Florence Nightingale led a team of young female nurses (none of them were nuns) to help care for wounded English soldiers. Upon returning to England, she began to advocate for the importance of nursing skills and subsequently established the first nonreligious nursing school in St. Thomas' Hospital, London in 1860. Perhaps the nursing profession would still have been established over time without this historical event. Nevertheless, the emergence of modern nursing in England is now inextricably linked with the Crimean War. Furthermore, the emergence of the nursing profession undoubtedly played a significant role in promoting the development of hospitals.

The industrial revolution of the late eighteenth and nineteenth centuries has also had a profound political impact. Numerous workers with fixed salaries who were gathered in cities established health insurance funds ("sickness funds") and supported the German Socialist Party (Deutschsozialistische Partei, DSP), which pledged to improve labor welfare. In the 1880s, Prime Minister Otto von Bismarck of the German Conservative Party (Deutschkonservative Partei, DKP) passed the world's first statutory health insurance act to compete with the DSP. This act reinforced health insurance funds, which continue to play an important role in the German healthcare system.

Colonialism has also influenced healthcare institutions of Asian and African countries that have now gained independence. European countries established the basic framework for public healthcare services to protect their overseas armies and colonists, as well as to facilitate the efficient exploitation of natural resources, originally established. For example, in the nineteenth century, the British-controlled Indian Medical Service (IMS) established a set of central-to-provincial healthcare institutions that managed hospitals and clinics and maintained environmental sanitation in urban areas. The IMS was a semimilitary medical service founded in the colonial era. Even after India gained independence in 1947, the newly established Ministry of Health was still influenced by the IMS, particularly in its designation of all physicians within the system as full-time civil servants, much like military agencies. Conversely, Latin American countries do not have such policies as their health ministries were unaffected by this type of political affiliation.

As for Africa, colonists were unable to recruit an adequate number of physicians and nurses from Europe. As such, they had no choice but to recruit and train locals as medical workers to assist in clinical work. These assistants were effectively apprentices, who received training and eventually became the most common healthcare workers in the colonies. Most African countries obtained their independence after World War II, after which these trained assistants and other auxiliary healthcare workers became the cornerstone of the new healthcare systems of these countries. The local healthcare schools under the new political systems of the African countries systematically trained the medical assistants. The current concept of healthcare assistants in Africa is, therefore, derived from the political system in the nineteenth century.

In the late nineteenth and early twentieth centuries, the emergence of labor unions and political labor parties during the industrialization of Western Europe catalyzed the development of social security, including health insurance. Public healthcare continued to expand with the growing strength of the labor unions, but their greatest impact was on the private healthcare market in Europe. The private market was affected by an increasing number of government health insurance schemes, such as those passed by the German Prime Minister Otto von Bismarck. After 1900, healthcare systems began to be included in the policy agenda of political parties in various countries. The First World War gave rise to the Russian Revolution and the emergence of the first healthcare system that covered all of society, which led to a clash of the mechanism of healthcare service provision and the market system.

After World War I, the famous Dawson's report published in the UK advocated for the provision of all healthcare services by governmental healthcare networks. This further demonstrates the importance of political events on healthcare systems in a capitalist society. Furthermore, in 1922, Japan became the first country outside of Europe to pass legislation that required compulsory health insurance schemes for employees. In 1924, the labor movement in Chile led to the issuance of the first health insurance legislation among developing countries and prompted other Latin American countries to follow suit.

Similar to early political movements, more recent political movements have also had a significant impact on health systems across the world. The Great Depression in the 1930s accelerated the implementation of statutory health insurance systems worldwide. In the US, the Great Depression led to the passing of the Social Security Act of 1935, which drove the development of national and local public healthcare services and laid the foundation for the introduction of Medicare in 1965. The Second World War also gave rise to some dramatic changes in the health systems, such as the UK National Health Service and the highly innovative socialist healthcare system in China.

In Southeast Asia, British colonists handed over control of the Malay Peninsula to the Islamic Sultans after the Second World War. These Sultans were well known as traitors during the Japanese occupation, which led to armed insurrections by guerrillas in rural areas. Unlike the French in Vietnam, the British Army carried out an effective repression in 1952. Nevertheless, a political question was raised after the establishment of the new Parliament of Malaysia: "Is it not necessary to gain the support of rural populations following such a bloody conflict?" Subsequently, hundreds of healthcare centers were constructed following the establishment of the Malaysian Rural Health Services Scheme in 1953, which has greatly improved disease prevention and treatment for millions of rural residents throughout the country.

Next, we will move on to the origin of Canadian health insurance and the post–Second World War outpatient health insurance. Although it was discussed by the Conservative Party of Canada in 1919, the health insurance scheme was not implemented until 1944, when a semisocialist party called the Co-operative Commonwealth Federation (CCF) won in the Saskatchewan municipal election and introduced the first universal health insurance scheme within the province in 1947. Over the next decade, the whole of Canada was covered by this new health insurance scheme. In 1962, Saskatchewan once again led the country by becoming the first province to establish a private health insurance scheme. In 1968, the Canadian government passed the private health insurance scheme despite the protests and strikes by a large number of physicians during the early stages of its promotion. By 1971, this private health insurance covered all 10 provinces of Canada.

We now focus on the political factors influencing healthcare services in Latin American countries. The political maturity and healthcare needs of urban voters are particularly worthy of attention, as they played a significant role in the development of the first statutory health insurance scheme in Chile in 1924 as well as the Uruguayan health insurance scheme in 1958, among others. Even when the economic demands have been met, the provision of advanced healthcare services in major cities would have been unfeasible without the enormous political power of the working class. The Cuban political movement in 1959 not only revolutionized the healthcare system of Cuba but also inspired the healthcare development plans in other Latin American countries.

The development of the health systems in Western Europe was essentially driven by the competition for votes under the parliamentary democratic system. The social democratic and labor parties of these countries were growing in popularity alongside the continual improvement of social security (healthcare and social welfare). Even conservative parties were more reluctant to reduce the allocation of funds to healthcare and social welfare to avoid losing votes. The British Labor Party launched the National Healthcare Service in 1948. After the Tories took office, the only significant adjustment they made was a slight increase in the copayment ratio of prescription medicines. On the other hand, in Eastern Europe, the socialist revolution after the Second World War inevitably gave rise to socialist healthcare systems that imitated the Soviet model after the First World War.

For political reasons, leaders in almost all countries pledge to protect citizens' right to basic healthcare. However, the definition of "suitable" or "reasonable" healthcare services differs according to the country's economic level and ideologies. Political ideology determines the prioritization of resources among different areas, such as health, military, transport, agriculture, and industry. Given the same level of priority, the performance of the health system still depends on its structure and policy, i.e., its efficiency and effectiveness.

Many of the aforementioned political events that have influenced health systems have been related to wars and revolutions. If the goal of the revolution is to achieve socialism, then the revolution would undoubtedly have an effect on the healthcare system. Nevertheless, even when revolutions are started for other reasons, a protracted and large-scale war will inevitably have an impact on the healthcare systems of multiple countries as well. Massive conscription is unavoidable for both sides of a large-scale military conflict. Furthermore, human and material resources (including healthcare resources) must also be gathered rapidly through multiple means to defend the homeland. A good example is the rapid establishment of local hospitals in Britain after its bombardment in World War II. Another example is the Middle East conflict between Israel and Egypt, which caused both countries to enhance their capabilities in organizing health systems during the conflict, not to mention the first aid, blood transfusion, nursing, surgical, and rescue techniques that were developed by battlefield hospitals. It is often easier to awaken a country's potential in effectively organizing social movements during a crisis (usually during the war). War is usually a consequence of failed political negotiations, but it is capable of reinforcing political willingness to initiate other implementations.

There are many more such examples that clearly demonstrate the significant impact of political events on health systems. However, it is extremely difficult to uncover a common theme from political events that took place several centuries ago. These political events, such as the French Revolution, the US Declaration of Independence, colonialism, the emergence of industrialization and urbanization, and the rise of labor unions and social movements have all influenced the governmental structure and have played different roles in the distribution of power between the state and the people.

A clear theme can be established if these social events are presented as part of a causal chain. There are varying sources of political pressure, but in the field of healthcare, the general direction of political forces have mainly been toward greater governmental intervention in the markets, in order to ensure access to healthcare services when needed. Market intervention implies the gradual transformation of healthcare services from commercialized products into public goods. This is an idea that is worthy of further discussion, but we must first consider a third set of factors affecting healthcare systems – cultural factors.

3. Cultural Factors

In addition to economic and political factors, the health system is also influenced by numerous other social and environmental factors, which are collectively referred to as cultural factors. Here, the definition of "culture" is not limited to the narrow scope of anthropology but covers a broader scope that includes various social customs. Important cultural elements include technological advancements, religion, social structure, language, family, and so forth. There are specific cases illustrating the effects of each of these elements on the healthcare system.

There are innumerable technological advancements that affect all the components of a health system. For example, pharmaceutical drugs are the foundation of many medical therapies, and pharmaceutical development forms the foundation of pharmaceutics. Therefore, the use of pharmaceutical drugs requires professional healthcare management policies, and it has also given rise to a large number of pharmaceutical companies, promoted legislation on drug administration, and led to innovations in insurance models.

Major scientific breakthroughs might alter the characteristics of health systems by broadening the scope of resource utilization and improving the capacity for disease control. For instance, consider the relationship of the therapeutic efficacy of streptomycin and isoniazid for tuberculosis with the occupancy rate of sanatoriums worldwide – a reduction in the number of tuberculosis patients naturally makes sanatoriums available for other purposes, such as general hospitals, nursing homes, or rehabilitation facilities. Another example is the application of DDT for the control of mosquitoes and malaria. These technological advancements have not only improved healthcare services but also enhanced the roles of healthcare institutions, enabling the full allocation and utilization of the limited resources in a system.

The discovery of pathogenic microorganisms and sterilization techniques has profoundly influenced the development of hospitals. Similarly, the discovery of anesthesia facilitated the development of surgery at hospitals. Many other inventions and discoveries have had similar impacts, such as the X-ray machine, biochemical and pathological tests, ECG, physiotherapies, hemodialysis, and so on.

Bacteriology and its related fields, such as virology, parasitology, and immunology, have contributed substantially to the development of public health. Although public healthcare institutions were established much earlier than the discovery of microorganisms by Pasteur

(1860–1890), the discovery of pathogenic microorganisms nevertheless catalyzed the development of public health. Vaccination has also seen a tremendous growth following the discovery of the smallpox vaccine in 1798. Approaches to the control of tuberculosis, STDs, and other infectious diseases have improved due to a solid foundation in environmental health and an increasing awareness of individual and community sanitation. Subsequently, the development of epidemiology, which includes infectious diseases and chronic noncommunicable diseases (e.g., cancer and cardiovascular diseases), has further broadened the scope of public health.

Technological advancements beyond the field of healthcare have also shaped many characteristics of health systems. As an example, let us explore the impact of rapid and efficient communication and transportation on healthcare services. The development of communication systems has facilitated easier communication between patients and doctors and has made long-distance medical consultation possible. Emergency medical services worldwide now rely on rapid communication and transportation systems, including marine, land, and air medical services.

The transportation system has also revolutionized the accessibility of medical treatment in health systems. Naturally, it is easier for patients to seek medical attention with a more convenient transportation system. Metropolitan transportation networks in both developed and developing countries have made it easier for most patients to seek medical attention, which has rendered the once-ubiquitous home-visit services obsolete in most countries. Additionally, in many developing countries, pharmaceutical drugs and other medical supplies are purchased in bulk and stored in central warehouses, from which they are delivered in batches to healthcare institutions throughout the country. Accordingly, the regionalization of healthcare facilities would have been unattainable without an appropriate transportation system.

Information technology has infiltrated all aspect of health systems. The popularization of printing and the mass publication of literature have accelerated the dissemination of scientific knowledge. In developed countries, computers are now capable of rapidly processing massive amounts of statistical data, thereby contributing to better healthcare management and are particularly effective for healthcare evaluations.

Religions and religious organizations have played key roles in the development of health systems since the earliest periods of human history. In ancient Egypt, priests assumed the role of physicians. Hence, most traditional medical schools have incorporated religious beliefs (with a certain degree of empiricism). In later chapters, we will explore how the modern hospital system originated in medieval Christian sanctuaries. Christianity emphasizes compassion and love for the weak and sick, and the hospital is where such an ideology can be put into practice. Similar ideologies can also be found in Buddhism and Islam, where followers also care for the weak and sick by building hospitals and conducting home visits.

In modern society, religious organizations continue to actively fund hospitals, as well as establish nursing homes and rehabilitation facilities for chronic diseases. Healthcare services as a whole, however, can also be affected by religious doctrines. For example, Judaism requires the circumcision of all newborn male babies, while the Roman Curia has consistently opposed "artificial" contraception and abortion (unless in cases where the mother's life is threatened), which undoubtedly influences both Catholic physicians and patients.

On the other hand, both Islam and Hinduism emphasize the subordinate role of women, regarding the wife as the property of her husband and considering it a desecration if other men touch or even look straight at her face. Although these beliefs are changing, they continue to influence the healthcare services in India and many Islamic countries. In some rural parts of India, only female physicians or assistants can treat female patients; therefore, both male and female physicians are required in rural healthcare centers. However, it is often difficult to recruit a sufficient number of female physicians because married women are supposed to spend most of their time at home to avoid being seen or seduced by other men. Additionally, they must cover their faces with scarves in public areas. Therefore, the religious beliefs and customs of these countries would undoubtedly limit the right of women to healthcare services.

To outsiders, the sacred cow is merely a symbol of Hindu religious beliefs. Although the situation has now begun to change, this symbol has had a major influence on the nutritional status of Indians in the past. Even though cattle can consume cereal and other foods, Hindus are prohibited from consuming beef. The prohibition of pork by some religious traditions can have similar outcomes despite being driven by the opposite logic. Furthermore, Hinduism respects all living creatures, from cattle to insects. Unfortunately, mosquito eradication is still required for the control of malaria. It is said that malaria was only effectively controlled in India after Mahatma Gandhi told the public that spraying with DDT would kill only the mosquitoes, instead of humans.

Preaching is perhaps the most effective way religions can influence health systems, especially in developing countries. Priests are responsible for comforting patients in nearly all religions. Religions have called on believers for fundraising in order to construct medical and healthcare facilities. Religious organizations worldwide, such as the Catholic Church, the majority of Protestant sects, Judaism and Islam, are still passionate about funding the construction of hospitals. The Catholic Church built the most important hospitals in Latin America, even into the nineteenth century. To date, hundreds of thousands of healthcare facilities have been built by religious organizations. These organizations also provide preachers that specialize in medical and healthcare services in Asia, Africa, Europe, and North America.

Religious ideologies can also influence the health system. The official religions in many countries affect all aspects of policymaking. The separation of church and state in the US is an exception. In Canada, public finances fund church schools; a similar practice is also seen in Latin American countries. The national affairs of Iran became dominated by religion following the Islamic Revolution of 1980. Even with the separation of government from religion, religions do continue to affect political parties, such as in the case of the Christian democratic parties of European countries. In term of public policies, the impact of religions usually manifests in favor of conservatives, who tend to emphasize personal and family obligations over social responsibilities.

Community structure forms a part of the cultural environment and does have an impact on health systems, but they are often overlooked. Hospital and outpatient services in almost all countries are primarily allocated and managed based on the geographical structures of cities, towns, and rural areas. It is necessary to flexibly utilize the communication and transportation systems between communities, to ensure the high efficiency of medical services throughout the entire region. Although urban lifestyles can potentially result in certain illnesses, cities also allow for greater resource mobilization to serve a large urban population.

Urban development is undoubtedly an important outcome of the industrial revolution. Crowded houses in industrial areas contribute to the spread of infectious diseases through human-to-human transmission, as well as transmission via food and water. However, there is always a solution to these problems. For instance, people have realized the necessity of sewage systems since ancient Rome, and therefore, have constructed underground sewers. Nowadays, the finest safe water systems in the world are only found in major industrialized cities. At the same time, the endless stream of occupational accidents due to industrialization has given rise to relevant laws on the responsibilities of employers and work-injury compensation acts to provide social insurance that covers medical expenses accrued for occupational accidents.

In our modern society, almost all major cities have communities of various social classes, and low-income communities are often considered slums. In industrialized countries, such slums are usually located in the center of cities and consist of dilapidated buildings. In developing countries, slums are more often located in suburban areas and are mostly occupied by unemployed farmers, who can only reside on the edges of urban areas. Regardless of their location, slums have a substantial impact on the health system. Slums serve as a breeding ground for the transmission of infectious diseases that require special surveillance from a public health perspective. Many basic healthcare services were originally established in slums before they were made widely available. This phenomenon remains prevalent in industrialized countries, where the development of national healthcare services is often opposed due to conflicts in commercial interests. For example, it is generally easier to establish community healthcare centers in other regions with better conditions if they have first been established in slums.

Language and cultural identity can also have an influence on health systems. There are hundreds of languages in many developing countries, such as India and Indonesia, where many citizens still do not speak the official language of the country. In such cases, the most basic communication issues often hamper healthcare services – health education materials must be made available in multiple languages, not to mention the barriers in oral communication. Linguistic issues are even more complicated among the different tribes of many African countries. Such a tribal system leads to long-term hostilities that might significantly restrict regional healthcare collaboration between hospitals.

Language differences can influence the implementation of healthcare policies even in highlydeveloped countries, such as Belgium or Canada. For example, bilingual government documents in French and Flemish are compulsory in Belgium, and the official languages of Canada are English and French. Language differences can also lead to different cultural identities. Some languages might be associated with particular religions or philosophical traditions. Although Canadians generally communicate in English, all health-related laws in the country must be made available to the proud French-speaking Québécois.

Family structure is another major cultural factor affecting health systems. Family is generally the strongest source of support for patients. In fact, studies have shown that single, divorced, and widowed individuals, who may lack familial support, tend to have the highest rates of hospitalization among adults. Similarly, among adults of the same age, patients with distant family relationships may not receive sufficient care, which implies that they are more likely to require hospitalization for medical treatment. Therefore, societies that emphasize family harmony tend to have lower demands from hospitals and social security institutions.

For the same reason, a family-oriented culture has a major influence on elderly care. Families with three generations living under one roof are commonly seen in Eastern cultures, which also tend to indicate greater respect for elders. The relative scarcity of nursing homes in China and other developing countries may not be due to their low economic development but may be a result of their family-oriented culture. Conversely, the high social mobility in Europe and the US has led to unstable family structures, where elderly couples with sufficient pension normally choose to live on their own. Most elderly individuals in these countries choose to live in nursing homes when they are incapable of self-care.

A wide range of intertwined social determinants can be found in national health systems, where economic, political, and cultural factors exert mutual influence and thereby determine the characteristics of the health system. Furthermore, these factors are in constant flux due to spatiotemporal variables. The discovery of important resources, such as oil, could enable the rapid development of all components of national healthcare systems. However, in general, these changes tend to occur gradually alongside the overall development of the country.

Health systems vary widely across different countries due to the vast economic, political, and cultural differences between them. We have previously mentioned that the healthcare services provided to different groups of people within the same country also vary considerably. Nation states play a key role in international affairs and the lives of civilians. Therefore, it is necessary to analyze the health systems of various countries based on their national characteristics.

SECTION III. ANALYSIS OF THE SOCIAL DETERMINANTS OF HEALTH

The WHO defines health as "not merely the absence of disease or infirmity, but a state of complete physical, mental and social well-being and perfection." The determinants of health refer to the multitude of factors that affect population health. In 1974, LaLonde reported that the main factors affecting human health status include lifestyle, environment, biological factors, and healthcare services. Since then, it has been recognized that the effects of medical and healthcare services have a fairly limited ability to determine human health. Thus, investment in medicine and healthcare is not likely to further improve human health. There are also a number of other factors that affect human health. The Canadian Ministry of Health has set forth the following determinants of health as a starting point for guiding the future direction of population health policies and research: income and social status, social support networks, education, employment and working environment, social environment, physical environment, personal hygiene behaviors and stress management skills, healthy child development, healthcare services, gender, culture, biology, and genetics. All these factors play decisive roles in health and affect one another. These determinants include both individual-level (e.g., personal hygiene behavior, biology, and genetics) and population-level determinants (e.g., education, employment, and income). The population-level determinants can indirectly influence the individual-level determinants.

There are two conventional perspectives on the determinants of health. One represents the mainstream perspective over the past 50 years, which considers health as a personal affair that can be addressed by the advancement of medical technology. The other perspective regards health as being primarily influenced by the living environment, including genetic, environmental, social, healthcare, and personal lifestyle factors. In recent years, the international community has increasingly focused on the latter, which is collectively known as the social determinants of health.

In 2005, the WHO established the Commission on Social Determinants of Health (CSDH) to work on the social determinants that affect health and to advocate the establishment of a "world that pursues health and well-being for everyone." The CSDH completed its work in 2008 and delivered a final report entitled "Closing the Gap in a Generation." As is evident from the history of development, the United Nations, WHO, and UNICEF have always had a major focus on health equality and the social determinants of health. Three of the Millennium Development Goals (MDGs) are related to health indicators, whereas the others are concerned with the social determinants of health, such as gender, education, globalization, and economics. The MDGs provide an excellent policy opportunity for all countries because they involve the commitment of 189 member states and international collaboration.

1. Conceptual Framework of the Social Determinants of Health

(1) Concept of the Social Determinants of Health

The WHO's definition of the "social determinants of health" (SDH) is by far the most widely recognized. SDH refer to factors influencing health that result from the basic structure of social stratification and social conditions in which people live and work, in addition to the direct causes of the diseases. They are, in other words, the "cause of cause" of diseases and include all the social conditions in which people live and work, such as poverty, social exclusion, and living conditions. Tarlov referred to them as "the social environment characteristics of human living" (Figure 3.2). They reflect the different statuses of class, power, and wealth in the social structure. This concept reflects the value orientation of health equality and human rights.

(2) The Action Framework for the Social Determinants of Health

Using the "causes of causes" of health as its starting point, the WHO established a complete conceptual framework of SDH, with the aim of instilling health equality as a basic value. Improvements in health equality and health development can be achieved by acting on the following two aspects.

1. Daily Living Environment   The daily living environment includes the health risk factors of early child development, social environment, and occupational environment determined by social stratification; the variations in the physical environment, social support networks, and psychosocial and behavioral factors across different populations; and the healthcare services received, such as health promotion, disease prevention, and treatment.

2. Social Structural Factors   Social structural factors refer to the status and level of social stratification; social culture, norms, and values; international and domestic socioeconomic policies; and political systems in different countries and regions.

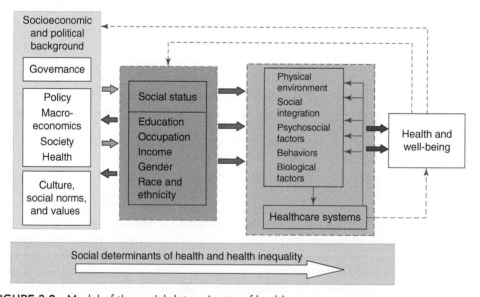

FIGURE 3.2 Model of the social determinants of health.

(3) The Action Areas for the Social Determinants of Health

A few of the SDH proposed in the WHO conceptual framework can be considered avant-garde when accounting for the present level of development in population health and healthcare policies. Therefore, based on the empirical evidence from multiple countries worldwide, the CSDH has compiled the key factors that influence the adoption of policy interventions in various countries into nine knowledge networks: (1) early child development, (2) employment conditions, (3) urban settings, (4) social exclusion, (5) women and gender equity, (6) globalization, (7) health systems, (8) priority public health conditions, and (9) measurement and evidence. In addition, other issues, such as food and nutrition, violence and crime, and climate have been considered important factors affecting health equality (called additional indicators) (Figure 3.3).

The Declaration of Helsinki was revised at the Eighth Global Conference on Health Promotion in June 2013. This conference reviewed the impact of health promotion since the Ottawa Conference; explored the establishment of effective mechanisms to facilitate cross-sectoral activities; and evaluated the economic, developmental, and social factors related to investments to achieve Health in All Policies (HiAP).

Based on the HiAP framework, the CSDH recommendations were implemented to resolve health issues and to build the capacity to integrate health in all policies. The conference reached the consensus that priority health conditions and health equality must be regarded as the core responsibilities of the government to its people and agreed that health policy coordination is imperative. The conference called for the government's commitment to integrate health into all social policies; prioritize the social determinants of health; ensure the establishment of organizational structures and procedures needed to integrate health into all policies; enhance the capacity of the Ministry of Health; and urge other government departments to achieve health outputs through policy implementation via various strategies, such as leadership, partnerships, advocacy, and mediation.

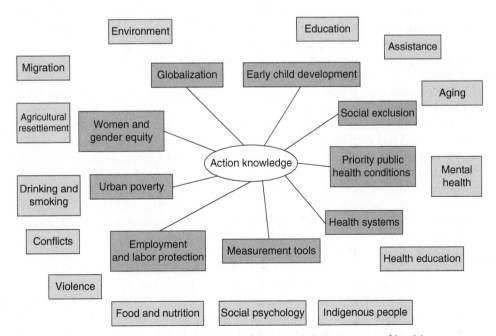

FIGURE 3.3 The nine knowledge networks of the social determinants of health.

2. Policy Values of the Social Determinants of Health

Our understanding of health has expanded considerably over the past half century. From the perspective of "capability approach" and "development as freedom" – concepts developed by the contemporary economist Amartya Sen – health is considered an important capability approach and "a very basic freedom" for humans. Based on this theoretical framework, the UNDP began to deliver Human Development Reports (HDR) in an attempt to reemphasize the initial concerns of economics in our understanding of development. Specifically, these reports proposed that human well-being is the actual objective of development, whereas economic growth is merely a developmental approach. Accordingly, one of the primary goals of human development is to live a long and healthy life, which is ranked first among the three foundations of human development, whereas economic growth (which has always been at the forefront of economics) only represents one of the developmental approaches.

Health must be regarded as an important dimension in assessing social development due to its profound intrinsic value. A healthy lifestyle is a good lifestyle and is generally considered an ultimate goal that is worth pursuing. The factors leading to the differences in health have become trending research topics, among which economic, social, cultural, and genetic factors appear to have an actual impact on health levels. Most of these studies, however, have focused on one of these factors while neglecting the interactions among them. In the 1990s, studies on the determinants of health began to consider the multifactorial interactions, which led to the generation of various theoretical models on the determinants of health, the most representative of which are as follows.

Grossman, who constructed a model of the demand for "good health," first proposed the health production function. The most important aspect of this model is that it views health as a durable capital stock that yields an output of healthy time. It is distinct from other forms of human capital in many respects. For instance, the model assumes that an individual can inherit an initial stock of health that decreases with age, but which can be improved via the investment of time and finances in healthcare services. In addition to medical expenses, this framework also incorporates nonmedical factors as the determinants of health, such as salaries, education, nutritional intake, and environmental conditions. Data has shown that there is a difference in the supply and demand curves of health capital.

Grossman's health production function provides three predictions, as follows. First, the rate of health depreciation increases with age once it passes some point in the life cycle, whereas the health capital required decreases over the life cycle. At the same time, if the elasticity of the marginal efficiency curve of health capitals is less than 1, the healthcare expenditure would increase with age. Second, consumers' demand for healthcare services is positively correlated with their wages. Finally, if education increases the output efficiency of health investments, then more educated individuals would demand a larger health stock.

One advantage of this model is that it considers the effects of demographic variables (e.g., age and education) on the cost or marginal efficiency of health capitals. However, a shortcoming of this model is its simplistic assumptions. For example, the model assumes that consumers can fully predict the temporal variations in the rate of depreciation and thus know their age of death with certainty, which is obviously impossible.

In addition, the effect of income on health has also been a topic of interest to scholars. The relationship between the two variables has been examined from different perspectives and has been intensely debated due to the presence of both consistency and disparity between them. The effect of absolute income on health is mainly manifested as the so-called "health–income stratification" phenomenon, in which health and personal income are directly proportional with one another, provided that all other variables remain constant.

At the same time, the effect of income on health diminishes as the income level increases. In other words, additional income of the same unit has a stronger impact on health in low-income groups than in higher-income groups. This is especially true with new medical advancements. Although numerous studies have confirmed the presence of health–income stratification with regard to the impact of health choices on the health–income relationship, other studies have proposed that income is endogenous when analyzing health choices in the health–income relationship. In other words, health leads to an increase in income, which in turn improves health. Hence, the structural effect of income on health is often overestimated. To this end, various approaches have been employed, such as instrumental variables estimation, to estimate the effects of income on health, in order to avoid the causal chain of overestimating the impact of income on health due to the endogeneity of the former. People are interested not only in the effect of income on health but also in the pathways of their causal relationship. Taken together, the results of previous studies reveal four main pathways: early child nutrition, accumulation of favorable or unfavorable factors in life, acquisition of healthcare resources, and behavioral factors (e.g., lifestyle differences).

Based on the preceding analysis, the value of improving the national healthcare policies is mainly manifested in the following aspects:

1. *An overall social policy framework toward health equality.* First, it is necessary to start by improving the environmental conditions of people's daily life and paying attention to their lifelong health issues. Second, measures should be taken in macroeconomic, social, and healthcare policies to mitigate social inequalities and advocate equality as a social value and norm. Relevant policy basis and data should be collected as a foundation for decision-making in government.

2. *Collaborative social, economic, and environmental developments.* Health is an important prerequisite of achieving social goals. The improvement of social inequalities and disparities can enhance health and well-being for everyone. It should be recognized that good health not only improves the quality of life, increases productivity and learning ability, and continuously improves the living environment of families and communities but also promotes social security, accelerates social integration, and reduces poverty. Presently, the interrelation between health and economic development has been included in the political agenda of nearly every country. People are increasingly looking to the government for concerted efforts to address issues related to the determinants of health, as well as to avoid duplication of effort and dispersion of resources.

3. *Basic ideas and concepts of health in all policies (HiAP).* The government could develop a strategic plan wherein the common cross-sectoral goals of all government departments are clearly defined. There is also a need for cooperation between civil organizations and the private sector. To manage issues related to health and well-being, the government must focus on the institutionalization processes that address cross-departmental issues and the balance of power, including providing leadership, delegation of authority, incentives, budget commitments, and sustainable mechanisms of supporting the collaboration between government agencies. The systematic intervention by the Ministry of Health is necessary to address health-related issues in activities organized by all levels of the government and other government departments. The Ministry of Health can also support the works of other government departments by actively promoting relevant policies and facilitating goal accomplishment. In terms of specific measures, there is a need for clear and coordinated authorization; systematic consideration of cross-departmental implications; an emphasis on the mediation of conflicts of interest; greater accountability, transparency, and sharing mechanisms for healthcare policies; active engagement of

nongovernmental stakeholders; and greater awareness of the importance of effective cross-departmental incentives in building partnerships and trust.

4. *Insights into the new responsibilities of the Ministry of Health in maintaining health.* The theory of SDH requires the Ministry of Health to understand the political agenda and management rules of other departments and to assume the responsibility for establishing a foundation of knowledge and evidence for policy decision-making and planning. The Ministry of Health must also evaluate the function of health outcomes from each program during the process of policy development. At the same time, the Ministry of Health should collaborate with other departments to establish a platform for discussion and problem solving, as well as to assess the effectiveness of cross-departmental collaboration and policy development. The Ministry of Health should also enhance its own capacities by seeking better mechanisms, resources, institutions, and skilled personnel. Finally, the Ministry of Health should work with other government departments to help them achieve their goals in conjunction with the promotion of health and well-being.

4

Basic Models and Evaluation of World Health Systems

 SECTION I. TWO-DIMENSIONAL CLASSIFICATION OF WORLD HEALTH SYSTEMS

1. Principal Models of International Health and Social Security Systems

In the comparative study of world insurance systems, domestic and foreign researchers have classified and categorized the various health insurance systems using different angles and criteria. Some have divided the health insurance systems of OECD countries into three types: National Health Service models (e.g., the UK), social health insurance models (e.g., Germany) and commercial health insurance models (e.g., the US). Other researchers have divided the health insurance systems of countries around the world into four models: national (government) health insurance models, social health insurance models, commercial health insurance models, and other health insurance models (e.g., savings-type health insurance, community-based health insurance, etc.). Some have also classified these systems according to whether the insurance liabilities fall into self-funded models, voluntary insurance, or compulsory insurance or public services. In addition, researchers have divided health insurance systems into six models based on different insurance methods: the self-funded voluntary model, the individual voluntary compensation model, the public compensation model, the individual voluntary contract model, the public contract model, and the unified public model.

By comprehensively considering the coverage of different income groups, the responsibilities assumed by the government, and the security levels and functions of various systems, Chinese researcher Wu Ri-Tu categorized the health insurance systems of different countries into five models (Table 4.1): national health service and social security systems, social health insurance systems, market-driven health insurance systems, personal savings health insurance systems, and social medical assistance systems.

TABLE 4.1 Comparison of the Primary Health Insurance Models in the World

Item	National Health Service and Social Security System	Social Health Insurance System	Market-Driven Health Insurance System	Personal Savings Health Insurance System	Social Medical Assistance System
Insured parties	Not based on income; covers all residents or specific groups	Mainly covers average-income groups; some countries also include high- and low-income groups	Mainly covers high-income groups	Mainly covers groups with any income	Low-income or no-income groups, elderly people, and people who have lost the ability to work
Government responsibility	Government-run health system	Legally mandated, socially-run health system	Government-supervised, socially-run health system	Government-encouraged, individual self-insurance	Government-run health system
Insurance functions	Includes medical and preventive healthcare; generally does not include sickness or maternity benefits	Generally includes medical treatment and maternity benefits; gradually expands to preventive healthcare	Generally includes hospital insurance and critical illness insurance	Generally includes inpatient medical costs and outpatient costs of specific diseases	Mainly insures medical costs of diseases
Insurance level	Insures basic health needs; relatively high insurance level	Insures basic medical needs; insurance level varies according to national economic level	Generally insures a relatively high level of medical needs	Insures basic medical needs	Insures medical needs
Status in the system	Generally forms the main body of the national system	Generally forms the main body of the national system	Generally complements the national system but also forms the main body in specific countries	Can serve as a basic component of the national system	Generally forms the basic system of the national system
Examples of typical systems	National health services in the UK, Canada, and Australia	Statutory health insurance in Germany, France, and Japan	Private health insurance in the US	Personal medical savings account in Singapore	Medicaid program in the US

Source: Wu Ri-Tu, *International Comparison of Health Insurance Systems*, Chemical Industry Press, 2003.

This system model classification can provide a general understanding of the characteristics of the health insurance systems in different countries. Nevertheless, in the study of institutional systems, using a system model to represent a country's health insurance system cannot fully reflect the overall picture or the specific characteristics of that country's health insurance system because the health insurance system of any country is composed of an organic combination of multiple systems. For example, based on the number of insured persons and the share of insurance funds in the healthcare market, commercial health insurance can be regarded as the primary or basic system in the US. However, this system does not reflect the overall picture of the US health insurance system, nor is it the US health insurance system's only defining characteristic, as the US also has health insurance systems for the elderly and the poor (Medicare and Medicaid) that are primarily administered by the government. Furthermore, current studies on system models have mostly focused on superficial comparisons of existing systems and are lacking in research on the deeper theoretical and historical evolution of the systems. In reality, different system models share a number of similarities.

For example, the Universal Healthcare System and National Health Service of welfare states such as Sweden and the UK share the same historical origin as the social medical assistance systems of other countries that only cover special or minority groups. Their evolutions into two different systems involve the process of quantitative to qualitative change. Similarly, one model type can also play different roles or manifest in different forms in different institutional systems. For example, the commercial health insurance system in the US is the basic system that covers the vast majority of residents. However, in other countries, this type of system is only a supplement to the basic or primary system or an alternative system for a small part of the population.

2. Selection of System Models for Countries with Different Development Levels

A two-dimensional classification was performed on the world health and social security systems based on the degree of socioeconomic development and the main type of health system (Figure 4.1). From this classification, the following five points were gleaned.

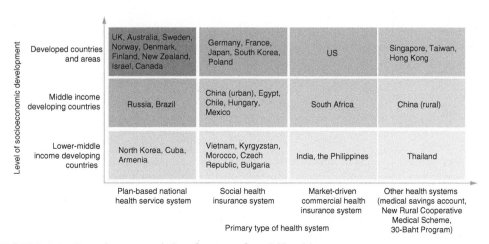

FIGURE 4.1 Two-dimensional classification of world health systems.

1. The health insurance systems of countries around the world are different. These differences indicate that a country's health insurance system is closely related to its institutional arrangements and political, economic, and cultural backgrounds. However, at the same time, countries at all levels of economic development can choose any type of health system. There is insignificant correlation or specificity between economic development and the health system type, and health insurance systems are highly localized.
2. The health insurance systems of countries around the world are not uniform. The formation of a multisystem, multilevel health insurance system is inevitable owing to the healthcare needs of different populations as well as the development and improvement of the system itself. In China, the three horizontal and three vertical tiers of the health security network are mutually complementary and constitute a multilevel security system with Chinese characteristics that strives to meet the medical needs of the majority of people.
3. The responsibility of the government is indispensable in the establishment and development of a health insurance system. However, the government plays different roles in different systems and different stages of development.

    For example, before the economic reform in China, the provision and financing of health services were both highly dependent on the government, which resulted in a heavy burden on the government. After the economic reform, the government was responsible for the bottom line and the daily administration of national healthcare (Figure 4.2).
4. Although the health insurance systems of countries around the world are complex and multilevel, one or more systems must exist as the basic or primary systems that cover the majority of the population. These basic or primary systems are mutually complementary with other systems and organically constitute a country's health insurance system. For example, the UK's National Health Service and Germany's statutory health insurance are the primary systems of their countries' health security systems and cover

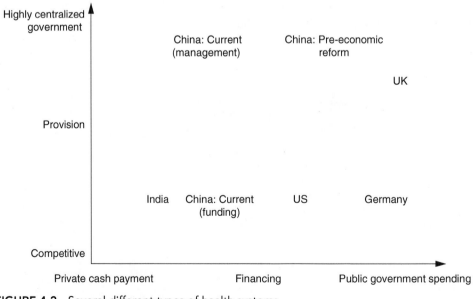

FIGURE 4.2 Several different types of health systems.

the vast majority of their countries' residents. However, the primary systems of the two countries are complemented by other health insurance systems that also play important roles. Another example is the US health security system, the main body of which is composed of Medicare, Medicaid, and the commercial health insurance system. However, there are also healthcare insurance systems for specific populations administered by the federal government, which are also crucial complements to health insurance.

5. The disparities in the health insurance systems of different countries imply that they are not comparable. Nevertheless, many aspects of the primary health insurance systems in some countries are identical or similar and, hence, can be compared with each other. For example, the public healthcare system of the commonwealth country Canada, the universal healthcare systems of Australia and Brazil, and the National Health Service of the UK share many common features that are mutually comparable. Similarly, Germany's and France's statutory health insurance, Japan's national health insurance, and Vietnam's compulsory health insurance share many similar characteristics. We refer to these identical or similar basic systems as the system models of health insurance.

SECTION II. SYSTEM MODEL OF THE NATIONAL HEALTH SERVICE

1. National Health Service and General Practitioner System

(1) National Health Service System

After World War II, the UK standardized the health system that took shape during the war. In 1946, the UK parliament passed the well-known National Health Service Act. In 1948, the UK government officially promulgated and implemented "hospital and specialist services" and "community health services based on the general practitioner system" that were funded by unified government taxation. All citizens, regardless of their individual abilities to pay, were entitled to free health services provided by the National Health Service (NHS) system. Thus, the first NHS, through which the government is responsible for raising health funds and directly providing services, was established in the Western world. From the 1970s to the 1980s, this system was successively adopted in other developed countries, including Denmark, Iceland, Italy, Portugal, Greece, Australia, and Sweden.

The purpose of the NHS is to provide all UK citizens or permanent residents, regardless of gender, age, education level, or religious beliefs, with the right to access the best level of free healthcare as permitted by the circumstances. The NHS includes general practitioner services, hospital services, community services, maternal and child healthcare services, emergency services, and dental care, optical care, and pharmacy services. The rights that patients are entitled to in the NHS (i.e., the main content of the NHS Constitution) include the following aspects:

1. Equal access to health services is based on clinical needs and not the patient's financial conditions, lifestyle, or any other characteristic.
2. Everyone can register with a general practitioner (GP) and has the right to change GPs quickly and easily.
3. Emergency patients can obtain ambulance and hospital emergency services through their GPs or directly from the hospital emergency service.

4. When a patient's registered GP deems it necessary, the GP can refer the patient to any hospital for a specialist or to a specialist hospital. Under general circumstances, patients will be referred to the nearest hospital for treatment.
5. Patients have the right to obtain clear explanations of their treatment plans, including any risks, side effects, and complications that the treatment may involve, before deciding which treatment plan to accept.
6. Patients can view their own health records and have the right, under statutory obligation, to keep their health records confidential.
7. Patients have the right to choose whether to participate in medical research experiments and the education of medical trainees.
8. Waiting times for services should be minimized. Ninety percent of patients should be referred to a specialist for diagnosis and treatment within 13 weeks, and the remaining should be referred within 26 weeks.
9. The waiting times for surgeries should generally not exceed 18 months.
10. Patients have the right to make any complaints they may have about the community health services or their GPs. If they are not satisfied with the outcome of the investigation, they have the right to appeal.

The UK has established a relatively complete management system for health administration, for which the corresponding administrative agencies have been set up. From the Department of Health to the primary healthcare teams, the health authorities all have clearly defined functions. The Department of Health is responsible for formulating the long-term development plan of the NHS, managing and allocating health resources, administering public funds, and formulating health service policies. Beneath it are eight regional health authorities that are responsible for monitoring and inspecting the program implementation of local health authorities and NHS trusts. The NHS trusts are composed of financial, medical, and nursing directors and mainly serve a supervisory role. There are 374 trusts nationwide, managing the respective service areas under their control. Clinical commissioning groups (CCGs) provide authoritative guidance based on local health needs. There are 99 CCGs nationwide, each of which is responsible for an average population size of 500,000. There are a total of 481 primary care teams, which are composed of a physician, a member of the community (e.g., a patient's relative), a nurse, a social worker, a nonexecutive staff member, and a director of the health sector. The basic framework of the UK health administration system is shown in Figure 4.3.

NHS funding mainly comes from three sources. The first is national tax revenues, which is the main avenue of NHS funding, accounting for 82% of funds. The second is various forms of insurance, accounting for 12% of funds. The third includes other income and accounts for 6% of funds. Hospitals and GPs report the funds utilized in a given year and the estimated budget for the coming year to the Department of Health, which then formulates a funding plan based on the budgets. The Treasury then allocates funds to the Department of Health, which, in turn, distributes the funds among the regional health authorities. The regional health authorities then allocate the appropriate funds to the hospitals and GPs.

Department of Health → Regional Health Authorities → {Local Health Authorities; NHS Trusts} → {Care Commissioning Groups; Primary Care Teams}

FIGURE 4.3   Basic framework of the UK health administration system.

According to the UK Department of Health, NHS spending has been gradually increasing each year. In 1949, total NHS spending was £4.37 billion; in 1969, it was £8.7 billion; in 1989, it was £17.72 billion; in 1996, it was £22 billion; and in 1997, it was £34 billion.

In 2000, NHS spending reached £55 billion, accounting for 11% of annual government expenditure. In 2010, total NHS spending was £103.8 billion, and it reached £106 billion in 2011, £108.4 billion in 2012, £111.4 billion in 2013, and £114.4 billion in 2014. The burden of healthcare costs has become the next target of future reforms by the government of the UK. According to an official from the International Division of the UK Department of Health, the scale of the NHS is increasing, which is accompanied by a greater number of problems. The cost per day is £150 million, and the annual cost per capita is £1,000–1,200. Hence, funding has become one of the major problems of the NHS.

(2) General Practitioner System

1. GPs and their services   There are 55,000 physicians in the UK, of whom 39,000 are GPs, and approximately 3 million patients receive treatments from GPs each week. All GPs are government employees. They provide a full range of primary healthcare services to registered residents from the cradle to the grave. These services include disease diagnosis, treatment, medical care, the prevention and monitoring of infectious diseases, health counseling, and patient referrals. GPs control the healthcare funds of registered residents and are the gatekeepers of residents' health and of NHS funding. They are essentially able to resolve 90% of health issues faced by registered patients. Unless they are visiting the emergency department, patients must be referred to NHS hospitals by GPs.

2. GP Mode of Operation   GPs are physicians who act as the first point of contact for patients. Each individual can choose to register with one GP. GP selection is a one-way choice in that residents are able to choose their GPs, but GPs are not able to choose the residents they serve unless they provide appropriate reasons. In general, one family unit will register with the same GP, and the GP will create health records for each individual in the family. Each GP has an average of 1,800–2,000 registered residents who can access various basic health services through that GP. A GP signs a service contract with the local health department and is paid according to the number and age structure of the residents served. The form of payment is fairly flexible. In 2010, the average per capita income of GPs was £57,300, which is equivalent to £40 per hour.

GPs can provide health and medical services independently. However, in recent years, the government has been encouraging GPs to set up joint clinics and to work as teams. This shift has arisen because even though every physician on a team is a GP, each GP may have his own specialty, and cooperating can help them to provide complementary services and resolve the problems of GP vacations and night shifts. The primary mode of contact between GPs and patients is letters or telephone, with less frequent face-to-face service. Patients have their GPs' telephone numbers and can contact them at any time. They can also arrange to see their GPs by appointment or can set up home visits by their GPs.

GPs are responsible for providing 24-hour service to their patients and are often overworked. The time taken to book appointments and the waiting times for treatments are very long, which also causes inconvenience for patients. To address this issue, the GPs under the Oldham NHS Trust in Manchester carried out an "after-hours clinic" community health service project, in which regional GPs covering over 300,000 patients formed a collaborative organization. Patients could contact their GP clinics via telephone, and the physician or nurse on duty recorded their telephone consultations by computer. The patients were then sorted according to the order of their calls and the severity of their conditions. Based on the times of their calls and their levels of medical need, the patients were referred to a GP or to a hospital for timely treatment and thus received better community health service. Patients did not have to wait in line to consult a doctor, and the number of GP visits was also reduced. Service efficiency was improved by providing about half of the patients with telephone consultations and half with home visits. Computers were used to retain and display health records, which facilitated the tracking of accountability. Furthermore, computers were also used by health authorities to conduct random checks on GP consultation rates, diagnosis accuracies, and misdiagnosis rates to control service quality.

3. GP Training   Becoming a GP in the UK requires at least nine years of medical education and on-the-job training. Individuals must first undertake five years of training in medical school followed by one year of clinical practice after graduation before they can apply to be a registered medical practitioner with the General Medical Council. After becoming registered medical practitioners, the general career paths of medical school graduates in the UK are as follows: GPs account for 48% of graduates, with hospitals, public health, medical schools, and others accounting for 25%, 13%, 3%, and 7% of graduates, respectively. Trainees require at least three more years of specialty training to become a GP. Within these three years, 18 months involve clinical practice in hospitals with rotations in at least three specialties, and the remaining 18 months involve training under an experienced, senior GP. Trainees can also choose to spend two years in hospital posts and one year in GP posts. Finally, trainees must pass the examinations run by the Royal College of General Practitioners to obtain their GP qualification and register as GPs. GPs can choose the communities they serve and must submit annual work reports for inspection and assessment. After registration, qualified GPs are also required to attend continuing medical education run by the Royal College of General Practitioners.

(3) Characteristics and Existing Problems of the UK Model

1. NHS characteristics and differences between countries   The first NHS established by the UK has the following three distinctive features. First, the NHS is implemented and safeguarded in the form of national planning. The funds for the NHS are mainly raised through national tax revenues, accounting for the vast majority of national spending on health services, whereas the proportion of cost-sharing by health insurance financing and copayments by individuals is very small. Second, the provision of medical and health services is dominated by public institutions. Public health and preventive services are provided by different levels of government, depending on the service content. Inpatient services are provided by public hospitals, which receive compensation from the government according to a planned budget. Hospital physicians are public servants who receive salaries. Outpatient services and primary healthcare are provided by GPs, who essentially act as private practitioners but are officially NHS employees who sign contracts with the government. They are compensated by the government based on the number of registered residents, which is a typical form of the capitation system. Third, all residents have free access to comprehensive healthcare services. Residents must first select and register with a GP and receive GP services, but they can switch to a new GP. In general, residents must be referred by the GP to obtain hospital services.

Countries that adopt the NHS also differ in their implementation of the service, mainly with regard to the degree of centralized management and the scope of health services included. The UK has a centralized system in which the central government provides funds and allocates budgets to regional health authorities. The regional health authorities, in turn, allocate budgets to hospitals and GPs to provide free healthcare services to the general public. In the early 1990s, the UK health administration attempted to implement reforms of internal market mechanisms, which aimed to form market buyers and sellers in the health system in order to promote service efficiency through competition mechanisms. In 1998, an assessment of the outcome of this reform showed that it was not ideal. Sweden follows a decentralized system in which county councils are responsible for financing the provision of services through local taxation. The central government only provides subsidies and consults with the local governments regarding the GDP ratio of healthcare costs. Denmark implements the NHS within the scope of local administrations and divides its residents into two groups on a voluntary basis. Residents in Group 1 receive free service and are required to register with their selected GPs for at least one year before they are permitted to change. Residents in Group 2 are free to choose any medical specialist but are required to pay part of the costs. Both groups have access to free inpatient services. Currently, only 6% of the population is in Group 2.

2. Main Problems of the UK model

1. *Inefficient health service.* As physicians receive a fixed salary that is unrelated to the quality of their work, their enthusiasm is limited, and they are unwilling to actively provide medical services. This issue has resulted in difficulties in accessing clinic visits, hospital services, and surgeries, as well as long waiting times.
2. *The impact of private healthcare on national healthcare.* Since the mid-1960s, the UK government has allowed private hospitals to be established and to undertake the healthcare tasks of some NHS hospitals. In addition, private providers also began setting up healthcare institutions such as elderly residential care homes and small nursing homes. Although the proportion of private healthcare is very small, it has a significant impact on the NHS due to the flow of NHS funds into private healthcare institutions through multiple channels, which has resulted in the rapid rise of healthcare costs. The uncontrolled flow of healthcare workers into private healthcare institutions has also eroded the technical strength of national institutions, and the weakening of public hospitals will impact overall national health to a certain extent.
3. *Insufficient national health funding.* This has resulted in relatively old and outdated hospital facilities and equipment.

2. The Social Welfare Model of Nordic Countries

Nordic countries, including Sweden, Finland, Norway, Denmark, and Iceland, have often been regarded as highly developed welfare states. These countries seem to have formed a widely accepted model of the welfare state that shares distinctive characteristics and commonalities. As most of these countries are Scandinavian countries, the Nordic welfare model is also known as the "Scandinavian model."

"Equality for all" is a fundamental social value held by Nordic countries, and, hence, their social welfare system is based on redistribution. After a standard for redistribution is set, needs above the standard are supplemented by social insurance, and additional needs below the standard are supplemented by means-tested social assistance. Therefore, the Nordic welfare model is essentially a universal public welfare subsidy scheme. This scheme includes all citizens in the welfare system and does not merely target specific groups for welfare. Furthermore, the funding of this scheme comes from the government's total tax revenues and employers' contributions, not the individual contributions of citizens. Therefore, the public welfare scheme is a third type of social welfare policy that is different from contributory social insurance schemes and non-contributory social assistance schemes targeting the poor. In theory, the welfare system of Nordic countries was established based on the principle of redistribution. However, within the public welfare subsidy scheme, the eligibility of welfare recipients does not fully comply with the principles of individual benefits and a minimum standard of a redistribution system. In this scheme, the state imposes high income taxes on individuals and employers and provides the same level of welfare funds or services to all citizens regardless of their living conditions, family property, or personal tax status. Thus, this redistribution system can have a considerable impact. With such extensive coverage, the number of individuals and families falling outside of the safety net is naturally much smaller. However, Nordic countries often call these welfare schemes "social insurance" instead of "social assistance" or "public funding." As this form of social redistribution that is based on equality is very similar to social insurance in terms of its payment methods, it is often mistakenly referred to as "social insurance." Thus, we need to make a conceptual distinction: public funding refers to universal aid given without means-testing, whereas social assistance refers to means-tested aid. Given this distinction, in Northern Europe, programs that fall under social assistance include the subsistence and housing allowances in Finland; the social assistance and housing allowance in Sweden; the financial assistance, transitional benefits, and housing allowance from the State Housing Bank in Norway; and the basic and housing benefits in Denmark. It should be noted that not all social assistance schemes target the poor, but all require means-testing of property or income, and most of them are given to low-income groups. In Nordic countries, the conditions for receiving welfare payments and services are more relaxed and are usually based on the principle of "universality" (without means-testing). Hence, the level of welfare provided is also relatively high. In other words, due to widespread and universal public funding, there is also a corresponding decrease in the need for social assistance.

In addition to public funding and social assistance, Nordic countries also have a small number of social insurance schemes in the traditional sense that are based on contributions. On top of an average annuity paid to the elderly and disabled (public welfare funding), there is also an insurance that is linked to the individual's original salary income that can only be received after paying contributions. Hence, this program is social insurance in its true sense.

Why do Nordic countries adopt such a large-scale model of redistribution? The earliest Nordic welfare systems originated from The Poor Relief Act. However, due to the Nordic value of "sharing hardships and prosperity," these countries have always had a cultural tradition of equitable distribution. Hence, social cohesion, social security, and equality are the basic principles of these countries' welfare provision. According to these principles, all citizens, regardless of their living conditions and social statuses, are entitled to a basic income and living security. Furthermore, since industrialization, the Nordic countries have historically been governed by social democrats. Social democracy advocates the key role of the state in the welfare model and believes that the actions of the government can be used to solve the inequitable distribution of wealth in society.

Nordic countries implement a two-tier management system in the administration of the welfare system. Universal benefits are paid by the state, and social assistance is provided by local governments. The payment of universal benefits on a national scale can reduce duplication and regional differences, whereas the provision of special social services by local governments can bring these services closer to the users and reflect the true needs of the citizens in a timely manner. Local governments hold substantial policy-making power at the level of local welfare. Welfare costs are shared between the central and local governments, with the central government bearing less than 50% and the local governments bearing more than 50% of the expenditures. The specific situations vary across different countries and years. Due to disparities in the financial resources of local governments, there are regional differences when formulating the standards for social assistance. However, the differences are not significant, due to the subsidies provided by the central government. Integration at the national level enables Nordic countries to attain a certain level of efficiency, whereas the individual service at the local level can satisfy "reasonable" requirements.

Based on the preceding introduction and analysis, we can summarize the typical features of the overall Nordic welfare model. To realize the social value of equality for all, Nordic countries provide the same level of welfare to all citizens, including vulnerable groups, and employ large-scale universal public welfare funding, which is supplemented by social insurance and social assistance, as their primary welfare systems. Doing so enables the governments of these countries to play a major role in this welfare model. The government guarantees the various basic needs of its citizens, and the state shoulders more responsibility for welfare provision, whereas the responsibilities of families, markets, and communities are more diminished.

In addition, based on these facts, we can see that there are ambiguous intersections among social insurance, social assistance, and public funding. A welfare policy introduced by the state may not necessarily belong to any one of these three schemes and could very well be part of an ambiguous area between the three schemes. Therefore, when analyzing the Nordic welfare model and its welfare policies, we should not stop at understanding its literal meaning but should explore its essence in greater depth.

3. Main Policies and Features of Developing Countries

(1) Main Policies of National Health Security Systems

1. Security coverage   The majority of developing countries that have adopted a national health security system are striving to provide free health services to all citizens. For example, Brazil has established a Unified Health System to provide free national healthcare, and the national health system in Cuba provides healthcare services to all citizens.

Among these countries, India is one of the representatives of this model and is characterized by providing free medical coverage for the largest population. The government is directly responsible for public healthcare institutions and formulates the public health and basic medical services that each level of public healthcare institution should provide. The government ensures that the most basic level of equipment and appropriate technologies are available for laboratory tests, examinations, and treatment. It also formulates a list of essential medicines that can be provided to patients free of charge. The Indian government fairly allocates its limited investment to areas where health services are most needed, and it not only supports the stable operation of government hospitals but also encourages the healthy development of private hospitals. The coexistence of public and private hospitals ensures that both rich and poor patients are provided for. The primary beneficiaries of the government's health subsidies and social security are poor and vulnerable groups, which is the fundamental reason for the relative equality of its healthcare system.

The core notion of India's health security system lies with the use of economic and administrative leverage to develop a series of effective public policies. Western researchers generally believe that developing countries cannot afford the cost of establishing a social security system due to poverty. However, the Indian government attaches great importance to the innovation of the public health system and has taken a new path in innovating its health insurance system that is applicable to developing countries. For example, the three types of health insurance schemes introduced by the informal economic sector in India have overcome the obstacles of insuring people with low or uncertain income who could not be accepted by conventional insurance schemes. This type of institutional innovation has opened up a new way of thinking.

2. Funding Sources and Payment Methods In the vast majority of countries that implement a national health security system, the government is the direct organizer of the system, and the security funds mainly come from the state's financial budget. Individuals bear no or only a small amount of healthcare expenses. Using the government budget as the basic financing channel guarantees the source of funding to a large extent. Furthermore, by administering healthcare institutions within the national health security system or purchasing private health services, the government can directly provide healthcare services to all citizens or specific groups without involving third-party payment.

Cuba implements a public health system, and its health financing relies solely on national taxation. Private providers are prohibited from supplying healthcare, and healthcare workers are government employees. All citizens have the right to access free preventive care, treatment, and rehabilitation services. Cuba's healthcare work falls entirely under the unified responsibility of the state. All treatment, prevention, healthcare, and rehabilitation activities and the salaries of healthcare workers are borne by the state treasury, which provides a strong material safeguard for the system's healthy development. The government is responsible for the establishment of health infrastructure; the construction of hospitals, clinics, medical schools, and medical research centers; the procurement of drugs and instruments; and the salaries of healthcare workers, teachers, and researchers.

Among South American countries, Brazil is the only one that has adopted a health financing system based on general taxation, which includes corporate tax, sales tax, consumption tax, social insurance tax, and so on. This system is similar to those of the UK and Sweden. The financing of Brazil's health insurance has progressed from occupation tax-based financing to a national tax mechanism based on general taxation. The health insurance funds are raised through centralized collection and decentralized distribution. That is, the central Ministry of Social Welfare raises funds through banks and the treasury. After a review and comprehensive balancing by the Ministry, the funds are then allocated to states according to the actual medical needs of each state and region based on the number of patient visits. Then, the states allocate the funds based on the budget after obtaining the approval of the governor. Brazil's health security system is composed of two parts. The first includes basic medical services, which are funded by the government through tax revenues. The other includes nonbasic medical services, which are funded by individuals through private health insurance agencies. Brazil's Unified Health System benefits 70% of the population, giving them free access to primary healthcare services. Aside from the costs of surgery, all other medical expenses are almost completely free. Hospitals even pay for meals during the hospitalization of patients and for parents accompanying a sick child.

(2) Common Characteristics across National Health Security System Models

The models of national health security systems in developing countries (Figure 4.4) share the following characteristics. First, the national health security system model follows a welfare-type system. Welfare is provided for free to all citizens in welfare states and is provided for free to specific populations in other countries. Second, in the vast majority of countries that implement a national health security system, the government is the direct organizer of the system, and the security funds mainly come from the state's financial budget. Individuals bear no or only a small amount of healthcare expenses. Third, by administering healthcare institutions within the national health security system or purchasing private health services, the government can directly provide healthcare services to all citizens or specific groups without involving third-party payments. Fourth, the covered services generally involve a health service package that includes prevention, healthcare, medical treatment, nursing rehabilitation, and various healthcare subsidies, which provide a relatively high level of security. Fifth, the allocation of health resources is highly planned, without the regulatory effect of market mechanisms.

The main advantage of the national health security model is that it addresses the negative effects of providing healthcare services and financing through a fully competitive healthcare market while also eliminating the root cause of market failure. First, the national health security model can overcome the market failure caused by information asymmetry, as healthcare providers are unable to use the advantage of professional knowledge to incentivize consumers. The medical advice provided to patients and the quantity and type of health services provided by healthcare providers are not affected by the prices set by the government. Healthcare institutions are compensated based on the government's budget review. Second, the government can set prices closer to marginal costs. Demand can be used to measure the marginal willingness to pay for healthcare services, which, in turn, can be used to measure marginal utility. Thus, based on the theory of marginal cost, the price can be set equal to the marginal utility, which also equals the marginal cost. Furthermore, in the national health security model, low-income earners pay lower taxes than high-income earners do and, hence, receive the same health services with lower expenses. This model benefits socially vulnerable groups and harms more affluent or healthier members of society.

Many developing countries, including Cuba, India, Brazil, and Malaysia, have adopted the national health security model. The Unified Health System, on which the poor are highly dependent, is the highlight of Brazil's national health security model. The Unified Health System is based on general taxation and has a unique financing system. The public service system mainly revolves around primary healthcare. The poor, who make up 30% of the

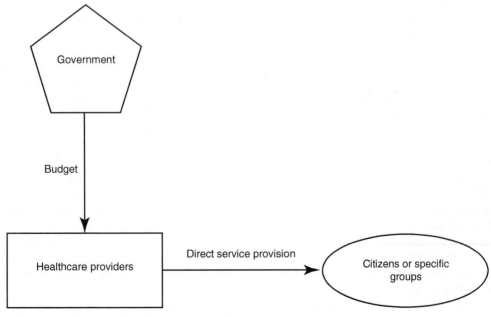

FIGURE 4.4 National health security model.

country, rely solely on the Unified Health System and do not purchase any health insurance. The implementation of the Unified Health System has drastically reduced Brazil's infant mortality rate and has controlled the spread of various infectious diseases and epidemics, thereby improving the health levels of Brazilians.

The main disadvantages of the national health security model are as follows. (1) Lack of incentive mechanisms. When health services are free, people are inclined to overuse health services, which increases society's overall healthcare costs. People also display risk-taking tendencies in their daily health behaviors because they know that they do not have to pay the price of the health consequences caused by their irresponsible behaviors. Thus, people use fewer preventive health services. (2) Lack of profit motive. Healthcare institutions or providers lack the motivation to continuously provide high-quality service in this model. (3) Increased public burden. When health services are free, the overall healthcare costs of society increase, which damages the welfare of the whole society. Hence, the costs of supporting this health system are high, which may easily lead to a shortage of resources while also affecting the short-term accessibility of medical treatment (i.e., creating overly long waiting times to access the health system).

SECTION III. SYSTEM MODEL OF SOCIAL HEALTH INSURANCE

1. National Health Insurance Systems of Germany and France

Social health insurance is another important model in the insurance system. Represented by Continental European countries, such as Germany and France, the emphasis of this system is on social insurance and the provision of services by private institutions or physicians. This system adopts the social health insurance system model, which combines market-driven and planned healthcare. The financing of national healthcare services mainly depends on social insurance. The system of health service provision is focused on private healthcare institutions and physicians, and the supply of health services is regulated by market demand. These countries have introduced mandatory health insurance schemes that finance the majority of their healthcare costs and provide basic health services to all residents. On top of this mandatory health insurance, individuals are also permitted to voluntarily purchase supplementary private health insurance to obtain better health services. The difference is that each country has its own funding policies for mandatory health insurance. The government of these countries only subsidizes the treatment costs of the military, the elderly, low-income earners, farmers, the disabled, and patients with chronic diseases, psychiatric disorders, and tuberculosis. The government grants different subsidies based on the economic conditions of the various health insurance organizations in order to achieve equality.

Germany was the first country to establish a health insurance system. It enacted the Health Insurance Bill, the Accident Insurance Bill, and the Old Age and Disability Insurance Bill in 1883, 1884, and 1889, respectively. Germany's health insurance system is centered on hospitals and insurance physicians. This type of social health insurance system that has been adopted in countries such as Germany and France is mainly financed by employees and employers in the form of payroll taxes. The major features of this system include the social pooling of funds, the market regulation of services, the purchasing of services from private institutions through public financing, and the regulation of service provision by market demand.

The advantage of this approach is that public financing can guarantee social equality, whereas service provision by private healthcare institutions according to market regulation can improve efficiency. Compared with the NHS, the management system of social health insurance is more focused on market regulation. Hence, the problems encountered include the neglect of preventive healthcare, the lack of healthcare quality management, and the rapid rise of healthcare costs. Therefore, countries implementing this type of health system have begun to focus on strengthening the regulation of insurance plans and rectifying the negative effects of market regulatory mechanisms. For example, France introduced a series of healthcare reform measures that would strengthen the supervision and management of healthcare expenditures, stabilize insurance expenditures, strengthen the price regulation mechanism, control the procurement of hospital infrastructure and equipment, and compress the range of services.

The German health industry is administered in a two-tier (federal and state) decentralized management system. The federal ministries in charge of healthcare work include the Federal Ministry of Family Affairs, Senior Citizens, Women, and Youth and the Federal Ministry of Health. These ministries are responsible for youth social work, family policy, women's policy, career guidance and training, public health, health coordination, drugs and anesthetics, welfare for the elderly and disabled, and related legislative affairs. In addition, there are three other ministries involved in health work: (1) the Federal Ministry of Labor and Social Affairs, which is responsible for healthcare, hospitals, rehabilitation and medical care, labor protection and other matters under social health insurance, and related legislative affairs; (2) the Federal Ministry of Education, Science Research, and Technology, which is responsible for health research and technology and related legislative affairs; and (3) the Federal Ministry of the Interior, which is responsible for environmental protection and related legislative affairs. In addition to implementing federal health laws, the state health ministries are also responsible for school health, oral hygiene, hospital management, the prevention and treatment of infectious diseases, emergency medical management, and other work. The state ministries enjoy independent legislative powers with respect to health. The states are subdivided into districts, which have their own health offices. In addition to implementing the health laws formulated by the Federal Ministry of Health and the state health ministries, the district health offices are also responsible for some primary healthcare work, such as health education, health guidance, vaccinations, and outbreak reports. The federal and state health ministries, the health administration executive teams, and the Federal Joint Committee coordinate the healthcare work of various health departments.

The German healthcare system consists of a combination of the public and private sectors that together form three pillars of healthcare: (1) public health institutions, (2) hospitals, and (3) private practice physicians. Public health institutions implement health protection, the prevention and management of infectious diseases, and some coordination work. Almost all outpatient care is undertaken by private practice physicians, and hospitals are responsible for inpatient care. There are three types of hospitals in Germany: public hospitals that are funded by the government, public organizations, and social insurance agencies, which account for 36.4% of hospitals; nonprofit private hospitals that are funded by donations to religious and charitable organizations or other foundations, which account for 34.2% of hospitals; and for-profit private hospitals that are run by private for-profit health service institutions, which account for 27.4% of hospitals.

The French health insurance system has also had a long history. It was established slightly later than that of Germany and has undergone major reforms since the mid-1970s. The history of health insurance in France began with the establishment of a social insurance program in 1928–1930. As with the development of old-age insurance, the historical development of health insurance varied according to occupation type and social status. The first step was the Social Insurance Law in 1930, which mainly benefited those who worked as employees, whereas the self-employed and farmers only received access to health insurance many years after World War II. In 1960, the French health insurance system included agricultural workers under its coverage. Thereafter, in 1966, France expanded the coverage of its four systems to accommodate self-employed professionals. In 1971, civil servants, agricultural workers, and railway workers were given medical compensation under the general system. Around the same time, in 1967, France implemented the reform of health insurance operators and management organizations. The universal coverage of health insurance for all residents was based on the Social Security Generalization Law in 1974. In December 1974, the Law for the Adjustment of Insurance Funds was enacted to implement the adjustment of funds between systems.

This model of health insurance has been developing steadily for more than a century, with different recipients and different degrees and levels of insurance at different stages of development. For example, Germany implemented mandatory insurance for blue-collar workers and has only recently permitted these workers to enroll in nonmandatory supplementary insurance. Under the 1973 energy crisis and the rapid deterioration of health insurance funds, France adopted certain legislative measures to control funding strategies and curb healthcare expenditures. In summary, the social health insurance model is better able to reflect the compatibility of the level of security and national economic development; the sharing of healthcare costs among the state, organizations, and individuals; and the combination of equality and efficiency. Thus, it reflects the mandatory, universal, protective, and welfare-oriented nature of social insurance. Based on the policy orientations of Continental European countries, social health insurance will become mainstream in world health insurance systems.

2. Health System and Insurance in Japan

Japan's Ministry of Health, Labor, and Welfare is the national-level health administration department. There are 47 health-related departments and bureaus in the country with different names, such as the Health Service Bureau, the Environmental Health Bureau, and the Environmental Sanitation Department. The administrative divisions below the prefecture level include cities, towns, and villages, which are local autonomous organizations. In terms of health administration, large cities with populations greater than 1 million generally have health and public cleaning bureaus; medium-sized cities with populations of 100,000 to 1 million have health bureaus (or departments); cities with populations smaller than 100,000 or towns (prefectures) have health divisions that are sometimes combined with national health insurance affairs and are known as the healthcare division; and villages often have health sections (units) or resident sections (units). Cities, towns, and villages have health centers where residents can engage in various health promotion activities.

The Japanese health system is mainly composed of the service system (healthcare institutions and healthcare workers) and the management system (the medical and healthcare management system). Since 1960, Japan has gradually established several high-level medical centers for special diseases, including the National Cerebral and Cardiovascular Center and the National Cancer Center. Many prefectures have also established prefectural cancer prevention and treatment centers and adult disease centers. A few large cities have also established children's medical centers and maternal and child health centers. Furthermore, dedicated healthcare facilities for individuals over the age of 65 have also been set up. There are 104 teaching hospitals in medical schools, of which 44 are state-owned, 11 are public, 49 are private, and 6 are affiliated with university research institutes. Teaching hospitals are generally equipped with a large number of advanced medical instruments and have an average of 486 beds per hospital. The main purpose of teaching hospitals is to train medical undergraduates and graduate students. The state has also designated 179 teaching hospitals for postgraduate medical residency training.

In 1961, Japan implemented the National Health Insurance (NHI) system, and all residents of Japan are required by law to have health insurance. Residents who enroll in the insurance program are free to choose any healthcare institution for treatment, and individuals are only required to pay a small portion of the total costs of treatment. After the formation of the NHI, Japan adjusted the system according to its economic conditions and medical needs. In the 1970s, free healthcare was provided to the elderly, tuberculosis patients, and patients with mental disorders. Since the 1980s, the acceleration of population aging, the continuous improvement of medical science and technology, and the diversification of people's demand for health services have led to an increase of healthcare expenditures. In particular, healthcare costs for the elderly accounted for an increasing proportion of the total costs, which led to health insurance facing increasingly prominent financial problems. Therefore, on the basis of the original NHI system, Japan has undertaken a series of adjustments to health insurance and the healthcare and welfare system for the elderly in order to ensure that citizens have equal access to and free choice in the health services they receive. In addition, Japan has also strengthened the containment of healthcare costs by exerting control over supply and demand through measures such as increasing the proportion of costs paid by individuals.

At the turn of the twenty-first century, under pressure due to the aging population, Japan began focusing on developing community-based care for the elderly as an important measure to ease the financial burden on the health insurance system. To further clarify the copayment ratio of healthcare costs, a piece-rate system was replaced by a quota system to implement managed health insurance. In terms of health insurance for the elderly, long-term care insurance, which aimed to transfer the long-term care of elderly patients from the hospital to the community (i.e., at home or in elderly welfare homes or elderly healthcare facilities), was introduced. Japan's long-term care insurance is a system in which the central government uniformly formulates policies to standardize service items and benchmarks, whereas its operation involves the joint participation of individuals, families, communities, and local and central governments. The service recipients of long-term care insurance are elderly patients who are bedridden or have dementia. This system is a major departure from the traditional family-care model for the elderly and has helped to realize the socialization of family care. In addition, the services are provided by the local governments of cities, towns, and villages and by civil society organizations. This aspect of the system not only helps the country to play a guiding role in care services but also promotes the enthusiasm of local governments and civil society organizations to provide better care services for the elderly. However, it should also be noted that the long-term-care insurance system is a product of declining birthrates and population aging and the inadequate provision of social security. As a result, it still has many deficiencies. Of these issues, the most controversial are whether the transition from the original social welfare approach to the social insurance approach for the elderly is a historical regression and whether the provision of high-quality, affordable, and accessible care for the elderly can be sustained. More investigation is needed to explore these issues, and further observations should be made over a longer period of time.

The most recent revision to Japan's Health Insurance Law was the Outline of Health System Reforms promulgated by the government in June 2006. This outline mainly involved amendments to the Health Insurance Law toward three goals: the rationalization of healthcare expenditures, the establishment of a new health system for the elderly, and the reorganization and integration of insurers.

3. Health System and Insurance in South Korea

South Korea's healthcare funds are not effectively allocated. Its mandatory National Health Insurance (NHI) program raises 70% of national healthcare costs. Although healthcare costs are shared between the government and patients, patients' out-of-pocket rates are relatively high (only 15.7% of inpatient costs and 36.9% of outpatient costs are paid by the government). This insurance program also forms the foundation of South Korea's national health system. The majority of national health spending (55.1% in 1996) is borne by families rather than by the state. The data indicates that in 2000, the proportion of healthcare costs paid by individuals was 55.1% and that paid by the government was 44.9%. In 2007, healthcare expenditure increased to 6.3% of total GDP (the average ratio in Asia was 3.6%), of which private health spending accounted for 45.1% of total spending and government spending accounted for 54.9% of total spending. In 2011, South Korea's total healthcare expenditure was 7.4% of GDP and government spending accounted for 55.3% of this total.

South Korea's public healthcare program covers a very limited range of benefits. Patients still have to pay the full cost of uninsured services, such as hospital meals, ultrasounds, and magnetic resonance imaging. Professor Ok-Ryun Moon from the Department of Health Policy and Management at Seoul National University proposed that high out-of-pocket rates for patients are a necessary measure to limit the overuse of health services. Before the implementation of the NHI in 1989, 87% of healthcare costs were borne by individuals, as opposed to only 46% in 1998. Based on this evidence, Professor Moon believes that the South Korean NHI is effective and can transfer the burden of payment from individuals to the public sector, which makes healthcare more affordable to individuals in poor financial situations.

For a long period of time, the state of healthcare in South Korea has been somewhat chaotic, and the national healthcare burden was too high, which led to the prevalence of rebates and resulted in more social problems. Prior to the implementation of reforms, South Korea's drug administration model was very similar to China's. Physicians had both drug prescription and drug sales rights. Hospitals and clinics had their own pharmacies and could sell drugs. Furthermore, consumers could purchase drugs directly from pharmacies without a prescription. Under this system, the drug sales practices of hospitals and pharmacies were extremely similar. In particular, when there was an almost 50% markup in drug prices, both physicians and drug retailers included unnecessary drugs in their prescriptions for their own economic purposes. These circumstances meant that South Korea's drug expenditures accounted for 30% of total healthcare costs, which was far higher than those of European and American countries. In order to reverse the above phenomenon and to reduce the burdens on patients and health insurers, South Korea was determined to reform its health system, and policies for the separation of drug dispensing and prescribing were an important part of this reform. However, due to strong opposition and concession by the governments, a series of reversals occurred after the separation of drug prescribing and dispensing was implemented, and the reform ultimately ended in failure.

South Korea's immense healthcare system is currently facing a crisis, and the Asian economic crisis has further exacerbated the situation. Despite the high out-of-pocket rates paid by patients, since its inception the NHI program has faced the problem of demand far exceeding service supply. As healthcare costs continue to rise, health-service providers and patients will both become increasingly disappointed in the NHI program. Service providers will not be adequately compensated for their services, but patients will complain about the high costs they pay for healthcare.

4. Main Policies and Features of Developing Countries

(1) Main Policies of Social Health Insurance Systems

1. Security Coverage   The social health insurance systems of most developing countries are mandated by law and do not provide individuals or insurers with the freedom of choice. This aspect is one of the key differences between these systems and market-driven health insurance systems. The main purpose of implementing mandatory coverage is to prevent the risk of adverse selection. The mandate guarantees that individuals with different income levels and health statuses can participate in the insurance scheme under the same conditions and also ensures sufficient health insurance funding to handle the level of risk and provide reciprocal aid. When determining the coverage of the insured population under the social health insurance systems of developing countries, the following issues should be taken into account: First, should the entire income-earning population, including, for instance, self-employed or high-income earners, be enrolled in the insurance program? Should retirees with income who are insured be obliged to contribute or exempted from contributions? Second, how should the base contribution be determined? Should it be determined according to actual income? Third, can the immediate relatives of employed persons have joint insurance, or should they also be obliged to pay contributions? Fourth, should the poor population with no income or low income be exempted from paying contributions, or should the government pay on their behalf? Alternatively, should the government set up a special social medical assistance system to address their health security issues? Fifth, should civil servants and other special occupations (e.g., the military) participate in a unified social health insurance system, or should they have a separate security system? Different countries have taken different approaches to address these issues. For example, Mexico has a diverse range of social health insurance schemes, a few of which cover workers in the formal economy who have relatively stable funding sources and provide a higher quality of service. There are several different types of coverage in Mexico's social health insurance system. The Social Security Institute, the Institute of Social Services for Civil Servants, the state oil company health insurance plan, and the public health insurance system all provide targeted coverage for different groups. Furthermore, the public health system is dominated by the Secretariat of Health and is financed by the federal Secretariat of Finance. It mainly provides health services to the poor who live in remote rural areas and areas around the city and who did not have access to social health insurance in the past. The private health insurance system provides services to individuals who are financially viable but who did not participate in the social health insurance system. This system's health services providers are more diversified and can provide higher-quality health services to the rich. In the Czech Republic, the population coverage of the health insurance system is extensive. Anyone who is a permanent resident of the Czech Republic is eligible for health insurance, and those who are not permanent residents but who are employed by a company registered in the Czech Republic are also covered by the health insurance system. All health insurance funds are obliged to accept the participation of any eligible person. Those who do not meet the statutory conditions for insurance may purchase contractual health insurance. Depending on the terms of the voluntary insurance and the range of health services covered, the customer can choose to have short-term or long-term health insurance.

2. Funding Sources   Social health insurance raises funds by collecting health insurance premiums from individuals with income. This financing model has the following primary characteristics. The first is that contributions are mandatory, meaning that anyone with a certain level of income must pay contributions. The second is reciprocity – that is, individuals with higher income levels must pay higher contributions. This characteristic implies that high-income groups support low-income groups (however, most countries have an upper limit for the contributions), the healthy support the sick, the employed share the obligations of retirees, and the single and childless share the obligations of individuals with families. Third, employees and employers share the obligation to pay contributions. Thus, although this system emphasizes the responsibility of self-care, it also reflects employers' responsibility for their employees. Fourth, the implementation of social health insurance funds follows the basic principles of determining revenue based on expenditure and achieving the balance of payments. All countries follow these principles in financing social health insurance, but they differ in the specific methods adopted. For example, in Mexico, the source of funding is contributions from beneficiaries or beneficiary households. The health insurance premiums of private- and public-sector employees are directly deducted from their gross salaries. The financial contributions of groups who had not been insured previously are also progressive, and the insurance premium payable by each household is directly proportional to its income. Social insurance is compulsory in the Philippines. Anyone who is employed is included in the social insurance system. Both the insured and their families then have access to basic health security. Most of those who are unemployed also participate voluntarily in this scheme. The employee program stipulates that it is mandatory for all government and private sector employees, including domestic workers and migrant workers, to enroll in the National Health Insurance Program. The National Health Insurance Act stipulates that 2.5% of the monthly wages of salaried workers should be used for health insurance, with the employer paying 1.25% and the individual paying 1.25%.

3. Payment Method of Healthcare Expenditures　The most prominent feature in the payment of healthcare institutions by social health insurance is third-party payments. That is, after an insured patient has received services from a healthcare institution and has paid the required proportion of the healthcare costs, all other expenses incurred are settled between the social health insurance agencies and the healthcare institution. Some countries have also adopted a reimbursement system. That is, individuals cover their healthcare costs upfront and then obtain a reimbursement from the health insurance agency. This approach has been gradually abandoned by social health systems due to the lack of cost control over the healthcare institutions and the inconvenience to patients accessing medical services.

The cost settlement of healthcare institutions by social health insurance is generally achieved through contracts or agreements. Numerous methods of settlement are available, including fees-for-service, capitation, diagnosis-related group (DRG)-based payments, and a global budget. In general, the settlement method used in social health insurance follows the principle of maximizing cost effectiveness. That is, given the premise of meeting patients' health service needs, on the one hand, healthcare institutions should be compensated reasonably and their enthusiasm for service provision should be encouraged, but, on the other hand, the cost of health services should also be minimized. Different countries have implemented different settlement methods for healthcare expenses. However, most countries do not adopt a single, fixed settlement model but rather a combination of various methods.

4. Management and Administration　In the majority of developing countries that are implementing a social health insurance system, all of the administrative agencies are public administrative agencies established according to law. These agencies are different from commercial health insurance agencies, mainly in that the former are not-for-profit. There are three types of administrative agencies that purely serve social health insurance. The first type is government-run public utility agencies, whose operating expenses and staff salaries are funded by the government. The second type is privately run statutory agencies, which are administrative organizations set up under management committees elected by the insured population. The administrative expenses of these agencies are obtained from the health insurance funds according to a proportion stipulated by the state. The third type is industry- and enterprise-run unions and associations. When the number of employees of an industry or enterprise reaches a certain level, the law permits the establishment of a health insurance agency within the industry (enterprise) that is responsible for administering the social health insurance of employees and their families within the enterprise. The administrative expenses can be deducted from the insurance funds, and the enterprises can also invest a certain amount of funds.

The following characteristics are shared among the social health insurance agencies of developing countries. First, the administrative agencies are not permitted to discriminate among insured persons covered by the law due to their age, health status, and number of family members supported. Second, the administrative agencies are responsible for taking appropriate measures to collect the prescribed health insurance premiums in full and do not have the right to exempt individuals who are obliged to pay contributions. Third, the scope and level of health insurance benefits stipulated by the law must be guaranteed. The administrative agencies do not have the right to reduce the scope and level of treatment. However, within the scope of the health insurance funds defined by the law, administrative agencies may take some measures to improve the benefits received by the insured. Fourth, it is the responsibility of the administrative agencies to ensure the balance of payments in the health insurance funds while also controlling the increase in healthcare costs. Fifth, the administrative agencies determine the payment methods and standards for healthcare costs in the form of contracts with healthcare institutions. Finally, the agencies are subjected to administrative and legal supervision to ensure that the interests of the insured are realized.

(2) Common Characteristics across Social Health Insurance System Models

The social health insurance system model is a health security system in which a country applies risk-sharing mechanisms and the principle of reciprocity in the form of social insurance in order to spread the risk of various diseases occurring at random in a minority of citizens across all members of society. In this model, employers and employees pay premiums at a fixed percentage, and statutory health insurance agencies act as third-party payment organizations that pay healthcare expenses on behalf of the insured to the institutions or individuals providing healthcare (Figure 4.5). The social health insurance model is mandatory, reciprocal, and compensatory. Such systems are generally financed based on the "pay-as-you-go" principle, and payment is made according to the principles of "determining revenue based on expenditure and achieving the balance of payments."

The social health insurance system model has the following characteristics:

First, social health insurance follows the general principles of social insurance, namely, it is mandatory, reciprocal, and compensatory. Mandatory refers to the fact that social health insurance is a national statutory insurance program in which all individuals who should be insured are required to enroll. Reciprocity refers to the mutual assistance provided by the health insurance funds within the scope of the insured population. Compensatory means that the social health insurance funds can only pay for part of the medical expenses incurred by the insured person and not the full cost. Second, the social health insurance funds generally come from special premium income. Funds are raised based on the pay-as-you-go principle, and payment is made according to the principles of determining

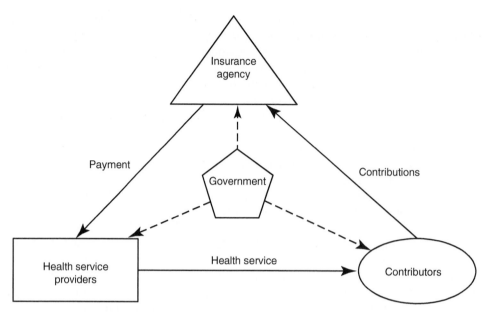

FIGURE 4.5 The social health insurance system model.

revenue based on expenditure and achieving the balance of payments. Third, social health insurance emphasizes the correspondence between rights and obligations. It requires both employers (including administrative agencies) and employees to pay health insurance premiums, whereas the state generally does not bear the costs or only provides some subsidies. Fourth, social health insurance is associated with employment and income. At first, the insured population is typically just the workers of certain industries, and it gradually expands to cover all members of society. Fifth, statutory health insurance agencies under socialized management act as third-party payment organizations, which undertake the unified management of health insurance funds on behalf of the insured and pay the medical expenses incurred to healthcare institutions that have provided health services to the insured. Finally, the level of treatment received under social health insurance is determined by ability of the health insurance funds to pay and generally ensures that the insured population can receive good healthcare services.

In summary, this system uses social cofinancing and establishes risk-sharing mechanisms to improve the equality and accessibility of the national health service. In addition, the health services provided are usually not completely free, and insured individuals still need to pay part of their healthcare costs. This feature constrains the demand for health services by increasing the cost awareness of individuals. However, this system also faces some existing issues. First, in the absence of strong constraints on the behaviors of health service providers and demanders, the financing and compensation method of social health insurance in which income is determined by expenditures will cause an upward spiral of rising income and expenditures in health insurance funds. Second, the social health insurance system uses a pay-as-you-go financial model, which generally lacks any accumulation of funds. Hence, with the acceleration of population aging, such systems are unable to resolve the intergenerational transfer of healthcare costs.

Compared with other health insurance systems, the social health insurance system has a longer history of development and is used as the basic or primary system within the health security systems of the greatest number of countries. Germany became the first country in the world to establish a social health insurance system in 1883, and this system gradually began to spread until most European countries had adopted the model as the main body of their health security systems. In addition, before and after World War II, this system spread to many countries in Asia, Africa, and America. At the end of the twentieth century, after the collapse of the Warsaw Pact, the Eastern European countries involved in the Warsaw Pact also began efforts to develop and establish health security systems, with the social health insurance system as its main body. Currently, developing countries implementing the social health insurance system include Egypt, Hungary, Iraq, Mexico, Paraguay, Peru, the Philippines, Vietnam, Thailand, Indonesia, Bangladesh, Kazakhstan, Russia, Bosnia, Romania, the Czech Republic, Cameroon, Ghana, and Kenya.

SECTION IV. SYSTEM MODELS OF COMMERCIAL HEALTH INSURANCE

1. Basic Characteristics of the Commercial Health Insurance Model in the US

Unlike the universal health system, the US health system does not have a stable source of income. As of 2010, 49.9 million people (16.3%) in the US were without health insurance, but healthcare costs were extremely high, the proportion of personal expenses was increasing and the burden on families was severe. Most of the expenses were spent on advanced and specialist medical services, whereas the state of preventive, primary and other comprehensive healthcare services continued to deteriorate, while the level of national health was not high. There was also a shortage of primary healthcare workers. Specifically, there was a shortage of 14,000 healthcare workers in 2008, and it has been estimated that this shortage will reach 50,000 in 2015. In 2009, total healthcare spending in the US was US$2.5 trillion, and per capita spending was US$8,047, which accounted for 16.8% of GDP. In 2011, the healthcare spending per capita of the US was US$8,467, and total healthcare costs accounted for 17.7% of GDP. China's current healthcare spending per capita is US$175, accounting for 4.96% of GDP. Hence, the healthcare spending of the US is approximately 46 times that of China.

Freedom of choice is a basic principle in American economic life, and consumers attach great importance to the availability of options. Hence, a wide variety of health insurance is available to satisfy the healthcare needs of different groups. However, some parts of the population are not covered by insurance. Based on population coverage, we can classify the US health insurance system into private insurance companies, Medicare, Medicaid, military and Indian insurance, and uninsured populations.

(1) Private Insurance Companies

The majority of people in the US are insured by private insurance companies, and this group includes 195.9 million people, or 64% of the population. Private insurance companies are relatively large in size and are often for-profit, but they can also be nonprofit, such as, for example, the Blue Cross and Blue Shield companies. Blue Cross is a well-known company of considerable size and accounts for 30% of US health insurance. Blue Cross and Blue Shield have branch offices throughout the US, and the two companies have shown indications of merging. Some states have already combined these two insurance agencies. For example, the national Blue Cross Blue Shield headquarters is located in Chicago and specializes in the health insurance business. For-profit insurance is provided by commercial insurance companies. Private insurance companies can take the form of fee-for-service, health maintenance organizations (HMOs), preferred provider organizations, and so on. The payment methods used are also diverse. For example, the insured may pay US$250 or 20% upfront at the time of treatment, with the remaining cost covered by the insurance company, or the insurance company can also set an upper limit and individuals who wish to spend less can opt for HMO insurance.

(2) Medicare

Medicare is government-run health insurance system for Americans aged 65 and older. By the end of 2008, 45.2 million people were covered by the program, accounting for 15.5% of the total US population. This program mainly provides healthcare services for acute diseases and predominantly includes short-term inpatient services, healthcare provision by skilled nursing units, and family health services. The Medicare system has two forms of payment.

(1) The first day of a hospital stay is paid for by the patient, and the subsequent days are paid for by the government, up to a maximum of 60 days. At this point, the government stops its payments for hospital stays, and the additional costs are borne by the patient. (2) For outpatient services, the government covers 80% of the cost for physician services, and patients pay 20% of the cost. The separation of hospitals and physicians by the US government is determined by their respective characteristics. The elderly population believes that relying solely on payments from the national healthcare system for health insurance is insufficient, as more than two-thirds of those covered by the national healthcare system have also enrolled in self-funded insurance. Funding for this program (Medicare trust funds) comes mainly from payroll taxes, total government tax revenues, and monthly premiums paid by beneficiaries. It is precisely because of federal health insurance that universal health insurance has truly been achieved for Americans over 65 years of age.

(3) Medicaid

Medicaid is a health insurance program that mainly targets the poor. In the US, citizens and legal residents with income up to 133% of the poverty line, including adults without dependent children, would qualify for coverage in any state that participated in the Medicaid program. The government provides health insurance assistance for this group of people. The federal and local governments each pay 50% of the costs. The local government first pays the full amount of the costs incurred and reports the costs to the federal government for compensation. In 2004, the population covered by this program was 43 million, which increased to 49 million in 2008.

(4) Military and Indian Health Insurance

The US Department of Defense provides health insurance service to active duty military personnel, veterans, and their families. The Department of Veterans Affairs provides health insurance service to military veterans. The US Department of Health and Human Services has a dedicated division responsible for providing health insurance services to Native American tribes and Alaska Native peoples. These groups include a total of 15 million people, accounting for 6% of the total population, and their health insurance is provided by the government.

(5) Health Security for Government Employees

The US government is responsible for providing healthcare services to government employees. The federal government has dedicated departments for collecting the healthcare expenses of all government employees in a specific area. These departments act as insurance companies and provide insurance to their employees. Government employees only need to pay one quarter of their premiums, and the remainder of the costs is settled with the hospitals by the government.

(6) Uninsured Population

In 2010, 49 million people were without health insurance, accounting for 16.3% of the total population. The US is a major economic power that is wealthier than all other countries, but a substantial proportion of its population does not have health insurance. The US government sees this issue as an embarrassment. In the US, the very poor (those living below the poverty line) and the population over 65 years of age are all basically covered by health insurance. The uninsured are often above the poverty line and under 65 years old. Within the uninsured population, 80% are employed uninsured people, some of whom are part-time workers (working less than 40 hours a week). For example, familiar fast-food restaurants generally employ part-time workers. However, since the government does not stipulate that employees working less than 40 hours a week must be insured, these employers have no obligation to purchase insurance for these workers. Another group of uninsured people are employees of small businesses with fewer than 15 employees. As these employers cannot afford to pay insurance premiums, they are more inclined to pay their employees more money so that they can purchase their own insurance. However, employees often do not purchase insurance after obtaining this money. In fact, more than half (54%) of the employed uninsured population are employees of small businesses.

2. Features and Existing Problems of the US Model

(1) Features of the US Health Services and Health Security

Before the healthcare reforms of the Obama administration, the US was the only country with a developed market economy that did not implement universal health insurance or a national health service system, where the demand and supply of health services were mainly determined by market regulation. The supply of healthcare is predominated by private hospitals, including private for-profit and nonprofit hospitals, and physicians mostly serve in private institutions. The majority of hospitals and outpatient physicians adopt a fee-for-service payment system. Despite abundant health resources and advanced medical technology, the cost of health services in the US is still high. In 2011, health spending per capita in the US was US$8,467, and total health spending was 17.7% of GDP. Due to the unbalanced geographical distribution of health resources, there is significant disparity in the levels of health services received by different populations.

The health insurance system is the primary method of financing health insurance funds in the US. A wide variety of health insurance covers most of the population in the US and plays a significant role in the health of the American people. Healthcare financing is mainly achieved through the voluntary purchase of private health insurance, which accounts for about 60% of the total amount. The government only establishes healthcare institutions and directly provides services for military personnel and veterans. It also provides health coverage for the elderly and the poor. The government enacted Medicare and Medicaid in the Social Security Amendments of 1965, which are funded by government taxation and social security payroll taxes to purchase services. Of the total healthcare costs in the US, 29% are paid by the federal budget, which mainly funds Medicare and Medicaid. The federal government also covers the healthcare costs of active duty military personnel, veterans, and their families through the Department of Defense and the Department of Veterans Affairs. State and local governments pay 13% of the total costs, of which 5% are spent on healthcare for the poor and 8% are spent on other state and local healthcare programs. Approximately 14% of the total population comprises low-income groups without health insurance.

The stratification of the US health security system is clear and mainly manifests in the following ways:

1. *The stratification of health programs.* In particular, Medicaid beneficiaries are almost completely excluded from mainstream health services and have no obligation to pay contributions. Hence, Medicaid's status is lower compared to that of Medicare, which is related to deep-seated cultural perceptions. As American society has inherited European traditions in its understanding of poverty and the poor, mainstream society does not pay much attention to this program.
2. *The stratification of healthcare institutions.* American researcher Diana Dutton believes that the US has a two-tier health system with private and public provision tiers. This situation implies that there are substantial differences in waiting times, accessibility of physicians, and quality of health services across tiers.
3. *The stratification among regions.* This discrepancy is first reflected in the uneven distribution of physicians between urban and rural areas. Some researchers have even found that among the 12 OECD countries, the US has the greatest lack of physicians in rural areas and the lowest quality of health services in poor areas. The lack of healthcare workers is not limited to rural areas. There are also very few private practitioners in poor and nonwhite areas.

(2) Main Problems of the US Model

1. High Healthcare Costs, Incomplete Insurance Coverage   The US health system primarily consists of voluntary health insurance. There are approximately 1,800 health insurance organizations nationwide, mainly taking the form of private and private group insurance companies. These private insurance organizations are essentially for-profit commercial organizations. The free competition in the health market and the for-profit services of healthcare companies have caused a rapid increase in healthcare costs in the US. In 2009, total health spending in the US reached US$ 2.5 trillion.

Due to the for-profit nature of private health insurance companies, expenditures on healthcare are far lower than the premiums paid by insured persons, and the remaining value is taken as profits for the insurance companies. To this end, private insurance companies often exclude individuals with low incomes or poor physical health. Nonprofit insurance organizations need to pay the salaries of managers and healthcare workers, purchase medical equipment, and so on, which incurs considerable expenses. Hence, their premiums are not low, and the insured receive limited compensation when they become ill. This situation has resulted in the inequality and incomplete coverage of the US health system.

The US is the only developed country that does not provide health insurance to all its citizens. Approximately 49 million (in 2010) US citizens do not have health coverage, including the unemployed, part-time workers, and individuals in between jobs. Furthermore, patients who are critically or terminally ill often lose their health insurance. At present, health and medical expenditures account for one quarter of total public welfare spending. Not only has this level of spending caused the budget deficit to reach unmanageable levels, but also, since part of private insurance is paid by employers, the burden on enterprises has increased, leading to rising costs. Thus, more low-income individuals and companies have begun to opt out of insurance, causing an increasing number of Americans to be excluded from health insurance coverage.

2. Serious Problems In Health Inequality Due to the high cost of healthcare in the US, including inpatient and outpatient services, seeking medical treatment can be prohibitively expensive without insurance, which creates an issue of inequality in US health services. The most obvious indication of this issue is the presence of 49 million uninsured people in the US. The healthcare reform plans of the Obama administration had two main goals: first, to expand health insurance coverage, and, second, to lower costs and improve efficiency. However, the process of reform has been full of obstacles, and making progress has been difficult.

3. Declining Health-Service Quality The increase in healthcare costs has caused the government and insurance companies to adopt a series of policies and measures to curb the surge in costs, which has also led to quality issues in health services. The declining level of health services has led to failures in providing basic healthcare services, which has endangered the basic rights of the insured and created public dissatisfaction. In concrete terms, this issue has manifested as the failure to perform necessary medical tests, the inability to provide good treatment, the shortening of hospital stays, significantly lower enthusiasm of physicians in their work, and so on.

3. Private Health Insurance in Developing Countries

India's commercial health insurance plans emerged in the 1980s and began developing at a rapid pace early in the twenty-first century. These plans accounted for 3% of the total healthcare costs in 2008–2009. The products provided by insurance companies are primarily intended for inpatient medical services provided by private healthcare institutions. The commercial health insurance market can be roughly divided into two broad categories: the group-buying market for employers and the retail market for individual and family plans. In 2010, commercial health insurance plans covered approximately 60 million people, accounting for 5% of India's total population. The health system of the Philippines is similar to that of the US, as the share of private insurance is relatively large. Government spending on health security has always been low in the Philippines. One of the paths to ensure the development of health security and the reduction of healthcare costs is to expand the regulatory role of the private sector in healthcare, such as in financing and setting up hospitals, thus enabling consumers to be charged for the use of public facilities. Charging a fee for the use of public facilities is the latest trend in the development of healthcare in the Philippines. With regard to health security, the trending reform in the international health insurance system is broadening health insurance coverage in order to include employees in the informal sector and the poor within the health security system, thereby improving the provision and quality of healthcare services. Under this general trend, the Philippines has also been promoting healthcare reforms and development.

In 2004, Armenia permitted the introduction and development of Voluntary Health Insurance (VHI). However, the public had limited awareness and understanding of this insurance program and was also skeptical about the quality and safety of the healthcare services under the terms of this insurance due to the traditional system. On top of these issues, the program had high commercial insurance premiums. Hence, the development of the VHI was largely limited.

In 1998, South Africa passed a new Medical Schemes Act that allowed the establishment of private health insurance schemes. Private health insurance schemes in South Africa take the form of mutual health insurance that is government-regulated, market-operated, and involves the purchase of professional management services. Individuals can participate voluntarily. Individuals and employers can share the insurance premiums, and the government allows part of these premiums to be deducted before tax. The schemes generally provide insured persons with medical services in private hospitals, which have better health quality and services. As of the second quarter of 2008, there were approximately 112 private health insurance schemes in South Africa, providing approximately 392 types of insurance plans. Currently, about one sixth of the population in South Africa has enrolled in private health insurance schemes.

Russia's voluntary health insurance was officially approved in 1991, and relevant regulatory laws were further introduced in 1992. These services can be provided to individuals or groups (e.g., corporate employees), and the insured population can receive additional services beyond the basic benefits package. Only private insurance companies (nominally joint-stock companies) can provide this service. These companies are for-profit, but there is no limit on nonprofit organizations entering this field. According to the Compulsory Health Insurance Act of 1993, voluntary insurance can be provided by private insurance agencies in the compulsory health insurance system. The "Concept of Development of Public Health and Medical Science in the Russian Federation" (Russian Government, 1997) proposed that voluntary insurance should be developed to encourage greater participation in this type of insurance. However, no further action was taken thereafter. Voluntary insurance plays a very limited role in the financing of healthcare in the Russian Federation. In 1999, it was estimated that voluntary insurance only accounted for about 3.5% of total healthcare financing. In general, only the rich and a small number of employers purchase this insurance for themselves or their employees (in addition to the compulsory premiums, foreign companies in particular are willing to provide private insurance for their overseas employees).

Brazil's private health insurance covers 25–30% of its citizens. According to the Association for Private Health Insurance Companies, 45–50 million people purchased various forms of private health insurance. Most of them were employees in the industrial and service sectors whose insurance was collectively managed by companies in that sector. Some households or individuals contract directly with insurance companies for private health services or receive double insurance coverage. Insurance companies determine the prices of services according to the insured amount and contracts with the private hospitals. The factors considered include the following. (1) The more individuals contracted with a hospital by an insurance company, the cheaper the unit prices are. (2) The prices for insured persons vary by age and gender; the contract prices of the elderly and women are higher. (3) Different prices are charged for different treatment measures, methods, and services. For example, the costs of individual surgeries and disease types must be negotiated with the insurance company.

In Chile, the commercial insurance and social insurance operate separately and independently. Social insurance is a type of compulsory insurance, but it is not mandatory for everyone, as only employees and retirees are required to be insured (employees contribute 7% of their salaries). The service targets of commercial insurance are high-income groups. Due to the lack of government supervision, the Chilean commercial insurance market has shown signs of "cream skimming," such that commercial insurers only cover low-risk individuals. Statistics have shown that in Chile, only 6.9% of individuals above 65 years of age are covered by commercial insurance. In contrast, about 26.7% of individuals aged 25–54 years are covered by commercial health insurance.

 ## SECTION V. SYSTEM MODELS OF SAVINGS-TYPE HEALTH INSURANCE

Singapore has a unique health insurance system with distinctive features, from its system design to its system implementation. In the mid-1980s, Singapore began implementing the unique Medisave health system reforms. Although this reform successfully contained healthcare costs, most of the more developed Asian countries and areas still had concerns about adopting this approach.

One of the first measures to be taken by the Singaporean government in 1959 was to introduce the new payment system of cost sharing among outpatients. Patients paid SG 0.50 (US$0.30) per outpatient visit at public hospitals and paid double the price per visit on public holidays (i.e., SG$1 (US$0.60)). Although the actual costs shared by individuals were negligible, this principle of cost-sharing made it necessary for people to directly invest cash in their healthcare and is therefore a key feature of Singapore's measures to contain healthcare costs.

The 1980s were an important period for Singapore's healthcare reforms. In 1982, the government began a comprehensive reform of the health system. The top priority of this reform was the introduction of a new financing methods based on compulsory savings. The National Health Plan was fully rolled out in 1983.

1. Establishment of 3M System Policies

Singapore has three different medical savings programs: Medisave, MediShield, and Medifund. Medisave is the predominant savings program that is compulsory for all employees, to which employers and employees each contribute half. MediShield is a voluntary, basic, low-cost insurance scheme for major illnesses. Medifund is a government-funded safety net intended to address the healthcare costs of the population not covered by Medisave or MediShield (e.g., the needy population). In 2000, Singapore began implementing a long-term care insurance scheme to solve the problem of population aging.

During the reforms of the 1980s, in addition to proposing the basic goals of healthcare for the next 20 years, the government also announced a major reform of the existing tax-financed health system and adopted a financing method based on medical savings accounts. This new scheme was known as "Medisave." Medisave stipulates that, depending on workers' ages, 6–8% of their income is set aside in a savings account to meet expenses beyond their healthcare budget. Medisave is capped at 10% of an employee's income and is tax-exempt. In the event that a saver dies with surplus funds in his Medisave account, the account can be used by his relatives.

Medisave initially only included hospitalization costs in public hospitals and the full costs of lower ward types (the wards of Singapore's public hospitals are divided into three classes: Class A is a single room, Class B is a four-bed room, and Class C is a six- to eight-bed room). In 1986, this scheme was expanded to include medical expenses in private hospitals. After two years, Medisave was further extended to include the expenses of all ward types. In 1995, a total of SG$12.7 million (US$7.62 billion) had been accumulated in 2.4 million

Medisave accounts, with an average of SG$5,400 (US$3,240) per account. In the same year, SG$311,000 (US$186.6 million) had been withdrawn from these accounts. These statistics indicate that the ratio of precipitation funds was relatively high, which is also the reason that Medisave has led to much controversy among experts and scholars has rarely been introduced in other countries and areas.

To supplement Medisave, the Singaporean government began implementing the basic, low-cost MediShield scheme for major illnesses in 1990. Based on the premiums paid by the insured, MediShield compensates SG$20,000–70,000 (US$12,000–42,000) to patients who are seriously ill or have a long course of disease. Premiums can be paid annually from a Medisave account. Since MediShield is a type of insurance policy, insured persons can opt to automatically transfer money from their Medisave accounts to pay for their Medifund premiums without having to pay additional premiums. By the end of 1995, the noncompulsory MediShield had 1.5 million policyholders, accounting for 87% of all eligible individuals. In 1995, a total of SG$25.6 million (US$7.9 million) was claimed for 43,919 insurance claims. Cancer and chronic kidney failure were the major disease claims. The MediShield policy is actually a correction of the defects in the Medisave policy in order to effectively utilize the excessive precipitation of funds in Medisave accounts.

Medifund is a government-funded safety net intended to address the healthcare costs of the population not insured by Medisave or MediShield (e.g., the needy population). Since this program was launched in 1993, 99% of individuals seeking help from Medifund received the financial assistance they needed. As of 1996, the total spending of Medifund was SG$30.7 million (US$18.42 million). In 1998, Medifund paid SG$14.6 million (US$8.76 million).

In addition, ElderShield is a special type of health insurance that was formulated and introduced by Singapore's Ministry of Health in 2002, and, as the name suggests, this scheme was intended for the elderly population. This program is a severe disability insurance scheme for the elderly members of the Central Provident Fund that provides financial insurance for those who require long-term care. In order to ensure that ElderShield could adapt to the changing needs of the population, this scheme underwent reforms by the Ministry of Health in 2007. The monthly payout amount and length were increased, and insured persons were able to purchase ElderShield Supplements.

2. Basic Evaluation of the Singaporean Model

Data from the World Bank indicate that the achievements of Medisave and MediShield over 15 years of implementation imply that they are effective means of savings in Singapore. About 90% of the funds invested in Medisave are unused. The net worth of the Medisave system has risen to 350% of total national health spending. The World Bank Chief Economist for the East Asia and Pacific region, Nicholas Prescott, summed up the achievements of the Medisave system as follows. If all current budgeted and household income is lost, an individual is still able to rely solely on funds from Medisave to pay for the same level of healthcare for three years. This is a phenomenal achievement that can cushion the impact from a sharp drop in income to a considerable degree.

The share of government investment in national healthcare spending has decreased gradually, from 51% in 1965 to 43% in 1984 and even further to 20% in 1995 after the implementation of Medisave. At the same time, the share of personal expenses in the total national healthcare cost has also increased.

Prescott believes that the healthcare approach in Asian economies should be divided into three levels. First, their health insurance systems should be allowed to partially or selectively resolve serious medical risks that individuals cannot afford, such as the financing of cancer treatments. Second, there should be an option of using personal medical savings accounts to supplement medium-level expenses (e.g., average hospitalization costs). Third, individuals should be required to pay for smaller expenses (e.g., outpatient care).

Due to concerns over the impact of tax cuts on Asian countries and areas, the World Bank is in favor of accumulating savings in medical savings accounts, such as Singapore's Medisave, which can be used to meet future needs.

Individuals with different opinions have claimed that when there are difficulties in raising the funding level of health insurance, the excessive precipitation of funds in Medisave is not conducive to maximizing the effects of scarce resources. This issue will reduce the level of health service, even affecting the level of health, and the reduction in government investment is also not ideal. Most researchers believe that since Singapore is a wealthy country, as long as the healthcare needs of its citizens are met, having a larger sum of special healthcare funds in the private sector is not necessarily a bad thing, especially since "saving up for rainy day" is a tradition in Eastern cultures. Therefore, the international community believes that Singapore's Medisave system has more pros than cons.

SECTION VI. OTHER HEALTH INSURANCE SYSTEM MODELS

1. Situations in Hong Kong, Macau, and Taiwan

(1) Health System in Hong Kong

In the early 1990s, the government funded hospital subsidies to cope with overburdened government hospitals, a mismatch between public hospital standards and social development, environmental distress, long waiting times, and poor staff attitudes. However, there was low morale, a severe loss of healthcare workers, strikes initiated by labor unions, and other conflicts. During this time, Hong Kong implemented the separation of ownership and management rights for its public hospitals. Thus, the ownership rights of public hospitals belonged to the government, and the management rights belonged to the Hospital Authority and its affiliated hospitals. The reform initiatives after the establishment of the Hospital Authority were as follows: in 1991, the Health Authority took over the management of 38 public hospitals and 50,000 employees and unified 16 different management systems, and in 2003, it took over the management of 59 general outpatient clinics under the Department of Health. In addition, the Health Authority built new hospitals to cope with the increase in urban residents; implemented a hospital network system to create regional synergistic effects; utilized the hospital referral system to expand the coverage of special services; unified the procurement of drugs and equipment to save resources; established a unified medical database and computer system platform; modified the hospital management structure and clarified the authority and responsibility involved; promoted large-scale, multilevel management training programs; organized relevant departmental experts in each hospital and established specialist commissions to plan service development and quality improvement; established a new patient-centered culture, including training employees' attitude and setting up a complaint mechanism; developed community-based medical teams to enhance community care; and enhanced staff enthusiasm through professional development and job satisfaction.

Furthermore, in accordance with Hong Kong's Hospitals, Nursing Homes, and Maternity Homes Registration Ordinance, registration and routine inspections were conducted for private hospitals. The registration and routine inspections that had previously been conducted by the Department of Health were more lenient. In recent years, there has been growing public demand for strengthening the management of private hospitals. In 2003, the Department of Health issued the Code of Practice for Hospitals, Nursing Homes and Maternity Homes, which sets a minimum standard of practice, including policies, organization, management, procedures, patient rights, risk management, and standards for certain clinical services. During registration and annual reviews, hospitals are assessed by a chief physician, a senior nurse, and a senior hospital administrator. In addition, the Department of Health encourages private hospitals to join in the British Trent Accreditation Scheme to improve management services. Furthermore, public and private hospitals in Hong Kong have also carried out a series of collaborations in staff training and patient referrals.

In Hong Kong, 82% of primary healthcare is provided by private hospitals or private physicians, whereas the Health Authority is responsible for 18% of primary healthcare. Both types of healthcare providers have referral systems. Patients must first have a referral from a general practitioner before they can access specialist outpatient services in public hospitals. The layouts of primary healthcare and inpatient services in both systems are that outpatient clinics do not have beds or inpatient services, whereas hospitals do not have general outpatient services and only have inpatient services and specialist clinics. In 2008, there were 12 private hospitals, 45 nursing homes, 74 clinics, 41 public hospitals and health-care institutions, 48 specialist outpatient clinics, and 74 general outpatient clinics, which were divided into seven hospital clusters. As of March 2010, the Health Authority had 57,713 employees, 68.5% of whom directly served patients; nurses accounted for 34.4% and medical staff (including medical staff, full-time medical staff, and medical support staff) accounted for 34.1%. In 2009, the actual expenditure of the Health Authority reached HK$36.6 billion. As the Health Authority has faced financial deficits since 2001, Hong Kong has carried reforms in such areas as repositioning public healthcare, adjusting public health charges to a limited extent, reducing operating costs, encouraging public-private record sharing, and so on.

Hong Kong has good health status and its various health indicators are on par with those of Western developed countries. In 2013, the life expectancy of men in Hong Kong was 81.8 years, that of women was 86.7 years, the infant mortality rate was 1.7 per 1,000 live births, and the maternal mortality rate was zero.

(2) Health System in Macau

In Macau, the governmental authority in the domain of healthcare is the Macau Health Bureau. Its functions include the direct organization and provision of public healthcare and disease prevention services to residents, the regulation of private health services, the administration of drug and food hygiene, and so on. The Macau public hospital (Hospital Conde S. Januario) is an integral part of the Health Bureau. Its ownership and management rights belong to the government, and its hospital staff are civil servants. Although there is no compulsory social health insurance in Macau, residents have access to free medical care in primary health centers. About 70% of patients in public hospitals (people aged under 15 years and over 65 years, civil servants, teachers, students, pregnant women, all patients with infectious diseases, poor individuals, cancer patients, etc.) can receive free treatment. As of 2010, Macau has a total of 2,022 physicians (including Western-style doctors, TCM doctors, and dentists) and 1,536 nurses. Hospital Conde S. Januario has a total of 549 beds. Macau's healthcare spending in 2009 was MOP$2.732 billion, and that in 2010 was MOP$2.974 billion.

At the end of 2001, Macau established a Healthcare Reform Advisory Committee to conduct a comprehensive evaluation and review of the existing healthcare system and to perform systematic and effective reforms of the health system. The study concluded that although the Macau health system designed in 1992 may appear effective on the surface, it still requires reforms of community care, accessible and comprehensive care, public health, the long-term viability of the system, the satisfaction of healthcare consumers, quality, communications, operational efficiency, financial performance and responsibility, and other areas. Based on the recommendations of the report, Macau established the Center for Disease Control and Prevention and implemented the far-reaching "Healthy City" project. The Macau Center for Disease Control and Prevention consists of the departments of disease surveillance, chronic diseases and health promotion, environment and food hygiene, occupational health, health planning, and tuberculosis prevention and treatment centers. The Center for Disease Control and Prevention also has community healthcare teams in seven grassroots community centers. In addition to disease prevention and control, these teams also perform the function of health supervision. For its next steps, the Center for Disease Control and Prevention will focus on capacity-building, including capabilities with respect to information, management, network building, communicable disease surveillance, community development, supported decision-making, emergency response, and on-site management.

Since 2005, the Macau Health Bureau has planned to expand the Hospital Conde S. Januario and health centers, increase the number of staff and advanced equipment, and strengthen services. The bureau plans to increase the recruitment and strengthen the training of medical staff as well as to encourage the exchange and cooperation of medical technology and scientific research. It also plans to retain a certain number of external experts and physicians. In addition, the Macau government also supports the continued training of Western-style private practice physicians and fully utilizes the strength of private healthcare institutions through cooperation between nonprofit and private institutions. Doing so can enhance the quality of medical services and the capabilities of healthcare workers, thus ensuring the balanced development of the health system in this region, which is composed of the government, non-profit, and private healthcare institutions, and safeguarding the safety and health of all residents in Macau. Since 2007, agenda has gradually started to include the drafting and amendment of the Medical Malpractice Act and related regulations, a prevention and control system for tobacco use, and professional requirements for physicians, TCM practitioners, and dentists.

(3) Situation in Taiwan

In 2011, the GDP per capita of Taiwan was US$37,403, and total health spending per capita was US$2,479. Total health spending accounted for 6.6% of GDP. As of the end of June 2008, the total number of people enrolled in the National Health Insurance (NHI) was 22,891,972, and the number of insurers was 644,589. Nearly all residents in Taiwan are insured. In 2006, the personal share of healthcare costs in Taiwan accounted for 3.74% of total household expenses on average. In 1998, total health spending in Taiwan grew by 9.4%, whereas the economy only grew by 7% in that year. In 1995, Taiwan launched the NHI, which had NT$50 billion (US$15 billion) of ample funding. By 1999, the NHI led to a deficit of NT$2 billion (US$700 million).

There are a few drawbacks to Taiwan's NHI. The insurance package offers too much coverage, including even minor illnesses like coughs and colds. 66% of health insurance costs in Taiwan are spent on outpatient services, which are usually for minor ailments that residents can resolve by spending a small sum of money. The low share of costs borne by patients is an issue that has only recently started to improve. Before 1998, patients only paid

8–9% of the costs of outpatient visits and only 7–8% of the costs of inpatient care. There is also a high rate of hospitalization in Taiwan, as 120 out of every 1,000 people are hospitalized per year, whereas only 77 out of every 1,000 people are hospitalized per year in South Korea. However, in 1998, Taiwan's low share of personal costs was increased to 16%, and residents were required pay an extra NT$10 (US$0.30) for prescriptions.

In recent years, the surge in healthcare costs in Taiwan has been controlled effectively because the Ministry of Health has implemented a point-based system to contain costs. The specific method involves dividing health services into individual units and assigning them a certain number of points based on an expert assessment. The value of the points is not known in advance. At the end of the year, the amount of NHI funding is divided by the total points across all health services provided in Taiwan to obtain the value of each point, and then healthcare institutions are compensated accordingly. The more services the healthcare institutions provide, the lower the value of a point. As a result, the total healthcare cost has been contained, but the hospital's enthusiasm for service provision has decreased and efficiency has declined, which has led to the dissatisfaction of Taiwan's residents.

As mentioned previously, Singapore's experience has shown that health savings accounts can curb the rise in healthcare costs and transfer the burden of expenses to individuals. South Korea and Taiwan both have comprehensive health insurance programs and are trying to address the issue of rising healthcare costs. Hence, they can benefit from the experiences of a health savings account system. Nevertheless, despite acknowledging the advantages of a health savings program, South Korea and Taiwan still refuse to adopt such a program, as it does not fit well with their concept of collective responsibility. Another key reason is the lack of funds and the excessive precipitation of the accounts. The philosophy of Singapore's healthcare system is to ensure quality and affordable basic medical services for all, but it also introduces the concept of efficiency and strives to achieve efficient equality. Singapore emphasizes that high social welfare borne by the government is unsustainable in the long run, because equality without efficiency cannot be maintained for long. This idea is a departure from the situations in South Korea and Taiwan.

2. The 30-Baht Universal Health Insurance Scheme in Thailand

The main distinguishing feature between developing and developed countries is that, due to low levels of overall economic development and uneven distributions of wealth, developing countries have larger numbers and proportions of socially vulnerable groups. In order to improve the accessibility of health services to these groups, in addition to introducing medical assistance to the lowest rungs of society, developing countries have also formulated various healthcare schemes for the vulnerable groups that make up the majority of these societies. Some examples include Brazil's Family Health Program and India's National Rural Health Mission. The most typical example is Thailand's 30-Baht Universal Health Insurance Scheme (the 30-Baht Scheme).

The community health services in Thailand have been described by the WHO as "a new idea of realizing healthcare reforms for all under the conditions of a market economy." The 30-Baht Scheme introduced in 2001 has further achieved health insurance coverage for 95% of the population.

(1) Health Security System Prior to Implementation

Before the implementation of the 30-Baht Scheme, Thailand's health security system mainly included the civil servant medical benefit scheme, the social health insurance system, the health card scheme, and the government medical assistance scheme. In the 1960s, Thailand established a medical benefit scheme for government civil servants and their families. In the 1970s and 1980s, it successively established a public medical benefit scheme and a rural voluntary health insurance scheme that covered the poor, the elderly, children, and the disabled. During the 10-year period from the 1990s to 2000, Thailand undertook the expansion of its health coverage. In 1991, it also established a social health insurance system that covered employees in the formal sector. In 1997, Thailand amended its constitution to emphasize that health is a basic right of its citizens. During this period, the coverage of the Workers' Compensation Fund expanded to include all employees of the private sector, and tripartite financing by employers, employees, and the government was implemented. Furthermore, a capitation system was adopted for the payment of hospitals. At the same time, the provision of free medical services for the poor was reformed into a public assistance system, and the hospital payment system was converted from a global budget to a capitation system. At this point, the total coverage rate of all health security schemes in Thailand was around 60%.

(2) Overview of the 30-Baht Scheme

In 2001, the Thai government proposed a universal health security system that covers all Thai citizens apart from civil servants, formal sector employees, and their families. This system, which was intended to replace the original public medical service system and the rural voluntary insurance scheme, was known as the 30-Baht Scheme. The central government preallocates funds to the provinces according to a set standard. The provincial health offices, in turn, distribute the funds to the appropriate healthcare institutions, where residents have access to free preventive healthcare services. Citizens participating in the scheme can seek medical care from designated healthcare institutions and only need to pay 30 baht (approximately RMB 6) to receive outpatient and inpatient services (excluding cosmetic treatments, organ transplants, and kidney dialysis). The poor, individuals over 60 years old or under 12 years old, the disabled, veterans, and monks can receive medical care for free. The 30-Baht Scheme initially only covered groups without health insurance and low-income groups, which accounted for more than 30% of the population. By 2002, coverage had been extended to 80%, making Thailand the first lower-middle-income country to achieve universal healthcare.

1. Conditions for Scheme Implementation   During the Thai general election in 2001, the Pheu Thai Party, represented by Thaksin Shinawatra, made three promises to the people, one of which was to establish universal health coverage.

When the Pheu Thai Party came into power, it began to fulfill its original commitments and embarked on the establishment of universal health coverage. At that time, Thailand's economy was just recovering from the financial crisis, and the opposition from the Democrat Party was fierce. Hence, implementing a high level of universal coverage seemed to be extremely risky. Shinawatra's governing philosophy was to serve the poor and improve their quality of life, thereby safeguarding every Thai citizen. Therefore, after weighing the pros and cons, it became more feasible to implement a basic, low-level 30-Baht Scheme.

Economically, in 2001, Thailand had just recovered from the financial crisis, and its state finances were more generous. In addition, Thailand increased the proportion of healthcare spending on health insurance and further diverted all alcohol and tobacco taxes to the 30-Baht Scheme. These measures provided the required financial support for the scheme.

2. Initiatives for Scheme Implementation

1. *Enactment of laws.* In April 2002, the National Health Security Act was enacted, which legally guaranteed the smooth implementation of the 30-Baht Scheme. The Guidelines for the Human Resource Management of National Health Security were formulated, which stipulate that hospitals with funding difficulties can apply for emergency funding but must manage the hospital, physicians, and patient diagnosis and treatment strictly in accordance with the guidelines. After a hospital submits an application, the government also arranges for healthcare experts to carry out investigations and research on the hospital in order to conduct an in-depth discussion on the management of the hospital's utilization of funds. The hospital's management staff also participate in the discussion, during which both parties cooperate to suggest improvements, and a recommendation report is written. There are also clear constraints in the utilization of emergency funds, which play a limiting role in regulating the actions of hospitals.

2. *Strengthening administration.* The National Health Commission was established, which is led by the Minister of Health. The National Health Security Office was set up to manage the funds of the 30-Baht Scheme. Health commissions were set up in each province, and they are responsible for contracting with participating healthcare providers.

3. *Reform of payment system.* A fee-for-service system was in use before the implementation of the 30-Baht Scheme. The state allocated funds based on the past healthcare expenditures of each provincial government. The factors affecting funding included the number of hospitals assisted, the number of beds, and the number of physicians. After the implementation of the scheme, the state preallocated funds based on the number of people served by each provincial government. The central government allocated funds according to the service population of each provincial government, and the provincial health offices distributed the funds to each hospital.

   After the implementation of the scheme, a capitation system was adopted for outpatient services and a DRG-based payment system was adopted for inpatient services. The amount allocated under the capitation system is determined based on the age, health level, and common diseases of the enrolled population and the local conditions of each province. The expenses are further adjusted according to annual price levels and changes in medical costs. The capitation system enables the effective containment of healthcare costs. It also improves the regional distribution of physicians, increases the fairness of budget allocation, and enhances the efficiency of healthcare institutions. Different payment methods are adopted for different services. For treatment services, outpatient care is paid using the capitation system, and inpatient care is paid using a global budget. Prevention and health promotion are paid using a performance-related capitation system. For accident and emergency services, outpatient care is paid using a fee-for-service system, and inpatient care uses a DRG-based payment system. The amounts and payment standards of the capitation system are adjusted on an annual basis according to costs and prices.

4. *Increased financial input and initiation of emergency funds.* After allowing for infrastructure and scientific research, the government has allotted the entirety of healthcare spending to the 30-Baht Scheme. This spending includes the day-to-day operations of all agencies, staff salaries, the physician salaries of all contracted hospitals, capitation payments, and reserve funds for public hospital operations.

   The government predicted that many public hospitals would face difficulties due to insufficient subsidies from capital flow. Hence, sufficient emergency funds were prepared to cope with this situation. This issue may arise because after the implementation of capitation, the funds received by each hospital correspond to the number of people the hospital serves, and the salaries of healthcare workers are also included in the capitation payment. Some hospitals have a large pool of healthcare workers but a small service population, and thus receive less funding.

These hospitals were unable to maintain daily operations or pay the salaries of their physicians and, hence, faced the risk of bankruptcy. Thus, the government started an emergency fund to help these hospitals overcome their difficulties.

5. *Establishing and improving the health system at all levels.* To further strengthen community health services and build up the government's capital investment, special emphasis was placed on the development of primary healthcare institutions, and a large proportion of the funds were allocated to provincial hospitals, rural clinics, and rural health-care centers.

The distribution of medical graduates to areas lacking in doctors was encouraged, and guidance was provided. Comparatively speaking, some areas had large service populations and received a large amount of funds but lacked healthcare workers and could not provide health services.

The government's solution to this issue was to actively guide medical graduates towards working in places that lacked doctors. Tuition relief, scholarships, wage compensation, and other policies were adopted to provide physicians in areas lacking healthcare workers.

These policies alleviated the unreasonable allocation of human resources.

(3) Advantages of the 30-Baht Scheme

1. Ample Compensation Mechanisms That Enable a Flexible System   Adopting a single payment method for health services, especially the fee-for-service system commonly implemented in China, can easily lead to soaring healthcare costs and the phenomenon of the poor subsidizing the rich in health insurance. Having a diversified compensation mechanism is one of the features of most foreign medical assistance systems. Thailand's 30-Baht Scheme encourages each province to adopted different compensation mechanisms based on their local conditions, which mainly involves DRG-based and capitation payment systems.

2. Timely Institutional Changes and Innovation   The formation of every system is based on continuous improvements and modifications. There is no system that is completely perfect. Thailand's 30-Baht Scheme originated from the Health Care Scheme for low-income residents in rural areas. On the basis of its free universal healthcare system, Brazil formulated the Family Health Program and Regional Management Plan based on its actual national conditions. In addition to its three-tier preventive healthcare network, the Indian government also began implementing the National Rural Health Mission in 2005.

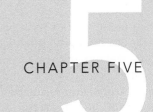

CHAPTER FIVE

Social Medical Aid System and Its Analysis

The social medical aid system is primarily the responsibility of the government, which is involved in organizing and coordinating charitable and social organizations to establish a health security system that provides healthcare services for patients living in poverty or other difficult circumstances. In the health security systems of developed countries, even those with universal health insurance (e.g., the UK and Canada) have established corresponding medical aid systems for vulnerable groups (e.g., impoverished individuals). The different forms of medical aid systems and policies were the earliest systems to take shape and currently remain the most fundamental form of health security policy. Healthcare spending in the US is considerable, and there is also a unique health security system wherein commercial insurance providers are exceedingly influential. However, the main beneficiaries of social health insurance are people living in poverty, the elderly, and children. In addition, there is compulsory admission to emergency departments.

SECTION I. THEORETICAL FOUNDATIONS OF SOCIAL MEDICAL AID SYSTEMS

The concept of a social medical aid system has a broad theoretical basis. In this section, we briefly introduce the most prominent of these theories, namely, baseline equality, social citizenship, Maslow's hierarchy of needs, and third distribution.

1. Theory of Baseline Equality

Since human societies began forming nations, governments have been engaging in public policy activities. Public policies have been developed alongside democratization, particularly with the establishment of democratic constitutionalism, which provides legal protection to these public policies. Equality is a measure of the social relations between individuals. Justice is the idealization of equality, whereas equality is the realization or concretization of justice. Both egalitarianism and welfare states have so far failed to achieve an optimal balance and baseline between the maximization of welfare and efficiency. Hence, baseline equality is a feasible option, particularly given that the limitations of a small welfare state have been overcome. In fact, the true discovery of this theory is that baseline equality is more conducive than other common types of equality to achieving social equality. How does one determine the baseline? We can refer to the principle of simplicity in scientific models and satisfy the minimum level of social security, or we can refer to the human development index (HDI) when providing social support. The main principles of baseline equality theory are universality, prioritizing the vulnerable, government leadership, and the persistent effects of social compensation. The institutional structure of baseline equality is as follows:

1. A baseline welfare system that embodies the consistency of rights and reflects the concepts of baseline equality in social welfare. It mainly includes the minimum livelihood guarantee system, public health and basic healthcare systems, compulsory education system, and public welfare services.
2. A nonbaseline welfare system that embodies the necessary diversity and reflects the concept of social welfare efficiency. It mainly includes various forms of personal savings account systems, a fully funded pension system, and a commercial insurance system.
3. An across-baseline welfare system that considers both consistency and diversity, which includes the health insurance system, pension insurance system, unemployment insurance system, and the social aid and services system.
4. The essential and nonessential components of the system are identified according to the theory of baseline equality.

2. Theory of Social Citizenship

Citizenship is a status bestowed on individuals who are full members of a community; all who possess this status are considered equal in terms of the rights and obligations with which the status is endowed. Citizenship is essential to ensuring social equality and consists of three basic dimensions or elements: civil rights, political rights, and social rights. It is essentially a social equality system that is developing continuously and exhibits the inherent potential of progressing toward more comprehensive and ample egalitarianism.

Civil rights are those rights that protect individual freedoms, including personal freedoms, freedoms of speech, thought and religion, the right to own property and sign valid contracts, and the right to seek justice. Courts are the institutions most directly associated with the maintenance of civil rights. Political rights, on the other hand, are the rights governing the participation in the exercise of political power as a member or voter of political authorities. Institutions dedicated to maintaining these rights include the national assembly and councils of local governments. Finally, social rights are those rights ranging from minor economic and security benefits to fully shared social heritage, as well as rights to a civilized living environment based on social contracts. The education system and social services represent the institutions most closely related to preserving these rights.

There are two major ideological traditions in the Western theories of civil rights. The first is liberalism, which is represented by the writings of John Locke. This tradition emerged in the modernernization of the West, in the wake of the monarchy being overthrown by the bourgeoisie. Liberalism advocates for the protection of personal and property security, as well as constitutional law, representative governments, and religious tolerance. The second is republicanism, which is represented by the Athenian model of democracy (i.e., direct democracy) and was championed in the modern era by Jean-Jacques Rousseau. It centers on the development of the quality and character of citizens, who in turn are responsible for protecting their own rights to equality and justice. It also emphasizes obligatory participation in political activities. As individuals constitute part of a nation or community, citizenship implies the right to participate in legislation and political decision-making, and to hold public office. Modern nationalism and socialism represent the new forms of republicanism.

From the perspective of conflict theories in sociology, the emergence of urban poverty can be considered a manifestation of the deprivation of civilian rights during the process of social change. Amartya Kumar Sen, an Indian welfare economist awarded the Nobel Memorial Prize in Economic Sciences, believed that entitlement refers to the "ability of people to command (goods) through the use of the legal means available in society," which does not solely refer to personal ability. From the perspective of social rights, the main poverty-related entitlements include rights to appropriate public resource allocation, work, healthcare, property, housing, education, preferment, recreation, reputation, alimony, custody, and gender equality. Individuals or groups are more likely to fall into poverty if they are deprived of these rights, leading to insufficient or hampered opportunities and means to exercise such rights. Therefore, a permanent solution to eliminating poverty would be strengthening social equality and justice. This theory is reflected in the current medical aid systems, such as the minimum livelihood guarantee system.

3. Maslow's Hierarchy of Needs

Maslow's hierarchy of needs is a theory proposed by Abraham Maslow, an American social psychologist, personality theorist, comparative psychologist, and humanistic psychologist (Figure 5.1). It is a theory of human motivation comprising a five-tier model of human needs:

1. *Physiological needs.* These are the most primitive and fundamental needs, which include food, clothing, housing, and healthcare. An individual's life is endangered if any of these needs are not met. In other words, they are the most fundamental and indispensable layer of needs that serves as a powerful driving force of human actions.
2. *Safety needs.* These include needs for labor safety, occupational safety, a stable life and secure future, and safety from disasters. Safety needs are placed at a higher level than physiological needs and take precedence once the latter have been satisfied. Every individual living in reality always desires a sense of security and freedom.
3. *Social belonging.* The need for socialization, also called the need for belongingness and love, refers to the individual's desire for the concern, care, and understanding of their families, social groups, friends, and colleagues. It refers to the need for friendships, trust, warmth, and love. The needs for social belonging are subtler and more elusive than physiological and safety needs. These needs are associated with personality, experience, living area, ethnicity, living habits, and religious beliefs, and are often difficult to fully comprehend and measure. They are difficult to detect and measure.
4. *Esteem needs.* These needs can be further categorized into the need for self-esteem, the need to feel respected, and the desire for power, and include the concepts of self-esteem, self-evaluation, and respect for others. Esteem needs are seldom fully satisfied, but basic satisfaction is sufficient to generate motivation.

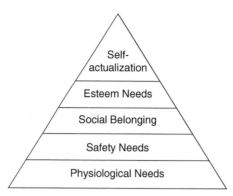

FIGURE 5.1 Maslow's hierarchy of needs.

5. *Self-actualization.* The need for self-actualization is the highest level of the hierarchy. Fulfilling this need requires the individual to accomplish work that is commensurate with their abilities, realize their full potential, and become the most that they can be. It is a need for creation. Individuals aiming to satisfy this need often try their best to achieve perfection. Self-actualization implies the desire to experience life fully, actively, selflessly, attentively, and empathetically.

Based on this theoretical system, Maslow postulated that physiological needs are the most fundamental and must be met to the extent that the individual can maintain survival before any of the other needs can become new motivating factors. Health security and personal safety fall within the scope of these basic needs.

4. Theory of Tertiary Distribution

Distribution is a crucial part of the national economy and refers to the dissemination of newly created goods or values (i.e., national income) within a certain period of time in a society. British economist Sir George Ramsay is considered one of the last representatives of classical (bourgeois) political economics. In his book *An Essay on the Distribution of Wealth*, he noted that there are two types of distribution: primary and secondary distribution. However, there is another type of distribution, known as tertiary distribution, which describes the practice of having wealthy individuals contribute more to social betterment than poor individuals. Wealthy individuals are specifically encouraged via legislation and taxation to donate to various social funds, charitable causes, scientific research, medical care, education, poverty reduction, medical aid, and so on. These three types of distribution have varying forms and properties and are interrelated with and complementary to each other.

 SECTION II. MAJOR POLICIES OF SOCIAL MEDICAL AID SYSTEMS

1. Recipients of Medical Aid

The main recipients of medical aid systems worldwide are people living in poverty, children, individuals with a disability, and patients with certain diseases (e.g., AIDS and tuberculosis). Recipients often seek medical aid for reasons closely related to their incomes. Furthermore, the scope of medical aid is closely associated with a country's level of economic development, and it is influenced by its traditional cultures, values, and demographic structure. However, the scope of medical aid is also constantly undergoing modifications based on economic and social development.

Medicaid, the medical aid system in the US, is a joint federal–state welfare program that is implemented by state governments. It is one of the two major public insurance programs in the US. In 1998, there were up to 40 million Medicaid recipients. The program covers not only those living in poverty but also all individuals who are supported in some form by the government or who need some form of care. Recipients can roughly be divided into four categories. The first category includes elderly adults living below the poverty line, who constitute more than half of the elderly population in the US. Many of these individuals are frail, living alone, and are dependent on others. Approximately one-fifth of elderly adults rely mainly on Medicaid to live in nursing homes before passing away. The second category consists of individuals with severe intellectual disability, blindness, or other forms of disability. The third category consists of children (and their parents) who are raised by single parents living in poverty; these individuals account for almost two-thirds of the total number of Medicaid recipients. The fourth category includes pregnant women and children from low-income families. During the Clinton administration, Medicaid was made mandatory for children in poor families.

The vulnerable groups who receive medical aid have different definitions across different countries. However, in general, the following sets of characteristics can be considered. The first are their social characteristics – for example, the National Health Insurance (NHI) in Japan requires an investigation of the employment status and job type of the applicants. The second are their economic characteristics – for example, in Singapore and the US, the incomes of medical aid recipients and their ability to pay premiums are considered. The third are their medical characteristics, as exemplified in South Korea, where medical aid recipients are assessed in terms of the presence of diseases or disabilities, the type of disease, and the severity of disabilities. The fourth are their demographic characteristics – for example, the elderly in Japan. The fifth are their insurance characteristics, whereby the government considers whether a recipient has been insured and their level of insurance.

The author believes that economic and medical characteristics should be prioritized as the basic criteria when defining vulnerable groups eligible for medical aid, while the other characteristics can serve as supplementary criteria. In other words, all patients unable to access basic healthcare for economic reasons should be considered vulnerable groups. Therefore, the medical aid recipients in each state can also be divided into three categories. The first category includes the uninsured. With the exception of those who are relatively well-off, these individuals are exposed to a greater degree of risk upon falling ill (especially severe illnesses) as compared to those covered by social insurance and/or commercial insurance, which may lead to hardships. Uninsured individuals are generally considered to be more vulnerable compared to insured individuals. The second category includes the disadvantaged, who are covered by a certain level of health insurance but whose basic standard of living is affected due to the impact of considerable medical expenses. The third category includes the impoverished, who live at or below the minimum standard of living, have no one to rely on, and have no source of subsistence. This category is mainly comprised of orphans, laborers without health insurance subsidies, patients with chronic diseases, and uninsured elderly adults without children or spouses.

In June 2002, Singapore launched the ElderShield scheme, which aims to provide basic financial assistance to 40- to 65-year-old Singaporeans with severe disabilities, in order to ensure that they receive long-term care services. In addition, the government of Singapore also established the Community Health Assist Scheme (CHAS) to provide elderly individuals living in poverty with convenient access to healthcare services.

Japan established its NHI for low-income earners, which mostly targets those with diverse sources of or unstable income. The premiums for NHI vary considerably, as they are determined by the income of insured persons. Therefore, the NHI is prominently characterized by the feature of self-help and mutual aid. However, with socioeconomic development and demographic changes, the NHI continues to suffer from a shortage of funds and operating deficits due to the increasing low-income and elderly populations (retirees are transferred from employer-sponsored health insurance to the NHI). Therefore, in March 1995, Japan revised the NHI system and established a new health insurance scheme for the elderly to reduce the burden on the NHI. However, this self-help and mutual aid system in Japan is restricted to those living in poverty, and thus has room for improvement in terms of its social equality.

2. Determining the Eligibility of Medical Aid Recipients

Social medical aid is mainly provided free of charge by the government. Therefore, the eligibility of medical aid recipients must be verified to prevent ineligible individuals from receiving such aid, which would aggravate health inequalities and put undue burden on public funds.

The social medical aid system of every country has a dedicated verification procedure to ensure recipients' eligibility. For instance, Medicaid applicants in the US are subject to investigations of their economic condition based on the Federal Poverty Guidelines to prove that their household income and assets fall below the limit for accessing medical aid. The Federal Poverty Guidelines released by the federal government on February 18, 2005, classified poverty levels into 100–250% of the federal poverty level (FPL), which is mainly determined by the number of family members. However, in some states, Medicaid eligibility is completely forfeited if the total household income exceeds the minimum standard. Therefore, although all Medicaid beneficiaries are living in poverty, more than half of those who live below the FPL are not eligible for Medicaid. Furthermore, no state provides Medicaid to all residents below the FPL. In the UK, the medical aid system has very strict approval and constraint mechanisms. Recipients who commit fraud are subjected to a penalty of five times the medical aid they received.

In Singapore, patients who cannot afford their medical expenses can request hospital staff to arrange for a meeting with a hospital social worker. The hospital social worker then works out a financial assistance plan based on the patient's financial situation. All public or restructured hospitals in Singapore have designated voluntary social workers who are familiar with the typical situations and needs of Singaporeans at the bottom of the society. These social workers have rich experiences; hence, appointing them to process applications and allocate funds not only helps those living in poverty but also prevents the misuse of funds. Singapore's Medifund is more helpful to the following two categories of recipients compared to others: The first are Central Provident Fund members who have continuously paid their Medisave premiums and participate in the MediShield Life scheme, and the second are elderly Singaporeans without a Medisave account or who have insufficient Medisave funds. In November 2001, the government of Singapore authorized nine unofficial Medifund institutions. Eligible patients admitted to these medical institutions may apply for medical aid from Medifund. Furthermore, since January 2009, government subsidies can be provided according to an assessment of inpatients' economic status. Individuals with an average monthly income of SG$3,200 or below can receive hospitalization subsidies of 65% or 80% in Class B2 or Class C wards.

In South Korea, medical aid recipients mainly consist of the following three categories: homeless individuals, unemployed individuals who are dependent on their families, and individuals with high medical expenses but who earn less than 25% of the national income per capita. Individuals who meet any of the above criteria are eligible for publicly funded medical aid. However, all three groups must be treated or hospitalized in designated medical institutions. Although all of them receive medical aid from the government, these groups enjoy different levels of benefits: The first group (homeless individuals) does not need to pay any medical fees. The second group must pay 20% of the hospitalization fees, and if the hospitalization fee exceeds ₩100,000, they can apply for an installment loan from medical aid funds. The third group must pay 20% of hospitalization fees and 44% of outpatient expenses.

3. Methods of Medical Aid

A country's social medical aid system is closely related to its health security system. In general, it might be affiliated with an existing health insurance system or be self-contained. The main types of social medical aid systems are as follows.

(1) Mandatory and Optional Medical Aid

Medicaid in the US primarily targets individuals living in extreme poverty, which include recipients of Aid to Families with Dependent Children (AFDC), children and pregnant women from poor families, beneficiaries of Supplemental Security Income (SSI), recipients of adoption assistance, certain protected groups, and some Medicare beneficiaries. Each state decides on the eligibility criteria for optional medical aid. Recipients of optional aid are typically poor children and women with incomes below a certain level who are provided with shelter by charitable organizations or receive aid from Family and Community Services (FACS); elderly, blind, and disabled individuals with incomes falling below the FPL, but who fail to meet the criteria for mandatory medical aid; beneficiaries of SSI state supplemental payments (SSP); disabled workers with incomes below a certain level; patients with certain diseases; individuals living in poverty due to illnesses; and so forth.

(2) Healthcare Subsidies for Impoverished Groups

Chile, for example, has established a public health insurance scheme (Fondo Nacional de Salud, FONASA) and a few private insurance agencies (Instituciones de Salud Previsional, ISAPREs), and it ranks its population in five groups in ascending order of income: A, B, C, D, and E. Group E represents high-income earners, who are generally required to subscribe to private health insurance. Individuals in Groups B, C, and D pay for public health insurance in order to access healthcare services; among them, Group B do not have high incomes but do not live in extreme poverty, and hence must partially cover their medical expenses. Group A are low-income earners, who do not have to pay premiums to social health insurance agencies and are given free access to the prescribed healthcare services that are fully covered by public funds. In Japan, families or individuals who benefit from the minimum livelihood guarantee system can only be admitted to healthcare institutions designated by the government. The government provides financial assistance to individuals whose medical expenses cause their incomes to fall below the minimum standard of living. The central and local governments assume three-quarters and one-quarter of their living expenses, respectively.

(3) Establishing Dedicated Health Insurance Schemes for Low-income Groups

These health insurance schemes, such as Medicaid in the US and Medifund in Singapore, are medical aid systems established for low-income earners living in poverty and incapable of covering normal medical expenses.

(4) Medical Aid Provided by Social Donations and Charitable Organizations

This type of medical aid primarily refers to healthcare services provided by nongovernmental organizations (NGOs) and charitable organizations to those living in poverty, or healthcare services for impoverished groups that rely on international aid. It involves a certain degree of randomness. Developed countries consider such aid supplemental to existing forms of medical aid for those living in poverty, whereas extremely poor countries that lack basic social security rely heavily on this type of unstable aid. This is more commonly seen in developing countries. In Bangladesh, for example, a considerable number of NGOs provide various healthcare services to those living in poverty, including health education, pediatric care, vaccination and immunization, and so on. Such healthcare services are mainly provided by trained volunteers and are funded via local and foreign fundraising efforts. However, due to the lack of a stable workforce and economic resources, the scope of service provision is relatively narrow and inconsistent, and its effectiveness is extremely limited. Therefore, this form of aid struggles to meet some of the basic healthcare needs of those living in poverty.

(5) Other Types of Medical Aid

There are other types of medical aid provided by special policies in other health security systems. For example, the social health insurance system in Germany stipulates that low-income earners are fully (social provisions) or partially (extraneous provisions) exempt from additional contribution obligations (where medical expenses must be covered by the insured persons in accordance with the health insurance scheme). In these cases, the health insurance agencies cover all expenses for the prescription drugs, first aid supplies, and ancillary supplies, and the insured persons are exempt from paying for medical expenses, including any additional contributions. In general, patients in countries with a National Health Service, such as the UK and Canada, must pay for prescription charges, whereas poor families who depend on subsidies are exempt from these charges.

4. Funding Sources for Medical Aid

The government is obliged to protect the right to health of impoverished individuals and other vulnerable groups, which can potentially act as a permanent means of breaking the causal chain between illness and poverty. This principle has been confirmed even in countries with well-developed healthcare markets, such as the US. Therefore, regardless of the type of medical aid, the government must play a leading role in this area, and public financing serves as the main source of funding for social medical aid.

In the US, all Medicaid expenses are shared between the federal and state governments. The funding sources for Medicaid include the federal government (generally accounting for 50–83%) and all levels of local government, which are used to provide financial assistance to eligible recipients. Medicaid employs the pay-to-provider method, where each state issues payments directly to providers depending on the healthcare services used or implements various prospective payment methods. The state governments decide on the method of payment and the ratio of reimbursement based on the upper limits and specific restrictions imposed by the federal government. This model has remained unchanged since Medicaid was first implemented. The federal government allocates matching funds to each state based on state income per capita, using a federal matching formula. For most states above the national income per capita, the minimum matching rate is 50%; for states below the national income per capita, the maximum matching rate is 83%. The federal government also covers 50% of the administration fees of each state.

Medifund is a government-sponsored health fund for impoverished groups in Singapore. It was established on April 1, 1993, with an initial government investment of SG$200 million, followed by annual investments of $100 million (contingent on sustained economic growth and budget surpluses). The current balance of Medifund is SG$700 million. The interest generated from the capital sum (rather than the capital sum itself) is used to pay for medical expenses. In Australia, about 80% of the expenses for prescription drugs for Medicare recipients are covered by the government via subsidies, and their healthcare funds are also mainly from government budget allocations.

According to the World Health Report 2005, in the UK, where medical expenses are borne entirely by the government, out-of-pocket health expenses as a share of total healthcare expenditure has reduced gradually from 19.6% in 1998 to 16.6% in 2002. Patients mainly pay for healthcare-related expenses not covered by the National Health Service (NHS), such as NHS prescription fees, dentist fees, ophthalmic fees, and travel expenses.

Japan's NHI was established by the government in an effort to combat poverty, which was a social concern at the time. The NHI is funded by the state treasure, local governments, and individuals. Since universal health insurance was made mandatory in 1961, out-of-pocket health expenditure has gradually reduced from 50% to 30%, as the percentage of expenses covered by the state treasury increased. Public funds are used to supplement the premium contributions of low-income groups; in general, the state treasury covers half of the expenditure, whereas the prefectural and municipal governments each cover one-quarter of the expenditure. The minimum livelihood guarantee fund is supported by national taxes, whereby the central government contributes three-quarter of the fund, and the local governments contribute one-quarter of the fund.

In South Korea, the central and local governments of South Korea contribute 80% and 20% to the medical aid fund, respectively. The Economic Planning and National Budget Administrations under the Ministry of Economy and Finance are directly responsible for managing social security policies and related budgets. Medical aid funds come from the revenues of general taxation and are administered through general accounting.

5. Treatment Standards for Medical Aid

The majority of social medical aid systems cover the most fundamental healthcare services. However, the treatment received by medical aid recipients is closely related to the country's level of economic development, and hence, there is a constant change alongside economic development. Only a handful of countries provide cash to medical aid recipients to pay for the basic healthcare services. For instance, Finland includes basic medical expenses as part of the minimum living allowance.

The services precisely covered under Medicaid in the US vary greatly across different states, with the exception of the following 10 major basic healthcare services: inpatient and outpatient services; X-ray and physical examinations; outpatient services and medical equipment in rural areas; elderly care services; physician services; family health plan services and equipment; nursing care services provided to eligible families; medical examinations, diagnosis, and treatment of children; and services provided by nurses and certified professional midwives. In addition, each state can also cover certain optional healthcare services, such as private nursing care, outpatient services, dentistry, physiotherapy, prescription, dentures, maintenance of medical equipment and eyeglasses; the associated expenses are paid for by the respective state governments. If the states decide to provide protection to other individuals lacking access to healthcare services, then despite their considerable flexibility in the provision of health services (state governments do not have to provide all the above-mentioned optional services), state governments are still required to cover all normal expenses. Since Medicaid is implemented by state governments, they are responsible for determining the payment of medical expenses. Medicaid funds obtained by recipients typically cover one-third to half of the healthcare expenses.

Social medical aid is often influenced by fiscal deficits. Since 1982, the US federal government has reformed the health insurance scheme and has progressively been reducing Medicaid expenses over the years, such as by reducing reimbursement standards, the number of healthcare services covered, and the number of family care services. On the other hand, the UK not only provides impoverished individuals with free medical treatment through the NHS but also subsidizes their travel expenses to NHS hospitals and provides free milk and vitamins to children and pregnant women.

In Japan, low-income families under the NHI are entitled to statutory convalescence benefits, specific convalescence expenses, high-cost convalescence expenses, other convalescence expenses, voluntary midwifery fees, funeral expenses, injury allowance, and parental allowance, all of which cover 70% of the actual cost. Low-income families are also entitled to access NHI-run healthcare facilities, health education activities, and various other activities. In the event of illness or injury, or when medical expenses cause an individual's income to fall below the minimum standard of living, medical aid recipients are entitled to free medical treatment at government-designated healthcare institutions or cash assistance. Furthermore, the daily supplies for hospitalized pregnant women, the elderly, single-mother families, and disabled individuals are also subsidized. In addition to financial assistance, the Japanese government provides ambulance facilities to individuals with severe physical or mental disabilities, as well as therapeutic facilities to those who need shelter and protection due to physical or mental disabilities.

The medical aid system in North Korea fully subsidizes the medical expenses of those living in poverty and covers 50% of the hospitalization expenses for individuals that are able to work.

The medical aid systems of some African countries, such as Zimbabwe, mainly provide free medical treatment for infectious disease.

6. Provision of Medical Aid Services

Social medical aid systems are generally administrated by the government or are entrusted to public agencies. Medical aid services are mainly provided to recipients through healthcare services at state-run healthcare institutions or private healthcare services purchased by the government. For instance, Medicaid in the US is primarily administered by the Health Care Financing Administration (HCFA), a federal agency under the Department of Health and Human Services (DHHS).

At the state level, Medicaid is generally administered by a specific healthcare or human resources department of the local government, although the precise administration agency varies across different states. Healthcare services provided to Medicaid recipients in the US tend to generate much lower revenues than do those provided to recipients of Medicare and persons covered by commercial health insurance. Therefore, most physicians refuse to receive Medicaid recipients, with only a handful being willing to participate in Medicaid programs; this has led to poorer outcomes for Medicaid.

SECTION III. MODELS AND FEATURES OF SOCIAL MEDICAL AID SYSTEMS

Poverty has always been the central focus of government policy in all countries. Governments are responsible for protecting the basic right of citizens to subsistence and promoting health equality. Medical aid is an indispensable part of any universal health coverage system and serves as a social safety net by supporting the access of impoverished groups to basic healthcare services. Both the government and society subsidize the medical expenses of low-income and impoverished groups or critically ill patients who are unable to cover their medical expenses, thereby achieving altruistic aid or income redistribution via fiscal transfers and social assistance. The medical aid system is a form of health security that requires minimal investment and yields substantial social benefits. It promotes social equality by helping low-income groups to access the most basic healthcare services.

The medical aid system in China was first introduced in rural areas. In October 2002, the State Council of China issued the "Resolution to Further Strengthen Rural Healthcare Work," which proposed "the implementation of medical aid to low-income families in rural areas." Medical aid in urban and rural areas of China has improved with the continuous increase in financial investment. The medical aid systems of some regions primarily focus on critical illnesses in conjunction with common diseases and outpatient services. The point at which medical aid is typically provided has gradually shifted from after treatment to during and before treatment. In terms of fund settlement, the application and processing procedures have been simplified by the Ministry of Civil Affairs, which directly settles payments with various healthcare agencies. The threshold for aid recipients has also been relaxed by eliminating or reducing deductibles and copayments. In terms of service provision, the feasibility of using community healthcare centers as platforms for the provision of medical aid services has been explored. In terms of institutional convergence, various approaches, such as advance payments and disbursements, have been adopted to ensure that disadvantaged groups who cannot afford the deductibles and copayments for the New Rural Cooperative Medical Scheme can receive compensation. Studying the experiences of other developing countries could serve as a reference for the development of the medical aid system in China.

1. Models of Social Medical Aid Systems in Developed Countries

Every country – both developed and developing – has vulnerable social groups, which serves as the impetus for the establishment of medical aid or similar policies in their health security system. Among developed countries, typical medical aid systems, such as Medicaid and Medicare in the US, are funded by the social security tax, in order to provide healthcare services to the poor, elderly, and disabled to meet their basic healthcare needs. In Singapore, a specialized fund has been established by the government to help those without Medisave accounts or those whose Medisave accounts are insufficient to cover their medical expenses fully. In countries with universal health coverage, such as the UK and Germany, preferential policies have been adopted to provide medical aid to the poor and elderly, such as the "Cinderella" system in the UK. Furthermore, in all countries, medical aid is also part of the social aid offered by charitable organizations, trade unions, mutual aid organizations, and various other social organizations. However, in general, these organizations provide only supplementary support to the social medical aid system led by the government. Given the nature of social medical aid, the presence of spontaneous medical aid from other institutions does not absolve the government of its responsibility in this regard.

Some scholars have summarized the main models and features of the medical aid systems in certain developed countries, which show the differences in their names, recipients, funding sources, and covered services, as seen in Table 5.1.

TABLE 5.1 Comparison of the Models of Medical Aid System in Developed Countries

Country	Name of Medical Aid System	Recipient	Funding Source	Covered Services
US	Medicaid	Low-income elderly, disabled individuals, minors in single-parent families, and children and pregnant women in low-income families	Public financing by federal and state governments	Healthcare services purchased from hospitals and physicians for eligible recipients
Canada	Medicare	Adults aged over 65 years and impoverished groups	Government budget allocation, with the federal government covering one-third of the expenses and provincial governments covering two-thirds of the expenses, and special tax subsidies	Community healthcare services, hospitalization, healthcare, free prescription drugs, family care, and long-term care services
UK	National Health Service (NHS)	The elderly, psychiatric patients, and children	Government budget	Nursing care, healthcare, and priority services
France	French National Health Insurance (NHI)	Impoverished groups	Government budget	Subsidies for medical expenses of patients via copayments
Japan	National Health Insurance (NHI)	Adults aged over 70 years and disabled individuals	Government budget	Elderly care services and other services related to geriatric diseases
Singapore	Medifund	Individuals living in poverty or individuals whose basic standard of living has been affected by considerable medical expenses	Government-established insurance fund and social donations	Medical expenses of those living in poverty

Source: Ren Ran and Huang Zhi-Qiang, *Framework & Strategies for the Development of China's Universal Health Coverage System*, Economic Science Press.

2. Features of Social Medical Aid Systems in Developed Countries

The medical aid system is a type of public good with an emphasis on the responsibilities of the government. In fact, it is impossible for organizations aiming to maximize profit to provide this type of public good through market exchange; hence, only the government can assume the responsibilities of medical aid. Although developed countries have established a variety of sources to fund health insurance, they continue to regard medical aid as the government's responsibility, whereby the government should provide funds to meet the basic healthcare needs of certain populations. Most governments attach great importance to the provision of medical aid to vulnerable groups. Equality in healthcare requires the government to take measures that improve social inequities in health and healthcare services to ensure that every member of the society can attain a basic standard of living. Medical aid serves as a social safety net for the bottommost level of the society, which supplements the health insurance scheme or social welfare system, thus providing help to those whose basic healthcare needs cannot be covered by either of these systems. Accordingly, the medical aid systems of all countries generally adopt lower standards, as its aim is to help vulnerable groups. The medical aid system also has a strictly regulated management system; hence, both policy formulation and implementation are equally important for an effective policy.

Medical aid systems typically work within a comprehensive financial management system with strict management procedures for fundraising, operation, utilization, and verification and monitoring of beneficiary applications. The law also ensures its normal operation and standardized development. Strict eligibility criteria for beneficiaries have been established in all countries, with varying criteria across different groups of people. Additionally, strict approval procedures with a heavy emphasis on supervision and management have been imposed to ensure the sustainable development of medical aid systems. In particular, to comply with the reforms of healthcare systems and curb the rapid increase in healthcare expenditure, corresponding adjustments are performed constantly on the medical aid policies of all countries, which involve more stringent criteria for eligibility and enhanced cost controls and management.

The models of social medical aid systems exhibit the following characteristics:

1. *The government assumes the main responsibilities for social medical aid.* These responsibilities include defining the eligibility criteria for medical aid, verifying recipients' eligibility, fundraising and managing medical aid funds, appointing healthcare institutions to provide medical aid services, settling medical expenses with those institutions, and providing guidance and assistance to charitable organizations and social groups for activities related to medical aid.
2. *Medical aid is primarily funded by public finances.* In most circumstances, expenses for social medical aid are shared between the central and local governments. Generally, medical aid recipients are not subject to any medical expenses or are required to assume a minor proportion of the medical expenses.
3. *Socially vulnerable groups are the main recipients.* In most cases, the recipients of social medical aid are mainly comprised of patients whose lives are below a given standard, including those living in poverty, the elderly, disabled individuals, and those living in difficult circumstances for other reasons.
4. *Types of social medical aid system.* Social medical aid is mainly provided directly to recipients via healthcare services at state-run healthcare institutions or via private healthcare services purchased by the government for the recipients.

5. *The nature of social medical aid differs from that of health insurance.* Social medical aid systems do not provide health security based on the principles of individual rights and governmental obligations; instead, they insure only the most basic healthcare needs according to specific needs and eligibility criteria.

3. Cost Containment for Social Medical Aid Systems in Developed Countries

(1) Measures and Implementation of Cost Containment for Medical Aid Systems

The social medical aid system is a type of institutional arrangement that targets specific disadvantaged groups. It is the most fundamental system within the health security systems of modern society. With the increasing healthcare needs of the impoverished and vulnerable groups, cost containment for medical aid systems has gradually become a key issue that has drawn widespread attention. In the following sections, we will illustrate the implementation of cost containment for medical aid systems in representative countries with four different funding systems.

1. Countries with NHS   The UK was one of the first countries to implement a social medical aid system. Before the promulgation of the National Health Insurance Act in 1911, medical aid mainly came in the form of the English Poor Laws, mutual aid organizations, and charitable organizations. Subsequently, the English Poor Laws gradually became obsolete, while mutual aid organizations have since been replaced by health insurance. Charitable organizations, on the other hand, continued to operate over a long period of time. With the promulgation of the National Health Service Act in 1948, medical aid was implemented through preferential policies within the framework of universal health coverage. Individuals with low or no income were legally exempt from the contributions or tax obligations, and they were incorporated under the health security system with the rest of the population. The law also stipulated that the government must not only provide free medical treatment under the NHS system, but also subsidize patients' travel expenses to NHS hospitals; provide free milk and vitamins for children and pregnant women; and give priority to the elderly, psychiatric patients, pregnant women and children in the provision of healthcare services (the so-called Cinderella system). Furthermore, eligible individuals are exempt from prescription charges at clinics operated by general practitioners and family nurse practitioners.

The medical aid policy in the UK has strict approval and constraint mechanisms, as well as detailed eligibility criteria for accessing various funds. The incomes and health status of recipients are subject to meticulous investigation to ensure that assistance is given only to those who are unable to afford their medical expenses, whereas those with the ability to pay should cover their own expenses. Recipients who commit fraud are subjected to a penalty of five times the medical aid they received.

2. Countries with a Social Health Insurance System   The social medical aid system in Germany is affiliated with the main health insurance scheme, where low-income groups are legally exempt from social welfare contributions or tax obligations. Low-income groups are also fully (social terms) or partially (extraneous provisions) exempt from additional contribution obligations (where medical fees must be assumed by the insured person in accordance with the health insurance scheme). For instance, in the past, individuals who earned below DM620 (in the former western territories of Germany) or DM520 (in the former eastern territories of Germany) were exempt from paying premiums under the statutory health insurance scheme. In recent years, the German government has increased the stringency of the approval mechanism to curb medical aid expenses, such that the eligibility of recipients is forfeited once their incomes exceed a certain level.

3. Countries with Market-Oriented Health Insurance Systems　As it is difficult for the commercial health insurance system to cover the elderly and the poor, the US government established Medicare specifically for the elderly and Medicaid for the poor. Medicaid is a joint federal–state welfare program, implemented by the state governments and administered by the HCFA, an agency under the DHHS.

Medicaid recipients are mainly: (1) Elderly adults living in poverty (more than half of the elderly in the United States have incomes falling below the FPL); (2) individuals with a severe intellectual disability, blindness, or other disabilities; and (3) children (and their parent) raised by single parents living in poverty. Together, these three categories of recipients constitute two-thirds of all Medicaid recipients. To access medical aid services, applicants must be investigated to prove that their household incomes and assets fall below the required limit. Therefore, although the beneficiaries of Medicaid are all living in poverty, more than half of those who live below the FPL are not eligible for coverage. Additionally, no state provides Medicaid to all residents who live below the FPL.

The services covered by Medicaid include inpatient and outpatient services, X-ray and physical examinations, outpatient services in rural areas, adult nursing services, and family health plan services and equipment. In addition, each state offers various optional healthcare services, such as private care, outpatient services, dentistry, physiotherapy, prescription, dentures, maintenance of equipment and eyeglasses; the associated expenses are paid for by the respective state governments.

Medicaid recipients account for one-third to half of the total healthcare expenditure in the US. However, medical aid is often affected by fiscal deficits. Since 1982, the US federal government has continually reformed the health insurance scheme, which has led to decreases in Medicaid expenses over the years through reductions in the reimbursement standards, number of healthcare services, number of family care services, and so forth.

In view of the increasing Medicare and Medicaid expenses, the US government introduced a payment system known as diagnosis-related groups (DRGs) in 1983. DRGs are based on a standardized disease classification system whereby patients are grouped according to their diagnosis, age, need for surgery, and so on, to determine the expenses for similar levels of healthcare services and standardize the utilization of healthcare resources. The DRG-based system uses fixed-amount payments to replace the retrospective fee-for-service system, thereby depriving hospitals of their autonomy in pricing and charging, replacing it with prices stipulated by the DRGs, and enabling the implementation of cost analysis. In addition, by controlling the expenses related to prescription drugs and reducing reimbursement for service providers, DRGs have gradually enhanced the role of managed healthcare (an innovative healthcare service model) as the main containment measure for Medicaid expenses.

Furthermore, in order to contain costs and reduce expenditure, beneficiaries in all states are also required to bear a minor proportion of expenses for certain healthcare services through deductibles, coinsurance, or copayments. However, pregnant women, minors under 18 years of age, inpatients, and individuals receiving emergency and family planning services are exempt from these policies. The cost-containment measures adopted in most states do not include groups with the highest medical expenses – the elderly and disabled individuals. Consequently, some elderly people transfer their assets to their children to become eligible for Medicaid. As such, it may be necessary to increase the stringency of asset monitoring and review.

In addition, budgetary constraints for Medicaid are needed to control the growth of medical expenses. For instance, in 2006, the New York State government placed an upper payment limit (UPL) on Medicaid reimbursements and shared the expenses with local governments. As a result, New York State and New York City saved about US$6.5 billion on Medicaid expenses.

4. Countries with Personal Savings Health Insurance Systems   In April 1993, the government of Singapore established the Medifund program for individuals living in poverty. Initially, the government allocated SG$200 million in startup capital for Medifund. Since then, fundraising for Medifund has been relatively stable, with the government investing an additional SG$100 million each year, given sufficient economic development. In order to access medical aid, individuals living in poverty who cannot afford their medical expenses or individuals whose basic standard of living has been affected due to large medical expenses must submit their application to the Medifund Committee, which is appointed by the government at each hospital, for investigation and approval. Singapore has also classified hospital wards using a tiered system with varying payment standards. This system has improved cost awareness among impoverished groups as patients can now select the most affordable ward type to prevent overutilization of hospital resources.

(2) Basic Features of Cost Containment for Medical Aid Systems

Although the designs of social medical aid systems vary considerably across countries, they share the following features in cost containment.

1. Enhancing the Investigation and Verification of Medical Aid Recipients   The main recipients of social medical aid include people living in poverty, children, disabled individuals, and specific patient groups. Various measures and approaches (e.g., classification or household surveys) have been adopted by all countries, from those with integrated health security systems (e.g., the UK and Germany) to those with independent medical aid systems (e.g., the US and Singapore) to ensure a strictly guarded "threshold of entry" and improve accuracy in identifying eligible recipients.

2. Emphasizing the Preferential Utilization of Community Healthcare Services at the Grassroots Level and Optimizing Allocation of Healthcare Resources   The UK employs the Cinderella system in prioritizing access of the elderly, psychiatric patients, pregnant women, and children to healthcare services. In the US, health maintenance organizations (HMOs) have been gradually introduced into Medicaid. Both systems advocate directing the flow of healthcare resources into community-based and primary healthcare services by systematically training primary healthcare physicians (i.e., general practitioners (GPs)), thereby reducing medical aid expenses.

3. Including Reimbursements for Public Health and Basic Healthcare Services in Medical Aid Systems   Preventive care and public health are considered the most cost-effective services, as they deliver long-term savings on medical aid funds by reducing the predicted probability of severe illnesses among impoverished and other vulnerable groups. Medical aid systems in all countries are constantly striving to develop mechanisms to control risks in advance, especially through the census of infectious and chronic diseases, strengthening the concept of tertiary prevention, and fully developing the effectiveness of primary healthcare services, thereby saving on expected expenses for major illnesses.

4. *Reforming the Payment System, Strengthening Control Over Providers, and Promoting Competition*   In the UK, GPs serve as the fund holders and charge on a capitation basis. Residents can register with the GP of their choice, while the regional healthcare administration allocates the majority of funds to GPs based on the number of registered patients and implements an independent budget. Thus, by connecting consumers with suppliers through contracts, the flow of funds is directed by the patients, which encourages suppliers to compete for service contracts. In the US, the introduction of the DRG-based payment system into Medicare and Medicaid programs has enhanced cost awareness among suppliers, as they must now seek maximum returns from each disease type by reducing costs and saving resources.

5. *Implementing Copayments to Raise Cost Control Awareness Among Medical Aid Recipients*   During the process of institutional change, Germany, the US, Singapore, and other countries have set certain deductibles and copayments such that beneficiaries are required to bear a minor proportion of expenses for certain healthcare services. These were implemented to raise cost awareness among impoverished groups, thereby reducing resource wastage due to excessive demands.

6. *Establishing Comprehensive Monitoring and Strict Penalty Mechanisms*   In Germany, the eligibility of medical aid recipients is forfeited once their incomes exceed a certain level. In the UK, the incomes and health status of medical aid recipients are subject to inspection, and recipients who commit fraud are subjected to heavy penalties.

4. Governmental Medical Aid Systems in Developing Countries

(1) Legal Protection and Social Support

The medical aid systems in developing countries mainly involve medical aid programs that are protected by state legislation and funded by the government, or the exemption of paying basic health insurance premiums. Some governments also adopt a joint cross-subsidization approach with other social groups or encourage social organizations to launch charitable programs. Most countries employ a number of approaches to sustain a comprehensive medical aid system. For example, the government of the Philippines provides free health insurance cards for medical aid recipients and also encourages the establishment of socially supported charitable organizations. The Indian government has not only established a tertiary healthcare network that provides free healthcare services to low-income individuals but has also launched the National Rural Health Mission (NRHM) to provide high-quality and efficient healthcare services to the poor, women, and children in deprived areas.

(2) Establishment of National Security Programs with Robust Institutional Mechanisms

In many countries, such as Kyrgyzstan, Armenia, and the Philippines, the institutional mechanism of medical aid systems is protected through state legislation. For example, the government of Armenia implemented a vertically managed and highly centralized health system to ensure universal access to medical aid via its institutional mechanism. Reforms in Armenia began after it gained independence. Among the laws and regulations promulgated by the Ministry of Health, the Medical Aid and Public Health Services Act introduced a wide range of fundraising approaches for medical aid to ensure on a national level that all Armenians had access to free medical care and services covered by the national health plan. In Kyrgyzstan, the Mandatory Health Insurance Fund (MHIF) was launched as a national health security program to provide medical and convalescent aid to Kyrgyz citizens.

Article VIII, Paragraph XI, of the 1987 Constitution of the Philippines states that the country must take comprehensive measures for health improvement and ensure that basic goods, healthcare, and other social services are sufficient to meet the needs of citizens at affordable costs. In particular, the healthcare needs of patients, the elderly, disabled individuals, women, and children should be prioritized. The National Health Insurance Program (NHIP) was established in the Philippines in 1995 with the passage of Republic Act (RA) 7875. The act stipulates that there are 18 basic principles of the Philippine NHIP, including universality, equality, responsiveness, and care for the indigents. The government is responsible for providing basic healthcare services to individuals living in poverty who need such services, which can be achieved by paying premiums on their behalf or directly providing them with healthcare services. Filipino residents with confirmed indigent status are provided with a free health insurance card. However, the medical aid program covers a different scope of services from other types of insurance. At present, it only covers inpatient services, and outpatient services are only covered in rural areas.

In some countries, such as Brazil and India, state-run public hospitals have been established to provide free basic healthcare services and pharmaceutical services to all citizens. Brazil provides free universal health care coverage as well as a private health insurance system. All Brazilians are entitled to free medical treatment, physical examinations, and preventive services at all public healthcare institutions. Poor families are exempt from consultation and prescription charges. In contrast, the government of India has developed a three-tier healthcare network comprising of subcenters, primary health centers, and community healthcare centers, which together provide free healthcare services to the vast majority of impoverished individuals. Free healthcare services include registration fees, physical examination fees, hospitalization fees, treatment fees, emergency care expenses, and even meals for inpatients. However, prescription charges are not covered under this network.

Some countries, such as Thailand, provide medical aid by paying premiums on behalf of the poor. In 1975, the government of Thailand implemented the Free Healthcare Program for Low-Income Individuals, and later expanded its coverage in 1992 to elderly adults aged over 60 years and primary and secondary school students not insured by other schemes. The government of Thailand issues "welfare cards" for low-income earners (similar to "medical aid cards") to eligible medical aid recipients who earn less than 1,000 Baht per month. These medical aid recipients must be registered with a public healthcare agency and must receive outpatient services at designated healthcare institutions, but may be referred to other institutions if necessary. The government allocates a certain amount of funds to healthcare centers or hospitals based on the number of registered medical aid recipients. In 1983, the government of Thailand introduced the Health Card Project (HCP) for low-income earners in rural areas, whereby each family voluntarily pays a certain amount of premiums annually, and the government subsidizes the remaining amount. Health card holders can access free healthcare services at public healthcare institutions under certain conditions. After introducing the 30-Baht Universal Health Insurance Scheme in 2001, the government of Thailand stipulated that eligible medical aid recipients are exempt from paying the 30-Baht premium. The institutional arrangements for registration, initial visit, and referral procedures remain unchanged.

(3) Cross-Subsidization Between the Government and Other Social Groups, with an Emphasis on Charitable Organizations

Chile is one of the countries where social security has been successfully implemented. The country also currently utilizes a medical aid model involving cross-subsidization between the government and other social groups. The current system is the result of the reforms made to an earlier system, wherein public financing was used to compensate for the deficits of the Ministry of Labor and Social Security. Furthermore, the social aid program, which was designed or tailored by the government for those living in poverty or with special needs, was integrated into the social insurance scheme. This made it exceedingly difficult to establish independent systems for both the funding sources and the management system. Following the reforms, the social aid program was gradually separated from the social insurance program through the establishment of relevant institutions. The government also implemented a unified management system for the social aid program involving coordination with various social organizations to form a comprehensive and systematic social aid system.

The medical aid system for impoverished groups in Chile utilizes the cross-subsidization approach between the government and other social groups. The government divides the population into five groups in ascending order of income: A, B, C, D, and E. Group E includes the high-income earners, who generally subscribe for private insurance schemes, whereas the other four groups generally participate in public insurance schemes. Group A consists of individuals who do not have to pay insurance premiums and whose medical expenses are entirely covered by public financing. Group B consists of individuals who only have to pay a certain percentage of the premiums while the remainder is subsidized by the surplus of premiums in the public healthcare system paid by individuals in Groups C and D.

The approach adopted in Chile ensures stable funding and the availability of highly comprehensive services that meet the healthcare needs of people living in poverty. The spirit of mutual aid has been embodied in the cross-subsidization approach between the government and other social groups adopted to subsidize those living in poverty.

The Philippines has also implemented a medical aid system that relies on social support. There are numerous philanthropic healthcare institutions in the Philippines, which usually provide healthcare services to impoverished groups free of charge or with minimal voluntary charges. For example, the Chinese community in the Philippines has organized various charitable healthcare institutions to provide medical aid for those living in poverty.

There are also countries that impose statutory medical aid obligations on social healthcare institutions. For example, the Brazilian government requires private healthcare institutions to provide a certain number of free healthcare services to low- and middle-income earners each year.

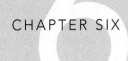

CHAPTER SIX

Features and Trends of Reforms in World Health Systems

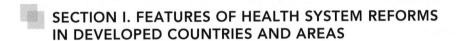

SECTION I. FEATURES OF HEALTH SYSTEM REFORMS IN DEVELOPED COUNTRIES AND AREAS

1. Common Features and Trends of Health Economic Policies in Developed Countries and Areas

(1) Common Features of Health Security Systems

1. Wide Health Coverage, High Security Level Apart from the US, most other developed countries have achieved universal health insurance, under which residents have equal access to various universal and comprehensive healthcare services.

2. High Proportion of Public Funding In Total Health Spending In 2008, public funding by the US government accounted for only 47.8% of total health spending, which was the lowest among all developed countries. Public funding in other major developed countries accounts for an average of 74.4% of total health spending, with most countries exceeding 70%. The socialization of health insurance is very high, and private insurance financing is a supplement to public financing plans.

3. Key Role of the Private Sector in Health Service Provision In countries implementing national and private health insurance systems, health services are mainly provided by the private sector, even in countries with a national health service, such as the UK. Although general practitioners (GPs) need to sign contracts with the government and are subjected to government management, the provision of primary healthcare services by GPs is still private in nature. In order to solve the problems of inefficiency in public health institutions and meet the needs of multilevel health services, private hospitals have undergone rapid development in recent years.

(2) Trends of Development in Health Policies

1. Pursuit of Fair Efficiency Goals   The health economic policies of all countries are centered on improving the equality and efficiency of health services, ensuring the fair allocation of health services, and maintaining the stable operation of the health economy. The vast majority of developed countries regard healthcare services as quasi-public goods, with an emphasis on the government's obligation to provide comprehensive medical services and health coverage for all citizens. Guidelines have also been formulated with the aim of both effectively financing and containing healthcare costs in order to maintain coordinated socioeconomic development.

2. Organic Combination of Planned Regulation and Market Regulation   In countries that implement universal health insurance and private health insurance systems, there is a trend of strengthened government intervention and planning in the health sector. Countries implementing national health service systems, by contrast, are undergoing reforms to introduce internal markets, thereby making using of market competition to positively impact efficiency.

3. Combination of Macro Control and Micro Autonomy   The governments of all countries implementing a universal health insurance system have stipulated that total health spending should maintain a relationship of coordinated development with national economic development (Germany) or the economic development of each province (Canada). These governments have reinforced their control over and regulation of the total budget for the long-term development and daily operations of hospitals while also preserving the hospitals' independence and autonomy. The governments' regulation of the actions of physicians also involves a combination of total income control and independent practice. An important measure in the reform of the UK's National Health Service is management decentralization, which permits the independent operation of certain large public hospitals according to market principles.

4. Legalization of Health Policies   The implementation, adjustment, and reform of health policies in developed countries all take the form of legislation, which is both authoritative and mandatory. In 1881, the German government enacted the world's first legal framework for the implementation of mandatory health insurance, which clearly stipulates the rights and obligations of all levels of government and all involved parties. After World War II, the legislature enacted a number of relevant laws and regulations. In 1983–1986, the German government passed five bills for the containment of healthcare costs alone. Thereafter, the Health Care Reform Act was enacted in 1988, followed by the Health Care Structure Act in 1993. These laws and regulations ensured that the German health security system became the most coherent part of the overall economy. The legalization of health policies can better reflect a country's long-term goals. The debates involved in the legislative process can help to prevent policy loopholes, reinforce all parties' understanding of the policy, and allow coordination among different sectors, thereby facilitating the comprehensive implementation of the policies.

5. Scientific Decision-Making in Health Economics   Increasing attention has been paid to the analysis and evaluation of the costs, benefits, and effects of policies in the decision-making processes of the health economies in developed countries. Extensive cost–benefit analyses have been conducted in these countries to prevent the excessive growth of advanced but expensive technical services nationwide. At first, such services are limited to a few major medical centers that employ specialists and have high utilization rates. The use of these services is usually concentrated in teaching hospitals. It is only when a given technology is perfected and becomes a basic part of modern medicine (e.g., diagnostic imaging) that it is allowed to be widely used throughout these countries. However, the use of these services is still funded through government budget allocations. The continual improvements in the methods for the analysis and evaluation of health economics have gradually expanded their scope of application.

2. Major Health Economic Reforms in Developed Countries and Areas

The development of the health industry, advances in medical science and technology, population aging, and improvements in living and educational standards have led to a corresponding increase in the public's healthcare needs. The health insurance costs of developed countries underwent rapid growth in the 1950s, and the pace of growth accelerated further in the late 1960s. From 1960 to 1975, the share of healthcare costs as a percentage of gross national product (GNP) increased from 4.8% to 8.4% in Germany, from 5.5% to 7.4% in Canada, from 5.3% to 8.6% in the US, and from 4.7% to 8.0% in Sweden. In the late 1990s, total healthcare spending accounted for 7.1% of GDP in the UK, 10.5% of GDP in Germany, 9.8% of GDP in France, and 14.3% of GDP in the US. By 2011, total healthcare spending had increased to 9.4% of GDP in the UK, 11.6% of GDP in France, and 17.7% of GDP in the US. This surge in healthcare costs has placed serious pressure on developed countries, and cost containment has become a common priority of health policies in all countries.

In addition to these objective reasons, the surge in costs is also related to the health insurance system itself. Due to the third-party payment system adopted by health insurance providers and the government, there is an absence of cost awareness among patients and physicians. This lack of awareness leads to unnecessary health demand and excessive health provision by hospitals and physicians, which stimulates the increase in healthcare costs. Countries have generally come to recognize the adverse consequences of the fee-for-service system. Starting in the mid-1970s, and especially after 1980, countries began to adopt a number of policies and measures with the aim of controlling costs. These policies and measures regulated both the supply and demand of healthcare.

(1) Adjustment of Short-Term Provision Policy

1. Reform Pricing Methods and the Implementation of Price Controls In countries implementing a national health service system, the government allocates funds to hospitals and GPs, and residents have free access to services. Hence, the provision of health services is not regulated by price signals. In countries implementing universal health insurance or private health insurance systems, charges for health services are jointly set by healthcare providers, and the prices set according to market demand tend to be relatively high. To control costs, these countries have modified this pricing method by implementing unified government pricing or negotiated pricing between healthcare providers and insurers.

In 1982, to contain healthcare costs, the US government enacted price control laws and regulations, which required hospitals and physicians to charge patients entitled to Medicare and Medicaid at government-prescribed prices (about 75% of conventional prices) or else reimbursements would not be issued. Consequently, the costs of Medicare and Medicaid could be controlled to a certain extent. However, these regulations also caused physicians to discriminate against patients with price limits, leading to the transfer of costs from price-limited to non-price-limited patients, which increased the healthcare costs of the latter. As a result, certain state governments mandated that hospitals should implement price control policies for all patients.

Germany, France, and Canada have formulated unified nationwide fee schedules for physicians. Canada also began to prohibit physicians from charging additional fees in 1984. Japan has even more stringent price control policies in place. All health insurance services must be charged according to the unified national point-based pricing system, and this system applies to all levels of healthcare institutions and clinics and to all physicians. As a result, all insurance agencies are required to pay all physicians according to the same fee standards, and individual agreed-upon rates are not permitted. Any changes to the fee standards must be made by the Central Social Security Council in the Ministry of Health and Welfare.

Drug prices are also strictly controlled in developed countries. Research and practice have shown that implementing uniform price controls is often more effective than only controlling part of prices. However, price controls may also stimulate providers to increase service provision to make up for the corresponding economic losses. Hence, price controls alone are still insufficient.

2. Reform of Hospital Payment Systems and Implementing Different Forms of Prepayment Systems   The cost of inpatient services consumes nearly half of the health resources in all countries. Among Organisation for Economic Co-operation and Development (OECD) countries, hospitalization costs account for about 60% of public health expenditures. All countries recognize that inpatient services are the costliest part of satisfying health needs, but not all services are indispensable. Thus, reducing expenditures on inpatient services is a common goal among all countries.

Countries with a national health service (NHS) have modified the budget allocation for hospitals from a fee-for-service system to a global budget (Australia) or a fixed budget (UK), which requires hospitals to operate within the limits of the budget. Strengthening budget constraints is more effective in controlling the rise in hospital costs.

Many countries with universal health insurance, such as Canada, Germany, France, and the Netherlands, have also changed their hospital payment systems by referencing the NHS countries and implementing a global budget system to replace existing payment systems based on lengths of hospital stays or services provided. This shift is because, under pay-per-diem or fee-for-service systems, hospitals are more willing to allow longer hospital stays for patients and do not provide strict treatments. In 1986, Germany began implementing a flexible budget that prescribes hospitals with a fixed number of inpatient days. Those hospitals that delivered fewer than the fixed number of inpatient days were rewarded, whereas those that exceeded that fixed number were punished. The global budget system requires hospitals to provide all necessary services to a specific population within a given budget and to absorb all losses and profits. Hence, this system encourages hospitals to reduce service costs and increase efficiency. According to OECD data, hospitals that implement global budgets have 13% higher cost-containment capabilities than those of hospitals that do not implement global budgets. A study in the US estimated that the global budget system can reduce inflation-adjusted healthcare expenditures by 9–17%.

The US introduced an alternative approach. In 1983, the federal government implemented the diagnosis-related group (DRG)-based payment system for Medicare patients, which pays hospitals according to predetermined rates for disease groups. This system is able to incentivize hospitals to reduce the service cost of each case and shorten the duration of hospital stays. DRGs have a significant effect on containing Medicare's hospitalization costs. In order to prevent the costs of implementing DRGs from being transferred to inpatients under private insurance, the inpatient costs for private insurance were also controlled. The US began to study the DRG system in 1984. Pilot projects were gradually implemented, and the system was widely promoted over the course of 20 years, which achieved good results. Although the number of cases increased by 18.5% from 1990 to 2006, the average length of a hospital stay decreased by 5.8 days, and the number of beds was reduced by 144,000 (21%). In 1987, the US implemented the DRG-based payment system nationwide. The main advantage of the DRG-based system is that it combines compensation for providers with the service volume determined by the features of diagnosis groups, which encourages providers to contain the costs of each case, rationally utilize treatments and drugs, and reduce the consumption of service resources. The disadvantages are that it requires extensive statistical data to measure the treatment costs for each level of each disease group. Providers are also more likely to select patients with milder conditions within a given disease group or to exaggerate the disease severity of their patients to obtain greater financial profits, which increases the management costs. Despite these shortcomings, however, the implementation of DRGs has led to significant effects. Hence, Europe and Japan have also begun investigating and piloting DRGs.

3. Changing the Remuneration Methods and Limiting the Reimbursement Level for Physicians   Physicians are health service providers and agents in health service consumption. Physician behaviors determine the efficiency of health expenditures to a large extent. As traditional payment methods can stimulate a rise in costs, many countries have changed the payment methods for their health service expenditures. In Italy, the capitation or salary system was implemented to replace the fee-for-service system. In France, the method of salary compensation for new physicians specifies that the salaries of specialists should increase together with GDP per capita. In Germany, a global budget system is implemented for the total service costs of all physicians affiliated with the German Medical Association, and each physician is paid according to service volume. This type of compensation mechanism encourages physicians to collectively control the total costs of services and ensures the mutual supervision of physicians, as any increase in service volume will lead to a reduction in the compensation of service units. This measure enabled a continuous decline in the average incomes of clinic physicians from 6.5 times the average wage in 1971 to 3.5 times the average wage in 1988.

Based on 10 years of research, the research group headed by William C. Hsiao of Harvard University has proposed the resource-based relative value scale (RBRVS), which is a new remuneration method for physician services. The US has been piloting the RBRVS since 1992. The fee standards for each specialty are adjusted according to the relative values of the actual costs of each specialty service (including physicians' time and labor intensity, practice costs, and opportunity costs for specialist training). Moreover, in order to contain the excessive service volume experienced by physicians, an expenditure target system is imposed on the total cost of physician services – that is, the growth rate is controlled. This evaluation system was successfully piloted in the US in 1992, and it has now become one of the measures adopted by the US to curb the rise in healthcare costs. Moreover, it has been applied in the US, Germany, Canada, and Japan for many years.

4. Peer Review of Services and Supervision of Service Use   The governments of many countries have appointed experts to perform regular examinations of physicians' behaviors in order to limit overtreatment or overprescription by hospitals and physicians through medical supervision. This practice helps to eliminate costly but ineffective or equally effective treatments and control the provision of health services while also ensuring quality. Denmark, Germany, Spain, France, Ireland, Portugal, and the UK have already formulated pharmaceutical regulations. In 1989, Germany imposed a statutory upper limit on drug costs, and the UK set an indicative budget for GP prescriptions to regulate physicians' prescribing behavior.

Belgium, Germany, France, and the Netherlands have implemented codes of medical conduct, but that of the Netherlands only targets specialists. Belgium, Spain, Luxembourg, and France have developed procedures for medical schemas, which involve comparing the materials provided by hospitals during the healthcare compensation process with predetermined standards for healthcare behaviors according to schemas, which are established based on specialty types to reflect medical activities and prescriptions. The Regional Medical Associations in Germany require physicians with 10% higher prescription costs than the average to provide a statement of reasons to a review committee. This group has also developed a system of penalties with different provisions for suggestions, advice, warnings, and fines. Recently, German sickness funds have been approved to hire physicians to investigate suspected fraudulent behavior.

In 1972, the US passed laws related to the review of professional standards and created Professional Standards Review Organizations (PSROs). PSROs frequently conduct random audits of physicians in hospitals to examine their prescription and treatment behaviors and whether their utilization rates are excessively high, thereby encouraging physicians to reduce waste. Research shows that PSROs do not reduce the service volume of physicians, as medical peers tend to protect each other during mutual audits.

The hospital insurance scheme in Canada frequently conducts unified analyses of various hospital services in the provinces in order to understand diagnosis and service volumes of inpatient services for various diseases and the length and cost of hospitalizations. These analyses can be used to prepare hospital budgets and control the cost of inpatient services. The hospital insurance scheme also reviews the service quality of hospitals and requires each hospital to retain complete medical records. The hospital insurance scheme then enters the medical records into a computer to analyze and evaluate the quality of inpatient services. If incomplete or erroneous medical records are found, the responsible parties are informed and asked to reflect on their mistakes. If malpractice is found, penalties ranging from warnings to fines are imposed according to the level of severity. This form of immediate control is effective in limiting physician-induced demand and controlling medical incidents.

(2) Adjustment of Long-Term Provision Policy

1. Controlling the Scale of Hospital Infrastructure and Valuable Equipment and Planning Resource Allocation Based on Regional Health Developments   In the past, investments in new hospital buildings and equipment were decided and funded by the owners of the hospitals in all countries. However, at present, in the majority of countries with mandatory universal health insurance systems and in those with NHS systems, capital investments for hospitals are directly controlled by the government and are funded primarily through government budget allocations (including private hospitals).

Although there are significant variations in the hospital sectors of countries in the European Community (EC), all of them adopt the principle of regionalization in the planning of provincial or regional healthcare institutions and facilities. Doing so enables them to avoid unnecessary duplications in healthcare institutions and costly technologies. In the UK, Sweden, and other countries that implement an NHS, government budget allocation is combined with healthcare network policies, and these countries currently have the most reasonable geographical distribution of health resources in the world.

In France, the Hospital Reform Act of 1970 set out a relatively detailed system for the planning and management of technologies. Under this law, the French Ministry of Health prescribes the maximum equipment-to-population ratio for specific items, including dialysis machines, linear accelerators, and CT scanners. Germany has implemented hospital planning since 1972. However, local governments failed to carry out these plans seriously and instead encouraged the expansion of hospitals, which led to excess health resources and vacant bed spaces. The 1985 Hospital Financing Act stipulated that the infrastructure costs of all hospitals would be funded by the federal budget but that only hospitals authorized according to hospital capacity planning would receive federal budget funding. In accordance with the Health Care Act of 1989, Germany established the Equipment Committee to reduce duplications in the purchase of equipment. Currently, all hospital hardware investments in Germany are completely controlled by the government. In the Netherlands, Article 18 of the Hospital Supply Act authorizes the Ministry of Health to grant permits for the quantity of high-tech services. This article aims to limit the quantity of high-tech equipment to improve service efficiency and quality.

A key feature in the hospital budget of the Canadian government is the separation between daily operational expenditures and capital investments. Procurement of new equipment by hospitals must be submitted to the Provincial Ministry of Health for approval in order to request funding. Lower-level hospitals that intend to expand their size, increase capacity, or introduce new technologies and equipment must be strictly vetted by the provincial Medicare system regardless of whether these hospitals have raised funds from individual and community donations or are directly applying for investments from the government. Newly added services that have not been vetted will not be subsidized, and the Medicare system will not adjust its budget to accommodate the unvetted service capacity. By law, Medicare administers the planning, scales, and levels of all provincial hospitals, which are divided into three tiers: general hospitals, regional hospitals, and urban health centers. Medicare has the authority to approve the renewal of equipment, the expansion of beds, and the replacement of fixed assets in each hospital. Therefore, hospital development in each province is planned according to a three-tier allocation criterion that strictly controls the introduction of costly and advanced technological capabilities in general hospitals and concentrates high-tech medical equipment in regional health centers. General and regional hospitals are allowed to use these expensive technologies and this equipment in the health centers. This practice enables resource sharing and prevents hospitals from blindly introducing technology, which can lead to low utilization rates, the waste of health resources, and even induced utilization.

Practice has shown that Canada has achieved excellent results in using economic instruments to regulate the scale and speed of hospital development. From the 1940s to the late 1960s, the US government attempted to promote hospital planning by providing states with funding according to the population size and per capita income of each region in order to invest in new hospitals and beds, thereby promoting the modernization of hospitals. However, since no parties were willing to abandon the principles of the free market, this measure ultimately did not succeed. In the 1970s, the US passed the more stringent certificate of need (CON) laws. These laws stipulate that all hospitals that need to purchase instruments and equipment worth more than US$100,000 must be reviewed and approved by the Health Planning Commission under the supervision of the municipal government (composed of local medical and nonmedical personnel). The aim of these laws is to control the rise in costs due to the overacquisition of equipment and beds. Studies have shown that

CON laws have virtually no impact on hospital costs and equipment investment but can provide control over the increase in hospital beds. Areas implementing CON laws reduced the number of hospital beds but not the total asset value of hospitals. Therefore, in 1984, Congress repealed the mandatory enforcement of these laws. On the one hand, the failure of CON laws was due to their imperfect nature, as they were only limited to the addition of hospitals, equipment, and beds and therefore still gave hospitals and private practitioners room to maneuver. On the other hand, since the decision-making for and financing of large-scale hospital equipment and the compensation mechanism of the fee-for-service system had remained unchanged, hospitals still had the impulse to invest. This situation is unlike those in countries such as Canada and Germany, where a unified third party (e.g., the government) invests in infrastructure and large equipment and controls service fees in order to regulate the long-term development of hospitals.

Japan has not intervened in hospital development and the acquisition of large-scale equipment in the past. As a result, Japan had the highest number of CT scans per capita and an oversupply of equipment. Japan's recent Health Care System Reform Law has set the ceiling for hospital beds in all districts. It has also proposed the shared utilization of expensive equipment and facilities and the liberalization of state hospitals.

Government control over investments in hospital infrastructure and equipment may lead to shortages and queues for certain expensive treatments in some countries. However, it also reduces waste caused by uncontrolled development and duplications in acquisition, thereby improving the utilization efficiency of limited resources.

2. Adjusting the Priorities of Health Services　In 1978, the WHO proposed the goal of "Health for All by the Year 2000 A.D." and formulated the Primary Health Care global strategy, which played an active role in promoting the identification of new priorities in health services.

In the late 1980s, faced by the challenges of increasing population aging and a changing disease spectrum, countries gradually began stepping up their adjustments to long-term healthcare provision policies in order to control healthcare costs. The related policies include revising inpatient medical services and emphasizing primary healthcare, nursing homes, day services, and home care services. From 1980 to 1988, the number of hospital beds in EC countries decreased by 30,000. At present, all countries are seeking stricter inpatient medical planning. Some countries, such as the US, have adopted the 3H policy, namely, home care, health service, and hospice, to deal with the increase in hospital beds by transferring hospital work to these intermediate facilities. Therefore, outpatient services, daytime surgery, and home care services have shown an increasing trend in all countries. In the US, the surge in healthcare costs has led to significant changes in healthcare organizations and their use of funds. Organizations such as HMOs, which focus more on preventive and primary healthcare, experienced rapid growth in the 1980s. Health promotion, disease prevention, and healthcare became the direction of development for US health services in the 1990s. The Public Commission of the Ministry of Health and Social Affairs in Sweden has developed a new, reformed health system that shifts the focus of healthcare from hospital treatment to primary healthcare and prevention. In Australia, public health and preventive healthcare have been garnering greater attention, and the role of the federal government is gradually expanding. To achieve the goal of Primary Healthcare for All by 2000, the government formulated a set of national primary healthcare goals and strategies. The federal government has also increased spending on prevention, healthcare, and education to promote research and personnel training for public health and preventive healthcare. In addition, many countries have also restricted the number of enrollments in medical schools. Japan has even conducted research on the most appropriate proportion of physicians.

(3) Adjustment of Health Security Policies

During the wave of free healthcare in the 1960s, the concept of patients sharing the costs of healthcare was gradually eroded. At present, in addition to making more effective policy adjustments in health service provision, countries have also turned to controlling the demand for health services as an important aspect of policy adjustments to curb the surge in healthcare spending.

1. Widespread Implementation of Cost-Sharing Systems   To strengthen the cost awareness of patients and reduce consumption, countries began widely implementing different forms of patient costsharing. A common practice is to increase the share of copayments by patients. In 1983, Japan abolished free elderly healthcare, and cost-sharing was implemented. In 1984, Japan introduced the partial sharing of healthcare costs by insured persons with salary income. Sweden implements a copayment scheme for healthcare expenses that sets a maximum value paid by patients for each prescription and does not require patients to pay the costs for clinic visits beyond 15 visits per year. In Norway, a patient's out-of-pocket expenses cannot exceed an annual ceiling, and copayments are primarily spent on drugs and dental care. In Denmark and Sweden, this ceiling is equivalent to a certain percentage of medication costs; in Germany, the Netherlands, and the UK, a fixed rate is charged in the form of prescription fees. The results in different countries have shown that the costsharing approach can have an impact on curbing patient overdemand to a certain extent. However, aside from genuinely low-income groups, many people pay for their shared costs using private health insurance, which influences the effects of costsharing.

2. Redefining the Scope of Mandatory Health Insurance   Countries generally distinguish between reimbursable and nonreimbursable drugs under mandatory health insurance. In 1982, Ireland developed a list of controlled drugs and was planning to formulate a list of reimbursed drugs. In 1983, Germany's statutory health insurance canceled the compensation of low-cost drugs. In 1985, the UK NHS stipulated that nonprescription drugs would no longer be covered. Belgium, Denmark, Italy, the Netherlands, and Portugal all developed lists of reimbursable prescription drugs to control the rise in healthcare costs.

Many countries changed the benefits provided and removed certain secondary benefits. Germany required both mandatory health insurance and private healthcare to guarantee basic health coverage. Certain secondary benefits were removed, and more preventive benefits were added, such as health check-ups for different age groups. Since 1985, the UK NHS no longer compensates adults for prescription eyeglasses, and it discontinued free dental and eye examinations as of 1988.

Through the implementation of these various policies and measures, different outcomes were achieved in controlling healthcare costs in different countries. The growth in healthcare costs was slower in the 1980s than in the 1970s. By the mid-1990s, the healthcare costs of the UK, Canada, Germany, and Japan began increasing at a stable rate and kept pace with GDP growth. In general, countries implementing an NHS had more effective cost containment than countries with universal health insurance. Among countries with universal health insurance, the most effective cost containment can be found in Canada, where the system is government financed, and in Japan, which implements uniform national fee standards. In the US, which is predominated by private health insurance, the local effects of cost containment are significant, such as, for example, shortening hospital stays and reducing costs for Medicare and Medicaid patients. However, the overall increase in national health spending remains high due to the transfer of healthcare costs from inpatient to outpatient services and from Medicare and Medicaid patients to other patients.

3. Exploration of Private Financing Initiatives

(1) Background to the Implementation of Private Financing Initiatives

The UK has implemented the NHS system for more than 60 years, and the main source of healthcare expenditures is national tax revenues. Although its share of GDP is below the EU average and is far lower than that of the US, it is also facing pressures from the continuous increase in national healthcare demand and growing healthcare costs. In the past 20 years, the UK has continually implemented policies to control and reduce hospital beds and avoid the stimulation of consumption in order to contain the growth of healthcare costs. Currently, the total number of beds in its 1,200 hospitals (of which 96% are public) is 190,000, and the number of beds per 1,000 people has been reduced to 27–30. Although hospitals have adapted to the shortage of beds by reducing the average length of stay, such as, for example, by reducing the average length of stay in public hospitals to six days, which is the lowest level in history, the waiting time for hospitalization has continued to increase. Hence, the problem of difficult access to hospitals has not been solved and is becoming increasingly prominent, which has led to strong societal dissatisfaction. In addition, the buildings and facilities of public hospitals are generally relatively old, as they cannot be updated in a timely manner. Hence, hospitals with buildings that have been in use for more than 10 years account for 83% of all hospitals. A large number of hospitals are urgently in need of expansion, and the addition of more beds is also required to satisfy patients' needs. The cost of new hospitals and building maintenance in the NHS capital building program has exceeded £1.7 billion and is expected to reach £3 billion in the next few years. The substantial funding gap and limited public finances have led to difficulties in satisfying the funding required to build a large number of hospitals and rapidly improve medical treatment by increasing public investment in the short term.

In contrast, the private sector in the UK possesses a large amount of idle funds and is keen to invest in the construction of public hospitals, which will provide a stable long-term return on earnings. With regard to the private sector's intentions, the UK government has adopted a willingness to introduce funds via the mechanisms of market competition under government administration while also drawing on private sector management practices to improve the public-sector performance of the government. This new market-based model of government administration is known as New Public Administration and focuses on transforming the government with market mechanisms, reshaping the government with entrepreneurship, encouraging competition, emphasizing results and performance, valuing consumer choice, and emphasizing efficiency.

The emergence of this new model of government administration is closely linked to the development of economic theories since the 1970s and especially with new institutional economics. The three major components of new institutional economics – public choice theory, principal-agent theory, and transaction cost economics – are precisely the knowledge foundation of New Public Administration. Starting with Thatcher's administration, the UK government has been actively attracting private institutions to invest in public infrastructure projects, such as schools, hospitals, roads, and waterworks. The private finance initiative (PFI), known also to some as public-private partnerships (PPP), is one such model and is primarily used for hospitals. The PFI mainly involves four components. First, private institutions invest in the construction of public hospitals. The ownership of the hospital building then belongs to the private investors for a certain period of time, and the hospital pays the investors a fixed fee every year. Second, in addition to investing in construction, the investor is also responsible for building repairs and maintenance and for providing the hospital with logistics support. Third, upon the expiration of the PFI term, the ownership of the building belongs to the hospital, and the hospital is no longer required to pay a fee to the private sector. Fourth, this length of this term is generally between 20 and 30 years. The amount invested and the annual fee payments are determined by negotiations among the investors, hospital, and government.

(2) Implementation Methods for Private Finance Initiatives

After the UK government opted for PFI, a large segment of public hospital construction was set aside for the introduction of private investment, which resolved the urgent need for funding, transferred the risk of investment, and accelerated the pace of construction. The NHS proposed the construction, renovation, and expansion of 100 hospitals and the addition of 7,000 beds by 2010, of which the construction operating under PFI will account for two-thirds of the total. By 2009, 8 newly built hospitals were already operating under the PFI model, 20 PFI projects had been approved, and nearly 50 projects were currently under review. The UK government hopes to break through the single model of public investment in public hospitals through the intervention of private capital. By introducing market mechanisms and advanced management and operations models in public hospitals, private methods can be used to change and improve the operating efficiency and business culture of public hospitals. This practice will drive the mechanisms of change, enhance business awareness, reduce cost, and enhance efficiency. The government also hopes that the PFI mechanism can overcome the widespread shortcomings of public investment, including budget overruns, late project completion, and inflexible mechanisms, thereby reinforcing the cost control of construction projects and improving construction quality.

To achieve this aim, the UK government has allowed private investors an annual return on investment of up to 20% in current PFI hospital construction projects. By subsidizing the cost of land replacement in relocation projects, the method of spending money to procure mechanisms is used to alter the culture and environment in which private institutions cannot participate in public hospitals and to change the traditional scenario in which hospitals are unable to reduce costs, reduce beds, or improve efficiency.

In the implementation of PFI, the government clearly defines the mode of operation and, hence, remains an important party that plays a leading role. The government regulations mainly include the following five components.

1. Consider Four Principles and Issues　All parties should abide by the following four principles. (1) Hospitals must clarify the purpose of the funds introduced and the method of repayment. (2) Investors must provide suitable projects and adequate services. (3) Both physicians and nurses must have the opportunity to participate in project design. (4) Investors must clarify the purpose of the investment. Issues that the investors and hospitals should consider include costs, repayment, partnerships, the utilization rate, risk transfer, the management culture, and management efficiency.

2. Establish Special Bodies and Clarify the Responsibilities of all Parties A special body should be established for each PFI project. This body is usually a board or committee that is responsible for the management, coordination, and implementation of the entire project. The board (committee) should consist of all parties involved in the PFI, including project investors, construction companies, the NHS, hospital operators, medical staff representatives, and community representatives. The relocation of the Royal Infirmary of Edinburgh is a PFI project commissioned by the Lothian University Hospitals Trust and designed and constructed by the Royal Infirmary of Edinburgh. The investor was the Consort Healthcare Consortium, and the facility manger was Haden Construction Limited. A special body consisting of 53 members was created for this project and was responsible for implementing the entire relocation project. Of these members, 39 were elected by hospital staff and included physicians, nurses, representatives of pharmaceutical companies, board members of Lothian University Hospitals Trust, and project members. The special body also included 14 external members, including representatives of NHS Lothian (where the hospital was located), GPs, and representatives of other NHS trusts. A professional project manager was solely responsible for the operations of this body.

PFI projects emphasize the use of contracts to clarify the responsibilities of all parties. As these projects last for 20–30 years and involve the interests of multiple parties, it is especially important to define the relationships among all parties and for all parties to fulfil their responsibilities. Hence, it is necessary to use contracts to establish the rights and responsibilities of all parties and to determine the funding sources and operational methods.

3. Implement Rigorous Project Actuarial Control In the UK, new hospitals generally take about 12 years to recover their investments and only begin to make profits in the thirteenth year. The fees paid by the hospital to the investor within the 20- to 30-year term are also related to the investment costs. Therefore, in infrastructure projects, both the investors and the hospitals try to minimize construction costs while ensuring quality in order to protect their own interests. Hence, both parties try to complete the project and begin hospital operations as soon as possible. In contrast, government-financed construction projects often have massive budget overruns and late completions. For PFI projects, rigorous project actuarial control ensures that construction costs are strictly controlled and that progress is clearly defined, which effectively prevents the overruns and late completions that are common in public investment projects. A hospital redevelopment project that involved a relocation from the city center to the outskirts and a building area of 100,000 square meters was originally projected to take at least 10 years under public financing. Moreover, late completion and overruns above 10% were almost inevitable. However, as a PFI project, the actuarial control meant that the entire project was completed in only four years, and the rigorous actuarial control also effectively constrained construction costs. The infrastructure costs of projects under PFI have been reduced by an average of 10%.

4. Bundle Investor Returns with Hospital Benefits After delivering the completed hospital for use, investors are still required to set aside sufficient maintenance funds for building repairs and maintenance and the provision of logistics support services such as hospital cleaning and catering. If normal hospital operations are affected due to the quality of construction, the returns obtained by the investors from the hospitals will be affected, and maintenance costs will increase. As investors' interests are closely related to building quality and hospital operations, the investors will avoid cutting corners during construction to protect their interests. Thus, the mechanisms in place effectively ensure the construction quality of hospitals. Construction engineering error rates have dropped by 20% among completed PFI projects.

5. Introduce Market Mechanisms and Efficient Management Models in Hospitals The requirement that hospitals pay an annual fee to their investors invigorates their business motivation and encourages them to introduce private-sector management models with the aim of reducing operating costs and improving efficiency. As an example, in one hospital relocation project, the hospital attempted to reduce costs by decreasing the number of beds from 1,200 to 857 and by trying to reduce the number of healthcare workers. The latter was achieved by not recruiting new physicians when senior physicians retired and sharing the workload among existing physicians. Moreover, part of the workload previously carried out by physicians was transferred to nurses, and part of the nurses' workload (e.g., delivering meals) was transferred to medical support staff. Despite the reduced number of beds and staff, hospital efficiency did not decline and instead improved, with significant increases in hospital bed turnover and utilization rates. Thus, we can see that the implementation of PFI has begun to introduce market competition mechanisms and advanced private-sector management models in public hospitals. This change has smoothly transformed the operating mechanisms of public hospitals and has improved the efficiency of operational management.

Under NHS planning, some of the hospitals relocated under the PFI have also reestablished their functional orientations. The service model has transitioned toward a newly emerging healthcare model in which the focus of service has shifted from inpatient services to daytime services and from secondary to primary healthcare. This shift has also led to the concentration of staff, expert, and equipment advantages; a reduction in the number of beds; and decreased costs, thereby ensuring that hospital resources can be more fully utilized.

(3) Effects of Implementing Private Finance Initiatives

To the UK government, the introduction of PFI made up for the shortcomings of public finances and enabled the government to achieve its goal of building and renovating public hospitals within a short period of time, thereby effectively adapting to the public's increasing demand for health services. In addition, it has also shifted the risk of investing in hospitals from the sole responsibility of the government to the shared responsibility of the government and private institutions. To the hospitals, the need to pay fees to private institutions has stimulated their business motivation and, thus, has encouraged them to convert mechanisms and improve efficiency. As for private investors, investing in new hospitals will lead to long-term, stable, and relatively high returns on investment. Therefore, by bundling the interests of investors with those of hospitals, PFI has achieved a triple-win effect. By controlling the appropriate proportions on a macroeconomic scale and emphasizing project actuarial control on a microeconomic scale, the UK government has made comprehensive improvements to the medical environment within a short period of time. The introduction of efficient management models and culture from the private sector into hospitals has facilitated the conversion of mechanisms, reduced costs, and increased efficiency.

SECTION II. FEATURES AND REFORM TRENDS OF HEALTH SYSTEMS IN DEVELOPING COUNTRIES

1. Features and Reforms of Health Systems in Asian Countries

It is widely known that the health system and security of any country are based on that country's specific social and political systems, level of economic development, and traditional cultural background, along with the influence of certain theoretical guidance.

In other words, the selection of health and security system models is constrained by multiple factors. There are undoubtedly many inherent logical links between the health and security systems of Asian countries and areas and their political, economic, social, cultural, and other local factors. However, there are also certain similarities among the health and security systems of countries and areas within certain regions. In the course of long-term development, these countries and areas have gradually formed certain key features that deviate from the conventional health system and security models of Europe and America.

(1) Centralized Power and Government Backing

Taking a broad view of the health management systems of developing countries reveals that these systems are mainly characterized by a centralized health administration, as the central governments of all countries have set up health administration departments that directly manage healthcare. At the same time, we can observe from the development trajectories of health security systems that the development of these systems is guided by the establishment and improvement of the systems together with exploration to improve management and service efficiency, thereby meeting the basic needs of coverage for the population. Thailand is a developing country in Asia, and its government attaches great importance to the equality of health security. In the 1970s, it began establishing a medical assistance system. In the 1980s, it implemented the Health Card system in rural areas and established a health security system that included preventive projects through enrollment in voluntary household contributions and government subsidies. In 2001, the 30-Baht Scheme, which aimed to establish a health insurance scheme with universal coverage, was implemented. Vietnam emphasizes poverty alleviation and social equality in guaranteeing healthcare. The government is trying to improve healthcare services to help the poor by implementing policies on hospital partial fees, free healthcare for the poor, and public health service support for the poor. The Philippines is a newly emerging democracy and is currently undergoing reforms in its health economic management system. Its health provision system includes the public and private sectors, and the private sector occupies a dominant position, especially in urban areas. In rural areas, the healthcare institutions are mainly government-run, and a provincial responsibility system is implemented to reinforce the authority and obligations of the local governments in rural health administration. In the early 1980s, the Indian government had already formulated the gradual establishment of a three-tier healthcare network in rural areas, which included healthcare subcenters, primary health centers, and community health centers. This network was intended to provide health services to the vast majority of the poor. India has also established various public health systems, such as the universal immunization program and the free treatment program in public hospitals, in order to ensure that vulnerable groups, especially the vast majority of farmers, have access to basic health security. China has also adopted certain aid measures for low-income and vulnerable social groups, such as the Minimum Living Standard Scheme, but overall support is not strong, especially in health security. With regard to difficult populations, vulnerable groups, rural residents, and certain groups with large healthcare costs and excessive personal burdens, there has been an increasing pace of research and the establishment of a social medical assistance system together with increased investment in special health insurance funds.

(2) Diverse Health Financing, Mainly Based on Personal Taxes

India's health financing mainly comes from the government and individuals. There are three levels of government health investment, which includes the central, state, and local governments; the state and local governments undertake three quarters of investment, and the central government undertakes one quarter of investment. Funding comes primarily from taxes, nontax revenues, and premiums from two social insurance schemes, the Employees' State Insurance Scheme and the Central Government Health Scheme. The source of health financing in Thailand also comes mainly from government taxes and individuals according to the scheme involved. One such example is the Civil Servant Medical Benefit Scheme, which provides free medical coverage to civil servants and their relatives. Currently, this scheme covers 6.6 million people, accounting for more than 10% of the total population. The funds come from national taxes and are administered by the Ministry of Finance. The second scheme is the health insurance provided by the Social Security Scheme. This insurance is a type of mandatory insurance that provides insured persons with non-work-related illness, disability, and death insurance. This scheme is financed by the Social Security Fund, which consists of contributions from employees, employers, and the government (each paying 1% of the employee's salary). The third is the health insurance provided by the Workers' Compensation Scheme, which is similar to work injury insurance. It provides insured persons with work-related illness, disability, and death insurance and is funded by the health insurance under the Social Security Scheme. The health insurance systems under both the Social Security Scheme and the Workers' Compensation Scheme are administered by the Social Security Office under Thailand's Ministry of Labor and Welfare. These two schemes currently cover 4.8 million people, accounting for 8% of Thailand's total population. China has confirmed that the responsibility of health security should be shared among the government, society, families, and individuals. The "Opinions of the CPC Central Committee and the State Council on Deepening the Reform of the Medical and Health Care System (No.6 [2009] of the CPC Central Committee)" clearly defined the health insurance system, which links payments and benefits, as the main body of the health security system and stated that multiple channels should be adopted to finance the purchase of basic health services. In addition, a health and social security model should be established that is consistent with China's current stage of economic development and health service market.

(3) Wide Coverage and Low Level of Social Security

At present, most developing countries in Asia have established health insurance and social security systems that cover urban and rural residents. After giving full consideration to their own characteristics, all countries strive to achieve multilevel, sustainable policies with broad coverage that guarantee the basics. These policies are based on social insurance, social assistance, and social welfare with a focus on basic pensions, basic healthcare, and a minimum living allowance system, and they are supplemented by charity and commercial insurance. These countries aim to consolidate and coordinate health insurance and social security, thereby achieving the sustainable development of the health insurance and social security industries. Although free universal healthcare is available in countries such as Vietnam and India, the emphasis is on wide coverage, and the level of security is relatively low due to limitations in economic development. China has already established various security systems, including the Urban Employees' Basic Endowment Insurance, Basic Medical Insurance, the New Rural Cooperative Medical Scheme, the Urban and Rural Minimum Living Standard Guarantee, medical assistance, and unemployment, work injury, and maternity insurance. In addition, the state has begun piloting the New Rural Endowment Insurance system in order to formulate and implement a voluntary pension scheme that is suitable for low-income, high-mobility migrant workers. China has also accelerated the resolution of health security issues for workers and retirees of businesses facing bankruptcy or difficulties. Furthermore, social security policies have also been implemented for land-expropriated farmers, and the scopes of the Minimum Living Standard Guarantee and medical assistance systems have also been expanded. By improving the unemployment insurance system and the urban and rural social assistance system, China has gradually enhanced the benefits levels of the Rural and Urban Minimum Living Standard Guarantee, the Five Guarantees in Rural Areas, and medical assistance, thereby ensuring the basic living conditions of poor rural and urban households, unemployed and retired workers, and impoverished undergraduates. However, the level of security is relatively low due to the large population and limited financial input.

(4) Late Start and Presence of Differences

Unlike the European health and social security systems, which have more 100 years of history, those of Asian countries and areas generally began developing after World War II. Due to their later starts and shorter histories, their overall levels of development are relatively low. In addition, unlike in developed countries in Europe, where the levels of the health and social security systems usually increase together with that of economic development, the development of health and social security systems in Asian countries and areas (except for Japan) tends to lag behind economic development, especially among developing countries. Thus, the level of social security tends to increase at a slower rate than economic growth does. This slower growth can be partially attributed to historical and cultural traditions as well as to the priority given to economic development. After World War II, Asian countries and areas regarded economic growth as their top priority and invariably chose low-welfare policy orientations that prioritized economic growth. These countries regarded social welfare as a burden on economic growth and believed that high-welfare policy systems would increase the burdens on and production costs of enterprises, which would weaken their global competitiveness and further affect their economic development. This situation is especially prominent in newly industrialized countries, including China, India, and the Philippines. As a result, a phenomenon has occurred in which the economies of these countries have been growing rapidly and their GDPs per capita have approached or reached those of developed countries, but their social security levels have not risen simultaneously with economic growth, and the share of social security expenditure in total government spending is far lower than that of developed countries. Hence, the standards and levels of social security are relatively low in these countries.

2. Features and Reforms of Health Systems in African Countries

(1) Concerns about the Poor

Africa bears one quarter of the global burden of disease but has only approximately 3% of the total global number of healthcare workers. This extreme imbalance is alarming. Millions of people die every day of malaria, tuberculosis, AIDS, and other preventable and treatable diseases throughout sub-Saharan Africa. This region accounts for 11% of the global population. However, when measured by the number of deaths from diseases and premature deaths, this region bears 24% of the global burden of disease. Health spending in this region accounts for less than 1% of the global total. The lack of healthcare workers is partially responsible for this tragedy. Currently, millions of people on the African continent do not have access to healthcare services provided by trained healthcare workers, which has resulted in unnecessary suffering. The crisis is the most serious in sub-Saharan Africa. At least 820,000 physicians, nurses, and midwives need to be added to offer even the most basic healthcare services. To remedy this shortage, most countries in this region must expand the size of their healthcare workforce by 140%. At present, African countries urgently need to formulate a scheme involving the market provision of health insurance and the government provision of partial subsidies. It is understood that Nigeria and Rwanda have already begun implementing a prototype that includes government subsidies and market provision to alleviate the burden of disease and the extreme lack of resources.

(2) Provision of Free Health Security and Assistance

The South African government sets aside a portion of its annual fiscal budget for social assistance for the poor and disabled. In 2000, R47 billion was allocated to assist 8 million people. Based on a national population of 47 million people, the amount per capita is R1,000; based on a population of 8 million, the assistance provided per capita is nearly R6,000. South Africa has adopted a three-tier management model at the central, provincial, and municipal levels. The central level is responsible for unified policy formulation and overall planning as well as for supervising, managing, and assessing whether the distribution of social welfare funds meets the requirements of the central government. The provincial (nine provinces nationwide) and municipal levels are responsible for implementation. The central government created the Department of Social Development mainly to provide social security services to the general population and services for vulnerable, disabled, low-income, and impoverished groups. The Department of Social Development has offices in all nine provinces to coordinate with the local development of social security work. In addition to the Department of Social Development, other governmental departments in South Africa are also involved in providing social security for its citizens. The first is the Department of Health, which is responsible for health and maternity insurance and for improving the residential and living environments of black citizens. The second is the Department of Labor, which is responsible for unemployment benefits; the unemployed are able to receive four to six months of unemployment benefits. The third is the Department of Transport, which is responsible for determining compensation for injuries from traffic accidents. As blacks live in black areas with a high rate of traffic accidents, the Department of Transport is responsible for setting up traffic accident insurance policies.

The South African and Egyptian governments also provide universal public health services, and all citizens can access free medical services in public hospitals. Egyptian law mandates participation in the government's healthcare system and also allows individuals who choose to participate in commercial health insurance to opt out of government health insurance. About 17 million people in Egypt participate in government health insurance. Of this group, the employed population is managed by the Social Insurance Agency under the Department of Labor, and the unemployed population is managed by the Medical Insurance Agency under the Department of Health. Civil servants mainly enroll in government insurance, but they are also free to enroll in insurance not provided by the government (mainly in the for-profit sector). The social security system of Egypt mainly consists of health insurance, work injury insurance, and pension insurance for retirees.

In addition, countries proclaimed by the UN as the least developed countries, such as Sudan and Burundi, have all implemented free universal health systems. The GDP per capita of Sudan in 2001 was US$442; Burundi is even poorer, with a GDP per capita of US$100 in 2003. Burundi, which has a weak economic foundation, implements a system with various levels of free healthcare. Medical assistance and health cards are used. Military personnel are completely exempt, civilians have partially free healthcare, and public officials contribute 10% of their monthly wages to mutual funds (6% from the individuals and

4% from government subsidies). Health cards can be used by an entire household, and card-holders pay 20% of medical expenses.

South Africa provides free, affordable basic healthcare services to all citizens but has yet to establish a clear health insurance system. However, the government has stipulated that all public hospitals have the obligation to provide free treatment to the poor, the elderly, orphans, and the disabled who are unable to pay, and all costs are settled uniformly by the Department of Health. As the fees are low, or even free, they are suitable for low-income households, and about 90% of the national population seeks medical treatment from public hospitals. There are also some civil servants and private business owners who seek medical treatment from private hospitals, and such treatment involves collaboration between the government and private hospitals, where individuals pay one-third of the costs, and companies pay two-thirds of the costs. High-income white people essentially do not seek medical treatment from public hospitals. The government is encouraging the development of commercial insurance. More than a dozen insurance companies throughout the country have introduced pension and health insurance. Premiums are paid by individuals with no government intervention, and the insured persons are essentially all members of high-income groups.

Public hospitals in Egypt provide free basic health security to unemployed persons who are not covered by health insurance. The unemployed can seek medical treatment from hospitals established by the government and managed by the Ministry of Health. The costs are settled by the government using the Health Insurance Fund. Unemployed persons can pay the relevant department to enroll in health insurance and can receive the same medical treatment as employed persons. In addition, the state also provides free basic health security for the unemployed who are not covered by health insurance. The unemployed can seek medical treatment from hospitals established by the government and managed by the Ministry of Health. The healthcare costs are funded by the 4% health fund collected by the government. There is approximately one health center for every three to four villages in rural areas, and these centers provide free services to rural residents.

Other African countries, such as Kenya and Zimbabwe, have also implemented free healthcare systems. In public hospitals, free healthcare is available to both adults and children. In February 1995, Zimbabwe launched the Poverty Alleviation Action Plan, which provides free healthcare to individuals with monthly incomes of less than Z$400. At that time, Zimbabwe's GDP per capita was only US$574.

(3) Encouragement of Commercial Insurance to Improve Security

South Africa has an advanced market economy and developed commercial health insurance. Public hospitals provide low-cost health services to all citizens. The government itself has not established a health insurance system, and this system is mainly operated by commercial insurance, with premiums paid by individuals and employers. Egypt issued a national decree that clearly requires all employed persons to enroll in the national basic health insurance system but also allows individuals or companies with the necessary means to enroll in commercial health insurance. Enrollment in commercial health insurance requires higher premiums than the national level for insurance coverage and implies that individuals do not need to participate in government-run health insurance. Companies or individuals are allowed to choose between government and commercial health insurance. After Egypt opened its economy to investment, the revenues of certain industrial systems, such as oil and banking, increased substantially. Thus, the old social insurance system could no longer meet the needs of some high-income groups, which led to the emergence of commercial insurance. Hospitals were originally all owned by the state. However, hospitals that could provide better services began to appear. After the implementation of economic policies and private ownership, the number of private hospitals rose sharply, and the equipment of certain private hospitals reached or exceeded that of public hospitals. Under these circumstances, some high-income groups began seeking medical treatment from high-end private hospitals. As a result, the consumer population began to increase, and the personal burden of healthcare costs also became very large. Therefore, insurance companies began to intervene in health insurance to compete with national health insurance. It should be noted that Egyptian women who do not participate in the labor force can only be enrolled in commercial insurance. However, upon the death of their husbands, wives can continue to contribute 3% of their husbands' salaries as a premium to enjoy the health insurance benefits previously received by their husbands.

(4) Implementation of the Separation of Prescribing and Dispensing

The healthcare institutions of South Africa and Egypt all implement the separation of prescribing and dispensing. After being diagnosed and treated in a hospital, patients proceed to a pharmacy with a prescription to obtain their prescribed medications. This practice eliminates the use of drug sales to fund hospitals and the abuse of medications. The separation of prescribing and dispensing ensures the stable operation of the health insurance system and also allows the public to enjoy higher-quality health services at lower costs.

3. Features and Reforms of Health Systems in European Countries

(1) Establishing a Social Health Security Model Aligned with Continental Europe

In the 1990s, following the transformation of the socioeconomic system, the healthcare systems of Russia, Hungary, Bulgaria, and other developing countries in Europe also underwent major reforms and changes. Hungary and Bulgaria transitioned from the original public healthcare system to a social health security system, and health financing shifted its main focus to social insurance. The outpatient services in both countries were mainly provided by GPs, and patients were free to choose another GP within six months or a year. The government manages and controls this system through lump sum contracts and specifying the maximum service volume. However, inpatient services are still provided mainly by public hospitals, and the number of private hospitals is still relatively small. Only about 10% of hospitals in Hungary are private, and there are almost no private hospitals in Bulgaria. Russia, on the whole, has inherited the free healthcare policies of the Soviet Union. Its health insurance services cover the basic drugs, medical treatment, and inpatient costs for the vast majority of common diseases. The current health security system in Russia is based primarily on statutory health insurance, which is supplemented by private health insurance. Due to the fundamental changes in the socioeconomic system, the goals of economic restructuring are now to achieve privatization and establish a market economy. However, healthcare reforms are still based on considerations for history and reality. Thus, the trends and goals of reform, which are essentially to establish a social health security model that is aligned with Continental Europe, are relatively clear.

(2) Gradual Progress in Healthcare Reform

Russia, Hungary, Bulgaria, and other countries have applied "shock therapy" to their economic restructuring. However, the difficulty and complexity of reforms in the field of healthcare have necessitated a long period of debate and the promotion of reform. Hence, countries are still relatively cautious in managing the progress of reform. Healthcare has undergone successive reforms since the 1990s, and each reform measure was adjusted according to continuous socioeconomic development. The pace of introducing market mechanisms has also been extremely cautious. Following gradual changes in the healthcare system, the reforms of the health service system all began with general outpatient services, which are more amenable to market regulation, and the role of GPs was introduced through clinic privatization. The public hospital service system has not undergone major changes. Complex medical services and inpatient services are mainly provided by public hospitals. With the development of the health market and the improvement of economic conditions over the past two years, the health service system has begun contemplating the introduction of market mechanisms and social capital. Although fundamental reforms have been undertaken in the security model of healthcare, the emphasis of health services is still on equality and accessibility. In Hungary, the implementation of the social health security system implies that healthcare costs are funded mainly by mandatory social insurance and partially by the government budget. Access to health security does not depend on contributions to premiums, and everyone has access to basic health services. Given the emphasis on social equality, the market factors that can come into play in the field of healthcare are relatively scarce. At present, some countries do not yet have private health insurance funds, and hospitals are primarily public healthcare institutions.

(3) Government Leadership and Market Participation

Following the socioeconomic transition, the governments of Russia, Hungary, and Bulgaria still play a major regulatory role in the field of healthcare. Public hospitals still provide the vast majority of health services. Apart from the services provided by general outpatient clinics, the health services of these countries are mainly provided by public institutions. The governments have strong policy control measures in place. The overall funding level, payment, and adjustment policies for health insurance are all proposed or formulated by the Ministry of Health. As independent legal entities, health insurance funds are only responsible for the specific operations of the funds. In addition, the governments also stipulate a maximum service volume for each healthcare institution and GP to prevent undue competition among healthcare institutions and GPs. Government budgets still account for a high proportion of healthcare expenditures. Apart from mandatory insurance, the government budget still accounts for 20% of total healthcare costs in Hungary and 40% in Bulgaria. Furthermore, the government selects and appoints the directors of public hospitals through a council, thereby maintaining a strong regulatory capacity over public hospitals.

4. Features and Reforms of Health Systems in South American Countries

(1) Emphasis on the Underpinning Role of Public Healthcare Institutions

The governments of Brazil and Argentina mainly depend on public hospitals to implement free universal health systems. Healthcare workers are also guaranteed relatively high levels of benefits. The system mainly relies on ideas, laws, and investment. Mexico's Secretariat of Health, Social Security Administration, and various health security administrative departments all have healthcare institutions under their direct management, and thus form a mutually independent and complementary healthcare system. In Mexico, healthcare is free for insured patients. The healthcare institutions managed by the Social Security

Administration apply budgetary management to separate physicians' incomes and practices. In addition, physicians are permitted to work part-time in their free time, which enhances the enthusiasm of physicians while also eliminating profit-seeking behaviors of healthcare institutions. The health system managed by the Social Security Administration implements a referral mechanism to effectively utilize various health resources, thereby further reducing healthcare expenditures. At the same time, various measures need to be adopted to encourage the society as a whole to increase its investment in the healthcare industry.

(2) Multilevel Health Insurance System

Although they implement free universal health systems, the governments of Brazil and Argentina have also stipulated that the costs of purchasing commercial health insurance by employers and individuals can be listed as pretax expenses. This system guarantees the basic interests of the poor while also meeting the high-end consumption needs of the rich. Therefore, this system embodies the principles of both guaranteeing the basics and adapting to multiple levels of health needs. Brazil's healthcare system is similar to the Nordic universal health system. The system was first established in the 1950s and gradually developed thereafter. Major changes occurred in Brazil's health security system in 1988. The 1988 constitution enshrines health as a citizen's right and requires the state to provide broad and equal access to healthcare services. In 1990, the Unified Health System (UHS) was formally established to implement free universal healthcare. The UHS benefits 70% of the population, giving them free access to primary healthcare services. In addition to the UHS, the Brazilian healthcare system also has a second subsystem, that is, the supplementary health system. The latter system includes certain self-funded private healthcare institutions and private health insurance companies, which cover 25–30% of the population in Brazil. Compared to public hospitals, private healthcare institutions provide better medical equipment, healthcare workers, and health services. The full development of private healthcare institutions has enabled the diversification of Brazil's overall healthcare system, which allows the population a greater freedom of choice. In terms of farmers in remote areas and the urban poor, the federal government has successively launched two important schemes: the Family Health Program (FHP) and the Regional Management Plan.

Established in 1994, the FHP is a primary healthcare system with a focus on families and communities, emphasizing the resolution of issues such as maternal and child health and disease control. The specific implementation of the program is carried out by individual Family Health teams, which include physicians, nurses, dentists, and other healthcare workers.

Argentina's Ministry of Health has relatively clear power and financial relationships with its local health administrations. The Ministry of Health is responsible for macro-level policies, disease prevention and control, food and drug supervision and administration, and the supervision and administration of local health work. Major decisions are implemented after full consultations between the Ministry of Health and provincial health administrations. The Ministry of Health mainly strengthens its macro control of local health work through the implementation of programs and plans, which mainly include drug plans and related health service plans. Argentina's health security roughly consists of three components: the free universal health system, a social health insurance system, and private commercial health insurance systems.

In Mexico, health insurance for employees of different industries and their families is mainly managed by the Social Security Administration. Urban residents and rural farmers without employers or employment have access to health security services. In addition, the People's Insurance was introduced to cover poor families excluded from traditional health security, thus addressing the health security issues of all groups in difficulty. Mexico has four main types of social security with different governing bodies. The most important of these types is the Mexican Social Security Institute, which mainly covers the private sector and civil servants of all states as well as a small number of independent participants. The Institute for Social Security and Services for State Workers mainly covers employees of the federal government. The public health insurance plan is administered by the Ministry of Health and serves individuals not covered by the social security system. The oil sector has its own independent health security system. These four systems each have their own healthcare institutions under their management.

(3) Establishing and Perfecting Tiered Health Service Systems

The establishment of primary healthcare institutions by the governments of Brazil, Argentina, and Cuba stemmed from the need to address the most common diseases faced by the public. Large and medium-sized hospitals and specialist hospitals could address a small fraction of healthcare needs, and a tiered healthcare system was strictly implemented. Mexico has established a three-tier health service system in which public and private healthcare institutions are mutually complementary. To improve the community health service system, great emphasis was placed on the expansion of community healthcare facilities and the training of numerous highly qualified GPs to take charge of primary healthcare. Only patients with referrals from primary care physicians can receive treatment in hospitals. The hospital emergency departments are open 24 hours and only accept emergency patients. Patients with minor illnesses must first be diagnosed and treated by their family doctors. If specialist treatment is needed, patients must also be referred to a specialist by their family doctors. This practice has greatly reduced healthcare costs and has contained their growth. On the basis of this system, patients are first required to receive treatment from community healthcare subcenters, for which the share of personal out-of-pocket expenses is the lowest. At the same time, the community referral system was gradually implemented and improved, eventually forming a mechanism through which minor illnesses are treated in the community and major illnesses in the hospital. This improvement enabled the full and reasonable use of existing healthcare resources and reduced healthcare costs. By the 1970s, the Cuban Ministry of Health had begun to form a three-tier system. Based on the functions and levels of the health service system, Cuba has established and refined a healthcare network with its own characteristics. This network is divided into three tiers: community-based primary healthcare institutions, mid-level healthcare institutions providing specialist medical services, and high-level healthcare institutions. In particular, the Cuban government began implementing the family doctor system in urban and rural areas in 1984, and this system was gradually expanded throughout the country in the 1990s. Doing so enabled the family doctor system to achieve a better form of organization for the primary healthcare network, which has its own unique appeal.

PART TWO

Characteristics of Health Systems in Developed Countries and Areas

CHAPTER SEVEN

Overview of Health Systems in Developed Countries and Areas

 ## SECTION I. STATUS OF HEALTH INVESTMENT IN DEVELOPED COUNTRIES AND AREAS

Health investment is one of the key indicators reflecting the level of support for health development in a country or area. It is generally expressed as the share of total health expenditure and government health investment, of which total healthcare costs and the payment structure are the most important components. Governments should increase their investments in healthcare and the proportion of compensation for public healthcare institutions in order to provide the necessary material basis for guaranteeing basic medical services. The experiences of developed countries have shown that a government can only play a substantial role in suppressing the rapid growth of total health expenditures by maintaining a relatively high level of investment in those expenditures. When government investment comprises a high share of total health expenditures, the government has relatively more capacity to guide and balance the direction of investment, thereby effectively reducing or eliminating disparities in the level of health consumption in the population.

Using the US as an example, total health spending was US$1.0928 trillion in 1997, leaped to US$1.553 trillion in 2002, and further increased to US$2.7467 trillion in 2011. Total health expenditure as a share of GDP has increased from 13.1% in 1997 to 17.7% in 2011 (Table 7.1). Thus, it is not difficult to see that the rise in total healthcare costs has been basically synchronous with economic growth. From 2000 to 2008, the US economy grew by US$4.4 trillion, one quarter of which was spent on healthcare. The Congressional Budget Office estimates that spending on healthcare will increase from its current level, 16% of GDP, to 30% of GDP by 2035.

In most European countries, healthcare costs make up a large share of government spending, as represented by the UK. In the UK, total health expenditure as a share of GDP was 7.6% in 2002, whereas in 2011, the share was 9.4%, health expenditure per capita was US$3,658.90, and personal out-of-pocket expenditures of residents comprised only 17.2% of total health expenditure. In Germany, total health expenditure as a share of GDP

213

TABLE 7.1 Total Healthcare Expenditure and GDP Growth in the US in 1997–2011

Year	Total Healthcare Expenditure (US$100 Million)	GDP (US$100 Million)	Total Healthcare Expenditure as a Percentage of GDP (%)
1997	10,928	83,180	13.1
1998	11,503	87,820	13.1
1999	12,226	92,740	13.2
2000	13,094	98,250	13.3
2001	14,207	100,820	14.1
2002	15,530	104,460	14.9
2003	16,582	108,379	15.3
2004	17,729	116,573	15.2
2005	20,210	123,761	16.3
2006	21,521	131,329	16.4
2007	22,835	140,108	16.3
2008	23,914	143,300	16.7
2009	24,863	148,000	16.8
2010	26,337	149,644	17.6
2011	27,467	155,179	17.7

was 10.8% in 2002, while in 2011, it was 11.3% and health expenditure per capita was US$4,474. In France, total health expenditure as a share of GDP was 9.6% in 2002, while in 2011 it was 11.6% and health expenditure per capita was US$4,128. The situation in Sweden is very similar, as total health expenditure as a share of GDP in 2011 was 9.5% and government spending accounted for 81.6% of total healthcare expenditure.

In Australia, total healthcare expenditure has remained at 8.5% of GDP since 1994. Australia's total healthcare expenditure in 1998–1999 was AUD$47.5 billion, of which the federal government accounted for 49%, state and territory governments accounted for 20%, and the nongovernmental sector accounted for 31%. The government plays a crucial role in health financing; the total expenditure of the federal government is AUD$23.5 billion, of which 31% is spent on the compensation of healthcare costs, 28% is spent on public hospitals, 13% is spent on drug subsidies, 13% is spent on elderly care, 4% is spent on private hospitals, 5% is spent on administration and research, and 6% is spent on other health services.

The total health expenditure of state and territory governments is AUD$9.4 billion, of which 69% is spent on public hospitals; 19% is spent on community and public health; 3% is spent on emergency, elderly, and dental care; and 3% is spent on administration and research. The total health expenditure of the nongovernmental sector is AUD$14.6 billion. In 2012, total health expenditure was 9.1% of GDP, and total health expenditure per capita was US$3,890.

SECTION II. STATUS OF HEALTH SERVICES IN DEVELOPED COUNTRIES AND AREAS

1. Equity in Health Outcomes

The standard for measuring the level of health services is the health status of all members of society. The US is the world leader in healthcare technology. However, not all Americans can enjoy these services. There are also disparities in the level of benefits among different types of health insurance, and, in practice, many individuals have incomplete health insurance. The residents of certain remote towns and rural areas still struggle with difficulties in seeking medical treatment. Furthermore, differences in wealth and race have also affected the accessibility and equality of healthcare. In summary, despite the massive sum of health investment in the US, the resulting utility is dissatisfactory. The main issue is inequality, as the rich can enjoy the best services in the world, whereas the poor are lagging very far behind. Compared to those of other industrialized countries, the basic healthcare conditions in the US can be summed up as having "two lows" and "two highs." The two lows are low average life expectancy and low health insurance coverage. The two highs refer to high infant mortality and high healthcare expenditure per capita.

In 2000, the WHO released a ranking of healthcare conditions in 191 countries. The US was ranked 37th in overall health system performance and 72nd in overall health level. Although the majority of Americans receive good healthcare services and are in good health, 23% of non-elderly poor Americans (the poverty line is defined as an annual income lower than US$11,000 for a household of three or a monthly income lower than US$1,000 for individuals over 18 years old) have average or poor self-rated health, whereas only 10% of the nonpoor population have the same complaint. The number of people with heart disease, diabetes, and psychiatric disorders among the poor is twice that among the nonpoor, and the total incidence among the poor is 2.5 times that among the nonpoor. Furthermore, the proportion of low-income households affected by AIDS, tuberculosis, and other infectious diseases is also especially high.

The health issues of impoverished children are even more serious. Inadequate prenatal care, coupled with environmental factors, has caused many children to suffer from poor health throughout their lives. A 2003 study conducted in New York showed that the incidence of low birth weight in the poorest areas was twice as high as that in the richest areas. Only 38% of children under two years old living below the poverty line receive comprehensive planned immunizations, compared to 61% of children living above the poverty line. In addition, living environments also have an adverse effect on poor children. A study conducted in 1986 found that 41% of children from households with annual incomes lower than US$6,000 had lead poisoning, compared with only 17% of children from households with annual incomes above US$15,000.

2. Accessibility of Healthcare Services

The accessibility of healthcare services is one of the basic elements of health management and can mainly be divided into geographical, service, and economic accessibility. Geographical accessibility refers to the distance and travel time to the nearest healthcare institution as well as the transportation conditions. In layman's terms, it refers to whether residents are able to seek medical treatment. Service accessibility refers to the service capabilities and effectiveness of healthcare institutions and healthcare workers. In layman's terms, it refers to whether residents can seek good medical treatment. Finally, economic accessibility refers to the level of local health insurance and the ability of residents to pay for health services. In layman's terms, it refers to whether residents can afford medical treatment. Due to differences in economic, cultural, demographic, and geographical factors, healthcare services differ to a certain extent across different regions. Studying the accessibility of healthcare services can reflect its equality to a certain extent.

The accessibility of healthcare services is affected by numerous factors, of which economic and demographic factors account for a large proportion. Major cities and more economically developed areas have populations that are larger and more concentrated, which results in greater healthcare needs. Thus, there is greater investment in health institutions and a denser distribution of healthcare outlets. In less economically developed areas, especially in poor mountainous regions, the population is more dispersed and has lower healthcare needs. Thus, the distribution of healthcare outlets is sparser. The transportation conditions in different regions can also affect the accessibility of healthcare services. Although the distance to healthcare is relatively far in some areas, the presence of convenient transportation can shorten the time taken to reach healthcare institutions. Therefore, analyzing the accessibility of healthcare services based on the distance to the nearest healthcare institution may not produce exactly the same results as analyzing accessibility based on travel time. This situation is also common in developed countries, but such countries generally perform better than developing countries do.

The distribution of health service institutions in the US is extremely imbalanced. There is a relative lack of healthcare institutions in villages, certain towns, and the South, and this lack of institutions has affected the medical treatment received by the residents of these areas. To reach a physician availability of 0.5%, which is the minimum standard required by the US government, these areas will need to add another 110,000 physicians engaged in primary healthcare services. In 1993, 70% of counties in the US were considered to have inadequate healthcare services. Of the 51 million Americans who lack healthcare services, approximately 43 million live in these counties. Among 11 states that are largely in the South, at least 20% of the population does not have access to comprehensive healthcare services. The reason for this uneven distribution is the lack of sufficient funding and the inability to retain physicians and other healthcare workers in these areas. In these relatively poorer areas, many people do not have health insurance. The federal government has funded healthcare programs to support poorer urban and rural areas. Services are provided through public hospitals, community health centers, and local health departments in order to establish healthcare facilities for those without health insurance. In 1991, more than 600 community and migrant health centers provided preventive and basic health services to six million children and adults without access to healthcare. In addition, 1,200 public hospitals, 2,932 local health departments, 2,310 community mental health centers, and a few healthcare centers provided preventive care, treatment, and care for critical illnesses, and other basic health services to those without access to healthcare. More than 400 school clinics also provided a series of healthcare services and health education to poor youth. However, as the healthcare needs increased, there was a shortage in funding for these public or charitable institutions, leaving many individuals without access to healthcare.

Generally speaking, richer countries spend more on healthcare than poorer countries do. In 2011, total healthcare expenditure as a percentage of GDP was 10.9% in Denmark, 9.4% in the UK, 11.3% in Germany, 11.6% in France, and 9.5% in Sweden. As for healthcare expenditure per capita in 2011, that of the US (US$8,467) was the highest, followed by those of Norway (US$6,106) and Luxembourg (US$6,020). In contrast, healthcare expenditure in Ukraine (US$528) and Vietnam (US$227) was relatively low, as these countries have lower levels of economic development.

Among European countries, the number of beds available per 10,000 people in 2006–2012 was 82 beds in Germany, 64 beds in France, 35 beds in Denmark, and 47 beds in the Netherlands. The number of available beds was lower in poorer countries, with Ireland having only 29 beds per 10,000 people. The number of physicians available per 10,000 people was similar across all countries. In 2006–2013, Italy had 40.9 physicians per 10,000 people, France had 31.8, Germany had 38.1, Spain had 37.0, Belgium had 29.9, Ireland had 27.2, and the UK had 27.9.

3. Differences in Health Service Utilization

In theory, due to their poorer health statuses, the poor, ethnic minorities, and rural residents should utilize health services more. However, this is not the case in reality. Using the US as an example, in 1997, researchers compared the utilization of health services between poor and nonpoor individuals under 65 years old and concluded that the difference was very significant. Statistical data from the US has also shown that 34.8% of the poor have never seen a doctor, compared with 27.4% of the nonpoor. The poor often seek medical treatment from community health centers, hospital emergency departments, public and nonprofit hospitals, and charitable heath service points. The proportion of poor individuals who receive health services from emergency departments is twice that of nonpoor individuals. The proportion of the poor with fixed avenues of healthcare is lower than that of the nonpoor. Specifically, 25% of nonelderly poor individuals lack fixed avenues of healthcare, compared with 18.6% of the nonpoor. Compared to whites, ethnic minorities have poorer health statuses but lower utilizations of healthcare services. In 1991, 33% of Hispanics and 22% of blacks did not have health insurance, compared with only 12% of whites. This difference exists across all income groups, even among patients with chronic diseases. For example, in 1986, 30% of black hypertensive patients had never measured their blood pressure, compared to only 19% of white hypertensive patients.

In addition, based on indicators reflecting the status of healthcare implementation, including vaccinations, cervical smear tests, and contraception, less economically developed countries have lower rates of administering required vaccinations before one year of age relative to richer countries (except for Portugal). The rate of cervical smear tests in women of a specific age is also related to the level of economic development and is higher in Denmark, France, Luxembourg, and the UK. Due to the constraints of laws and religious beliefs, there is a north–south divide with regard to contraceptive measures. The utilization rates of southern Europe and Ireland are much lower.

4. Impact of Health Insurance on Health Services

Health insurance is an important way to ensure that Americans have access to healthcare services. However, as of 2010, 49.9 million people in the US, or 16.3% of the population, did not have health insurance. Many Americans also face the risk of losing their health insurance. For example, in 1987 and 1989, at least 25% of Americans had previously discontinued their health insurance. It is difficult for Americans without health insurance to receive appropriate treatments and preventive healthcare services in a timely manner. There are also racial differences in health insurance coverage; 11.7% of whites do not have health insurance, compared to 20.8% of blacks and 30.7% of Hispanics. The percentage of white children without health insurance is 6.9%, whereas the respective percentages for blacks, Asians, and Hispanics are 11.0%, 8.9%, and 16.3%. Health insurance coverage also differs by wealth. Only 8% of households with annual incomes of US$75,000 do not have health insurance, compared with 26.9% of households with annual incomes of US$25,000. Among poor children, 15.4% do not have health insurance, which is significantly higher than the average level of 9.8%. Regional differences also exist, as 19.1% of people in southern states do not have health insurance, compared to 12.4% in eastern states.

The US currently has various forms of health insurance. Private insurance accounts for 64% of coverage (195.9 million people), but this percentage has been declining steadily since 2001. The percentage of direct purchases by individuals is 9.8% (30.1 million people). The coverage of government-funded insurance is 31% (95 million people). The percentage of insurance purchased by companies decreased from 56.1% (170.8 million people) to 55.3% (169.3 million people) within 2009. The ratio of individuals receiving medical assistance is 15.9% (48.6 million people). The high cost of purchasing health insurance is a key factor affecting the voluntary provision of insurance by employers to their employees. Furthermore, to avoid the impact of large claims, insurance companies have adopted the practice of requiring the bulk purchase of insurance. Moreover, insurance companies charge high premiums for high-risk individuals or small companies or simply refuse to sell their insurance to these parties. Therefore, nearly two million Americans have been denied insurance coverage for various diseases.

SECTION III. STATUS OF HEALTH INSURANCE IN DEVELOPED COUNTRIES AND AREAS

There are differences in the health insurance structures and systems across developed countries that reflect differences in the institutional arrangements of each country under the influence of their social, political, and economic characteristics. In the section below, we analyze the health insurance systems of each country across different income groups, government responsibilities, and security functions.

1. Health Insurance Systems for Different Income Groups

During the establishment of a health insurance system, most countries must consider differences in the healthcare needs of different income groups and must create different health insurance systems based on these differences. In general, different systems are established for high-income, average-income, and low-income groups to satisfy the healthcare needs of these different income groups. Having different systems by income group is a very prominent feature in some countries. The high-income group has greater healthcare needs than other groups and a greater resistance to risk. Thus, most countries provide more freedom of choice in this group's health system. However, some countries also emphasize the role of social solidarity and require this group of people to fulfill more obligations for society.

Therefore, the health insurance system for the high-income group generally falls into one of three situations. The first is mandatory enrollment in the basic or main national health insurance system. The second requires members of this group to choose between the basic or main national health insurance system and private health insurance. The third allows voluntary enrollment in various types of health insurance schemes.

Mandatory requirements for high-income individuals to enroll in the basic national health insurance system are generally found in countries implementing a universal national health service system, such as the UK. Among countries and areas implementing a social health insurance system, there are also examples of mandatory participation for the high-income group. Examples include the insurance for exceptional medical expenses in the Netherlands and the "National" Health Insurance in Taiwan. In countries that mandate the enrollment of high-income individuals in the basic national health insurance system, these individuals also have the freedom to choose to purchase private health insurance. Hence, the health insurance systems of these countries generally consist of a health security system with universal coverage and private health insurance that covers a small group of high-income earners. For example, in the UK, the National Health Service covers all citizens, including those with high incomes. However, at the same time, 12% of the population also purchases private health insurance, and most of these individuals are high-income earners who enroll in private health insurance to receive better healthcare services.

In most countries that implement a social health insurance system, the law stipulates that high-income individuals may choose between the state-administered social health insurance system and private health insurance. Those who earn a certain level of income cannot revert back to social health insurance once they have opted for private health insurance. For example, German law stipulates that all citizens below the insurance limit (annual income less than €49,500 or monthly income less than €4,125 in 2011) are obliged to participate in social health insurance. Private business owners and employees with monthly incomes exceeding €4,125 are free to choose between the statutory health insurance and private health insurance. However, once they have opted for private health insurance, they can no longer participate in social health insurance. Therefore, the German health insurance system is mainly composed of two system types. The first is the statutory health insurance system, in which more than 90% of residents participate, and the second is the private health insurance system, in which about 10% of the population participates.

The size of private health insurance coverage for the high-income group in a country is determined by the level of security provided by the basic health insurance system for the average-income group. In general, the higher the level of security and the wider the scope of the basic health insurance system, the smaller the scale of enrollment in private health insurance by high-income individuals, and vice versa. This rationale also explains why the private health insurance markets in welfare states, such as the UK and Sweden, are relatively small, whereas that of the US is more developed.

The health insurance system for the average-income group often forms the basic or main body of the health insurance system in a country or area. The scale of its development mainly depends on the level of economic development or the economic capacity of most residents in the country. Statutory health insurance in Germany, the basic healthcare insurance in the Netherlands, Employees' Health Insurance in Japan, and National Health Insurance in Taiwan are all the primary or main body of the health insurance system in these countries and areas.

There are substantial differences among countries and areas in the institutional arrangements of health insurance for low-income groups. Not only does security take different forms, but there are also significant variations in the level of security, which can roughly be divided into three types.

1. An independent medical assistance system funded and established by the government. A typical example is the Medicaid and Medicare programs in the US for low-income individuals.
2. A health insurance system that exempts low-income individuals from premium or tax obligations through government legislation and unifies the inclusion of average-income individuals. For example, German law stipulates that the spouses and children of employees with no income, disabled individuals, and those earning less than DM620 (€ 314, former West Germany) or DM520 (€263, former East Germany) can enroll in the statutory health insurance and are exempt from the obligation to pay premiums. All health insurance funds must accept these individuals. The UK, Sweden, Finland, Italy, and other countries implementing a national health service system have included low- and no-income groups in their coverage regardless of their ability to pay taxes.
3. A health insurance system with enrollment for the general population and government subsidies of premiums. This approach has been adopted in countries and areas implementing social health insurance, where the government pays premiums to the health insurance funds on behalf of low- or no-income groups. For example, the National Health Insurance in Taiwan stipulates that the premium amounts for low-income

households are based on average contributions (about NT$925 per month) and are fully subsidized by the central and local governments.

2. Responsibilities of the Government in the Health Insurance System

The establishment and implementation of a health insurance system that can promote the improvement of national health quality is one of the socioeconomic development goals of most countries. However, the governments of different countries have different roles and responsibilities in the establishment and implementation of health insurance systems, and these roles can roughly be divided into the following categories. The first is direct government administration, the second is government support and administration by society, the third is government encouragement and market operations, and the fourth is government guidance and personal self-funded insurance.

There are two approaches for direct government administration. The first type includes the National Health Service in the UK, the public healthcare system in Canada, the universal healthcare system in Australia, and the health insurance systems for federal employees (civil servants), the military, and Native Americans in the US. The other type refers to medical assistance systems that target specific groups in society, such as the long-term care system for individuals over 65 years old in Canada, the elderly care systems in the Netherlands and Japan, and the Medicare and Medicaid programs in the US. The most prominent feature of direct government administration is the clear involvement of welfare benefits. This approach is mainly achieved through the establishment of public hospitals to directly provide free or virtually free healthcare services to the groups mentioned above. Under this system, the government is both the health insurer and the provider of healthcare services. The government undertakes a series of responsibilities, including the formulation of policies and regulations, the provision of funds, and specific administration.

Typical examples of government-supported and society-administered systems are the statutory health insurance of Germany and France, the Employees' Health Insurance and National Health Insurance in Japan, and the employees' health insurance and family healthcare insurance in South Korea. In this form, the government's responsibilities are to plan, regulate, and supervise the strong development of the health insurance industry according to national laws. Doing so mainly involves formulating the rules and regulations for social health insurance and safeguarding the legitimate rights of insured persons, health insurance agencies, and healthcare providers. The government generally does not provide insurance funds or only provides a small subsidy. The specific insurance operations are administered by the nongovernmental sector or health insurance agencies.

Market operations under government encouragement are primarily adopted by the private health insurance systems of most countries and include both for-profit and nonprofit health insurance organizations. The most typical example of this approach is the private health insurance system of the US. Under this system, the government's responsibilities primarily include the formulation of laws, regulations, and market rules; the supervision of the insurance market; and safeguarding the legitimate rights of insurers and the insured. The government does not assume any economic responsibility within the scope of the insurance contract. Health insurance companies conduct their operations and management according to market rules and share the risks with the insured parties.

The most typical example of the government-guided and self-funded approach is Singapore's medical savings scheme. Singapore emphasizes the sharing of the healthcare burden between individuals and the government. On the one hand, this approach promotes active prevention and healthy lifestyles to ensure the health and productivity of the population while also continuously improving the efficiency of healthcare services and reinforcing the individual's responsibility in health maintenance. On the other hand, despite the emphasis on personal responsibility in Singapore's system, the government has also been creating favorable conditions for the effective operation of the system and implementing the sharing of responsibility among the government, individuals, and the community. Doing so ensures that Singaporeans can afford the healthcare expenses incurred by diseases.

3. Functions of the Health Insurance System

There are currently several different views on the functions that the health insurance system should fulfill. The first view regards the system as life insurance, that is, as insurance against the hardships caused by diseases. The second view regards the system as insurance against healthcare expenses. That is, the main role of health insurance is to pay for the healthcare expenses of patients to ensure that they will not be impoverished by these expenses. The third view regards the system as insurance for health. That is, health insurance does not merely pay for healthcare expenses but should also be expanded to cover insurance for health. By analyzing the health insurance systems of different countries and areas, we can see that a relatively complete health insurance system usually consists of all three functions: (1) a compensation system for the loss of income due to the temporary or permanent loss of the ability to work caused by illness; (2) a compensation system for the healthcare expenses incurred in the course of the treatment of illness; and (3) a comprehensive health insurance system that includes treatment, prevention, care services, rehabilitation, and so on.

The compensation system for the loss of income due to illness was the primary function of the early health insurance system. Its purpose was to prevent impoverishment caused by illness. In modern health insurance systems, it aims to safeguard the basic subsistence of the employed population and is generally known as a sickness allowance. Most countries set up a sickness allowance system when establishing a health insurance system, and this system usually takes one of two types. The first type is to include the sickness allowance as part of the insurance content of the overall health insurance system. For example, Germany requires employers to pay their employees up to six months of sick pay, and a sickness allowance exceeding six months is compensated by the statutory health insurance based on 70–90% of the employee's normal salary. Insured women can receive a maternity allowance of up to DM25 per day for six weeks before their due date and eight weeks after they have given birth as well as a fixed grant of DM150 during hospitalized childbirth. The second type involves the establishment of a separate insurance system or levies from the social security tax for the sickness allowance. This approach is mainly adopted by countries implementing a national health insurance system, such as Ireland, where employers and employees each contribute 1% of an employee's salary to sickness allowance funds.

The sickness allowance system, which protects against the loss of income due to illness, developed into the medical insurance system, which covers expenses on healthcare services, and the system gradually shifted its focus to healthcare expenses. This shift was an important step in the development of the modern medical insurance system, as it marks the evolution of the health insurance system from simply functioning as relief from poverty in its initial stages into a more advanced stage of protecting against the risk of disease. In general, outpatient, inpatient, and drug services are all included within the scope of health insurance funds. However, the health insurance systems in different countries have different provisions for the specific healthcare services that are covered. Some are determined by the cost of healthcare services, and others are settled based on the health services provided.

For example, most countries have clear regulations for prescription drugs covered by health insurance, whereas nonprescription drugs are generally not included in the scope of medical insurance payments. Some countries have also stipulated that drugs are not covered by medical insurance payments, as in the case of the Medicare program in the US.

Based on the modern concept of health, the inclusion of prevention, healthcare, disease treatment, and rehabilitation within the scope of health insurance represents a key milestone in the development from medical insurance to health insurance. This shift marks the evolution of the medical insurance system into an even more advanced stage of development. On the one hand, this change is the result of the expansion in the contents of the medical insurance system and the influence of changes in biomedical models that are permitted by the economic conditions of economically developed countries. On the other hand, due to population aging, the governments of all countries have no choice but to reconsider the methods and measures for the efficient use of limited health resources. Most countries have gradually included prevention, care, and nursing services within the scope of health insurance. Some countries have also established new care and insurance schemes. For example, Germany enacted the Long-Term Care Insurance Act in 1994, which established a long-term care insurance system for the elderly and separated it from the statutory health insurance system. Some countries have also established separate systems for medical insurance and public health. Such governments fund the establishment of a public preventive and care service system to provide free or low-cost care services.

CHAPTER EIGHT

The Role of the Government in the Health Service Markets of Developed Countries and Areas

SECTION I. HEALTHCARE MARKET FAILURES AND GOVERNMENT INTERVENTION

1. Basic Concepts of Healthcare Markets

Conventional healthcare markets are generally believed to be influenced by three main factors: (1) healthcare service providers (physicians or healthcare institutions); (2) healthcare service demanders (patients or service recipients); and (3) healthcare services and prices. Healthcare services are related to health, which is affected when a patient does not seek medical attention in a timely manner when necessary. Healthcare needs (i.e., health status) are closely correlated with income in real life. In other words, high-income earners often have better health status and a higher ability to pay for healthcare expenses but have lower healthcare demands. Conversely, low-income earners have poorer health status and higher healthcare demands but have a lower ability to pay for medical expenses. To improve the equality of and accessibility to healthcare services, so that those living in poverty can enjoy equal access to healthcare services, the modern healthcare market has seen the emergence of a third party, that is, the payers of healthcare expenses, which are typically health insurance agencies.

2. Significance of Government Intervention in Healthcare Markets

(1) Main Characteristics of Healthcare Markets

1. Physicians Hold a Dual Position as Both Providers and Agents, Leading to Information Asymmetry in Healthcare Markets   Physicians hold a dual position as both the providers and agents of healthcare services. More specifically, in the healthcare market, physicians are, first and foremost, the providers of healthcare services, but due to the particularities of the healthcare market, the physician–patient relationship also follows a principal–agent model. Hence, physicians also act as agents who can decide on the patient's behalf regarding the types of drugs, the therapeutic methods, and the need for hospitalization. Their power of agency is derived from the consumers' lack of knowledge of healthcare services. Consumers have a much greater understanding of the products in general markets than in healthcare services. For example, when visiting a grocery store, consumers generally not only know what they want to purchase but can also easily compare the quality of products and prices and can even visit other stores before making a final decision. However, consumers tend to lack sufficient medical knowledge and are generally incapable of identifying the diseases they have contracted, the healthcare services they need, and the medical expenses they must cover. Patients are also relatively passive in healthcare consumption because they are unable to bargain with the healthcare service providers and must let the physicians decide on their behalf. Consumers tend to be active in seeking medical attention from physicians, but passive in receiving healthcare services because they are incapable of selecting from among different treatment options and have to let physicians decide on their behalf.

From the perspective of information economics, physicians tend to hold a greater power, which leads to a degree of information asymmetry between physicians and patients; that is, patients are a disadvantaged group for medical information, whereas physicians are the advantaged group. From a subjective standpoint, information asymmetry can be attributed to the differences in the information received by different individuals; from an objective standpoint, it can be attributed to the social division and specialization of labor. Information asymmetry is an objective phenomenon that is present in general markets. However, due to the dual position held by physicians, it is particularly prominent in the healthcare market and cannot be overcome by relying solely on market forces. In general markets, consumers who have insufficient information can delay or refuse their consumption. However, such bargaining is often not possible in the healthcare market, as patients who refuse treatments recommended by physicians due to a lack of sufficient information might delay their treatment time and endanger their lives.

2. The Healthcare Market is a Highly Specialized Market with Strict Market Entry Requirements, Leading to an Imbalance in Physician Supply and Demand   General markets have lower entry requirements, such that investors with sufficient capital can quickly enter without needing to acquire professional validation. Healthcare services are distinct from other types of services as they are closely related to people's lives and rights to healthcare. Therefore, a prerequisite for entry into the healthcare market is attaining healthcare professional qualifications. The legality and safety of the healthcare market can only be guaranteed by the compliance of healthcare professionals with relevant laws and regulations and the strict review of physician licensure. The strict market entry system is reflected in the high opportunity cost of the medical profession; that is, it takes several years to become a qualified physician. All countries have similar practices regarding the mode of market entry for physicians. US law stipulates that after passing the qualifying examination, a physician must undergo three- to seven years of medical education and training depending on their specialty, followed by a national specialist examination to obtain a specialist certificate. In the UK, an individual must undergo at least nine years of medical education and on-the-job training to become a general practitioner (GP). This includes spending at least five years in medical school and participating in one year of clinical practice after graduation in order to register with the General Medical Council (GMC) as a physician. The Japanese law stipulates that after the acquisition of a medical license, physicians must complete five to six years of clinical or postgraduate studies, followed by two specialist examinations, in order to be awarded a specialist certificate by the relevant specialist society. The Hong Kong law stipulates that after graduating with a Bachelor of Medicine and Bachelor of Surgery, physicians must undergo another six years of training and examinations to become a fellow of the Hong Kong Academy of Medicine, in order to be recognized as a specialist. Therefore, before attending the specialist qualifying examination, it is usually necessary for physicians to undergo specialist education and training courses, which have been strictly developed by the specialist society or health authorities. Physicians must also complete their education and training courses within the stipulated time period before they can take part in the qualifying examinations. The examinations typically involve written and oral examinations, on-site assessments, and research dissertations, which aim to comprehensively evaluate the physicians' professional knowledge, skills, and problem-solving ability. After completing several years of education, training, and examinations, qualified physicians are equipped with a very high degree of professional skill, which is the entry threshold for medical professions.

This strict entry system of the healthcare market can hamper the correction of regional imbalances in physician supply and demand. The availability of the healthcare workforce varies considerably across different regions in developed countries, with higher levels in some regions (e.g., urban areas) and lower levels in other regions (e.g., rural areas). The economic development of urban areas has given rise to well-established medical training systems with an abundant supply, or even a surplus, of physicians. On the other hand, the supply of physician is highly limited in rural areas, despite the high demand in such areas, due to poorly established medical training systems. For example, in the US, the relatively short supply of physicians in rural areas has long been a serious issue for healthcare policymakers at both the federal and state levels, as well as for medical educators. Around 20% of the US population (more than 50 million) lives in rural areas, whereas only 9% of physicians serve in these areas.

In September 1998, the US federal government designated 1,879 districts in nonurbanized counties as areas lacking in primary healthcare physicians. These districts needed a total of 2,370 primary healthcare physicians to meet the minimum standards, while 5,355 physicians were required to achieve the ratio of one physician per 2,000 people. On the one hand, the imbalance in physician supply and demand in rural areas cannot be solved by simply training more physicians in rural areas due to the strict entry requirements of the healthcare market; that is, medical licensure is impossible without first completing the professional training for physicians, and local hospitals reject quack doctors. On the other hand, most qualified physicians graduate from medical schools in urban areas, where they spend several years interning in hospitals to attain medical licensure. The majority of physicians prefer to settle in urban areas because of the higher and more attractive remunerations in these areas. Therefore, it is also unfeasible to transfer the surplus physicians in urban areas to rural areas with a high demand for physicians. For example, in 1967, the US established new medical schools or campuses of existing schools in urban areas to recruit a large number of physicians, in the hope that some physicians would choose to settle in the countryside, thereby resolving the regional imbalance in physician supply. The outcome of this measure was that, as of 1997, there were 736,264 registered physicians (about twice that of 1970) in the US, and the number of physicians per capita had risen from 130 per 100,000 people in 1970 to 276 per 100,000 people in 1997. However, the number of rural physicians showed limited growth, which was mostly attributed to the large rural communities of neighboring cities. Furthermore, the number of physicians per capita was virtually unchanged in remote rural areas where the population is less than 10,000.

In light of these two reasons, there are several obstacles to allocating the healthcare workforce through market forces, and it has always been particularly difficult to improve the regional imbalances in physician supply and demand in developed countries. This phenomenon has, in turn, led to various issues in health inequality.

3. The Healthcare Market is an Industry-Controlled Market that Leads to Monopolies, Inefficiencies, and Restricted Technological Advancements   The healthcare market is industry-controlled, whereby a handful of authoritative healthcare institutions form a healthcare network that covers the local healthcare market of an entire administrative area (e.g., a city). The overall healthcare market is divided by these healthcare institutions based on their geographical location and operational capacity. In other words, the local healthcare industry tends to be controlled by a small subset of healthcare institutions. The formation of this industry-controlled market can be attributed to the following aspects.

First, the life and health of patients are directly influenced by medical practices, and the government of any country is responsible for ensuring safe medical practices based on the principle of "the prioritization of life and health." Therefore, the medical profession is strictly regulated by the government, and the administrative approval of healthcare institutions for healthcare market entry represents the starting point and foundation of governmental healthcare regulation. All healthcare institutions must be approved and registered with the level of health authority that corresponds to their scale, function, and impact before proceeding with their operations, regardless of their investment channels, affiliations, sector, ownership, and economic properties. Additionally, the strict system of market entry serves as an effective barrier to medical malpractice and helps to control the number of healthcare institutions.

Second, the consolidation of hospitals has become commonplace since the 1990s. For example, 20% of hospitals in the US were involved in mergers and sales in 1995. The total number of inpatient institutions distributed across 37 states in the US, UK, and Switzerland declined from 6,701 in 1975 to 6,376 in 1996. In the UK, hospital consolidation not only serves as a strategic alliance in the general sense but also enables resource restructuring within the mergers, which brings together independent hospitals on an institutional level. The hospital consolidation in the UK and US eventually caused the entire healthcare industry to be controlled by a handful of healthcare institutions.

Finally, the benefits from the economies of scale imply that large-sized hospitals are more competitive than small hospitals. These benefits manifest as lower marginal costs for hospital operations with increasing scale. For example, even a small clinic catering only to a single patient must set up a registration area, consultation room, cashier area, and dispensary for registration, consultation, prescription, payment, and drug dispensing, respectively. On the other hand, large-sized hospitals are visited by numerous patients each day, which enables them to fully utilize their own medical facilities and reduce costs. In other words, the healthcare services provided by large-sized hospitals have lower unit costs because they serve a larger number of patients. Therefore, the benefits from the economies of scale have consistently led to the concentration of capital in large-sized hospitals, eventually giving them control over healthcare resources and markets.

Monopolies have always been associated with inefficiency, as they significantly reduce the efficiency of resource allocation in markets. The oligopoly of the healthcare market by a few large-sized healthcare institutions will eventually lead to a rise in medical expenses, as they might collude to suppress industrial competition and increase the prices of healthcare services and drugs.

(2) Manifestation of Healthcare Market Failure

Certain conditions need to be satisfied before market mechanisms can exert a positive effect on optimizing resource allocation; not meeting these conditions will result in market failure. Market failure occurs when the regulatory outcome of market mechanisms fails to ensure the normal operation of the market economy, which instead leads to economic imbalances and confusion. In certain sectors or under certain circumstances, market mechanisms may not have a positive effect or may completely fail to fulfill its role in optimizing resource allocation, and may hamper the optimization of resource allocation instead.

1. The Nonexcludable and Nonrivalrous Nature of Public Goods Leads to "Free-Riding" Public healthcare services are special service products for disease prevention and health promotion. From an economic perspective, they are considered public goods and exhibit significant positive externalities. Unlike private goods, public goods are considered goods for collective consumption, making them both nonexcludable and nonrivalrous. Nonexcludability refers to the fact that once the public good is made available to the public, anyone can access it without exception, and that no one can prevent others from consuming that good or extremely high costs are associated with preventing others from consuming that good. Examples include disinfected clean water and health and safety measures at public places. Nonrivalry implies that the same unit of public good can be consumed by multiple individuals simultaneously, and supply to one individual does not reduce the supply to other individuals. Examples include publicity of health knowledge, the protective effects of infectious disease control, and prevention of local diseases. In light of these two characteristics, the consumption of public healthcare services will inevitably give rise to a phenomenon known as "free-riding." This refers to how some individuals are unwilling to pay for the production costs of public healthcare services despite using these services, leading to the absence of market transactions and prices. Hence, the private sector is often reluctant to provide public healthcare services as they are unable to control market transactions and prices. Therefore, the demand is much greater than the supply of public healthcare services and market mechanisms are unable to ensure the optimal allocation of such public healthcare resources.

2. Positive Externalities of Public Healthcare Services Lead to an Insufficient Supply Product externality refers to the effect of an economic activity on a third party unrelated to the activity. Externality can be divided into positive externalities (wherein an economic activity has a beneficial effect on the third party but the economic agent does not receive any compensation) and negative externalities (wherein the economic activity causes harm on the third parties but the economic agent does not have to compensate for the damage caused). Public healthcare services have significant positive externalities, which manifest as social welfare. For instance, planned immunization not only stimulates the production of antibodies in immunized persons (consumers) to protect them against infectious diseases but also establishes immune barriers in the population, thereby reducing the risk of nonimmunized persons (third parties) from being infected. Another example is interventional measures, such as smoking cessation, which reduces the risk of chronic diseases among smokers and the risk of passive smoking among surrounding nonsmokers, thereby ensuring the health of the overall population. However, the positive externalities of public healthcare services can cause its demand to exceed its supply, even when the balance of supply and demand has been achieved via market regulation. Although private and social costs are considered equal, social benefits are generally considered greater than private benefits. Thus, optimized resource allocation has been achieved from a social perspective, but not from an individual perspective.

3. Heterogeneity of Healthcare Services Leads to a Lack of Competition in the Healthcare Market   Generally speaking, the healthcare market lacks product homogeneity due to differences in medical facilities, techniques, and services among healthcare service providers, as well as the varying health statuses, disease severities, and complications among consumers. For example, appendectomies are not entirely homogenous and have low product substitutability among different hospitals. As for more complicated healthcare services, such as the medical treatment of myocardial infarction and coronary artery bypass surgery, there are even greater differences in terms of service content, quality, therapeutic efficacy, and patient risks during treatment, which lead to even lower product substitutability. The low homogeneity of healthcare services raises the search costs for patients when seeking out "high-quality and low-price" services and limits patients' range of choice, thereby reducing the competitive pressure among different healthcare institutions and forming a weak competitive environment in the healthcare market. It should be noted that the substitutability and competitiveness are variable among different medical services. For example, therapeutic services for common or frequent diseases exhibit greater substitutability and competitiveness, thus enabling the greater role of market competition mechanisms. On the other hand, emergency services and therapeutic services for complicated diseases tend to exhibit lower substitutability and demand elasticity, thus requiring government intervention due to the limited role of market competition mechanisms.

4. Moral Hazard, Adverse Selection, and the Crowding out Effect Lead to the Failure of Health Insurance   Information asymmetry between healthcare service demanders and healthcare financing agencies lead to moral hazard and adverse selection among consumers. Private insurance companies are for-profit, and hence charge higher premiums for high-risk groups. As a result, those who are most in need of insurance (e.g., the elderly, patients with chronic diseases, and children) are often excluded from commercial insurance because they are unable to afford the high premium rates (a phenomenon known as the "crowding out effect"). Additionally, moral hazard is also present in insured persons, as they conceal their actual health status to reduce their insurance premiums, leading to an increase in the average premium rate. This can cause healthy individuals to withdraw from health insurance plans due to the artificially high levels of premium rate (adverse selection). Insurance companies have to raise the average premium rate to remain sustainable, which further aggravates the crowding out effect and creates a vicious cycle.

3. Consequences of Government Nonintervention in Healthcare Markets

(1) The Government Not Considering the Impact of the Nonexcludability, Nonrivalry, and Positive Externality of Public Goods on Service Providers Will Lead to an Inadequate Supply of Public Health and Basic Healthcare Services

Healthcare services comprise healthcare (mainly basic and special healthcare) and public health. Both the government and the market have significantly different degrees of impact on these two facets. In health economics, public health is generally considered a public good or quasi-public good, whereas basic healthcare is considered a quasi-public good, and special healthcare is considered a private good. As noted earlier, the consumption of public goods is nonexcludable, nonrivalrous, and places limited demands on market mechanism. Hence, the private sector is not motivated to provide public goods. Similarly, the supply of quasi-public goods does not meet the optimal demand under market mechanisms. However, investment in public health and basic healthcare gives rise to excellent input–output effects (where output is measured based on health). The *World Development Report 1993* estimated that the disease burden of developing countries can be reduced by one-quarter if 50% of their medical expenses on services with poor cost-effectiveness are reallocated to public health and basic healthcare. The government should be responsible for providing public health and basic healthcare services with inadequate supply. As for the issue of positive externalities, we can use the treatment of infectious diseases as an example: the outcome of treatment is twofold; that is, the recovery of patients from the disease and the prevention of disease transmission. Patients are generally more concerned about the former but not the latter. However, if positive externalities are not considered and the market is allowed to demand higher prices, the supply of therapeutic services will be inadequate, as exemplified by the recent increase in the incidence of tuberculosis in China. Therefore, the provision of basic healthcare services with positive externalities must be subsidized by the government.

(2) If the Government Does Not Resolve the Issue of Information Asymmetry, Basic Healthcare Demands Will Turn into Special Healthcare Demands, Leading to Higher Medical Expenses

As mentioned earlier, physicians hold a dual position, serving as both healthcare service providers and agents. Thus, the issue of information asymmetry is even more prominent than that in the general market. Therefore, the focus of government intervention should be to facilitate the communication between physicians and patients, thereby ensuring that physicians will respect the patients' rights to consent and autonomous choice. Additionally, the government should establish a mechanism for the release of healthcare information to allow patients to make an autonomous choice regarding their physicians and therapeutic methods. If the government continues to neglect the issue of information disadvantage among patients and does not compensate for this information asymmetry in the healthcare market, it could easily lead to "incentive incompatibility," whereby physicians induce healthcare demand and sacrifice patients' interests for their own benefit. More specifically, incentive incompatibility refers to a situation wherein agents have their own interests, and when there is a conflict of interest between agents and principals, the agents prioritize their own interests over those of the principals. In other words, a conflict of interest will lead to incentive incompatibility between the two parties. For instance, if healthcare services are charged on a fee-for-service basis and the income of physicians is linked with the medical fees, then physicians might provide unnecessary healthcare services (e.g., overprescription, unnecessary medical examinations, and prolonged hospitalization) in the pursuit of profits for the hospitals and themselves. One example of the overprovision of healthcare services comes from the US, where 8% to 10% of surgeries are unnecessary, which may result in physical impairment or even death of the patient. Some physicians also serve as "salespeople" who earn a commission by persuading patients to purchase drugs, healthcare products, and medical equipment. Hence, there is a conflict of interest between physicians (agents) who aim to pursue their own profits and patients (principals) who aim to spend the least amount to treat their disease. Under such circumstances, physicians can use their advantages in information and status to erode the interests of the patients. The immediate consequence of this action is that the demand for unnecessary special healthcare services will be required for some patients with basic healthcare needs, which will result in an unreasonable rise in healthcare expenditure and the waste of scarce healthcare resources.

(3) The Government Not Restraining Monopolies Will Give Rise to Expensive and Inadequate Healthcare Services, Which Is Contrary to the Goal of the Healthcare Industry to "Provide High-Quality Services at Low Prices"

The healthcare industry is a public utility that is intimately related to human life. Consequently, the price of healthcare services is intrinsically associated with the healthcare costs of the society as a whole. Monopolistic healthcare institutions transfer a large proportion of the benefits to patients in their pursuit of profits by setting monopolistic prices, which are much higher than competitive prices, thus leading to increased healthcare costs for the entire society. Healthcare institutions can obtain excessive profits via monopolies, which hinder the improvement in their efficiency and enthusiasm to provide better healthcare services to patients. In addition, such monopolies also forbid market entry for other investors, greatly dampening their investment enthusiasm and depriving the public of access to a diversified healthcare market. When physicians induce healthcare demands by capitalizing on the information asymmetry between physicians and patients, it undermines patients' interest. Therefore, an industry monopoly not only leads to overconsumption but also elevated prices, causing patients to suffer a double loss with respect to the quantity and price of healthcare services. This is contrary to a major principle of the healthcare industry, which is to "provide high-quality services at low prices."

(4) The Sustainable Development of Healthcare Systems Is Unattainable Without Governmental Healthcare Planning

A healthcare system is fraught with many issues related to health, and these issues must be gradually adjusted and resolved through careful planning and guidance. In contrast, regulation through market mechanisms is spontaneous and post hoc, which cannot be used to resolve the balance or long-term development on a macroeconomic level or achieve industry restructuring. Therefore, the lack of governmental medium- and long-term healthcare planning, as well as its administration, planning, and guidance of regional healthcare systems, will inevitably lead to the disorderly development of the healthcare system, thus rendering the sustainable development of healthcare systems unattainable.

4. Goals and Policy Orientations of Government Intervention in Healthcare Markets

Healthcare is a unique industry that emphasizes equality over efficiency. The spontaneous self-regulation of the healthcare market can ensure its operational efficiency but not healthcare equality, which can expose the lives and health of patients to considerable risks. On the other hand, market failure will reduce the operational efficiency of the healthcare market. Therefore, in developed countries, government intervention in the healthcare market is not only related to the balance between efficiency and equality in healthcare services but also associated with factors related to healthcare market failures, such as industry monopoly, information asymmetry, and public goods.

(1) The Objective of Government Intervention Is to Maintain The Balance Between Equality and Efficiency

The first priority of the government is to ensure healthcare equality. For example, health insurance should allow for "national treatment" of all patients, thereby achieving balance in the delivery of healthcare services between poor and wealthy individuals. Given the premise of maintaining equality, the government should also strive to overcome market failures and improve the operational efficiency of the healthcare market through various measures, such as optimizing the allocation of healthcare resources and controlling the growth of healthcare expenditure.

(2) Policy Orientations Under Established Objectives

1. Compensating for Information Asymmetry in the Healthcare Market via Health Insurance Private health insurance and social (universal) health insurance are beginning to play a greater role in the supervision and restriction of hospitals and physicians. Scholars have predicted that insurance agencies might become the greatest or even the only constraining force for hospitals in the future. Most health insurance agencies have full-time personnel that work with specific hospitals over a long period. These personnel may even have a background in medical education or at least be familiar with basic medical knowledge and hospital operating procedures. Entrusting the responsibility of regulating the medical practices of hospitals and physicians to these health insurance personnel will exert a strong constraining force due to the low level of information asymmetry between them and healthcare workers. Additionally, as a collective and spokesperson acting on behalf of patients, health insurance agencies have sufficient incentive to protect the interests of patients, especially in restraining physician-induced demand.

2. The Government Encourages the Use of Private Healthcare Resources to Reduce the Burden of Social Health Insurance

1. *Governments generally turn to private health insurance when social health insurance fails.* The health insurance system in Australia consists of both universal and private health insurance. The universal health insurance system is jointly funded by federal and state governments to ensure that all citizens receive the necessary healthcare services at reasonable prices. Aside from this system, Australia has also encouraged the development of private health insurance. Together, these two systems form the healthcare and insurance system of Australia.

   Universal health insurance provides comprehensive protection and coverage and has helped to achieve healthcare equality. Hence, it is generally well-received by the majority of citizens. However, in recent years, universal health insurance systems have become overwhelmed by the substantial increase in healthcare expenditure due to increasing immigration, population aging, and widespread application of advanced technologies in clinical practice. This situation can also be attributed to loopholes in the existing system, such as false reports or fraudulent claims of medical expenses by a minority of insured persons; physicians in private practice dividing patient consultation into multiple visits for more insurance claims; patients' optional participation in health insurance and overtreatment for minor illnesses; and the overuse of expensive large-scale medical equipment in public hospitals. To reduce the burden of universal health insurance, governments are actively publicizing the advantages of private insurance and encouraging citizens to buy private insurance using the following measures: (1) prohibiting the arbitrary transfer of private health insurance funds to ensure its security. (2) Combining universal health insurance with private health insurance companies to allow private health insurance agencies to become agents of universal health insurance. (3) Encouraging the early purchase of private health insurance, as the premium rate of private insurance increases with age, whereas the premiums for young adults decrease over the years. (4) Extending the period before the insurance coverage becomes effective and stipulating that insurance benefits can only be claimed after one year of premium contributions, in order to prevent patients from purchasing insurance only after contracting a major illness. Concerning the last measure, patients often prefer to receive insurance claims as early as possible. On the other hand, patients also prefer liquidity, as they want to have more cash in the event of unexpected expenses during illnesses. Therefore, this measure increases the time costs for insurance claims and reduces liquidity during illnesses, thereby prompting the early purchase of private health insurance to avoid future losses due to illnesses.

2. *Governments have begun guiding private healthcare funds to play a leading role since the establishment of social security systems.* At present, the social security systems of most countries operate based on the principle of joint responsibility among the government, private enterprises, and individuals. However, in some countries, such as Singapore, Malaysia, Indonesia, and other Southeast Asian countries, social security is jointly funded by individuals and private enterprises, whereas the government only takes on a supervisory role. Singapore introduced "Medisave," which is a national medical savings scheme that uses individual or family savings as the main source of future medical expenses. In addition to this government-managed scheme, individuals can also obtain funds from private health insurers, who cover more than 750,000 employees and their dependents in Singapore. The premiums for such private health insurance are paid by the employers.

Since the 1980s, the government of Singapore has shifted the financial burden of healthcare to the private sector, such that the government now contributes about 30% of healthcare expenses, which only account for less than 1% of the government's total expenditure. The resulting financial surplus is used for healthcare subsidies or the provision of free healthcare services to those living in poverty. In 1993, the government of Singapore issued a health policy report in a White Paper entitled "Affordable Health Care," which pointed out that the expenses for health insurance premiums will eventually be passed on to the citizens regardless of the fundraising approach (payroll deduction or taxation). Therefore, the government's main task is to guide private health insurance to play a more effective role in social security.

3. Measures Adopted by the Government Against the Shortcomings of Private Health Insurance Private health insurance harbors certain shortcomings, such as moral hazards, risk selection, and adverse selection. Although the government cannot address the issue of moral hazards, it can be very effective in curbing both risk selection and adverse selection. Specifically, the government plays two major roles in this regard. First, it passively compensates for the financial gap in private health insurance. That is, the private health insurance companies are free to choose individuals they are willing to insure, and the government is responsible for the health coverage of the remaining high-risk populations. These measures are commonly seen in countries dominated by private health insurance, such as the US. Second, it actively eliminates risk selection behavior among private health insurers. For example, the government typically prevents insurers from excluding those with unfavorable health conditions by requiring them to insure all potential clients using the same policy and premium rate. The government can also require insurers and individuals to sign a long-term contract that ensures low premiums for the insured persons, even when they age and fall into high-risk groups. These measures are commonly observed in countries dominated by social health insurance, such as Australia.

1. *Governments passively compensate for the financial gap in private health insurance.* The US is the only developed country in the world that does not provide health insurance to all citizens. About 150 million people, or 60% of the US population, are covered by private insurance. Freedom of choice is one of the basic principles of American economic life, whereby consumers attach great importance to the availability of choices. The American health insurance industry is a free competitive market where private insurance companies are allowed to compete with each other to attract clients by providing them with high-quality services. Such competition has led to high efficiency and optimized resource allocation. However, private insurance companies also have limited coverage as they charge high-risk-based premiums to high-risk groups in order to make a profit. As a result, those most in need of insurance (such as the elderly and patients living in poverty) are often excluded from commercial insurance because they are unable to afford the high premiums (i.e., the crowding out effect). In order to compensate for this gap in private health insurance and protect the right of all citizens to equal access to healthcare, the US government introduced Medicare and Medicaid.

   Medicare refers to the public health insurance program administered by the US federal government for Americans over age 65. Currently, there are about 32.5 million Medicare enrollees, which accounts for 13% of the US population. The main services provided by Medicare are hospital insurance, healthcare insurance, and prescription drugs. The funding sources of Medicare include payroll tax levied on employers and employees under 65 years of age, general taxes, premiums paid by enrollees, and the medical costs borne by enrollees. At present, 89% of the Medicare fund is made up of general taxes and payroll tax levied on employers and employees, while the premiums paid by enrollees contribute to the remaining 11%. Medicaid, on the other hand, is a public health insurance scheme for low-income earners; it has about 17.5 million recipients, accounting for approximately 7% of the US population. Both the federal and state governments contribute equally to the Medicaid fund via general taxes and income taxes.

2. *Governments actively eliminate risk-selection behavior in private health insurance.* The Australian government has implemented the community rating system, whereby everyone in a given community, regardless of their gender, age, or health status, pays the same premium for their health insurance based on the average probability of disease in that community. The primary aim of developing this policy was to ensure that all Australians can purchase private health insurance, regardless of their age and health status, thereby achieving health equality.

   In addition, the government has also established a regional reinsurance (group) system to bear risks. Due to the implementation of the community rating system in Australia, some insurance companies might be overburdened because of structural issues, such as the aging of insured members. In response, the Australian government implemented a regional reinsurance system in an attempt to redistribute the burden among insurance companies due to the differences in expenses arising as a result of the varying age structure of insured members. Under this system, a reinsurance fund is established in each state, and both private health insurance companies and the federal government pay a certain amount into this fund. The allocation of the reinsurance fund to private health insurance companies is adjusted annually based on their medical expenses for chronic diseases. The reinsurance fund also partially subsidizes the medical expenses of patients aged over 65 years who have been hospitalized for more than 35 successive days. The reinsurance fund is administered by the Private Health Insurance Administration Council (PHIAC), and the federal government maintains an intervening role via the negotiation between the Minister of Health and PHIAC.

5. Failures and Rectifications of Government Intervention

(1) Failures of Government Intervention

Government intervention is necessary to fully exert the effects of market mechanism due to the presence of market failures. However, the regulatory mechanism of government is not invincible, which means that there are instances of "government failures." Government failure is a situation in which policy measures and government interventions fail to rectify market failures, and instead lead to the deterioration of resource allocation, inefficient resource utilization, or even more damaging consequences than market failure. For example, the government-led National Health Service (NHS) of the UK caused what is known as the "British Disease," which is characterized by a rise in healthcare expenditures, inefficient healthcare services, and long waiting times for medical treatment. Similarly, the market-oriented model in the US that combines commercial insurance with Medicaid has led to a similar "American Disease," characterized by high medical fees and healthcare inequalities. The root causes of these problems are related to governmental failures. The main reasons for government failures are as follows:

1. Government Policy Mistakes　　There are numerous difficulties and obstacles that lead to mistakes in the policymaking process. The most prominent are as follows:

1. *Limited information.* Limited market information is an important reason contributing to market failures. In policymaking, the government requires comprehensive and accurate information as a scientific basis for policies. However, it is often infeasible for the government to obtain all the necessary information.
2. *Limitations of public policies.* Although government policies are universal and authoritative, it is impossible for the government to develop policy measures that suit everyone's preferences. In the end, government policies often embody the values of the dominant social groups. This is because policies are generally developed by a small group of individuals who consciously or unconsciously serve the interests of the class or group they represent. Even elected policymakers often serve special interest groups.
3. *Uncertainty in the process of policy implementation.* Even when the government has formulated the correct policies, various factors can interfere with the actual implementation of a policy, which may render it incapable of achieving the expected outcomes. Such factors include coordination challenges in large-scale government agencies, shortcomings in the policy itself, inherent difficulties in implementing targeted measures due to the complexity and variability of the interventional targets, the uncertainty of "time lags," and the interest and supervision of government officials.

2. Overexpansion of the Government
1. *Pursuit of scale maximization.* Government officials are examples of "economic man," who often pursue selfish goals, such as reputation, status, power, and remuneration, rather than "altruism." According to the now-famous Parkinson's law, the reputation,

status, power, and remuneration of government officials are often proportional to the scale of the government agencies to which they belong. Accordingly, government officials tend to make every effort to expand the government agencies they belong to and strive to attain expanded roles and greater budgets, in order to enhance their reputation, social status, authority, and remuneration.

2. *The behavior of government officials is not governed by property rights or profits.* Both private entrepreneurs and consumers are subject to budget constraints because they must act in accordance with private property rights. They will strive to reduce costs to maximize their profits with the smallest budget for their own interests, such as job promotion and profit sharing. However, the constraints of property rights are almost nonexistent for government officials, whose earnings tend to be proportional to government budgets rather than their own work efficiency. As government budgets are publicly funded, budget deficits are permissible and budget amounts can be increased through the legislature to raise taxes. Therefore, the behaviors of government officials are not driven by profits, which have led to the pursuit of budget maximization and excessive government expansion.

3. *Lack of supervision for government departments.* In a democratic system, government officials cannot act arbitrarily because they are subject to the political supervision of elected representatives. In a political appointment system, however, the effectiveness of supervision is greatly reduced because the information used for exercising supervision is provided by the supervisees. In other words, the supervisees can utilize their information advantage to deceive or manipulate supervisors.

4. *Monopoly of government agencies.* The state is a natural form of monopoly characterized by government agencies that serve as the sole provider of various public goods. Monopolistic government agencies are capable of concealing the actual production costs of public goods, which is not only unfavorable to the reduction of production costs but might also lead to the expansion of government agencies and their budgets.

3. Inefficiency of Bureaucracies   Bureaucracies are widely known for their inefficiency, which stems from the following characteristics. (1) Lack of competition: Bureaucracies monopolize the supply of public goods, and thus lack the pressure to reduce costs and improve efficiency. (2) Lack of profit-based incentive mechanisms: It can be difficult to determine the cost and output of public services due to their nonmarket-driven nature. In addition, it is impossible for government officials to keep the profits to themselves. Therefore, the aim of bureaucracies is not to maximize profits but to maximize the scale of the agencies to which they belong, in order to increase their opportunities for personal advancement and to expand their scope of influence. This inevitably leads to public overproduction, bloated government agencies, and inefficiency. (3) Lack of supervision: Bureaucracies have an information advantage in public production, and supervisors are prone to be manipulated by the supervisees. Even in the presence of supervisory agencies, the information advantage allows the supervisees to develop policies that best suit their own interests.

4. Unequal Distribution   Market mechanisms can lead to income or wealth inequalities. Government intervention aiming to overcome unequal market allocation might itself create an unequal distribution of power and income. This is because any form of government intervention involves the imposition of power by one group over another, and this power is always deliberately delegated to some people and not to others. The unequal distribution of power inevitably results in the phenomenon of "rent-seeking," which leads to the transfer of economic resources and the failure of government interventions.

5. Rent-Seeking Activities   The activities of human beings in pursuit of their own economic interests can be divided into two categories: productive activities, which can improve social welfare; and nonproductive rent-seeking activities, which do not improve, and might even reduce, social welfare. In a broad sense, rent-seeking activities refer to nonproductive activities in human society that are solely for the pursuit of economic interests. Rent-seeking activities also refer to nonproductive activities that protect vested economic interests or redistribute these vested interests. In a narrower sense, rent-seeking activities refer to the most common nonproductive pursuit of interests in modern society. They involve the use of administrative and legal approaches to impede the free flow and free competition of productive factors among different industries to maintain or seize vested interests (e.g., bribery and lobbying). Rent-seeking activities do not increase overall social wealth, but instead lead to the transfer and redistribution of social wealth, as well as the nonproductive consumption of resources.

The consequences of rent-seeking activities include: (1) distorted allocation of economic resources and preventing the implementation of more efficient production methods; (2) wasting of economic resources in the society that could have been used for productive activities; and (3) further rent-seeking or "rent-avoidance" activities. Therefore, the behavior of government officials can be distorted by the special interests they derive from rent-seeking activities, as these special interests trigger further wasteful rent-seeking competition in the pursuit of administrative power.

(2) Rectification of Government Failures

The prevalence of government failures suggests a problem; that is, government failures cannot be fully equated with government irresponsibility. Government irresponsibility, policy mistakes, and market failures that cannot be resolved by the government and structural defects within government organizations may eventually lead to government failures in the health insurance sector. The main strategies for rectifying government failures in the healthcare sector include (1) introducing market mechanisms and profit motives, and (2) improving the scientific nature of policies.

1. Introducing Market Mechanisms into the Public Sector   Economists have envisaged that government efficiency can be improved by introducing market mechanisms into the public sector. Specifically, they propose that two or more government agencies should be established to provide the same public goods or services to improve their efficiency via competition. Furthermore, incentive mechanisms in the private sector can be implemented. This involves issuing special "bonuses" to senior government officials based on their performances and allowing the heads of government agencies to use the "financial surplus" for "extrabudgetary investment" in order to motivate government agencies and their respective officials. Additionally, the production of certain public goods can be subcontracted to private producers to increase the reliance of public goods production on market economies. Furthermore, the competition among local governments can be enhanced and encouraged to improve their performances.

2. Introduction of Profit Motives   This refers to the establishment of incentive mechanisms in public healthcare agencies to cultivate profit-seeking among government officials and grant them the power to decide the use of fiscal surplus.

3. Improving the Scientific Nature of Policies   To improve the scientific nature of government healthcare policies, on the one hand, it is necessary to provide policymakers with reliable and sufficient information, which will provide a scientific basis for policymaking. On the other hand, it is also necessary to improve the quality of their policymaking by enhancing their skills and literacy in policymaking.

SECTION II. MACRO-LEVEL PLANNING BY GOVERNMENTS IN DEVELOPED COUNTRIES AND AREAS TO STRENGTHEN HEALTHCARE INSTITUTIONS

1. Implementation of Regional Healthcare Planning

(1) Adjusting the Distribution of Healthcare Institutions

Healthcare institutions in Japan can be divided according to their ownership into state-owned hospitals (run by the central government), public hospitals (run by local governments), and private hospitals. The Ministry of Health, Labor, and Welfare (MHLW) of Japan can undertake major institutional reforms (including merging, closure, and transfer of ownership) of state-owned healthcare institutions to achieve a reasonable distribution. The specific methods adopted are: state-owned healthcare institutions incapable of fulfilling their roles due to the presence of similar public or private healthcare institutions within the same area are subjected to closure. Similar state-owned healthcare institutions located close to each other are subjected to merging. State-owned healthcare institutions that have a certain impact on the healthcare activities of local residents but will be more effective if operated by local governments or nongovernmental organizations are subjected to a transfer of ownership. Using these measures, the MHLW of Japan can adjust the distribution of state-owned healthcare institutions in order to improve their efficiency.

(2) Promoting the Rational Division of Work Among Healthcare Institutions

The MHLW of Japan has called for the gradual delegation of primary and general healthcare services to public and private healthcare institutions, while state-owned healthcare institutions are instructed to focus mainly on policy-oriented healthcare activities. In other words, state-owned healthcare institutions are tasked with overcoming major public health threats by playing a leading role in the treatment of diseases and conducting clinical trials; providing sophisticated medical and scientific equipment, laboratories, and technical support to public and private healthcare institutions; educating and training clinicians, specialists, and hospital management personnel for hospitals at all levels; collecting and disseminating medical information and research outcomes.

The government of Singapore has adjusted the division of work in a similar manner as Japan's MHLW. Currently, 80% of primary healthcare services are provided by private healthcare institutions, with the remaining 20% provided by public polyclinics. Conversely, public hospitals are responsible for providing 80% of relatively expensive hospital services, while the remaining 20% is provided by private healthcare institutions. The implementation status of this division can be seen from the ratio of hospital beds to the number of patients admitted to public hospitals. As of the end of 2006, Singapore had 29 hospitals and specialist centers, among which 72% of the country's hospitals beds were found in 13 public healthcare institutions, including seven public hospitals (five general hospitals, one women's and children's hospital, and one psychiatric hospital) and six state-owned specialist centers. From 2006 to 2013, Singapore had 20 hospital beds per 10,000 people, 6,380 physicians, 18,710 nursing and midwifery personnel, 19.2 physicians per 10,000 people, and 63.9 nursing and midwifery personnel per 10,000 people.

2. Government Intervention in the Formulation of Healthcare Service Contracts via Market Coordination Mechanisms

In countries with an NHS or social health insurance service, all citizens receive healthcare services as a whole, and all healthcare institutions provide services as a whole. In order to improve the efficiency of cost settlement, both healthcare service providers and payers are generally asked to sign a presale contract for healthcare services that includes service prices, service standards, and compensation methods. The governments can play the following two roles in the formulation of these contracts.

(1) The Government Does Not Participate as a Contracting Party During Contract Formulation and Is Only Responsible for the Final Contract Approval

France is a typical example of such a case. The healthcare service providers are the unions of professional physician associations that negotiate as labor unions and strive for their own best interests. The payers are representatives of the National Health Insurance Fund for Salaried Workers, the Central Agricultural Social Mutual Fund for farmers, and the National Health Insurance Funds for Self-employed Persons. The health insurance contract is decided and signed by both parties without government intervention. After reaching a consensus on all matters related to the revision of healthcare prices, both parties sign the contract with the consent of the Minister of Health and Welfare, who then announces the contents of the contract. The Minister of Health and Welfare also has the right to intervene if the contracting parties fail to reach an agreement.

In Japan, health insurance contracts are made between health insurance agencies and healthcare institutions. The contract includes the service content, region covered, and validity period, and it is jointly approved by the health insurance agencies and local governments. In Canada, a Schedule of Medical Benefits (i.e., a fee schedule) is formulated through negotiations between the provincial and quasi-provincial health insurance agencies and physicians. The government will only formulate the contract if both parties fail to reach an agreement.

(2) The Government Participates Directly in Contract Formulation as Contracting Party

The UK is a typical example of this approach. Following the country's introduction of an "internal market," national health administration agencies became buyers of healthcare services – specifically, they are responsible for analyzing the healthcare needs of UK citizens and signing contracts with service providers to purchase healthcare services, rather than directly managing hospitals and providing healthcare services. The direct involvement of the government in contract negotiations is essentially a form of market coordination mechanism.

3. Vertical Integration of Healthcare Resources via Clusters

(1) Prerequisites and Roles of Medical Clusters

Over the past two decades, the integration of healthcare institutions has become an important trend in health reforms worldwide. "Medical clusters" refers to the integration of high-level specialist hospitals with community healthcare institutions located within certain areas to form vertical clusters. Residents can choose to register with their nearest medical cluster, where they can receive their first visit in the community and can be referred to other healthcare institutions when required. Professor Liu Yuanli, of the Harvard T. H. Chan School of Public Health, stated that the essential qualities of regional medical clusters are "coordination and homogeneity." Medical clusters must be equipped with interconnected information platforms, standardized collaborative service procedures, and clearly defined benefit distribution mechanisms. In addition, entry/exit rules and risk-sharing mechanisms are key prerequisites for the effective operation of regional healthcare clusters.

The policy functions and value of promoting regional healthcare clusters are mainly embodied in the following: (1) medical clusters are conducive to the improvement of vertical integration and efficiency of resource allocation, thereby saving costs and reducing resource wastage caused by disorderly competition among healthcare institutions and duplicate medical treatments. (2) Medical clusters are often associated with specific prospective insurance schemes that can promote a shift to low-end, preventive healthcare services, thereby enhancing preventive healthcare and improving the control and saving of medical expenses. (3) Medical clusters allow for the provision of technical support by higher-level hospitals to facilitate the improvement of service provision at primary healthcare institutions; this ensures that patient demands can be fully addressed within a medical cluster, thereby reducing the occurrence of medical disputes. (4) Medical clusters can promote competition among different regional clusters to improve the efficiency and economies of scale of healthcare resources, while also reducing the loss of efficiency caused by monopolies. (5) Medical clusters serve as the basic platform for promoting the concept of family doctors, thus providing both supplies and support in this regard.

(2) Policies and Operations of Medical Clusters in Developed Countries

1. In the 1960s, the managed healthcare system emerged in the US, which is mainly represented by health maintenance organizations (HMOs), points of service (POS), and preferred provider organizations (PPOs). The core purpose of the managed healthcare system is to achieve cost containment via the reduction of unnecessary healthcare services. In particular, insured persons have lower cost-sharing rates when seeking services within the provider network than outside it. The managed healthcare system has the following key elements: selection of healthcare service providers (hospitals, clinics, and physicians) based on clearly defined criteria; grouping of the selected service providers together to provide services for insured persons; formal regulations to ensure the quality of healthcare services and regular reviews on the utilization of healthcare services; and the provision of economic benefits to insured persons who seek medical treatment from designated healthcare service providers in accordance with the prescribed procedures. Currently, there are four major types of representative "managed healthcare" systems in the world: market-oriented healthcare, national welfare, public contracts, and public–private partnership, each of which has clear management implications and effects that are worthy of reference.

   In 2009, the Obama administration's Patient Protection and Affordable Care Act (also called Obamacare) promoted the development of medical clusters that are known as "Accountable Care Organizations" (ACOs). There were two main objectives in promoting medical clusters in the US: (1) to improve healthcare quality through systematic management and coordination of the entire patient treatment process, and (2) to prevent medical errors and control healthcare expenditure by improving healthcare quality and reducing the rates of unnecessary tests and treatments. These are important elements of Obamacare, which suggest that not only can healthcare clusters help to resolve the issues in seeking medical attention but also play a greater role in health reforms. The fact that medical clusters in the US are called ACOs implies that healthcare service providers are responsible not only for the treatment of diseases, but also for the entire treatment process and patients' overall health. Thus, medical clusters must be of a certain scale to cover the entire treatment process, especially for patients with chronic diseases, who require a wide range of healthcare service, including the treatment of acute diseases, the management and care of chronic diseases, and pharmacotherapies.

2. In Russia, the medical cluster system was implemented mainly to provide high-quality healthcare services to residents; reduce the incidence of diseases, disability, and death by organizing regular preventive services for employees and residents; and organize health education and dissemination of health information among residents. To accomplish these major tasks, the cluster must: (1) determine the needs of residents for ambulance and healthcare services; (2) develop and improve the quality of medical services by strengthening preventive services and utilizing advanced methods in the diagnosis, treatment, and management of healthcare institutions; (3) ensure continual development of the medical cluster by creating a modernized material basis, improving production efficiency, establishing the conditions to give workers adequate rest, and building a system for the fair division of labor; (4) ensure the economic independence of the medical cluster, enhance the work enthusiasm of each worker, and paying attention to collective and national affairs; (5) guarantee the health of the population by combining material benefits for workers with high-quality productive labor.

   The payroll fund of medical clusters is generally determined according to income generated from the provision of healthcare services and paid services and is adjusted proportionally as the total income from healthcare services increases. Workers are paid by a cluster payroll fund and their salary standards are determined based on their contribution. The production development fund, social development fund, and material incentive fund can be withdrawn from the collective economic revenues. Medical clusters can incorporate preventive medical institutions (e.g., clinics, healthcare departments, disease control centers, hospitals, and sanatoriums), preventive healthcare agencies, and other healthcare agencies, which enable the centralized allocation of all or some of the roles, materials, technologies, funds, and workforce within the cluster.

3. In Canada, there are three models of hospital organizational structure: the conventional pyramidal model, horizontal model, and vertical model. The conventional pyramidal model refers to the organizational structure of individual hospitals and healthcare service providers, where those with higher positions are located higher on the pyramid, such that hospital management information is delivered to the vice president before being passed on to the chief executive officer (CEO). Functional sectors or departments that are organized based on this pyramidal structure have a clear chain of command, such as the pediatric department, obstetrics department, and public sector. This model leads to a fragmented and duplicated organizational framework, which is also expensive and inefficient. It also tends to attach little importance to patients' interests and the government pays physicians for the number of services provided. This is in conflict with the goals of healthcare services, as the physicians do not have a salary; instead, they receive more remuneration from the government by providing more services.

   The horizontal model has a decentralized structure and is based on a project management system; that is, horizontal management is implemented for each project.

This model deviates from the models of conventional departments and community healthcare management, and cross-departmental integration. Its reliance on separate payment mechanisms can lead to fragmentation and inefficiency but also allows the establishment of cross-departmental ties, which improves efficiency and concretizes the rules. However, this model harbors some problems during cross-referrals of patients, such as the referral of patients from community healthcare centers to hospitals. The common feature of both the conventional pyramidal and horizontal models is the dual-reporting system.

The third type of organizational structure is the vertical model, whereby healthcare service providers are organized according to region and provide comprehensive services to a designated population. In this model, hospitals are gradually integrated with other healthcare service providers. This is arguably the best model, as noted by the CEO of Providence Medical Group, Mr. Carl Roy, "This vertical organizational model keeps our services seamless." In Canada, patients are generally not allowed to seek medical attention directly at hospitals, which also lack a registration area or department. Instead, they are first required to visit "family physicians," who usually have their own clinics with one or two secretaries or assistants. These physicians deliver various healthcare services, ranging from obstetrics and gynecology to psychiatry but do not specialize in any particular area of medicine. Hence, they are capable of treating minor illnesses, whereas patients with major illnesses must be referred to hospitals or specialists. The Providence Medical Group, which originally had eight CEOs and 20 vice presidents, has been reorganized to have one CEO and four vice presidents. This type of model requires systematic development and teamwork, as well as mutual communication and cooperation to reorganize resource allocation within the medical group. It is established on the basis of advanced information technology, whereby CEOs can monitor the situation in other departments from their office using computers. This model is different from the former two models in that the former models are established based on information asymmetry, which leads to poor cross-departmental or cross-project communication and multiple reporting lines.

With regard to the current healthcare reforms in China, it is worth exploring the application of this vertical model, which is suitable for such large-sized healthcare institutions as the Providence Medical Group, to a nonprofit public welfare system.

4. Since 2002, the Hong Kong Hospital Authority, which is responsible for the construction and management of public hospitals, has implemented the hospital cluster system. The system divides Hong Kong into seven areas according to regional and population needs, and each area operates as a cluster. The Hospital Authority is the sole statutory body for public healthcare institutions in Hong Kong, and a Cluster Chief Executive is appointed for each cluster. Hospitals within each cluster are divided into emergency and rehabilitation hospitals based on the nature of their service. There are one- to two rehabilitation hospitals and various auxiliary facilities in the vicinity of every emergency hospital. Hospitals within each cluster have their own specialties and characteristics that do not overlap with other facilities, and services are provided to patients through mutual referral, thereby improving the service efficiency of each hospital. In addition, large equipment is not duplicated between hospitals within the same cluster, thereby reducing the operating costs through resource sharing.

Singapore divides public healthcare institutions into two groups based on their geographical location and size: the institutions in the eastern region are collectively referred to as the Singapore Health Services (SHS), while those in the western region are the National Healthcare Group (NHG). The aim of this division is to promote internal competition among public healthcare institutions. These two medical groups are of equal size and receive an equal amount of government subsidies. The SHS consists of four hospitals, seven general clinics, and four healthcare centers, while the NHG consists of four hospitals, nine general clinics, and two healthcare centers. The president of each medical group is appointed by the Ministry of Health while the heads of the member institutions constitute the board of directors. Both medical groups have different management and incentive mechanisms. The Ministry of Health also imposes "total revenue control" on each medical group; that is, once the total expenditure of the group exceeds an upper limit, the subsidies given by the government will be reduced in proportion. Studies have shown that the operation of these two groups has played an important role in controlling healthcare expenditure and improving the efficiency of resource utilization.

(3) Relevant Experiences and Insights

1. The worldwide trend in the integration of healthcare institutions has witnessed a general shift away from horizontal integration toward vertical integration. In other words, there has been a transition toward vertical clusters that consist of different levels of healthcare institutions and emphasize the "seamless convergence" of healthcare services, rather than powerful cooperative medical groups.

2. In general, the establishment of regional vertical medical clusters involves three developmental stages, starting with "loose integration" before progressing to "tight integration" and then to "complete integration," eventually achieving a scientific and reasonable corporate governance structure. Experiences from various countries have suggested that the ultimate developmental model of medical clusters is the implementation of a standardized management and allocation model and a uniform hospital culture, which centers on medical clusters in the appointment of legal representatives and uses assets and skills as organizational ties. In addition, an integrated governance structure can be adopted, whereby all hospitals within the medical cluster are controlled via a centralized system that integrates the management, functions, personnel, and information of all constituent hospitals, thereby forming a horizontally and vertically integrated service network.

3. Within "tightly integrated" medical clusters, where a council is responsible for standardized operations management and resource allocation, each hospital within the cluster must have its own legal representative. A strict contractual relationship with clearly defined benefit and risk-sharing mechanisms is especially necessary within this organizational form in order to regulate and restrain the behaviors of member hospitals, the absence of which might cause the cluster to revert to the "separate and loosely integrated" stage.

4. The establishment of a new healthcare service model must be supported by corresponding health insurance payment methods. According to the developmental trajectory of health insurance systems in developed countries, future reforms in the method of health insurance payment in China will most likely involve the implementation of standardized prospective payments (determined based on the number of patients who register with the cluster) or payments to family physicians within the cluster (who purchase the necessary specialist healthcare services).

SECTION III. GOVERNMENT REGULATION OF HUMAN RESOURCES IN DEVELOPED COUNTRIES AND AREAS

1. Regulating the Total Supply of Physicians Based on Healthcare Demand

The overall demand for healthcare services changes constantly alongside continuous socioeconomic development. To keep up with these changes in demand, the governments of developed countries, such as the US, various Western European countries, and Japan, have established necessary interventional approaches to provide a suitable number of physicians, the most important of which is the adjustment of the number of medical students. On the one hand, governments generally believe that great importance should be attached to service safety in the healthcare industry; hence, the increase in physician supply must be achieved through medical education. On the other hand, when the government needs to limit the number of physicians, reducing the enrollment in medical schools tends to have less impact on social stability than laying off staff in healthcare institutions, as the former does not result in unemployment. For example, in the UK, the total number of students enrolled in medical schools each year is determined by the Ministry of Health according to the demand for physicians. The number of students enrolled might be reduced due to concerns about unemployment of healthcare workers or increased to utilize the resources of medical schools fully. However, enrollment must sometimes be capped to avoid straining their resources and to optimize the training of physicians.

In the late 1960s, the governments of many developed countries began adjusting the supply of physicians. In 1967, the federal advisory committees of the Health Resources and Services Administration (HRSA) in the US released an influential report pointing out a physician shortage, which contributed to the expansion of the physician training program. Since then, numerous new medical schools have been established nationwide and existing schools have been expanded, in order to increase the supply of physicians substantially. According to the American Medical Association (AMA), there were 736,264 registered physicians in the US in 1997, which was twice the number in 1970. The number of physicians per capita increased from 130 physicians per 100,000 people in 1970 to 276 physicians per 100,000 people in 1997. Nevertheless, while the shortage of physicians has been solved in terms of the total supply, there are still issues with distribution. The Nordic countries also have a history of physician shortage. In order to overcome this issue, Sweden established three new medical schools after World War II, which led to a sevenfold increase in the number of physicians from 1947 to 1972. In Finland, two new medical schools were established in the early 1970s, and student recruitment was expanded. In addition to expanding education, governments have also adopted policies to recruit foreign physicians in an effort to increase the physician supply.

Since the 1980s, there has been a rapid growth in the physician supply in nearly all countries, leading to a surplus in some cases; this surplus has in turn led to a rapid increase in the unemployment rate among physicians. Therefore, governments began to emphasize the surplus of physicians and adopted measures to control the number of physicians. The most commonly used approaches are as follows.

(1) Limiting the Number of Medical Students

Denmark reduced the number of enrolled students by 23% from 1982 to 1987. France imposed a stringent examination system to control the number of medical graduates, and in recent years, the number of graduates has been significantly lower than the number of enrolled students. The number of enrolled students in Italy showed a 62% reduction from 1980 to 1989, following the implementation of various control measures. Singapore has also begun limiting the number of newly recruited specialists by 40%, with the remaining physicians being trained as GPs.

(2) Layoff of Surplus Healthcare Workers

Spain, Italy, and Ireland have implemented a number of control measures for the healthcare workforce. In 1983, Ireland stopped filling the positions of retired physicians. In Italy, the number of healthcare workers was reduced by 12,000 from 1983 to 1985. In 1982, the government of Spain stipulated that there will be no new vacancies for physicians, with the exception of newly established hospitals. In 1983, the UK government proposed laying off 8,000 employees in the healthcare system. Furthermore, nine months before 2010, the NHS eliminated 15,000 healthcare jobs in the UK. In the US, 100 hospitals undertook large-scale layoffs in 2003, followed by another round of layoffs in 117 hospitals from January to November 2008.

(3) Control of Market Entry via Medical Licensure Management

The US government has imposed a series of measures to limit market entry, mainly by implementing national qualifying examinations and employing different medical licensure standards across different states. Similarly, medical licensure in Germany and Canada is governed by the state and provincial governments, respectively, while in the UK, it is conducted by the central government.

(4) Restricting the Entry of Foreign Physicians

In 1975, Canada's Royal Commission on Health Services (also known as the Hall Commission) proposed controlling the entry of foreign physicians. Prior to the proposal, 1,200–1,300 foreign physicians were hired annually between 1965 and 1974, accounting for 56%–57% of all new physicians in Canada. However, only about 300 foreign physicians were hired each year after 1975 (about 15% of new physicians). Before the implementation of immigration controls in 1974, there was a total of 2,657 foreign physicians and medical graduates in Canada, which declined to about 2,000 in 1977. Although the drastic growth in physician supply has been curbed, the current number of physicians has not significantly declined compared to that in 1965–1972. Therefore, there appears to be no other solution than to reform the enrollment quota.

(5) Restricting Medical Training of Foreign Medical Graduates at Local Hospitals

The US initially allowed foreign graduates to complete residency training at local hospitals in the hopes that they would serve in rural areas where local physicians were reluctant to practice. While some foreign graduates did, in fact, choose to serve in rural areas, on the whole, the number was similar to that of local physicians. Furthermore, studies have even shown that some metropolitan hospitals rely on foreign graduates for residency work. There are no reliable data suggesting that foreign graduates are more likely to serve in rural areas than local medical graduates. Studies have also shown that the geographical distribution of foreign graduates is similar to that of local medical graduates, both of which show a slight bias toward metropolitan hospitals. The US Government Accounting Office reported that the attempt to solve the regional imbalance in the distribution of physicians by employing foreign graduates has not only failed but also aggravated the surplus of physicians in the US and led to a loss of talented clinicians in other countries. As a result, the US government began to limit the quota for the residency training of foreign medical graduates through strict visa procedures.

2. Government Efforts and Outcomes in Improving the Regional Imbalances of Physician Supply and Demand

Governments across the world have made various efforts to address the physician shortage in rural and impoverished regions. The main approaches are as follows.

(1) US Government-Funded Programs

There are numerous government programs in the US that directly target medically under-served areas (MUAs). For example, the Family Medicine Residency Program, which is funded by both the federal and state governments, is considered useful because family physicians are more likely to serve in rural areas than specialists. However, this approach alone cannot resolve the physician shortages in rural areas.

The National Health Service Corps is another influential program. Prospective physicians who participate in this program sign contracts with a specific government department, which then pays their medical school tuition fees and residency training expenses. In exchange, physicians agree to serve in government-designated MUAs for a certain period of time. Since its establishment in 1970, the National Health Service Corps has spent more than US$2 billion to appoint more than 15,000 physicians. In the late 1980s, members of the National Health Service Corps constituted about a quarter of the newly recruited primary healthcare physicians serving in MUAs. This program has provided an important safety net for the shortage of physicians in rural areas.

Furthermore, as a means of nurturing rural physicians, Thomas Jefferson University proposed the Physician Shortage Area Program (PSAP) in 1974. The program works as follows: each year, the program recruits 15 Jefferson Medical College students who are from rural areas and willing to serve in the rural areas of Pennsylvania. These medical students must then complete a family medicine internship in a rural area during their third year and an advanced internship at a family medicine clinic (also usually in a rural area) during their fourth year. This program aims to increase the affection of medical students for rural areas and provides a preliminary understanding of primary healthcare work, while also providing students with some study allowance. Upon graduation, these students must complete residency training as a form of postgraduate education to become GPs, before they begin serving in the rural areas of Pennsylvania. A survey carried out in 2008 revealed that 79% of physicians training from this program continued to serve in rural areas.

Another program worth mentioning is the Area Health Education Centers (AHEC) program, which was established in 1970 to provide healthcare services to underserved communities. Since then, the AHEC program has been established in many regions and states. Hynes and Civner studied the extent to which the number of physicians per capita in rural areas was affected by the AHEC program. They found that from 1975 to 1985, among counties with a population of less than 50,000, the number of physicians per capita in counties with an AHEC program was 3%–5% higher on average than in counties without such a program.

(2) Effects of Changes in the Medicare Compensation Strategy on Rural Physicians in the US

Medicare was introduced in 1966 for elderly adults over the age of 65 years in the US. Given its wide coverage, any policy change in Medicare will have far-reaching implications for the entire healthcare system. One notable change pertaining to rural healthcare systems was the Medicare Bonus Payment Program (also known as the Merit-Based Incentive Payment System, or MIPS) established in 1989. The MIPS provides significant economic incentives for physicians who serve in rural MUAs. The bonuses offered by this program increased from 5% in 1989 to 10% in 1991 and has remained the same to date. It is apparent that these bonuses serve as important incentives for physicians who reside in MUAs, as they have had clear stabilizing effects in the number of physicians in at least some regions.

(3) Japan Has Established a Medical University That Trains Physicians for Rural Areas

Jichi Medical University was proposed by the central government and established by government agencies in charge of community healthcare in 47 prefectures, each of which contributes an equal amount of funds to this medical university each year. This university targets students who intend to serve in their respective prefectures after graduation. Upon admission, each student must sign an agreement with the university stipulating that the university will provide a loan to the student for the course of their study but that this loan might be waived if the students serve at a designated rural healthcare institution for a certain period of time after graduation (1.5 times the duration of their university course). The medical university was built in a rural town located 100 km north of Tokyo, in order to allow students to experience rural life and prepare them for serving in rural areas in the future.

Since its establishment in 1972 to 1995, Jichi Medical University has produced a total of 1,871 physicians, among which 1,434 (77%) are currently working in rural areas; the majority of the remaining graduates are enrolled in postgraduate training or graduate schools. Approximately 792 (42%) graduates are currently working in rural areas designated by prefectural governments. Furthermore, 858 out of 924 graduates (93%) from the first to the ninth batch of graduates have completed their nine-year service in government-designated areas according to the contract, 619 (67%) are still serving in their respective prefectures, and 305 (33%) are serving in other rural areas. Based on the geographical distribution, these graduates are distributed almost evenly throughout the country. Only 75 graduates (4%) failed to fulfill their contracts and had to repay their study loans. Almost all the graduates (96%) fulfilled their obligations according to the contract. Therefore, the regional imbalance in physician supply has been solved by the large number of medical graduates now serving in rural areas.

(4) The UK Government Has Limited New GP Practices Based on the Number of Registered Patients at Existing GP Practices in Each Region

To avoid a biased distribution of GPs, the UK government has divided the country into four types of geographical region based on the number of registered patients at existing GP practices. (1) Designated regions: in regions with an average of more than 2,500 registered patients per GP, family physicians are free to open new medical practices and are given special allowances. (2) Vacant regions: in regions with an average of 2,200–2,500 registered patients per GP, family physicians are free to open new medical practices. (3) Intermediate regions: in regions with an average of 1,800–2,200 registered patients per GP, new practices must first be reviewed before they are permitted to practice. (4) Restricted regions: in regions with fewer than 1,800 registered patients per GP, the opening of new practices is only permissible when there are job vacancies.

SECTION IV. GOVERNMENT INTERVENTION IN DRUGS AND THE CONTROL OF HEALTHCARE QUALITY IN DEVELOPED COUNTRIES AND AREAS

1. Government Intervention in Drugs

(1) Direct Price Control

There are three types of direct control over drug prices in different countries: the first type is imposed on all drugs, such as the direct drug pricing systems in France and Japan. The second type is based on the class of drugs, such as the reference pricing system in Germany. The third type is based on drug prices in other countries, such as the international reference pricing systems of Italy and the Netherlands. A major limitation of supply-side price control is that it cannot restrict drug consumption on its own, and price reduction may lead to an increase in consumption. In addition, some forms of price control, especially the reference pricing system, might distort drug parity prices, prescription behavior, and rewards for drug innovators.

(2) Quantity Control

In addition to price control, some countries, such as France, have adopted measures to control the quantity of drugs entering the market. At the drug manufacturer level, governments often directly restrict the number of drugs entering the market. Governments can also influence the number of drugs at the physician level by issuing prescription drug lists and strict prescribing codes. The prescription drug lists might be formularies, positive lists, or negative lists, while the prescribing codes specify when or how to use a particular drug.

Some European countries and the US control the use of drugs by physicians via the "separation of prescribing and dispensing." After consulting the community-based physician (GP or family physician), the patient obtains their drugs from a retail pharmacy using a prescription issued by the physician, and the medication instructions are given by the pharmacist. The UK government prohibits family physicians from dispensing drugs. After a family physician issues a prescription, the patient must obtain the drugs from a pharmacy with NHS-approved pharmacists. In rural areas or for drugs that are not readily available in pharmacies, family physicians can both prescribe and provide the drugs to patients. However, the lack of supervision of these family physicians might induce patients to purchase more expensive or unnecessary drugs. Therefore, since 1983, the UK government has stipulated that drugs dispensed by family physicians in remote areas must be approved by the Dispensing Doctors' Association. Similar measures have been adopted in France, where pharmacists and family physicians operate independently. Pharmacists can relay their opinions to physicians or even refuse to dispense medicines if the physician's prescription is deemed inappropriate.

Total drug consumption can be effectively controlled by limiting the quantity supplied. However, a key question that remains is what constitutes an "appropriate" total amount of drug consumption, which is an issue that is still being investigated.

(3) Consumption Control

In recent years, many countries have paid increasing attention to intervening in the pharmaceutical market at the level of total drug consumption. The UK Pharmaceutical Price Regulation Scheme (PPRS) is one such mechanism that attempts to control the pharmaceutical market by regulating the profitability of pharmaceutical manufacturers. The PPRS gives pharmaceutical companies a certain degree of freedom in pharmaceutical pricing but also links the total pharmaceutical sales with the company's investment in the UK, return on capital, and long-term risk level. According to the latest PPRS, pharmaceutical companies are free to set prices for patented prescription drugs but must maintain a profit margin of 17–21% for drugs sold to the NHS. France, by contrast, has taken a different approach, which involves signing a revenue-limiting agreement with every pharmaceutical company. These methods give some freedom to market participants but are unfavorable to the development of new products in the market. This is because, while the sales of a breakthrough product increase exponentially in a few years, the aforementioned measures restrict the sales of a product based on its sales history and investment level. In conjunction with supply-side control, many countries are also turning to demand-side consumption control, such as controlling the budget allocated for physician-prescribed drugs or total healthcare expenditures.

2. Government Control of Healthcare Quality

Healthcare quality should be a matter of concern for healthcare workers. However, many healthcare workers have poor self-regulation due to their information advantage over patients. Therefore, the governments of developed countries place greater emphasis on the quality control of healthcare services provided by healthcare institutions at all levels. The methods of quality control include the certification of healthcare workers and healthcare institutions, use of medical guidelines, release of healthcare outcomes from government inspections (including the public release of healthcare quality outcomes), involvement of patients and communities in quality assessment, and handling of medical disputes. These methods are applicable to both market-based and public healthcare systems.

(1) Certification of Healthcare Workers and Healthcare Institutions

Certification is a commonly adopted method of ensuring that healthcare workers meet the minimum requirements. There are two types of certifications for healthcare institutions: (1) the government directly establishes a set of standards that serve as prerequisites for healthcare institutions to continue operating and receive funding; (2) independent industry self-regulatory bodies are established to determine the supervision standards of their members.

The US has primarily adopted the second type of certification system, by establishing a single nonprofit organization – the Joint Commission (JCAHO) – to assess and certify more than 18,000 healthcare institutions and programs nationwide. The regulations of federal and state governments are performed based on standards established by the JCAHO.

In Canada, the certification of physicians is conducted via a peer review system that is supervised by an independent committee, in which healthcare workers constitute no more than 50% of committee members. However, healthcare workers in Canada generally have little incentive to meet the standards established by this committee because public funding is not allocated based on whether they are certified. This type of organizational structure places a greater emphasis on education and self-development.

In contrast to Canada, certification in Australia is a prerequisite for healthcare institutions to receive public funds. In Australia, the certification agency is an independent body primarily composed of healthcare workers. It focuses on reviewing the use of internal quality assurance systems in healthcare institutions and aims to promote the provision of healthcare services that meet certain standards, rather than simply penalizing healthcare institutions for not upholding these standards.

The UK utilizes different regulatory structures between private and public healthcare institutions. The King's Fund, headquartered in London, focuses on improving the quality management of the universal healthcare system. To this end, the fund has helped formulate the existing certification standards. The UK also utilizes peer review, which is intended to promote self-improvement rather than eliminate offending physicians.

(2) Government Use of Medical Guidelines

Governments use medical guidelines to influence medical decision-making. These guidelines are usually developed based on a review of the actual situation, sometimes complemented by expert advice. These guidelines may be utilized in conjunction with a merit/demerit system, and can be mandatory or voluntary, and flexible or rigid. However, physicians often resist the implementation of guidelines, as they believe that the guidelines are intended to constrain them. In fact, medical guidelines alone are insufficient to alter the norms of medical practice. Physicians generally become more motivated to comply with medical guidelines if doing so is linked with some form of economic compensation.

(3) Government Release of Healthcare Quality Outcomes

The monitoring of healthcare outcomes is arguably the most effective method of ensuring the quality of healthcare services. In the US, information on healthcare outcomes is not only widely collected and supervised, but also sometimes made publicly available. For example, the US Medical Funding Committee published the mortality rate of elderly patients in the 30 days after hospitalization for each hospital in the country from 1986 to 1992. Furthermore, in 1988, the committee published the ranking of hospitals by mortality rates for heart disease, stroke, and pulmonary diseases. The release of certain healthcare outcomes can effectively improve healthcare quality. For instance, in New York City, the release of data on coronary artery bypass graft (CABG) was closely associated with a 41% reduction in operative mortality rates over the subsequent four years. Another study has reported that some hospitals have taken direct measures to reduce mortality in response to the published data.

(4) Involvement of Patients and Communities in Quality Assessment

The involvement of patients and communities in the technical assessment and individual quality assessment of healthcare services has become increasingly important because patient satisfaction is a key factor in determining the quality of healthcare services. A report released by the Managed Care Organization (MCO) recommended that multiple methods are required to ensure healthcare quality. The report particularly emphasized the importance of patient-focused interventions.

(5) Handling of Medical Malpractices

The handling of medical malpractice is the most conventional approach to ensuring that healthcare workers are responsible for their medical practice and uphold a certain level of healthcare service quality. The most severe penalty for malpractice is revocation of medical license. In the US, the Board of Medical Licensure and Discipline in each state is responsible for handling complaints and taking disciplinary action against physicians involved in malpractice. However, these boards often lack credibility because they are primarily composed of healthcare workers. In the UK, the GMC is responsible for receiving and handling complaints against healthcare workers. The UK has far fewer medical lawsuits than the US. However, since January 1990, the Ministry of Health began compensating for the costs of lawsuits against all hospitals and community healthcare workers, which has led to a rapid increase in the number of medical lawsuits.

SECTION V. GOVERNMENT MEASURES FOR HEALTHCARE COST CONTAINMENT IN DEVELOPED COUNTRIES AND AREAS

The irrational increase in healthcare expenditure is a common problem faced by many developed countries. To reduce these expenditures and make efficient use of limited healthcare resources without compromising the quality of healthcare services, these governments have introduced various policies to ensure consistency between the increase in healthcare expenditure and economic growth.

1. Managed Healthcare and Managed Competition

Healthcare reform is inevitable in the US due to the fatal flaw in its healthcare system, namely, the contradiction between the US ranking first in healthcare expenditure among developed countries and the limited improvement in the health status of its population. The higher healthcare expenditure in the US compared to other countries is not due to the widespread and frequent use of advanced healthcare services, but can be attributed to the high fees for each service item. Patients in the US are charged on a fee-for-service basis, and treatment fees are reimbursed by a third party – the insurance companies. Hence, there is no incentive mechanism for cost optimization, and healthcare institutions often attempt to attract patients by providing high-quality services without considering the overall healthcare expenditure. Furthermore, the allocation of healthcare resources to the market without ensuring that patients are fully informed of relevant healthcare services has led to significant issues in efficiency. The increase in healthcare expenditure is generally caused by overallocation of resources to advanced and specialist healthcare, as well as underallocation of resources to primary and long-term care. In light of this issue, the US government has introduced two reform measures that target the personal insurance of patients and the overall insurance market.

(1) Managed Healthcare Predominates Personal Insurance

"Managed healthcare" is a system of providing integrated healthcare based on a very simple principle: limit unnecessary or excessive expenses under the premise of quality assurance. "Managed healthcare" relies on organizations known as HMOs, a payer-led competitive arrangement consisting of an optional combination of healthcare units and insurance companies. It provides a series of predefined healthcare services prepaid by registered members.

No additional charges are incurred after the provision of these healthcare services. The prepaid fee varies according to age, gender, medical history, and the number of HMO members.

HMOs sign contracts with numerous healthcare units and physicians or have their own hospitals and physicians to provide healthcare services to all members. Members of an HMO must first choose an HMO-accredited GP to access the necessary healthcare services. The GP can refer the patient to specialists whenever necessary.

Previously, both hospitals and physicians only incurred service charges after the provision of healthcare services. However, hospitals and physicians or medical groups within the HMO system receive monthly payments from HMOs based on the number of registered patients. In other words, hospitals and physicians with more registered patients receive higher monthly payments. Consequently, hospitals and physicians can generate more profits by reducing patient visits and incurring lower costs. Therefore, hospitals and physicians strive to reduce healthcare costs by improving their healthcare services to reduce incidence and visit rates.

GPs play a key role in the HMO system as gatekeepers who manage, coordinate, and provide healthcare services, and refer patients to relevant specialists when necessary. Patients can access specialized healthcare services, hospitalization, or surgery only if these are deemed necessary by their GP. This is believed to significantly minimize the misuse of healthcare services. However, a disadvantage of this approach is that hospitals might suppress reasonable demands of patients to save costs, while GPs might reduce the service volume for patients to ensure a balanced budget or to increase their profits.

(2) Introduction of Managed Competition into the Insurance Market

"Managed competition" refers to the use of competitive pressure in the market to reduce healthcare expenditure and insurance premiums under the control of the federal government. State governments have to establish one or more Health Insurance Purchasing Cooperatives (HIPCs), also known as Regional Health Alliances (RHAs). Every American citizen must participate in one of these government-established and government-run alliances. These alliances are actually buyer clubs that purchase health insurance from insurance companies and negotiate with physicians and hospitals on behalf of their members. In addition, they also help standardize medical fees, collect health insurance premiums, and pay insurance companies and hospitals on behalf of their members. The competition rules stipulated by these alliances promote competition among insurance companies in terms of insurance content, criteria, and prices. On the other hand, these rules also create competition among healthcare units in terms of service quality and price. Furthermore, healthcare plans must provide basic services to insured persons according to the basic insurance premiums of HIPCs. If they wish to obtain profits from these services, the prices must be stated explicitly and separately in the form of supplemental insurance. HIPCs require a degree of statistical transparency in all rival agencies, which is achieved through the collection of clinical data for each healthcare plan, including mortality, incidence of complications, re-hospitalization rate, and six-month or one-year survival rates. Additionally, service user satisfaction surveys are carried out for each healthcare plan. The resulting data and findings must be made publicly available by the HPST regularly. These data can then be used to improve the service quality at healthcare agencies and control their healthcare expenditure. Therefore, the integration between the free market and government-related policies has created a competitive health insurance market to ensure that citizens enjoy a certain quality of healthcare services with relatively lower insurance premiums.

With the aging of the US population, the government is striving to control health insurance prices and healthcare expenditures. Hence, "managed healthcare" and "managed competition" are likely to become the core aspects of the US healthcare system in the future because of their important roles in this regard.

2. Hospital Global Budget System

Health Canada is responsible for the reimbursement of medical expenses. This organization has implemented a "global budget system," which requires each hospital to provide free inpatient services to all residents living in the community. Health Canada negotiates with hospitals regarding the total budget based on the actual expenditures in the past year and their growth rate in the current year. After reaching an agreement, the budget allocation among physicians is resolved by the Canadian Medical Association (CMA). Physicians' income is based on service points: physicians with more service points receive greater budget allocations. The CMA reserves the right to take disciplinary action against physicians who fail to comply with the CMA's rules and regulations.

In France, the annual budget allocated to each hospital is determined by multiplying the number of patients by the average daily expenses in the past year. This budgeting method was loosely implemented in the past due to the lack of strict budget management in hospitals. Since 1984, however, the government of France has controlled the inpatient medical expenses via a global budget system, which requires stricter budgeting and implementation compared to the previously adopted method based on average daily expenses. Since 1985, the outpatient department of hospitals has also been included in this new budgeting method. The new budgeting system has the following stipulations: (1) Strict budgeting is required for the coming year, but deficits in the previous year are not transferred to the budget of the coming year. (2) Complete rationalization of hospitals is necessary and the budget is allocated based on the degree of rationalization. (3) The annual budget is divided into 12 parts and allocated on a monthly basis, regardless of expenditure variations between different months. (4) In order to address the arbitrary, irresponsible, and inefficient aspects of each department at hospitals, a director general (nonphysician) is appointed and authorized for budget management to control each department through the global budget allocated to hospitals. In general, the global budget system has been shown to be effective in curbing the rise of inpatient expenses.

3. Regulating the Provision of Elderly Healthcare Services

Empirical studies in developed countries have revealed that the rapid growth in healthcare expenditure is mainly attributed to the increase in inpatient expenses, while the inpatient expenses for the elderly constitute a large proportion of the total inpatient expenses. In addition, the governments of developed countries have begun to realize that a wave of population aging will sweep the world in the near future. Therefore, some countries have proposed a reduction in healthcare expenditure by altering the methods of elderly healthcare service provision, which includes home-based therapy and home-based care.

(1) Home-Based Therapy

Home-based therapy is also known as home care. In France, home-based therapy is characterized by treatments conducted at the discharged patient's home by attending physicians in collaboration with hospital physicians and nurses. A total of 32 healthcare institutions provide home-based therapy services in Paris, including 10 public hospitals (e.g., the Assistance Publique–Hôptiaux de Paris) and 22 nonprofit incorporated associations. The average age of home-based therapy users is 63 years, and 45.6% of users are elderly adults over the age of 70 years. The main targets of home-based therapy are elderly individuals with chronic diseases. In 1982, the ranking of diseases based on the use of home-based therapy was as follows: cancer (47.6%); circulatory system diseases (14.7%); sports injuries, including fractures (8.8%); and neurological and sensory disorders (8.1%).

There are several reasons for governments to promote home-based therapy: Patients might recover faster if they receive treatment in their daily living environment; terminal care can be effectively provided at home for incurable diseases; and home-based therapies are less expensive than hospitalization.

(2) Home-Based Care

Home-based care is equivalent to home-visit nursing system. Specifically, it is a form of medical social work that seeks to improve the quality of life of elderly adults following the completion of inpatient treatments. Home-based care is provided by nurses based on physicians' prescriptions, but might also involve collaboration with other practitioners, such as massage therapists and physiotherapists. Home-based care is now considered a vital component of home assistance services for the elderly in France. Incorporated associations are the predominant provider of home-based care services (57%), followed by public agencies (31%), social security funds (9%), and other organizations (3%). Regarding the payment of medical expenses for home-based care, beneficiaries generally bear none of the expenses as insured persons are covered by health insurance funds while uninsured persons are covered by their respective counties according to law. In 1984, the medical expenses covered by health insurance amounted to F67.7 million.

The statistical data released by Japan's MHLW in 2004 showed that 23,418 nurses worked in home-visit nursing stations. Each station had an average of 4.7 designated nurses, each of whom visited 69 patients per month.

There are several reasons for the government to promote home-based care: hospitalization can be avoided whenever the medical and social conditions allow, which will reduce the medical expenses; it can facilitate the transition to living at home after hospitalization; it enables the monitoring of users' physical conditions to alleviate possible deterioration after discharge; and it can prevent the need for elderly adults to visit social welfare facilities.

SECTION VI. GOVERNMENT MEASURES TO ADDRESS HEALTH SERVICE PROBLEMS IN DEVELOPED COUNTRIES AND AREAS

1. Measures to Address Long Waiting Lists for Inpatient and Outpatient Services

(1) The UK Government's General Practitioner Prescribing Budget and Publicly Funded Overseas Medical Treatment

Despite its excellent guarantee of healthcare equality, the UK NHS is largely inefficient. In addition, medical fees at private hospitals in the UK are often unaffordable to the general population. Therefore, the majority of patients choose to join the NHS's long waiting list. At present, there are about 600,000 patients on the waiting list for hospitalization in the UK, which peaked at 680,000 patients in 1978 and has gradually declined thereafter. Waiting lists vary across departments and regions, but those for surgical departments are often the longest. In general, the waiting times for hernia surgery, vascular tumor surgery, and tonsil hypertrophy surgery are 15–20 weeks, 20–25 weeks, and 10–23 weeks, respectively. Hence, the UK government has been attempting to shift the care of inpatients to outpatient departments, which in turn has increased the number of outpatients. Based on the number of first visits, it is clear that the number of outpatients has increased over the years, ranging from 1.37 million patients in 1954 to 2.12 million patients in 1981. Similar to inpatient services, the number of waiting days for outpatient services has increased alongside increasing demand, which has also led to the problem of a long waiting list. To help resolve this issue, in July 1986, the UK government launched a three-year plan to shorten the inpatient and outpatient waiting lists and improve hospital efficiency.

The UK government introduced the General Practitioner Prescribing Budget program in the NHS to enable healthcare associations to allocate the budget directly to GPs with a greater number of registered patients, which allows them to purchase certain services from hospitals for their patients, including specialist consultations, diagnostic tests, inpatient treatments, and outpatient surgeries (except for expensive and complicated inpatient treatments). In April 1991, 306 GPs became the first budget owners under this program. Another 300 GPs joined the program in April 1992. As of 1995, the number of patients registered with these budget-holding GPs accounted for more than 50% of the total number of registered patients. The program has also improved the efficiency of treatment, as patients who have registered with budget-holding GPs usually receive treatment within shorter periods of time without a long waiting list for treatment, compared to those who have registered with nonbudget-holding GPs.

As of 2002, there were approximately one million patients on the waiting list for medical treatment in the UK, among which 42,000 patients had been waiting for more than a year. It is common for British citizens to wait months or even years for nonurgent operations. The European Union (EU) has stipulated that patients in an EU member state have the right to receive treatment at hospitals in other member states when the expected treatment is unavailable in their own countries. Coupled with the recommendations and pressure of local medical communities, in October 2001, the Minister of State for Health finally allowed patients who have been waiting more than six months for surgery to receive treatment at a local private hospital or overseas using public funds. On January 18, 2002, the first batch of British patients traveled to France for medical treatment using public funds. Given the limited number of physicians and hospital beds, patients can greatly benefit from the opportunities to receive treatment overseas with advanced equipment and less stringent eligibility criteria, despite being an expedient measure during an urgent situation.

Since April 2004, the NHS has implemented a new service contract, known as the General Medical Service (GMS), to improve both healthcare equality and the quality of basic healthcare services. This contract introduced a new salary system for GPs, to replace the previous system, which determines salaries based on the number of patients. GPs can also receive additional remuneration based on their Quality of Outcomes Framework (QOF) scores. Taking into account the service workload of GPs, higher QOF scores indicate higher service quality and remuneration. These changes in the salary system induced the motivation of GPs.

(2) The Government of Singapore Solved Problems by Establishing Rigid Standards

In 2001, the Ministry of Health of Singapore signed an agreement with each medical group that not only clearly stipulates the right of each group to receive subsidies from the Ministry of Health, but also established rigid standards regarding the quantity and quality of services to be achieved by each group. For instance, the agreement has established acceptable ranges of appointment waiting time and the waiting time in the healthcare facility: the average appointment wait time for subsidized patients is 14 days and appointment waiting time of more than 42 days is considered a failure; similarly, the average waiting time in the facility is 30 minutes and waiting time of more than 75 minutes is considered a failure. This agreement also strictly enforces fines against hospitals that fail to meet the set standards.

2. Introduction of the "Community Healthcare over Inpatient Treatment" Policy

It is estimated that the annual operating cost of a hospital is six times that of a community healthcare center, as the latter can significantly improve the health status of residents, thereby reducing the necessity of treatments and medical expenses. Therefore, many countries have shifted their policy priorities from inpatient treatment to community healthcare services.

The UK government has implemented the "community healthcare over inpatient treatment" policy to encourage elderly patients and patients with physical and mental disabilities to receive treatment at home by increasing their reliance on community care. This policy requires ample primary community healthcare workers whose core members are family physicians. However, health visitors (including female health visitors), district nurses, and midwives are also highly valued by the government.

(1) Healthcare Workers Who Cooperate with Family Physicians

1. *Health visitors.* Much like district nurses and midwives, health visitors work under regional health authorities. They visit the elderly and families with disabled individuals (specifically children) to understand and advise on their health issues, as well as contact family physicians, hospitals, and the social welfare departments of local authorities whenever necessary. To become a health visitor, a licensed nurse must complete a three- to six-month midwifery course and a one-year health visitor course, after which they must pass the licensure examination. Additionally, a licensed health visitor must receive continuing education every four- to five years. In 1980, there were approximately 9,800 health visitors who performed a total of 3.82 million visits each year.

2. *District nurses.* District nurses are responsible for visiting elderly adults and families with disabled individuals to assist them in body cleansing, bathing, changing bedsheets, changing wound dressing, injections, drug administration, blood and urine tests, and so forth. To become a district nurse, a licensed nurse must complete a three- to four-month practical training program and pass the licensure examination. In 1980, there were approximately 13,000 nurses who carried out a total of 3.42 million visits in the UK each year.

3. *Midwives.* Midwives are responsible for performing home births, as well as providing prenatal and postpartum guidance and care. A licensed nurse needs to complete an 18-month practical training program to become a midwife. In 1980, there were approximately 2,800 midwives providing community healthcare services in England.

(2) Introduction of a Community Physician (Public Health Physician) System

The Report of the Royal Commission on Medical Education 1968 advocated for a class of physicians specialized in community healthcare issues, rather than personal health issues.

Based on this report, a system for organizing community physicians (also known as public health physicians) was introduced in 1974. Community physicians are local medical officers affiliated with local health authorities, regional medical officers affiliated with regional health authorities, and specialist physicians employed by local or regional health authorities. The local and regional medical officers supervise their respective subordinate specialist physicians. Community physicians are responsible for analyzing the healthcare needs and services in regions or districts within their jurisdiction, as well as the environmental health, social welfare, housing, and education of local autonomous communities. Community physicians are also responsible for communicating and coordinating with relevant agencies, as well as conducting research. In reality, however, administrative affairs account for 60% of the scope of their job. To become a community physician, a practicing physician needs to register with the GMC, complete a practical training program, and pass the relevant examination. In 1982, there were only 500 community physicians in the UK.

Previously, the government of Canada had focused on providing healthcare services in healthcare facilities such as hospitals when meeting the demand for long-term convalescent care. However, reforms became necessary when factors, such as population aging, emergence of new diseases, advancement of medical technology, and the increase in medical expenses, were taken into account. Therefore, the government has also been making the effort to implement regional services (community health services) as well as expanding existing facilities, in order to ensure the efficient use of resources as well as more effective and efficient care. To achieve this, the government requires the cooperation of healthcare practitioners, NGOs, and individuals to improve community healthcare services. Furthermore, a supportive network of family and friends must be established as the implementation of this policy is expected to face a shortage of professionals. The promotion of home-based care as the center of long-term convalescent care has become a major issue in Canada due to the increase in demand for elderly care.

3. Adjustments for Reasonable Compensation Policies

Health insurance in Canada consists of medical insurance and hospital insurance. Medical insurance refers to the universal social health insurance that covers necessary healthcare services and specific dental surgeries. According to the Canada Health Act, patients are entitled to free healthcare services for items covered by this insurance. In other words, the Act did not recognize requests by GPs and dentists for additional charges. Five provinces requested for additional charges to be covered under this insurance from 1984 to 1987. To maintain the main purpose of their social medical insurance system, the government has deducted a total of US$240 million in federal subsidies for four of these provinces, where medical expenses are borne by the patients. As of 1987, all provinces and quasi-provinces have abolished the request for additional charges and medical expenses borne by patients, and have accepted the insurance reimbursement for reduced medical expenses.

4. Improving Service Quality by Increasing the Number of Healthcare Workers

The healthcare system in Japan once faced a prominent issue, namely, a decline in patient satisfaction due to low service quality. According to a survey conducted by Harvard University on Japan, Canada, Germany, the UK, and the US, Japan had the lowest overall patient satisfaction (67%). Among the remaining four countries, the UK had the lowest patient satisfaction (87%), but this was still higher than Japan's by 20 percentage points. The low quality of hospital services in Japan is manifested by the number of healthcare workers assigned to each patient. In Japan, each inpatient is allocated an average of 1.0 healthcare worker (including physicians, nurses, administrative staff, and technicians), while the average length of hospital stay for each inpatient is 30 days. In contrast, each inpatient in the US is allocated an average of 4.5 healthcare workers (excluding physicians), while the average length of hospital stay for each inpatient is 5.5–5.6 days. In other words, the number of healthcare workers in the US is 4.5 times that of Japan, and the length of hospital stay is only one-sixth that of Japan. Each inpatient in the UK is allocated an average of 3.0 healthcare workers, while the average length of hospital stay is approximately 10 days. Each inpatient in Germany and France is allocated 2.5 healthcare workers, while the average length of hospital stay is 12–13 days. Therefore, the average number of healthcare workers allocated to each inpatient appears to be inversely proportional to the length of hospital stay.

Japan is the only developed country in which the average number of physicians and nurses allocated to each patient is the same as it was 30 years ago. This is attributed to the continuous increase in the number of hospital beds, the rate of which is two to five times that of other countries. On the other hand, the average numbers of physicians and nurses allocated to each patient in the US, France, Germany, and the UK have almost tripled in the past 30 years. An increase in the number of healthcare workers can reduce the length of hospital stay and improve healthcare efficiency. The unit cost of medical expenses will increase but the total cost remains unchanged due to shorter hospital stays. Therefore, the MHLW of Japan proposed the following reform measures in 1997: increase the standard number of nurses allocated to general wards from one nurse per four inpatients to one nurse per three inpatients, and reduce the number of hospital beds and the length of hospital stay.

5. Regulatory Roles in Stabilizing National Healthcare Needs

Singapore's Medisave is a national mandatory medical savings scheme that assists Singaporeans in saving a portion of their income into Medisave accounts, which can be used to cover the future inpatient expenses and some of the most expensive outpatient expenses for themselves or their family members. The government has adopted several measures to prevent the fluctuation of healthcare needs when implementing this scheme.

(1) Prevention of Excessive Healthcare Demands Due to Overfunded Savings Accounts

The Medisave contribution rate is configured not only to meet the basic healthcare needs of Singaporeans but also to prevent an improper increase in healthcare needs, excessive utilization of healthcare services, and wastage of healthcare resources due to "overfunded" Medisave accounts. Therefore, the government has imposed an upper limit on the monthly contribution to Medisave accounts.

(2) "Deficit" Measures Against Insufficient Demands

In order to ensure access to basic healthcare service for families whose Medisave funds are insufficient to cover their medical expenses, the government allows "deficits" in their Medisave accounts to be repaid afterward at the same interest rate as the Central Provident Fund.

6. Compensation Measures for the Inadequate Supply of Public Health and Basic Healthcare

(1) Government Provision

In countries with well-developed market economies, the provision of public goods (including public healthcare services) through taxation is one of the responsibilities of governments. The establishment of nonprofit healthcare institutions by the government not only prevents monopolies but also is favorable to fulfilling the population's demand for public health and basic healthcare. Nonprofit healthcare institutions do not aim to maximize profits in the provision of public goods; hence, when positive externalities are generated or when consumers are unwilling to cover the production cost of public goods, these institutions will still prioritize the meeting of consumer demand and not cause a shortage of public health and basic healthcare.

(2) Government Purchases

When private providers are reluctant to provide services due to a lack of compensation from external benefits, nonprofit healthcare institutions can purchase public health and basic healthcare services at prices that are equivalent to the positive externalities and then provide them to the public, thereby indirectly compensating for the inadequate supply.

(3) Subsidizing Private Producers

The government can also subsidize producers that generate positive externalities to internalize those externalities. As a result, the external benefits become part of producers' incomes, such that the private income is increased to the point where it is equal to the social benefits. This in turn motivates producers to increase productive activities with positive externalities. The effects of this measure are similar to that of government purchases. Therefore, the injection of greater capital into public healthcare institutions and reasonable compensation to private healthcare institutions are important strategies to increase the supply of healthcare services.

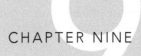

CHAPTER NINE

Basic Drug Administration Policies in Developed Countries and Areas

SECTION I. GOVERNMENT POLICIES RELATED TO DRUG MANUFACTURING IN DEVELOPED COUNTRIES AND AREAS

The governments of developed countries typically focus on two issues with regard to the administration of drug manufacturing: (1) drug safety and efficacy, and (2) cost. Most developed countries have formulated fairly detailed and complicated regulations for the administration of drug safety and efficacy. In this chapter, we introduce the administrative policies that have a significant influence on drug manufacturing in developed countries. The administrative objectives of drug manufacturing in developed countries have gradually shifted in its emphasis along with continued socioeconomic development and improvements in health insurance, which can roughly be divided into three stages.

1. Stage 1: Market Management and Legal System Improvements

Mid-1960s to mid-1980s. This stage involved the legalization of the comprehensive reinforcement and improvement of drug market administration. The thalidomide (Immunoprin) tragedy of the early 1960s prompted developed countries to review and enhance their administration of the quality of drug manufacturing. During this stage, developed countries progressively established a marketing licensing system that includes six licenses – raw materials, products, manufacturing, clinical trials, sales and advertising, and promotions. The market entry of new drugs, generic drugs, and biological products is permissible only if they meet the stringent standards established by the government and relevant drug administration agencies. Furthermore, these countries have also enacted laws banning or sanctioning the sale of counterfeit and substandard drugs.

From the 1980s, most developed countries have begun carrying out inspections of the side effects of clinical drugs as part of their drug administration. Furthermore, European and North American countries began granting patent terms or market exclusivity to protect the marketing of new drugs (the average terms are 8.5 years in the US, 7–10 years in Canada, and 6–10 years in European countries).

2. Stage 2: Reduction of Drug Costs

Mid- to the late 1980s. In this stage, governments began enacting policies that encouraged and promoted the development of new drugs. Furthermore, in response to the heavy financial burden caused by the rapid increase in drug costs, governments also began loosening restrictions on generic drugs, in order to reduce drug costs by increasing the production of generic drugs.

(1) Development of New Drugs

The majority of research-based manufacturers are headquartered in developed countries (the US, the UK, France, Germany, Sweden, etc.) with high export rates. Hence, policies regarding the development of new drugs are a key area of drug administration in these countries (e.g., in France, the expenditure on new drug development was ranked third among different research areas). The number of new drug applications (NDAs) has been decreasing consistently since the mid-1970s due to scientific and political pressure on pre-clinical trials and the consequent economic pressure. For example, in the US, the license for the manufacturing of new drugs can only be obtained after the entire NDA process has been completed, and each NDA requires an average capital injection of approximately US$231 million, which has objectively led to the decrease in NDAs.

Nevertheless, since the mid-1980s, governments began to adopt various preferential policies for the development of new drugs. In 1984, the US Congress enacted the Drug Price Competition and Patent Term Restoration Act (also known as the Hatch-Waxman Act, and does not apply to biological products). This act allows for the extension of patent terms for up to five years to compensate for the delay caused by the NDA procedures of the Food and Drug Administration (FDA). In 1985, the US adopted stronger policies that encourage and protect the development of new drugs for the treatment of rare diseases (i.e., diseases with only about 200,000 target patients), which included: (1) tax incentives and (2) seven years of market exclusivity (which is longer than the patent term). These policies had a crucial impact on the development of new drugs in the US and were applicable to almost all research-based pharmaceutical companies. In 1987, the European Communities enacted a market protection directive for biological products and highly innovative drugs. The directive required data protection for these two types of drugs (including those without patent protection), and the second license application can only be submitted after 6–10 years.

Since January 2, 1993, the member states of the European Communities permitted the application of supplementary protection certificates (SPCs) from the European Patent Office (EPO), which allows the extension of the patent term by up to five years for patented drugs (including pharmaceutical compounds and drugs and their preparation methods or applications) if the remaining patent term is less than five years after being granted a manufacturing license by the relevant health authorities. Subsequently, the Uruguay Round Agreements Act (URAA) was enacted on December 8, 1994, which extended the patent term to 20 years from the earliest filing date instead of 17 years from the issue date. Patents issued after June 8, 1995, followed the new regulations, while unexpired patents issued prior to June 8, 1995, followed either the old or new regulations, whichever has the longer patent term.

(2) Production of Generic Drugs

The patent expiration of a new drug that has generated high profits will attract more manufacturers to produce and sell "similar" products. Experience has shown that there are cost differences of 40% to 70% between new and generic drugs due to the difference in their cost structures. Therefore, governments have been adopting policies that encourage the production of generic drugs for cost control since the mid-1980s in order to promote the competition of drug prices. The US Drug Price Competition and Patent Term Restoration Act of 1984 stipulates that upon the expiry of the patent term or market exclusivity period, generic drugs can be manufactured after a simple NDA procedure that does not require repeating previous animal and clinical trials. In other words, the FDA does not need to further review its efficacy and safety. Furthermore, a provision in the Drug Price Competition and Patent Term Restoration Act, known as the "Bolar" amendment, even allows generic drug manufacturers to research generic counterparts of brand-name drugs even before the expiry of patent terms. However, the production of generic drugs prior to patent expiration is only permissible for research purposes and not for commercial purposes. Consequently, the production of generic drugs has increased substantially in the US. In 1987, the European Communities simplified the application procedure for manufacturing generic drugs, such that the production of "a product that is comparable to" its brand-name counterpart is exempt from providing pharmacological, toxicological, and clinical data contained in the "first filed application" after the patent expiration for that drug.

3. Stage 3: Emphasis on Health Economic Benefits

1990s to the present. In this stage, governments (or insurance agencies) adopted an active role in stimulating the production of substitute drugs by abolishing the restrictions on the types of alternative drugs. In the US, for example, the proportion of generic drugs out of all prescription drugs increased from 29% in 1979 to 40% in 1990, and the goal is to ensure that this share is at least 50% in the future. In addition, the integrated licensing regulation for drug manufacturing came into effect in the European Communities in 1993. The worldwide trend toward license integration has positive implications for the reduction of healthcare expenditure, as it further enhances the competition in the drug market, reduces drug administration costs, and delays the marketing of new drugs.

In recent years, developed countries have begun to attach greater importance to the legislation of premarketing health economics (e.g., cost/benefit analysis) of new drugs. It is expected that the results of these analyses can be used to guide the selection and utilization of new drugs. Although there are still some problems with the current evaluation techniques, they are soon expected to be applied to the manufacturing licensing procedures of new drugs. In August 2011, the Phys.org internet news portal reported that American scientists have begun, for the first time, to use computer models and genomic information to find new applications for existing drugs. They found that the drugs used in the treatment of ulcers and epileptic seizure can also be used to treat lung cancer and inflammatory bowel disease. Dr. Rochelle M. Long, the Director of the NIGMS Division at the Pharmacogenomics Research Network (PGRN) of the National Institutes of Health (NIH), has stated that the discovery of new applications for approved and marketed drugs could decrease the time taken for a new drug to proceed from laboratory testing to clinical trials, reduce the associated costs, and improve therapeutic efficacy.

SECTION II. GOVERNMENT POLICIES RELATED TO DRUG MARKETING IN DEVELOPED COUNTRIES AND AREAS

The pricing of drugs is different from that of general products due to their specificity. Pharmaceutical companies may exploit their information advantage and system flaws to charge higher prices for drugs, which increases the medical expenses of patients and reduces the operational efficiency of the national healthcare system. Therefore, drug pricing is of great importance to the governments of all countries worldwide. Broadly speaking, the pharmaceutical industry encompasses not only drug manufacturers but also drug distributors and retailers. The primary channel of drug marketing is as follows: manufacturers → distributors → retailers (approximately 80%). There are also several branch channels in drug marketing. In general, governments have two primary means of controlling drug distribution: (1) Distributors and retailers must obtain licenses from relevant government agencies, and their operational scope and eligibility criteria are strictly limited. (2) Due to the widespread implementation of universal health insurance systems, the government is the only body that has the right to raise health insurance funds. Therefore, most developed countries (or insurance agencies) are capable of implementing various cost control measures on drugs, i.e., the control of profits or prices of manufacturers, distributors, and pharmacies (or pharmacists). In addition, governments have also developed policies and regulations that indirectly influence drug distribution, such as drug classification and administration acts, as well as policies that encourage the importation of drugs.

Next, we focus on policies related to drug distribution in developed countries.

1. Price Control on Manufacturers

Most European and American countries have established their own price control systems for prescription drugs as part of their health insurance system but with varying degrees of freedom in pricing, as shown in Table 9.1.

(1) Price Control System

This is the most direct approach to price control. Countries such as France and Sweden have implemented this approach on outpatient prescription drugs. In this system, the prices and price increases of new drugs are directly controlled by the government, and the prices are based on negotiations between the government and each manufacturer. There are three pricing criteria: the therapeutic value of the new drug, the price of comparable treatment,

TABLE 9.1   Methods of Drug Price Control Adopted by Five Developed Countries in Europe and America

Price Control Method	US	UK	France	Germany	Sweden
Price			+		+
Profit		+			
Reference price				+	+
Market competition	+				

Note: + indicates that the price control method is adopted in the country.

and the economic contribution of the drug. Sweden also uses prices in other countries as a benchmark when setting the prices for new drugs. Currently, the prices of all drugs registered in the reimbursement list of the French National Health Insurance are set by the government. These drugs account for approximately 95% of all marketed prescription drugs and 78% of the total pharmaceutical sales.

In France, the Transparency Committee and the Economic and Public Health Evaluation Committee under the French National Authority for Health are responsible for the pricing of new drugs. An evaluation is first carried out by the Transparency Committee, after which the Economic and Public Health Evaluation Committee use the value-based evaluation results and price recommendations of the Transparency Committee to conduct negotiations with drug manufacturers on the wholesale prices, retail prices, and reimbursement ratio, and sign relevant the agreements with manufacturers. Once a price agreement is reached, the agreed prices and reimbursements are valid for four years. Generally speaking, the prices of drugs will be reduced by 1–2% after every price adjustment. The Swedish government has attempted to synchronize drug prices with inflation rates.

(2) Reference Price (or Reimbursement Price) System

This is an indirect approach to price control. Reference pricing is based on the principle that a common reimbursement level can be determined for a specific group of drugs that have equivalent therapeutic efficacies and are clinically interchangeable. In other words, the government (or insurance agencies) imposes a price ceiling (i.e., a reference price) for reimbursable drugs covered by insurance. In 1989, Germany became the first country to introduce the reference pricing system. The German legislation stipulates that the reference price is based on the average price for a given drug and similar products. Pharmaceutical companies are free to set their own prices, but consumers must pay the difference between the retail price and the reference price. Hence, the prices established by pharmaceutical companies are restricted by consumers' willingness to pay. The reference pricing system lowers drug prices by reducing the demand for high-priced medicines and encouraging companies to reduce prices voluntarily, rather than imposing direct price control. However, as of July 1993, about 50% of drugs in Germany lacked reference prices. Even more than a decade later, in 2005, about 40% of drugs lacked reference prices in the German market. In Sweden, the reference prices are set at 10% higher than the cheapest generic drugs. In New Zealand, the lowest price for the same group of drugs is selected as the reference price. In Canada, the health insurance scheme for the elderly and impoverished individuals in each province has also adopted policies for drug reimbursement prices.

(3) Profit Control System

This is another form of indirect price control that has been adopted by the UK and Spain. In addition to cost-plus pricing for pharmaceutical products, Spain has further restricted the profit margins of pharmaceutical companies to 12–18%. In the UK, the price regulation system for patented prescription drugs (known as the Voluntary Price Regulation Scheme) was initiated in 1957 and was renamed the Pharmaceutical Price Regulation Scheme (PPRS) in 1978. The PPRS is revised every five years. According to the latest PPRS, pharmaceutical companies are free to set prices for patented prescription drugs, but the profit margin of drugs sold to the NHS must be maintained at 17–21%, with an allowable margin of tolerance of 25%. The profits of manufacturers are related to their levels of investment (production and development). When the actual net profit exceeds the target profit by 25%, pharmaceutical companies must reduce the prices of one or several drugs to ensure that their net profits fall within the target level, or they must transfer the excess profits to the Ministry of Health. However, companies earning 50% or less of the target profit can request permission from the Ministry of Health to increase their drug prices, such that their profits will reach 80% of the target. In addition, the NHS also limits the amount used by manufacturers for promotional purposes to less than 9% of the total sales. Pharmaceutical manufacturers in the UK are free to set the prices of new drugs, but any price increase must be approved by the government. The NHS has limited profits margins for generic drugs due to their much lower initial investments compared to new drugs. Generic manufacturers primarily generate profits by reducing manufacturing costs and increasing sales. Japan has adopted the fee schedule system since 1996 for drug supplies, whereby the price of each drug is set according to its average purchase price and reasonable profits. Since the implementation of this fee schedule system, pharmaceutical profits have reduced from 15% in 1992 to 5% in 1998 and further to 2% in 2000.

(4) Free Price System

Health security in the US is predominated by commercial health insurance and the country lacks nationwide universal health coverage; hence, the government has a relatively low capacity for intervening in drug pricing. Therefore, a free price policy has been adopted for drugs, which does not involve nationwide price control measures, a national formulary, or integrated policies on consumer copayments. Under this system, drug pricing is mainly determined by the overall trend of supply and demand in the market. Companies tend to raise pricing benchmarks intentionally when pricing new drugs, which leads to higher prices in the US than in Europe for the same drug. Therefore, pharmaceutical companies outside the US prefer to market new drugs in the US before any other country. This free price policy provides a powerful incentive for the development of the pharmaceutical industry in the US. The main forces for curbing drug prices in the US are nongovernmental managed healthcare organizations (e.g., HMOs). HMOs provide services via healthcare institutions contracted by insurance companies. HMOs also establish lists of reimbursable drugs for physicians and reimburse for drugs listed therein. Hence, the inclusion of a drug in this list will directly affect its sales. HMOs have much room for price reduction in negotiating with pharmaceutical companies because of their close ties with physicians and patients. Hence, powerful nongovernmental organizations in the US can impose relatively strong restrictions on drug prices.

Price control policies imposed on manufacturers in developed countries rely on both executive orders and market forces with varying points of balance between the two – namely, governments have varying degrees of reliance on executive measures and market mechanisms. France places greater emphasis on executive measures and the enforcement of one-to-one price controls. Germany, however, places greater emphasis on market regulation and has adopted the reference pricing system, which can have two major effects: on the one hand, manufacturers will compete with each other to reduce prices in order to include their products in the reimbursement system; on the other hand, patients are encouraged to choose less expensive drugs. The UK has adopted a more compromising and relatively flexible administrative strategy – namely, a combination of profit control, executive orders, and market competition, which gives manufacturers considerable freedom in pricing. In contrast, Sweden has integrated the approaches adopted by France and Germany.

2. Policies for Distributors

(1) Encourage Competition

In 1992, the European Communities promulgated the distributors licensing law, which came into effect on January 1, 1993. The implementation of this law increased competition among distributors (both domestic and international) by reducing the barriers to pharmaceutical trading among the member states of the European Communities. Governments also imposed policies that encourage competition among manufacturers, distributors, and pharmacies, thereby reducing the profits of drug sales in the member states of European Communities to about 6.5–8.5%.

(2) Government Monopoly

European countries (except for Denmark) have uniformly adopted one of the following measures for the distribution industry: profit controls, policies for enhancing competition, or a monopoly on drug procurement. Within the European Communities, some small-sized distributors were susceptible to elimination due to low competitive profits, whereas large-sized distributors tended to undergo organizational restructuring (e.g., mergers, acquisitions, and joint ventures) to become major international companies. Since 1993, the government of Canada has forced distributors to limit their profits to a percentage of their sales. The profit margin in 1993 was 9.5%, and parts of their net incomes were used to support pharmacotherapeutic and clinicopathological studies, as well as establishing internationally comparable pharmacostatistical studies.

The sales commission of distributors is reduced through reimbursements based on the maximum allowable cost (MAC) and the bulk purchase of drugs; that is, the government negotiates wholesale prices with distributors via contracted pharmacies to control distributors' profits. At present, the sales commissions of distributors are 10–15% and 40–60% for new drugs and generic drugs, respectively.

(3) Reimbursement Limits for Pharmacies

In the US, HMO interventions (i.e., agreements between HMOs and pharmacies) have defined the MAC for reimbursement. Hence, wholesale prices for drugs are more important to pharmacies than their own service charges. This is because pharmacy service charges do not change with time, whereas the sales commission of distributors does. Therefore, pharmacies strive to gain more profits by reducing the sales commission of distributors. In the US, the wholesale profits made via market mechanisms are higher than that in Europe.

3. Policies for Pharmacies (or Pharmacists)

The member states of the European Communities (except for Denmark) have established an upper limit on the drug price markup for pharmacists, which is calculated using a fixed service charge per prescription. In France, the fees charged by pharmacists are calculated at 30% of the retail price. The number of pharmacists is limited by national legislation to one per 2,500 people, which also stipulates that nonprescription drugs must be purchased at pharmacies. Pharmacies in Germany earn nearly 30% profit and are taxed at about 50% of their total income. There is no limit on the number of pharmacies (the current number of pharmacists in Germany is one per 4,000 people), and nonprescription drugs can be sold at other stores. The newly established Danish Competition Council is experimenting with the liberalization of pharmacies in order to enhance drug price competition. In the US, HMO-contracted pharmacies charge US$2.50 for each prescription. In Australia, pharmacists charge different markups based on the wholesale prices of drugs. Specifically, the markup of drugs with wholesale prices below AU$180 is 10%; the markup for drugs priced at AU$180–450 is a flat rate of AU$18; the markup for drugs priced at AU$450–1,000 is 4%; the markup of drugs priced above AU$1,000 is AU% 40 (which is similar to price differentials). In addition, pharmacists charge prescription fees of AU$5.44, with additional charges of AU$2.71 and AU$2.04 for dangerous drugs and compounded medications, respectively.

4. Policies for Hospitals

The direct sale of products from pharmaceutical manufacturers to hospitals also constitutes a certain share in the distribution channels of drugs, for example, by accounting for 5–19% of sales in the UK, France, and Germany. Prices are based on agreements between the hospitals and manufacturers. In terms of commodity flow, the governments (or insurance agencies) of European countries (except for Denmark) exercise greater intervention on pharmaceutical manufacturers and distributors. Most European countries have established price control systems. In addition to directly controlling the prices or profits and drug markups, these countries have also adopted various measures to promote market competition. The overall effect is that both manufacturers and distributors have higher degrees of centralization. In contrast, governments impose relatively weak interventions on pharmacies (or pharmacists), which has led to lower degrees of competition among pharmacists. Despite government control over drug price markups, pharmacists remain one of the highest paid occupations.

Although drug prices have been controlled to a certain extent through the aforementioned cost containment measures, this does not imply that the overall drug expenditure has been sufficiently controlled. The increase in drug expenditure can be attributed to the following: the increase in drug prices, the increase in drug consumption, and the increase in drug expenditure due to changes in product mix. Changes in the product mix refer to the replacement of low-priced drugs (usually conventional generic drugs) with high-priced drugs (usually new drugs). Numerous studies investigating the increase in drug expenditure have indicated that the main reasons are the increase in drug consumption and the change in product mix, rather than price increases. For example, Berndt analyzed US prescription drug data and found that the average annual growth rate of drug expenditure in the country in 1994–2000 was 12.9%. Of which, the increase in drug prices accounted for only 2.7%, while the remaining 10.2% came from the increase in drug consumption and the change in product mix. Addis and Magrini analyzed the increase in drug expenditure in Italy and found a 13.5% increase from 2000 to 2001, 9.5% of which was attributed to the increase in drug consumption and 4.8% to the change in product mix; over the same period, drug prices fell by 1%. The average annual growth rate of drug expenditure in the UK in 1992–2000 was 8.7%, of which 4.9% was derived from the increase in drug consumption and 5.4% from the change in product mix, whereas drug prices fell by an average of 1.8% during the same period. Similarly, expenses for patented drugs in Canada increased by 13.9% from 2001 to 2002. During the same period, the price of patented drugs fell by 1.2%, whereas its consumption increased by 15.5%. These practical experiences in developed countries show that the key to reducing drug expenditure is not through price control, but through guiding physicians toward the rational use of drugs.

SECTION III. DRUG REIMBURSEMENT POLICIES IN DEVELOPED COUNTRIES AND AREAS

Most developed countries have established a prescription drug reimbursement system as part of their national health insurance systems. In the early- to mid-1980s, the goal of drug cost containment in all countries was confined to drug prices, especially at various segments of the marketing channel (manufacturers → distributors → pharmacies). These conventional policies appeared to restrict drug prices to some extent, but drug expenditure continued to rise across all countries due to the substantial overuse of drugs and high-priced new drugs. Under these multiple factors that began placing new pressure on healthcare budgets, the governments (or insurance companies) of these countries began to establish a series of supplementary policies around 1990 – known as Prescription Drug Reimbursement Policies – in order to further enhance conventional price control. On the one hand, these policies have extended the control to physicians and consumers. On the other hand, they have also reinforced the control over manufacturers. These policies were established with the following objectives: (1) controlling the overuse of drugs and (2) transferring the increased financial burden of governments to consumers, physicians, and manufacturers.

In the US, HMOs and other insurance agencies have adopted integrated approaches to control the reimbursement costs of prescription drugs, such as maximizing the use of generic drugs, employing MAC-based reimbursement, and stipulating the range of reimbursement, so that physicians prescribe the most cost-effective drugs.

Next, we focus on specific approaches to drug reimbursement policies in developed countries.

1. Increasing Consumer Copayment of Drug Expenses

The aim of increasing consumer copayment of drug expenses is to reduce the overuse of drugs by raising cost awareness among consumers, thereby alleviating the country's financial burden (Table 9.2).

2. Encouraging Physicians to Prescribe Cheaper Drugs

As physicians are first-level decision makers regarding the use of drugs and play an important role in their selection, governmental (or insurance company) reforms to drug policy have, to varying degrees, linked economic incentives for physicians with their selection of prescription drugs in order to raise cost awareness, thereby promoting competition in drug prices. For instance, the UK has encouraged physicians to act as agents for the reduction of drug expenses using two strategies. First, the government provides physicians with information about the safety and cost-effectiveness of drugs, along with periodic reports on the quantity and cost of physicians' prescriptions for comparison with the norm. Second, the government established financial targets for physicians' prescriptions in 1991. The determinants of these targets include historical expenditures; the demographic composition of patients; local, social, and epidemiological status; and drug price inflation. Currently, these budget targets are not strictly implemented, and GPs who exceed the targets will not be penalized. However, this situation may change in the near future.

TABLE 9.2 Increase in Patient Copayment of Drug Expenses in Four European Countries in 1989–1993

Country	Drugs	1989	1991	1993
France	"Essential" medicines	30%	30%	35%
	"Sedative" drugs	60%	60%	65%
	Chronic diseases	0	0	0
Germany	Drugs with reference prices	Patients pay the amount exceeding the reference price	Patients pay the amount exceeding the reference price	(1) Copayment of 10% for drug expenses exceeding DM30 (2) Progressive increase in copayment of amount exceeding the reference price for patients with chronic disease
	Drugs without reference prices	Copayment of DM3 per prescription	Copayment of DM3 per prescription	(1) Copayment of DM5 for drug expenses between DM30 and DM50 (2) Copayment of DM7 for drug expenses above DM50
UK	Fixed copayment 80% of the population (the elderly, impoverished individuals, children, and pregnant women) Patients who require long-term medication can purchase medical cards	£2.8Free £14.5 per 4 months £40 per 12 months	£3.4Free £14.5 per 4 months £40 per 12 months	£4.25 85% £22 per 4 months £60 per 12 months
Sweden	Fixed copayment	SEK 90	SEK 90	Copayment of SEK120 for the first prescription for a maximum prescribing period of 90 days Patients pay the amount exceeding the reference price

Since 1993, Germany has implemented a "global budget for outpatient expenses," which, if exceeded, is compensated by a reduction in the budget for outpatient physicians. This budgeting system was first implemented when a sum of DM280 million (or 1% of total physician income from patients covered by statutory health insurance) was deducted from the budget for physicians' salaries as a penalty for exceeding the budget. As a result, the number of prescriptions decreased from 795 million in 1991 to 712 million in 1993. The total drug expenditure in Germany in 1993 was lower than that in 1991, and the government's drug expenditure in 1993 was 25% lower than that in 1992. However, the number of prescriptions has increased gradually since 1994, eventually reaching its original level, but the official budget control program has saved about 10% of the pharmaceutical budget. Canada, on the other hand, controls the reimbursement of drug expenses for inpatients via a similar global budget approach.

3. Strict Control Over Manufacturers

(1) Implementation of Further Drug Cost Reduction Policies on Manufacturers

Across-the-board price cuts: In 1991, the French government ordered that drug prices be reduced by 2.5%. In 1993, the German government ordered a 5% reduction in the prices of drugs not covered by the reference price system and a reduction in prices for all prescription drugs to 2% below the prices in May 1992. In addition, the government ordered a price freeze on all drugs, which remained in effect since 1994. In 1993, the UK government ordered a 2.5% reduction in the price of all drugs, followed by a three-year price freeze.

(2) Limiting the Scope of Reimbursable Drugs

In order to control the expenses of prescription drugs, governments (or insurance agencies) have excluded drugs from reimbursement if they have ambiguous therapeutic efficacies or prices that exceed other drugs with equivalent therapeutic efficacies. The use of a reimbursement list further enhanced the competition among pharmaceutical companies as the inclusion of a drug in the reimbursement list is closely associated with its commercial success. The majority of new drugs are no longer automatically included in the reimbursement list. This list is taking on an increasingly prominent role in health economic evaluation.

Almost all countries have adopted drug formularies to identify the reimbursement status of a drug: positive lists include reimbursable drugs, whereas negative lists include nonreimbursable drugs. The criteria for the inclusion of a drug in the positive list involve its absolute therapeutic efficacy, relative therapeutic efficacy, range of social applications, expected sales volume, and manufacturing costs. On the other hand, negative lists usually include drugs with very weak therapeutic efficacies. Negative lists are not less widely applied than positive lists, and are mainly employed in Germany, the UK, and Hungary. The UK has also adopted a "grey list," which contains drugs that are reimbursable only for specific diseases. Governments or insurance companies must constantly revise and update these lists to ensure their applicability in the market environment. The frequency of these revisions varies considerably across countries: some countries revise them frequently; for example, Belgium, France, and Ireland revise their lists on a monthly basis, while Denmark revises its list once every two weeks. On the other hand, Germany and the UK seldom revise their negative lists. Germany has only made three amendments since 1991, while the UK has not made any major changes to its list since it was created in 1984.

(3) Limiting the Reimbursement Prices of Insurers

New market incentives – specifically, the increase in patient copayments and the implementation of a global budget system for physicians or healthcare institutions – can undoubtedly facilitate drug cost containment by reducing unnecessary drug consumption through the increased cost awareness of patients and physicians. However, the sharing of drug costs does not include all drugs and/or patients. Furthermore, the copayment rate and budget determination are far from being problem-free. The scope of reimbursable drugs and the prices of reimbursement are another important source of government control over the pharmaceutical industry through their respective health insurance systems, which ensure healthcare quality using the appropriate techniques. This approach is desirable, but there are still two problems. First, health economic analysis and evaluation methods for the list of reimbursable drugs require further optimization. Second, the majority of drugs not included in this system are high-priced new drugs, which could lead to a two-tier system that gives rise to new healthcare inequality. Therefore, it is still too early to draw any conclusion about the outcomes of the cost containment mechanisms for new drugs in the different countries.

In summary, over the past three decades, the pharmaceutical market in European and American countries has shifted from moderate to strict management and from competitive generic alternatives to mandatory generic substitution. Furthermore, the goal of governments (or insurance companies) has shifted from drug price control to expenditure control (i.e., by limiting both the price and quantity of drugs). Currently, the drug prices in European countries are under control, but the new cost containment mechanisms must be further improved. Although the pharmaceutical industry is still maintaining a high level of profits, their return on investment has been substantially reduced.

SECTION IV. POLICIES FOR ESSENTIAL MEDICINES IN DEVELOPED COUNTRIES AND AREAS

1. Conceptual Development and Impact of Essential Medicines

(1) Conceptual Development of Essential Medicines

The concept of "essential medicines" has been developing for more than 20 years. Prior to the release of the first WHO Model List of Essential Medicines (EML), some countries had already adopted similar models in their drug supply systems. Sweden, the Netherlands, and Switzerland, for example, selected 300–500 medicines for the procurement and usage in public healthcare institutions. Although these countries did not use the term "essential medicines," they implemented the concept of "essential medicines." In 1975, the WHO published an analytical report on pharmaceutical issues in various countries and introduced the concept of essential medicines. Its intention was to serve as a guideline for promoting the use of key medicines, thereby reducing global gaps in the access to medicines. In 1977, the WHO Expert Committee on the Selection and Use of Essential Medicines released the first WHO EML and a technical report in their first meeting. The WHO Technical Report Series (No. 615) defined essential medicines as medicines "that satisfy the priority healthcare needs of the population" and developed the first WHO EML. The WHO initially recommended the concept of essential medicines to underdeveloped countries with low pharmaceutical manufacturing capacity, so that they could use their limited resources for the purchase and rational use of essential medicines that have guaranteed quality and efficacy based on the respective healthcare needs of each country.

In 1985, the WHO convened the Nairobi conference, which introduced new content to the concept of essential medicines. During that conference, essential medicines were defined as medicines that meet the priority healthcare needs of the population, and governments were required to guarantee their production and supply, and to attach great importance to the rational use of drugs. That is, the concept of essential medicines should be combined with the rational use of drugs. Furthermore, governments were recommended to combine the selection of essential medicines with the development of formularies and guidelines for standard treatments. The International Network for Rational Use of Drugs (INRUD) was established, which was funded by the WHO in 1989, and was headquartered at the Health Management Science Center in the US. In July 1990, the INRUD held its first international meeting in Indonesia, followed by several workshops aimed at promoting the rational use of drugs. INRUD is an international and representative organization that works closely with the WHO Essential Drugs and Medicines Policy (EDM) program to promote the concept of essential medicines and the rational use of drugs worldwide. The rational use of drugs has been widely promoted and implemented worldwide. With the support of INRUD, many developing countries have established their own centers for ensuring the rational use of drugs.

In 2002, the term "essential drugs" was renamed "essential medicines" by the WHO to provide a more accurate description, and the following definition was adopted: essential medicines are those that satisfy the priority healthcare needs of the population. The selection of essential medicines should take into account public health relevance, evidence on efficacy and safety, and comparative cost-effectiveness. In the context of functioning health systems, quality-assured essential medicines with sufficient information should be always available in adequate quantities and proper dosage forms, at individually and socially acceptable prices.

The WHO concept of essential medicines has evolved from 1975 to 2002 in the following ways: (1) a more systematic method of selecting essential medicines was adopted, whereby selection is based on evidence-based treatment guidelines and identification of priority diseases. (2) Prior to 2002, expensive drugs were considered impractical and thus excluded from the WHO EML. However, according to the new definition, cost-effective drugs with high unit prices can be included in the EML.

(2) Impact of Essential Medicines

From an ethical standpoint, medicines should not be divided into essential and nonessential. Regardless of the type and incidence of diseases, a high-priced drug can serve as an essential medicine for patients if it can treat or alleviate the disease. However, a large number of drugs have been marketed in various countries, many of which can be used to treat the same disease and vary considerably in their therapeutic efficacies and prices. Moreover, the medical and healthcare resources available in each country are limited. Given its budgetary constraints, no public or private healthcare system can afford to purchase all drugs on the market. Therefore, when resources are limited, it is necessary to limit the variety of drugs used from both a medical and an economic perspective. From a medical standpoint, a certain number of essential medicines can result in high-quality healthcare services and better health outcomes, as well as facilitate targeted quality control, dissemination of drug information, and provision of prescription training and clinical audits. The "efficacy and safety" of drugs should be considered when selecting essential medicines. Hence, the use of essential medicines is one of the means of promoting the rational use of drugs. From an economic perspective, essential medicines can help to maximize the value of funds used; reduce drug costs via the economies of scale; simplify the procurement, supply, distribution, and reimbursement systems; and reduce inventory and operating costs.

The concept of essential medicines has had an enormous impact. Certain international organizations did not recognize the importance of this concept when it was first introduced. In 1977, only about 10 countries had a list or program of essential medicines. By contrast, currently, 156 out of the 193 WHO member states have developed a list of essential medicines based on the WHO's model list in order to organize drug-related activities and promote healthcare development. Among which, 29 countries have had a list of essential medicines for more than five years, and 127 countries have updated their lists over the past five to 10 years. Currently, more than 100 countries have developed or are developing national drug policies. More importantly, an increasing number of countries are moving from policy to action. National drug policies are increasingly becoming a framework wherein stakeholders can commit to pharmaceutical reforms in their countries. In 1977, objective information on the rational use of drugs was extremely limited. At present, at least 135 countries have developed their own treatment and prescription manuals to update healthcare professionals with the most accurate and objective recommendations on the rational use of drugs. The WHO Program for International Drug Monitoring was established upon the release of the first WHO EML. There is also a network of 83 countries involved in the monitoring of adverse drug reactions (ADRs) worldwide, which regularly collects information on potential drug safety issues. Three decades ago, price information was rarely available to the public, and only a few countries actively encouraged the use of generic drugs. As of 2007, at least 33 countries have conducted surveys on the availability and prices of drugs and disclosed the relevant information to the public.

The impact of essential medicines is not limited to poor and developing countries. Issues concerning the increase in demand, the rapid rise in expenses, and the irrational use of drugs also exist in developed countries. Therefore, it is equally relevant for developed countries to maximize their limited funds via the systematic selection of essential medicines. Many developed countries have established "formularies," which essentially function as "lists of essential medicines" (despite not being called by that name). As the core of national drugs policies, formularies have been integrated into nearly every aspect of pharmaceutical manufacturing, purchasing, sales, and utilization. The WHO often recommends the policies adopted by developed countries such as Australia. Statistics have shown that more than 70% of drugs in developed countries are funded by public agencies through reimbursement schemes and other mechanisms, such as the Pharmaceutical Benefits Scheme (PBS) in Australia, which covers 90% of drugs available in the market.

2. Selection and Utilization of Essential Medicines in Developed Countries and Areas

(1) Selection of Essential Medicines (Formularies)

1.Who Standards for the Selection of Essential Medicines   The WHO standards and procedures for the selection of essential medicines have evolved over time and undergone continuous improvements based on systematic analyses and scientific evidence. The WHO Expert Committee on the Selection and Use of Essential Medicines has adopted the following criteria for selection: (1) Medicines with adequate data on efficacy and safety from clinical studies. (2) Factors related to disease incidence and prevalence, genetic and demographic changes, environmental factors, conditions of healthcare institutions, financial resources, and technical capabilities should be taken into account. (3) The "relative cost/benefit ratio" is a major consideration in the selection of essential medicines within the same therapeutic category. The selection should be based on the relative safety, efficacy, quality, price, and availability of the drug. In addition to the unit price, the cost of treatment should also be considered. (4) Most essential medicines should be formulated as single compounds. Fixed-dose drug combinations are acceptable only if they have a proven advantage in terms of therapeutic efficacy, safety, and patient compliance, or can reduce drug resistance in the treatment of malaria, tuberculosis, and AIDS.

The WHO has pointed out that the selection of essential medicines is an ongoing process, and it is necessary to consider the emergence of new therapies, new diseases, and drug resistance in this selection process. The EML should also be updated regularly based on ADR and adverse event data. Only then can essential medicines maintain their representativeness. However, updating the list of essential medicines too frequently would undoubtedly increase the cost of supervision and management and its operational difficulty. Therefore, the stability of the list should be considered while increasing its flexibility. The WHO EML is

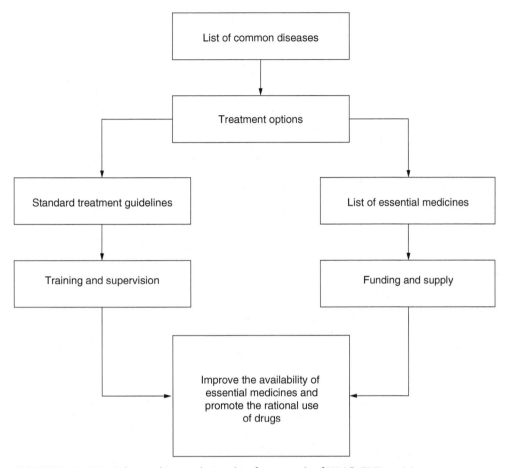

FIGURE 9.1 Principles and interrelationship framework of WHO EML revision.

revised every two years. Other countries with a list of essential medicines also adjust their lists at intervals of no more than two years. The principles and interrelationship framework used in the revision of the WHO EML are shown in Figure 9.1.

2. Formulary Selection Procedure in the UK First, priority drugs and medical devices in the selection procedure are identified. The National Institute for Health and Care Excellence (NICE) assesses the "appropriateness" of a list of candidate drugs submitted by the relevant agencies (e.g., pharmaceutical and medical device manufacturers). This assessment includes whether the drug falls within the purview of NICE, whether it is an interventional measure in response to sudden public health crises, and whether it is a clinical treatment or interventional approach for orphan diseases. Subsequently, the list of candidate drugs is further reviewed to generate a temporary and recommended list according to the standards established by the Ministry of Health, including disease burden (patient-to-population ratio, mortality, morbidity, etc.), impact on the health financing system, clinical significance, and political significance (i.e., whether it is included in the government's priority development strategy). Second, the National Coordinating Center for Health Technology Assessment (NCCHTA) appoints a qualified external third-party assessment organization to generate the assessment report along with the list of assessors to monitor each step of the selection process. Third, relevant issues related to the drugs and medical devices to be assessed are identified. These include a clear definition and detailed description of the drug or medical device, an understanding of the information needed by healthcare policymakers, the development of a schedule for the selection procedure, and a detailed description of the selection techniques. Fourth, pharmaceutical manufacturers that intend to participate in the selection submit a written application, which includes clinical laboratory and cost-effectiveness analysis (CEA) data, to the third-party assessment organization. Fifth, this assessment organization generates a selection assessment report on the drug and medical device; this step usually takes about 36 weeks. In addition to the information submitted by pharmaceutical manufacturers, other relevant organizations, such as other assessment organizations, patient organizations, and healthcare workers, can also submit factual data to the appointed organization. Sixth, the NICE forwards the selection assessment report to the Technology Appraisal Committee (TAC) to generate a preliminary selection report, which provides preliminary opinions on the formulary inclusion. Subsequently, the preliminary selection report is released to the public and opened up to questioning for four weeks. Seventh, the NICE provides its final opinion on the formulary selection using the results of the preliminary selection report; this process should be completed within 14 weeks.

The entire selection process takes at least 14 months. In case of disagreements, the consultant or pharmaceutical manufacturer may appeal the decision. In addition, the NICE has designed a selection channel dedicated to urgently needed or highly innovative medicines to ensure that they are available to patients as soon as possible.

3. Public Selection Procedure in Australia   The transparency of the selection procedures for essential medicines and the openness of its selection basis not only protect the widespread participation of relevant interest groups, but also play an important role in establishing an open and transparent regulatory mechanism. All departments must have clearly defined responsibilities and work under public supervision in order to limit "rent-seeking space" in the selection of essential medicines. Ultimately, a public selection procedure is conducive to the establishment of a more scientific system of selecting essential medicines. For example, the Pharmaceutical Benefits Advisory Committee (PBAC) regularly updates the PBS formularies via strict procedures and requirements, and this entire updating process is open and transparent. Enterprises, consumers, pharmaceutical workers, and other relevant interest groups can learn and download the formularies from the official website of the PBS. The selection is currently implemented in accordance with the 2008 "Guidelines for Preparing Submissions to the PBAC," which have been updated multiple times. These guidelines clearly state the responsibilities and operating procedure of the Pharmaceutical Benefits Pricing Authority (PBPA) of the PBAC, and explain how to apply, prepare, and submit evidence. Additionally, the guidelines also clarify other important information, such as the PBAC cycles, the type and timeframe of submissions, and the technical details of evidence assessment. The procedure for the public selection of essential medicines in Australia is shown in Figure 9.2.

(2) Use of Essential Medicines (Formularies)

The concept of essential medicines is currently widely applied in various areas, such as the training of healthcare workers, the reimbursement of health insurance premiums, the formulation of guidelines for the rational use of drugs in clinical practice, the development of standardized treatment guidelines, the manufacturing and supply of drugs, the quality assurance of drugs, the public procurement system, the reimbursement system, the

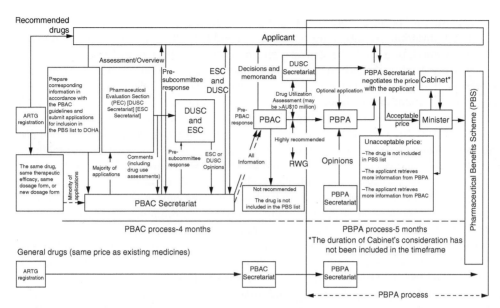

FIGURE 9.2 Workflow to list registered drugs in the PBS list of essential medicines in Australia.

establishment of primary healthcare, pharmaceutical donations, postmarketing research, surveillance against antimicrobial drug resistance, public education, and other health-related activities. In addition, lists of essential medicines have also been used to guide multiple pharmaceutical programs organized by the United Nations (UN), bilateral cooperation between countries, and nongovernmental organizations (NGOs).

Many developed countries have established "formularies" to serve as the core of their national drug policies. The main objective of formularies is to improve the availability, affordability, rational use, and safety of drugs.

Taking the S. Martino Teaching Hospital as an example, which is the largest hospital in Italy (approximately 2,500 beds), a cost-benefit analysis (CBA) showed that the length of hospital stay did not vary significantly from 1997 to 1998 (727,641 days and 707,280 days, respectively). However, following the implementation of a formulary in 1998, the expenses for antibiotics reduced by 10.5% compared to 1997, saving €345,000. Furthermore, the average daily expenses of antibiotics for inpatients decreased by 8.5% from €4.53 in 1997 to €4.18 in 1998. The greatest decrease was for the expenses on cephalosporins, which decreased by 52% from €741,000 in 1997 to €356,000 in 1998. In addition, the formulary system had a substantial impact on drug quality control and can reduce the incidence of prescription errors and medical accidents.

SECTION V. SEPARATION OF PRESCRIBING AND DISPENSING POLICIES AND RELEVANT INSIGHTS IN DEVELOPED COUNTRIES AND AREAS

1. Conceptual Definition of the Separation of Prescribing and Dispensing

The concept of the separation of prescribing and dispensing (SPD) is internationally advocated and mainly requires the division of labor between physicians and pharmacists based on their unique specializations and tasks: physicians are given the authority to diagnose and issue prescriptions according to patients' conditions but have no right to review or dispense prescription drugs. In contrast, pharmacists are given the authority to review and dispense prescription drugs and provide pharmaceutical consultations but have no right to perform a diagnosis. This is the result of a more refined social division of labor required by social development and technological advancement. The purpose of SPD is to standardize the professional behavior and technical services of physicians and pharmacists in such a way as to establish a cross-checking system for prescriptions, thereby ensuring good pharmacotherapeutic and healthcare quality. In addition, SPD also enforces accountability for the pharmacotherapeutic outcomes of patients and improves their quality of life by preventing, reducing, or alleviating harmful effects related to the drug usage.

The concept of SPD emphasizes that physicians and pharmacists are distinct professions with a clear division of labor that are nevertheless intimately associated; this is especially true of clinical pharmacists, who are equipped with modern pharmaceutical expertise as well as basic knowledge of clinical medicine. They are capable of participating in pharmacotherapies and assisting physicians in drug selection and usage but are not allowed to perform diagnosis or provide treatment for patients in place of physicians. Physicians, on the other hand, can provide diagnostic and treatment advice based on diagnostic imaging or clinical examination results and their knowledge of modern medicine and can also prescribe medications. Pharmacists are a part of the medical team. Given the technological advancement, physicians must rely on the participation and advice of pharmacists on drug usage for clinical pharmacotherapies. Physicians cannot review or dispense prescription drugs in place of pharmacists. SPD enables the optimization of medical and pharmaceutical skills and emphasizes specialized technical services, thus forming a cooperative, complementary, and interventional mechanism that promotes the rational use of drugs.

2. Rationale and Policy Implementation of the Separation of Prescribing and Dispensing in Western Developed Countries

(1) Rationale for SPD in Western Countries

SPD policies proposed in Western countries, Hong Kong, Macao, and Taiwan are associated with the properties and structure of their healthcare services. SPD is implemented primarily to regulate the professional behaviors of physicians and pharmacists, as well as to define the scope and responsibilities of professionals, especially for clinics and independent practitioners, who might be more prone to professional misconduct. Some private clinics and independent practitioners have pharmacies without licensed pharmacists, and there is no division of labor between physicians and pharmacists. In such circumstances, physicians perform diagnosis, issue prescription, and provide treatment, while physicians or nonpharmaceutical technicians dispense prescription drugs. The lack of pharmaceutical expertise by these individuals increases the risk of medical error or accident. Additionally, profit-driven overprescription and prescription of irrelevant drugs often occur in private practices as well.

Therefore, most developed countries have enacted a Physicians' Act and a Pharmacists' Act to clearly define the scopes, responsibilities, and behaviors of these professions. These acts require healthcare institutions with pharmacies to employ registered pharmacists; otherwise, they are barred from setting up pharmacies or dispensing drugs. These acts typically prohibit clinics from setting up pharmacies (but they are permitted to offer first aid medicines), while independent practitioners are not allowed to dispense drugs. Any drugs prescribed by physicians must be retrieved or purchased from a registered or licensed pharmacist at community or hospital pharmacies. Pharmacies are not categorized as health-care institutions despite the fact that the practice of community pharmacies and pharma-cists is considered a form of healthcare behavior. Therefore, community retail pharmacies are not allowed to establish clinics that offer diagnostic services and issue prescriptions for patients. Patients must consult clinicians at community healthcare centers, clinics, or hos-pitals for diagnosis, prescription, and treatment.

Based on the evolution of the healthcare service systems in Western countries, physi-cian services are conventionally separated from hospital services in most countries. Patients consult community generalists (i.e., GPs or family physicians) to obtain prescriptions, based on which retail pharmacies dispense and provide medication instructions. Healthcare insti-tutions typically have pharmacies that serve only inpatients; due to the smaller number of outpatients or emergency patients, these patients can often obtain prescriptions from community pharmacies without causing too much inconvenience. However, some hospitals also provide pharmacy services and facilities for patients' convenience. There is no economic link between healthcare institutions and drug marketing in these countries. Furthermore, the economic link between physician income and prescriptions has not drawn social attention due to external constraints, such as health insurance and high incomes among physicians in general. An issue that remains to be solved is the enhancement of professional communication between physicians and pharmacists in order to improve the healthcare quality associated with medication.

(2) SPD Systems in Western European and American Countries

1. The US Most hospitals in the US have a pharmacy department. Some medium- and small-sized hospitals do not have outpatient pharmacies; thus, patients must consult physicians at community healthcare centers and obtain prescriptions from community pharmacies. The Durham-Humphrey Amendment, which was adopted in 1951, strictly distinguishes between the roles of pharmacists and physicians in the provision of healthcare services: Physicians are specialized in diagnosis, treatment, and drug prescription, whereas pharmacists are specialized in dispensing drugs and providing medication advice based on the physicians' prescriptions. In order to address the severe information asymmetry between physicians and patients, the US has employed an effective market equilibrium mechanism to restrain physicians' professional behavior. Specifically, a comprehensive mechanism of ex-ante, ex-dure, and ex-post supervision by health insurance agencies, pharmacy benefit managers (PBM), and pharmacists, respectively, has been established. This manifests the prevalence of market mechanisms that is advocated by the US and vividly embodies the pro-motion of rational drug use via a market approach.

1. The separation of drug dispensing from healthcare services has partially affected the information advantage of physicians in the process of diagnosis and treatment. However, the review and audit of prescriptions carried out by pharmacists is merely a type of ex-post supervision, which might not be effective against physicians.
2. Health insurance agencies serve as agents of patients that have employed their professional advantages in the utilization and management of healthcare services and in cost containment (e.g., strict medication audits, supervision, and analysis of physi-cians' professional behaviors), thereby further standardizing the professional behaviors of healthcare institutions/physicians and altering the physician–patient information asymmetry to a considerable extent. However, the scope of healthcare services and the list of reimbursable drugs are considered ex-ante interventional approaches. Due to the

complexity of drug and disease information and the differences in clinical treatments, health insurance agencies are not equipped with detailed information on drugs, diseases, and clinical treatments. Therefore, they are still unable to exercise strong restrictions on how physicians prescribe and what types of healthcare services patients need.

PBMs further isolate the function HMOs in drug administration and expand the professional advantages of HMOs in drug administration, disease management and clinical diagnostic management, thus enabling the ex-dure supervision of physicians and pharmacists through drug administrative services. PBMs share their extensive database of pharmaceutical and disease information with health insurance agencies and provide the most effective prescription solutions in real-time according to the diagnosis and treatment of different diseases. This measure allows patients to receive an appropriate treatment regimen while achieving lower medical expenses borne by insurance agencies.

2. European Countries

1. Germany was one of the earliest countries in the world to implement the SPD system. Healthcare services have been separated from drug sales since the era of Rudolf von Goldenbaum in the twelfth century. The attempts and explorations made over several centuries have resulted in a distinctive, clear, comprehensive, and valuable healthcare system that meets basic healthcare needs and guarantees basic healthcare for low-income and critically ill patients. Germany is currently implementing a two-tier consultation system in hospitals and clinics, where medical consultations with physicians have been separated from drug sales at pharmacies. The vast majority of hospitals do not have an outpatient pharmacy due to the low number of outpatient visits. However, all hospitals do have an inpatient pharmacy to serve inpatients and emergency patients. Revenues generated from drug sales at these pharmacies belong to the hospital. On the other hand, clinics provide community healthcare services and outpatient services. Regardless of which facilities they use, all Germans seek medical attention using designated health insurance cards. Aside from the copayment specified in patients' health insurance policy, hospitals or clinics do not charge patients with prescription or medical consultation fees, and they cannot sell drugs to patients. Patients must purchase drugs from community pharmacies using their health insurance cards. Physicians employed by these hospitals and clinics can then claim compensation from the insurance companies that issued the health insurance cards, while community pharmacies can claim compensation for drug sales from insurance companies based on the prescriptions. Therefore, there is no direct financial transaction between patients and hospitals/pharmacies, which prevents any cooperation or conflict among physicians and patients, pharmacies and physicians, and pharmacies and patients. The success of SPD in Germany is attributed to its health insurance system. This system, which has existed since 1883, offers a comprehensive range of services and 100% coverage for the population. German law requires all Germans to enroll in statutory or private health insurance schemes based on their income level. Although their premium contributions may differ, all insured persons receive essentially the same benefits under the health insurance scheme.

2. France also has a comprehensive health insurance system with 100% coverage. It has adopted a family physician system, where each citizen must register with a family physician, who in turn can refer the patient to a corresponding hospital for further treatment whenever necessary. Hospitals in France are only responsible for issuing

prescriptions, which allows patients to purchase prescribed drugs from pharmacies. Data show that 84.7% of drugs in France are sold at pharmacies, while the remaining 15.3% are sold directly from manufacturers to hospitals. Hence, retail pharmacies are the main channels for patients to purchase drugs. Pharmacies are widely distributed throughout France and can be found on nearly every street in every town. To avoid a vicious competition and ensure the quality of pharmaceutical services, pharmacies are distributed according to the population of residents living on a given street, and setting up new pharmacies must be approved by the national pharmaceutical department. In addition, all pharmacy workers must be professionally trained. France has a very strict drug administrative system with a clear division of labor in the pricing process. The system is highly transparent and allows for collaboration between the government and experts, thereby demonstrating a high level of scientificity and equality. Accordingly, drug prices do not vary significantly across pharmacies. To increase their revenues, pharmacies can only improve their own reputations and services.

3. Sweden is a welfare state, where the reduction in healthcare expenditure relies on the improvement of social welfare. In the mid-1960s, Sweden established a pharmacy company that markets drugs using a model similar to franchising. Hospital pharmacies throughout the country are uniformly controlled, supplied, and operated by this company, which negotiates and signs agreements with pharmaceutical manufacturers for relatively low drug prices and high discount rates. Swedish hospitals lack pharmacy departments, and thus, the various roles and tasks of hospital pharmacies have been eliminated, and hospital pharmacy does not exist as a discipline. However, the pharmacy company still attaches great importance to drug consultations at pharmacies. It can be said that Sweden has implemented a relatively thorough system of SPD.

4. Norway, Iceland, and Switzerland have all implemented an SPD system in which medical consultation is strictly separated from drug sales. Healthcare institutions are mainly responsible for medical consultations, while inpatient pharmacies only provide drugs for inpatients that cannot be sold to external parties. Community pharmacies are responsible for drug sales and do not provide medical consultations. In general, healthcare institutions in these three countries implement the two-tier consultation system of hospitals and clinics. Patients seek medical attention from private physicians, who in turn refer them to hospitals for medical conditions that cannot be resolved at the private clinics. Patients diagnosed with minor illnesses do not require hospitalization and can purchase drugs at community pharmacies using prescriptions issued by physicians. In contrast, patients with severe illnesses must be hospitalized for treatment. All drugs required by inpatients are provided by the hospital pharmacy, and their drug expenses are included as part of their total medical expenses. Aside from the common SPD measures, these countries also implement stricter management and control over drug prices through various measures.

5. Belgian hospitals do not have pharmacies, and therefore, patients are required to purchase drugs at community pharmacies using prescriptions issued by physicians. Belgian pharmacies also sell drugs (e.g., a box of aspirin) at three different prices; this is not fraud but is a requirement of the Belgian social security system. Patients who are not enrolled in social security must make a full payment for drug purchases and medical consultations, whereas those who are enrolled must make only a partial payment. Pensioners and unemployed individuals are required to pay the lowest price, which can be reimbursed.

3. Reforms and Evaluation of the Separation of Prescribing and Dispensing in Asian Developed Countries and Areas

(1) South Korea

1. Reform Process   Only East Asian countries with similar healthcare service systems have begun to implement SPD. South Korea was the first country to enforce SPD.

South Korea originally lacked cross-checking and supervision mechanisms for prescriptions, as physicians and drug retailers were considered mutually independent in their sale of drugs, which led to widespread drug misuse and abuse. In 1994, South Korea began to consider the implementation of an SPD policy using a somewhat radical approach. However, the radical approach taken by the original reforms – scheduled to be implemented in July 1999 – led to a physician strike. After a long period of negotiation with relevant stakeholders, such as physicians, pharmacists, and hospitals, the government eventually relented under the pressure and made substantial concessions by supplementing the original, more reasonable, policy with several measures: Health insurance premiums will be raised by 40% within a year to compensate for a possible decline in physician incomes; the proportion of expenses for prescription drugs out of the total drug expenses will be increased from 50% to 75%; physicians are allowed to charge prescription fees (in addition to treatment fees) and pharmacists are allowed to charge dispensing fees; and pharmacists are prohibited from replacing brand-name drugs prescribed by physicians with their generic counterparts.

The SPD reform was therefore postponed until July 1, 2000, when it was officially implemented in all healthcare institutions, including clinics, district hospitals, municipal hospitals, and hospitals affiliated with the Ministry of Health. The core measures of this reform included abolishing outpatient pharmacies at hospitals; requiring outpatients to purchase drugs directly from pharmacies using prescriptions issued by physicians; only permitting the purchase of prescription drugs (particularly those administered via injection) with the written prescription of physicians; and requiring patients to purchase injection drugs and then return to hospitals for injections, with the exception of patients with severe illnesses, such as anticancer drugs and injections that require refrigerated storage.

In theory, pharmacists' review of the prescriptions issued by physicians can reduce medication errors and improve medication safety. Furthermore, dispensing prescribed drugs at community pharmacies can also increase the transparency of healthcare services, reduce the distribution costs of drug, improve the resource allocation efficiency of the pharmaceutical industry, and increase patients' right to medication information. The initial purpose of the SPD policy was to reduce the economic incentives for overprescription by physicians and improper drug dispensing by pharmacists. The additional prescription and dispensing fees charged by physicians and pharmacists, respectively, are expected to reduce the proportion of their income derived from the profit margin of drug sales, thereby reducing overall drug expenditure and increasing drug accessibility to the public. Other expected benefits include reducing the irrational use of drugs and the emergence of antibiotic resistance.

2. Implementation Outcomes and Lessons Learned   Some studies have analyzed the use of drugs in South Korea following the implementation of the SPD policy. Taking the treatment of peptic ulcer as an example, the implementation of SPD increased the prescription volume and drug expenses (especially for high-priced and brand-name drugs) for this condition by 13.9% and 98.4%, respectively. In addition, other studies have also found that the number of prescriptions for all drugs (including antibiotics) and the irrational use of antibiotics for the treatment of viral infections have been reduced after physicians were restricted from dispensing drugs.

However, the implementation of SPD policy led to distortions in the healthcare system, largely due to the massive opposition to this policy and the government's subsequent concessions to it. Overall, these distortions have made the government face an even worse situation: (1) Physicians and pharmacists can now work together to deceive consumers in the pursuit of common economic goals, which not only leads to the failure of the cross-checking system for prescriptions, but also compromises the control of drug overuse. (2) The increase in the proportion of prescription drugs has elevated patients' actual drug expenses. Patients and insurance companies not only have to pay for drug expenses but also prescription and dispensing fees, thereby increasing their financial burden. (3) Since the replacement of brand-name drugs with their generic counterparts is prohibited, most physicians now specify brand-name drugs in their prescriptions. Therefore, the issue of overprescription remains because physicians earn "commissions" from pharmaceutical manufacturers based on the brand specified in their prescriptions. For example, the prescription volume declined slightly from 95.2% in January 2000 (prior to the reform) to 92.6% in January 2002. In addition, the number of drugs per prescription also decreased. However, the proportion of high-priced drugs increased from 29.8% to 38.5% while the duration of medication specified in the prescription increased from 5.1 days to 7.5 days.

The problems that have risen in response to the progress and outcomes of the SPD reform in South Korea are worthy of further study. Specifically, researchers might examine adjustment of interests among multiple stakeholders, which reflects, to some extent, the political resources of stakeholders and their roles in the political structure that in turn determine their relative influence on policymaking. The most crucial lesson is that in future policymaking, it is essential to evaluate the status of each stakeholder when proposing and implementing policies, the potential benefits they might receive from these policies, and to what extent they will fulfill their responsibilities after policy enactment.

Pharmaceutical companies are the most direct beneficiaries of South Korea's SPD policy, and as such, they have heavily exercised their political influence by lobbying the government to promote its implementation. Conversely, physicians will suffer the loss of their dispensing authority. However, given their significant social status and political influence, physicians are capable of negotiating with the government as well, and can participate in policy revision or altering the policy orientation to ensure that the vested interests of their community are maintained.

It is hard for patients to completely change their habits within a short period of time. In addition to the increased complexity of the dispensing procedure compared to before the reform, the implementation of the SPD policy did not generate actual benefits for patients. Instead, patients now bear even greater drug expenses. The initial aim of the government was to protect the rights and interests of the public; in this case, however, it adopted a radical strategy without the proper coordination of interests among all parties. As a result, the policy has invited massive opposition from the public and has damaged the image of the government.

(2) Japan

1. Reform Process　In Japan, provisions related to SDP first appeared in the Medical Care Act enacted in 1874. In 1956, the principle of prescription release became an obligation following the revision of some clauses in the Medical Practitioners' Act, the Dentists' Act, and the Pharmacists' Act. However, it was difficult for SPD to develop successfully due to the ingrained habit of obtaining drugs directly from physicians. Hence, SPD was not officially implemented in Japan until 1974, when Japan began to increase prescription fees.

Subsequently, Japan further increased the prescription fees and introduced the copayment system for prescription drugs in 1994 and 1997, respectively. In addition to maintaining physicians' prescribing authority, the government took measures to ensure the safe and effective use of medications. In 1996, more than 200 million prescriptions were issued in Japan, which then had an SPD rate of 22.5%. The number of prescriptions issued increased in 1997, as did the SPD rate (27.3%); by 2002, the SPD rate had increased to 48.3%. In 2004, more than 610 million prescriptions were issued and the average annual SPD rate was 53.8%. The latest "Insurance Pharmacy Trends" released by the Japan Pharmaceutical Association reported that the SPD rate of Japan was 59.7% in 2007. In addition, geographical variation in the progress of SPD implementation was observed. The SPD rates of Akita prefecture, which ranked first (79.2%), and Fukui prefecture, which ranked last (18.7%), both exceeded 50% in 2004.

Japan adopted a gradual strategy for the implementation of SDP, in the hopes that progress could be accelerated by increasing prescription fees and introducing a copayment system for outpatient prescription drugs. It was believed that these efforts would lead to the gradual separation of drug dispensing from healthcare services. The SPD policy in Japan was implemented by the Ministry of Health, Labour and Welfare (MHLW). In 1985, this ministry established a model area for promoting SDP, and by 1992 had begun to establish centers for drug storage, dissemination of pharmaceutical information and promotion of SDP. These centers focused on the collection and dissemination of drug information, and provided guidelines to conduct research on pharmaceutical services. Specialized agencies, such as the SDP Working Group (consisting of representatives from the Tokyo Medical Association, Tokyo Pharmacy Association, and Tokyo Dental Association), are responsible for studying and discussing issues related to the establishment of an SPD system.

2. Reform Outcomes   The prices of drugs (covered by social health insurance) approved by the MHLW often differ from the actual purchase prices paid by healthcare institutions. Therefore, for-profit healthcare institutions are motivated to reduce the purchase prices of drugs. In the unique supply-and-demand relationship between patients and physicians, the latter has an absolute advantage in being able to reduce the purchase price of drugs by increasing drug use. This "drug price margin" has led to the widespread issue of "overreliance on drug sales to support healthcare institutions," which has hampered the smooth development of the social health insurance system in Japan. To ensure the rational use of drugs in healthcare institutions, control the growth of healthcare expenditure, and reduce the proportion of income attributed to drug sales, Japan has implemented a proactive and effective drug price control system: that is, all drugs covered by health insurance are priced by the government. The MHLW has continuously reduced drug prices and introduced new drug pricing standards in order to gradually reduce the drug price margin. In addition, the ministry has also increased the remuneration of physicians for their healthcare services, particularly for technical services. This reform has given rise to some notable outcomes for drug expenditures: Drug expenses accounted for more than 30% of the total healthcare expenditure from 1975 to 1984, peaking at 38.7% in 1981. However, the proportion declined to 20–30% in 1985–2000, fell below 20% in 2001, and reached 18.4% in 2002. Furthermore, the proportion of inpatient drug expenses in the total healthcare expenditure has been reduced to 9.7%.

In recent years, Japan has been advocating for the development of community healthcare. Patients are guided to seek medical attention at community clinics and obtain drugs from pharmacies using prescriptions. Patients who seek medical attention at hospital outpatient departments can obtain drugs from hospital pharmacies or pharmacies outside the hospitals. However, most patients still prefer to obtain drugs from hospital pharmacies. Nevertheless, the reform in Japan has led to an increase in the SPD rate and a decrease in the proportion of drug expenses out of the total healthcare expenditure. It has also led to some increments in the number of pharmacies and pharmacists. However, SPD reform is still ongoing in Japan.

(3) Taiwan

1. Reform Process Statistics show that as of 2010, there were 7,558 pharmacies (including 5,049 pharmacies with licensed pharmacists and 2,509 pharmacies with unlicensed pharmacists), 5,388 Western medicine sellers (pharmacies or drugstores), and 11,308 traditional Chinese medicine sellers (Chinese pharmacies) in Taiwan. In 1989, Taiwan's administrative authorities proposed the universal health insurance scheme as an important governmental approach to expanding social welfare and narrowing the gap between the rich and poor. The health insurance scheme was officially implemented in 1995 after several years of planning. Two years after the implementation of this universal health insurance scheme, an SPD policy was introduced in Taipei City and Kaohsiung City. This policy prevented healthcare institutions from establishing pharmacies. It also designated physicians as specialists in medical treatment and prescriptions, while the pharmacy staff of community pharmacies were given authority over dispensing drugs and providing medication advice. However, the SPD policy in Taiwan was controversial from the very beginning and was protested by the two major interest groups (the Taiwan Medical Association and Taiwan Pharmacist Association). Both associations took to the streets to protest on who could have prescribing and dispensing authorities. Ultimately, Taiwan's authorities passed a multiphase "two-track" approach to implementing SPD, which aimed to help balance the interests among all parties. The "two-track" approach allows hospitals and clinics to establish pharmacies with designated pharmacists for drug dispensing while also giving community pharmacists the same dispensing authority. As a result, a large number of "front-door pharmacies" were established by hospitals and clinics in front of healthcare institutions.

According to experts from the Chinese Stores Development Association and the Taipei City Pharmacists Association, only about 35% of hospital prescriptions are dispensed by pharmacies outside healthcare institutions in Taiwan. After excluding prescriptions for chronic diseases, only 7% of prescriptions are dispensed by district pharmacies. These statistics have shattered high hopes for SDP, and many people in Taiwan now consider this SPD model an "utter failure."

Experts believe that the main reason for the implementation of the "two-track" approach in Taiwan is the presence of interest factors, whereby healthcare institutions are reluctant to give up their interests. Under such circumstances, community pharmacies, which mainly rely on prescriptions covered by health insurance, have to establish a rapport with physicians in order to attract an outflow of hospital prescriptions. However, community pharmacies are still unable to compete with hospitals; their disadvantaged position is mainly attributed to: (1) institutional factors: After medical consultations, patients tend to be asked by physicians to retrieve their drugs directly from pharmacies affiliated with their respective healthcare institutions. (2) Social factors: Physicians generally have a higher social status and authority than do pharmacists. (3) Interest factors: There are differences in prices among certain drugs (those commonly known as essential medicines). (4) Legal factors: In the event of any medication errors, the responsibility often falls on physicians rather than pharmacists.

2. Reform Outcomes and Evaluation Previous studies have shown that following the implementation of the SPD policy, around 60% of clinics in Taiwan employed pharmacists. There was no significant change in drug use and most prescriptions were still prescribed by physicians rather than community pharmacists. The policy did not significantly influence clinics with pharmacists, but the proportion of outpatient prescriptions at clinics without pharmacists declined rapidly. The outpatient prescribing rate and drug expenses per outpatient service in those clinics were 17–34% and 12–36% lower than those of control clinics, respectively, suggesting that the policy has changed physicians' prescribing behavior to a certain extent. However, the dispensing and consultation fees increased in conjunction with the reduced drug expenses, so the overall medical expenses per outpatient service did not decrease. Other studies have indicated that most pharmacy prescriptions were still derived from clinic physicians. Some clinics have established pharmacies nearby to compensate for the economic losses due to the abolition of their dispensing authority. The SPD policy was intended to enhance the prescribing and dispensing autonomy of pharmacists in order to protect the rights and interests of patients by increasing the transparency of the prescription process. However, data analyses indicated a high degree of market concentration, with most clinic prescriptions only being dispensed at a particular pharmacy in a given region. Therefore, while the SPD policy has not caused much social turmoil in Taiwan, it has not had a remarkable outcome thus far either.

Various factors, such as the incomplete SDP, unbalanced physician–pharmacist competition for profits, and unfair competition at the fringes of the law, have forced many pharmaceutical retailers in Taiwan to expand into nonpharmaceutical sectors and adopt a composite business approach based on nonpharmaceutical products. Drugstores, which now sell diverse products, such as drugs, health foods, cosmetics, and baby products, are developing rapidly in Taiwan. Presently, drugstores in Taiwan are in the process of product diversification but are still hoping for the achievement "complete" SDP. Indeed, Taiwan is struggling with its incomplete SPD and physician–pharmacist competition for profits, and its situation is similar to the SPD policy in Japan. However, it is believed that SPD in Taiwan will become fairer and more reasonable with further policy improvement. Currently, the majority of developing countries is exploring or will be implementing even more unique SPD policies. These policies may involve the government (or health insurance agencies) designating the geographical scope from which patients can obtain drugs or healthcare institutions and even prescribing physicians who can recommend pharmacies relevant to their own interests. As for which conditions will determine the direction of future developments, these will undoubtedly be driven by the respective interests of each party: Government administrative agencies will focus on administrative convenience and social equality, while healthcare institutions or physicians will focus on their own interests. It is much harder to accomplish SPD in developing countries compared to developed countries due to the complexities of their national circumstances.

4. Value of and Insights for the Separation of Prescribing and Dispensing in China

(1) SPD Helps Control the Disorderly Growth of Healthcare Expenditure and Improve the Quality of Healthcare Services

According to the practice of SPD in developed countries, the purpose of SPD is to form a "cooperative, complementary, and interventional mechanism for clinical medication," promote the rational use of drugs, and improve the quality of healthcare services. It embodies the concept of advanced healthcare management. On the one hand, the SPD policy helps to control healthcare expenditure, especially the rapid growth of drug expenses. On the other hand, the dispensing of physician prescriptions at community pharmacies has improved the transparency of healthcare services and effectively prevented commercial bribery in pharmaceutical purchasing and sales activities. Moreover, it has reduced the distribution costs of drugs and improved resource allocation efficiency in the pharmaceutical industry. Pharmacists can reduce medication errors and improve medication safety by reviewing the prescriptions issued by physicians. SPD can provide physicians with guidelines on the rational use of drugs and pharmaceutical information, which in turn can facilitate the monitoring of ADRs. In particular, SPD avoids increasing the financial burden of patients due to repeated visits at different hospitals.

(2) The Core Motivation of SPD Is to Break the Economic Ties Between Physicians and Pharmacists

The scientificity and rationality of SPD have long been confirmed by health economics theory and the practical experience of many countries. SPD has been implemented in European, North American, and South American countries. There is a clear division of labor between medicine and pharmacy, but they are inseparable professions. In other words, they both cooperate with one another and restrict each other, which is an inevitable outcome of technological advancement and healthcare development. Medicine and pharmacy are inseparable in the development of healthcare, but are, in fact, separable in terms of economic operations and benefits. For example, in the US, community pharmacies are the main pharmaceutical marketing channel. In 2006, a total of 3.4 billion prescriptions were sold and dispensed at community pharmacies, with an average of >11 prescriptions per patient. Furthermore, hospital drug expenses accounted for only 15% of the total healthcare expenditure. Hospital drug expenses in European countries were maintained at 12% to 31%, which is an example worth studying in China. The share of hospital drug expenses out of the total healthcare expenditure in several developed countries is shown in Table 9.3.

It is particularly important to emphasize that the main purpose of implementing SPD is to break the economic ties between the professional behaviors of healthcare institutions/physicians and the income from pharmaceutical sales. This can help to change the incentives of healthcare institutions/physicians to prescribe drugs that exceed the scope of rational

TABLE 9.3 Share of Hospital Drug Expenses in the Total Healthcare Expenditure of Developed Countries

Country	Share of Hospital Drug Expenses out of Total Healthcare Expenditure	Country	Share of Hospital Drug Expenses out of Total Healthcare Expenditure
US	15%	Netherlands	19%
Belgium	27%	Poland	12%
Finland	25%	Spain	29%
France	26%	New Zealand	20%
Germany	13%	UK	26%
Hungary	19%	Canada	11%
Italy	31%	Japan	38%

treatment for patients. That is, SPD aims to transform the incentive structure of physician behaviors rather than focusing on the formal separation of healthcare institutions from pharmacies in terms of their immediate relationship and/or income and expenditure accounts.

(3) SPD Must Be Implemented in Accordance with the National Circumstances and Health System in China

A generalized approach to implementing and operating SPD is inadvisable, as each country has its unique national circumstances and health system. SPD in European and American countries is mainly related to the structure of their healthcare institutions. There are a large number of private hospitals, especially small-sized hospitals, clinics, and self-employed physicians, in these countries, most of which do not have professional pharmacists. Nonpharmacy professionals can easily cause medical errors or accidents in drug dispensing due to their unfamiliarity with or lack of pharmacy knowledge. Therefore, patients must purchase drugs using prescriptions issued by physicians at community pharmacies or hospital pharmacies with designated licensed/registered pharmacists. Japan has adopted a gradual strategy for the implementation of SDP. However, as of 2007, it has an SPD rate of only 59.7%, despite almost a century of development, and there is significant geographical variation in the progress of the implementation. South Korea had previously adopted a mandatory approach to implement SDP. However, the reform did not achieve desirable outcomes, leading to street protests by healthcare workers, public discontent, and social instability due to poor management.

In contrast, in China, healthcare institutions at all levels are generally equipped with pharmacies for historical reasons. There is considerable resistance and a number of obstacles to the complete separation or trusteeship of these pharmacies. Moreover, the reforms implemented in some regions in previous years have not achieved notable outcomes or have gradually petered out. In view of the existing policy environment and operability, it is more feasible to implement a zero-markup policy on pharmaceutical products under the premise of increased capital injection and social security funds.

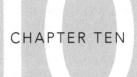

CHAPTER TEN

Models and Policies of Healthcare Cost Containment in Developed Countries and Areas

SECTION I. BACKGROUND OF HEALTHCARE COST CONTAINMENT IN DEVELOPED COUNTRIES AND AREAS

1. Changes in Healthcare Costs in Developed Countries and Areas

The US has the highest healthcare expenditure in the world. In 1960, its total healthcare cost was only US$26.9 billion, accounting for less than 6% of GDP. By 1993, this indicator had doubled in size, reaching 13% of GDP. In 1996, total healthcare costs exceeded US$1 trillion for the first time, reaching US$1.0351 trillion. By 2011, this figure had increased to US$2.7 trillion, accounting for 17.7% of GDP, and healthcare expenditures per capita were US$8,467. From 1999 to 2009, Canada's total healthcare costs increased by an average of US$9 billion per year, reaching US$193.8 billion by 2011 and accounting for 10.9% of GDP. Canada's health expenditures per capita in 2011 were US$4,541.

Germany's total healthcare costs as a share of GDP shrank by 0.1% from 1985 to 1993 and were 8.6% in 1993. However, healthcare costs as a share of GDP began to grow thereafter, reaching 10.3% of GDP in 2000 and further increasing to 11.3% in 2011. As France has universal health insurance, most of its healthcare expenditures are covered by social health insurance (the average compensation rate of the general system is 90%). The growth rate of healthcare costs in France far exceeds that of its GDP. In 1980, total healthcare expenditures were only 7.0% of GDP, but this share increased to 10.1% in 2003 and further to 11.6% in 2011. In 1950, Sweden's total healthcare costs as a share of GDP were 3.4%, which increased to 6.1% in 1970, 8.9% in 1981, and 9.5% in 2011.

In 1973, as Japan gradually became an aging society, the government announced that free healthcare would be provided to individuals over 70 years old, which led to a sharp increase in healthcare costs for the elderly. Thus, dispersing the healthcare risk of the elderly formed a major component of Japan's health insurance system reforms. In 1955, Japan's healthcare costs as a share of GDP were 3.42%, which increased to 5.22% in 1975, 7.7% in 2000, and 10% in 2011.

A direct consequence of the growth in healthcare costs is increasing difficulty in paying medical bills. As shown in Figure 10.1, among developed countries in 2009, the US had the highest percentage (20%) of individuals who had serious problems paying or were unable to pay their medical bills, far exceeding that of other countries. The US was followed by France (8%) and Australia (9%), and the UK had the lowest percentage at only 2%.

2. Causes of the Rapid Growth of Healthcare Costs

For more than 50 years after World War II, four major causes have led to the continuous expansion of the global demand for health services and the sharp increase in healthcare costs.

1. *Revolutionary changes in medical technology, especially in the development of diagnosis and treatment methods.* Half a century ago, the duties of physicians were limited only to recognizing diseases, predicting possible outcomes, and providing patients with a certain extent of care. Physicians were usually helpless in the face of most diseases. Today, however, physicians are not only able to diagnose the vast majority of difficult diseases using ultrasounds, CT scans, MRIs, genetics, and other techniques, but they can also use antibiotics and other effective drugs, as well as pacemakers, renal dialysis, organ transplants, microsurgeries, gamma knives, proton knives, and other methods to effectively cure diseases or control their progression. The emergence of new and expensive medical technologies after the twentieth century has led to the rapid rise in healthcare costs, which is a common problem among Western developed countries. The promotion of medical technology is growing especially rapidly in the US, with a particularly wide range of applications. Economists and insurers have long recognized that the annual growth in healthcare costs stems largely from the use of new technologies.

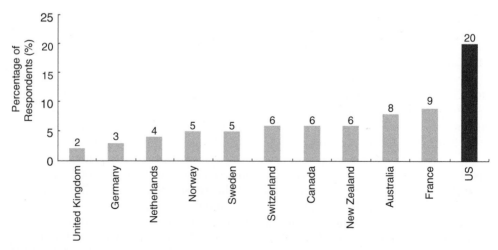

FIGURE 10.1 Percentage of individuals who had serious problems paying or were unable to pay medical bills among developed countries in 2009. *Source:* 2010 Commonwealth Fund International Health Policy Survey.

2. *Establishment of third-party payment mechanisms.* National health services (NHSs), social health insurance, and other systems have uncoupled patients' access to free healthcare and the number and extent of health services they receive from the amounts of patients' individual contributions. This mechanism reduces patients' financial risk from diseases and increases the accessibility of healthcare services. However, it also drastically increases the demand for healthcare services, which leads to a sharp rise in healthcare costs.

3. *Impact of population aging, disease spectrum changes, and other biological factors.* Western developed countries successively became aging societies in the 1970s. The sharp increase in the elderly population led to the formation of a sizeable demand for "silver" medical and nursing care. The rapid rise in the morbidity and mortality of cardiovascular diseases, cancers, and other chronic diseases led to fundamental changes in the disease spectrums of residents in these countries. Furthermore, as the rate of international urbanization continued to accelerate, the pace of life quickened, and the pressure of work increased, thus resulting in the rise of mental disorders. A substantial increase in investments was needed to cope with these changes, which led to the rise in healthcare costs.

4. *Rapid economic development, popularization of health knowledge, and other social causes.* Rapid economic development and the popularization of health knowledge have resulted in a fundamental transformation of people's understanding of health. The public is no longer satisfied with low levels of healthcare, and the demand for high-quality services is increasing. These factors have caused healthcare expenditures to rise continuously. Additional factors influencing the rise in healthcare costs include increasing enrollments in health insurance, massive management costs, increases in physicians' salaries due to inflation, and the rising prices of healthcare services.

The continuous and rapid rise in healthcare costs has already placed a heavy economic burden on many countries. In the 1970s, the economies of Western developed countries began to experience long-term stagnation and high levels of fiscal deficit. Thus, health service models characterized by high benefits, low obligations, and all-inclusive payments gradually began to face difficulties caused by successive years of overspending and unsustainability. Since the 1990s, many types of advanced medical equipment and new technologies have been introduced, and these advancements have also caused the majority of developing countries to face the problem of ever-increasing healthcare expenditures. To ensure that healthcare costs could be kept within the limits of the national economy, both developed and developing countries began to undertake reforms of their health service and insurance systems. These reforms aimed to control the overexpansion of healthcare costs, resolve the contradiction between low economic growth and high healthcare costs, balance the relationship between the health security level and economic development, reduce the waste of health resources, and improve the allocation and utilization efficiency of health resources.

With regard to implementation, the most problematic issue commonly faced by governments across the world is as follows. On the one hand, a government needs to continually meet the health needs of its people, improve their health levels, and promote the development of medical science. On the other hand, the government also needs to maintain a fiscal balance, reduce the burden on companies, guarantee the balance of payments in health insurance funds, and achieve social stability. By taking a broad view of the health reforms in various countries over recent years, we can see that the focus has always been on finding a balance between these two roles.

Governments and scholars have reached a consensus on a few ideas. (1) The mainstream view of reform is to limit the growth rate of healthcare costs by determining total healthcare expenditures according to a country's socioeconomic capacity. (2) Countries should reduce waste, lower the cost of healthcare services, and promote the application of appropriate technologies and services. (3) Long-term mechanisms for the shared control of healthcare costs that involve hospitals, physicians, and patients should be established. An internal market with appropriate competition mechanisms should be introduced among hospitals and among physicians. Third-party payments, such as social health insurance, and cost-sharing mechanisms, such as copayments, should be implemented to improve service efficiency, lower costs, and reduce waste. (4) The equality, accessibility, and efficiency of health services should be continuously improved. Both equality and efficiency should be taken into consideration. The focus on efficiency is based on consideration for the scarcity of health resources. However, the international community currently has placed a greater emphasis on improving efficiency under the premise of guaranteeing equality, which is considered from the perspective of human rights. Within this context, a variety of models for the containment of healthcare costs has been introduced over the past 20 years. (5) Healthcare services can be stratified to meet the healthcare needs of different groups. The social health insurance or NHS provided by governments is not all-inclusive and only ensures that basic healthcare needs are met. The scope of basic healthcare needs is determined based on the economic ability of each country. The participation of social funds and commercial insurance agencies is encouraged in order to act as partial buffers for this discrepancy.

3. Three Stages in the Economic Model of Health Service Development

By examining the relationship between healthcare costs and socioeconomic capacity from the perspective of health economics, we can see that the model of health service development can be divided into three stages, namely, the expansion stage, the containment stage, and the coordination stage (Figure 10.2). At the beginning of the expansion phase, healthcare expenditures are lower than the socioeconomic capacity. As the level of medical technology and service capabilities continues to improve, there is a rapid rise in healthcare expenditures, and the rate of increase gradually surpasses the level and capacity of economic development.

The discrepancy continues to intensify and results in government intervention, and the economy thus enters the containment stage. In the containment stage, control is exerted over healthcare expenditures, and the growth of healthcare costs surpassing the country's socioeconomic capacity will begin to decrease and gradually revert back to the limits of the socioeconomic capacity, thus resolving the existing discrepancy. In the coordination stage, the rate of increase in healthcare expenditures is consistent with the level and capacity of socioeconomic development.

The most typical method adopted during the expansion phase is the fee-for-service system. This system is the most traditional model of health services and is a type of retrospective payment. It originates from the general principle of market exchange; that is, payments are made according to the service volume, whereby more services incur greater remuneration. The fee-for-service system is still commonly used by most countries today. This method plays an active role in promoting the development of the health industry during the initial stages of health service development, especially in states or regions lacking medical services and drugs. However, it is precisely because the incomes of healthcare providers are linked

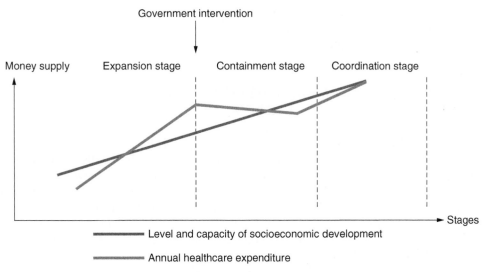

FIGURE 10.2 Three stages in the economic model of health service development.

to the service items and levels provided that the providers have an economic incentive to provide healthcare services. This fact, coupled with the information asymmetry between providers and consumers and the ineffective supervision of third-party payments, leads to the overprovision of services when the level and scale of healthcare development reaches a certain stage. Thus, the providers may add unnecessary healthcare expenditures to increase their financial benefits, which will result in the waste of health resources.

The crux of the problem is as follows. First, the criterion for judging the overprovision and waste of healthcare services is a variable that changes according to improvements in the level of socioeconomic development and in medical technology. Overprovision and waste of services is a concept that is defined relative to economic capacity. Second, the technical requirements for and management costs of constraining the overprovision and waste of services are relatively large. Under this model, it is very difficult to rely on the government's health administrative department to constrain overprovision. The strong driving force from the economic interests of healthcare institutions makes it difficult to unify the competing needs of the government and hospitals, between hospitals and residents, and between residents and the government.

Maintaining to a certain extent the driving force of economic interests, which drives competition among healthcare institutions and improves efficiency, while also controlling the unreasonable growth of healthcare costs is a problem faced by all countries. Thus, the governments of all countries began to intervene and introduced new policies and measures such that the health service model transitioned from the expansion stage to the containment stage. There are two basic approaches that are typically adopted in the containment stage. (1) Global budget systems, such as health maintenance organizations (HMOs), diagnosis-related groups (DRGs), and global control, are one approach. The main feature of this method is that the total service price for service recipients is determined prospectively, and, hence, the level of service provided by healthcare institutions is unrelated to total postservice revenues. (2) Revenue obstruction, such as regional health planning (the Resource Allocation Working Party, or RAWP), individual medical accounts (IMA), and the expansion of the copayment ratio (ECPR), is the second approach. Revenue obstruction is mainly characterized by constraining the development scales of healthcare institutions or enhancing the cost consciousness of patients, which will restrict the revenues of healthcare institutions, thereby controlling the rapid growth of healthcare costs.

SECTION II. MAIN MEASURES OF HEALTHCARE COST CONTAINMENT IN DEVELOPED COUNTRIES AND AREAS

The rise in healthcare costs due to the use of high technology and population aging has resulted in heavy economic burdens on many countries. Since the 1970s, the economies of developed countries have experienced long-term stagnation and high levels of fiscal deficit. Thus, health security systems characterized by the all-inclusive payments of welfare systems gradually faced difficulties caused by successive years of overspending and unsustainability. All countries began to reform their health security systems to coordinate the relationship between the security level and economic development, thereby containing the unreasonable growth of healthcare costs.

1. Strict Control over the Allocation of Large Medical Equipment

During the course of half a century, people gradually came to realize that the clinical safety and efficacy and cost effectiveness of novel high technology could not be guaranteed in the development stage. Hence, it was necessary to strengthen the technical evaluation and allocation management of such technologies. Countries generally implement regional health planning for the allocation of resources, including large and expensive medical equipment. Strict access systems are in place to reinforce control over management and allocation quantities.

In 1976, amendments to the Food, Drug, and Cosmetic Act gave the Food and Drug Administration of the US the power to review and approve equipment entering the market. Magnetic resonance imaging (MRI) was the first imaging product to enter the US market after being approved for certification. The Healthcare Committee of the German Federal Standing Committee of Physicians and Sickness Funds is responsible for reviewing whether new technologies can be included within the scope of payment. This committee is also responsible for evaluating existing medical technologies. In Portugal, legislation enacted in 1998 provided the Ministry of Health with full control over the acquisition of large medical equipment, and equipment acquisitions by the private sector are also included under its administration. The UK government stipulated that the CT and MRI scanners owned by the whole country should be allocated at the levels of 4.3 units and 0.9 units per million inhabitants, respectively. In 1970, France established an extremely strict planning and control system, which implemented a planned ceiling for large equipment. Japan did not previously impose policies to restrict the amount of large-scale hospital equipment, which caused it to have the highest number of CT scans per capita. In recent years, Japan has begun planning caps on the number of hospital beds in each district. It has also proposed the shared utilization of expensive equipment and the liberalization of state hospitals. In the 1970s, the US passed Certificate of Need (CON) laws, which required all hospitals intending to purchase equipment worth more than US$100,000 to be reviewed and approved by health administrative departments. However, due to the strong opposition of healthcare institutions, CON laws were terminated after being implemented for several years. Nevertheless, access to large-scale medical equipment in the US has become more stringent in recent years.

2. Establishing Healthcare Cost-Sharing Mechanisms

A comparative study of intentions conducted by the RAND Corporation in the US showed that, compared to the free-care group, 95% of the copayment group showed a 60% decrease in per capita expenses. Furthermore, the number of healthcare services and the amount of medication provided also decreased with the increase in the copayment ratio. However, the overall health status of the insured persons was not affected. To increase the cost consciousness of patients, many countries have gradually implemented cost-sharing mechanisms. Commonly used methods mainly include deductibles, copayments, ceilings, and different combinations of the three.

In terms of drug use, from 1982 to 2000, the UK gradually increased the copayment rate from £1.30 to £3.80 for each drug prescription. Germany introduced the Health Care Reform Act in 1989, which stipulated that fixed reimbursements were made for drugs with reference prices, with the difference being paid by patients, whereas, for drugs without reference prices, patients paid DM3 for each prescription. The copayment ratio for drugs was raised in 1993. Starting in 2000, the hospitalization fees for inpatients paid by Germany's statutory health insurance were reduced from DM25 to DM17 per day in West Germany and from DM20 to DM14 per day in East Germany, which, in turn, increased patients' out-of-pocket expenses. In 1984, 1986, and 1988, Portugal successively stipulated and adjusted the copayment ratios of four categories of drugs covered by health insurance. Since 1979, the NHS in the UK increased the out-of-pocket costs for eyeglass prescriptions and dental treatment. In 1987, the price ceiling for dental treatment was set at £115, and patients had to pay 40% of routine treatments exceeding £17. Patients requiring long-term medication could purchase prescription prepayment certificates, which cost £14.50/4 months and £40/12 months in 1989 and were adjusted to £22/4 months and £60/12 months in 1991. Since 1999, Japan increased the individual copayment ratio of the government-administered health insurance from 10% to 20%. In 2004, France's healthcare reform increased the copayment for each outpatient visit by €1. In addition, health insurance agencies were given the right to determine the ratio of drug reimbursement based on the rate of economic growth of that year.

3. Strengthening the Management of Healthcare Services

The prices of healthcare services are traditionally set by the service providers. Such supplier-led, freely fluctuating prices were one of the major reasons for the rise in healthcare costs. Many countries have reformed their pricing methods for healthcare services. Government pricing or negotiated pricing between insurance agencies and healthcare institutions has been implemented to guide the standardization of healthcare behaviors using unified prices.

Germany introduced the Health Care Reform Act in 1989, which required the establishment of a drug reference pricing system and formulated implementation rules regarding drug reference pricing and the list of drug prices. In July 1993, about 50% of drugs in Germany did not have reference prices. By January 1, 1997, the reference prices of approximately 339 drugs and 27 pharmaceutical compounds (about 60% of the market) were set. This act also clearly stipulates that all sickness funds must pay the prescribed prices of drug costs and that the pharmaceutical industry receives compensation from the statutory health insurance. To curb the continued growth of drug costs, Germany undertook the first direct intervention in drug prices in 1993. This intervention mandated decreases in the prices of prescription, quasi-prescription, and nonprescription drugs by 5%, 2.5%, and

2%, respectively. In 1983, the UK selectively reduced the prices of certain drugs and implemented a price freeze scheme. Japan's Ministry of Health, Labor, and Welfare revises the Treatment Remuneration Point Fee Schedule and the Drug Price Standard once every two years according to the development of medicine. Points are assigned to clinical examinations, treatments, and drug prices, and healthcare institutions are paid according to the number of points corresponding to the services provided.

4. Implementing a Global Budget System

The traditional approach to health insurance involves retrospective payments based on the volume of healthcare services (fee-for-service). The overprovision of healthcare services by physicians occurs frequently due to the pursuit of their own economic interests, which leads to a rapid rise in healthcare costs. When investigating the best practices for the reasonable control of healthcare costs, countries have attempted various methods for settling healthcare expenses, and the global budget system has generally been accepted by most countries. This method is characterized by the formulation of standards and total amounts of prospective payments to restrain the healthcare behaviors of providers. Doing so enables the sharing of economic risks, the standardization of healthcare behaviors, and the conscious and voluntary use of appropriate technologies rather than the blind pursuit of expensive technologies, thereby achieving healthcare cost containment. The practices of different countries indicate that the payment of healthcare costs has shifted from the fee-for-service method to the global budget system, which mainly involves a DRG-based payment system for hospital services and a capitation system for community services. This shift has now become a major developing trend in the payment systems for health insurance costs in all countries. A summary report indicated that after five years of implementing a DRG-based system within the US Medicare program, the hospitalization rate of individuals over 65 years of age decreased by 2.5% each year, and the average hospital stay length decreased from 10.2 days in 1982 to 8.9 days in 1987.

In Germany, the emergency Health Care Structure Act came into effect on January 1, 1993. This act imposed global budget management on the outpatient fees of 109,000 health insurance physicians. The global budget was calculated based on total outpatient expenditures in 1991 and would only be increased if the total amount of health insurance funds increased. However, the act also provided for exceptions, such as an increase by 10% in the annual budget for outpatient surgery and 6% in the annual budget for preventive treatment. As for the costs of inpatient services, Germany implemented a pay-per-diem system, which is based on the cost per bed-day and hospitalization rates, for the payment of hospital costs prior to 1993. This payment system does not encourage hospitals to rationally utilize healthcare resources, nor does it facilitate the effective containment of inpatient healthcare costs. Therefore, in the 1993 Health Care Structure Act, the pay-per-diem system was removed and was gradually replaced by a case-based payment system. Budget caps were gradually implemented for healthcare expenses that could not be settled using the case-based system. By 1996, one-off case-based payments had been implemented for 76 types of surgery. In 1998, Japan began piloting case-based payments for 183 types of diseases in 10 hospitals. The system was assessed in 2003 and was further promoted nationwide. In addition, Denmark, the Netherlands, Italy, and Costa Rica have primarily adopted the global budget system, which provides lump-sum prospective payments based on the service population; Argentina, Australia, and Hungary have primarily adopted the case-based system in settling inpatient healthcare costs; and the UK, Canada, and Ireland have implemented a global budget system for their healthcare institutions.

SECTION III.COMPARISON OF MODELS FOR HEALTHCARE COST CONTAINMENT IN DEVELOPED COUNTRIES AND AREAS

1. Five Models of Healthcare Cost Containment

In the context of the overexpansion of healthcare costs, maintaining the reasonable growth of health expenditures to ensure the coordinated development of the health security industry with society and economy has become the common goal of all developed countries in the world.

Currently, the following approaches have primarily been adopted in the cost containment of healthcare services.

(1) Health Maintenance Organization (HMO)

An HMO is a typical capitation system that is implemented in the US. Under this system, a healthcare provider uses premiums prepaid by each insured person to compensate for all health services stipulated in the contract within a fixed period of time, with no additional charges. Thus, the provider consciously adopts cost-containment measures while also carrying out disease prevention, health education, regular checkups, and other activities in order to minimize disease incidence and reduce expenditure. This approach presents providers with economic incentives to reduce costs in order to widen the difference between revenues and expenditures. However, this approach may also induce providers to opt for low-risk insured persons to reduce service costs and to limit the quantity and quality of services provided, thereby affecting the equality and accessibility of health services. Recently, the US government has taken measures to reduce the negative impact of HMOs through the uniform charging of premiums by insurance agencies and public registration.

HMOs have played a positive role in controlling healthcare costs and improving the accessibility of health services in the US. Nearly 40 research articles have reported that, compared to the fee-for-service system, the capitation system has decreased healthcare costs per capita by 10–40% and the rate of hospitalization by 25–45%; the number of outpatient visits and the average length of hospital stays have essentially remained the same.

(2) Diagnosis-Related Group-Based System

The Diagnosis-Related Group (DRG)-based payment system for healthcare expenditures has mainly been adopted in the US, Australia, and Argentina. Recently, Canada, certain European countries, and some developing countries have also begun to implement this approach. Under this system, the healthcare provider predetermines all of the costs for the healthcare services of each case or treatment stage. The main advantage of this system is that it combines the provider's compensation with the service volume determined by the characteristics of the DRG, thus encouraging the provider to control the costs of each case and reduce the waste of service resources. Its main disadvantage is that it can easily induce providers to select patients with milder conditions in the same disease group or to exaggerate the disease severity of patients to obtain greater financial profit, thereby increasing management costs.

(3) Resource Allocation Working Party

The Resource Allocation Working Party (RAWP) employs planning as the main means to achieve the rational allocation of health resources. It was first proposed by UK scholars according to the basic principles of the NHS and was later adopted by the government. Its theoretical basis is to improve equality in the provision of health services and avoid the duplication of allocations to reduce the waste of healthcare resources. The RAWP aims to balance the conflicting interests among social needs, economic development, and health-care costs by adjusting the allocation of regional healthcare resources. Areas with excessive healthcare resources and unreasonable growth in healthcare costs are controlled by placing constraints on healthcare institutions, the number of physicians, medical equipment, the number of beds, and funding. This approach has been accepted by the governments of most countries. Its main disadvantage is the lack of market competition and low efficiency, which limits the benefits brought about by competition and efficiency. To address this issue, the UK government proposed reform measures in 1991 known as the "internal market." RAWP was used to allocate healthcare providers (i.e., the planning and allocation of providers to achieve equality). On the demand side, each resident was able to choose a general practitioner (GP) for the treatment of common diseases, and in the event of a serious illness, the GP was able to choose a hospital for the resident (i.e., the market regulation of the demand side to achieve competition and increase efficiency). Unfortunately, an evaluation performed in 1998 revealed that the effects of this reform measure were not significant in the UK. Thus, the hypothetical "half-market" that took both equality and efficiency into account did not achieve the expected results in the UK.

(4) Individual Medical Account (IMA)

The IMA was first proposed by American scholars but was comprehensively implemented by the Singaporean government. It takes the form of a medical savings account that takes the financial risks arising from the occurrence of diseases at a given age and disperses the risk vertically across the entire course of the person's life. It may even disperse the risk across a few generations through the inheritance of the IMA. The main advantage of the IMA is that it can significantly enhance patients' awareness of demand-side savings in healthcare costs. Compared to social pooling (social health insurance), which involves the horizontal dispersion of disease-induced financial risk across the population, its disadvantage is that it has limited abilities in dispersing the financial risks of disease. After studying the advantages and disadvantages of these two methods, Chinese experts have designed a "two-in-one" urban basic medical insurance model. That is, the financial risk of minor outpatient illnesses is dispersed vertically using the IMA, whereas that of major inpatient illnesses is pooled across society and dispersed horizontally. Doing so enables the control of healthcare costs while also avoiding the impoverishment of patients with serious illnesses to a certain extent.

(5) Expansion of the Copayment Ratio (ECPR)

The ECPR was a recommendation proposed by the WHO in 1987 to control the overly rapid growth of healthcare costs in all countries. This recommendation was especially targeted at developing countries. The WHO believed that when the economic development of a country had not yet reached a certain level and its healthcare needs had also exceeded its economic capacity, then the expansion of the copayment ratio was an effective means to control healthcare costs. The WHO also pointed out that it is only by exerting effective control over the rapid growth of healthcare costs that a country is able to expand its health insurance coverage.

2. Comparison of Models for Healthcare Cost Containment and Conclusions

To summarize the five models of healthcare cost containment, a comparative analysis was performed on the following seven characteristics: cost containment of physician behaviors, reduction of average costs, containment of patients' out-of-pocket costs, containment of the number of health services, the overall effect of cost containment, the management cost of cost containment, and the promotion of competition among hospitals, as shown in Table 10.1. Based on the background analysis and international comparisons of various containment-type health service models, the following preliminary conclusions and recommendations were obtained.

1. Countries should select and formulate simple and effective restrictive healthcare models that are in line with national conditions.
2. No restrictive healthcare model is perfect, and each has its own pros and cons. The shortcomings of most models can be controlled using other measures.
3. Adopting a composite restrictive healthcare model is superior to choosing a single model. A composite model not only facilitates implementation and management but can also eliminate the negative effects of a single model.
4. Countries should explore the implementation of the capitation system for community health services and the DRG-based system for hospitals under health insurance. Although this approach involves larger management costs, it is more scientific, and the benefits from having greater cost containment and reduced wastage far outweigh the management costs. This approach can facilitate competition among hospitals and promote the positive development of hospitals, and, hence, it has been adopted by the vast majority of developed countries.
5. Regardless of which restrictive healthcare model has been adopted to control the unreasonable growth of healthcare costs, the quality of healthcare services cannot be sacrificed. Hence, the quality of healthcare services must also be guaranteed while controlling healthcare costs.

TABLE 10.1   Comparison of Five Healthcare Cost-Containment Models

Item	HMO	DRG	RAWP	IMA	ECPR
Containment of hospital cost behaviors	+ +	+ + +	+	–	–
Cost containment of physician behaviors	+	+ + +	–	+	+
Containment of patients' out-of-pocket costs	–	–	–	+ + +	+ +
Containment of the number of health services	+ +	+ + +	+	+ +	+
Overall effect of cost containment	+ +	+ + +	+	+ +	+
Management cost	+	+ + +	+ + +	+ +	–
Competition among hospitals	+	+	–	+	+

Note: + + + indicates a strong effect; + + indicates a moderate effect; + indicates a weak effect; – indicates no effect.

SECTION IV. POLICIES OF HEALTHCARE COST CONTAINMENT AND THEIR TRENDS IN DEVELOPED COUNTRIES AND AREAS

1. Policies of Healthcare Cost Containment in Developed Countries and Areas

The continuous rise in healthcare costs is a worldwide universal problem that affects the growth of national economies to a certain extent. Healthcare spending in developed countries has generally reached the upper limit of 7% of GDP, and its rate of growth has far exceeded that of GDP in most countries. This increase has led to a new round of financial crises in the health security systems of some countries. Hence, countries have implemented various policy measures to control the excessive growth of healthcare costs. The main policies for healthcare cost containment adopted by developed countries are shown in Table 10.2.

Germany adopted an income-oriented expenditure policy in 1976 to achieve balance and stability in its health insurance funds. In 1977, it implemented the Health Care Cost Containment Act, which included an increase in patients' copayments, the reform of remuneration for physicians, and the adjustment of bonuses among sickness funds. In 1981, Germany formulated the Supplementary Cost Containment Act and the Hospital Cost Containment Act. The latter mainly involved controlling the building of hospitals and the acquisition of medical equipment, limiting the hospital daily average increase in healthcare expenditures, and so on.

The cost-containment policies adopted by Sweden mainly included stronger macro-control by the government, with the decentralization of management power to the 26 counties and the reinforced fiscal autonomy of all counties; the introduction of market mechanisms and organized competition among suppliers; greater control over providers, including more control over hospital budgets, scale, development, healthcare manpower, and healthcare cost-effectiveness as well as the formulation of drug use regulations; and stronger control over healthcare demand, including an increase in patients' copayments and greater insurance fund management.

TABLE 10.2 Healthcare Cost-Containment Policies in Developed Countries

Country	Main Cost-Containment Policies
Germany	(1) Income-oriented expenditure policy (1976). (2) Health Care Cost Containment Act (1977). (3) Supplementary Cost Containment Act and Hospital Cost Containment Act (1981).
Sweden	(1) Stronger macro-control by the government. (2) Introduction of market mechanisms. (3) Greater control over providers and the formulation of drug use regulations. (4) Increase in patients' copayments. (5) Stronger insurance fund management.
France	(1) Healthcare cost-containment policy and new sources of insurance funds (1979). (2) New drug price regulations and restrictions (late 1980s). (3) Improved health insurance rates (1990s). (4) Unification of the health insurance system and the global healthcare cost planning system (2000). (5) Health system reform program (2004).
US	(1) Implementation of a payment method based on disease diagnosis and fee standards (1983). (2) Cost management plan. (3) Regulated health service plans.
Japan	(1) Optimization of healthcare institutions (1996). (2) Reform of drug pricing system (1996). (3) Increase in patients' copayments; elderly healthcare delayed until 75 years of age (2001). (4) Case-mix payment system (2003). (5) Introduction of market mechanisms.

As France has universal health insurance, most of its healthcare expenditures are covered by social health insurance (the average compensation rate of the general system is 90%). The healthcare cost-containment policies mainly involve controlling the healthcare costs of hospitals, increasing the ratios of individual copayments, reducing examination fees, and so on. In the late 1980s, France implemented new regulations and restrictions for drug prices. In the 1990s, the aforementioned cost-containment measure complemented the addition of new funding sources, including an increase in insurance premiums, levying health premiums from retirees (1% of basic pensions and 2% of supplementary pensions), a special sales tax levied on pharmacies equivalent to 1.5% of annual net income (limited to once a year), a 2.5% special tax on advertising costs levied on pharmaceutical companies, and so on. In 2000, the unification of the health insurance system and the global planning system for healthcare costs was implemented. In early 2004, health system reforms that mainly included the establishment of the attending doctor system, a reduction in the compensation rate for outpatient services, control of the scope of drug use, the promotion of electronic health records for patients, and changes in the budgeting methods of public hospitals were introduced.

The US attaches great importance to macro-control by the government and emphasizes market competition mechanisms. There are three main approaches to the management and supervision of healthcare costs: institutional and service management, effectiveness management, and premium and benefit management. Based on these three management approaches, the federal government introduced three types of cost management plans at different periods in time: the Certificate of Need, the Professional Standards Review Organization, and the prospective payment system.

In 1983, the US began implementing a payment method based on disease diagnosis and fee standards (i.e., the DRG-based payment system). As a competitive prospective health security model, HMOs applied the following three methods for cost containment: (1) establishing incentive mechanisms to stimulate the restructuring of healthcare institutions and to shift various healthcare channels from more expensive inpatient treatments to cheaper outpatient services, thereby achieving the integration of healthcare; (2) introducing competition into the traditional healthcare delivery system, thus encouraging mutual competition among healthcare institutions; and (3) choosing the best prices among HMOs through market mechanisms.

The drastic increase in Japan's healthcare costs is mainly due to population aging and the corresponding rise in elderly care and healthcare costs. The main direction of healthcare cost-containment policies for the elderly lies in controlling the provision of healthcare, expanding healthcare facilities for the elderly, promoting self-care efforts, and utilizing the proactiveness of the population. Japan's cost-containment policies mainly include optimizing healthcare institutions, reforming the drug pricing system, increasing patients' copayments, delaying "elderly healthcare" until the age of 75 years, implementing the case-mix payment system, and introducing market mechanisms.

2. Future Trends and Directions

Developed countries have adopted a variety of policies and measures to control the excessive growth of healthcare costs. These include strengthening drug administration, increasing patients' copayments, implementing the regional planning of health resource allocations, budget control, reforming the payment system, introducing market mechanisms, and increasing competition. Future trends are primarily as follows.

(1) Development of System Reforms from Simple Microeconomic Control to Comprehensive Macroeconomic Management

Different health insurance management systems and payment models involve different economic benefits and management costs, which in turn affect the consumption of health resources and have significantly different healthcare cost-containment effects. Countries such as the UK and Canada implement national, unified health insurance management and payment models. Germany and France implement the multichannel financing of health insurance funds, which ultimately funnels into the quasi-unified payment model of certain social health insurance agencies. These two models have been verified after many years of practice as having significant cost-containment effects. In the US, which is predominated by market-based health insurance, multiple payers use different methods and standards to reimburse healthcare providers, which consumes a large amount of management costs and accounts for about 15% of health expenditures. It has been estimated that health insurance management costs as a share of insurance premiums among OECD countries are less than one-third those of the US. Hence, an increasing number of health economists have recommended the implementation of a unified management system and centralized single payer system to reduce management costs and save on health spending.

(2) Shifting from Demand-Side to Supply-Side Orientation and Taking Both Sides into Consideration

During the initial stages of development in the health insurance system, it was generally believed that the rapid rise in healthcare costs was due to the excessive demand for healthcare, and, hence, the control measures were mostly directed at the demand side. As a greater understanding was gained of the particularities of the health service market, such as information asymmetry and technological and geographical monopolies, this market became a supply-side-oriented market with imperfect competition, in which the quantity, price, and quality of healthcare consumption were determined by the suppliers. The implementation of health insurance also reduced the demand-side sensitivity to costs, which resulted in the expansion of consumption. In other words, the overprovision of healthcare services drove excessive demand for healthcare services, and healthcare cost containment shifted toward the supply side while also taking the demand side into account. Demand-side control mainly took the form of cost-sharing mechanisms and setting up individual accounts, whereas supply-side control mainly involved implementing the regional planning of health resource allocations, budget control, and reforming the payment system.

(3) The Focus of Control Is on Reforming and Improving the Payment System for Suppliers

The health insurance reform practices of many countries have shown that imposing constraints on suppliers is the key to and the core of healthcare cost containment, whereas the payment method for suppliers is, in turn, the most effective way to control suppliers' behaviors. At present, health insurance payment methods include the fee-for-service, DRG-based, capitation, case-based, and global budget systems. Following the continuous appearance of various shortcomings in retrospective payment systems, combinations of prospective settlement methods, including the DRG, capitation, and global budget systems, gradually became the mainstream reforms to the health insurance payment methods of all countries. The mainstream payment method is the global budget system in Germany; the global budget and capitation systems in the UK; the case-mix payment system in Japan; and the DRG-based and capitation systems in the US. Overall, the use of DRG-based systems for inpatient services and capitation systems for outpatient services will become the mainstream method of payment in the future and also represents the developing trend in payment methods.

(4) Transforming from a Subject–Object Relationship to a Collaborative Relationship

The traditional mode of operation in health insurance is a triangular four-party relationship. That is, an insured person pays premiums to an insurance agency; a healthcare institution provides services to the insured person; the insurance agency pays the contracting healthcare institution as a third-party payer; and the government performs macro-control and management of the recipient, provider, and insurer. Although healthcare institutions face the threat of being removed as "designated" providers, this threat is insufficient to promote effective competition among healthcare institutions and does not facilitate the containment of healthcare costs. Such traditional cost-containment systems consist of the controlling subject, health insurance agencies, and the controlled object, healthcare institutions.

Since the 1970s, the rapid development of HMOs and preferred provider organizations in the US has broken the traditional triangular relationships. HMOs combine health insurance providers and healthcare providers into one body, thus converting the controlled object into a self-controlling subject. This body, on the one hand, competes with traditional insurance in terms of premium levels, insurance coverage, convenience, and service quality. On the other hand, it also attempts to provide healthcare services at the lowest possible cost and competes with hospitals and physicians under the original fee-for-service system. This development not only reduces the friction cost between medical insurance agencies and healthcare providers but also provides healthcare providers and physicians with an incentive to control costs so as to obtain cost advantages in the insurance market. This kind of management-oriented healthcare model has a positive impact on the cost containment of medical expenses.

(5) Developing from the Simple Control of Healthcare Expenditures to Comprehensive Healthcare Cost Containment

The control of health insurance costs is a system-wide undertaking that requires the full cooperation of all sectors of society and necessitates the application of multidisciplinary knowledge, including insurance, actuarial science, medicine, pharmaceutical economics, and management science. The continuous rise in healthcare costs involves both "demand-pull" and "cost-push" and is a form of "mixed demand-cost inflation" that is predominated by cost-push. Since the 1980s, the control of healthcare expenditure in developed countries gradually extended to comprehensive control over the cost of healthcare services, which mainly targeted the costs of labor and drugs. The control of labor costs mainly involved limiting the number of physicians, removing redundant healthcare workers, and restricting the access of physicians to health insurance. The control measures for drug costs mainly included increasing the copayment standard for drugs, stipulating the yearly deductible for drugs, formulating drug use regulations, and implementing various control measures for drug prices.

(6) Transitioning from Retrospective Control to Dual Retrospective and Prospective Control

There are two possible approaches for the economic regulation of health insurance operations, namely, retrospective and prospective risk regulation. Prospective risk control can strengthen prevention and promote community healthcare and services, which greatly reduces the incidence of diseases, especially that of chronic diseases, thereby effectively controlling healthcare expenditures. In the reforms of countries throughout the world, the emphasis has gradually shifted from the retrospective and passive payment of insurance premiums in the past to prospective risk control, which is based on strengthening prevention and community services. Thus, a dual insurance mechanism has been established, involving the prospective reduction of risk frequency and the retrospective provision of risk security, which is manifested in the formulation of laws related to health promotion and the reinforcement of primary healthcare.

(7) Transitioning from Planned or Market-Based Measures to an Organic Combination of Both

Both planned and market-based measures for resource allocation have their own advantages and disadvantages. It is only by fully utilizing their respective strengths to compensate for their individual weaknesses that we can improve the efficiency of resource allocation. Healthcare cost containment essentially determines the flow and distribution of health and financial resources, which also requires an organic combination of planned and market-based measures. For example, the US, which has an extremely well-established market economy, has also implemented health planning for medical equipment resources. The UK government has introduced market-style incentive mechanisms and management functions to establish an "internal market" that separates the buyers and providers of health services, thus enabling healthcare funds to follow the patients. In order to improve service efficiency and control healthcare costs, market competition mechanisms have also been introduced to Singapore's savings-type healthcare system. Internal competition is encouraged between two public healthcare groups within a given maximum limit of total healthcare spending, thereby fully utilizing the collaborative and complementary functions of planned and market-based measures.

PART THREE

Health Systems in Developed Countries and Areas

CHAPTER ELEVEN

National Health Service Systems of Representative Countries

 ## SECTION I. THE HEALTH SYSTEM IN THE UNITED KINGDOM

The United Kingdom (UK) is a Western European country, which comprises the island of Great Britain, the northeastern part of Ireland, and many surrounding islands. It covers an area of 244,000 km^2 and is divided into four regions: England, Wales, Scotland, and Northern Ireland. The full name of this country is the United Kingdom of Great Britain and Northern Ireland. The total population of the UK in 2013 was 64.097 million, which ranked third in Europe after Russia and Germany. The socioeconomic level, health status, and other indicators of the population in England are highly representative of the entire UK as its population accounts for 83.2% of the total UK population. For historical reasons, each of the four regions of the UK has relatively independent legislation and management systems, but the principles and basic form of their National Health Service (NHS) systems are essentially the same. The socioeconomic and health indicators of the UK population are shown in Table 11.1.

TABLE 11.1   Socioeconomic and Health Indicators of Residents in the UK in 2013

Indicators		Indicators	
Total population	64,097,085	Percentage of population aged over 65 years	17.5%
Average life expectancy (male/female)	79.5/83.6 years*	Annual population growth rate	0.6%
Infant mortality rate	3.9 per 1,000 live births	National income per capita	US$41,680
Percentage of total healthcare expenditure of GDP	9.4%*	Maternal mortality rate	8.0/100,000 live births

* Based on 2012 data.

Demographic characteristics of the UK: The UK has a large elderly population, high average life expectancy, high population density (246 people per km^2), high urban population ratio (80%), low birth rate, low mortality rate, and low rate of natural increase. Population aging is currently a prominent social issue in the UK.

The UK was the first country to adopt the two-party system of government. The current opposition party (at the time of writing), the Labour Party, adheres to the principles of Fabianism, which seeks to reconcile the conflicts between the public and the ruling party via a reformist approach. It promotes inter-class cooperation, advocates the nationalization of large enterprises, and emphasizes "social welfare." The Conservative Party (now in power), on the other hand, advocates for market competition, free enterprise, and market regulation. It does not advocate for government intervention but strives to protect the interests of the monopoly capital. As the ruling party has mainly alternated between the Labour Party and the Conservative Party, the aims and policy orientations of both have had a significant impact on the healthcare policies of the UK. The NHS program was formulated by the Labour Party as part of its focus on welfare policies.

An important feature of healthcare regionalization in the UK is its separation from administrative division. In terms of administrative division, the country is divided into 61 counties, 39 of which are located in England. These counties are further subdivided into 444 districts, with 369 districts in England and Wales, 49 districts in Scotland, and 26 in Northern Ireland. Each district can be further divided into communities or parishes. In terms of healthcare regionalization, the country is divided into four regions: England, Wales, Scotland, and Northern Ireland, each of which has its own health department that works directly under the Cabinet. In England, specifically, there are eight regional offices of the NHS Executive and 221 District Health Authorities (DHAs) under the jurisdiction of the Department of Health and Social Care (DHSC). Each regional office covers several counties, while each DHA covers two to three administrative districts. Healthcare regionalization in the UK is mainly implemented according to population distribution, geographical characteristics (e.g., mountains and rivers), distribution and catchment areas of healthcare facilities, and so on. It fully considers the convenience and objective demands for healthcare services, especially community healthcare services.

When the NHS was first established, public financing covered 90% of its funds, and the resultant heavy financial burden became one of the greatest challenges facing the country. Therefore, the Conservative Party attempted to abolish the NHS multiple times after it came to power. However, the NHS has strong public support, and the opposition party often uses government policies on the NHS as a basis for criticizing the ruling party. Since the NHS is a major issue of concern to the public, candidates have always made policy commitments to resolve issues related to the NHS at every general election. As a result, a change in power inevitably led to reforms in NHS policies.

In May 1997, six months after the Labour Party came to power, it released a white paper to affirm the long-standing principles of the NHS – namely, that state-owned healthcare agencies shall provide free and comprehensive healthcare services as needed to the general public at the taxpayer's expense. The government firmly believed that the NHS in the UK is an efficient and fair healthcare service system compared to other countries. In the more than 50 years since the NHS was implemented, policies in all sectors have undergone significant changes with the shift in political power; however, the NHS is regarded as one of the major exceptions. Although the government has always been determined to reform the NHS and has carried out extensive reforms to various aspects, such as service delivery and management measures, the basic elements and principles of the NHS have not changed. This makes the NHS one of the most continuous administrative systems in existence.

1. Establishment of the National Health Service

(1) The Origin of the National Health Service

1. The Origin of the National Health Service in the UK   The National Health Service (NHS) and community health services (CHS) are the basic features of the healthcare services in the UK. The government budget allocation for healthcare accounts for more than 80% of the total healthcare expenditure in the UK, and the public is provided with access to free healthcare services. The implementation and management of healthcare are characterized by the centralized control of healthcare resource allocation, and community healthcare is considered the centerpiece of healthcare services. In fact, the UK is the birthplace of modern CHS, which continues to hold a high status in the UK healthcare system and plays an important role in health protection.

The healthcare system in the UK was established on the basis of the National Health Service Act 1946, which aimed to ensure comprehensive healthcare services for UK citizens, including disease prevention and health protection. The creation and implementation of the National Health Service Act was not only a major event in the British society but also triggered a strong response from the international community and was called "one of the greatest achievements of the twentieth century." The key aspects of this act are as follows.

1. *Nationalization of all hospitals in the UK.* The government took over all hospitals, while hospital physicians and administrators were employed and salaried as civil servants.
2. *Implementation of the general practitioner system.* Each resident was required to choose and register with a general practitioner (GP), who would provide basic healthcare services for health protection, common illnesses, and frequently occurring diseases. GPs were responsible for contacting hospitals on behalf of patients requiring hospitalization. They signed an agreement with the relevant government departments and receive remuneration according to the number of registered patients. They were free to choose the location of their clinics, but the government encouraged them to establish their clinics at government-run CHS centers.
3. *Accountability of the health authorities.* The health authorities of local governments were responsible for the management of CHS centers and ambulances, along with public health, school health services, and obstetric services.
4. *Free services.* All healthcare services were free of charge and covered by public financing through tax revenues.
5. *Residents' right of choice.* Residents retained the right to choose their physicians.

The most distinctive features of the NHS were as follows: first, it covers all UK residents, even foreigners who have lived in the UK for at least six months, thereby fully embodying the principle of equal access to healthcare for everyone. Second, it provides free healthcare services, regardless of wealth, race, gender, occupation, and income differences, and all healthcare expenditures are publicly financed. Third, it standardizes healthcare services through a centralized management system, which makes it more effective at reducing regional and interpersonal variations.

There have been several revisions to the healthcare system, including the implementation of patient copayment policies for medicines (1949) and dentures (1951), the introduction of charges for foreigners in 1982, and the implementation of policies that promote private healthcare since 1979. However, the NHS has still retained its basic structure to date.

2. The Origin of the UK Medical Aid System   The UK is one of the first countries to implement a social medical aid system. The UK government promulgated the Poor Relief Act (the Old Poor Law) during the Elizabethan era in 1601 and the Poor Law Amendment Act (the New Poor Law) in 1834. The biggest difference between the old and new laws was the transition from outdoor relief (relief given outside workhouses) to strict indoor relief (relief given within workhouses). However, outdoor relief was not completely abolished after the implementation of the New Poor Law. In fact, both outdoor and indoor relief were implemented up until 1948. The medical aid provided under the poverty relief system for patients and individuals with physical disabilities can be divided into two categories: livelihood relief and provision of healthcare services. Under this system, healthcare services were primarily provided by "hospitals for the poor" to low-income earners who were unable to afford medical expenses and to recipients of indoor relief.

At that time, due to the overall shortage of medicines and beds in the "hospitals for the poor," the medical aid system imposed stringent restrictions on those seeking medical attention, even their personal conduct. Hence, only the most basic health protections could be provided to meet the healthcare needs of a small handful of medical aid recipients. It should be noted that in addition to the poverty relief system, there were other channels of social medical aid, including worker mutual aid societies (e.g., trade unions and friendship associations), which provided medical aid to their members, and charitable organizations, which provided various healthcare services. The former is now regarded as a rudimentary form of health insurance, which gradually evolved into the existing social health insurance system; the latter were independent entities that even now provide various social aids, including medical aid, in many countries.

(2) Preliminary Organizational Structure

The preliminary organizational structure of NHS is shown in Figure 11.1. For historical reasons, the services provided by the NHS were divided into three areas: GP services, hospital services, and CHS, which are administered and operated separately by the Executive Committee, local hospital committees, and local governments, respectively.

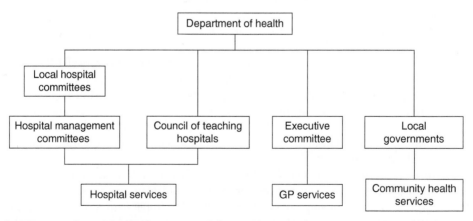

FIGURE 11.1   Organizational structure of the NHS (1948–1974).

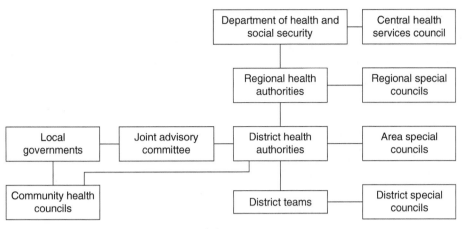

FIGURE 11.2 Organizational structure of the NHS (1974–1982).

2. Developments and Changes in the NHS Management System

(1) First NHS Reform

The separation of the three areas of the NHS led to a lack of cooperation among their constituent departments, which posed significant obstacles to the planning and integrated continuity of healthcare services.

Both the Guillebaud Report of 1956 and the Porritt Report of 1962 pointed out the serious problems faced by the administrative agencies of the NHS.

Following these reports, the government began placing greater emphasis on these issues. In April 1974, the three areas were integrated and reorganized into a three-tier management model, composed of the regional, area, and district levels, as shown in Figure 11.2. Since then, the CHS run by regional governments has been implemented as part of the NHS.

(2) Second NHS Reform

The first NHS reform focused on the integration of healthcare services but led to a more complicated accountability system due to the three-tier management model. Hence, more effort was spent on management than on service provision. For example, the Department of Health and Social Security issued up to 200 government documents per year to its affiliated organizations.

Therefore, the second reform was launched in April 1982 to simplify the three-tier management model. It was reduced to a two-tier model by abolishing the Area Health Authorities (AHAs), as shown in Figure 11.3. This two-tier model has been in place ever since.

(3) Third NHS Reform

In 1991, the Conservative Party conducted a substantive reform of the NHS, with the greatest changes being made to two aspects: First, the government abolished all 17 regional health authorities and replaced them with eight offices under the NHS Committee of the Department of Health. This not only simplified the organizational structure but also

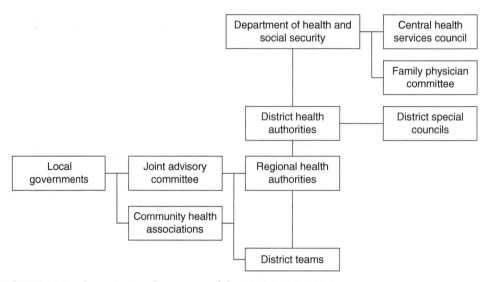

FIGURE 11.3　Organizational structure of the NHS (1982–1991).

enhanced the control of the central government over the NHS, especially over health budget goals. Second, market competition mechanisms were introduced to form an internal market for the NHS. Purchaser–provider split was implemented in the delivery of healthcare services, leading to the emergence of various trust agencies and funds that formed contractual relationships with the Health Administration Department (Figure 11.4).

(4) Fourth NHS Reform

After taking over the office in 1997, the Labour Party halted most reform measures adopted by the Conservative Party, with the exception of the purchaser–provider split. They believed

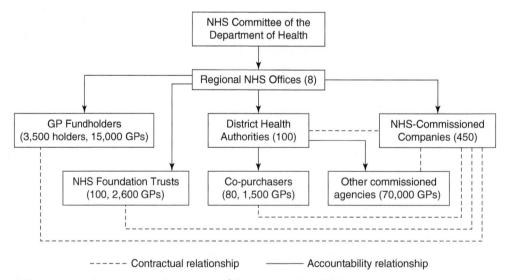

FIGURE 11.4　Organizational structure of the NHS (1991–1997).

that the NHS reforms made by the Conservative Party raised commercial awareness of healthcare services, which was detrimental to the continuation of the basic principles and policies of the NHS.

The Labour government placed particular emphasis on the partnership between healthcare providers and users, and among providers, especially extensive coordination and cooperation for CHS. One of the most important changes made during this health reform was the integration of various community healthcare management organizations, as shown in Figure 11.5.

The main purpose of the reform is to achieve extensive coordination within the community, in order to create a genuine partnership between healthcare providers and users.

1. NHS Reform Orientation The aim of the reforms was to provide fast, convenient, and patient-centered healthcare services, thus improving service quality and eliminating the main causes of diseases and healthcare inequalities.

2. Six Principles of NHS Reform and Development
1. The NHS shall become a truly national health service that enables equal access to high-quality healthcare services nationwide.
2. Healthcare services provided by the NHS shall not only meet national standards but also emphasize the responsibilities of local authorities owing to their greater awareness of the needs of patients.
3. The NHS shall emphasize internal partnerships and break down interdepartmental barriers to provide more patient-centered services.
4. The NHS shall overcome bureaucracy and strive to improve the efficiency of healthcare services.
5. The NHS shall strive to improve the quality of health services.
6. The NHS shall reshape its public image.

3. Main Focus of NHS Work
1. Reduce the waiting time for outpatient and inpatient appointments.
2. Help patients understand their health status and the healthcare services they receive and actively participate in healthcare-related activities, healthcare measures, and policies that improve healthcare service quality.

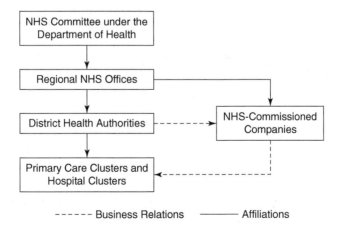

FIGURE 11.5 Organizational structure of the NHS since 1997.

3. Establish more one-stop centers and walk-in centers to make the CHS more convenient for the public.
4. Renovate GP clinics.
5. Improve the food and environmental sanitation at hospitals.
6. Enhance the preventive and therapeutic measures against chronic diseases, such as cancer and cardiovascular diseases.
7. Enhance mental health services, drug abuse control, tobacco control, health education, pediatric healthcare and so on.

(5) Fifth NHS Reform

In July 2000, the UK government introduced "The NHS Plan: A Plan for Investment, A Plan for Reform," which sought to increase investment in the universal healthcare system. This was the first major NHS reform by the Labour Party since 1997, and it laid out a plan for the direction of the NHS over the next decade. In particular, it outlined a new implementation system for patient-centered healthcare services. It also introduced several changes to the relationships between healthcare and social public services, and between the NHS and the private sector.

1. Core Principles of the Reform
1. Provide free and basic healthcare services nationwide.
2. Provide comprehensive, integrated, and patient-centered healthcare services to meet the needs of different groups of patients.
3. Continue to improve service quality and minimize the occurrence of errors and problems.
4. Support and respect NHS staff and their contributions.
5. Allocate public healthcare funds that are dedicated to NHS patients.
6. Cooperate with relevant departments to ensure comprehensive services.
7. Help the population to stay healthy and reduce inequalities in health and healthcare.
8. Respect patients' privacy and provide them with information about healthcare services and treatments.

2. Specific Reform Measures
1. Integrate self-employed GPs into the NHS through contract management, thereby greatly enhancing the role of GPs as healthcare service providers.
2. Strengthen the ability of the UK healthcare system to provide nonhospital healthcare services.
3. Enhance the inspection and evaluation of healthcare quality and the supervision of healthcare institutions.

(6) Sixth NHS Reform

In December 2005, the UK government released a report entitled "Health Reform in England: Update and Next Steps" as part of further reforms to the NHS. This report summarized the first half of the 10-year plan, and further refined the NHS reforms for the next 5 years. The key focus of the reform was to introduce incentives into the healthcare system in order to promote sustained improvements in healthcare quality, healthcare output, and financial utilization.

TABLE 11.2   Health Reform Timeline in the UK

Time	Major Reforms
1980–1981	5% reduction in the short-term allowance of patients
1982	Proposal to reduce public expenditures, including on private health insurance schemes and the NHS
1983	Privatization is proposed as a useful alternative to the NHS, as it would relieve the burden on the NHS
1985	A green paper entitled "Reform of Social Security" is released, which proposes that social security should be the shared responsibility and obligation of both citizens and the government
1989	A white paper entitled "Working for Patients (NHS Reforms)" is published, which emphasizes the introduction of market mechanisms to reform the health insurance system and expand patients' rights of independent choice
1991	The Conservative Party promulgates the new National Health Service and Community Care Act, which introduces an "internal market" for the supply of healthcare
1992	The GP Fundholding policy is established, allowing GPs to control the budget
1996	Regional health authorities are abolished and replaced with 9 regional offices of the NHS Executive
1997	The Labour Party came to power and vowed to "work 24 hours to rescue the NHS"
1999	The GP Fundholding policy is abolished
2000	The government promulgates a new plan with the goal of improving healthcare services and reducing waiting times
2001	Introduction of hospital rankings
2002	Government announces a substantial increase in funding for healthcare services
2002	PCTs take over the responsibility of service commissioning
2002	100 regional health authorities are replaced with 28 strategic health authorities (SHAs)
2004	The first basic hospital network is approved
2005	Implementation of the pay-for-performance policy
2005	The government announces a policy whereby hospital services are commissioned by primary care staff
2006	The number of PCTs falls from 302 to 152. The number of SHAs reduces from 28 to 10
2006	Abolition of hospital rankings
2008	New NHS Constitution
2009	The healthcare regionalization system is abolished, allowing citizens to "vote with their feet" by exercising the right to choose their preferred GPs

Specific reform measures:

1. Patients have more choices and a stronger right to make decisions (demand-side reform).
2. Diversified providers have more freedom to innovate and improve their services (supply-side reform).
3. The flow of funds is directed by the patients, such that the best and most effective providers are rewarded, which provides incentives to others to make improvements (business reforms).

In addition, there were also some minor policy changes interspersed among these major NHS reforms. Please refer to the health reform timeline in the UK shown in Table 11.2.

3. NHS Funding

(1) NHS Funding

In 2002, the NHS had approximately £32.1 billion in funding, of which 83.3% came from direct tax revenues, 8.9% from indirect tax revenues from government budgets, and only 7.8% came from payments made by patients. In 2009, NHS funding reached about £100 billion, of which 82% came from tax revenues, 12.2% from national insurance contributions, 2% from medical expenses paid by patients (mainly prescription fees and dental and ophthalmic expenses), and 3.8% from other sources of income and donations from charitable organizations.

Out of the total healthcare expenditure, personnel expenditure accounted for 60%, drug expenditure accounted for 20%, and home appliances, training, medical equipment, reception, and logistics accounted for 20%. About 80% of the healthcare funding was allocated directly to local primary care trusts (PCTs), which establish service items and service content standards, as well as pay GP clinics according to the number and quality of primary healthcare services provided. PCTs also pay for the referral fees involved in sending patients to corresponding referral hospitals. Equal funding was allocated to GP clinics and hospitals.

The capital flow of the UK NHS in 2009 is shown in Figure 11.6.

(2) Patient Copayment in the NHS

1. Prescription Fees Patients are charged for each prescription as part of their copayment. The prescription fee has gradually increased over the years: for instance, it was £1.06 in 1984, after which it increased to £3.80 in 1996 and £5.20 in 2004. The prescription fee is imposed on all patients except for the following:

1. Drugs needed by inpatients
2. Drugs needed for the treatment of sexually transmitted diseases (STDs)
3. Patients under 16 years of age or students under 19 years of age
4. Elderly adults aged 65 (males) or over 60 (females) years

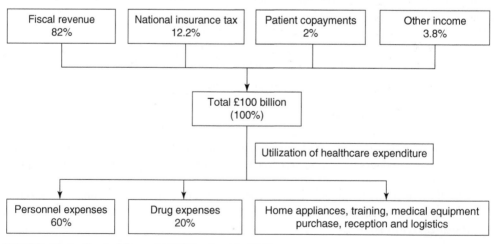

FIGURE 11.6 Capital flow of NHS England in 2009.

TABLE 11.3 Dental Services Requiring Patient Copayment in the UK

Dentures	Dental Composite Resins	Dental Metals or Porcelain
1–3 teeth	£22	£40
4–8 teeth	£23	£42
More than 9 teeth	£24	£44

5. Pregnant women or women in the first postpartum year
6. Patients who require continuous treatments due to epilepsy, pernicious anemia, and other diseases
7. Disabled individuals incapable of traveling without assistance
8. Unemployed individuals or benefit recipients and their dependents
9. Treatment for diseases and disabilities due to military affairs

Furthermore, individuals requiring continuous medication can be exempted from 4 or 12 months of copayments if they pay a certain amount to the Family Council.

Since April 1985, over 2,000 drugs (including analgesics, sedatives, and cold medicines) have been excluded from the reimbursement list by the NHS in order to reduce the rapidly increasing drug expenses.

2. Dental Services Patients must pay copayments for some dental services (Table 11.3). Dental crowns with over 45% gold charged £50 per tooth, while dental fillings with other materials are charged at £26 per tooth (up to a maximum of £95).

However, for inpatients, those under the age of 16 years, students under the age of 19 years, and pregnant women or women in the first postpartum year are exempt from patient copayments.

3. Self-Paid Hospital Beds Chief physicians at hospitals can make use of NHS hospital facilities to treat patients as if they are self-paying patients. Facilities that can be used for this purpose are called "self-paid hospital beds." This unconventional system was created in the context of opposition to the NHS by hospital physicians and helps meet the needs of some users who require the services of chief physicians but do not want to join the long waiting list.

Patients who self-pay for hospital beds must bear all expenses; physician consultation fees are added to the personal income of physicians while facility fees are paid to the hospitals. All fees are priced according to the law.

4. Amenity Beds An "amenity bed" is a single-patient ward with good conditions that patients can access for personal reasons rather than medical reasons. Amenity beds cost significantly more than do the ordinary beds and must be fully covered by the patients.

5. Hospital Services for Foreigners People with foreign passports who have lived in the UK for less than six months have been required to pay for hospital services since October 1982. This is due to fiscal challenges facing the NHS, which have gradually drained the NHS of surplus to provide free hospital services to foreigners. Moreover, many considered it unfair for non–tax paying foreigners to receive priority for free emergency treatment, while many British citizens have to contend with long hospital waiting lists. However, foreigners who have resided in the UK for more than six months, employed or self-employed foreigners in the UK, or citizens of countries that have signed reciprocal healthcare agreements with the UK, are not subject to these charges.

(3) NHS Expenditures

The expenditure of the NHS in the UK has increased rapidly over the years. In 1949, the total expenditure was approximately £400,003,700, which increased to £16,900,008,500 in 1984 and £50 billion in 2003. As a share of the GDP, NHS expenditures accounted for 3.9% in 1949, 4.6% in 1970, 6.2% in 1984, 7.6% in 2002, 8% in 2004, and 9.4% in 2012. These expenditures have continued to increase and were £103.8 billion in 2010, £106 billion in 2011, £108.4 billion in 2012, £114.1 billion in 2013, and £114.4 billion in 2014.

NHS expenditures have been increasing due to population aging and the advancement of medical technologies, which has caused the government to become more committed to the efficient use of resources. For example, the 1984 budget required hospitals to reduce their expenditure by 0.5% through the efficient use of funds.

As for the efficient use of healthcare resources, the government has also shifted their policy orientation from hospital services to CHS. Nevertheless, hospital services still account for 51% of the total healthcare expenditure.

4. Community Health Services

(1) Characteristics of Community Health Services

Although the UK has a market economy, its Community Health Services (CHS) and the entire NHS essentially operate according to a planned model.

Many departments are involved in the development of CHS in the UK. The relationships between CHS agencies and main government departments are shown in Figure 11.7. The main features of CHS are as follows.

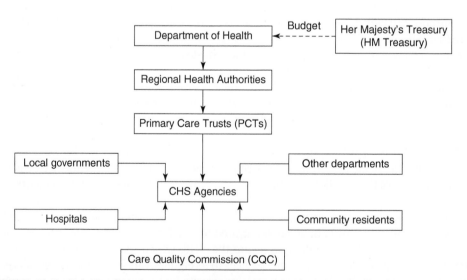

FIGURE 11.7 Relationships between CHS agencies and other departments.

1. Implementing Regional Health Planning and Emphasizing Equitable Healthcare Resource Allocation The UK has implemented policies for allocating healthcare resources according to its regional demographic characteristics, and the balanced allocation of healthcare resources is strictly regulated according to the saturation of healthcare services (e.g., number of GPs per capita) within a given region.

Regional health planning, commonly known as the Resource Allocation Working Plan (RAWP), was first proposed by British experts in the 1970s and was later adopted by the government. The core element of the RAWP is a resource allocation formula known as the Crossman formula or RAWP formula, which serves as the foundation of healthcare resource allocation. Some of the major parameters included in this formula are the population size, age, gender, marital status, birth rate, and mortality rate in each district. The RAWP formula has undergone continuous revisions over the past three decades, but its basic parameters have remained the same. The RAWP formula has also been adopted as the primary basis for current policies on healthcare funding allocation.

2. Implementing Preferential Policies for "Cinderella" Services in Healthcare Social demand for healthcare services is in a state of constant growth. The relative inadequacy of resources is always a consistent challenge, regardless of whether the country implements a health insurance system or NHS system. Healthcare resources in the UK are almost entirely dependent on national taxes, but it is impossible for public funding to fully meet the healthcare needs of the entire population. Furthermore, a tremendous burden has been placed on the healthcare industry over the past 20 years due to population aging, rapid medical advances, and rising medical costs due to the use of expensive devices and drugs, which have forced the government to make policy adjustments with relatively limited resources in order to adapt to the changes in social development.

These insufficient resources have driven the preferential allocation of healthcare resources to disadvantaged groups, which has been a key direction of many government healthcare policies. Since the 1970s, both the Labour Party and the Conservative Party have implemented this preferential allocation policy during their administration in order to prioritize the elderly, disabled individuals, psychiatric patients, and women and children in healthcare services. Hence, there is a degree of consensus among different political parties and the public that these social groups are most in need of healthcare. This preferential policy has been referred to as "Cinderella" services, after the character in the fairy tale, who is neglected by society and desperately needs help. The "Cinderella" service policy has promoted the development of CHS to a significant extent.

3. Competition and Partnership The Labour Party believed that although the NHS is split between the providers (healthcare institutions) and the purchasers (health authorities that represent the residents), a partnership should be established between the two, in order to form continuous and integrated healthcare services. The current direction of health reform is to reduce profit-seeking and commercial competition in the healthcare system and to enhance a sense of partnership, thereby promoting broad, community-wide coordination of healthcare services.

4. User Involvement in Healthcare Decisions User involvement is a healthcare strategy advocated by the World Health Organization (WHO). In recent years, the NHS and CHS in the UK have begun placing increasing emphasis on user involvement in healthcare decisions. Users not only help to identify issues related to community health and healthcare services but also participate in discussions on how to address these issues. In the past, the government obtained user opinions about healthcare services mainly through complaints and only addressed these issues when the supply-demand relationship was sufficiently tense. Users are now involved in the decision-making process and have now shifted from passive to active participation in problem-solving.

5. Patient's Charter, Patient's Rights, and Complaint Mechanisms　The Patient's Charter was enacted in 1991 with the aim of protecting patients' rights and interests. The main elements of the Patient's Charter include rules for changing GPs, referral rules, and maximum waiting time for nonemergency and surgical services. The current Patient's Charter also includes specific quality indicators for various operational items in clinical and community healthcare services, which were included in order to draw patients' attention and interest. Patients can lodge complaints regarding dissatisfaction with services but must do so within one year after the event; otherwise, the complaint will be deemed invalid. In general, complaints are mainly processed by the Community Health Committee rather than resolved by the judicial system. There are officials specialized in investigating medical disputes in health authorities at all levels.

6. "Money Following Patients" and Continuous, Accountable Physician–Patient Relationships　A continuous and accountable physician–patient relationship is one of the main characteristics of CHS in the UK and represents a major contribution of the UK to the international healthcare industry. When the NHS was established in 1948, UK citizens aged 16 years and above and foreigners who resided in the UK were eligible to register with a GP of their choice (parents and guardians registered on behalf of children under 16 years of age) to establish a permanent physician–patient relationship. Each person is given a medical card with a unique registration number. Patients are required to seek medical attention from their respective GPs and subsequently retrieve drugs from pharmacies using prescriptions issued by GPs. Patients pay only a small amount for prescription fees and do not have to pay drug expenses. Furthermore, patients could be admitted to specialist hospitals through referrals from their GPs whenever hospitalization is needed or when the GPs are unable to manage their medical conditions. The hospitals inform GPs of patients' medical condition upon discharge, thereby allowing GPs to take over the rehabilitation process.

　　Users are free to register with another GP without notifying the original GP, and the health authorities will transfer their registration numbers to the new GP accordingly. GPs can reject patient registrations but must provide good reasons for doing so, and the health authorities must provide the necessary explanations to the patients within two days. Users residing temporarily in a new place can temporarily register with a local GP while keeping their registration with the original GP. Users who are traveling for a short period of time can choose to pay for healthcare services first, after which they can make a reimbursement claim to their respective local health authorities or other NHS organizations when they return home. This practice has further enhanced the "money following patients" policy, which is a health reform measure adopted in recent years for the convenience of patients.

7. Health Improvement Program　The health improvement program is a community health project that aims to improve healthcare equality, utilization, and quality through coordination and cooperation among local governments, community health organizations, and other government departments. The main measures adopted include the accomplishment of national health goals via healthcare regionalization and the signing of three-year service contracts, both of which have improved the responsiveness and standards of the health service system. In addition to healthcare institutions, the local governments, relevant government departments, and voluntary organizations are also required to assume prominent roles and duties in the healthcare industry.

8. Care Quality Commission   The Care Quality Commission (CQC) is the highest body of quality management for healthcare services in the UK and is fully responsible for improving the quality of healthcare services throughout the country. Each year, the CQC assesses the quality of all UK healthcare institutions (including CHS organizations) and releases the outcomes of this assessment to the public, thereby promoting the proactive quality improvement of CHS organizations and ensuring user access to high-quality CHS.

(2) GP Services

1. General practice   GPs are required to sign a contract with the General Practitioners Committee (GPC) to provide NHS-related services. The government has divided the UK into four types of regions in order to prevent uneven GP distribution.

1. *Designated regions.* Each existing GP has an average of more than 2,500 registrants. New GPs are free to open new practices and are given special allowances.
2. *Vacant regions.* New GPs are free to open new practices in regions with 2,200–2,500 registrants per GP.
3. *Intermediate regions* New practices must be reviewed prior to opening in regions with 1,800–2,000 registrants per GP.
4. *Restricted regions.* New GP practices must wait for vacancies in regions with fewer than 1,800 registrants per GP.

In 1982, England and Wales had 1% of GPs working in designated and 32% working in vacant regions. In addition, there were 525 intermediate regions and 155 restricted regions.

GPs tend to perceive metropolitan areas as poor residential and educational environments for their children. On the other hand, their workloads tend to be heavy due to the high healthcare demand in these areas. Therefore, only a few GPs are willing to open new practices in metropolitan areas, while existing GPs in those areas are aging.

Hence, the government released a green paper on GP reform entitled "Primary Health Care" in April 1986, which proposed a three- to five-year short-term contract that offered GPs higher remuneration if they set up practices in metropolitan areas, in order to promote the establishment of new GP practices in those areas.

Each GP may accept up to 3,500 registrants and serve as their family physician. GPs may accept up to 4,500 registrants if they have partnered with other GPs. In 1995, there was an average of 2,147 registrants per GP in England and Wales.

2. Operation of General Practice
1. *24-hour service.* GPs work under the principle of 24-hour service, but each GP performs 60–200 consultations with 20–30 visits weekly. Over 60% of GPs spend an average of more than 60 hours per week on the provision of healthcare services.

A substitute GP might be appointed at nighttime or when the original GP is on vacation. There are currently about 60 agencies that specialize in the substitution of GPs throughout the UK. However, substitute GPs from these agencies can lead to numerous issues with respect to the quality of healthcare services due to their lack of information on the routine health status of the users.

2. *GP team.* The majority of GPs worked alone when the NHS was first established. However, general practices with two or more GPs had some advantages, such as being able to discuss their treatments and support each other during nighttime or vacation. Furthermore, they can share various resources, such as facilities and assistants. Therefore, GPs are encouraged to provide team-based care services. The increasing trend in GP team-based care services is shown in Table 11.4.

   Community health centers are being integrated as venues for team-based care. In the UK, there were 1,385 community health centers in 1982 and 1,572 centers in 2003, where one-fifth of all GPs served patients.

   There are other healthcare workers who work in community health centers, including health visitors, district nurses, midwives, social workers, and clerks. They work in cooperation with GPs and engage in the management of residents' health. Community health centers also serve as venues for various regional health-related activities (except for environmental health), such as medical consultation, vaccination, maternal classrooms, and mental health facilities, as well as healthcare services such as elderly care and health guidance, ophthalmology, dentistry, and otolaryngology.

3. *GP tasks.* GPs are responsible for managing the routine health of users and the capitation-based expenditure on healthcare workers. UK users who feel unwell seek medical attention from their GPs, who are responsible for providing healthcare guidance, including the necessity of inpatient treatment and the use and management of healthcare funds. Therefore, GPs are also known as "gatekeepers" of healthcare expenditure for users. This gatekeeper system is a core element of GPs' tasks in the UK and is one of the keys to the success of the NHS.

GPs issue prescriptions that patients can use to retrieve drugs at pharmacies. However, GPs can also prescribe and dispense drugs to patients in remote areas or for drugs that are not readily available at pharmacies.

GPs engage in a wide range of health management for users, such as medical consultation, vaccination, and health counseling. The healthcare expenditures incurred by GPs

TABLE 11.4   Changes in GP Team-Based Care Services in the UK (1970–2000)

Year	Alone (10,000)	Team-Based Care (10,000)					Total (10,000)
		2 GPs	3 GPs	4 GPs	5 GPs	6 GPs	
1970	5,037	5,970	6,081	3,748	1,631	1,230	23,697
1975	4,362	5,344	6,264	4,584	2,489	2,148	25,191
1980	3,729	4,941	6,442	5,291	3,345	3,159	26,907
1985	3,325	3,461	6,632	5,571	5,427	4,376	27,792
1990	3,307	3,452	6,637	5,683	5,445	4,621	29,045
1995	3,254	3,393	6,623	5,599	5,471	4,884	29,224
2000	3,101	3,276	6,638	6,626	5,492	5,291	30,424

are sometimes much lower than hospitals, which has prompted the UK health authorities to promote CHS and GP systems. The total number of cases handled by GPs has reached an average of four services per year per UK resident.

3. User Registration　Users can register with their preferred GPs, but GPs reserve the right to refuse additional registrations when there is an overload of registrants. The GPC might intervene to help patients who cannot find a GP. Parents can register with a preferred GP on behalf of children under 16 years of age. In addition, GPs must issue a notice one week prior to canceling the registration of any enrolled registrant.

Registration with GPs is permanent. Patients who wish to change their GPs must send their registration cards to the GPC, which will implement the change after two weeks.

Previously, anyone who lived in the UK was eligible to register with a GP. However, since the introduction of the NHS charges for foreigners in October 1982, and based on a notice issued by the Department of Health in May 1984 to the GPC, the GP registration of foreigners who have resided in the UK for less than six months (with the exception of foreign employees and citizens of countries that have signed reciprocal healthcare agreements with the UK) will no longer be accepted, and they are subjected to healthcare charges.

It has been estimated that one in four UK citizens has not registered with a GP, and that 30% of existing registrants are either deceased or have migrated.

Among foreigners who fall ill while traveling to the UK, those who visit for a short period (less than three months) are considered "temporary residents," whereas those who stay for less than 24 hours are considered "emergency patients"; only the latter is eligible to receive GP services.

4. GP Remuneration　The Review Body on Doctors' and Dentists' Remuneration (DDRB) advises the DHSC on the standard remuneration for GPs. The standard remuneration for GPs is determined by first calculating GPs' average income (e.g., the average annual income in June 2000 was £29,418). Then, the deviation from the average income is calculated based on the number of registrants and the services provided by the GP. For example, the income of GPs who work alone and who serve 550 registrants is less than £10,000, whereas the income of GPs who work in a team and serve more than 3,000 registrants is more than £30,000.

Expenditure required for GP consultation can be reimbursed via the following methods: (1) direct reimbursement for the actual amount incurred (e.g., the amount required to pay substitute physicians, healthcare assistants, and rental fees of healthcare facilities), and (2) indirect reimbursement via various allowances (e.g., processing fees for vaccination, which include vaccination expenses and physician incomes). GP remuneration items can be divided into the following four categories: (1) remuneration based on the number of registrants; (2) various allowances (e.g., basic care allowance, team-based care bonus, overtime allowance); (3) service processing fees (vaccination, endometrial cytologic examination, maternity services, etc.); and (4) fixed expenditures (e.g., pharmaceutical charges).

The relationship of each item with GP income and reimbursement is as follows:

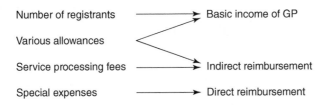

Number of registrants ⟶ Basic income of GP

Various allowances

Service processing fees ⟶ Indirect reimbursement

Special expenses ⟶ Direct reimbursement

In 2000, each GP earned an average of £58,908, of which £29,418 came from their basic income, £14,560 came from indirect reimbursements, and £15,200 came from direct reimbursements. A 2006 report noted that a British GP earned an average of £95,000 a year (52 weeks).

Under the current GP remuneration system, the number of registrants contributes a much greater share to their income, whereas high-quality services provided by GPs are not correctly reflected in their remuneration and instead may lead to economic problems due to their higher costs. Therefore, a green paper was issued to reform the remuneration system of GPs by introducing a policy of "medical allowance for good-quality services." According to this policy, allowances are determined according to the implementation of certain services (e.g., medical consultation service, healthcare services, and vaccination) as well as postgraduate medical education. In addition, the GP contract implemented in 2005 introduced performance standards and established the Quality and Outcomes Framework (QOF) to link payment schemes directly to the quality of healthcare services. The theoretical basis of this system has since become the "new favorite" of payment schemes worldwide – namely, pay-for-performance (PFP). The QOF has revolutionized the payment schemes for physicians by establishing a direct relation between performance and income, in order to improve the quality and maximize the cost-effectiveness of healthcare services.

5. GP Training   The Royal Society of Medicine defines a GP as a licensed medical graduate who offers comprehensive healthcare services to various types of patients at their clinic or patients' homes. GPs combine physiological, psychological, and social factors when making a diagnosis and providing preliminary treatments. Additionally, GPs seek to improve the health status of patients and their families through therapeutic and preventive care, as well as health education.

British medical education typically takes five years, and medical students are awarded a Bachelor of Medicine, Bachelor of Surgery (MBBS) upon graduation and passing an examination. General practice education is a type of postgraduate education, and medical graduates who wish to become GPs must complete another three years of training. They must serve as resident physicians in the first year of training, while in their second year, they undergo training at a GP training base and become a trainee GP at a healthcare center. Finally, in their third year, they continue their training at hospitals or community healthcare centers. The clinical training covers a range of fields, including general medicine, geriatrics, pediatrics, psychiatry, emergency medicine, general surgery, obstetrics and gynecology, and so on. Trainees can focus on certain fields depending on their interest. The content of GP training includes the management of acute, chronic, rehabilitative, and terminal patients, preventive care and health promotion, continuity of care for patients and their families, and the knowledge and skills required for teamwork and coordination with other community healthcare workers.

In addition to the aforementioned training programs, medical graduates can also obtain GP certificates through sabbatical training, which is designed to provide physicians with more opportunities to become GPs. The participating physicians must have rich clinical experience, undergo an interview, and accumulate at least six months of sabbatical training. Regardless of the training approach, physicians must pass a qualifying examination to acquire a GP certificate and register as a member of The Royal College of General Practitioners (RCGP) before they can start their own general practice.

The GP qualifying examination is a comprehensive examination that includes multiple-choice questions, medical record writing, special reports, and practical skills. The examination covers the knowledge and skills of clinical medicine, communication skills, and comprehensive analytical capabilities that are required for general practice.

The funding for GP training is provided by the Department of Health, and medical graduates who undertake GP training are treated similarly to resident physicians.

The number of GPs in the UK has increased rapidly over the last few decades, rising from 29,220 GPs in 1980 to 34,051 GPs in 1990, 37,981 GPs in 2000, and 49,184 GPs in 2009, with an average of 29.83 GPs per 1,000 people.

Despite the central role of GPs in CHS, other healthcare workers that work closely with GPs, such as health visitors, district nurses, midwives, and school nurses, are also equally important in CHS.

(3) Other Healthcare Technicians

1. Health Visitors　Health visitors, like district nurses and midwives, are affiliated with District Health Authorities. They are responsible for visiting the elderly and families with disabled individuals (children) to understand and provide recommendations about health issues. When necessary, they also contact GPs, hospitals, and the social welfare departments of local governments.

A licensed nurse must complete a three- to six-month midwifery course and a one-year health visitor course, followed by passing the licensure examination, in order to become a health visitor. Additionally, licensed health visitors must receive continuing education every four to five years. There are approximately 9,800 health visitors, who perform around 3.82 million visits annually.

2. District Nurses　District nurses are responsible for visiting the elderly and families with disabled individuals to assist them in body cleansing, bathing, changing bed sheets, changing wound dressings, injections, drug administration, blood and urine tests, and so on.

A licensed nurse must complete a three- to four-month field training program and pass the licensure examination in order to become a district nurse.

In the UK, there are approximately 13,000 district nurses, who make around 3.42 million visits each year.

3. Community Midwives　Community midwives are responsible for performing home births, as well as providing prenatal and postnatal guidance and care. A registered nurse must complete 18 months of practical training to become a licensed midwife. There are approximately 2,800 midwives providing CHS in England.

4.Community Physicians　The Royal Commission on Medical Education Report (also known as the Todd Report) released in 1968 advocated for the development of physicians who are specialized in community-based preventive services rather than personal health issues. In response to this report, the community physician (public health physician) system was introduced in 1974.

Community physicians are public health physicians (who receive the same treatment as hospital consultants) who serve as officials of District Health Authorities or are employed by District Health Authorities to lead or direct community health activities.

Community physicians are responsible for providing recommendations, from a medical perspective, on the analysis of healthcare needs and services, as well as environmental health, social welfare, residence, and education in the areas within their jurisdiction. Furthermore, they are also responsible for communicating and coordinating with relevant agencies and for conducting investigations and research. However, administrative affairs account for about 60% of their jobs.

In order to become a licensed community physician, a physician must register with the GMC, complete practical training, and pass an examination. Currently, there are only about 500 community physicians in England and Wales.

5. Hospital Services

The NHS Act 1977 defined hospitals as facilities that provide patients with hospitalization, diagnosis and treatment, fertility services, rehabilitation, and other healthcare services; often, their premises consist of medical facilities, dispensaries, and outpatient departments. Hospitals have no formal legal classifications. In the UK, only a handful of private hospitals are not affiliated with the NHS. With the exception of the section on private healthcare institutions, the remaining discussion below pertains to NHS hospitals.

Patients must make an appointment through their GPs to receive treatment at NHS hospitals, except for emergencies. Hospital physicians are responsible for visiting and treating patients who cannot be transferred to hospitals for medical reasons.

(1) Inpatient Services

The average length of hospital stay has decreased significantly over the past few decades, from 30 days in 1965 to 18 days in 1981, 11 days in 2002, and 6.8 days in 2009. This is especially true in geriatric departments, which decreased from 128 days to 52 days over that same period. Apart from factors such as the improvement of medical technologies, this reduction in hospital stay can be attributed to a government policy stipulating that community healthcare should be prioritized over inpatient treatment. This policy aimed to prioritize elderly individuals with mental illness and individuals with physical and mental disabilities, thereby ensuring that they can lead a normal life at home while also receiving treatment. Naturally, this policy requires the support of numerous primary healthcare workers, such as GPs, district nurses, and health visitors, as well as social workers affiliated with local public bodies. The policy also requires cross-sectoral collaborations between primary healthcare workers and social workers. Therefore, its implementation requires the NHS budget to be used for the improvement of social welfare.

Despite the decline in the number of hospital beds, the delivery of inpatient services has become more efficient with the reduced length of hospital stay. The number of discharged patients (including deaths) increased significantly from 3.7 million in 1951 to 5.01 million in 1961, 6.44 million in 1971, 7.18 million in 1982, and 15.94 million in 2002. Concurrently, the number of hospital beds decreased to 206,000 beds with an average of 3.4 beds per 1,000 people in 2008 (Table 11.5).

Waiting time is one of the most important issues related to hospitalization. The number of patients awaiting hospitalization in England tends to remain at around 600,000 patients; this figure peaked at 680,000 patients in 1978, and gradually declined thereafter. The waiting lists might vary across departments and regions, but surgical departments often

TABLE 11.5 Number of NHS Hospital Beds in the UK (1950–2008)

Year	Number of Available Beds (1,000 Beds)	Average Number of Hospital Beds per 1,000 People	Year	Number of Available Beds (×1,000)	Average Number of Hospital Beds per 1,000 People
1950	542	10.8	1990	453	8.1
1955	561	11.0	1995	486	8.3
1960	559	10.7	2000	481	8.2
1965	551	10.2	2002	236	3.98
1970	536	9.7	2004	231	3.87
1975	497	8.9	2006	216	3.61
1980	458	8.2	2008	206	3.4
1985	449	8.0			

have the longest waiting lists. In general, the waiting time for hernia surgery is 15–20 weeks, vascular tumor surgery is 20–25 weeks, and tonsil hypertrophy surgery is 10–23 weeks.

Nevertheless, the adequacy of the hospital supply system should not be assessed based on the length of the waiting list. In fact, nonacute patients accounted for 90% of patients on waiting lists, which also include patients who have been treated in other hospitals. Since July 1986, the UK government has implemented a policy to shorten waiting lists. Some of the most important measures adopted as a result of this policy include improving the efficiency of public hospitals and purchasing services from private hospitals. An assessment in 2002 showed that this policy has achieved excellent outcomes but has still not solved the fundamental problem.

(2) Outpatient Services

There is an increasing trend in the number of outpatient visits at hospitals (excluding visits to community GPs). Due to policies encouraging a shift from inpatient to outpatient care, the number of new outpatient cases increased from 1.37 million in 1954 to 2.12 million in 1981 and 7.23 million in 2002. However, the increasing demand for outpatients at hospitals prolonged patient waiting times. Therefore, the government began to systematically reduce outpatient waiting times in 1986, as it did with the inpatient waiting list. An assessment in 2002 revealed consistencies in waiting times between outpatient and inpatient services.

(3) Day Hospitals

In the 1970s, a day hospital model was proposed. Day hospitals are defined as hospitals where patients receive treatment during the day and return home at night, which compensated for the shortcomings of home-based care compared to inpatient care. These hospitals mainly targeted the elderly and individuals with physical and mental disabilities. This model is currently being implemented as a policy. An ambulance service is typically used to transport patients between their homes and hospitals.

(4) Hospital Staff

In 1951, there were 410,000 hospital staff; by 2002, this figure had increased by more than threefold to 1.55 million. Although there has been an increase in the number of personnel in several professions over this period, the number of management and assistant personnel has decreased due to recent policies to prioritize professions that are directly involved with patients.

In general, hospital physicians must receive five to six years of education at a medical school and undergo one year of clinical training as house officers before they can register with the General Medical Council (GMC) as independent physicians. Subsequently, these physicians will need to serve as senior house officers for one to two years, registrars for two to three years and senior registrars for four to five years before they can be promoted as associate specialists and consultants.

Due to the aging of hospital physicians, their demographic structure resembles an inverted pyramid, whereby consultants account for 37% of the physician population, senior house officers account for 28%, and registrars account for 17%. This demographic structure hinders the preferment of physicians at lower levels, leading to numerous issues, such as lower work motivation and work overload among physicians.

(5) Regional Planning of Hospitals

Areas with a population of about 200,000 people generally have hospitals with 800 beds that are equipped with internal medicine, surgery, pediatric, geriatric, and psychiatric departments. Other specialist hospitals, such as ophthalmology and neurology hospitals, may also be established according to local demand.

Although the hospital development plan has not been fully implemented, the modernization of hospital facilities is still ongoing. Despite the persistence of district general hospitals, the government proposed policies emphasizing community hospitals as early as 1974. Community hospitals are small-sized, lightly-equipped hospitals with 50–150 beds that serve as bridges between general hospitals and GPs, and are typically established in residential areas. It is expected that community hospitals will also be able to assume the role of general practices, especially for elderly care, chronic diseases, rehabilitation after discharge from large hospitals, and minor surgeries.

(6) Private Healthcare Institutions

The vast majority of healthcare services in the UK are delivered by the NHS, but there is still a small number of private healthcare institutions and nursing homes, providing a total of 34,000 beds. The construction of private hospitals must align with the NHS Act 1976, which stipulates that the establishment of a private hospital with more than 20 beds or in designated regions must be approved by the Secretary of State for Health to ensure that it will not adversely impact the NHS. Nuffield Health Leeds Hospital is currently the largest private hospital in the UK, with around 100 beds. It is situated near the largest public hospital – St. James Hospital, which has nearly 1,800 beds.

Healthcare services at private healthcare institutions are entirely paid for by patients, with an exception of services purchased by the NHS to reduce the waiting time for NHS services.

The existence of private hospitals in the UK is attributed to the following reasons.

1. Dissatisfaction with the NHS   Under the NHS, users often have to wait a long time before they can be admitted to hospitals. Additionally, they are typically unable to make appointments at their own convenience, even for outpatient services. Moreover, worn-out NHS facilities can also lead to dissatisfaction among inpatients. Therefore, some users prefer to seek medical attention at private hospitals at their own expense.

2. Presence of Private Health Insurance Private health insurance companies are nonprofit organizations that can share the financial burden of patients seeking medical attention at private healthcare institutions, among which Bupa, AXA PPP Healthcare, and WPA Healthcare are the most representative companies in the UK. There is an increasing trend in the number of individuals with private health insurance. In 1982, there were 4.18 million insured persons across these three companies, which doubled to 8.26 million in 2002. Another factor supporting the growth of private health insurance is the fact that many enterprises are now paying insurance premiums as a benefit for their employees, which has led to a gradual increase in their participation. At present, BUPA has more than four million insured persons and provides health insurance services for more than 40,000 enterprises in 190 countries and regions worldwide.

The premiership of Margaret Thatcher introduced policies that promoted healthcare privatization, which is consistent with the basic philosophy of the Conservative Party – that is, reducing the administrative scope of the government and maximizing the involvement of civil society. Furthermore, the demand for the NHS can be partially transferred to private healthcare institutions, thereby stimulating NHS services through the high-quality resources and services provided by such institutions.

There are two approaches to promoting this healthcare privatization policy: (1) private health insurance companies are given tax concessions, and the insurance premiums of employees are treated as business expenses; (2) cooperation with the NHS is enhanced via the purchase of services. For example, NHS patients can be transferred to private hospitals whenever surplus beds and equipment are available in order to reduce the waiting time at NHS hospitals, while also expanding the scope and methods of NHS funding.

6. Other Healthcare Services

(1) Pharmaceutical Services

Drugs can sometimes be dispensed by GPs in remote areas, but in general, patients must retrieve drugs at NHS-contracted pharmacies using prescriptions issued by GPs.

The remuneration for pharmacists is paid by the GPC according to the prescriptions submitted to the Accounting Office of the DHSC for review.

Pharmacists' remuneration is calculated by subtracting the average allowable discount (usually a percentage) for wholesalers from the wholesale prices of drugs. The resulting amount is marked up with the average processing fee for each drug (£1.5 in 2002) and an additional cost equivalent to the pharmacist's profits. This additional cost is calculated as 23% of the wholesale price if there are 249 or fewer dispensed items per month and 8.4% of the wholesale price if there are 5000 or more dispensed items per month, with more than 80 intermediate grades between these two values. In addition, the basic operating allowance (usually £3,500), services provided beyond normal business hours, oxygen mask services, and training of pharmacist trainees must be included and paid based on their performances.

In order to prevent pharmacy overcrowding in metropolitan areas, the government stipulates that pharmacies that begin a contract with the NHS after July 1980 are not entitled to the basic operating allowance if there are other pharmacies within a kilometer radius.

The number of NHS-contracted pharmacists in 2002 was 13,884 and that in 2010 was 39,715.

(2) Dental Services

The NHS stipulates that users must make an appointment with NHS-contracted dentists to access dental services. Unlike for GPs, users seeking dental services are free to choose their preferred NHS-contracted dentists without prior registration. However, dentists may also refuse to provide treatment in exceptional circumstances. A list of dentists is made available in most post offices, libraries, community health associations, public advisory councils, and the GPC. Users who receive treatment must show the dentists their NHS registration number and sign the necessary dental service bills.

NHS-contracted dentists are required to obtain prior approval from the General Dental Practice Committee for gold dentures or fillings, more than two dental crowns, and large-scale, long-term treatments. In addition, high-priced treatments beyond what is medically necessary also require prior approval from the General Dental Practice Committee and are only permitted when users can bear the additional costs.

Patients can seek treatment from the dental department at hospitals if they require highly technical dental services. NHS-contracted dentists can also perform special self-paid dental services. As dentists have a propensity to prioritize these highly profitable self-paid dental services, it can sometimes be difficult to find a dentist who is willing to provide dental services covered by the NHS.

In view of this, the government released a green paper in April 1986 proposing the reform of general practice, which mandated a minimum period that an NHS-contracted dentist must spend providing NHS-covered services. The green paper further stipulated that the GPC must assist users who are unable to find an NHS-contracted dentist.

The NHS remuneration for dentists is based on a fee-for-service system. Dental services are classified into 150 service items, each of which has a clear fee standard. The fee schedule is determined using a coefficient for each item, which is based on the overall pretax income and invested capital of the dentist. The deserved income standard for dentists is determined by the DHSC based on the recommendations of the Royal Commission on Doctors' and Dentists' Remuneration. The annual income standard for dentists in June 2002 was £38,765, but it was reported that the actual annual income of dentists in 2006 was 1.2 times that of the standard, or £44,860.

NHS payments to dentists in 2002 were analyzed according to operating costs and dentist income. (1) For operating costs, the percentages were as follows: salaries for assistants, 21%; dental consumables, 11%; inspection costs, 8%; facility maintenance, 7%; and others, 13%. (2) For dentist income, the percentage was 40%.

The dental fees of dentists are paid by the GPC according to dental bills submitted to the General Dental Practice Committee for review.

In 1983, there were 16,010 NHS-contracted dentists in the UK, with an average of 28.4 dentists per 100,000 people. This figure has shown an increasing trend, as by 2002, there were 19,584 dentists with an average of 32.1 dentists per 100,000 people, and in 2010, there were 22,799 dentists with an average of 37.0 dentists per 100,000 people. Although the UK has a sufficient number of dentists, many of them are older in age. Hence, the aforementioned green paper also proposed the introduction of the same retirement system for dentists as for GPs.

(3) Ophthalmic Services

Users who experience problems with their eyes usually contact their GPs, who then refer them to hospitals or ophthalmologists. Cataracts or other eye diseases are treated in the ophthalmology department of a hospital.

Ophthalmologists are physicians trained to perform eye examinations (optometry) and prescribe spectacles to customers. Spectacles are fabricated by optometrists or spectacle manufacturers. Optometrists can also perform eye examinations for their customers. In 2002, there were 1,236 ophthalmologists, 6,478 optometrists, and 2,631 spectacle manufacturers in the UK. The remuneration of ophthalmologists or optometrists is paid by the GPC according to their performance.

The NHS used to provide free eye examinations and optician services, but the majority of users preferred to purchase spectacles at their own expense over the unattractive spectacles supplied by the NHS. Therefore, free spectacles were abolished in April 1985, except for low-income earners and children. Policies for low-income earners are likely to be further reformed and made more humane by providing more options using a coupon system instead of benefits in kind.

7. Settlement of Medical Disputes

(1) Regulatory System for Healthcare Services

1. Three Stages of Regulatory Reforms for Healthcare Services in the UK

1. *The rise of regulation (1990–1997).* During this period, the main government supervisory agency was the Health Advisory Service (HAS), which was established by the DHSC in 1969 and was responsible for the professional regulation of healthcare services. The HAS is accountable to the DHSC, and the head of the HAS is appointed by the Principal Secretary of State for Health and Social Care. The budget and funding of the HAS are from the DHSC, but it still has a certain degree of independence, primarily to maintain and improve the administrative and organizational levels of healthcare institutions (especially sanatoria and psychiatric hospitals), as well as to examine issues in long-term care institutions (sanatoria and psychiatric hospitals). The Audit Commission and National Audit Office (NAO) play important roles in the financial supervision of healthcare institutions. The Health Service Ombudsman receives complaints about the NHS not only from members of parliament (MPs) but also directly from the public. Local inspection offices perform similar functions under the supervision of local authorities.

    In addition to the governmental regulatory agencies, some NGOs in the UK are also involved in supervising NHS agencies, including the Academy of Medical Royal Colleges, which primarily monitors medical education and training. In 1995, the UK launched the Clinical Negligence Scheme for Trusts, which is run by the NHS Litigation Authority to monitor the management risks of NHS agencies.

2. *Regulatory expansion (1997–2002).* In the "New Labour" era beginning in 1997, the government adopted an internal market approach, which sought to improve the quality of the NHS through competitive mechanisms. The government established two new regulators: the National Institute for Health and Care Excellence (NICE), which provides national guidance on clinical practice and technical assessments; and the Health Promotion Council, which monitors NHS agencies. Additionally, the government also established three new regulatory agencies: the National Clinical Assessment Service (NCAS), the National Patient Safety Agency (NPSA), and the NHS Modernization Agency.

3. *New regulatory reforms (2002 to the present).* In April 2002, the DHSC announced a comprehensive regulatory reform program, which involves the separation between the regulation of healthcare and social care. Two new super-regulators were established as part of this reform: the Commission for Healthcare Audit and Inspection and the Commission for Social Care Inspection. In addition, the Health Promotion Council, the

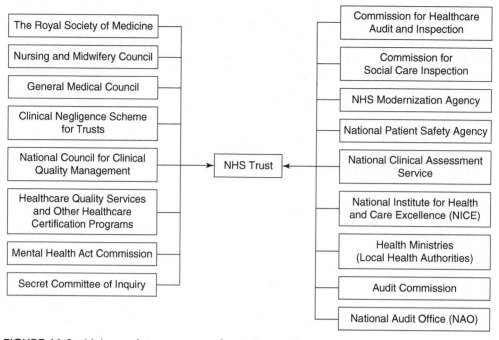

FIGURE 11.8 Main regulatory agencies for NHS agencies.

National Care Standards Commission, and the Health Service Ombudsman were abolished, while the size and jurisdiction of the Audit Commission were greatly reduced, such that it provided only financial and performance audits for local governments.

2. Current Regulatory Status of Healthcare Services in the UK The existing regulators of healthcare services in the UK can be divided into two categories as shown in Figure 11.8: Government regulators (right) and nongovernment regulators (left).

(1) Government regulators
1. *Industry regulators.* The UK DHSC assumes the role of the central government in dealing with issues related to healthcare and public health, as well as coordinating and monitoring local healthcare services in England and Wales. The specific roles of the DHSC include: (1) clearly defining the direction of development for healthcare and social care services; (2) establishing standards for healthcare and social care services and monitoring their implementation; (3) ensuring the availability of necessary resources in the NHS and social care organizations; and (4) ensuring that patients and the public are able to choose their healthcare and social care services.

   The primary industry regulator – the Commission for Healthcare Audit and Inspection – has taken over all the roles that were previously filled by the Health Promotion Council. These include reviewing the quality of healthcare management in NHS agencies, conducting in-depth investigations on serious issues related to the NHS and performing nationwide reviews of healthcare services, and providing advice and guidance to NHS agencies on healthcare management. In addition, it is also responsible for the regulation of private healthcare services (National Care Standards Commission), performance auditing (NHS Audit Commission), and some previous duties of the DHSC (e.g., providing statistics and ratings on the performance assessment of healthcare services).

The responsibilities of the Commission for Social Care Inspection are as follows: regulation of private social care (National Health Standards Committee); previous responsibilities of the Health Service Ombudsman; performance audits of social care (Audit Commission); and statistical analysis on performance assessments and ratings (DHSC and Audit Commission).

The responsibilities of the NICE are as follows: assessing existing and emerging medical technologies; guiding the rational use of these medical technologies at NHS agencies by patients and physicians; and recommending clinical guidelines for key health areas and patient groups.

The NHS Modernization Agency is not an independent agency but is affiliated with the DHSC. Its main objective is to comprehensively improve the healthcare quality of the NHS. Therefore, it has a wide range of authorities, and there are often no intrinsic ties between its regulatory activities.

(2) Financial regulators

The Audit Commission and the National Audit Office (NAO) play important roles in the financial supervision of healthcare institutions. The responsibilities of both agencies include approving the accounts of public healthcare institutions, inspecting the implementation of financial norms and standards, imposing penalties for the violation of financial rules and fraudulent behaviors, and examining the efficient and effective use of public funds in NHS agencies. It is worth mentioning that the financial regulation of NHS agencies only constitutes a small part of the regulatory purview of these agencies. In fact, both are responsible for the financial auditing of all public agencies.

The NAO was established in 1983 to ensure that public funds are spent in accordance with the intentions of the British Parliament, thereby enhancing financial control over the government and public agencies, as well as improving the efficiency of public resource utilization. The NAO is responsible for financial and performance assessments of all government departments and agencies. In the healthcare industry, the NAO is primarily associated with the DHSC. The Audit Commission is a public agency that is not affiliated with any government ministry. It was founded in 1983 through legislation and is run by a council consisting of members that are jointly appointed by the Principal Secretary of State for Health and Social Care and the Principal Secretary of State for the Environment, Food and Rural Affairs. The objectives of the Audit Commission include improving the management of public funds, promoting the improvement of public services, and assisting local authorities and the NHS in the provision of cost-effective and efficient public services.

(3) Nongovernment regulators

Besides government regulators, there are several nongovernment regulators in the UK that supervise NHS agencies, including the Royal Society of Medicine (RSM), Clinical Negligence Scheme for Trusts (CNST), and National External Quality Assurance Services (NEQAS). These regulators have neither formal statutory authority to monitor NHS agencies nor the authority to request NHS agencies to cooperate with their investigations and meet their requirements. However, they do have a certain degree of informal authority. For example, NHS agencies will not be able to recruit junior physicians if the RSM withdraws their medical training accreditation, which would affect their delivery of healthcare services.

The RSM is primarily responsible for regulating the education and training of junior physicians. It has established the accreditation process for physician training of NHS agencies, and the accreditation standard is revised every five years by its members and senior physicians. The RSM will withdraw its accreditation of NHS agencies if they fail to meet the accreditation criteria for physician training.

The CNST is operated by the NHS Litigation Authority and mainly regulates the management risks of NHS agencies. It has established a certification mechanism for risk management and a series of risk management standards. NHS agencies that comply with these standards bear lower costs in medical litigations.

The NEQAS is responsible for conducting external quality assessments on the services provided by NHS pathology laboratories. It examines the performance of these laboratories by testing a series of control samples.

Clinical Pathology Accreditation (CPA) is a program founded by the Royal College of Pathologists to regulate pathology services, which has established a series of accreditation standards and investigation procedures. The participation of pathology laboratories in this accreditation is voluntary, but a pathology laboratory must be accredited in order to participate in the national pathology program.

The Healthcare Quality Service was founded in the 1980s by the Queen's Trust in order to regulate the NHS and private healthcare service providers. It is now an independent agency providing quality accreditation services to NHS agencies and private hospitals. The Secret Committee of Inquiry was established in 1987 to review and generate a general report on surgical quality via secret inquiries on postoperative mortality rates.

(2) Disputes Over Hospital Services

Broadly speaking, disputes over hospital services can be divided into medical disputes not directly related to professional behaviors, such as hospital operational efficiency, and medical disputes directly related to professional behaviors. The former is first presented to the person involved, but if the patient remains dissatisfied, the dispute is presented to the head of the respective hospitals. Finally, the issue is presented in writing within one year after the event to the Director-General of the District Health Authorities if patients remain dissatisfied.

The Director-General obtains the opinion of the person involved and issues a resolution response letter with the consent of that individual. If the resolution fails, the case is transferred to regional teams, which are responsible for the regional operation of healthcare services. Major cases are handled by the Director of District Health Authorities.

The handling of healthcare-related disputes by the Department of Health Administration can be divided into the following three stages.

1. Dissatisfaction with the professional behavior of a hospital physician must be presented to the physician concerned, who can respond to the patient through the District Health Authority.
2. In cases where the patient is dissatisfied with the physician's response, the complaint is made in writing to the Department of Health Administration of the District Health Authority, which issues comments after reviewing statements made by both the physician and patient. The Department of Health Administration can clarify the patient's doubts if the physician is found to have conducted appropriate medical care. However, ex-post services will be provided to minimize harm to the patients in the event medical malpractice is found.
3. If the complaint remains unresolved after the above stages, the health administration officer must entrust the case to two hospital consultants for investigation, one of whom

has to be a consultant from another hospital. The health administrative officer will reply to the complainant upon the receipt of the investigation report. A committee comprised of more reviewers will be established to address more complicated cases.

There are approximately 12,000 disputes related to hospital services in the UK each year.

(3) Disputes Over GP Services

Any disputes over GP services must be presented in writing within eight weeks after the event to the GPC instead of the British Medical Association (BMA).

First, the Director-General of the GPC will handle the dispute. However, if the case is complicated and cannot be resolved by the Director-General, it will be entrusted to a medical dispute resolution committee consisting of three physicians and four nonphysicians (one of whom must be a consultant). After considering opinions from both the complainee (GP) and the complainant (patient), the committee will generate an investigation report, based on which the GPC will come to one of the following conclusions.

1. The GP concerned did not commit any misconduct.
2. The GP concerned made minor mistakes that need not be considered a problem.
3. The GP concerned committed medical malpractice and shall be penalized by reducing the number of registrants.
4. It is recommended that the health authority issue a warning to the GP.
5. It is recommended that the health authority deduct the remuneration of the GP.
6. The GP concerned shall be disqualified while the case and opinions are submitted to the NHS Review Board for adjudication.

The investigation is conducted by the GPC in a nonpublic manner according to the requirements of the DHSC established in 1968.

There are approximately 800 disputes over GP services in the UK each year.

(4) Complaints Lodged to the Health Service Commissioner

The Health Service Commissioner (HSC), commonly known as the Health Service Ombudsman, was established in 1974 to handle all NHS-related complaints, including those concerning hospital operational services, emergency services, hospital meals, nursing services, and health administrative authorities.

There are 500–800 disputes in the UK each year. Complaints are lodged to competent health authorities and the HSC (if the complainant remains dissatisfied) within one year of the event. The following matters, however, do not fall within the jurisdiction of the HSC.

1. Matters related to medical judgment
2. Matters related to the professional behavior of GPs
3. Matters related to legal trials and litigations

(5) Complaints Lodged to the BMA

Users might request that the BMA penalize GPs and hospital physicians who have violated their professional ethics, including the following.

1. Medical negligence
2. Breach of patient privacy
3. Anesthetic drug abuse
4. Making false claims to patients and charging inappropriate fees

Complaints lodged to the BMA are investigated by the Medical Ethics Committee (MEC). These investigations take the form of formal lawsuits, and the BMA either issues a warning or revokes the concerned physician's medical license.

Physicians whose behavior is considered to have strongly influenced the health status of the complainant are subject to a one-year period of probation for investigation by the MEC.

No specific action is taken for cases that do not need to be handled by the MEC.

(6) Tasks of Community Health Councils

Community Health Councils (CHCs) represent the interests of users at the community level and deliver users' opinions to District Health Authorities in meetings held several times per year. District Health Authorities must also seek advice from CHCs in the case of policy changes.

CHCs take the side of users when receiving user complaints and introducing approaches and relevant policies in order to resolve disputes. In addition, CHCs provide support to users when lodging complaints to the GPC.

CHCs typically comprise 18–24 members, including representatives from local governments (1/2), voluntary organizations (1/3), and local health authorities (1/6).

8. NHS Reforms and Future Policies

(1) Outcomes of the NHS Plan 2000

There are numerous challenges facing the development of the NHS, such as insufficient funding, long waiting times for patients, relatively poor therapeutic outcomes for some major diseases compared to neighboring countries, human resource shortages, and worn-out facilities. Therefore, the UK government launched a major modernization program in 2000 to revitalize and reconstruct the NHS. Program funding has increased gradually by 5.8% each year since then, and the program has resulted in several remarkable outcomes.

The program mainly focuses on the following four aspects of reform: (1) Redesigning healthcare services to improve their efficiency. (2) Reforming the operating mechanisms of the health system, such that greater authority is delegated to local NHS agencies, while also introducing external competition and new economic incentives. (3) Restructuring the roles of employees, as well as improving their working conditions and remuneration. (4) Exploring new pathways of knowledge acquisition and the application of new science and technology.

This health reform also aimed to prioritize patients and local users by implementing the following four reform strategies: (1) Contract management reform – using funds to reward outstanding performers, in order to improve the incentive mechanism. (2) Demand-side reform – improving preventive care via enhanced accountability and providing diversified choices for patients. (3) Supply-side reform – improving provider diversity and providing users with a greater degree of freedom in service selection in order to achieve supply-side service innovation and improvement. (4) Management system reform – altering the management, supervision, and decision-making frameworks to better ensure safety, quality, equality, and efficiency of services.

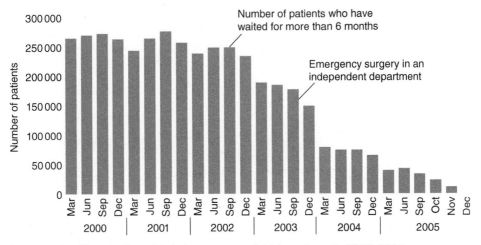

FIGURE 11.9 Changes in waiting times among British patients in 2002–2005.

The outcomes of the reform are as follows:

1. *Shorter waiting times.* Figure 11.9 shows that the number of patients who spent more than 6 months on the waiting list decreased from 250,000 patients in 2000 to fewer than 50,000 patients in 2005. As a result, more patients were able to have timely access to healthcare services, which improved the control of certain diseases.
2. *Significant improvements in emergency services.* Figure 11.10 shows that in 2003–2006, the percentage of patients admitted within four hours increased from approximately 80% in early 2003 to 98% at the end of 2006 – that is, 98% of emergency patients received treatment within four hours, which improved treatment delivery to patients.
3. *Lower mortality rates for major diseases.* Figure 11.11 shows that the mortality rates for coronary heart disease, tumors, and cerebrovascular disease in the UK population declined from 1992 to 2002, while the mortality rate for liver disease increased slightly over that same period.

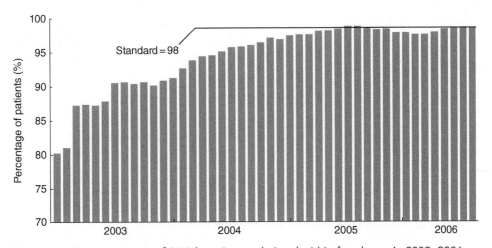

FIGURE 11.10 Percentage of British patients admitted within four hours in 2003–2006.

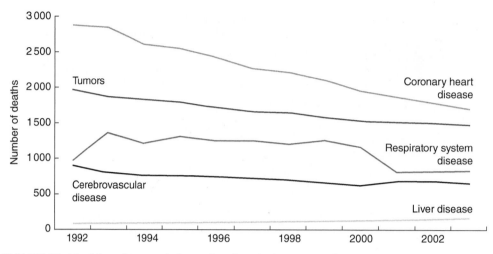

FIGURE 11.11 Mortality trends for major chronic diseases in the UK (1992–2002).

4. *Improved patient satisfaction.* Figure 11.12 shows that the degree of satisfaction among emergency patients, inpatients, outpatients, and GP patients increased each year from 2002 to 2006. The degree of satisfaction among inpatients showed a curved increase. In addition, the overall satisfaction with the NHS improved gradually over the same period.

(2) New NHS Act

In June 2008, the UK Secretary of State for Health, Lord Darzi, proposed a new NHS program known as "High Quality Care for All: NHS Next Stage Review." This program replaced the management by objectives (MBO) model with a model of quality management and laid out the development plan of the NHS over the following decade. Since the proposal of this program, patients' rating of healthcare institutions has become an important reference for public funding allocation.

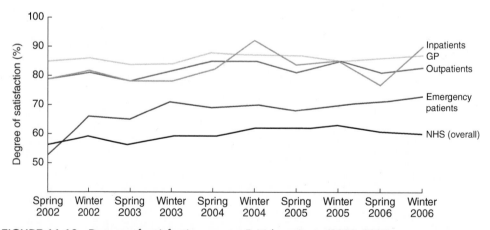

FIGURE 11.12 Degree of satisfaction among British patients (2002–2006).

The core elements of the new program are (1) patient-centered care, whereby patients are given more rights and control over their own health and treatment, and (2) quality management, which seeks to improve the quality of healthcare services.

1. Specific Measures for Ensuring Patient-Centered Care
1. Expand the choice of GPs available to the public.
2. Clearly outline the new right to choose in the new NHS Act.
3. Ensure that every UK citizen has a personal long-term healthcare service program.
4. Control personal health budgets (PHBs).

2. Specific Measures for Quality Management
1. Determine the basic scope of care.
2. Determine independent quality standards and clinical priorities.
3. Perform the first systematic survey of healthcare quality and publish the relevant information.
4. Use the assessments of patients' initial perceptions and satisfaction as the basis for budget allocation among hospitals.
5. Reward outstanding healthcare performance.
6. Facilitate information acquisition via a professional network among NHS healthcare workers to improve their service quality.
7. Take measures to ensure continuous improvement in the quality of primary and community healthcare services.
8. Analyze new tax systems in different regions and adopt those that encourage the improvement of service quality.

(3) White Paper for New Health Policy

In July 2010, the UK coalition government, consisting of the Conservative and Liberal Democrat parties, introduced a new health policy via a white paper that clearly outlined a five-year NHS development plan.

1. Main Reform Objectives
1. Prioritize the interest of patients (patient-centered care).
2. Improve healthcare outcomes.
3. Further increase the qualification requirements for healthcare workers and enhance their sense of responsibility.
4. Limit bureaucratic behaviors to improve the efficiency of healthcare services.

2. Main Reform Measures
1. Ensure that healthcare funds follow the patients and allow GPs to administer the fund.
2. Enhance patients' right to choose and influence care.
3. Reduce the number of inpatients to improve the efficiency of healthcare services.
4. Reduce administrative waste.
5. Focus on community healthcare and vulnerable groups.
6. Establish hospital-led partnerships in community health to overcome NHS monopoly.

SECTION II. THE HEALTH SYSTEM IN CANADA

Canada is located in the northernmost part of North America and is the second-largest country in the world by area (9,976,000 km²). As of 2013, its total population was 35,158,304, the vast majority of which are descendants of British and French immigrants. The country is divided into 10 provinces and two federal territories. The federal government has adopted the cabinet system. Canada is a Commonwealth country with a similar administrative system as the UK.

Data from the World Bank show that the average life expectancy of Canadians in 2012 was 81.2 years (79.1 years for men and 83.4 years for women). In 2013, the maternal mortality rate was 11 per 100,000 live births, and the infant mortality rate was 4.6 per 1,000 live births. The total healthcare expenditure in 2012 was US$ 198.5 billion, accounting for 10.9% of its GDP, and the healthcare expenditure per capita was US$ 5,740.70.

Canada has adopted a national healthcare system, whereby the government is not only the main provider of healthcare funds but also imposes strong regulation and control over healthcare services. Health Canada is the planning and administrative agency for the national healthcare service. The provincial health administrations have similar institutional settings to Health Canada. Their primary responsibilities include planning, organization, provision, financing, administration, and regulation of healthcare services, as well as conducting assessments of public healthcare services. In addition, they are also responsible for formulating various payment systems to regulate and control the growth of healthcare expenditure.

The Canadian national healthcare system (known as Medicare) is closely associated with the socialized health insurance system known as the "universal health insurance," and is structured around a framework of statutory rights granted to local authorities by the national constitution. Medicare is regarded as a national healthcare system because the provincial and community healthcare services and health insurance schemes were established in accordance with a state-regulated framework of healthcare principles. Each province and territory is responsible for providing and managing its own healthcare services.

Medicare stipulates that all Canadians have equal access to national healthcare and health security, regardless of their economic abilities. All Canadians need only pay a small amount of medical expenses to receive the necessary outpatient and inpatient services. Thus, Medicare has achieved a significant extent of healthcare equality, which guarantees the basic right to healthcare for all. Despite the continuous improvement in the equality and accessibility of healthcare services, health reform and development are still hampered by health disparities among different population groups, a rapid increase in healthcare expenditure, and an insufficient supply of healthcare services in remote and rural areas.

In order to further improve the equality and accessibility of healthcare services, Canada has developed five basic healthcare principles that govern its health reforms and health policymaking: (1) Uniformity of Public Administration: The state is responsible for the planning and administration of healthcare services on a nonprofit basis. (2) Comprehensiveness: The available services must include hospital services, primary care services, and community healthcare services. (3) Universality: All residents in the community must have equal access to healthcare services covered by health insurance. (4) Portability: Healthcare expenses incurred when the resident travels to another province or country can be reimbursed in accordance with the standards of the Canada Health Act (CHA). (5) Accessibility: Residents must have timely access to the necessary healthcare services without being affected by economic factors or other obstacles.

TABLE 11.6 Total Number of Registered Physicians in Canada in 2000–2009 (Excluding Resident Physicians) (Unit: Person)

Year	2000	2001	2002	2003	2004	2005	2006	2007	2008	2009
Total	57,806	58,546	59,412	59,454	60,612	61,622	62,307	62,307	65,440	68,101
GPs	29,113	29,627	30,258	30,662	31,094	31,633	31,989	32,598	33,712	34,793
Specialists	28,690	28,919	29,154	28,792	29,518	29,989	30,318	31,084	31,728	33,306

Source: Canadian Institute for Health Information (CIHI, 2011a).

1. Establishment and Development of the Health System

(1) Physician System

1. Historical Evolution   Canada has long adopted the provincial autonomous certification system for physicians. Thus, the origin, allocation, and licensure of physicians are administered independently by each provincial government. Since the establishment of the Medical Council of Canada in 1912, it has adopted a uniform standard for the physician qualifying examination. However, the medical qualification and licensure of physicians are determined by the individual provincial certification agencies rather than by the federal government.

The Royal Commission on Health Services (also known as the Hall Commission) established in 1961, put forth a proposal in 1965 to greatly enhance the training of physicians. Its recommendations mainly involved increasing the number of medical students enrolled in existing universities and establishing four new medical universities, with the goal of ensuring that the number of physicians per capita in the 1970s and 1980s was on track with a blueprint developed in 1961. The Hall Commission also recommended that the federal government establish the Health Resources Fund in 1966 in order to subsidize educational research institutes. In addition, the commission also encouraged the recruitment of foreign physicians.

These measures led to a rapid increase in the number of physicians in the late 1980s, which exceeded their initial expectations and has gradually resulted in a surplus of physicians. As a result, the government shifted from the previous intensive training policy to a suppression policy in the 1990s.

2. Current Qualification System for Physicians   Currently, there are 16 medical universities in Canada (5 of which are in Ontario) that provide four-year courses, as stipulated by the government. These medical universities were established by their respective provinces and receive subsidies from provincial funding. Students are recruited among graduates from other universities for the four-year medical course, which consists of basic medicine in the first two years and clinical education in the last two years. However, some of these universities also provide three-year courses consisting entirely of clinical education. Medical graduates must pass a qualifying examination held by the Medical Council of Canada before participating in their first year of residency in hospitals. To become a specialist, the medical graduate must then serve as a resident physician for four years and pass the qualifying examination of the Medical Council of Canada, before they can be approved by the respective

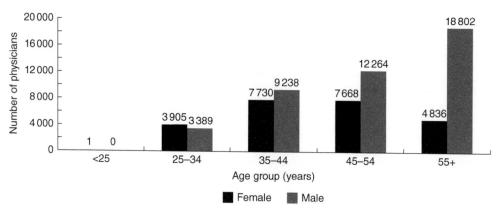

FIGURE 11.13   Gender and age composition of Canadian physicians in 2009.

provincial medical associations. The total number of registered physicians (excluding resident physicians) in Canada is shown in Table 11.6. The number of physicians per 100,000 people was 150 in 1979 and 201 in 2009. The difference in ratio between male and female physicians shows an increasing trend with age (Figure 11.13).

In Canada, a physician must meet the following criteria in order to become a family physician, medical specialist, or surgical specialist: (1) Obtain a Doctor of Medicine through accredited courses; (2) Complete an accredited residency program in family medicine, a surgical specialty, or another medical specialty; (3) Pass the qualifying examination held by the Royal College of Physicians and Surgeons of Canada or the College of Family Physicians of Canada; (4) Pass the first and second parts of the qualifying examination held by the Medical Council of Canada; (5) Register with their respective provincial regulatory agencies. Physicians certified by the Royal College of Physicians and Surgeons of Canada or the College of Family Physicians have portable medical licenses. They do not have nation-wide medical licenses but may apply for licensure in different provinces without additional examinations or training.

Physicians who have received their medical education overseas and wish to practice medicine in Canada must meet the following criteria: (1) Contact the respective provincial regulatory agencies for assessment and certification, which includes language proficiency and other criteria; (2) Submit their medical credentials to the Medical Council of Canada; (3) Pass the qualifying examination held by the Medical Council of Canada and complete an accredited residency program in family medicine or another medical specialty; (4) Pass the first and second parts of the qualifying examination held by the Medical Council of Canada; (5) Pass (in some cases) the qualifying examinations held by the Royal College of Physicians and Surgeons of Canada or the College of Family Physicians of Canada, in order to obtain a medical license from the respective regulatory agencies; (6) Register with and obtain a license from the respective provincial regulatory agencies. All provinces reserve the right to request additional qualifying assessments on physicians who apply to practice medicine or undergo residency in the province.

3. Current Status and Issues   In 2000, there were 61,134 physicians in Canada, among whom 25–30% were hospital physicians, while the remaining were private practitioners. Most received fee-for-service payments, and the amount was decided via negotiation

TABLE 11.7 Trends in the Population of Canadian Physicians in 1960–2000

Year	(1) Number of Immigrant Physicians	(2) Number of Canadian Medical Graduates	(1) + (2) Total	Percentage of Immigrant Physicians (%)	Percentage of Medical Graduates (%)
1960	445	839	1,284	34.7	65.3
1965	792	1,032	1,824	43.4	56.6
1970	1,113	1,108	2,221	50.1	49.9
1975	1,221	1,546	2,767	44.11	55.9
1980	1,302	1,747	3,049	42.7	57.3
1985	745	1,835	2,580	28.9	71.1
1990	326	1,853	2,179	15.0	85.0
1995	227	1,920	2,147	10.6	89.4
2000	231	1,976	2,207	10.5	89.5

between provincial governments and the respective medical associations. The average income of physicians in Canada is about four times that of the salaried class.

As for the supply of physicians, the number of medical universities and medical students increased as a result of the proposal of the Royal Commission on Health Services in 1965. Thereafter, the supply of physicians was reassessed and replanned as recommended by the Health Human Resource Strategy in 1987.

The Health Human Resource Strategy first proposed to restrict the recruitment of foreign physicians. Table 11.7 shows the annual increase in the number of physicians. Following the recommendations by the Hall Commission in 1965, there were 1,200–1,300 new foreign physicians annually, accounting for 42–50% of the total number of new physicians. However, the number of new foreign physicians fell to 231–326 physicians annually after 1990, accounting for only 10–15% of the total number of new physicians.

In 1990, the physician-to-population ratio was planned according to the recommendations made in 1987, as follows: (1) one GP per 2,300 people; (2) one internist per 8,200 people; (3) one neurologist per 90,000 people; and (4) one psychiatrist and general surgeon per 11,000 people.

In light of this plan, the Hall Commission generated a report on the Canadian national and provincial healthcare system in 1995, and proposed the establishment of the Federal/Provincial/Territorial Advisory Committee on Health Delivery and Human Resources in 1999, with the following recommendations: (1) Reduce the enrollment of medical degrees by 10% after 2000; (2) further enhance the restriction against the recruitment of foreign physicians; (3) reduce the training opportunities for specialists; and (4) encourage foreign physicians who are trained and interned in Canada to return to their home countries.

Over the past decade, each province has adopted and implemented policies in accordance with these recommendations. For example, Ontario reduced the training opportunities for specialists, while British Columbia not only reduced the training opportunities but also reduced the number of practicing physicians.

As for the uneven regional distribution of physicians, physician salaries have been adjusted as a countermeasure to address this issue. In other words, physicians residing in rural areas are given ample income security. This issue has also given rise to the opportunity to introduce a health insurance scheme. The authorities believe that the introduction of health insurance that ensures equal access to healthcare services for both low-income earners and wealthy individuals might better secure the income of physicians. This, in turn, could resolve the uneven distribution of physicians, especially in areas with an inadequate number of physicians.

Naturally, this measure alone is incapable of resolving this uneven distribution. Hence, each province has sought other solutions. In most cases, policies which provide subsidies to physicians serving in remote areas were introduced. However, Canada is still facing some challenges concerning the supply of physicians and healthcare services. On the one hand, the waiting time for medical consultations is too long. As the service fees of physicians are determined by the negotiation between medical associations and local governments, there is a lack of price competition mechanisms, which in turn has led to an insufficient supply of healthcare services, and hence a long waiting list. For instance, a patient might need to wait for one or two years for a surgical operation. On the other hand, Canada is also facing a shortage of physicians. The majority of physicians in Canada serve in private practice, which gives a greater degree of independence and a higher income level. These physicians do not have to accommodate more patients into their schedules in order to earn a living. For example, a hospital clinic in Montreal may claim to provide 24-hour service, but its actual service time may only be 12 hours. In order to reduce healthcare expenditure due to high operating costs, the government has drastically reduced expenditure on physician income (currently, the government must pay up to C$500,000 per physician annually), the number of employed physicians, and expenditure on physician service charges. Furthermore, the Canadian government has decided to reduce the enrollment of medical students, which has further aggravated the shortage of physicians. Currently, there are more than 1,200 vacancies in some provinces, such as Quebec, where up to one-third of the Medicare card holders are unable to access the contracted services. As a result, Quebec has become the most medically underserved region of Canada. Therefore, it is becoming increasingly difficult for disadvantaged groups, such as impoverished individuals, recent immigrants, and individuals with substance addictions, to access the healthcare system.

(2) Hospital System

1. Historical Evolution Provincial governments assume frontline responsibilities in the healthcare supply system, while the federal government is responsible only for indirect administration (except in certain designated hospitals). However, historically speaking, hospitals were not originally established by provincial governments. Hospitals in Canada have a long history of being established and administered by religious organizations, and their primary goal was to treat impoverished patients.

The development of the medical industry after World War I attracted increasing attention to inpatient treatments and the popularization of hospitals. In the 1930s, numerous hospitals, including tuberculosis sanatoria, psychiatric hospitals, and clinical facilities, were established in each province.

After World War II, the number of hospital beds increased significantly alongside the expansion of general hospitals and the major transformation of the hospital system. In particular, there was a substantial increase in the number of hospital beds in 1948–1960. This can be attributed to the National Health Grants Program (implemented in 1948 by the federal government), which subsidized the construction of almost all hospitals in each province.

Subsequently, in 1970, the federal subsidy scheme was suspended because the federal government considered that the further expansion of hospital construction was no longer needed. However, the federal government continued to use the Health Resources Fund to subsidize the continuing education and training of healthcare practitioners, as well as the expansion of research-based hospitals.

2. Current Status and Issues In 1999, there were 126 federal hospitals, 1,054 public hospitals, and 75 private hospitals. Of the 175,058 hospital beds in Canada, the aforementioned hospitals account for 4,895 (3%), 169,714 (94%), and 3,453 (2%) beds, respectively. Thus, public hospitals account for the vast majority of hospital beds. Most public hospitals are in fact operated by private institutions. However, according to the law, they must be open and available to all those who require medical attention.

Based on the aforementioned figures, in 1999, there was an average of six to seven beds in public hospitals per 1,000 people, half of which were hospitals for short-term treatment and surgery. Approximately one-fourth of the hospital beds were for long-term care. More than half of public general hospitals had less than 100 beds for long-term care to ensure the availability of hospital beds.

Federal hospitals include hospitals for special groups, such as veterans' hospitals and marine hospitals. Currently, there are only two veterans' hospitals left in Canada, while the rest have been sold to nonprofit organizations. Healthcare services for veterans are provided by Veterans Affairs Canada (VAC).

There are 62 teaching hospitals in Canada that are affiliated with medical universities. Many patients prefer to seek medical attention at these hospitals due to their advanced technologies and are willing to participate in medical education. Patients who seek medical attention at teaching hospitals may refuse to participate in medical education, but such patients would normally avoid teaching hospitals. Some, but not all, teaching hospitals run medical universities. However, like other hospitals, they still rely on health insurance for their income.

Canada has 18 rehabilitation hospitals, 132 hospitals for chronic or long-term care, and more than 300 acute general hospitals containing beds for long-term care. Many small-sized local hospitals have a higher proportion of long-term inpatients than large-sized urban hospitals.

The federal government subsidized the establishment of hospitals from 1948 to 1970. In order to obtain federal subsidies, a hospital had to obtain approval from the provincial government by meeting facility standards and highly technical regional healthcare planning standards (uneven distribution of facilities, which necessitates the sharing of some tasks across the region). The subsidy scheme resulted in the reconstruction and modernization of numerous hospitals throughout Canada within two decades. Many provinces expected a dramatic increase in healthcare demand when the general hospital insurance was first introduced, and hence constructed many emergency hospitals. This, however, became one of the major obstacles of regional healthcare planning. Nevertheless, by the 1970s, the provincial governments had taken control over health insurance and hence could effectively implement regional healthcare planning. Many provinces have successfully confined CT and MRI services to regional healthcare centers or tertiary referral hospitals. Some have noted that the efficiency of Canadian regional healthcare planning has facilitated the control of healthcare expenditure.

Provincial governments have established standards for the allocation of hospital facilities and human resources. Annual financial assessments are performed on hospitals through the subsidy scheme for hospital construction, in order to ensure their compliance with these standards. In addition, provincial governments have encouraged hospitals to voluntarily seek accreditation from various agencies. One of the agencies established for this purpose is the Canadian Commission on Hospital Accreditation. It is evident that this form of autonomous hospital management is gaining increasing attention in Canada.

(3) Regulatory System of the Healthcare Industry

The general principles of industry regulation include the delegation of regulatory authority to various medical, accounting, engineering, and legal professions, and creating a system of industry self-regulation. Regulatory authority is delegated by provincial governments through the enactment of relevant laws, which include the scope of authority available to the regulators; for example, the Health Profession Act applicable to the healthcare industry. The regulators might establish subsidiary provisions under the regulatory act.

The mission of regulators is to serve and protect the public interest. They are responsible for ensuring that industry members fulfill all professional qualification criteria and comply with professional standards and ethics. For example, there are 25 self-regulated medical professions in British Columbia, each of which is regulated by one of 22 colleges (note that these are not government agencies), such as the College of Physicians and Surgeons of British Columbia, College of Dental Surgeons of British Columbia, College of Massage Therapists of British Columbia, College of Pharmacists of British Columbia, College of Psychologists of British Columbia, and the College of Traditional Chinese Medicine Practitioners and Acupuncturists of British Columbia. These colleges are authorized to establish standards for industry entry, practice standards, codes of professional conduct, and regulations for implementing the standards of practice (professional competence) and codes of behavior (professional conduct). These authorities are all codified in law. The colleges are funded by industry members via annual membership fees; members must pay these membership fees to maintain both their memberships and licenses. New members entering the industry have certain rights, such as the right to use professional titles and the right to practice. Otherwise, the above-mentioned rights cannot be exercised.

The regulatory procedures include determining the procedures for industry entry, investigating and resolving medical complaints, and permitting healthcare workers to appeal against a complaint decision. The College of Physicians and Surgeons of British Columbia, as an example, was founded in 1886 to regulate the licensure of physicians and surgeons in British Columbia. The college is authorized by the provincial government to establish, regulate, and enforce strict standards for professional certification and medical practice. In addition, the college itself realizes that self-regulation is a unique right and that its ultimate purpose is to serve the public interest. The college is run by a committee of 15 members, among whom 10 are peer-elected physicians while the remaining 5 are civil representatives appointed by the provincial health department. The college is responsible for establishing the professional qualification standards to which physicians and surgeons must adhere for licensure in British Columbia; ensuring physicians' compliance with the strict standards of practice and professional conduct; and handling public complaints against physicians and penalizing physicians who engage in misconduct. The college is also responsible for ensuring the compliance of healthcare facilities (e.g., private surgical clinics, laboratories, and imaging diagnostic centers) with established standards by implementing formal certification procedures; responding to public inquiries about policies, guidelines, patient care, medical records, and so on; and providing physicians with practice guidance at all levels, especially in terms of ethical codes, professional conduct, compliance with legal norms, and so on. In addition, the college collaborates with the government, universities, hospitals, and other organizations to address issues regarding the improvement of public access to healthcare services, improvement of healthcare quality, and the protection of patient privacy and medical records. In accordance with the requirements of the Health Professions Act, the college also handles public complaints and doubts, evaluates and communicates about ethical issues, and establishes and maintains

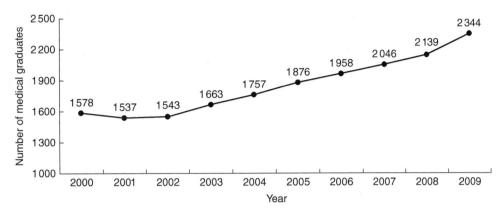

FIGURE 11.14   Number of medical graduates in Canada in 2000–2009. *Source:* The Association of Faculties of Medicine of Canada (AFMC), 2011.

stringent standards for physicians' professional ethics and performance. Based on the regulations stipulated by the provincial government, the college issues licenses to qualified and competent physicians, as well as coordinating quality assurance and facility improvements, in order to enforce and maintain stringent healthcare standards. It also adjudicates public complaints against medical misconduct by physicians. Complaints against physicians must be lodged in writing, and be accompanied by the complainant's address, telephone number, and signature. The college's inquiry committee reviews the documents relevant to the complaint and then communicates with the complainant and the physician concerned. Physicians found to have committed misconduct might be formally requested by the inquiry committee to improve their practice or take part in continuing education. If the physicians fail to meet the current professional standards or have violated the relevant codes of ethics and conduct, the college can lodge a complaint or recommend remedial action. Under certain exceptional circumstances, the college might implement formal disciplinary procedures to restrict or completely prohibit the physician concerned from continuing their practice. For this to occur, there must be sufficient evidence prior to the restriction or prohibition, which proves that the physician concerned has clearly engaged in misdiagnosis or misconduct, lacks the latest knowledge and skills, or has health issues that render them unsuitable to continue their practice. All evidence must be submitted to the Discipline Committee with the consent of the physician concerned. The physician can appeal to the court if they refuse to accept the verdict.

The role of the court in industry self-regulation relates to the college's use of its authority. The court ensures that the college does not overreach its authority and exercises its authority in an impartial manner. The court tends to respect the professionalism of self-regulatory bodies and consider that professional qualification, competence, and conduct are best judged and determined by industry regulators.

2. Healthcare Providers

(1) Education and Regulation of Healthcare Providers

Health education programs are available in every province of Canada. Most such programs have been accredited to ensure that they meet specific standards and are effective in preparing students for a future career in the healthcare industry. As shown in Figure 11.14, the number of medical graduates in Canada has increased over the past decade.

TABLE 11.8 Number of Health Education Programs in the Provinces and Territories of Canada in 2010

Profession	Newfoundland and Labrador	Prince Edward Island	Nova Scotia	New Brunswick	Quebec	Ontario	Man-itoba	Saskatchewan	Alberta	British Columbia	Yukon	Northwest Territories	Nunavut	Canada
Audiologists	0	0	1	0	1	2	0	0	0	1	0	0	0	5
Massage therapists	0	0	0	0	0	1	0	0	0	0	0	0	0	2
Dental hygienists	0	0	1	1	8	20	1	1	1	7	0	0	0	40
Dentists	0	0	1	0	3	2	1	1	1	1	0	0	0	10
Dietitians	0	1	3	1	3	4	1	1	1	1	0	0	0	16
Health information management specialists	1	0	1	1	4	6	1	1	1	1	0	0	0	17
Licensed practical nurses	2	2	3	4	42	22	4	2	8	16	1	0	1	107
Medical examiners	1	0	1	2	10	5	1	1	3	2	0	0	0	26
Medical physicists	0	0	0	0	1	2	1	0	2	2	0	0	0	8
Medical radiographer	1	1	1	4	4	10	2	2	3	1	0	0	0	29
Midwives	0	0	0	0	1	3	1	0	1	1	0	0	0	7
Nurse practitioners	1	1	1	2	6	10	1	2	3	4	0	1	0	32
Occupational therapists	0	0	1	0	5	5	1	0	1	1	0	0	0	14
Optometrists	0	0	0	0	1	1	0	0	0	0	0	0	0	2
Pharmacists	1	0	1	0	2	2	1	1	1	1	0	0	0	10
Physicians	1	0	1	0	4	6	1	1	2	1	0	0	0	17
Physiotherapists	0	0	1	0	4	5	1	1	1	1	0	0	0	14
Psychologists	0	0	1	1	4	9	1	2	2	3	0	0	0	23
Registered nurses	1	1	3	2	9	15	4	2	6	13	0	1	1	58
Registered psychiatric nurses	n/a	n/a	n/a	n/a	n/a	n/a	1	1	1	3	0	n/a	n/a	6
Respiratory therapists	1	0	1	2	7	6	1	0	2	1	0	0	0	21
Social workers	1	0	1	2	8	12	1	2	1	7	0	0	0	35
Speech-language pathologists	0	0	1	0	3	3	0	0	1	1	0	0	0	9

Source: Health Workforce Database (HWDB), CIHI, 2012.

TABLE 11.9 Regulatory Environments of Healthcare Professions in the Provinces and Territories of Canada in 2010

Profession	Newfoundland and Labrador	Prince Edward Island	Nova Scotia	New Brunswick	Quebec	Ontario	Mani-toba	Saskatchewan	Alberta	British Columbia	Yukon	Northwest Territories	Nunavut
Audiologists				Y	Y	Y	Y	Y	Y	Y			
Massage therapists	Y	Y	Y	Y	Y	Y	Y	Y	Y	Y	Y		
Dental hygienists	Y	Y	Y	Y	Y	Y	Y	Y	Y	Y	Y	Y	Y
Dentists	Y	Y	Y	Y	Y	Y	Y	Y	Y	Y	Y	Y	Y
Dietitians	Y	Y	Y	Y	Y	Y	Y	Y	Y	Y	Y		
Licensed practical nurses	Y	Y	Y	Y	Y	Y	Y	Y	Y	Y	Y	Y	Y
Medical examiners			Y	Y	Y	Y	Y	Y	Y				
Medical radiographers			Y	Y	Y	Y		Y	Y				
Midwives			Y	Y	Y	Y	Y	Y	Y	Y		Y	Y
Nurse practitioners	Y	Y	Y	Y	Y	Y	Y	Y	Y	Y		Y	Y
Occupational therapists	Y	Y	Y	Y	Y	Y	Y	Y	Y	Y		Y	Y
Optometrists	Y	Y	Y	Y	Y	Y	Y	Y	Y	Y	Y	Y	Y
Pharmacists	Y	Y	Y	Y	Y	Y	Y	Y	Y	Y	Y	Y	Y
Physicians	Y	Y	Y	Y	Y	Y	Y	Y	Y	Y	Y	Y	Y
Physiotherapists	Y	Y	Y	Y	Y	Y	Y	Y	Y	Y	Y		
Psychologists	Y	Y	Y	Y	Y	Y	Y	Y	Y	Y	Y	Y	Y
Registered nurses	Y	Y	Y	Y	Y	Y	Y	Y	Y	Y	Y	Y	Y
Registered psychiatric nurses	n/a	n/a	n/a	n/a	n/a	n/a	Y	Y	Y	Y	Y	n/a	n/a
Respiratory therapists			Y	Y	Y	Y	Y	Y	Y	Y			
Social workers	Y	Y	Y	Y	Y	Y	Y	Y	Y	Y			
Speech-language pathologists				Y	Y	Y	Y	Y	Y	Y			

Note: Y indicates regulated occupations in 2010.
Source: HWDB, CIHI, 2012.

347

Some education programs, including those for registered nurses and radiologists, are available in every province, whereas education programs for other healthcare professions are only available in some provinces. For example, as of 2010, the chiropractic education program was only available in Quebec and Ontario. Understanding the number and location of education programs throughout the country is important because it provides information on the potential supply and flow of fresh graduates entering the healthcare industry. Table 11.8 summarizes the number of education programs for certain healthcare professions.

Some professions, such as dentists, pharmacists, physicians, optometrists, and registered nurses, are regulated in every province and territory of Canada. In other words, practitioners must register with the respective provincial or territorial regulators in order to serve in a given administrative area. Other professions, such as medical laboratory technicians and radiologists, are only regulated in certain provinces. Table 11.9 summarizes the regulatory environments of healthcare professions in each Canadian province (territory) in 2010. The geographical mobility of these healthcare professions might be affected by the differences in regulatory policies across administrative areas.

(2) Supply and Distribution of Healthcare Providers

The ratio of healthcare providers to the population served reflects the relative number of a specific category of healthcare worker within a geographical area. The number of healthcare providers in Canada showed an increasing trend from 2005 to 2009, with the precise growth rate varying by profession. For example, the number of registered psychological nurses increased by 5.0%, whereas that of midwives increased by 58.8% (Figure 11.15).

In 2006, the average age of healthcare workers in Canada was 42 years old, which was 3 years younger than the average Canadian workforce. The workplace distribution of healthcare providers depends on the population served and their healthcare needs, region of practice, and funding sources. Hospitals function as a critical venue for different healthcare professionals, despite the substantial variation in their specific workplaces. In 2009, 23% of healthcare workers worked on a part-time basis.

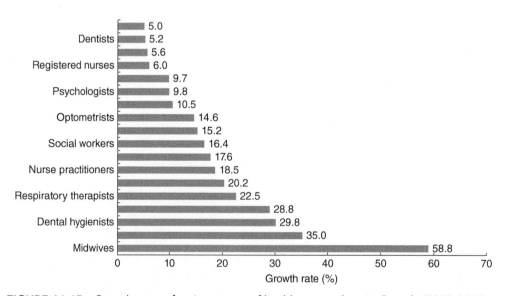

FIGURE 11.15 Growth rates of various types of healthcare workers in Canada (2005–2009).

The planning and management of the healthcare workforce are crucial as it guarantees the access of all Canadians to healthcare services. The Canadian Institute for Health Information (CIHI) has predicted the future demand for the healthcare workforce by comparing the current healthcare workforce with the expected healthcare services needed by the population in the future.

(3) General Practice System

In Canada, regions with a greater number of specialists tend to have populations with relatively poorer health status. The same is true of populations residing in regions with fewer primary care physicians. GPs are exceedingly important in communities with a wide gap between the rich and poor. Each year, every GP is required to provide approximately 2,500 healthcare services, diagnose 450 diseases with different clinical manifestations, and issue 20,000 prescriptions that cover 833 drugs for about 1,500–2,000 residents. GPs are the first point of contact practitioners, who provide patients with vertically integrated, universal, coordinated, family-centered, and community-oriented healthcare services. Hence, the training of Canadian GPs places heavy emphasis on understanding the community and patients. Medical students are often placed in communities and clinics in the early stages of their medical education, in order to bring them into close contact with local residents and patients. Consequently, the contact between medical students and community residents increases with the progression of their medical education. Since private practice (accounting for 24%) cannot fully meet the diverse healthcare needs of local residents, general practice services are mostly provided by GPs in cooperation with various professionals, such as secretaries, nurses, physiotherapists, social workers, community psychiatric nurses, district nurses, registered nurses, and midwives.

Broadly speaking, general practice education in Canada can be divided into three major stages: undergraduate education, postgraduate education, and continuing education. Medical graduates can take part in the national examination upon graduation, followed by a practical examination in the next year. They become nationally licensed GPs after passing both qualifying examinations, after which they may apply to practice anywhere in Canada. Their clinical practice covers 90.5% of patients with chronic diseases, 89.5% of patients requiring psychological interventions or treatment, 86% of patients requiring preventive care, 83.1% of other psychiatric patients, and 74.7% of patients requiring hospice care. They also respond to 73.9% of telephone inquiries from families of patients.

3. Current Status and Future Trends in Health Insurance

The current Canadian healthcare system was established according to the CHA of 1984 and is composed of hospital insurance and health insurance. The former has been implemented since July 1, 1958, in accordance with the Hospital Insurance and Diagnostic Services Act introduced in April 1957. The latter has been implemented since July 1, 1968, in accordance with the Medical Care Act introduced in December 1966.

These two systems are implemented by each province according to certain standards and are subsidized by the federal government. Both systems have relatively wide coverage, as they are available to almost all citizens. The processes involved in establishing these two systems are outlined in the following sections.

(1) The Birth of the Health Insurance Scheme

Canada's quest for nationwide health insurance can be traced back to before World War I. For instance, in 1928, an inquiry committee answering directly to the House of Commons began to collect information on sickness insurance via a population survey. In addition, the Employment and Social Insurance Act of 1935 gave the supervisory committee the responsibility of collecting information related to building a health insurance system. However, the development of the Canadian health insurance system was hampered for several years as the court found that one of the provisions in the act related to unemployment insurance was unconstitutional. In 1938, the nationwide health insurance system was officially proposed by the Social Security Commission of the House of Commons. The report released by the commission outlined in detail a comprehensive health insurance plan, but its implementation was temporarily suspended due to the outbreak of the Second World War.

After the end of World War II, in August 1945, the federal government proposed a social security plan with a broader scope of coverage to the provincial governments. The plan advocated for cost-sharing and collaboration between the federal and provincial governments in the establishment of a comprehensive health insurance system. In this system, preselected family physicians (GPs) in each region would be responsible for providing healthcare services for their registrants, and their remuneration would be based on a capitation system. In addition, the provincial-level administration and operation of the health insurance system were entrusted to committees composed of the representatives of consumers and healthcare service providers. Each committee was monitored by designated medical officers in each region. Despite receiving substantial support from the general public and major healthcare service providers, this proposal was not immediately implemented due to fears of its encroachment on provincial autonomy. However, the concept of cost-sharing between the federal and provincial governments had already been accepted. In 1947, Saskatchewan took the lead in piloting free healthcare services at public hospitals. In 1957, the federal government of Canada introduced the first health act (i.e., the Hospital Insurance and Diagnostic Act, HIDS), which proposed a 1:1 cost-sharing mechanism between the federal and provincial governments in disease diagnoses and inpatient treatment. However, there were still cases of poverty or even bankruptcy due to illness, as most Canadians still had to bear the physician and drug charges, with the exception of those whose employers (companies) were willing to cover these charges. The HIDS mandated the allocation of tax revenues for the required funds, which are administered by the Department of Public Administration based on the principles of universality and public administration. Then, in 1964, the federal government enacted the Medical Care Act, which stipulated 1:1 cost-sharing between the federal and provincial governments for out-of-hospital services and the inclusion of physician services in universal health coverage. This enabled Canadian residents to receive healthcare services covered by the health insurance fund in all regions across Canada, thereby achieving the full portability of healthcare services. The act also outlined the responsible administrative departments and their principles, with a focus on portability and comprehensiveness. In 1984, the federal government passed the momentous CHA, which more clearly defined the responsibilities and tasks of the federal and provincial governments in the provision of healthcare services. More specifically, the federal government is charged with the legislative enactment, and the provincial governments are responsible for the administration and provision of healthcare services, while both share the cost of financing healthcare services. It further ensured that all medically necessary services are covered by universal health insurance regardless of the patients' ability to pay.

At this point, the Canadian healthcare system was already well-established and centered around five basic principles: universality, public administration, portability, comprehensiveness, and accessibility.

Funding Sources. The health insurance fund of Canada relies heavily on taxes: specifically, personal and corporate income taxes, and basic insurance premiums levied by both federal and provincial governments.

Cost Sharing. The federal government bears 50% of expenses for the statutory hospital insurance and health insurance, whereas expenses for other items, such as retirement homes, drugs, and mental healthcare, are borne solely by the respective provincial governments. In reality, the federal government contributes only about 25% of the actual expenses for all publicly-funded healthcare services, and the remaining 75% is borne by provincial governments. Since 1997, the federal government began providing funds to provincial governments through tax transfers and cash allocations through Canada Health and Social Transfer (CHST). In British Columbia, for example, the healthcare expenditure in 2010 was C$19.5 billion, of which C$15.7 billion came from the budget of the provincial government, while the remaining C$3.8 billion came from the federal government's healthcare capitation-based healthcare transfer fund. The contribution of the federal government was far below the stipulated percentage (50%), which is related to the better fiscal performance of British Columbia. Alberta had a similar situation.

(2) Hospital Insurance

1. Status of Each Province Before the Implementation of Hospital Insurance The government of Saskatchewan had already implemented an independent provincial insurance scheme for hospitalization long before the rest of the nation. In 1914, Saskatchewan developed a prototype of Canadian health insurance known as the Municipal Doctor Plan, which provided health insurance coverage for urban employees for unforeseen illnesses and accidental injuries. In 1947, the Co-operative Commonwealth Federation (CCF) came into power in Saskatchewan and created the Saskatchewan Hospital Service Plan (SHSP), which covered hospitalization costs for all residents using personal insurance premiums and provincial taxes. This plan clearly stipulated that all Saskatchewanians are entitled to inpatient healthcare services provided by the SHSP, regardless of their political ideologies and economic status.

On the other hand, the Cottage Hospital and Medical Care Plan was introduced in 1934 by the government of Newfoundland (which, at that time, was not part of Canada) to provide hospital and healthcare services for geographically and economically disadvantaged residents. Physicians and nurses received monthly salaries under this system. After Newfoundland became a province of Canada in 1949, the system was further expanded.

Health insurance systems were subsequently established in other provinces, such as British Columbia, Alberta, and Ontario, which suited their unique situations. However, relying solely on provincial systems caused the Canadian healthcare system to be fraught with difficulties. Hence, the Canadian government promoted the establishment of various schemes through provincial hospital associations and the private insurance industry in order to complement and improve the provincial systems. Unfortunately, the private sector had limited effects – even in Ontario, which had a well-established private hospital insurance scheme, only about 40% of residents participated in the hospital insurance in 1956. In addition, there were numerous flaws regarding the reimbursements covered by private insurance, and the continuous increase in hospital expenses eventually led to private insurance payments becoming overstretched. After the war, the federal government implemented the General Health Grants Program for provinces facing these circumstances, which functioned as a transitional measure during the establishment of a health insurance system.

2. General Health Grants Program   This program was implemented in 1948, and as stated by Prime Minister Mackenzie King, its primary objective was to lay the foundation for the implementation of a national health insurance system. It proposed that the federal government would subsidize the surveying, hospital construction, improvement of medical facilities, and medical education conducted by provincial governments. This program gradually attained a number of prerequisites for implementing a nationwide health insurance system in Canada.

3. Federal–Provincial Agreement Process   Independent provincial health insurance systems had been implemented in certain provinces (e.g., Ontario) prior to the establishment of the national health insurance system. In 1955, the premier of Ontario, L. M. Frost, successfully began a discussion on issues related to health insurance in federal–provincial consultation meetings.

At the beginning of one meeting, L. M. Frost stated that health insurance is a vital issue that deserves in-depth discussion at the meeting. Moreover, the implementation of any type of health insurance system requires the participation and cooperation of federal and provincial governments. Health-related issues are also one of the major goals of human progress. Therefore, reaching an agreement is worthwhile to establish a better system. In response, the Canadian prime minister, Louis St. Laurent, clearly stated his intention to strive towards establishing a health insurance system. Subsequently, he proposed a concrete federal program to provincial governments in January of the following year (1956). This program focused on establishing guidelines for the priority implementation of health insurance for hospitalization and diagnostic services. By the end of that year, several joint meetings were held by both federal and provincial health ministers and finance ministers to discuss the major components of the HIDS in depth. As a result, the act was passed unanimously by the House of Commons, ratified on April 1, 1957, and officially implemented on July 1 of the following year.

4. Basic Standards and Coverage of Hospital Insurance   The primary objective of hospital insurance is the provision of assistance to hospitals and related services by the federal government through provincial governments, in order to improve the accessibility and quality of healthcare services. The nationwide hospital insurance is composed of the hospital insurance schemes from all provinces. Naturally, each province has its own unique scheme that does not overlap with those of other provinces. However, to be eligible for federal subsidies, provincial schemes must meet the basic standards established by the federal government.

1. *Basic federal standards.* (1) Universality. All eligible individuals are insured according to the same set of terms and conditions, regardless of age, gender, physical condition, and economic status (with the exception of the military and Royal Horse Guards). (2) Nonprofit. Hospital insurance must be administered and operated by nonprofit organizations. (3) Comprehensiveness. The hospital insurance must have

comprehensive reimbursement coverage. (4) Accessibility. Appropriate standards should be established for insurance premiums and co-payments. (5) Portability. Residents that move permanently or temporarily from one province to another retain their insurance coverage. Provincial schemes that meet the above standards are eligible for financial assistance from the federal government.

2. *The scope of insurance coverage.* (1) For inpatient services, coverage includes but is not limited to the following nine domains: incidental charges for hospitalization and meals, nursing services, diagnoses, drugs, surgeries and anesthetic use, routine surgical supplies, radiotherapy, physiotherapy, and the healthcare workers employed by hospitals. (2) For outpatient and emergency services, coverage was initially limited to accidental and emergency cases, but this has inevitably and gradually expanded. Each province is responsible for determining the types of outpatient and emergency services covered by insurance, which are also subsidized by the federal government.

3. *Reimbursement procedures.* Insured persons in all provinces (except for Alberta and Ontario) are automatically registered for insurance reimbursement. In Ontario, companies with more than 15 employees must pay the insurance premiums for both the employees and their dependents, while other companies are free to choose. This is because Ontario levies premiums on insured persons in advance and reimburses their medical expenses later whenever applicable. In reality, only a handful of Ontario residents do not participate in the insurance scheme.

     On the other hand, provinces are free to choose whether to participate in the Canadian hospital insurance system according to their unique situations.

4. *Timeline of participation in hospital insurance.* Prior to the ratification of the HIDS in 1957, independent hospital insurance schemes had already been implemented in several provinces, such as Saskatchewan, Newfoundland, Alberta, and British Columbia. However, the establishment of this federal act contributed greatly to the development of these provincial schemes, particularly in provinces where the scheme was poorly developed. The timeline of the participation of each province in the Canadian hospital insurance scheme is shown in Table 11.10.

5. Other Characteristics of Hospital Insurance   Prior to the implementation of hospital insurance, patients in tuberculosis sanatoria, psychiatric hospitals, nursing homes, and geriatric hospitals were excluded from receiving federal medical aid. Hence, these institutions were mainly funded by the provincial governments and charitable organizations.

TABLE 11.10   Timeline of the Participation of Canadian Provinces and Territories in Hospital Insurance

Province/Territory	Date of Participation	Province/Territory	Date of Participation
Newfoundland	July 1, 1958	Ontario	January 1, 1959
Saskatchewan	July 1, 1958	New Brunswick	July 1, 1959
Alberta	July 1, 1958	Prince Edward Island	October 1, 1959
British Columbia	July 1, 1958	Northwest Territories	April 1, 1960
Manitoba	July 1, 1958	Yukon	July 1, 1960
Nova Scotia	January 1, 1959	Quebec	January 1, 1961

Source: L. Soderstrom, *The Canadian Health Care System* (London: Croon Helm, 1978).

However, with the establishment of the Canada Assistance Plan in April 1966, the federal government began bearing half the expenses of these institutions. Furthermore, due to the establishment of the hospital insurance system in 1957, funding for inpatient and outpatient services began to be covered by the nationwide insurance scheme. However, the scheme did not cover the consultation fees of physicians.

(3) Health Insurance

1. General Conditions of Canadian Healthcare Before the Establishment of Health Insurance In 1920–1930, the private insurance industry began offering health insurance to residents. By the 1940s, nonprofit insurance organizations began to emerge with the support of physician groups. After the Second World War, the relationship between medical associations and the private insurance industry led to the rapid growth in various voluntary insurance schemes, each of which had its own restrictions. For instance, insurance companies were reluctant to sign insurance policies with the elderly or individuals with poor health conditions, unless they were willing to pay extremely high premiums. The eligibility criteria for coverage were slightly less stringent for group insurance plans, such as company-based plans. Therefore, the majority of Canadians were not prepared for the risk of future disease. The nonprofit voluntary insurance organizations also had numerous shortcomings, such as coverage limited to inpatient or surgical treatments and an upper limit for reimbursement.

2. Independent Provincial Health Insurance Schemes
  1. *Newfoundland.* In January 1957, Newfoundland implemented a children's health service, whereby the reimbursement for inpatient and outpatient services for children was covered by general taxes. As a result, since 1958, public funds have been used to cover hospital healthcare expenditures (including medical and surgical treatments) for children under the age of 16.
  2. *Saskatchewan.* In early 1959, the premier of Saskatchewan, Tommy Douglas, began vigorously promoting a comprehensive health insurance program based on five fundamental principles: prepayment, universal coverage, comprehensive reimbursement standards, public administration, and acceptability (for both service recipients and providers). The comprehensive health insurance program was formulated in November 1961 in keeping with these principles and implemented on July 1, 1962.

     During this process, the provincial government admitted that physicians were not directly affiliated with the health insurance program and that patients (instead of the provincial government) reserved the right to directly apply for the reimbursement of medical expenses. This momentous event in Saskatchewan not only affected other provinces but also contributed to the subsequent establishment of universal health coverage in Canada.

3. Hall Commission Since the establishment of the hospital insurance system in 1957, inpatient, outpatient, and emergency services have been the major targets of nationwide coverage. However, nationwide coverage for physician consultation fees had not been established.

Following the Second World War, Canada conducted several large-scale nationwide surveys to improve its healthcare system, among which the report of the Hall Commission (Royal Commission on Health Services) has arguably had the greatest impact on the establishment of the Canadian health insurance system. The commission was established in 1961 under the Diefenbaker government, and was chaired by Emmett Matthew Hall (E. M. Hall).

The commission was established with the goal of providing universal, high-quality health-care services to Canadians, as well as advising the federal government on expected future health-care needs based on surveys of the current healthcare system. The reports of the Hall Commission published in 1964 and 1965 focused on the training of physicians and healthcare experts, the expansion and improvement of healthcare institutions, the establishment of new medical education institutions, and the improvement of mental health services. Of particular note were its recommendations regarding the services not covered by the hospital insurance system. It proposed that there was a clear need for financial subsidies from the federal government for the independent provincial health insurance that offered "equal reimbursement conditions for all residents." In 1965, Prime Minister Lester B. Pearson accepted the Hall Commission's recommendations and proposed the Canadian universal health insurance system to the provincial governments. This led to the federal government's passing of the Medical Care Act in 1966.

4. Federal Standards for the Health Insurance System   Prior to the federal–provincial summit in 1965, the Canadian health insurance scheme proposed by Prime Minister Lester B. Pearson was discussed in advance among federal and provincial health authorities. These authorities ultimately agreed that all provinces should prioritize the establishment of a healthcare system that provides residents with prepaid services. Subsequently, Prime Minister Pearson announced during the federal–provincial summit in 1965 that the federal government would share half of the expenses on services covered by the health insurance for provinces that complied with the following "four points." Note that these points applied to both health insurance and hospital insurance.

1. *Comprehensive coverage.* Health insurance must cover all medically necessary services provided by physicians, including facial plastic surgery. The health insurance only covers services deemed necessary from a medical perspective.

   In addition, health coverage for dental services was mainly confined to oral surgeries at hospitals, but some provinces also covered general dental treatments. Other provinces also covered specialist services, such as eye examinations, foot treatments (e.g., blisters), and chiropractic treatments.
2. *Universality.* Several provinces promoted the universality of social health insurance in order to restrain the growth of private health insurance. The federal health insurance act stated that "over 95% (90% in the first two years of the enactment) of individuals who are eligible for insurance must be covered by the provincial schemes."
3. *Public administration.* Provincial health insurance schemes had to be administered and operated by provincial governments or their affiliates on a nonprofit basis.
4. *Portability.* The eligibility of recipients must not be affected by travel or relocation to another province.

   Nevertheless, despite the basic federal standards for health insurance described above, provincial schemes still varied considerably across different provinces due to their socioeconomic status.

   There was a need for federal–provincial agreement regarding the detailed requirements of service types and cost-sharing mechanisms prior to the implementation of the hospital insurance system. In contrast, the health insurance system only required a general federal–provincial consistency, which made its implementation more flexible.

TABLE 11.11 Timeline of the Participation of Canadian Provinces and Territories in Health Insurance

Province/Territory	Date of Participation	Province/Territory	Date of Participation
Saskatchewan	July 1, 1968	Ontario	October 1, 1969
British Columbia	July 1, 1968	Quebec	September 1, 1970
Nova Scotia	April 1, 1969	Prince Edward Island	December 1, 1970
Manitoba	April 1, 1969	New Brunswick	January 1, 1971
Newfoundland	April 1, 1969	Northwest Territories	April 1, 1971
Alberta	July 1, 1969	Yukon	April 1, 1972

Source: L. Soderstrom, *The Canadian Health Care System*. Croon Helm, London, 1978.

5. Reimbursement of Health Insurance The federal health insurance act stipulates that all eligible insured persons shall be reimbursed in accordance with the health insurance scheme, with the exception of the military and Royal Horse Guards. Although the residents of Alberta, British Columbia, and Ontario had the right to choose whether to enroll in the health insurance scheme, the vast majority of them still chose to become beneficiaries of the provincial schemes. Residents in other provinces must register with the relevant social health insurance agencies in order to obtain insurance coverage. As mentioned previously, the health insurance covered various medical treatments provided by physicians and dentists (including those provided at hospitals).

6. Timeline of Participation in Health Insurance of Each Province As with the hospital insurance, each province in Canada was free to decide when they participate in the health insurance system. The timeline of the participation of each province in the health insurance system is shown in Table 11.11.

7. Main Features of the Current Payment System for Health Insurance
1. *Single-payer system.* Both the federal and provincial governments have shared the payment of health insurance for a long period of time, but the responsibility ultimately falls to the provincial governments. In 2002, federal allocations and the fiscal budget of provincial governments accounted for 71% of the total healthcare expenditure. Private insurance agencies, on the other hand, mainly covered items beyond the scope of government insurance for inpatient, medical, and dental services and prescription drugs.
2. *Implementation of an unbundled fee-for-service payment system for physicians.* The fee-for-service system is the main payment method by which provincial health insurance pays for physician charges. For example, this payment method accounted for 91% of health insurance payments to physicians in Ontario. In general, hospital physicians, such as radiologists, pathologists, and anesthesiologists, are paid in the form of wages.
3. *Implementation of global prepayments for most hospitals.* Health insurance payments made to hospitals strictly follow the "global budget system for hospitals." A global budget is calculated and negotiated between the provincial health authorities and hospitals based on the hospitals' actual expenditure in the previous year and expected growth rate. The global budget does not guarantee payment for overruns. Furthermore, it does not include long-term capital investments, such as the maintenance and procurement of

hospital facilities, which must be assessed and approved by the provincial government according to the hospitals' needs, and hospitals must contribute 10–40% of such expenditures.

4. *Implementation of fixed-price healthcare services.* The price of each healthcare service covered by Canadian universal health insurance is regularly negotiated between provincial governments and medical associations. Thus, all physicians who serve in the same province must charge the same price for the same healthcare service. In Ontario, the Ontario Medical Association (OMA) annually revises the OMA Schedule of Fees and recommends service items to the Ministry of Health that have yet to be covered by health insurance. However, the final payments are negotiated according to the scope and standards of the Ontario Health Insurance Plan Schedule of Benefits (OHIP Schedule of Benefits) based on extensive expert advice. Physicians may impose charges based on the OMA Schedule of Fees for services that fall beyond the coverage of health insurance. Currently, the OHIP Schedule of Benefits covers about 59% of the OMA Schedule of Fees.

5. *Demand-side access to free basic healthcare services.* An important feature of the Canadian health insurance system is to ensure that Canadians are free from the economic risks caused by illnesses. The CHA of 1984 explicitly prohibits provinces from overcharging or levying additional charges on patients. The federal government penalizes provinces found to permit service charges or additional charges by hospitals or physicians for items covered by public health insurance. The revenues obtained from these illegal charges are also deducted from the province's federal allocation.

(4) Extended Healthcare Services

The federally subsidized Extended Health Care Service (EHCS) program was introduced in the Established Programs Financing (EPF) Act of 1977. Prior to the introduction of this program, each province implemented extended healthcare services beyond the coverage of health insurance at their own expense.

The EHSC program covers: (1) elderly care and convalescence care, (2) nursing home care, (3) home-based care, and (4) rehabilitative care in rehabilitation centers. The federal subsidies are allocated according to healthcare expenditure per capita. For instance, the federal allocation in 1998 was C$150 per capita, which subsequently increased with the growth of the gross national product (GNP). There are two prerequisites for the allocation of federal subsidies: the recognition of the need for federal subsidies, as well as the provision of necessary information and the acceptance of supervision.

4. Management of Health Insurance

(1) Funding and Financial Assistance of Health Insurance

Health insurance funding was shared equally between the provincial and federal governments prior to the enactment of the EPF Act on April 1, 1977. Following this Act, the federal government changed its contribution, which was based on the insurance premiums of each province, to capitation-based funding, whereby the amount is increased annually based on the average annual growth rate of the GNP over the past three years. This measure was adopted for the following objectives: (1) to ensure stable funding; (2) to allow each province to make flexible funding adjustments; (3) to ensure the equality of healthcare expenditure and services among provinces; (4) to enable joint discussions on policies; and

(5) to standardize healthcare services in Canada. The asset liability management of health insurance is based on the 1977 (renamed in 1984) Federal–Provincial Fiscal Arrangements and Established Programs Financing Act.

The Canada Health Act stipulates the following principles of health insurance: (1) nonprofit, public administration; (2) comprehensiveness; (3) universality; (4) portability; and (5) acceptable insurance premiums and patient copayments. Implementation of these principles is made possible by federal subsidies, which in turn require the following: the provision of information about the operation and management of health insurance to the insurance and welfare department; the recognition of federal subsidies; and the abolition of patient copayments.

The amount of federal subsidy is determined using the following methods: (1) The average amount of federal subsidies per capita is first calculated. This is standardized across the different provinces by summing up the average amount of federal subsidies per capita in 1995 and the average annual growth rate of the GNP over the past three years. (2) The total federal subsidy received by each province is the average amount of federal subsidies per capita multiplied by the total population of the province.

The federal subsidy is provided to provincial governments via cash payments and balanced tax-transfer payments. In 1998, the federal subsidy for health insurance and extended healthcare services was C$22.1 billion (cash payment: C$10 billion; balanced tax-transfer payment: C$12.1 billion) and C$2.8 billion, respectively, totaling C$24.9 billion. The total federal subsidy was C$26.6 billion in 1998, based on an average of C$845 per capita.

Health insurance mainly relies on the general tax revenues of federal and provincial governments. However, there are also a handful of provinces that impose supplementary labor insurance premiums or patient copayments. For example, Ontario, Alberta, and British Columbia levy insurance premiums, but Alberta and Ontario subsidize the insurance premiums for low-income earners and exempt the premiums of elderly adults aged over 65 years. Thus, it can be seen that each province can determine the means by which it raises health insurance funds, but the amount collected from patient copayments is deducted from the federal subsidy. The health insurance premiums and patient copayments in each province are shown in Table 11.12.

(2) Organizational Management of Health Insurance

Hospital insurance, health insurance, and extended healthcare services are operated and administered by provincial governments or their affiliated public agencies on a nonprofit basis. These administrative agencies vary across the different Canadian provinces/territories. For instance, hospital insurance in Newfoundland, Nova Scotia, Quebec, Saskatchewan, and British Columbia is administered by provincial insurance departments or health and social services departments, while health insurance is administered by a health insurance committee or health services committee. In most of the other provinces/territories, both insurance systems are administered by insurance services committees or health departments. On the other hand, extended healthcare services are provided by nursing homes under the supervision of provincial health departments or social services departments (this system is administered by provincial health departments, regional health authorities, and social services departments).

TABLE 11.12   Health Insurance Premiums and Copayment Status of the Provinces and Territories of Canada (Including Extended Healthcare Services) in 1994

Province/Territory	Health Insurance	Hospital Insurance
Saskatchewan	No insurance premiums or copayments	No insurance premiums or copayments
New Brunswick	No insurance premiums or copayments	No insurance premiums or copayments
Nova Scotia	No insurance premiums or copayments	No insurance premiums or copayments
Prince Edward Island	No insurance premiums or copayments	No insurance premiums or copayments
Northwest Territories	No insurance premiums or copayments	No insurance premiums or copayments
Yukon	No insurance premiums or copayments	No insurance premiums or copayments
Quebec	No insurance premiums or copayments	No insurance premiums or copayments
Newfoundland	No insurance premiums or copayments	No insurance premiums or copayments
British Columbia	Some insurance premiums but reduced for low-income earners. No copayments.	No insurance premiums or copayments
Alberta	Some insurance premiums, but waived or subsidized for those aged over 65 years. No copayments.	Some insurance premiums, but waived or subsidized for those aged over 65 years. No copayments.
Ontario	Some insurance premiums, but waived or subsidized for those aged over 65 years. No copayments.	Some insurance premiums, but waived or subsidized for those aged over 65 years. Patients with chronic diseases must pay for their convalescence but low-income earners are waived.
Manitoba	No insurance premiums or copayments	Patients must pay US$21.9 per day (extended healthcare services) for admission to a personal care home (PCH) to receive personalized care that is deemed medically unnecessary by hospitals.

(3) Payment Methods for Healthcare Expenditures

Most physicians receive fee-for-service payments. The price list (fee schedule) varies across provinces and is determined via negotiation between provincial health insurance agencies (committees) and physicians. In addition to fee-for-service payments, physicians also receive salaries and capitation payments. The remuneration of hospitals is performed through budget allocation, and their operations are based on these budgets.

(4) Private Health Insurance

In Canada, private health insurance is used to supplement the coverage of provincial health insurance. Private health insurance is primarily operated by private insurance companies and various nonprofit organizations (e.g., Canadian Life and Health Insurance Association, and Blue Cross Canada).

The number of private insurance policyholders began to increase after 1970, from 2.7 million in 1970 to 6.5 million in 1985 and 7.95 million in 1995 (accounting for nearly

TABLE 11.13 Number of Physician Services Provided in the Provinces and Territories of Canada in 2007–2008

Service Item	Newfoundland and Labrador	Prince Edward Island	Nova Scotia	New Brunswick	Quebec	Ontario	Manitoba	Saskatchewan	Alberta	British Columbia	Yukon	Total
Number of consultations	197,360	38,600	306,306	361,291	4,180,748	5,796,229	349,423	424,858	1,852,349	2,207,714	Not Reported	15,714,878
Number of key assessments	139,010	54,538	161,094	105,520	7,708,439	7,969,281	833,116	344,104	1,727,637	11,444,911	Not Reported	30,487,650
Number of other assessments	2,090,763	358,303	3,596,595	2,283,502	26,816,152	43,760,048	3,722,727	4,035,907	12,860,420	8,128,230	Not Reported	107,652,648
Length of hospital stay (days)	268,234	86,396	324,159	280,213	1,591,001	4,470,936	926,758	572,815	1,448,812	1,327,427	Not Reported	11,296,751
Number of telephone consultations	36,033	19,598	66,191	30,303	466,057	2,988,567	194,687	123,262	537,583	942,210	Not Reported	5,404,491
Number of psychotherapy/counseling sessions	92,780	33,109	141,542	117,380	3,402,977	7,404,878	299,478	212,634	1,929,882	1,401,356	Not Reported	15,036,016
Total number of consultations and Visits	2,824,180	590,544	4,595,887	3,178,209	44,165,375	72,389,940	6,326,190	5,713,580	20,356,683	25,451,848	Not Reported	185,592,434
Major surgeries	43,945	8,297	67,945	78,691	630,455	1,458,998	118,635	104,018	376,783	354,199	Not Reported	3,241,966
Minor surgeries	57,198	5,538	26,770	15,173	635,030	957,565	77,630	90,990	295,747	270,982	Not Reported	2,432,624
Surgical assistance	4,026	6,134	19,668	16,305	44,727	407,103	20,912	34,060	246,380	197,106	Not Reported	996,421
Anesthesia	**	**	**	**	**	**	**	**	**	**	Not Reported	**
Obstetric services	2,877	1,534	12,587	7,649	158,801	386,502	26,197	15,396	174,005	79,951	Not Reported	865,499
Diagnostic/therapeutic services	485,852	183,254	560,285	817,994	5,187,058	19,234,887	960,371	1,166,185	2,624,172	4,197,541	Not Reported	35,417,598
Special services	81,590	43,441	431,563	245,415	38,859	6,177,521	419,942	160,400	885,269	596,157	Not Reported	9,080,209
Other services	313	7,275	35,355	336,361	856,789	7,922,183	260,387	523,608	138,959	1,015,738	Not Reported	11,096,968
Total number of consultation sessions	675,801	255,473	1,154,173	1,517,588	7,551,719	36,544,759	1,884,074	2,094,716	4,741,307	6,711,674	Not Reported	63,131,284
Total number of services	3,499,981	846,017	5,750,060	4,695,797	51,717,094	108,934,699	8,210,264	7,808,296	25,097,990	32,163,522	Not Reported	248,723,718

Source: National Physician Database (NPDB), CIHI, 2010.

TABLE 11.14 Clinical Service Fees Paid to Physicians in the Provinces and Territories of Canada in 1999–2008 (Unit: C$1,000)

Fiscal year	Newfoundland and Labrador	Prince Edward Island	Nova Scotia	New Brunswick	Quebec	Ontario	Manitoba	Saskatchewan	Alberta	British Columbia	Yukon	Northwest Territories	Nunavut	Canada
Unit: C$1,000														
1999–2000	153,047	38,916	309,604	205,965	1,995,615	4,103,523	328,449	272,463	840,227	1,392,630				9,640,439
2000–2001	156,442	36,162	318,591	204,053	2,117,383	4,274,114	375,530	321,693	906,592	1,463,859				10,174,420
2001–2002	171,547	37,206	329,806	229,104	2,264,173	4,458,579	403,467	354,524	1,047,262	1,693,013	8,050			10,996,730
2002–2003	181,196	40,941	359,901	255,182	2,345,356	4,530,445	425,597	379,325	1,223,614	1,812,306	9,578			11,563,442
2003–2004	217,040	43,951	404,075	281,889	2,570,703	4,896,254	450,683	391,538	1,270,431	1,858,765	10,644	31,146		12,427,120
2004–2005	239,260	45,682	427,759	303,874	2,632,717	5,169,037	485,037	437,885	1,364,047	1,893,752	12,023	31,185		13,041,759
2005–2006	244,487	46,250	450,912	320,119	2,727,587	5,766,526	513,225	467,031	1,512,813	1,981,913	12,579	31,185		14,074,627
2006–2007	238,956	51,716	476,370	347,622	2,801,522	6,076,564	556,106	487,026	1,589,344	2,144,271	14,943	30,260		14,814,698
2007–2008	250,257	58,911	495,172	367,510	3,032,484	6,685,286	591,757	523,979	1,790,223	2,281,835	16,342	30,651		16,124,408
Annual Rate of Change														
1999–2000	–	–	–	–	–	–	–	–	–	–	–	–	–	–
2000–2001	2.2	-7.1	2.9	-0.9	6.1	4.2	14.3	18.1	7.9	5.1	–	–	–	5.5
2001–2002	9.7	2.9	3.5	12.3	6.9	4.3	7.4	10.2	15.5	15.7	–	–	–	8.1
2002–2003	5.6	10.0	9.1	11.4	3.6	1.6	5.5	7.0	16.8	7.0	19.0	–	–	5.2
2003–2004	19.8	7.4	12.3	10.5	9.6	8.1	5.9	3.2	3.8	2.6	11.1	–	–	7.5
2004–2005	10.2	3.9	5.9	7.8	2.4	5.6	7.6	11.7	7.4	1.9	13.0	0.1	–	4.9
2005–2006	2.2	1.2	5.4	5.3	3.6	11.6	5.8	6.8	10.9	4.7	4.6	0.0	–	7.9
2006–2007	-2.3	11.8	5.6	8.6	2.7	5.4	8.4	4.3	5.1	4.7	18.8	-3.0	–	5.3
2007–2008	4.7	13.9	3.9	5.7	8.2	10.0	6.4	7.6	12.6	6.4	9.4	1.3	–	8.8

Note: Blank space indicates that the province/territory did not submit data for that year.
Source: NPDB, National Health Expenditure Database (NHEX), 2010.

one-third of the total Canadian population). The number of policyholders for dental insurance is especially high, and dental insurance has become an important part of private health insurance. In 1998, the reimbursement of private health insurance accounted for 24% of total healthcare expenditure.

The fee-for-service payment method has been adopted for the vast majority of private health insurance schemes. However, the capitation payment method is sometimes adopted for dentists.

(5) Utilization and Payment of Physician Services

Table 11.13 shows the number of physician services in the various provinces and territories of Canada between 2007 and 2008.

A total of 72 million consultations and visits were delivered in Ontario, which ranks first and far exceeds that of all other provinces and territories, followed by Quebec, British Columbia, and Alberta. Ontario is also significantly higher than the other provinces and territories in terms of the total number of services provided, accounting for about 57.9% of the total number in Canada (except for Yukon). Ontario accounted for about 43.8% of the total number of physician services delivered in Canada (except for Yukon), followed by Quebec (20.8%), British Columbia (12.9%), and Alberta (10.1%).

Table 11.14 shows the clinical service fees paid to physicians in the provinces and territories of Canada from 1999 to 2008. Ontario also had the highest healthcare expenditure each year, followed by Quebec, British Columbia, and Alberta, which was consistent with the number of physician services. In 2007–2008, the expenses on clinical services in these four provinces accounted for more than 85% of the total expenditure in Canada (except Nunavut), among which expenses in Ontario peaked in 2005–2006 (with a growth rate of 11.6%), followed by 2007–2008 (with a growth rate of 10.0%). The growth of expenses for clinical services in Alberta is also worthy of attention, as the growth rate exceeded 15% in two consecutive years (2001–2003), after which it was 10.9% in 2005–2006 and 12.6% in 2007–2008.

5. Trends in Healthcare Expenditure and Containment Policies

(1) Trends in Healthcare Expenditure

1. Total Healthcare Expenditure   In 2009, the total healthcare expenditure in Canada was C$182.1 billion (equivalent to C$134.4 billion after correcting for inflation), which represented an increase of 3% compared to 2008. In 1975–1991, the average annual growth rate of total healthcare expenditure was 3.8% (Table 11.15). In 1991–1996, the growth of total healthcare expenditure was somewhat attenuated and showed a growth rate of 0.9%. In 1996–2009, the average annual growth rate was 4.5%. From 1997, the total healthcare expenditure saw a rapid growth, which was only attenuated in 2009. This trend can mainly be attributed to the increase in government investment after the fiscal austerity in the early and mid-twentieth century (Figure 11.16).

2. Healthcare Expenditure Per Capita   In 2009, the health expenditure per capita in Canada was C$5,401. After correcting for inflation (calculated at the price in 1997), the average annual growth rate of healthcare expenditure per capita in Canada was 2.6% in 1975–1991.

TABLE 11.15 Growth in Total Healthcare Expenditure in Canada in 1975–2009 (Calculated at Current Prices)

Year	Total Healthcare Expenditure (C$ 1 million)	Annual Growth Rate (%)	% of GNP
1975	12,199.4	–	7.0
1980	22,298.4	16.3	7.1
1985	39,842.4	8.4	8.2
1990	61,026.3	8.8	9.0
1995	74,086.4	1.3	9.1
2000	98,589.1	9.1	9.2
2005	140,653.4	6.7	10.2
2009	182,112.7	5.7	11.9

The healthcare expenditure per capita decreased at an annual rate of 0.2% from 1991 to 1996. However, there was a considerable rebound in the growth rate in subsequent years. In 1996–2009, the healthcare expenditure per capita increased by 3.5%, as shown in Figure 11.17.

3. Healthcare Expenditure and Economic Growth In 2009, the total healthcare expenditure in Canada accounted for 11.9% of the GDP (Table 11.15). Over the past decade, the total healthcare expenditure has increased by an average of C$9 billion annually. The GDP also showed an increasing trend over that same period, except for during the economic recession in 2009.

In 1975, the total healthcare expenditure in Canada accounted for 7.0% of GDP. In the late 1970s, the total healthcare expenditure and GDP increased at almost the same rate. However, from the early 1980s, the GDP and total healthcare expenditure began to increase

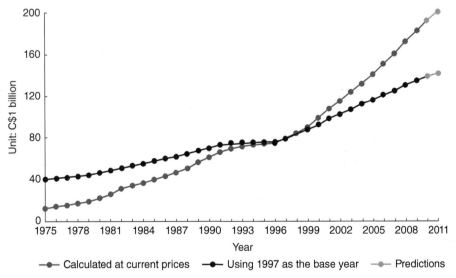

FIGURE 11.16 Growth of healthcare expenditure in Canada in 1975–2011. *Source:* CIHI, NHEX, 2011.

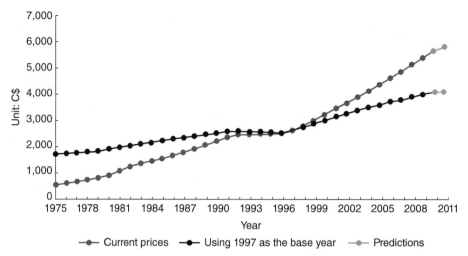

FIGURE 11.17 Healthcare expenditure per capita in Canada (1975–2011). *Source:* CIHI, NHEX, 2011.

at different rates. The former fell during the economic recession of 1982 and did not recover to its prerecession levels until 1984, whereas the latter showed a continuous increasing trend. As a result, the total healthcare expenditure as a share of the GDP increased significantly from 6.8% in 1979 to 8.3% in 1983.

Canada experienced another economic recession from 1990 to 1992, which led to a significant increase in the total healthcare expenditure as a share of the GDP, reaching 10% for the first time in 1992. In 1993–1997, the total healthcare expenditure increased at a lower rate than the GDP, thus resulting in a gradual decrease in the total healthcare expenditure as a share of the GDP and reaching 8.9% in 1997. However, from 1998, the total healthcare expenditure increased at a higher rate than GDP, resulting in a continual increase of total healthcare expenditure as a share of the GDP over the past decade, which peaked in 2009 (Figure 11.18).

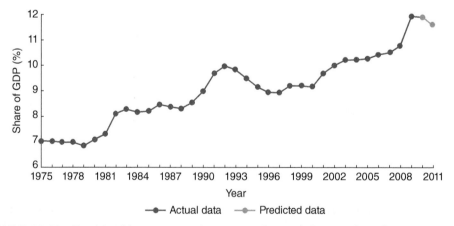

FIGURE 11.18 Total healthcare expenditure as a share of GDP in Canada in 1975–2011. *Source:* CIHI, NHEX, 2011.

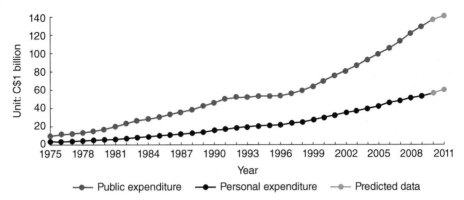

FIGURE 11.19 Healthcare expenditure in Canada by funding source in 1975–2011.
Source: CIHI, NHEX, 2011.

(2) Funding and Utilization of Healthcare Expenditure

1. Funding Sources In 2009, the Canadian government and various government agencies (i.e., the public sector) spent C$129.1 billion on healthcare, while commercial health insurance companies and households (i.e., the private sector) spent about C$53 billion. Since 1997, the public sector has contributed about 70.0% of the total healthcare expenditure, which increased to 70.9% in 2009 (Figure 11.19).

In 1975–1991, the average annual growth rate of public healthcare expenditure was 11.0%. However, the trend in the healthcare expenditure of the public sector changed significantly during the economic recession in 1990–1992, when the government employed austerity measures that significantly influenced healthcare and social care expenditures. During this period, the healthcare expenditure of the private sector increased at a higher rate than that of the public sector, leading to an increase in the share of the private sector, which reached 29.9% in 1997 and remained stable thereafter.

1. *Public healthcare expenditure.* The funding sources of public healthcare expenditure include the provincial governments, federal direct healthcare expenditure, municipal governments, Workers' Compensation Boards, and the Quebec Drug Insurance Fund. The composition of funding sources from the public sector is shown in Table 11.16. In 1975, provincial governments contributed C$8.7 billion to healthcare, accounting for 93.6%, while other funding sources contributed C$600 million, accounting for 6.4%. In 2009, the provincial governments spent C$118.9 billion on healthcare, accounting for 92.1% of public expenditure.

Table 11.17 summarizes the federal, provincial, and local shares of public healthcare expenditures. It can be seen from the table that Canada's public healthcare expenditure has been relatively well contained in recent years, accounting for about 86% of the total healthcare expenditure in 2000. Ontario and Quebec accounted for about 61% of the total healthcare expenditure. The average healthcare expenditure per capita in 2000 was C$3,168. However, there was a substantial difference between the provinces with the highest (Ontario, C$3,861) and lowest (Prince Edward Island, C$2,167) healthcare expenditure per capita.

Canada is also experiencing rapid population aging. It is estimated that by 2040, individuals aged over 65 years will account for about 22.5% of the total Canadian

TABLE 11.16   Composition of Funding Sources of the Public Sector in Canada in 1975 and 2009

	1975		2009	
Funding Sources	Amount (C$1 Million)	Percentage (%)	Amount (C$1 Million)	Percentage (%)
Provincial governments	8,709.3	93.63	118,900.5	92.1
Federal direct expenditure*	398.3	4.3	6,871.9	5.3
Social security fund	121.1	1.3	2,378.2	1.9
Municipal governments	71.6	0.8	938.8	0.7
Total expenditure	9,300.3	100.0	129,089.4	100.0

* Healthcare expenditures transferred from the federal government to provincial governments are regarded as provincial expenditures.
Source: CIHI, NHEX, 2011.

population. Given this demographic trend, it is estimated that the share of public healthcare expenditure spent on the population aged over 65 years will increase from 57.4% in 2000 to 70.2% in 2040. It is also expected that the healthcare expenditure per capita in 2040 will be 1.8 times that in 2000.

2. *Private healthcare expenditure.* Private healthcare expenditure is comprised of three distinct components: household expenditure, commercial and nonprofit insurance expenditure, and nonconsumption expenditure (including hospital revenues unrelated to patients and health studies). In 1988, household expenditure accounted for 58.1% of the private healthcare expenditure; this decreased to 48.4% by 2009 due to the rapid increase in the expenditures of commercial insurance companies (Figure 11.20).

Commercial health insurance expenditure per capita increased at a higher rate than other funding sources. Within 20 years, it had grown from C$139.40 per capita in 1988 to C$648.90 in 2009. During the same period, the household expenditure

TABLE 11.17   Federal, Provincial, and Local Shares of Public Healthcare Expenditure in Canada in 1960–2000

Year	Public Healthcare Expenditure (C$1 Million)	Annual Growth Rate (%)	Share of GNP (%)	Healthcare Expenditure Per Capita (C$)	Share of Total Healthcare Expenditure (%)
1960	904	–	2.4	50	42.2
1965	1,779	14.5	3.2	90	52.1
1970	4,392	19.8	5.0	206	70.2
1975	9,263	16.1	5.5	408	76.2
1980	16,695	12.5	5.5	694	74.7
1985	29,618	6.3	6.4	1,167	75.6
1990	33,422	6.4	6.6	1,586	77.3
1995	39,664	6.8	6.9	2,214	81.5
2000	41,643	7.3	7.1	3,168	86.9

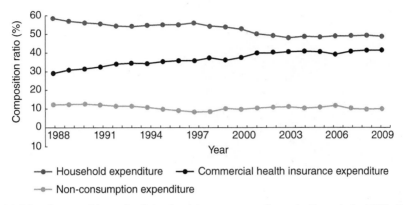

FIGURE 11.20 Composition of private healthcare expenditure in Canada in 1988–2009.

per capita increased from C$277.50 to C$761.60, while the nonconsumption expenditure per capita increased from C$60.70 to C$161.90 (Figure 11.21).

2. Capital Flow Healthcare funds are used for a variety of purposes, which can be divided into nine categories, including the purchase of healthcare products and services, provision of capital investment, management of public and commercial insurance plans, maintaining public health programs, and supporting research and development, and so forth. In 2009, hospitals accounted for the largest proportion (29.1%) of healthcare expenditure, followed by drugs (16.2%) and physicians (13.6%), as shown in Figure 11.22.

Figure 11.23 shows the dynamic changes in hospital, physician, and drug expenditures (calculated based on current prices) from 1975 to 2011. It is apparent that since 1997, the expenditure on hospital consumption has been increasing at a higher rate compared to physician and drug expenditures.

1. *Hospitals.* Hospitals play a leading role in the delivery of healthcare services. In the mid-1970s, hospitals accounted for approximately 45% of the total healthcare expenditure

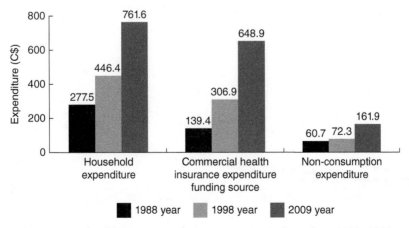

FIGURE 11.21 Private healthcare expenditure per capita in Canada in 1988, 1998, and 2009.

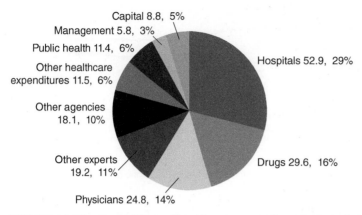

FIGURE 11.22   Capital flow of healthcare expenditure in Canada in 2009.

and 56% of the provincial healthcare expenditure. Over the past three decades, the share of hospitals in the total healthcare expenditure has decreased somewhat and has remained stable at about 29% since 2001. In 2009, provincial governments spent about C$47.4 billion on healthcare, accounting for 89.5% of hospital revenues, while the private sector spent C$4.85 billion, accounting for 9.2%.

2. *Drugs*. In 2009, the expenditure on prescription and nonprescription drugs (excluding drugs dispensed at hospitals and other healthcare institutions) was C$29.6 billion, of which prescription drugs accounted for 83.9%. In 1975, private-sector expenditure accounted for 79.5% of the expenditure on prescription drugs, which decreased to 52.3% in 1992 and remained relatively stable thereafter. Private-sector expenditure can be further divided into household and commercial health insurance expenditures. The latter accounts for a higher share and has increased gradually over time, whereas the former has decreased from 44.5% in 1988 to 32.4% in 2009.

3. *Physicians*. In 2009, C$24.8 billion was spent on physician services, which accounted for 13.6% of the total healthcare expenditure. Since 1975, the public sector has con-

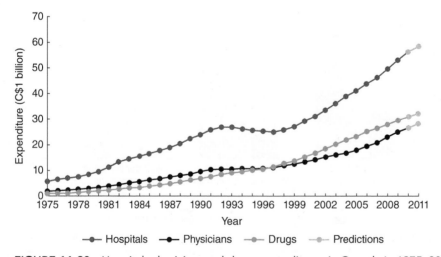

FIGURE 11.23   Hospital, physician, and drug expenditures in Canada in 1975–2011.

tributed more than 98% of the healthcare expenditure for physician services, which reached C$724 per capita in 2009. Private expenditure was almost completely dominated by household expenditure.

(3) Containment Policies and Priorities of Healthcare Expenditure

To date, Canada has not yet adopted a strong containment policy for healthcare expenditure, as its growth rate and share of GDP have been deemed to be more reasonable compared to other developed countries.

However, Canada has taken the following measures as part of a moderate healthcare cost-containment policy: (1) budgetary restrictions; (2) reassessing and continuously expanding the applicability of the private sector; (3) shifting healthcare delivery from facility care to regional care, and coordinating community-based healthcare services with social care services; and (4) enhancing health promotion activities.

Collaboration between governments, healthcare practitioners, NGOs, and individuals is necessary to meet the future needs of institutional reforms caused by various factors, such as population aging, the emergence of new diseases, advancement in medical technology, and the rise in medical expenses. Previously, the focus was on inpatient care in order to meet the demand for long-term care. However, the government is currently encouraging the expansion of out-of-hospital care services for the efficient use of limited resources in long-term care. Furthermore, a support system of family and friends is also needed because the implementation of this policy has led to a shortage of healthcare professionals. Due to the increasing demand for elderly care, the promotion of home-based care as a core element of long-term convalescent care has currently become a major issue in Canada.

SECTION III. THE HEALTH SYSTEM IN AUSTRALIA

Australia is a Commonwealth country located between the southwestern Pacific Ocean and the Indian Ocean. Its territories include Mainland Australia and Tasmania. Australia covers a total area of 7.682 million km² and consists of eight states. Among these, Western Australia is the largest state in terms of area. The Australian population grew rapidly after World War II. A census in 1981 reported that the total Australian population was approximately 14.92 million; by 2009, this had increased to 21.293 million. However, the distribution of the population is uneven across the country, with New South Wales having the largest population, accounting for about 35% of the total. In 2013, the total Australian population reached 23.13 million.

Australia has a well-developed economy. World Bank data showed that its GDP per capita in 2013 was about US$67,500. In 2012, the total healthcare expenditure in Australia accounted for about 9.1% of the GDP. The health status of its population is excellent. In 2012, the life expectancies of males and females were 79.9 and 84.4 years, respectively; in 2013, the maternal mortality rate was 6 per 100,000 live births, and the infant mortality rate was 3.4 per 1,000 live births. Australia also has relatively low crude birth rates, crude mortality rates, and 28-day neonatal mortality rates compared to other countries.

Australia previously implemented a universal, compulsory social health insurance scheme known as Medibank. However, following health reforms in 1984, a new health insurance system known as Medicare was established. Medicare funding is partly covered by general tax revenues and partly by the Medicare levy, the latter of which accounts for 1.5% of an individual's taxable income. In addition, private health insurance constitutes a large market share, accounting for about 11% of the total healthcare expenditure in Australia.

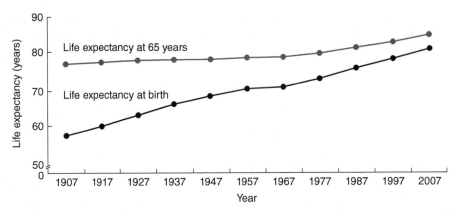

FIGURE 11.24 Trends in Australian life expectancy at birth and at 65 years from 1907 to 2007.

1. National Health Status and Current Challenges

(1) Overall Health Status

The life expectancy at birth in Australia has increased rapidly over the past century. Similarly, the life expectancy among elderly adults has increased significantly over the past few decades. Presently, the average life expectancy of males at 65 years is about 84 years, which is equivalent to the life expectancy at birth of females. The average life expectancy of females at 65 years old is 87 years. The trends in Australian life expectancy at birth and at 65 years from 1907 to 2007 are shown in Figure 11.24.

Australia's Health 2010 reported that the country was in the top one-third of the 29 Organisation for Economic Co-operation and Development (OECD) countries in terms of national health status, which was determined by the comparison of 30 health indicators. Specifically, Australia was in the top one-third for the majority of health indicators, with a few exceptions, such as obesity and infant mortality rate.

Moreover, Australia is a top-ranking country for some indicators, such as life expectancy, stroke mortality rate, and smoking prevalence among adults.

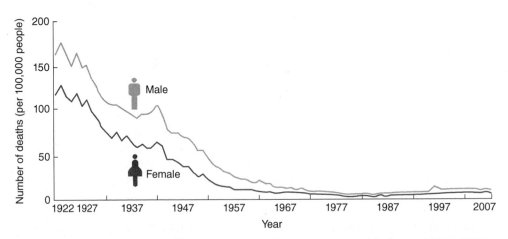

FIGURE 11.25 Trends in the mortality rates from diseases in Australia from 1922 to 2007.

For disease-related mortality, that of infectious diseases showed the most prominent, long-term trend of decline over the past few decades, largely due to improvements in living conditions and nutrition, vaccination, antibiotics, and other control measures. In the twentieth century, the mortality rate from infectious diseases fell by about 96% and dropped to the lowest point in history in the late 1970s, during which infectious diseases caused only about 5% of all disease-related deaths.

After the 1980s, the mortality rate from infectious diseases increased slightly due to the increase in the number of deaths from sepsis, AIDS, and hepatitis but has essentially remained stable after the late 1990s. In 2007, deaths from infectious diseases accounted for only slightly more than 1% of the total deaths in Australia compared to 15% in 1922 (Figure 11.25). However, infectious diseases remain common and still have the potential to become more severe.

(2) Health Distribution in Different Populations

The overall mortality rate varies considerably among the different populations in Australia. For instance, the mortality rate of Indigenous Australians is almost twice that of the entire Australian population. Furthermore, the mortality rate of the bottom one-fifth of the population in terms of socioeconomic status is 13% higher than the national level, and the mortality rate of the population living outside capital cities is 8% higher than the national level. In contrast, the mortality rate of foreign-born Australians is 6% lower than the national level, whereas the mortality rate of the top one-fifth of the population in terms of socioeconomic status is 17% lower than the national level, as shown in Figure 11.26.

The overall mortality rate of Indigenous Australians indicates that there is a ubiquitous and substantial disparity between their health status and that of other Australian populations. The mortality rates of indigenous males and females for several major diseases are significantly higher than that of males and females from other Australian populations. For instance, the mortality rate from cancer/tumors is 20% higher than that of other Australian populations, while the mortality rate from diabetes is six times the rate in other populations. In addition, the higher disease-related mortality rates among Indigenous Australians are not limited to just a few diseases; the life expectancies of indigenous males and females are 12 and 10 years shorter than those of their counterparts in other Australian populations.

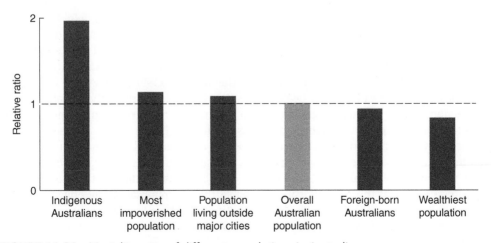

FIGURE 11.26 Mortality rates of different populations in Australia.

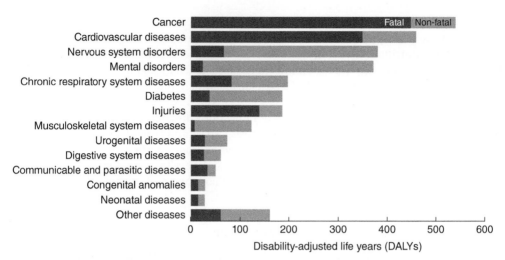

FIGURE 11.27 Predicted fatal and nonfatal burden of major disease types in Australia in 2010.

The health status of Australians in different socioeconomic groups also varies significantly. In addition to the significant disparity in health between the lowest and highest socioeconomic groups, the health status of the middle-class population also shows a clear stratification. As with the Indigenous Australians, the range of health vulnerabilities is very broad. Australians of low socioeconomic status, in particular, pose serious challenges to public health and society because of the large size of its population.

Using individuals aged 15–64 years in 2002–2006, as an example, the mortality rate of the lowest socioeconomic group was 70% higher than that of the highest socioeconomic group.

The most impoverished groups also have a significantly higher prevalence for many diseases and health risk factors compared to the wealthiest. Social stratification has a strong effect on health status in most circumstances, and the latter appears to improve linearly with socioeconomic status. One exception is alcohol consumption, which is a risk factor that is not significantly correlated with socioeconomic status.

(3) Healthcare Challenges

In 2010, cancer was the main burden of disease and injury in Australia, which was even significantly higher than that of cardiovascular disease. The fatality of cancer and cardiovascular disease are still much more severe than diseases that are ranked third and fourth. However, mental disorders, which are ranked fourth in disease burden, have a much greater prevalence and disability burden than do any other disease, as shown in Figure 11.27.

The main purpose of primary healthcare is to help people maintain their health and life satisfaction. From a systems perspective, it also prevents patients from being admitted to the hospital. Under normal circumstances, health issues must be appropriately managed to prevent unnecessary hospitalization. These include infectious diseases that can be prevented through vaccination, acute diseases (e.g., ear infections and severe gastroenteritis), and chronic diseases (e.g., diabetes, emphysema, and related complications). Although the prevention of hospitalization due to these health issues is possible, their hospitalization rates have increased from 2002–2003 to 2007–2008. It is worth noting that these increments were associated with geographic remoteness and low socioeconomic status, as shown in Figure 11.28.

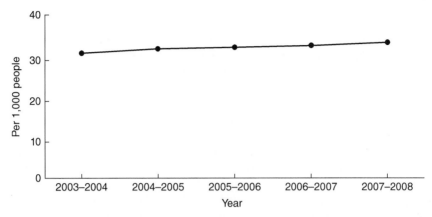

FIGURE 11.28   Trends in avoidable hospitalization rates in Australia from 2003–2004 to 2007–2008.

The median waiting time for elective surgeries rose from 28 days to 34 days within the five years from 2003–2004 to 2007–2008. Patients living in remote areas had the longest waiting time by far, while the top one-fifth of the population in terms of socioeconomic status had the shortest waiting time. Furthermore, coronary artery bypass surgery had the shortest median waiting time (14 days), whereas knee replacement had the longest median waiting time (156 days). The median waiting time for tumor surgeries is 20 days, as shown in Figure 11.29.

In recent years, Australia has performed poorly in terms of the following aspects of healthcare: (1) the incidence of unsafe needle-sharing among injecting drug users; (2) utilization rate of antibiotics for the treatment of upper respiratory tract infections among GPs (upper respiratory tract infections are generally caused by viruses, which do not respond to antibiotics); (3) screening rates for breast cancer and cervical cancer; (4) waiting time for emergency care at hospitals; and (5) incidence of adverse events at hospitals.

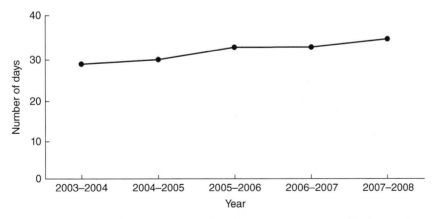

FIGURE 11.29   Median waiting time for elective surgeries at public hospitals in Australia from 2003–2004 to 2007–2008.

2. Health Service System

Australia is a federal state where the Department of Health (affiliated with the federal government) is responsible for overseeing the country's healthcare system. It is responsible for not only providing public health services, such as quarantine but also formulating and implementing nationwide healthcare service plans and policies, providing specialized scientific services, and financially supporting some healthcare services provided by other agencies. All eight states have health departments, known as public health associations, which are charged with overseeing healthcare in their respective regions.

These associations have the following four functions: healthcare management at the state level, construction of healthcare networks in small- and medium-sized cities and rural areas, community healthcare centers, and private healthcare services. Each of these functions is delegated to a corresponding society affiliated with the public health association. These societies engage in government healthcare planning, which is then implemented by their subordinate units after being reviewed by the State Council. Each society is composed of members of various disciplines that represent the interests of different population strata. They serve as organizations for the coordination between healthcare institutions and governments.

(1) Community Health Services

Community health services have a long history in Australia, which initially originated from infant healthcare. Australia established its first infant healthcare center in 1914, after which the Australian states began carrying out campaigns to promote the establishment of healthcare centers. School health services can be traced even further back to 1907. However, community health services only began to gain support from other government departments in the early 1970s. In 1972, the government began to engage in community health planning and to emphasize public health work. By 1973, community health services in Australia truly began to undergo rapid development alongside the formulation of the Australian Community Health Plan, which advocated for the establishment of multidisciplinary healthcare service systems to provide health protection for people living in designated areas.

There are various types of community healthcare agencies in Australia, the largest of which are known as integrated community healthcare centers. Other types of community healthcare agencies include women's healthcare centers, maternal and child health centers, Indigenous Australian healthcare centers, community mental health centers, and community care centers.

Australia is divided into communities, based on geographical location, population size, and traffic, for the purpose of establishing healthcare agencies. These agencies include community healthcare centers, rehabilitation centers, children's healthcare centers, geriatric care centers, mental health centers, prenatal clinics, nursing homes, and so on. The aforementioned agencies may or may not provide beds depending on their service functions. In some places, community healthcare centers are established in general or specialist hospitals, which ensure that community health services form a major component of hospital work.

1. Management of Community Healthcare Centers   Community healthcare centers are planned and constructed by the government and administered by management committees elected by the residents of the respective communities. The management committee appoints the person-in-charge of the center once every five years. Each year, the government organizes relevant personnel to review these centers.

2. Staffing of Community Healthcare Center Each community healthcare center serves a population of 20,000–60,000 people and generally comprises 40–100 workers, who are mainly multidisciplinary healthcare workers such as physicians, dentists, nurses, social workers, public health advocates, project staff, and administrative staff. In addition, some centers also provide interpreters for immigrants. Physicians, nurses, and dentists are licensed medical practitioners employed by these centers as nonpermanent workers and remunerated according to the services they provide and their performance. Community healthcare centers aim to protect and improve the health of residents living in their respective communities. Although the scale, content, and administrative agencies of community health services vary greatly across different states, they share the same core principles and values. Community healthcare centers are mainly responsible for meeting the healthcare needs of residents living in the respective communities; ensuring the equality and accessibility of services; bringing services closer to people's lives and work; overcoming economic, geographical, and cultural barriers; and providing comprehensive and integrated services. Community healthcare centers are also required to encourage residents and community groups to actively participate in discussions and decision-making on public health issues and their own healthcare issues, and to establish a coordination mechanism for multidisciplinary collaboration.

3. Content of Community Health Services Community healthcare centers are typically the closest healthcare venues for residents. The main services they offer are simple treatments for diseases and general healthcare services for community residents; setting up home-based hospital beds for general nursing care; providing geriatric care and home visits for the elderly; providing preventive care services, such as vaccinations for children and medical examinations for pregnant women; providing various forms of health consultations and health education that are informative and practical for different groups at different periods in time; conducting healthcare-related, community welfare services, such as referrals, regular physical examinations, and follow-ups; providing health education for adolescents, such as psychological counseling and sex education; and providing education and psychological counseling for drug addicts.

4. Characteristics of Community Health Services As the public health component of the primary healthcare system in Australia, community health services have the following characteristics:

1. *The simultaneous development of community health services and the economy in Australia.* Both federal and state governments jointly share the expenditure for the construction and operation of community healthcare centers in Australia. The state governments plan and organize the establishment and distribution of community healthcare centers. All constructions or renovations of community healthcare centers proposed by the state public health associations (i.e., the state health departments) that meet the requirements of regional health plans are included in the government's annual fiscal plans. The government also allocates operating budgets to these centers annually based on the service scope and population size. Healthcare expenditures are borne by the government, such that residents can access a series of free services, such as medical treatment, healthcare, and preventive care, by using a medical card at any community healthcare center in Australia.
2. *Community healthcare centers have a comprehensive and standardized management system.* Every community healthcare center in Australia has a strict staffing system, whereby

GPs employed by the centers can be freely transferred to other centers at any time, whereas other staff members are relatively permanent. Every staff member in the center has clear responsibilities and duties. The affairs of each center are managed by a director who is appointed and supervised by the administrative committee comprising representatives of local residents. The committee may decide to continue or discontinue the director's appointment based on an annual assessment of their performance. Other staff members of the center are paid according to their performance.

3. *Diversified community health services.* About one-third of the staff members of community healthcare centers are involved in the delivery of health education to residents. Many of them are health advocates, such as advocates for chronic noncommunicable diseases, drug abuse counselors, adolescent counselors, or health policy advisors. Community healthcare centers are also equipped with educational materials, such as cameras, video recorders, and sound players and produce hundreds of thousands of dollars' worth of color-printed advocacy materials. Each center is also equipped with vehicles that enable staff to travel to every corner of the community for advocacy work. In addition to healthcare-related tasks, these centers also provide basic healthcare services (simple treatments) for residents; psychological counseling for the elderly, children, women, and individuals with mental disorders; and services for individuals with disabilities and drug addicts.

4. *Bridging patients and hospitals.* Community healthcare centers are frontline contact points that are located within the community, directly providing residents with health-care services, serving as gatekeepers of general and specialist hospitals. Residents who need referrals or other healthcare services must be referred by their respective community healthcare center or GP in order to receive treatment at higher-level hos-pitals and to access the healthcare benefits provided by the government. As GPs are located within the community, they tend to have a close relationship with residents as a result of their long-term contact, which gives GPs a better understanding of residents' healthcare needs. Residents, in turn, place much greater trust in these centers and their own GPs than in other healthcare institutions and physicians. Regardless of their place of residence, residents first consult their GPs when necessary before deciding whether to seek further medical attention and medication. Community healthcare centers and GPs then refer patients to higher-level hospitals for medical treatment and provide follow-up care services for discharged patients, thereby serving as a bridge between the patients and hospitals.

5. *Implementation of preventive care.* These centers and their affiliated GPs are responsible for providing prenatal and postnatal check-ups for, and visits to, pregnant women living in communities; vaccinations for infants and one-time physical examinations for children; and annual physical examinations for residents or periodic physical examina-tions entrusted by hospitals. These preventive care services have been institutionalized and effectively implemented.

6. *Separation of medical and preventive care services.* Community GPs provide the more basic healthcare services, whereas community healthcare centers provide other healthcare services, such as preventive care, health protection, rehabilitation, and health edu-cation. The majority of these centers neither have designated GPs and nor provide therapeutic services. Furthermore, GPs and community health services have differ-ent funding sources: The former are independent practitioners funded by the federal government via the health insurance scheme, while the latter are funded by state and local governments. Hence, it can be difficult to achieve the organic integration of the

TABLE 11.18 Number of Public and Private Hospitals in the States (Territories) of Australia In 2009–2010 (Unit: Hospitals)

Category	New South Wales	Victoria	Queensland	Western Australia	South Australia	Tasmania	Australian Capital Territory	Northern Territory	Total
Public hospitals	226	150	17	95	80	24	3	5	753
Private hospitals	173	161	106	55	56	8	12	2	573
Total	399	311	276	150	136	32	15	7	1326

two. GPs receive remuneration based on the fee-for-service (FFS) payment system, which is not conducive to preventive services because it encourages the overprovision of therapeutic services.

5. Funding System for Community Health Services   The healthcare expenditure in Australia is mainly supported by the following three sources. (1) Medicare levy: Taxpayers who earn above a certain income level must pay a Medicare levy of 1.4% of their taxable income as part of the social health insurance (public sector). (2) Supplementary health insurance: Each person can choose a health insurance scheme that best suits them and pay the corresponding insurance premiums (private sector). (3) Federal and state health-care funds: The federal and state governments allocate a certain percentage of various taxes each year to subsidize the health insurance system. However, the federal and state funds are intended for different purposes. The former is mainly used for primary healthcare services provided by GPs; emergency care services at hospitals; and supporting basic, clinical, and public health research. In contrast, the latter is used for secondary and tertiary services at hospitals (including specialist services). The healthcare resources are allocated in accordance with the resource allocation formula. For example, New South Wales implements an allocation system in which healthcare resources are allocated by the state health department to district health service management centers, which in turn allocate these resources to each healthcare institution.

(2) Hospital Services

1. Overview of Healthcare Institutions and Service Utilization   There are two types of hospitals in Australia. (1) Public hospitals: There are 753 federal-, state-, or district-owned hospitals funded by the government, which account for 80% of hospital beds. (2) Private hospitals: There are 573 private hospitals founded by individuals or cofounded by several individuals, which account for 20% of hospital beds in Australia.

In 2002, the number of hospital beds per capita was relatively high, at around 8.26 beds per 1,000 people. By 2008, this had decreased to about 3.78 beds per 1,000 people, with a total of 81,163 hospital beds (Table 11.18 and Table 11.19).

In 2009–2010, there was a total of 54,812 beds in public acute hospitals, 2,088 beds in public psychiatric hospitals, 2,260 beds in private day-only hospitals, and 25,778 beds in other private hospitals in Australia. The number of hospital beds in Australia increased

TABLE 11.19 Statistics on Different Types of Public Hospitals in Australia in 2009–2010

Type of hospital	Location			Number of Hospitals Total	Service Provided				Average Number of Beds	Average Number of Discharged Patients	Average Length of Hospital Stay (Days)	Non-emergency Workers (%)	Number of Ar-Drg (5+) Cases Per Hospital
	Major Cities	Designated Areas	Remote Areas		Emergency Department	Accident and Emergency Care	Outpatient Services	Elective Surgeries					
Core hospitals responsible for admitting referral patients	50	24	1	75	75	75	74	74	413	43,591	3.3	8.4	454
Maternal and child health specialist hospitals	11	0	0	11	9	9	11	11	199	20,635	3.1	0.4	231
Large-sized hospitals	26	16	1	43	41	41	38	36	142	15,190	3	13.9	265
Medium-sized hospitals	23	69	0	92	30	76	8	46	64	5,899	3.1	23.2	143
Small-sized acute hospitals	0	116	38	154	20	146	2	20	22	1,218	3.1	9.1	51
Psychiatric hospitals	13	4	0	17	0	0	0	0	123	658	58.8	52.4	10
Rehabilitation hospitals	6	2	0	8	0	0	1	1	69	975	21.8	90.8	13
Nursery schools	8	0	0	8	0	0	0	0	26	1,681	3.7	0	9
Small-sized nonacute hospitals	16	54	13	83	3	61	1	3	32	805	11	71.8	30
Integrated care agencies	0	45	33	78	0	70	0	0	12	346	3.9	29.1	13
Others	28	86	70	184	6	122	0	1	11	284	9.7	79.3	7
Total	181	416	156	753	184	600	135	192	76	6,716	3.6	17.1	98

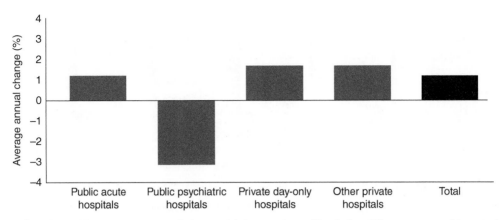

FIGURE 11.30 Average annual change in the number of beds for different types of hospitals in Australia from 2005–2006 to 2009–2010.

by 3.3% from 80,828 beds in 2005–2006 to 84,938 beds in 2009–2010, with an average annual growth rate of 1.2% (Figure 11.30).

In 2002, Australia had 1,796 days of hospital stay per 1,000 people, with a hospital bed utilization rate of 81.5%. In the same year, the average hospital stay per 1,000 self-pay patients was 318 days, with a hospital bed utilization rate of 61.7%. Private hospitals consist entirely of self-pay patients, whereas 50% of patients at public hospitals are self-pay patients with special healthcare needs. As of 2008, the average length of hospital stay in Australia was six days.

The service volume of hospitals in Australia, especially private hospitals, increased steadily in the decade before 2007–2008. During this period, the number of hospital stays in private and public hospitals increased by 67% and 23%, respectively, with an overall increment of 37%. After correcting for population growth, the hospitalization rate in private and public hospitals also increased by 40% and 5%, respectively (Figure 11.31).

Aside from hospitals, other institutions provide similar services in Australia, such as nursing homes. Nursing homes operate in compliance with federal regulations, whereby their standard fees are set by the Department of Health. Nursing homes are jointly

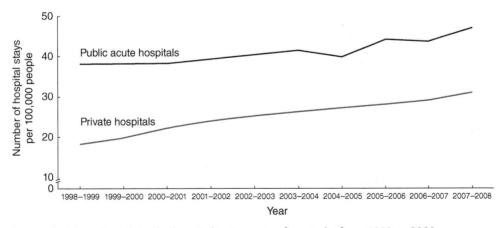

FIGURE 11.31 Trends in the hospitalization rate of Australia from 1998 to 2008.

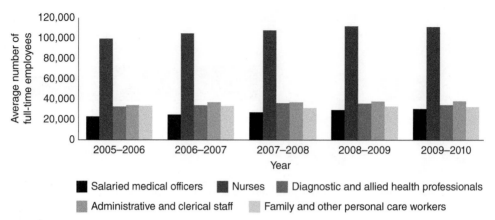

FIGURE 11.32 Number of full-time employees at public hospitals in Australia from 2005–2006 to 2009–2010.

administered by the federal and state governments, but only the latter are responsible for supervising, licensing, and providing funds to these institutions. In Australia, the expenditures devoted to the elderly are allocated for pensions (63%), inpatient care (15%), nursing homes (10%), and community-based elderly care (3%) (Kendig and Duckett, 2001).

Most nursing homes are run by the private sector and mainly serve chronic patients and the elderly. These institutions must comply with various rules and regulations laid down by the Parliament of Australia, such as the minimum number of hours and staff for nursing care. Nursing homes are usually established within rehabilitation facilities to serve as places for long-term inpatient care.

Nursing homes are gradually being regarded as the most suitable places for providing medical services to chronic patients and the elderly in Australia. The degree of population aging is very high in Australia, where the elderly aged over 70 years account for nearly 15% of the total population. Nursing homes attach great importance to elderly care services, including therapeutic services, psychological counseling, domestic care, functional exercises, and so on. The government spends approximately A$158 per hospital bed-day for each elderly inpatient.

2. Healthcare Workforce In 2009–2010, there were approximately 251,000 full-time employees in Australian public hospitals. In 2008–2009, there were more than 52,000 employees in private hospitals. Hospital staff include medical officers (e.g., surgeons, anesthetists, and other specialists), nurses, diagnostic and allied health professionals (e.g., physiotherapists and occupational therapists), administrative and clerical staff, and family and other personal care workers. However, the data here do not cover short-term contracted physicians or most medical officers working in private hospitals (Figure 11.32).

In 2009–2010, nurses constituted the largest proportion (45%) of full-time employees at public hospitals, while medical officers and diagnostic and allied health professionals accounted for 12% and 14%, respectively.

From 2005–2006 to 2009–2010, the number of salaried medical officers increased at an average annual growth rate of 7.5% to 31,000, while the number of nurses increased to 114,000 at an average annual growth rate of 3.6%.

The composition of employees at private hospitals differs from that in public hospitals because most healthcare services in the former are not provided by hospital staff. Additionally, public hospitals have a different scope of healthcare services. In 2008–2009,

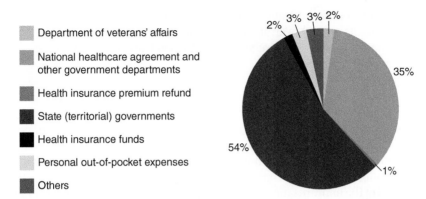

FIGURE 11.33   Funding sources of public hospitals in Australia in 2008–2009.

nurses constituted the largest proportion (60%) of full-time employees at private hospitals, while medical officers and diagnostic and allied health professionals each accounted for 7%.

3. Funding Sources of Hospital Expenditures   Public and private hospitals in Australia have different compositions of funding sources, which reflects the differences in target patients and services provided. Emergency and outpatient services are mainly funded by the government, whereas inpatient services are generally jointly funded by private (nongovernmental) and governmental agencies.

The statistical data here are mainly based on the original funding sources rather than the direct source. For example, the federal funds allocated to state (territorial) governments or tax credits granted by the federal government to commercial health insurance companies are considered federal funds.

In general, the majority of funding for public hospitals comes from the state (territorial) governments and the federal government of Australia. The proportion of federal funds declined from 2004–2005 to 2006–2007, and then increased in 2008–2009. On the other hand, commercial health insurance and patient out-of-pocket expenses are mainly spent in private hospitals (Figure 11.33, Figure 11.34).

(3) Public Health and Other Services

Federal, state, and local governments are all responsible for providing public health services, predominantly the latter two. However, in recent years, the federal government has expanded its role, mainly by formulating and coordinating national policies, legislation, planning, and

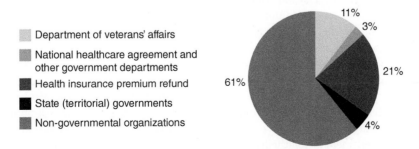

FIGURE 11.34   Funding sources of private hospitals in Australia in 2008–2009.

health standards through the National Health and Medical Research Council (NHMRC), thereby enhancing its control over disease surveillance, disease prevention, rational use of drugs, occupational health, environmental health, food nutrition, poisoning, pesticides, and so on.

1. Prevention and Treatment of Infectious and Chronic Diseases   The government of Australia is placing increasing emphasis on health promotion and disease prevention. Specific preventive services include infant and child care, school health, dental and ophthalmic services, water fluoridation, immunization programs, antismoking campaigns, national AIDS programs, and national drug abuse prevention programs, as well as health education and health promotion programs administered by state health departments. In terms of the immunization programs for children, the child immunization rate in Victoria is over 70%, whereas areas such as Kirra (Queensland) have a more desirable child immunization rate of up to 96%. Primary school children must be immunized at schools for the prevention of rubella, while women are required to be immunized at least three months before conception to prevent congenital damage to the brain, eyes, ears, and heart of the fetus due to rubella infection in pregnancy. All immunization services are provided free of charge.

Common infectious diseases are rare in Australia. Therefore, there has been a shift in focus towards the prevention and control of chronic diseases that are closely related to social factors and lifestyles, such as heart disease, cerebrovascular diseases, malignant tumors, chronic obstructive pulmonary disease (COPD), and diabetes. The Department of Health, nongovernmental healthcare agencies, and public organizations are enhancing the screening and early diagnosis of these diseases, while also actively implementing health advocacy and educational activities for the public.

2. Environmental Health Services   Australia provides a number of environmental health services, including water quality, air quality, noise control, waste disposal, food hygiene, and consumer product safety, in order to control health-related environmental factors. All levels of government in Australia employ health inspectors who are responsible for carrying out these tasks. In recent years, environmental health services in Australia have been expanded to include urban planning, architectural design, transportation systems, factories, housing density, and so on.

3. Occupational Health Services   According to the Australian Bureau of Statistics, there are nearly 400 work-related deaths each year in Australia. In order to reduce occupational hazards, state governments have adopted several interventional measures, such as establishing workplace mandatory health and safety (WHS) standards, implementing the Comcare and Seacare Legislation Amendment, and enacting various laws and regulations for work-related injuries. In addition, state governments have also enhanced the education and training of occupational health and safety for both employers and employees.

4. Health Promotion Services   In addition to the public health programs for diseases, the government of Australia attaches great importance to interventional measures for health risk factors, such as smoking, alcohol consumption, drug abuse, poor dietary habits, and physical inactivity. The government of Australia is clearly aware that investing in health promotion not only helps to improve population health and the labor force but also directly reduces the government's healthcare expenditures. Joint efforts among the federal, state,

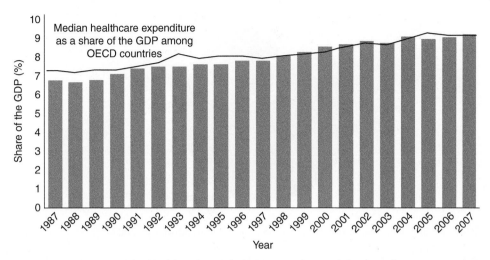

FIGURE 11.35 Australia's healthcare expenditure as a share of the GDP from 1987 to 2007.

and territorial governments in health promotion have yielded significant outcomes, mainly reflected in the decline in the mortality rates from chronic diseases, such as cardiovascular and cerebrovascular diseases, the control of blood-borne infections, and the decline in the mortality rate from road traffic accidents.

5. Healthcare Services in Remote Areas   Australia has a vast and sparsely populated inland region. To provide healthcare services to residents living in these areas, the government founded an agency with the first air medical service in the world. This agency was founded in 1928 and has since established an air medical service network consisting of "flying doctors" to cover the vast inland areas of South Australia and northeastern Queensland. These flying doctors either fly by themselves or take a flight from the central base, during which they communicate with patients via radio equipment. The agency is equipped with 40 light aircraft at 17 bases across the country, and physicians can reach the majority of patients within two hours. Most patients can be treated by the flying doctors themselves, but patients who are critically ill or who require inpatient treatment can be transported by the flying doctors to nearby hospitals by air. The service team travels about 12 million km each year to serve about 200,000 patients. Australia's air medical service is the oldest, largest, and most experienced air emergency center in the world.

(4) Healthcare Expenditure and Flow

In recent years, Australia has seen a very steady increase in healthcare expenditure as a share of the GDP. In the fiscal year 2007–2008, the healthcare expenditure in Australia was A$103.563 billion, accounting for 9.1% of the GDP. In the past decade, Australia has shown a medium level of healthcare expenditure as a share of the GDP among OECD countries. In 2007–2008, Australia's healthcare expenditure as a share of the GDP was higher than that of the UK (8.4%), lower than that of the US (16%), and close to the median of OECD countries (Figure 11.35).

As of 2007–2008, hospitals have consistently shown the greatest contribution to total healthcare expenditure. Specifically, hospital expenditures accounted for 39% of recurrent healthcare expenditure, which in turn accounted for 95% of the total healthcare expenditure. This is followed by the healthcare services provided by individual practitioners

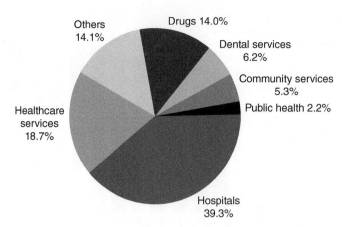

FIGURE 11.36 Recurrent healthcare expenditures in Australia in 2007–2008 (calculated at current prices).

(including GPs and specialists), which accounted for 19% of the recurrent healthcare expenditures, while drug expenditures accounted for about 14% (Figure 11.36).

The Australian health authorities have clearly recognized the importance of public health, which includes preventive care and health promotion. Government expenditure on public health has continued to rise over the years, reaching A$2.159 billion in 2007–2008, which accounts for 2.2% of recurrent expenditures of that year and represents an increase of 2.0% compared to the previous year. This increase was mostly attributed to immunization programs, especially against human papillomavirus (HPV). The government spends a considerable share of public health funding on immunization and control measures against other infectious diseases; this share was 45% in 2007–2008. In addition, the government spent approximately A$367 million on health promotion activities, which accounted for about 17% of the total public health expenditure (Figure 11.37).

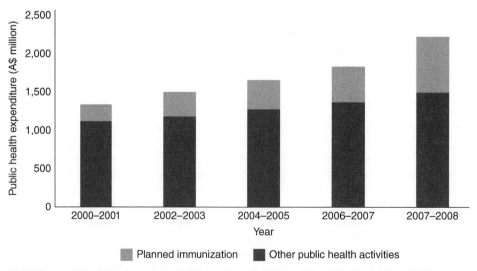

FIGURE 11.37 Government public health expenditure from 2000–2001 to 2007–2008.

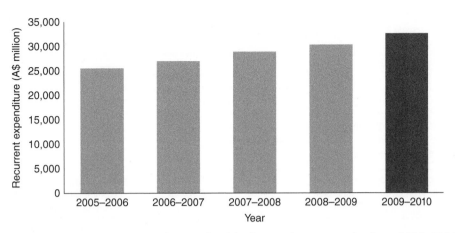

FIGURE 11.38 Recurrent expenditure of public hospitals in Australia from 2005–2006 to 2009–2010 (after adjusting for inflation).

Hospital expenditures consist of recurrent and capital expenditures. The former refers to annual expenses on goods and services, such as salaries, whereas the latter refers to expenses for construction and large-scale equipment.

In 2009–2010, the recurrent expenditure of public hospitals in Australia was A\$33.706 billion (excluding currency depreciation), which represents an increment of 3.7% compared to 2008–2009 (after correcting for inflation). More than 62% of this expenditure (A\$21.099 billion) was spent on salaries. About 70% of the recurrent expenditure could be attributed to inpatient services rather than emergency, outpatient or nonhospitalization services or other hospital activities (Figure 11.38).

In 2008–2009, the recurrent expenditure of private hospitals was A\$8.137 billion (excluding currency depreciation), of which A\$4.124 billion (about 51%) was used to pay salaries. From 2005–2006 to 2009–2010, the average annual growth rate in recurrent expenditure for private hospitals was 2.4% (after correcting for inflation).

3. Universal Health Insurance System

Australia's health insurance system is comprised of two components: the universal health insurance system, Medicare, and commercial health insurance. Medicare is a form of universal insurance that guarantees access of all residents to essential healthcare services at reasonable prices. It is primarily provided by government-affiliated healthcare institutions (i.e., public hospitals), which are administered by the respective state health departments. They are jointly funded by the federal and state governments mainly through federal and state taxes, as well as National Health Insurance (NHI), which is supported by payroll taxes. In addition to implementing Medicare, the Australian government has also encouraged the development of commercial health insurance. Currently, there are nearly 50 commercial health insurance agencies, among which 18 operate nationwide, while the rest are limited to one or two states. Together, Medicare and commercial health insurance form the healthcare and insurance systems of Australia, as shown in Figure 11.39.

In the 1970s, Australian law stipulated that permanent residents or citizens and lawful residents of Australia, whether rich or poor, are entitled to Medicare coverage. This gave them access to free essential healthcare services and inpatient services at public hospitals, as well as free services provided by community healthcare centers. Medicare recipients can

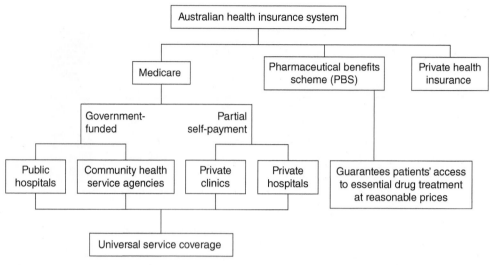

FIGURE 11.39 Australian health insurance system.

only be admitted to public hospitals and do not have the right to choose specific hospitals, physicians, facilities, and wards. Additionally, with the exception of emergency cases, such as road traffic accidents, they are not entitled to priority treatment and hospitalization and hence must queue in order of appointment. However, Medicare has received widespread approval as it guarantees the access of Australians to basic healthcare services.

(1) Medicare Institutions and Their Functions

In 1984, the Parliament of Australia established the universal, socialized Medicare scheme, to be administered by the Health Insurance Commission (HIC). The HIC was established by the Parliament in August 1974 and is an independent legal institution that initially administered the Medibank program (the predecessor of Medicare), which came into effect on July 1, 1975. At that time, the Australian government aimed to develop the private health insurance industry in order to enhance the competitiveness and vitality of the private health insurance market, thereby addressing the shortcomings of public socialized health insurance. As a result, the private Medibank was officially established on October 1, 1976, and placed under the administration of the HIC. Following the abolition of the national Medibank in November 1978, the private Medibank became the sole health insurance program under the administration of the HIC. However, when the new government took office in 1983, they began to seek the restoration of public health insurance. On February 1, 1984, it officially launched the Medicare scheme, which was administered by the HIC. Since then, the policy orientation of Medicare and other relevant government plans must be jointly formulated by the Department of Health and HIC, while the HIC is responsible for formulating and implementing the operational strategies of Medicare. In contrast, the private Medibank must compete directly with other private health insurance agencies without government financial subsidies.

The HIC (renamed Medicare Australia in 2005) is an independent functional department working in parallel with the Department of Health, but the managing director of the HIC is not a cabinet member. The organizational structure of the HIC consists of chief executives and general and state managers. Currently, the HIC employs approximately 4,800 staff members, of whom about 750 work in the National Office headquartered in Canberra, while the rest work in state offices. The number of staff members assigned to state offices is based on the population size of each state, as the workload is directly proportional to the population size (i.e., the number of insured persons). There are six branch offices (one in each state) and seven divisions under the National Office: the Financial Management Division, Human Resource Division, Information Technology Services Division, Consultancy Services Division, Program Review Division, Government Program Division, and Private Medibank Division. Each division is headed by a general manager, who is assisted by several managers in completing daily managerial tasks and program implementation. The National Office also has an Office of the Commission Secretary and the Audit and Risk Assurance Services Branch that are directly affiliated with the Managing Director. The National Office serves to provide Medicare with the following support services: corporate support, information technology support, and consultancy services.

The primary roles of the HIC are as follows: (1) establish and administer federal healthcare programs; (2) oversee financial operations and management of Medicare (i.e., publicly funded healthcare); (3) administer the Pharmaceutical Benefit Scheme (PBS); (4) manage the Medicare computer system; (5) review and reimburse personal medical subsidies; (6) engage in epidemic prevention and registration management (including child immunization programs); (7) implement overseas student health coverage (via the private Medibank); (8) perform GP registration; (9) conduct licensure and approval of inspection centers; and (10) coordinate among relevant commissions in related departments. The newer roles of the HIC include the management of childcare plans for employment issues, as well as the prevention, investigation, and handling of misconduct.

Each state office of the HIC is headed by a state manager, who is charged with overseeing the operation of all service points and processing centers in the state. The main roles of these state offices are to ensure proper usage of healthcare funds, formulate regional health plans, and supervise the registration of healthcare workers.

There are 268 service centers and 10 processing centers throughout Australia, which are responsible for the reimbursement of medical expenses, cash transfers, and processing of relevant affairs.

The Program Review Division is a special agency that works independently under the Managing Director. It has branches in all states to assist state managers in investigating misconduct. The primary role of this division is to investigate and supervise inappropriate claims made by policyholders (residents) and misconduct by healthcare workers during the delivery of healthcare services. The ultimate goal of the Program Review Division is to prevent and rectify misconduct related to health insurance through supervision and education, and thereby encourage reasonable practices.

(2) Payment Methods for Medicare Premiums

Health insurance in Australia mainly takes the form of national insurance, which is supplemented by private insurance, thus achieving the coexistence between public and private health insurance agencies. It is mainly supported by public funds. The Health Insurance Act 1973 stipulated that every citizen has equal opportunity to enroll in health insurance, and that it is compulsory for every resident to participate in public health insurance, which gives them access to basic healthcare services free of charge at public hospitals. However, owing to the large disparities in the income of insured persons, the insurance premiums they contribute should also vary accordingly. The specific approach adopted is as follows: First, each insured person must pay a fixed amount (base premium) as part of the "insurance fund"; second, each insured person must contribute 3% of their salary as a "basic premium"; finally, insured persons must pay a variable "progressive insurance premium" based on their salary, whereby high-, medium-, and low-income earners contribute 5%, 3%, and 1% of their salaries, respectively. The government then subsidizes 30% of health insurance expenses.

(3) Medicare Benefits

Australia has established a GP network wherein patients with minor illnesses must seek medical attention from contracted GPs, who in turn may refer patients to specialists or public hospitals whenever necessary. All medical expenses incurred are paid by the federal Medicare Benefits Advisory Committee.

Both public and private hospitals in Australia have comprehensive facilities, advanced technology, and first-class services. At public hospitals, outpatients and inpatients are entitled to all facilities and services free of charge (including meals during hospitalization). However, since public hospitals only provide basic healthcare services, nonemergency and chronic patients often have long waiting times.

Patients with greater financial means may opt for private physicians or private hospitals for faster and better healthcare services. However, they are entitled to only 75% of reimbursement, with the remaining amount being borne by private insurance or the patients themselves. The government imposes strict regulations on the fee standards of all service items at private hospitals and does not permit overcharging. The fee standards are jointly formulated by the Department of Health, HIC, and Australian Medical Association.

In addition, the Australian law prohibits the sale of drugs at private hospitals and clinics. Therefore, the government introduced the PBS, which provides pharmaceutical subsidies to all residents. All residents aged over 18 years are eligible for a Medicare card, which they can use to obtain discounted prices when purchasing drugs. There are two types of PBS recipients. The first type consists of ordinary individuals who do not receive government aid. They must pay for prescription drugs costing ≤A$20; as for prescription drugs costing >A$20, patients must make a copayment of A$20, and the remaining balance is covered by the government. The second type of recipients are low-income earners who receive government aid. They must pay A$3.2 per prescription but no more than A$166.40 per year.

(4) Scope of Medicare Coverage

Medicare covers a wide range of healthcare services.

1. Services Covered by Medicare

1. All outpatient services at public hospitals are provided free of charge.
2. 85% of the medical expenses for inpatient services listed in the Medicare Benefits Schedule (MBS).
3. 385% of the medical expenses for outpatient services listed in the MBS. The MBS lists government-set prices based on the principle of fairness for both patients and physicians. Here, out-of-hospital healthcare services refer to services provided by registered practitioners (e.g., GPs, consultant physicians, specialists).
4. All inpatient expenses for a "public" patient (who is entitled to free services) at designated public hospitals, and all expenses for therapeutic services provided by designated physicians (this implies that the patient does not have the right to choose a preferred physician or hospital, the time of admission, or the time of surgery).
5. All laboratory tests and X-rays for "public" patients at public hospitals.

6. 75% of the expenses for MBS-listed healthcare services for "private" patients (patients with special needs) at public hospitals.
7. According to the MBS ophthalmology reimbursement list, the expenses for vision examinations by an optometrist are partially reimbursable, but the patient must pay for glasses or contact lenses.
8. 75% of the treatment and operational expenses incurred by oral surgeons at hospitals (excluding services provided by general dentists).

2. Services not Covered by Medicare
1. Hospitalization expenses for private patients, such as inpatient fees, theater fees, and certain pharmaceutical fees
2. Dental treatment fees
3. Ambulance service fees
4. General care fees
5. Acupuncture (unless prescribed by a qualified physician), speech therapy, chiropractic services, podiatry services, medical nutrition therapy, physiotherapies, clinical psycho-therapy, and so on
6. Equipment such as eyeglasses or contact lenses, prosthetic limbs, and hearing aids, and medical devices such as medical air compressors and blood glucose meters
7. Medical and inpatient expenses incurred overseas
8. Surgeries solely for cosmetic purposes
9. Healthcare services that are clinically unnecessary
10. Physical examinations for life insurance, superannuation, or memberships of certain organizations

Expenses that fall beyond the scope of Medicare coverage are reimbursable under private health insurance.

Additionally, the Australian Medicare system includes a medical aid scheme for those with long-term or multiple illnesses, or those requiring more extensive services. Although 85% of the expenses for public patients are reimbursable, the remaining 15% is not borne entirely by the patients themselves. There is an absolute cap on the amount paid by the patient, whereby they only pay A$29.30 for each service (corrected for inflation on November 1 of each year), equivalent to a cumulative cap of A$2,712 per year (corrected for inflation on January 1 of each year). Patients do not have to pay the remaining balance, which is covered by the medical aid scheme. Individuals who utilize Medicare are automatically registered for the Medicare Safety Net, and eligible individuals do not need to pay any fees. The Medicare Safety Net is primarily designed for low-income earners who are unable to purchase commercial health insurance or afford the copayment for medical expenses under the Medicare scheme. Families can register as a Medicare Safety Net family by filling in and submitting a registration form to a Medicare customer service center. A Medicare Safety Net family refers to a married couple and children under the age of 16 or full-time students under the age of 25. According to this scheme, Australian citizens whose annual income is lower than the threshold do not need to pay out-of-pocket expenses incurred at healthcare institutions (e.g., general practice), which are covered under this scheme through bulk-billing.

(5) Medicare Eligibility and Reimbursement Methods

The eligibility criteria for Medicare are very simple. All legal permanent residents of Australia are eligible for enrollment. Furthermore, the citizens of certain countries that have signed reciprocal health care agreements with Australia are also eligible for Medicare coverage during their stay in Australia. There are currently seven such countries: the UK, New Zealand, Finland, Malta, Italy, the Netherlands, and Sweden.

Eligible applicants can become members of Medicare and receive a Medicare card by completing an application form at a nearby service center to prove their legal status. Individuals residing in remote areas can request an application form and then send the completed form together with a photocopy of their ID card. The service center then delivers the Medicare card with the relevant information. Medicare cardholders are entitled to the aforementioned reimbursable healthcare services mentioned. Specifically, the Medicare card can be used for the following: (1) seeking medical attention at a hospital as a public patient; (2) seeking medical attention from bulk-billing physicians or optometrists; (3) visiting a Medicare customer service center for reimbursement; and (4) retrieving one's Medicare number as needed for reimbursement. Medicare cards must be renewed every five years. Cardholders must promptly notify Medicare service centers if there is any change in their address or family members (for Medicare Safety Net families) during this period.

Medicare uses a simple reimbursement method whereby medical bills can be mailed or directly delivered to Medicare service centers in person. Medicare cardholders who intend to mail medical bills for reimbursement must send along a completed form, the original receipt, and their own account numbers to the Medicare processing center in their state capital. The reimbursement outcome is then sent back to cardholders as a check. In addition, Medicare cardholders can deliver their medical bills in person to the customer service centers along with their cards, completed forms, original receipts, and account number. Although cardholders may prefer cash, there are certain limits on the amount of cash reimbursement for safety reasons. Medicare service centers also have mailboxes where cardholders can simply drop a completed set of documents in an envelope. The reimbursement outcome is sent back to cardholders in the form of a check after a few days. However, when applying for reimbursement by mail, cardholders should include only the completed forms, never their Medicare cards, as cardholders must always carry their Medicare cards.

There are two types of physicians and three reimbursement methods available to Medicare cardholders seeking medical attention. The first type is "bulk-billing" physicians, who do not conduct any transactions with their patients. The cardholders need only present their Medicare cards and sign a form (of which cardholders should keep a backup copy). The physicians then send this form in batches for reimbursement from Medicare. The bulk-billing approach has become increasingly popular in Australia. The second type of physicians are "non-bulk-billing" physicians, who receive payments in two forms: (1) patients can pay in cash and be reimbursed later; (2) patients can claim the reimbursement on behalf of the physicians from state Medicare processing centers using the physicians' account number. The patient then receives a check for the reimbursement and forwards this check to the physician.

(6) Medicare Benefits

Australians are generally entitled to proper inpatient and outpatient treatment at public hospitals. All public hospitals in Australia are Medicare-contracted hospitals that implement policies and provisions laid down by the HIC. These public hospitals implement global budgets for their healthcare expenditure. In contrast, general healthcare services are provided by private physicians. The healthcare services provided by public hospitals and private practices are both covered by Medicare. Medicare stipulates precise payment standards on the basis of a precise disease classification system known as the diagnosis-related group (DRG) system.

The DRG system was developed in the US in 1970 for the classification and grading of diseases. In 1983, health insurance agencies in the US adopted DRGs as part of the budgetary control system to pay management fees to hospitals. Healthcare institutions in Australia took a keen interest in this method, and therefore organized several research institutions and development units to study it. From 1988 to 1995, the federal, state, and local governments focused on promoting the use of DRG software in practice. Specifically, hospitals began to conduct disease classification and coding based on disease information, and to determine treatment regimens and drug dosages. Hospitals in all states and territories in Australia, with the exception of New South Wales, began employing the DRG system to manage special funding allocations for public hospitals.

The federal government of Australia reimburses the recurrent expenditures of hospitals via a DRG-based reimbursement system, wherein the specific subsidy for each disease is determined based on its DRG classification and coding. Specifically, the Australian Refined DRGs (AR-DRGs) classify diseases into 24 major diagnostic categories and 661 DRGs. Subsequently, the Guidelines for Case Classification further subdivide these diseases into 11,450 minor diagnostic categories and 3,624 procedure categories. Each disease course is assigned a DRG code. The disease is also assigned a cost weight, which is determined based on discussions and analyses of its severity, diagnostic complexity, and expenses incurred. For example, if the mean cost weight for all diseases is 1 (i.e., 1 point), then the cost weights of lobar pneumonia, vaginal delivery, and coronary artery bypass grafting are 0.9536, 0.3876, and 4.3592, respectively, when compared to the DRG standard. The government provides a fixed amount of subsidy to hospitals based on the cumulative cost weight of the diseases treated. Private insurance companies have also adopted this method for paying hospital expenses on behalf of patients. The earliest DRG system is known as AR-DRG version 6.0, and was introduced in December 2008.

Under the constraints and guidance of this allocation and payment method, hospitals must implement rigorous management, with a particular emphasis on optimizing the cost and efficiency of each task, thereby accelerating the turnover of hospital beds, reducing the length of hospital stays, overcoming drug abuse, and preventing the overprescription of medical examinations and treatment. This payment method also aims to maximize the economic benefits for hospitals in order to achieve a good balance between the social and economic benefits of healthcare; otherwise, it would be impossible for healthcare institutions to survive and develop.

(7) Existing Issues and Reform Measures

Most Australians are satisfied with the existing Medicare scheme because of its advanced management approach, governmental financial strength, and a high degree of protection. However, in recent years, Australia has witnessed a substantial increase in medical expenses due to an increasing number of immigrants, gradual population aging, and widespread application of advanced technologies in clinical practice. The growth in medical expenses can also be attributed to the exploitation of loopholes in the existing system, such as false reports and fraudulent claims of medical expenses by a minority of insured persons; and private practitioners who divide the patient consultation into multiple visits in exchange for more insurance claims. Additionally, other factors, such as elective health insurance, overprescription for minor illnesses (e.g., hospitalization), and overuse of expensive medical equipment in public hospitals, have also greatly increased healthcare expenditure. In light of these drawbacks, the government has adopted certain reform measures to reduce waste and ensure universal access to basic healthcare services. The government has also actively publicized the benefits of private insurance and encouraged its purchase among residents, which would help reduce the government's burden while also allowing policyholders greater freedom in choosing their preferred hospitals, physicians, and insurance coverage. The Australian government has implemented a variety of incentive measures for this purpose: (1) The premiums for private insurance increase with age, while the premiums offered to young adults decrease over time. (2) The government no longer arbitrarily mobilizes commercial health insurance funds to secure the insurance compensation of policyholders. (3) The government has extended the period before insurance coverage becomes effective to one year, in order to prevent elective insurance (i.e., patients purchase insurance only after major illnesses). (4) The government has integrated Medicare with commercial health insurance companies, thus allowing these commercial agencies to become Medicare agents.

4. Commercial Health Insurance

Commercial health insurance serves as a supplement to Medicare, and thus occupies an important position in the Australian health insurance system. It comprises two parts: (1) reinsurance of some hospital services covered by Medicare, primarily out-of-pocket expenses for inpatient treatments; and (2) supplementary or additional insurance for expenses falling beyond Medicare coverage. Commercial health insurance is an optional scheme that citizens can purchase voluntarily. Policyholders of commercial health insurance can not only be admitted to private hospitals, which usually have better services than do public hospitals but also choose their preferred physicians and be reimbursed for auxiliary services, such as eyeglasses and dental implants. In addition to voluntary commercial health insurance, there are also certain mandatory insurance programs, such as workers' compensation. Specifically, the law requires employers to purchase labor insurance for permanent employees who work more than 10 hours per week. Medical expenses incurred due to work-related injuries and time-loss compensation are borne by insurance companies, which must also offer one-time compensation if a permanent employee loses the ability to work due to work-related injuries. This statutory labor insurance is operated by insurance companies that charge processing fees.

Commercial health insurance agencies are required to operate in strict accordance with national policies and provisions. To ensure this, the government has established the Private Health Insurance Administration Council (PHIAC). The PHIAC supervises the operations of commercial health insurance agencies and ensures the value-added and effective utilization of private insurance funds.

(1) Characteristics of Commercial Health Insurance

1. High-Income Earners are the Main Target Group   Although the Australian government has stipulated that commercial health insurance companies must accept the voluntary participation of all citizens, it primarily encourages the participation of high-income earners. In 1996, the government stipulated that an additional levy, known as the Medicare Levy Surcharge (MLS), will be imposed on individuals earning more than A$50,000 annually or couples earning more than A$100,000 who do not have commercial health coverage. Additionally, families with minors will also face an additional MLS of A$1,500 for each minor.

2. Serving as a Supplement to Medicare   In Australia, commercial health insurance serves as a supplement to Medicare by covering items that fall beyond the scope of Medicare coverage. Since the introduction of Medicare in 1984, commercial health insurance companies are not permitted to cover out-of-hospital physician services. Instead, they can only cover fees incurred by policyholders receiving hospital services (e.g., accommodation fees and theater fees) and physician services at private or public hospitals. Currently, there are two major types of schemes offered in private hospital insurance: basic hospital insurance and supplementary hospital insurance. The former is a prerequisite for participating in the latter. In addition to hospital insurance, there are also supplementary health insurance schemes that cover out-of-hospital physician services, including oral therapy, physiotherapy, eyeglasses, and so on.

At present, the basic benefits of private hospital insurance are as follows: (1) It covers out-of-pocket expenses incurred by public hospitals other than Medicare-covered inpatient fees, and partially covers inpatient fees incurred by private hospitals and day hospitals. (2) It covers the 25% gap between physician fees incurred by public and private hospitals and Medicare benefits for policyholders of commercial health insurance. Basic commercial health insurance cannot cover out-of-hospital service fees or surcharges. Supplementary commercial health insurance, on the other hand, usually provides additional allowances to cover the higher accommodation fees charged by private hospitals, as well as the high fees incurred for single-bed wards at public hospitals. However, the supplementary insurance does not cover additional fees incurred for physician services.

At public hospitals, patients can choose to seek medical attention as public patients covered by Medicare or as self-paying private patients. The former is served by hospital-assigned physicians free of charge, whereas the latter pays a certain amount of the physician service fee and is given the right to choose their preferred physicians, treatment regimens, and accommodation conditions.

3. Strict Regulatory and Management Policies   The government of Australia has imposed a number of strict regulations on commercial health insurance. Firstly, a strict certification system has been put in place, such that health insurance agencies must be registered in accordance with the Australian National Health Act and are only allowed to operate after obtaining a series of certifications. Secondly, a community-wide flat premium rate has been established, which implies that everyone within a community pays the same premiums, regardless of gender, age, and health status; the premiums are based on the average prevalence of diseases in that community. This policy was developed by the government to ensure health equality, such that all Australians can purchase private health insurance regardless of age and health status. Thirdly, there are strict reserve requirements, meaning that commercial health insurance funds are required to have at least A$1 million or the equivalent of two months of ordinary expenses in cash reserves; if the fund fails to meet either of these conditions, it faces temporary suspension.

4. Establishment of Regional Reinsurance (Groups) Schemes for Risk-Sharing   Some insurance companies might be overburdened by the community-wide flat premium rate due to demographic factors, such as the aging of insured members. As such, the Australian government introduced the regional reinsurance scheme in an attempt to reduce differences in the burden among insurance companies resulting from the age structure of insured members. A reinsurance fund has been established in each state, which receives joint contributions from private health insurance companies and a partial subsidy from the federal government. Allocation of these reinsurance funds to private health insurance companies is adjusted annually based on their expenses for chronic diseases. Furthermore, the reinsurance fund partially subsidizes the medical expenses for patients aged over 65 years and who have been hospitalized for more than 35 successive days. The reinsurance fund is administered by the PHIAC, but the Minister of Health (federal government) reserves the right to intervene via negotiations with the PHIAC.

(2) Fee Settlement with Commercial Health Insurance

Private hospitals are able to join Medicare, but must first be certified and approved by the Medical Services Advisory Committee (MSAC). The following two approaches to fee settlement are used by such private hospitals: (1) Private hospitals or physicians charge according to the standard reimbursable fees of policyholders. For example, dental extraction, which has a standard fee of A$100 and a reimbursement cap of A$75, is charged at A$75. (2) In cases where the standard fees exceed the reimbursement cap, the reimbursable portion is paid by the MSAC based on the MBS, while the remaining balance is borne by the patients. In this case, a dental extraction with the same standard fee and reimbursement cap as the previous case will be charged at A$100, but the patient must only pay A$25. Currently, the majority of private hospitals or private physicians choose the former approach, which can help to attract more patients.

(3) Commercial Health Insurance Rebates

On January 1, 1999, the federal government of Australia introduced the Federal Government 30% Rebate, which subsidizes 30% of the premiums paid by Australian citizens with commercial health insurance. Since April 1, 2005, the federal government has increased the premium rebate to 35% for commercial insurance policyholders aged 65–69 years, and 40% for policyholders aged 70 years and above. These incentives have greatly boosted the development of commercial health insurance in Australia. In 2006–2007, there were approximately 5.1 million commercial health insurance policyholders who were eligible for the 30% rebate. This figure increased by 3.9% in 2007–2008 to 5.3 million policyholders. In 2007–2008, the Australian government spent a total of A$3.62 billion on these rebates.

Presently, the main commercial health insurance companies in Australia include Australian Unity, HBA, HBF, HCF, MBF, Medibank Private, NRMA, SGIC, and SGIO. Medibank Private is currently the largest among these.

(4) Existing Problems in Commercial Health Insurance and Their Causes

1. Considerable Reduction in the Number of Policyholders and a Reversal in Demographic Structure   The establishment of Medicare has made many healthcare services free of charge. Thus, in many circumstances, patients covered by commercial health insurance not only lack additional benefits but also might have to pay a significant amount of out-of-pocket expenses, thereby rendering commercial insurance "unnecessary." Furthermore, the establishment of Medicare has hindered the purchase of commercial health insurance because taxpayers who have paid the Medicare levy (which they regard as a health insurance premium) are unwilling to purchase commercial health insurance. In addition, the community-wide flat premium rate has meant that insurance companies are now incapable of attracting young and healthy individuals. Therefore, the number of commercial health insurance policyholders has declined continuously since the establishment of Medicare in 1984. In particular, the percentage of commercial health insurance policyholders out of the total population has decreased from 50.0% at the end of June 1984 to 31.6% in 1997. Currently, there are only about five million private insurance policyholders, accounting for around 29% of the total population. The demographic structure of commercial health insurance policyholders has also shown a reversed trend and has begun to age – that is, there has been a decline in the proportion of young, healthy policyholders and an increase in the proportion of elderly individuals with multiple illnesses. In 1992, the ratio of policyholders under the age of 45 years to those over 45 years was 60:40; this ratio decreased to 51:49 in 2000. Therefore, private insurance companies issued a new regulation in 2000 whereby policyholders aged over 45 years are charged an annual premium three times that of policyholders below that age. Additionally, the waiting period for health insurance is generally not longer than the waiting time at public hospitals. As a result, some individuals purchase insurance before hospitalization or surgery, while others plan to purchase it only during their old age, thereby effectively delaying the initial enrollment age.

The above trends have increased the burden placed on private health insurance companies, forcing them to raise premium rates to maintain their funds. The increase in premium rates has prompted the withdrawal of young and healthy individuals, thereby leading to a vicious cycle. Furthermore, the continuous decrease in the number of commercial health insurance policyholders has led to increased cost pressure on Medicare. The government healthcare budget is estimated to increase by A$100 million for every percentage point reduction in the number of commercial health insurance policyholders.

2. Increased Cost Pressure in Commercial Health Insurance   Cost pressure has been a continual problem affecting both the healthcare budget of the Australian government and commercial health insurance. Aside from the reduction in the number of policyholders and the reversal of demographic structure, the cost pressure faced by the commercial health insurance industry can be attributed to the following three factors.

1. *Continuous increase in public expectations.* The demand for healthcare services has expanded from disease needs to health needs. In other words, there is a much stronger demand for the healthcare system to help people achieve healthy living, and not merely to cure diseases. This expectation is continuing to increase along with income levels and technological advancement.
2. *Supply-side cost-push inflation.* Healthcare workers occupy a monopolistic position in the healthcare market due to information asymmetry. Furthermore, the ultimate goals of hospitals, especially private hospitals, are to increase business revenues and promote the improvement and development of their health protection capabilities and medical technologies. Physicians are remunerated on an FFS basis, which motivates them to provide expensive services and to use expensive medical equipment. Similarly, hospitals compete with each other by adding sophisticated facilities and equipment, thereby attracting and encouraging physicians to use these facilities. The resulting costs are passed on to the government and commercial health insurance companies.
3. *Transfer of public expenditures to commercial health insurance.* A series of measures adopted in the 1980s and 1990s have led to the partial transfer of the public fiscal burden to commercial health insurance companies. These measures include terminating a capital injection of about A$220 million per annum into the reinsurance fund by the federal

government; terminating a subsidy of about A$235 million per annum for private hospital beds by the government; raising the standard fees incurred by public hospitals for commercial health insurance policyholders via cost-based pricing; and reducing the reimbursement level of medical aid schemes for healthcare services.

It is estimated that from 1994 to 1995, the government transferred a fiscal burden of about A$900 million per annum to the commercial health insurance industry, which is equivalent to a 42% increase in the premium rate. The transfer of public fiscal burden has increased the burden of commercial health insurance, which has prompted further increase in premiums and further reduced the number of young and healthy policyholders, thus aggravating the demographic structure of policyholders.

3. Barriers to Fair Competition in the Insurance Industry

1. Some commercial health insurance companies in Australia believe that a number of policy factors are affecting the fairness of competition and the efficiency of the insurance industry. First, the presence of a state-owned Medibank Private Limited is questionable. From the perspective of fair competition, it is not necessary for the federal government to own a commercial health insurance company, given that the private sector is capable of successfully operating health insurance companies. In addition, this government-owned commercial health insurance company is not fully commercialized and is not subject to the control of the financial market. It may also enjoy explicit or implicit government protection and may not be subject to the same taxes or charges as other private insurance companies. As it is operated by the government, it has an advantage over fully private companies given its close association with the medical aid scheme. For example, Medibank Private is the sole agent of the medical aid scheme, which provides customers with integrated services concerning the processing of insurance benefits; this clearly violates the principle of fair competition.

2. The reinsurance funds are regional, whereas the registration, coverage, and reimbursement of insurance companies are nationwide. The financial burden imposed by the community-wide flat premium rate must be balanced on a nationwide basis rather than a regional one, as the latter could give rise to unfair competition due to the over-burdening of insurance companies in some states. In addition, the reinsurance should also cover certain less expensive but more appropriate healthcare services, such as the general care of the elderly.

3. The government of Australia offers tax incentives to commercial health insurance companies, whereas nonprofit commercial agencies are exempt from income tax. This has led to an increasing trend among insurance companies towards business activities unrelated to insurance; as these activities still enjoy tax incentives, this hinders fairness in the insurance industry.

4. The current reserve system allows government departments to exempt some insurance companies from the minimum reserve requirement. This has further hindered the rational allocation of resources in the insurance industry.

5. Reforms in Healthcare Services and Payment Systems

(1) Reform Background

Long waiting times are a common phenomenon and may be the biggest problem facing the Australian healthcare system. The root cause of long waiting times is the lack of any effective incentives in the funding and payment systems for improving the efficiency of healthcare services. This is because the payments made by the federal government are not linked to the performance of hospitals.

In 1993, the casemix funding model was first introduced in Victoria as part of the public health service reform program. Subsequently, in 1994, South Australia adopted a casemix funding model very similar to that of Victoria. Since then, most Australian states, such as Western Australia and Queensland, have reformed their payment systems based on the casemix funding model. New South Wales is the only Australian state that has implemented reforms towards a population-based payment system in healthcare services rather than the casemix funding model. However, the health authorities in New South Wales have also attached considerable importance to the casemix model in budgeting and providing information on healthcare services for patients living in different regions of the state. Other more remote states have integrated only some of the important aspects of the casemix model into their reform programs due to their small populations and lack of healthcare service providers.

The initial casemix model involved the classification of complex healthcare services into several major categories: inpatient services, outpatient services, and teaching and research. Despite having the most complicated definition and description of service categories and items ("products"), the casemix model was first introduced into the payment reforms for inpatient services.

(2) Single-Disease Management in Inpatient Services

The casemix-based payment system for inpatient services has a simple core idea – single-disease management. The payment for hospitals is determined based on types of inpatients and the corresponding services provided by the hospitals. In addition to being a well-developed clinical disease classification system, DRGs are also an excellent clinical classification for inpatients. Therefore, DRGs can be applied in the design and implementation of a casemix-based payment system. This type of payment system allows for performance- and outcome-based funding of hospitals, rather than funding that is solely based on negotiations and historical or political factors.

Although the casemix models adopted by each Australian state are not exactly the same and may even differ significantly in some respects, they still share certain basic characteristics and core elements: (1) a universal nomenclature system, that is, AR-DRG version 6.x. (2) Consistency in payment reforms and budget cuts. Essentially every state has introduced capped fees that are generally combined with specific goals for hospitals. However, some states have relatively flexible control goals that allow only partial payments for hospitals with budget overruns. (3) As the DRG system is based on coded diagnostic and treatment procedures, all states have established code review systems to ensure the accuracy of the casemix-based model, especially the classification of diseases and clinical services.

(3) Payment Systems

There are two casemix funding models used in Australia. The initial Victoria model included both fixed and variable rate payments, which were improved in 1990 and subsequently adopted by Queensland. The former uses a fixed budget to subsidize the recurrent expenditures of hospitals (indirect or fixed costs of medical consultation services), while the latter is determined according to the variable cost of each patient admitted to the hospital. The theory of this type of payment system holds that hospitals reach a critical level of motivation in providing a new service when the marginal cost of providing more services is equal to the marginal reimbursement from the government; hospitals will be reluctant to provide additional services after exceeding this critical level. Hence, this maximizes their service efficiency while preventing overprescription. Here, marginal reimbursement refers to the variable reimbursement from the government, which is determined by the respective state health departments. This payment system, which combines fixed and variable rates, has effectively reduced the motivation to overprescribe hospital services. In addition, when the service capacity of the healthcare system has been fully utilized and needs to be expanded (e.g., additional hospital beds), hospitals can request a corresponding increase in the amount of fixed-rate reimbursement from the government. However, these newly included fixed costs can only be partially subsidized, thus allowing the government to control the capital investment in the healthcare system.

The other casemix-based model is the integrated reimbursement model, where the government provides an overall reimbursement for both variable and fixed costs spent on the hospital services for each inpatient. This model has mainly been adopted in Western Australia and Tasmania. South Australia has adopted a similar system, but the state health department must negotiate with hospitals to determine the hospital's requisite service volume. The reimbursement for the hospital will be reduced at a certain rate if the hospital fails to achieve the predetermined service volume. This is because the failure to meet the required service volume indicates a reduced marginal cost (or variable cost) spent by the hospital.

(4) Differences in Reimbursement Levels

In general, within a specific DRG system, different hospitals provide the same service for the same type of patients. Therefore, logically speaking, different hospitals should be provided with the same amount of reimbursement for the same type of diseases. However, state governments in Australia have noted that there are clear certain differences in the actual costs incurred. Hence, the state governments of Victoria, Queensland, Western Australia, and South Australia have established their own disease subclassification systems with varying reimbursement amounts.

Additionally, these states have different interpretations of the economies of scale. The policymakers in Victoria and Western Australia do adhere to the economies of scale, meaning that the state governments provide less reimbursement for patients at large hospitals than at small hospitals for a particular DRG. Conversely, policymakers in Queensland and South Australia do not believe in the presence of economies of scale in the healthcare system. Hence, the governments of these states provide greater reimbursement for patients at large hospitals than at small hospitals.

The DRG systems in these states provide varying payment levels due to differences in the definition of cost weights and baseline prices among the casemix-based models. There might be up to a 40% difference in the DRG reimbursement level across states adopting the integrated reimbursement model. Additionally, differences in reimbursement level are also reflected in the treatment and reimbursement of patients with abnormal conditions. The conventional DRG classification system describes the typical situation of a disease, that is, a routine case. However, for nonroutine cases, the classification criteria and reimbursements vary across states. For example, the maximum funding baseline of urban hospitals in Melbourne was A\$3,153 in 2006 (adjusted to A\$3,279 in 2008), whereas that of rural hospitals was A\$3,589, which represents a difference of A\$436 between the two.

(5) Reform Outcomes and Prospects

Most Australian states have reformed, or are in the process of reforming, the casemix-based payment system; however, there are significant variations in their existing payment models. Therefore, after reviewing the Victorian and integrated reimbursement models, healthcare service providers believe that there are still many problems with the reforms to the current payment system. Although the design of reforms to the payment system is mainly focused on ensuring that healthcare service providers receive the appropriate incentives to promote service efficiency, consideration should also be given to ensuring greater fairness for healthcare service providers in the payment system. The disparities in the reimbursement of different Australian states for a specific DRG clearly demonstrate the presence of inequalities in the reimbursement for healthcare services.

In addition, the design of casemix-based payment systems entails a series of complex, technical problems that require a balance between competing policy objectives. Furthermore, given the premise of maintaining a relatively stable payment system, this design must also consider the impact of advancing medical technologies and other factors on healthcare costs, in order to avoid any possible side effects of the system design. In sum, designing a payment system is a complicated undertaking, and it is necessary to recognize that no casemix-based payment system is perfect.

Nevertheless, the international academic community has expressed high praise for the reforms to the hospital payment system in Australia. In general, scholars believe that the casemix-based payment system has significantly improved the service efficiency of the public healthcare service system. In the past, health insurance funding for the elderly was allocated by the federal government to state governments, which in turn reimbursed hospitals directly based on their budgets. After the reform, the health insurance fund for the elderly is now allocated by the federal government directly to hospitals based on casemix-adjusted costs. This payment system has been proven to not only improve service efficiency but also inhibit cost transfer, such as the transfer of patients covered by health insurance for the elderly to the private healthcare sector.

6. Plans for a New Round of Healthcare Reforms

(1) Basic Ideas and Principles of the Reform

The Australian healthcare system is currently ranked among the best in the world. However, due to population aging, the increase in chronic and preventable diseases, the emergence of new therapeutic approaches, and rising healthcare expenditures, the residents of Australia have been imposing a greater demand on the healthcare system. State (territorial) governments will eventually become financially overwhelmed without national health reforms. It is estimated that healthcare expenditure alone will exceed the total income of state and local governments by 2045–2046. The federal government of Australia is cooperating with state (territorial) governments to address these challenges. In August 2011, a nationwide agreement was made (known as the National Health Reform Agreement), which promised to meet the funding needs of public hospitals with unprecedented transparency and accountability, in order to reduce the wastage of resources and waiting time for patients.

1. Basic Ideas of the Reforms

1. *Improve the rationality and efficiency of funding.* The federal government of Australia has made an additional major capital injection of around A\$16.4 billion to public hospitals. The investment from the federal government is expected to achieve an effective growth of 45% from 2014 and 50% from 2017.

   The Australian government has also established the Independent Hospital Pricing Authority (IHPA), which has set national standards for public hospital services and developed an activity-based national funding system. The IHPA seeks to set appropriate reimbursements at a reasonable price for the services provided by public hospitals. This is expected to considerably improve the efficiency of capital injection for hospitals and prevent price deviations from the actual hospital expenditures.

2. *Improve transparency and accountability.* The state (territorial) governments have agreed to enhance the transparency of the healthcare system in order to improve its funding arrangements. Furthermore, the government of Australia has also established the National Health Funding Pool (hereafter, the Pool) to improve the transparency of funding for public hospitals. The administrator of the Pool must report to both the federal and state (territorial) governments regarding the flow of funding and the delivery of healthcare services. The Pool also ensures that all hospitals have access to the same funding channels and that citizens have a full understanding of how the government utilizes taxes.

The state (territorial) governments have also begun establishing a network of local hospitals that will enable the handover of decision-making for hospital management to local authorities.

The National Health Performance Authority (NHPA) releases hospital performance reports and community health reports in an effort to improve national health status and the transparency of hospital performance. These reports will help Australians to make informed choices about their healthcare based on the performance of all hospitals in Australia.

3. *Reduce patient waiting time.* The federal government has allocated A$1.8 billion to state (territorial) governments, which is intended to incentivize hospitals, in order to achieve newly-established objectives concerning emergency departments and elective surgeries. Additionally, the federal government provided another capital injection of A$1.6 billion and 1,316 hospital beds for sub-acute care or similar services to capital cities.

The new objectives are as follows. (1) To reduce the waiting time at emergency departments to within four hours. This involves the completion of examination, treatment, and hospital admission or discharge approval for 90% of triage-classified patients within four hours. (2) To ensure that all patients undergoing elective surgery will wait no longer than the clinically recommended period of time.

The first objective is expected to be implemented within four years after 2012, while the second is expected to be implemented within five years after 2012.

The federal government's new capital injection program mainly focused on primary healthcare, in order to reduce the burden of public hospitals. These primary healthcare services include overtime services, new training bases for GPs, and new general practices.

To promote the reform of elderly care, the federal government has directly funded all essential community healthcare services for individuals aged over 65 years in all states (territories), with the exception of Western Australia and Victoria.

This funding is expected to increase the scope and accessibility of healthcare services for the elderly population. The reforms will also clarify the healthcare boundaries between young individuals with disabilities and elderly people in need of care.

The federal government has also made a new commitment to allocate A$2.2 billion over five years to reform the mental health system. Specifically, the federal government allocated A$624 million to the mental health sector as part of national health reforms and election commitments, followed by A$1.5 billion as part of the 2011–2012 Budget for National Mental Health Reform.

Aside from the National Health Reform Agreement, the government of Australia has continued to focus on other aspects of health reform, which include reducing public demand for hospitals by promoting preventive care; enhancing the healthcare workforce to ensure an adequate supply of physicians and nurses; and applying new technologies to provide more coordinated and flexible healthcare services, such as by establishing electronic health records (EHRs) and health informatization.

2. Contents and Objectives of the Reforms Since April 2010, the government of Australia has put tremendous effort into reforming the following eight healthcare areas: hospitals, GPs and primary healthcare, elderly care, mental health, national standards and performance, healthcare workforce, preventive care, and health informatization.

In July 2010, the Australian federal government released a bulletin entitled "A National Health and Hospitals Network for Australia's Future: Delivering better health and better hospitals for all Australians." This bulletin outlined a plan for implementing the aforementioned health reforms. The National Health Reform Agreement enacted on August 2, 2011, also concretized the responsibilities of both the federal and state (territorial) governments in Australia in promoting health reforms.

According to this agreement, both the federal and state (territorial) governments have agreed to initiate major reforms in the organization, funding, and provision of healthcare and elderly care services. Through increased federal budget allocation, these reform measures are expected to improve the accessibility of healthcare services, while also increasing the responsibilities and transparency of local health authorities. The reform measures also enable the delivery of community healthcare services that can meet local needs and may improve the financial sustainability of the Australian healthcare system.

The health reforms outlined in this agreement seek to achieve the following objectives:

1. To improve the accessibility of healthcare services and the efficiency of public hospitals via activity-based funding (ABF) at reasonable prices.
2. To ensure the financial sustainability of public hospitals by increasing their share of federal budget allocation.
3. To improve the transparency of public hospitals via the Pool.
4. To improve the clinical healthcare, performance reporting, and accountability standards in the healthcare and elderly care systems.
5. To improve how local authorities exercise their responsibilities and their responsiveness to meeting the local healthcare needs of various communities.
6. To improve the delivery of GP and primary healthcare services.
7. To improve the elderly care services and healthcare services for individuals with disabilities.

The federal government has also reiterated its commitment to preventive care delivery, mental health reform, and health informatization programs, some of which are jointly provided by both the federal and state (territorial) governments.

3. Principles of the Reforms The aforementioned agreement states that the national health reform must be implemented based on the following principles:

1. Both the federal and state (territorial) governments agree that a healthcare system that can best meet community healthcare needs requires the collaboration between hospitals, GPs, primary care, and elderly care institutions in order to minimize the duplication and dispersion of services.

2. Australians should be able to access transparent and nationwide comparative performance data and information about hospitals and healthcare institutions providing primary healthcare, elderly care, and other healthcare services.
3. The government should continue to support the diversification and innovation of healthcare systems, which will serve as a key mechanism for achieving better health outcomes.
4. All Australians, including those living in remote areas, should have equal access to high-quality healthcare services.
5. Both the federal and state (territorial) governments agree that the Australian healthcare system should encourage social integration and reduce the population of disadvantaged groups, especially Indigenous Australians.

(2) Hospital Reform Plan

The federal government has promised to provide strong financial support for the Australian healthcare system. According to the new National Health Reform Agreement, the federal and state (territorial) governments have reached a consensus on hospital payment and operational systems to ensure the sustainability of comprehensive healthcare services for Australia's future generations.

On June 1, 2012, the government of Australia launched a nationwide hospital reimbursement method for basic services to increase the transparency of hospital funding and reimbursement, while also improving the technical efficiency of hospital services. This payment method provides reimbursement for public hospitals according to their service types and volumes. The federal government also planned to inject A\$4.8 billion from 2010 to 2017 to address key issues in public healthcare institutions. This measure is in accordance with the opinions of the Council of Australian Governments (COAG) expert panel on routine surgeries and emergency services. Currently, all state or territorial governments in Australia have achieved a consensus on the National Partnership Agreement on Improving Public Hospital Services (NPA IPHS) and agreed to jointly work under the framework of this agreement. The NPA IPHS aims to provide better healthcare services for patients, including more hospital beds, faster emergency services, and more convenient routine surgeries and subemergency services. The specific objectives are as follows:

1. *Four-hour target for emergency departments.* Emergency departments need to complete examination, treatment, and hospital admission or discharge approval for 90% of the triage-classified patients within four hours.
2. *Target for routine surgeries.* All patients who require routine surgeries should wait no longer than the clinically recommended period of time; this includes reducing the number of patients on the waiting list and the length of waiting time.
3. Additional investment of A\$1.6 billion for the installation of 1,316 emergency beds and related healthcare services, in order to improve the health status, physical function, and quality of life of all Australians

(3) GP and Primary Healthcare Reform Plan

One of the federal government's concerns is ensuring the delivery of high-quality primary healthcare, such that patients can access required services near their place of residence.

The federal government has placed special emphasis on the reforms of GPs and primary healthcare, mainly through the following measures:

1. Establish Local Healthcare Organizations (i.e., independent primary care organizations) throughout Australia and integrate their services with general medicine and community healthcare services, in order to improve the accessibility of primary care services and promote service integration.
2. Ensure the availability of general healthcare services to local residents during non-working hours.
3. Try new service delivery models for primary healthcare, including the treatment and ongoing management of patients with diabetes, with the aim of improving the flexibility of service delivery.
4. Establish 64 general practices and implement 425 reform items related to general medical services, primary healthcare, and community services, and aboriginal healthcare services, in order to integrate GP services with primary care services, thereby improving service accessibility.

(4) Elderly Care Reform Plan

The acceleration of population aging in Australia implies that increasing numbers of elderly individuals require healthcare services tailored to the characteristics of their age group. The current elderly care system in Australia is relatively fragmented, with inconsistent arrangements in elderly care services. Hence, it is necessary to reform its service delivery to cope with the increasing demand for elderly care. The federal government provides policy and financial support for the elderly care system throughout the country. In particular, the elderly care systems in states other than Western Australia and Victoria are supported by the federal government instead of the Family and Community Services (FACS). This shift in responsibilities has facilitated the establishment and development of a centralized elderly care system that covers services ranging from home-based primary care to advanced healthcare services offered in elderly care facilities. Additionally, this has also enabled the federal government to promote the integration of emergency services, public hospitals, GPs, primary care services, and elderly care facilities. The federal government also assumes policy and funding responsibilities for elderly care services targeting nonresidents over the age of 65 years, as well as Indigenous Australians and Torres Strait Islanders aged over 50 years.

The federal government has conducted extensive expert consultations in implementing elderly care reforms on the following key issues:

1. The shift in responsibilities between the Home and Community Care (HACC) program and the federal government.
2. The allocation of an additional A$120 million to install 286 hospital beds, in order to expand the sub-emergency care capacity of multifunctional healthcare services in remote areas, and increase the number of remote communities that can apply for the establishment of multifunctional healthcare services.
3. The allocation of an additional 2,000 beds for elderly bedridden patients and financial support to state (territorial) governments. This is equivalent to allocating A$277 million to each state (territorial) government over the next three years.

4. The allocation of A\$1.6 billion for the addition of 1,300 beds for sub-emergency care at hospitals and community healthcare centers, in order to improve patients' health status, physical function, and quality of life, while also freeing up hospital beds at public hospitals and emergency departments.

(5) Mental Health Reform Plan

In the fiscal year 2011–2012, the federal government introduced a new mental health reform plan worth A\$2.2 billion. In line with the National Mental Health Reform of 2011–2012 and its assessment criteria announced in 2010, the federal government has attempted the comprehensive reform of the Australian mental health system. It aims to achieve more timely clinical or nonclinical support for Australians with mental illnesses, secure the best opportunity for recovery, and stabilize patients' conditions. After a comprehensive review of the data and focus group interviews, the government has focused on the following five key areas in reforming the mental health system:

1. Improve the services for patients with severe mental illnesses, who also belong to the most vulnerable group in society.
2. Enhance the basic services for mental health.
3. Promote the prevention and early intervention of mental illness for youths.
4. Encourage the participation of individuals with mental illnesses in economic and social activities, including providing them with job opportunities.
5. Improve the quality of mental health services, build a robust accountability system, and encourage innovation.

(6) Healthcare Workforce Reform Plan

The training of healthcare workers represents a core element in health reforms to better meet future challenges. In order to improve the shortage and uneven distribution of the healthcare workforce in the Australia, the federal government has allocated A\$1.8 billion from fiscal years 2010–2011 to 2014–2015, in order to recruit more GPs and medical experts, and to provide better support for general medical services, elderly care, nursing staff in rural areas, and healthcare technicians in rural areas.

(7) Preventive Care Reform Plan

Due to the rapid spread of chronic, preventable diseases in Australia, it has become necessary for the national health reform to focus on preventive care. Preventive care can help in preventing diseases and hospitalization, as well as in improving the quality of life of the general population. The federal government has attached great importance to preventive care in the present health reform, in order to alleviate the burden placed on other healthcare areas and to manage the risk factors of chronic diseases due to lifestyles and living habits. Current measures by the federal government to reform preventive care in Australia include curbing the worsening obesity crisis, reducing smoking and alcohol consumption, encouraging a healthier lifestyle, and launching health education programs for Australians on the harmful effects of chronic diseases.

(8) Electronic Health Records (EHR) Plan

The federal government has recognized the importance of EHRs for establishing a responsive and patient-centered healthcare system. The government's recognition is evident in its implementation of two milestone funding programs. First, the federal government has planned to allocate A$467 million from 2010–2011 to 2011–2012, in order to establish a nationwide Personally Controlled Electronic Health Record (PCEHR), which is an interface allowing all Australians to access their own health records. This reform offers a wide range of benefits to residents and the entire healthcare system, particularly in that it will reduce medication errors and duplication of medical tests in the long run. Second, the federal government has planned to allocate A$621 million over the next five years to support and expand electronic health services, with the aim of increasing the accessibility of clinical and expert services, especially among those living in remote areas. Additionally, the government has also increased funding allocated to the National Broadband Network program. These reform measures will enable residents to actively engage in health management without being constrained by their place of residence and time.

SECTION IV. THE HEALTH SYSTEM IN SWEDEN

Sweden is a long, narrow Scandinavian country in Northern Europe; it has a total area of 450,000 km², more than half of which is covered by forests. The total population of Sweden in 2013 was about 9.593 million, with an average of 23 inhabitants per km². The country is divided into 23 county councils and 290 municipalities. Sweden is an aging country: In 2013, the elderly population aged over 65 years accounted for 19.3% of the total population. Like the other four Nordic countries, Sweden is highly industrialized, lying at the forefront of economic development, welfare, and health status worldwide.

The GDP per capita of Sweden in 2013 was US$ 60,430. Sweden has a very low agricultural output as a percentage of the gross national product (GNP), as a very low proportion of the Swedish population engage in agricultural production. The level of education is generally quite high among the Swedish. In 2012, the average life expectancies of Swedish women and men were 83.6 years and 79.9 years, respectively. In 2013, the maternal mortality rate in Sweden was 4 per 100,000 live births, and the infant mortality rate was 2.4 per 1,000 live births. The total healthcare expenditure of Sweden accounted for 9.6% of its GDP in 2012.

Sweden has a comprehensive social welfare system covering the following five aspects: health insurance, work injury insurance, unemployment insurance, basic pension, and supplementary pension. Social insurance is mainly funded by taxation, and the government bears more than 60% of the expenses for unemployment insurance. The Swedish health insurance system provides universal coverage. The country has also enacted laws and regulations to guarantee the access of all Swedish residents to necessary treatments at very low costs. The fundamental purposes of the health insurance system are to protect population health and ensure the equal rights of all Swedish residents to healthcare services. The government is responsible for providing fair and appropriate healthcare services for all Swedes.

Sweden is a constitutional monarchy, and its legislative power is held by both the King and the Riksdag. The government is divided into three levels: central government, county councils, and municipalities. At the county level, there are 18 county councils, 2 regional councils, and 1 county administrative board; at the local level, there are 290 municipalities. The Swedish healthcare system is also administered at the national, county, and local levels, with a high degree of decentralization. The central government and Riksdag establish overall health goals and policies, while county councils and municipalities are primarily responsible for the funding and management of healthcare services. At the national level, the healthcare system is administered by two health authorities: the Ministry of Health and Social Affairs and the National Board of Health and Welfare (*Socialstyrelsen*). The Ministry of Health and Social Affairs is a government department accountable to the Cabinet. It is mainly responsible for establishing various health programs, including healthcare, social welfare, and health insurance programs. The Health Planning Committee is a subordinate department of this ministry that is responsible for the coordination of national healthcare plans. The National Board of Health and Welfare, on the other hand, is a relatively independent government agency primarily responsible for the management of healthcare services, pharmaceutical supplies, and social welfare. Its specific functions include planning and designing (i.e., providing basic information related to planning to the Cabinet, Riksdag, and county councils, as well as supervising and assisting county councils in the implementation of these plans); supervising the healthcare services for outpatients and inpatients; supervising the business operations in the healthcare sector; and collecting health information.

In Sweden, both the Ministry of Health and Social Affairs and the National Board of Health and Welfare must collaborate with other central government agencies, the most important of which are the Medical Responsibility Board, the Medical Products Agency (MPA), the Swedish Agency for Health Technology Assessment and Assessment of Social Services, the Dental and Pharmaceutical Benefits Agency, and the Swedish National Institute of Public Health.

Integrated funding and service delivery have long been a prominent feature of the Swedish healthcare system. County-level public authorities (county councils and municipalities) are responsible for the delivery of healthcare services, which are funded through taxation. County councils are mainly responsible for healthcare, the training of healthcare workers, social welfare, and cultural works. Healthcare is directly administered by various medical boards affiliated with the county council. The municipal authorities are mainly responsible for disease prevention; the public health advisors to municipal authorities and other related agencies are appointed by the medical officers in the county councils.

This planning model for healthcare services has long been effective for ensuring universal access to primary care, preventive care, rehabilitation, and emergency care. However, it has been difficult for the Swedish healthcare system to adapt to the increase in healthcare demands, shortage of funds, and rapid changes in social concepts, demographic structures, and medical technologies. A survey in 1990 showed that 58% of participants believed that the Swedish healthcare system should be reformed. In fact, due to the long tradition of local self-government in Sweden and the relative independence of local authorities in the healthcare system, healthcare reforms were gradually rolled out in some regions in the 1990s.

Sweden's demographic indicators (birth, mortality, and infant mortality rates) are all low, and it has one of the highest life expectancies at birth in the world. Infectious diseases are no longer a major healthcare issue; the main causes of death are circulatory system diseases, malignant tumors, and accidents.

1. Healthcare Provision System

(1) Provision of Healthcare Services

The Swedish healthcare provision system is publicly owned. In 2000, there were nine regional (provincial) hospitals (which declined to eight hospitals in 2001), accounting for only 0.9% of the total hospital beds in Sweden; 26 county hospitals, accounting for 34.7% of total hospital beds; community hospitals that accounted for 57.8% of the total hospital beds; and private healthcare institutions that accounted for 6.8% of the total hospital beds. Before 2000, there were only a handful of nonpublic hospitals in Sweden; by 2003, however, there were about 300 private hospitals out of the 1,100 community hospitals in Sweden. In 2003, there were approximately 12 million visits to physicians at primary care centers, of which 27% were visits to physicians at private healthcare institutions, and about 29% of outpatient consultations were delivered at private institutions. By 2010, there were 60 public hospitals providing specialist healthcare services and 24-hour emergency services in Sweden, of which 8 were regional hospitals providing highly specialized healthcare services, while also serving as teaching and research hospitals.

In 2000, the total number of physicians was 18,669, including 856 private practitioners, which was less than 5% of the total. The number of physicians in Sweden increased to 29,122 in 2005 and 32,495 in 2010. Private practitioners are not widely distributed throughout Sweden, and tend to be found only in Stockholm, Gothenburg, and Malmö.

Regarding the sharing of responsibility for healthcare services, Sweden is divided into 290 municipalities, 18 county councils and 2 regional councils (i.e., the Västra Götaland and Skåne regional councils). Municipal, county, and regional councils have their own local authority for self-governing and are responsible for various matters of state; they do not have a hierarchical relationship among them. Healthcare services constitute about 90% of the work of Swedish county councils, but they also cover other areas, such as culture and infrastructure construction. Swedish municipal councils are charged with family care and residential care for the elderly; the delivery of healthcare services for individuals with physical disabilities and mental disorders; as well as service delivery and support for discharged patients and school health services. The considerable cross-border mobility among European Union (EU) countries has substantially increased the need for cooperative healthcare services. In recent years, there has been an increase in the number of Swedish patients seeking treatment in other EU countries. Furthermore, the number of Swedish medical professionals employed in other EU countries has also increased continuously. Hence, Sweden is actively collaborating with other EU countries to improve the delivery of healthcare services, particularly in the areas of specialized care, medical safety, and patients' rights.

The planning and budgetary management of the Swedish healthcare system are made possible by the publicly owned healthcare system. The Swedish healthcare system that exists today was implemented in the 1980s, based on an initial proposal by the National Board of Health and Welfare in 1975. The Swedish healthcare system is administered on three levels: primary care, county, and regional, as shown in Figure 11.40.

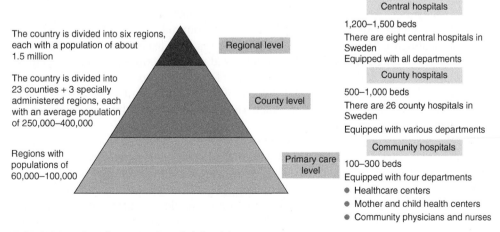

FIGURE 11.40   Three-tier Swedish healthcare system.

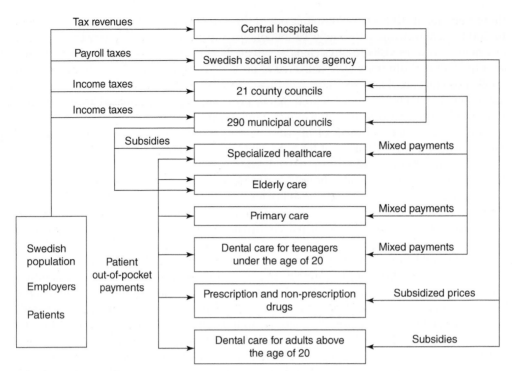

FIGURE 11.41 Funding and payment process in the Swedish healthcare system.

(2) Healthcare Funding

Healthcare expenditures in Sweden are primarily funded by taxes levied by county and municipal councils. Another source of funding is subsidies by the Swedish central government; out-of-pocket expenses paid by patients account for a very small proportion of the healthcare expenditure. Generally speaking, Sweden's healthcare expenditure is mainly funded by the following four sources of income: tax revenues (including all taxes levied at national, county, and municipal levels); the national social insurance system (statutory contributions from employers); private cash payments; and private health insurance (Figure 11.41). In 2002, the Swedish healthcare expenditure was mainly funded by resident taxpayers (61.6%), followed by government subsidies (10%) and health insurance (8.4%); patients' out-of-pocket expenses only accounted for 7.6% (Table 11.20). In 2003, the healthcare funds of county councils were mainly from tax revenues (72.2%), followed by government subsidies (12.8%), sales and other revenues (5.9%), and general government funding (5.4%), while patients' out-of-pocket expenses only accounted for 2.8% (Table 11.21). In 2008, the total income of Stockholm County was SEK65 billion (80% of which was from local taxes), of which 18% was allocated to the delivery of healthcare services and 9% to drug expenses.

The main funding source of the Swedish healthcare system is tax revenues, which include direct taxes levied at the county and municipal levels, as well as indirect taxes levied by the central government. The provision of healthcare services in Sweden is delegated to local governments, whereby each county and municipal council reserves the right to levy taxes proportional to residents' income for various public services. The tax rate is determined by the local government. The Swedish resident tax comprises county and municipal taxes,

TABLE 11.20 Composition of Healthcare Expenditure in Sweden in 2002

Item	Share (%)
Tax revenue	61.6
Government subsidies	10.0
Health insurance	8.4
Equalization grant	7.6
Patient out-of-pocket payments	7.6
Others	4.8

both of which are fixed taxes unrelated to the income of taxpayers. The county tax rate has increased alongside the rise in total healthcare expenditure over the years; after adjustments by the relevant departments, this rate has increased from 9.3% in 1974 to 13.4% in 1986, 15.8% in 1994, and 17.2% in 2002. The resident tax (comprising of county and municipal taxes) has also increased considerably, from 24% in 1974 to 35% in 2002. These taxes have become the main cause for the large financial burden of Swedish residents. Tax revenue contributes to about 70% and 60% of the county and municipal income, respectively. In 2010, each county and municipality had average tax rates of 10.6% and 21.56%, respectively. However, the Swedish government does not impose taxes specifically for healthcare services; these are instead funded by the general taxes intended for all public services.

Public expenditure makes up the largest proportion of the total healthcare expenditure of Sweden, although this share is currently lower than those in the 1970s and 1980s. Furthermore, medical expenses account for the largest share of expenses for all healthcare services. Statistics from the final settlement from the Swedish county council assembly (*Landstingsfullmäktige*, LF) in 2002 showed that inpatient, outpatient, and other expenses accounted for 63%, 13%, and 24%, respectively, of the total healthcare expenditure of county councils. As of 2008, the Swedish county councils have spent a total of SEK186 trillion on healthcare (excluding dental care), representing an increase of about SEK9.2 trillion (or 5.2%) compared to 2007. Basic healthcare services accounted for the largest share of the expenditure, with increased demand for general medical treatment and physiotherapy in 2008 compared to previous years. Unsurprisingly, with the increase in the

TABLE 11.21 Composition of Funding Sources of Swedish County Councils From 1998 to 2003 Unit (%)

Income sources	1998	1999	2000	2001	2002	2003
Tax revenue	68.5	68.3	69	70.4	70.8	72.2
Subsidies	13.0	13.6	14.0	13.5	13.4	12.8
Sales and other income	5.7	4.5	5.0	6.4	6.6	5.9
General government funding	6.8	7.6	7.0	6.3	6.0	5.4
Patient and other out-of-pocket payments	3.4	3.4	3.0	2.8	2.7	2.8
Others	2.6	2.6	2.0	0.7	0.6	0.9
Total funding	100	100	100	100	100	100

Source: Swedish County Councils (2004).

number of private healthcare institutions in Sweden, county councils are now paying for healthcare services provided by these institutions. More specifically, the councils pay about 10% of the expenses for services provided by private healthcare institutions. This is protected by an agreement to ensure that patients have access to the same treatments at both public hospitals and private healthcare institutions.

2. Health Insurance System

(1) Overview of Health Insurance System

After more than 70 years of development and reform, Sweden has developed a comprehensive and universal health insurance system that ensures basic health coverage and expense reimbursement.

The Swedish social insurance system provides universal coverage and is mandatory for all residents. It partially compensates for the loss of income during the course of treatment for illnesses, and also reimburses the medical expenses and the cost of prescription drugs as part of its high-cost protection schemes. A large percentage of health insurance premiums is borne by employers, with the remaining balance being borne by the central government via transfer payments. Private employers and state-owned enterprises pay premiums at a fixed rate for each employee. In 2004, about 11% of the total salaries of employees went towards the payment of insurance premiums. It is worth noting that the above two methods of compensation (i.e., compensations for the loss of income and reimbursement of medical expenses) are relatively independent. Furthermore, compensation for income and production losses can be further increased in the event of inappropriate or delayed delivery of healthcare services. The Swedish health insurance system also covers injury benefits, pharmaceutical costs (via the PBS), and medical and dental expenses (via high-cost protection schemes with cash benefits).

The Swedish healthcare system is mainly characterized by its decentralized system. The Ministry of National Health and Social Affairs is an important government agency responsible for national healthcare administration, health planning, and supervising and coordinating all aspects of healthcare in Sweden. The National Board of Health and Welfare is a relatively independent governance body mainly responsible for healthcare, drugs, social welfare, and so on. The responsibility of local healthcare services is delegated to the 26 county councils and three large municipalities (i.e., Gothenburg, Malmö, and Gotland Islands), which hold considerable authority in the decision-making of local social issues such as health, education, and economic development. The Swedish Social Insurance Agency is a government agency affiliated with the national budget allocation unit, and is headquartered in Stockholm. The agency has 21 regional offices, 240 municipal offices, and five computer centers, with more than 16,000 employees.

(2) Funding and Payment of Health Insurance

The Swedish social insurance system stipulates that all insured persons are required to contribute nearly 10% of their income as insurance premiums, while their employers must contribute the equivalent of 32.82% of their salaries. Of these funds, nearly one-third is used to cover healthcare expenses and sickness benefits. The central government subsidizes the remaining balance of healthcare expenses not covered by the social insurance. Hence, all insured persons are entitled to healthcare services (e.g., diagnostic services, treatment, hospitalization, and surgeries), as well as sickness benefits, work injury benefits, and treatment-related travel allowances.

TABLE 11.22 Income and Expenditure of Swedish Health Insurance System in 2002

Income/expenditure	Item	Amount (SEK100 Million)	(%)
Income	Insurance premiums	1,924	79.3
	Government subsidies	481	19.8
	Others	21	0.9
	Total	2,426	100
Expenditure	Injury benefits	828	32.8
	Parental benefits	260	10.3
	Drug expenses	290	11.5
	Public healthcare Services	448	17.8
	Private healthcare services	58	2.3
	Other healthcare services	180	7.2
	Dental care services	240	9.5
	Inpatient services	49	1.9
	Patient transfers	29	1.1
	Administrative fees	140	5.6
	Total	2,522	100
Balance of payments		-46	

In 2002, the Swedish social insurance fund raised a total of SEK242.6 billion, of which SEK192.4 billion (79%) came from employers, SEK48.1 billion (19.8%) from government subsidies, and SEK2.1 billion (0.9%) from other funding sources. During the same year, the Swedish social insurance fund spent a total of SEK252.2 billion, leading to a deficit of approximately SEK4.6 billion. Cash benefits, such as sickness benefits (SEK82.8 billion) and parental benefits (SEK26 billion), accounted for 51% of the expenditures (Table 11.22).

Sickness benefits compensate employees with injuries or illnesses for about 75–90% of their income during the course of treatment. These sickness benefits also provide a living allowance of SEK8 per day for unemployed persons. The average length of sickness benefits per person was 22.9 days in 1979, 20.9 days in 1985, and 25.6 days in 2002. Patients must pay a certain proportion of out-of-pocket expenses, but the remaining balance is covered by the insurance agency. Inpatient care is essentially free of charge, but with a maximum length of hospital stay of 365 days for elderly adults aged over 70 years, and patients must pay for all inpatient charges incurred after exceeding this limit. Since January 1982, all retirees are entitled to coverage for a certain proportion of their inpatient charges after hospitalization for one full year, as stipulated by their respective counties. However, there is a lower limit to inpatient charges, which was set at SEK150 per day in 2002.

Inpatient charges used to vary across counties, with the highest being about SEK400 per day. Four counties had inpatient charges of more than SEK300 per day, while the majority of counties (about 72%) charged less than SEK160 per day, and only 6% of counties charged more than SEK190 per day. These inconsistencies in inpatient charges and scope of services led to public dissatisfaction and criticism. Therefore, in April 1986, the government of Sweden decided to standardize inpatient charges. By 2002, the maximum inpatient charge was set at SEK150.

In the past, patients had to pay registration fees for outpatient services, but since July 1981, the government has implemented a system whereby patients are given a card with 15 blank spaces. Each time an individual pays the outpatient registration fee, a space is stamped; a fully stamped card can be submitted to the relevant administrative agency to obtain a free slip. Patients with free slips are exempt from paying registration fees, and the free slip is valid for one year from the date of the first stamp.

The payment of registration fees for children under the age of 16 years can also accrue stamps for cards held by their parents. As a result, families with more children can obtain free slips more frequently.

In 2002, the average inpatient expenses for general hospital beds (internal medicine) were SEK1,550 per day (including bed charges, medical expenses, drug expenses, nursing charges, food expenses, and so on) and that for long-term care beds was SEK765 per day, while the charges for outpatient services was SEK320 per visit. The Swedish health insurance system pays counties to provide these medical services (i.e., medical remuneration). The Swedish government has implemented standardized outpatient (SEK250 per service) and inpatient charges (SEK500 per day) (in 2002) rather than adopting the methods adopted in other countries, such as fee schedules. Based on the average inpatient expenses of SEK1,550 per day, we can see that the reimbursement (SEK500) paid by insurance agencies only covers about one-third of the actual expenses.

The central government and county councils have been negotiating to determine the standards for increasing the reimbursement rates for county councils. In principle, the reimbursement rate should increase automatically with the rise in the price index.

The government currently employs a cost-based reimbursement system according to the healthcare services provided by county councils (length of hospital stay and outpatient visits), such that expenditures are reimbursed in proportion with the county's population size. This reimbursement system not only allows for partial reimbursement of medical expenses but also for the implementation of preventive care programs. It also shifts the responsibility for health promotion to county councils, as required by the 1983 Health Care Act.

(3) Medical Benefits and Income Allowances

1. Medical Benefits

1. *Outpatient care.* In Sweden, patients are required to pay only a small amount of outpatient and drug fees at public hospitals. Hospitals in different regions have different outpatient charges, but these differences are minor (between SEK100 and SEK140). However, specialists might impose slightly higher charges, ranging from SEK120 to SEK260; for example, the specialist outpatient charge in Stockholm is SEK260. In order to reduce the burden of residents who are frequently ill, those who have accumulated over SEK900 in outpatient charges per year are exempt from these charges. Children and teenagers under the age of 20 years are also exempt from paying outpatient charges. Aside from the outpatient charges, patients do not need to pay for other service items, such as laboratory tests and drugs administered in the hospital.

   Drug expenses tend to be higher than outpatient charges. The new regulations implemented in 1999 stipulate that patients must pay for prescription drugs that cost less than SEK900 within 12 months. For drug expenses between SEK900 and SEK1800, patients are entitled to a reimbursement of 50–90% as part of the PBS. If their cumulative drug expenses over 12 months exceed SEK1,800, the remaining balance is borne entirely by the government.

2. *Inpatient care.* The inpatient charge in Sweden has been standardized at SEK 80 for current employees and SEK 75 for retirees; this mainly covers food expenses during hospitalization. Medical treatments, such as surgeries, are completely free of charge. The government of Sweden stipulates that physicians who perform these treatments have to be employees of public healthcare institutions and licensed practitioners.

3. *Dental care.* In Sweden, patients receive partial subsidies for dental care services, but the out-of-pocket expenses are much higher than those for medical and drug expenses. Patients are entitled to a 30% subsidy if their dental expenses exceed SEK 3,500, and the subsidies may be up to 70% for procedures costing more than SEK 13,500. However, Swedish residents under the age of 19 years are entitled to free dental care and treatment. Currently, the government of Sweden is considering reforming the dental insurance scheme to improve dental care services.

2. Sickness Benefits   One of the most distinctive features of the Swedish social insurance system is the wide diversity of benefits. There are more than 50 different benefits or subsidies that are meant to ensure good welfare and humanistic care. These benefits include the following: (1) Sickness benefits: Employees are entitled to receive 80% of their salaries from their employers from the second to the fourteenth day of sick leave. From the fifteenth day onwards, they are also entitled to sickness benefits equivalent to 80% of their salaries from the Swedish Social Insurance Agency. (2) Maternity benefits: Pregnant women receive 11 months of maternity benefits equivalent to 80% of their salaries from the Swedish Social Insurance Agency. Additionally, the fathers of newborn babies are entitled to 10 days of paternity leave, during which they receive 80% of their salaries. (3) Work injury benefits: Employees who suffer from work-related injuries or diseases are entitled to receive work injury benefits. Employees with work-related disabilities are entitled to lifetime disability benefits. As for work-related deaths, in addition to funeral benefits, the children of these employees are also entitled to survivors' pensions until the age of 19 years. (4) Disability benefits: All individuals over the age of 16 years with a partial loss of working capacity are entitled to care and disability allowances. The amount of these allowances depends on the severity of the disability.

(4) Characteristics of the Swedish Health Insurance System

1. *Universal coverage.* The government's social health insurance covers all Swedish residents for a wide range of services. Swedish law stipulates that all residents who work or reside in Sweden have equal access to basic health insurance and the comprehensive "cradle-to-grave" social security system.

2. *People-oriented.* The Swedish social security program fully embodies the people-oriented principle, offering comprehensive benefits such as sickness benefits, maternity benefits, disability benefits, overseas medical treatment, dental care, even benefits for patients' dependents, and transportation allowance.

3. *Three-party funding.* The Swedish social insurance premiums are mainly from the government, employers, and employees. The government contributes about one-fourth of the total premiums, while the remaining balance is covered by employers' social security contributions and employees' income taxes. Overall, the premiums are mainly covered by the employers. At present, the Swedish social insurance premiums account for 17% of the GDP.

4. *Government-administered.* All affairs related to Swedish social insurance are administered by the Swedish Social Insurance Agency; local governments have also established their own social insurance agencies, whose operations rely on government funding.

3. Formulation and Value Orientation of Health Policies

(1) Formulation Process of Health Policies

In Sweden, the county councils are primarily responsible for the establishment of hospitals. As the main providers of healthcare services, county councils play a vital role in the formulation of policies related to healthcare services. They tend to have a considerable degree of autonomy as well as independent powers of taxation. Since the early twentieth century, there has been a gradual shift in Swedish healthcare management practices from a centralized system to a decentralized one. This decentralized system has since characterized both the government administration and healthcare system of Sweden. The 1982 Health Care Act stipulates that all Swedes have the legal right to access basic healthcare services. Additionally, it also stipulates that county councils have the authority to formulate and implement local health regulations based on their specific local conditions and healthcare needs. This enables the councils to supervise, administer, and coordinate local healthcare programs, as well as ensure the normal operation of healthcare institutions, in order to meet the ever-growing demand for healthcare in Sweden. In Sweden, the responsibility for healthcare is shared among the 26 county councils and three large municipalities (Gothenburg, Malmö, and Gotland).

The process by which Sweden formulates health policies is shown in Figure 11.42. Counties are the main bodies of the healthcare supply system. Each county is responsible for establishing both five-year midterm plans and annual plans that are subordinate to these five-year plans.

The principles and policies for planning and budgeting in each county are established by the county council assembly (i.e., the LF).

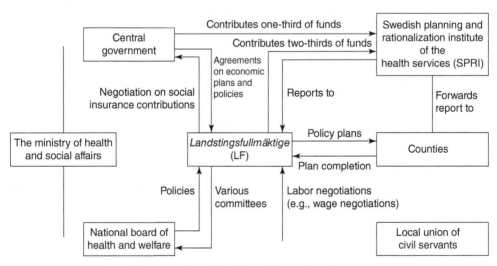

FIGURE 11.42 Formulation process of health policies in Sweden.

The LF is a joint assembly of local leaders (county governors), who are the appointed presidents of the county councils rather than elected local leaders. Hence, the LF is a joint assembly of county governors forming a large-scale permanent agency known as the "county administrative board." Together, the LF and county administrative board play vital roles in the following major tasks related to formulating and administering health policies.

1. Coordination Between the Central and Local Governments The LF established a national five-year plan based on the budgetary and five-year plans of each individual county, in coordination with the central government's economic policies, budgetary structure, and economic plans. The LF can also propose general principles, guidelines, and policies to each county based on the coordinated plan. As a result, the budgetary and five-year plans of each county are aligned with the economic policies of the central government.

2. Formulation of Health Policies Some of the LF's most important tasks are assigning special committee members to various healthcare-related committees, receiving reports from these committees, and commenting on the recommendations made in these reports. The LF also assigns special members to committees established by the Ministry of Health and Social Affairs, in order to exchange opinions on the healthcare affairs of the National Board of Health and Welfare and participate in the formulation of government policies.

3. Coordinate the Interests of all Parties The LF serves as the representative of healthcare providers and insurance agencies. Hence, it focuses on the following aspects when coordinating the interests of all parties: (1) negotiating with county councils on issues related to the funding and payment of healthcare expenditure; and (2) negotiating with the Swedish Medical Association (and the associations of other medical professions) on the remuneration and working conditions of healthcare workers, in order to find a balance of interests among all parties.

4. Investigate, Study and Participate in Healthcare Industry The LF plays various roles in the healthcare industry. However, as the representative of hospitals in Sweden, the LF also requires professional knowledge or information about healthcare or related technologies, which led to the establishment of the Swedish Planning and Rationalization Institute of the Health Services (SPRI). SPRI is a think tank jointly funded by the central government (which contributes one-third of the funding) and LF (two-thirds of the funding) to investigate and disseminate results on issues related to basic healthcare, healthcare institutions, staff management, goods management, information systems, hospital buildings, and so on. It focuses on pragmatic, policy-oriented research topics and methods, such as determining which healthcare services can help reduce overall healthcare expenditure.

In addition, the counties, LF and municipalities of Sweden have organized a public procurement center for making bulk purchases of medical products. The SPRI has also established various companies, such as medical supplies inspection companies, SPRI Material Proving Company (a material quality inspection company), and SPRI Consult Company (a commissioned investigation and evaluation company).

(2) Value Orientation of Health Policies

1. Emphasis on Primary Healthcare Sweden has seriously considered the drawbacks of overconcentration of healthcare resources in large-sized hospitals, which has led to its gradual shift in policies and resources to support community healthcare services. Sweden is gradually resolving the imbalance of supply and demand in healthcare services due to physicians' preference for serving at large-sized hospitals and the excessive division of labor. A survey in 2006 showed that 49–63% of Swedes highly trusted primary care providers.

2. Installment of Long-Term Care Beds Due to the increasing demand for elderly care, Sweden is seeking to install more long-term care beds for the following reasons: To enable the transfer of elderly patients who require less intensive care to long-term care beds, thereby alleviating the problem of hospital beds at general healthcare institutions being occupied by such patients; to reduce overall healthcare expenditure by installing long-term care beds with lower average unit prices per day; and to enable a shift in responsibilities from the welfare sector to the healthcare sector, thus meeting the demand for elderly care beyond the scope of welfare coverage. The demand for elderly care is expected to increase considerably in the future alongside the aging of the Swedish population.

3. Reduction in the Number of Inpatient Beds at Psychiatric Hospitals Following the greater public openness and socialization of mental health, Sweden has reconsidered the drawbacks of large-scale inpatient care and, thus, has reduced the number of psychiatric hospital beds from 34,000 in 1973 to 21,000 in 2000 and 18,000 in 2005.

In 2002, there was a total of 31 million outpatient visits, with an average of 2.45 visits per capita (excluding the 1.2 million visits to women and children health centers).

The annual growth rate of outpatient visits from 1980 to 2000 was 1.9%. It is worth noting that the proportion of outpatient visits to community clinics increased from 45% in 1980 to 52% in 2000. As of 2005, the number of outpatient visits to facilities other than hospitals, such as healthcare centers and community physicians, has increased by 3.2% per year, whereas the number of outpatient visits to large-sized hospitals has only increased by 0.3% per year. These statistics suggest that Sweden attaches great importance to primary care.

4. Healthcare Cost-Containment Policies

(1) Total Healthcare Expenditure and Its Growth Trends

Since the 1930s, Sweden has implemented a universal health insurance scheme and has gradually expanded its healthcare and welfare benefits. However, since the 1960s, Sweden has contended with slow economic growth, market depression, increasing fiscal deficits, a large unemployed population, and a low inflation rate. In addition, the implementation of the universal health insurance policy substantially increased its healthcare expenditure, leading to a shortage of health insurance funds, overstaffing of the healthcare industry, and a lack of social insurance funds, which caused a severe socioeconomic crisis.

Statistics show that in 1950, the total healthcare expenditure of Sweden accounted for 3.4% of the GNP, which increased to 4.6% in 1960, 6.1% in 1970, and 8.9% (SEK51 billion) in 1981. In 2003, the total healthcare expenditure was 8.7% of the GNP, and the healthcare expenditure per capita was US$2,270, which increased to US$2,828 in 2004 and accounted for 9.1% of the GDP). Currently, the total healthcare expenditure in Sweden accounts for 9% of the GDP, and this share has remained stable since the early 1980s.

From 1970 to 1928, healthcare expenditure in Sweden increased by 15.4% and then by 16.8% from 1981 to 2001, during which the healthcare expenditure per capita increased by 3.7% (after correcting for inflation). During the same period, Sweden's GDP growth rate was 110%. Currently, Sweden spends approximately SEK150 billion per year on healthcare services. The government also spends around SEK102 billion per year on sickness benefits (about one-eighth of the annual government expenditure). Although inflation is a major contributing factor to the increase in healthcare expenditure, there are undoubtedly several shortcomings in the Swedish social security and health insurance systems that have contributed to this rise. As a result, the reform of the social security system, the reform and improvement of the healthcare systems, more rational allocation and utilization of resources, and the improvement in healthcare service efficiency have become major social issues that urgently need to be resolved by the government.

An increasing number of Swedish health policymakers and health economists are recognizing the need to reform the prescriptive planning model that has been in use in Sweden for some time. Many regions of Sweden are seeking and experimenting with several reform measures. For instance, some are attempting to adapt health reform models and concepts from the UK, the US, and Canada, in order to implement reforms that are best suited to the unique conditions of Sweden. This will enable the discovery and development of specific approaches to ensure the rational exploitation and utilization of healthcare resources, and to impose strict limits on or even reduce healthcare expenditure.

(2) Macro-Level Regulation by the Government

The Swedish government is re-examining its role in healthcare services, and has defined its main responsibilities as the formulation and implementation of health policies and legislation, as well as the supervision of healthcare funding. The government must withdraw from the frontline in healthcare funding and medical services, as allowing the independent operation and administration of healthcare funding agencies and healthcare service providers can improve their operational efficiency and service quality.

The government has enhanced its macroprudential regulation and clarified that the principle of Swedish health reform is based on the integration of financial and operational autonomy, whereby operation autonomy is delegated to the 26 counties, and their financial autonomy is further enhanced.

(3) Health System Reforms

Sweden's current attempt at health reform was initiated primarily to substitute the former rigid and inefficient planning model with a market-based mechanism, in order to foster the development of an internal market and allow orderly competition among suppliers. This reform has influenced the Swedish healthcare system. Currently, some regions and hospitals are experimenting with the US DRG system, whereby payments to healthcare institutions are made by a third party based on a fixed amount that is determined according to the DRG classification of patients. These regions and hospitals have effectively controlled the growth in healthcare expenditure and improved the quality of healthcare services they provide.

In 1990, certain hospitals in Kopparberg county initiated the Dalarna reform, whereby patients are given the freedom to choose their preferred hospitals and orderly competition is promoted among hospitals. This reform prompted medical institutions to reduce their costs and operating expenses in order to improve the cost-effectiveness and efficiency of their healthcare services. In 1992, the Stockholm County Council passed a healthcare funding and organizational reform bill (known as the Stockholm model), which proposed the separation of services from fundraising by allocating healthcare resources according to the population needs (based on population size, age structure, and socioeconomic status) in the region. The freedom of patients to choose their preferred healthcare institutions and physicians without geographical restriction was found to encourage competition among healthcare institutions and more effective utilization of local healthcare resources, thereby restricting the rise in healthcare expenditure and improving healthcare service efficiency. Overall, the Swedish government has reformed its healthcare system using a number of reform models, multichannel investments, internal markets, orderly competition, and enhancing hospital cost-effectiveness.

Since 2003, Swedish residents have been free to choose where to receive healthcare services. This means that they are able to access healthcare services in all regions of the country. In February 2009, the Riksdag approved the development of a preliminary selection system for basic healthcare in all counties, giving patients the freedom to choose between private and public medical centers; this system has been in operation since January 2010. All healthcare providers that meet the requirements of the county councils can establish medical centers with financial support from the county public funds. These medical centers must employ social workers or psychologists and provide family health services and emergency services until 9.00 p.m. All medical centers receive a standard reimbursement based on the number of visits.

(4) Enhance Supply-Side Control in Healthcare

Supply-side control refers to effective macroprudential regulation by the government to effectively manage and control healthcare expenditure, enhance the cost-effectiveness of the healthcare sector, allow for the rational exploitation of healthcare resources, and improve the accessibility and equality of healthcare services.

To achieve this, the Swedish government has assumed greater control over the budget, the scale and development of hospitals, the size of hospital healthcare workforce, and the cost-effectiveness of healthcare services. For instance, the total number of hospital beds in Sweden has decreased by nearly 40% from 1985 to 1997, which is equivalent to a decline from 4.4 beds to 2.7 beds per 1,000 people. The scope of outpatient services was also been actively expanded to reduce the number of inpatients. In addition, the number of healthcare practitioners was reduced from 451,000 in 1990 to 326,000 in 1996 (a reduction of 27.7%). The control of the healthcare workforce and the improvement in healthcare service efficiency has curbed the growth in healthcare expenditure.

The government of Sweden also established specifications for drug use to prevent overprescription and to curb drastic increases in drug expenses. The government has also been establishing relevant review bodies to assess new medical technologies, drugs, and devices; provide advice on new technologies, devices, and drugs that are ineffective or expensive and hence deemed as unsuitable for reimbursement by health insurance; and to strictly limit the addition and utilization of new medical devices and equipment. In addition, the government has strictly limited the enrollment of medical students and is actively encouraging medical graduates to serve in remote, impoverished, and sparsely populated areas. Several measures have been also been adopted to optimize the allocation of health resources and control hospital expenses.

(5) Enhance Demand-Side Control in Healthcare

As another approach to controlling the rise of healthcare expenditure, the Swedish government has been striving to enhance demand-side cost-containment mechanisms for healthcare services. Specifically, it has focused on patient cost-sharing, increasing patients' awareness of healthcare expenditure, cultivating an understanding of health economics among patients, helping them develop a proper attitude towards healthcare services, and supporting patient self-care. For example, before 1990, all Swedish employees were entitled to receive sickness benefits equivalent to 90% of their salaries from the Swedish Social Insurance Agency from the first day of sick leave. Unfortunately, this provision led to malingering or overtreatment among some employees, which placed a greater financial burden on the government. Thus, the provision was reformed so that employees are entitled to 65% of their income losses from the second to the third day of sick leave, and 70% of their income losses from the fourth day onwards. However, the maximum amount of sickness benefits is SEK 587 per day, and the benefits are taxable. Furthermore, the first two weeks of sick leave are covered by the employers, rather than the government.

Moreover, the government has enhanced its own supervision and control over healthcare expenditure via spot checks and audits of the rationality of prescriptions and treatments at hospitals. It has also reformed the unreasonable payment system, increased the proportion of patient out-of-pocket expenses for healthcare services and certain drugs, and reduced the coverage and service content of health insurance.

In addition to enhancing healthcare cost containment, the Swedish government has also improved the management of health insurance funds. Specifically, the government proposed that healthcare expenditure in all regions should match the amount of health insurance funds raised. Thus, all local councils must strictly examine and approve the health insurance budget and stipulate the annual increase in the health insurance expenditure in order to strictly control its growth rate.

The purpose of such demand-side reforms is not only to alleviate the financial pressure on healthcare services but also to promote their efficiency by ensuring patients' freedom of choice and promoting competition among healthcare service providers, thereby also achieving healthcare cost containment

These reform measures have yielded certain outcomes, but the financial overburden of the health insurance has not yet been resolved. Hence, new reform measures are still being discussed and anticipated.

5. Difficulties in the Healthcare System and Reform Attempts

(1) Difficulties Facing the Healthcare System in the 1980s

1. User Dissatisfaction   In October 1983, the SPRI published a total of four promotional advertisements, once every other week, in every Swedish newspaper with the aim of promoting the improvement of healthcare services. The slogans of those advertisements were as follows: "Why is the best healthcare in the world being criticized?"; "Why is it easier to see the Prime Minister than to see a doctor?"; "It takes too long to see a doctor"; and "Healthcare is not comprehensible and not informative." Through these advertisements, the SPRI noted the essential problems with the healthcare system, and solicited feedback from the general public via telephone or written letters on how to improve the system.

These slogans mainly focused on the following reform issues: (1) improving the ease of public access to healthcare resources; (2) shortening patient waiting time; and (3) eliminating suspicions of healthcare among patients. These are precisely the key problems in the Swedish healthcare system.

These advertisements intended to emphasize that many Swedes were dissatisfied with healthcare services, even though Sweden had arguably the best healthcare quality and utilization rate. In addition, how to improve the services of Swedish public and private healthcare institutions was often a subject of debate and concern among the public.

However, in the past, the Swedish government focused solely on the establishment, expansion, and financial security of the healthcare system, and had little interest in consulting public opinions on healthcare issues. Moreover, the government never emphasized the importance of healthcare services or committed itself to improve their quality. Accordingly, improving healthcare services became a key direction of healthcare development throughout the 1980s.

2. Issues in the Health Insurance System and Healthcare Services

1. *Constant adjustments are needed for health insurance policies.* The health insurance system of Sweden is predominated by cash benefits, particularly sickness benefits. The sickness benefits system involves a benefit rate of 90% from the date of disease onset. In 1976, the average length of sickness benefits was 22.9 days per person. This system not only placed a considerable financial burden on the government but also invited strong criticism from members of the public, particularly business owners, who considered this as "excessive" social security.

   Perhaps due to the controversy over sickness benefits or due to changes in the terms of employment such that long-term absenteeism was no longer allowed, the length of sickness benefits peaked in 1976, after which it decreased for seven consecutive years to 18.8 days in 1983. This figure only increased after eight years in 1984, reaching 20.9 days by 1985.

   The increase in 1984 was attributed to an extra day of sickness benefits among women, which had exceeded the 1981 level (i.e., the average numbers of days were 17 days and 20 days for men and women, respectively).

2. *Increased input with reduced efficiency.* Although Sweden does not have the highest healthcare expenditure among developed countries, this expenditure did increase by 145% from 1980 to 1990, during which the healthcare output was reduced. During the same period, the number of healthcare workers in Sweden increased from 300,000 to 370,000, among which the number of physicians and nurses doubled while the number of administrative staff tripled. A possible explanation for these statistics is that the Swedish healthcare system does not fully and reasonably utilize its healthcare resources. Furthermore, the healthcare expenditures per capita in Sweden vary considerably among the different regions, and charges for the same surgical operation were significantly different among healthcare institutions. In summary, suppliers play a dominant role in the Swedish healthcare system due to the relative absence of competition among hospitals. This is related to the government's funding system, whereby the government budget for hospitals is allocated based on their budgets for the previous year. As a result, there is a lack of incentives for hospitals to increase service efficiency and enhance their responsiveness to consumer demand. According to the 2007 statistics for the EU, Sweden and Portugal occupied the bottom two positions in a ranking of the accessibility of healthcare services.

3. *Weak primary care system.* The Swedish healthcare system has a weak primary care system compared with other countries. Despite the high salary for physicians at community healthcare centers, it is still difficult to recruit qualified physicians for these positions. This is potentially because GPs lack high social status, which causes them to lack enthusiasm and motivation. Additionally, there is a lack of links between healthcare services, social care services, and sickness insurance with primary care and hospital services. There are also no "gatekeepers" at the local level who can help control the irrational use of resources. Patients may seek medical attention directly from specialists at general hospitals because of an absence of GPs, which increases the utilization rate of healthcare services at such hospitals. However, this practice is not beneficial to healthcare cost containment, as there are differences in the service costs between general hospitals and community primary care institutions. Moreover, the increased use of hospital services has prompted an increased input of healthcare resources to hospitals. In the 1950s and 1960s, the government allocated a major share of the healthcare funds (approximately 75% of total healthcare expenditure in Sweden) to a minority of large-sized hospitals with a greater number of beds.

4. *Funding shortfalls in healthcare institutions due to budget cuts.* Due to Sweden's poor economic performance, its tax-based public healthcare services, much like other welfare systems, are increasingly vulnerable to government budget cuts. Due to the government's incomplete attempts at reforming the hospital reimbursement system, certain large-sized public hospitals are facing severe losses. This is caused by a lack of specific regulations on the types and quality of services that these hospitals should deliver, thus leading to confusion regarding their service provision.

5. *Issues in the efficiency of service delivery.* A serious problem facing the Swedish healthcare system is the long waiting time for surgery. Although this problem had been addressed in the past, it reemerged in 1995. There are long waiting lists not only at large general hospitals but also at community primary care institutions, which have led to some patients seeking medical attention at large hospitals, thus leading to an increase in healthcare expenditure.

6. *Relative lag in the development of medical technologies.* The Swedish healthcare system provides first-class healthcare services compared to other developed countries. Nevertheless, Sweden is lagging behind other developed countries in adopting new technologies, especially the introduction and promotion of large, expensive medical equipment and cutting-edge surgical techniques, due to strict budgetary controls.

7. *Lack of coordination and integration in healthcare services and management.* The Swedish healthcare system has long been a conventional hospital-based healthcare system. Compared to other countries, it has a larger proportion of physicians serving in hospitals. In the 1970s, Sweden was already committed to improving the quality of primary care and enhancing the cooperation between hospitals and primary care institutions. However, Sweden's decentralized healthcare system has impeded the adequate cooperation among different healthcare tiers. Additionally, issues related to the operational performance of the primary care sector and cross-tier healthcare cooperation vary across different regions. Current structural reforms to the healthcare system, such as the concentration of emergency hospitals, specialization of treatment, the transition from inpatient care to primary and home-based care, and the improvement of primary care, represent major challenges facing the allocation efficiency of healthcare resources. Therefore, the government of Sweden should strive for a more rational distribution of physicians in hospitals and primary care institutions and continue to enhance cross-tier cooperation.

3. Overlap Between Social Welfare and Healthcare Services   The cooperation between social welfare and healthcare services is arguably the most problematic aspect of the current Swedish healthcare system. This stems from the fact that social welfare is administered by districts, whereas healthcare is administered by counties. The former are responsible for the social welfare of healthy elderly individuals, while the latter are responsible for elderly individuals who require medical attention.

Social welfare, which is centered on home-based care and residential services, generally focuses on the care for healthy elderly adults. Healthcare services, by contrast, have devoted a large number of hospital beds to elderly patients requiring long-term care.

Given the importance of the cooperation between social welfare and healthcare services, the government of Sweden has been working towards merging nursing homes with county hospitals (including long-term care wards), such that the first floor of the nursing homes would offer traditional nursing home services, while the second floor would house long-term care wards (as in the newly built facilities in Stockholm). However, some scholars are skeptical as to whether long-term care wards can take good care of elderly adults, as they are considered a new measure in elderly care. Furthermore, even with 24-hour services, home-based care is still preferable to inpatient care from an economic perspective. Therefore, the establishment of long-term care wards might be restricted in favor of home-based care services.

In Stockholm, for example, the County Healthcare Center has cooperated with the district government to organize teams consisting of home healthcare nurses and home helpers. These teams have attempted to create a new home-based care system by adopting night care services. These teams have since transferred about 30 inpatients back to their homes, thereby reducing the county expenditure by SEK 6.5 million per year. Furthermore, their home visit services increased the district expenditure only by SEK 2 million. Therefore, the teams have reduced the overall healthcare expenditure by SEK 4.5 million. Considerable attention has been paid to these beneficial, exploratory reforms since the 1980s, and they seem capable of addressing the gap between social welfare and healthcare services to some extent.

4. Controversies over the Introduction of Private Healthcare Institutions   The monopolization of the healthcare system by the public sector has been criticized. Indeed, conservative and centrist parties are dissatisfied with the current healthcare system and its lack of GPs, and have compared Swedish hospitals to factories. They pointed out that the public sector's monopolization of the healthcare system is worth reforming.

In February 1983, a private emergency clinic was opened in the city center of Stockholm. The clinic had served about 100 patients by the afternoon of its opening day, which was a clear indication that Swedes found the long waiting list at public hospitals unbearable. One year later, this private clinic was ranked fifth nationally in the number of visits.

The controversy over the liberalization of the Swedish healthcare system began in 1983. Since then, the introduction of private healthcare institutions has become a major issue.

(2) Swedish Health Reforms in the 1990s

1. Reform Background   The Swedish universal healthcare system is funded by taxation; hence, public funds cover the largest share of Sweden's total healthcare expenditure. The total healthcare expenditure continued to rise alongside population aging and the advancement in medical technologies. At the same time, the unemployment rate in Sweden had risen continually since the late 1980s because of economic stagnation. From 1991 to 1993, the negative economic growth in Sweden reduced the government tax revenues, while the rising unemployment rate increased public expenditure to 73% of the GDP in 1993. The Swedish government recognized the need to reduce its public expenditure in order to balance its income and expenditure, and thereby promote economic development. To this end, the Riksdag passed a law prohibiting any increase in local taxes between 1991 and 1994. In addition, the county councils were forced to reduce their expenditures by 2% annually since 1992. These financial difficulties prompted local governments to explore reforms in their healthcare systems. Moreover, Sweden also recognized the need to reduce its tax revenues to better compete in the coming era of economic globalization and to meet the standards for joining the EU.

Numerous issues have hindered the Swedish healthcare system from adapting to environmental changes. Nevertheless, public dissatisfaction has accelerated the government's efforts to reform the healthcare system. Some of Sweden's the traditional welfare policies were questioned or reformed, but as a welfare state, the principle of universality in Swedish healthcare was not extensively challenged. Based on this principle, an increasing number of provincial and county governments sought to provide more flexible healthcare services in the 1990s. Therefore, it became necessary to reform the traditional healthcare system.

In general, most local governments in Sweden introduced new approaches to funding and service delivery as reform measures. These reforms were based on the internal market reforms of the NHS in the UK and sought to introduce market competition into a healthcare system that has traditionally been characterized by a high degree of planned control. Patients now have the right to choose their preferred healthcare institutions, thus forcing these institutions to compete with each other. Healthcare institutions have also established market-based budgets to maintain their revenues and the salaries of their employees. Healthcare institutions were also given the right to determine their prices based on the number of visits, which in turn depended on their service quality. In summary, Swedish healthcare institutions shifted from traditional budget execution and service provision to acting as semi-independent, nonprofit companies.

The traditional prospective payment system for hospitals was abandoned by most regions, and replaced by an FFS system for hospital services and a capitation system for general medical services. In addition, 14 provinces introduced the purchaser–provider split model in 1994 to reduce their healthcare expenditures. Hospitals in these provinces are reimbursed based on their performance, such as the number of patients and service quality. This is similar to HMOs in the US, but the hospitals in Sweden were reimbursed via DRG-based payments based on a predetermined number of medical consultations and surgeries.

The Swedish health reforms of the 1990s were based on a number of reform models. This was because Sweden consists of self-governing, highly independent counties, and county councils are primarily responsible for the delivery of healthcare services. Among these models, the Stockholm model and Dalarna model are of particular importance; both of which focus on improving the service efficiency of healthcare institutions, controlling healthcare expenditure, and reducing the financial burden on the government.

2. Stockholm Reform Model
(1) Objectives, basic principles, and content of the reform In January 1992, the Stockholm County Council (population: 1.7 million) began proposing new funding and organizational models to enhance the effective use of county healthcare resources and improve patients' overall status. These models were fully implemented in 1995. The specific objectives of the Stockholm model were as follows: (1) to improve patients' freedom of choice; (2) to improve healthcare quality; (3) to ensure healthcare continuity; (4) to improve the

accessibility of healthcare services; (5) to improve public health; (6) to improve the productivity of the healthcare system; and (7) to enhance the participation of healthcare workers.

The Stockholm model was based on the following basic principles: (1) purchaser–provider split; (2) providers are reimbursed via a pay-for-performance model and are permitted to charge for necessary items; (3) providers are encouraged to provide services in the most competitive environment possible. Naturally, the adequacy of each of these principles is questionable.

In the previous system, the government allocated funds to hospitals and healthcare centers based on global budgets. The greatest drawback of these global budgets is the lack of coordination between service delivery and resource allocation.

The Stockholm model created an internal market for hospital services. Health districts purchase hospital services on behalf of their residents or patients via an FFS system (the payment rate for inpatient acute care is determined based on DRGs, while that for out-of-hospital services is determined by another outcome measurement system). Patients have the freedom to choose their preferred GPs, healthcare centers, and hospitals (including private hospitals) located not only within their region of residence but also in other regions. The role of the government has also changed in this new model. Although the governments are still responsible for serving the local residents, allocating and utilizing healthcare resources, and determining the budget of each health district, they are no longer involved in managing day-to-day operations.

Apart from scientific research, hospital development, medical education, and employee training, the incomes of acute care hospitals were entirely from the services provided in health districts. The fee amount was determined using a capped fixed fee schedule. All free items and services were abolished, while the prices of X-rays, laboratory tests, and other medical and administrative services were determined using an internal pricing system. Additionally, clinics could provide opportunities for patients to purchase other hospital services. Through these means, the Stockholm model has given rise to a competitive healthcare environment.

The contracts between local health districts or primary care departments and acute hospitals are renewed annually via negotiation. The scope, price, quality, and accessibility of services within each acute care hospital, as well as the extent of collaboration between providers, must also be negotiated.

A capped fee schedule for inpatient services was also implemented; this fee schedule was consistent with the structure of DRGs. A fixed fee schedule was established for mobile healthcare services as well, and the prices were higher than were those for clinical specialist services. In 1994, the Stockholm County Council proposed the establishment of a family physician system and allocated funds for primary care, geriatric care, and mental health care based on a composite demographic and socioeconomic index (similar to the RAWP formula adopted in the UK). As a result, the reimbursement system for geriatric and mental health care is expected to be further improved.

The Stockholm model has brought about considerable changes in the division of functions and responsibilities among the various departments of the Stockholm County Council. In fact, the model has influenced the entire county council to a certain extent, from county elections to the staffing of healthcare institutions.

(2) Reform evaluation
1. *Patients' freedom of choice.* Consumers usually have limited ability to determine the need for preventive and therapeutic services, as some of their questions require medical knowledge to answer. The Stockholm model stipulates that consumers have the freedom to choose in matters they are capable of deciding and can choose between GPs and hospital specialists (who impose higher fees). However, physicians are reluctant

to let patients choose different treatment regimens because hospitals are reimbursed according to the type and number of patients.

In order to make a rational and effective choice, consumers need to understand the types of services available and their therapeutic efficacies. The availability of such information must be ensured by implementing a comprehensive regulatory system that is supervised by an independent party. These measures could help increase the number of consumers who wish to exercise their rights to choose.

2. *Efficiency.* Health districts serve as purchasers in the Stockholm model, which allows the allocation of healthcare expenditure to be based on the population's overall health status and risk of diseases. In addition, purchasers might prioritize primary care by allocating healthcare resources in a way that maximizes health outcomes but minimizes the use of resources in the long term.

The health districts are responsible for signing healthcare service agreements with healthcare providers. In order to prevent increases in service charges due to institutional changes, there must be true competition among providers, which will ensure that they pay greater attention to the wishes and needs of the patients. This may also improve their service volume and quality. However, it is worth noting that the increase in service volume does not necessarily reflect the actual situation because providers might induce demand or engage in cost shifting to increase their revenues.

To prevent issues such as cost shifting and quality reduction, purchasers may explain in advance to providers that their charges, services, and therapeutic outcomes are subject to strict supervision. Such supervision may be more effective when used in conjunction with quality control. Purchasers' knowledge of the service quality of providers can reduce the latter's tendency to engage in fraud. As a result, the Stockholm model can increase productivity without sacrificing healthcare quality.

3. *Equality.* Healthcare systems that give patients the freedom of choice may also give rise to healthcare inequality. This is because highly educated individuals are more likely to emphasize their own interests compared to less educated individuals. Thus, highly educated individuals are more likely to actively and consciously select their family physicians, which may imply that less educated individuals are more likely to receive low-quality healthcare services. In addition, the high fees incurred for hospital outpatient services might suppress healthcare demand among low-income earners. To prevent such inequalities, it is important that patients' rights and physicians' responsibilities be clearly defined; health districts provide reimbursements with greater consideration of the effect on patients' freedom of choice; patients are diagnosed by GPs (gatekeepers) before being admitted to hospitals; and standardized fees are incurred for outpatient services.

4. *Cost containment.* Costs can be strictly controlled under the Stockholm model because providers compete for patients or contracts and a fixed price is established for each discharged or scheduled patient. However, some practices associated with the Stockholm model can actually increase healthcare expenditure. In particular, the freedom of patients to choose between GPs and hospital outpatient departments might lead to an increase in the demand for specialist and inpatient services. Similarly, the freedom of providers to meet the healthcare demands of patients, including their demand for non-essential care, might also increase the overall demand for healthcare services. A dearth of contracts or patients might also induce providers to make more cost-driven decisions. These risk factors for increased expenses can be prevented via the following approaches: enhancing the role of GPs as gatekeepers to help regulate basic healthcare demand, thereby limiting service volume, and rectifying increased expenses via price reduction when a certain threshold is exceeded.

Preliminary statistics generated by the financial officers of Stockholm County Council have illustrated the vitality of the Stockholm model. In particular, the county council has lowered prices continuously due to increases in healthcare service productivity, freedom of choice among patients, cost awareness, and service volume, thereby controlling healthcare expenditures to a certain extent. However, more effort is still required in this regard. It can be concluded from the Stockholm experience that an internal market is insufficient for effective cost containment in the healthcare industry. It should be noted there has been no report on the quality and performance of healthcare services before and after the implementation of the Stockholm model.

3. Dalarna Reform Model   The Dalarna model sought to create an integrated public/private market in which public and private healthcare institutions compete with each other. The model also shifted the financial responsibilities from the county level to the community level, so that the latter can directly manage their healthcare service delivery. These communities can directly negotiate and sign healthcare service contracts with local providers, while residents are given the freedom to choose their preferred healthcare centers, including those located beyond their place of residence. Furthermore, the budget originally allocated to hospitals was allocated to the primary care sector instead. The advantage of this model is that primary care centers can reduce hospital workloads and supervise the necessity of specialist services. Additionally, the model also forced hospitals to improve the efficiency and rationality of their services due to budgetary control.

The two key elements of the Dalarna model are the freedom of patients to choose healthcare institutions and the establishment of a business incentive mechanism. The model stipulates that patients can seek medical attention at healthcare agencies within and beyond the region of their residence, and that the expenses incurred are borne by their respective community management committees. Patients seeking medical attention at private practices must bear part of their medical expenses, but a large proportion of these expenses are still borne by the primary care centers in their place of residence.

In the Dalarna model, the actual healthcare demand in a certain area is determined based on demographic factors, such as the gender and age of residents, and the budgets of primary care centers are allocated via capitation-based methods. Additionally, community primary care centers must also be reorganized in terms of cost and quality, such that they are in a less vulnerable position during competition. As such, the form of service provision and internal work efficiency of community primary care centers are the keys to their success.

Theoretically speaking, the Dalarna model relies on macro- and micro-level policymaking processes that are separate but still closely associated. At the macro-level, the Dalarna model seeks a cooperative form of market to improve the efficiency of healthcare services and the responsibility of various social groups. Therefore, market mechanisms have been incorporated into the planned system to form a "planned market." This special "planned market" combines profit and nonprofit organizations to achieve a balance between the equality and efficiency of healthcare services. The key factors that determine the success of market-oriented reforms under the conventional planned system lie with defining the goals of the new market, determining how to achieve these goals, and formulating measures and standards for organizational assessment and incentives.

Under this macro-level "planned market," nonprofit companies are established at the micro-level as main players in marketized operations. Community primary care centers are a type of nonprofit company that plays a crucial role in the Dalarna reform model. In practice, however, there are four types of nonprofit companies in the Dalarna model: primary care centers with capitated budgets; hospital outpatient departments with FFS budgets;

TABLE 11.23 An Overview of the Major Health Reforms and Policy Measures in Sweden in the 1990s

Year	Name of Act	Specific Policy Measures
1992	Ädel Reform	Municipalities took over the responsibilities for running long-term care and social welfare services for the elderly and disabled individuals
1992	National Guarantee of Treatment	Limited waiting times for treatment
1993/1994	Disability Reform	Extended rights of people with functional impairments
1994	Family Doctor Act	Residents could choose their preferred family physicians
1994	Act on Freedom to Establish Private Practices	Encouraged the establishment of private practices
1995	Abolishment of Family Doctor Act and Act on Freedom to Establish Private Practices	Decreased ability to establish private practices and choose family physicians
1995	Psychiatric Reform	Municipalities took over the responsibility for fully treating psychiatric patients
1997	Act on Supervision	Established a supervisory mechanism for supervising all healthcare institutions
1997	Quality Systems	General rules addressing healthcare quality systems
1997	Guarantee of Medical Treatment	Promoted the utilization of primary and specialist care
1997	Act on Priorities	Introduced the healthcare priority system
1997	Pharmaceutical Reform	Implemented the new pharmaceutical benefits scheme
1998	Pharmaceutical Reform	County councils will pay for the expenses on prescription drugs
1999	Act on Professional Activities in Health and Medical Services	All healthcare activities must be reported to the National Board of Health and Welfare
1999	Patients' Right Reform	Increased obligations for county councils regarding patients' rights
1999	Dental Care Reform	Fixed subsidies for different types of services and free pricing system for healthcare institutions

nursing homes and long-term care institutions that adopt the quality-cum-cost-based selection (QCBS) method; and county-administered auxiliary and hotel services that compete in the market as limited for-profit companies.

4. Other Health Reform Policies Swedish health reforms began in the 1980s, but the government only established relevant health reform programs for those with special needs, such as the elderly and disabled individuals, in the 1990s, as shown in Table 11.23.

From 1991 to 1993, the ruling conservative/center-right political alliance introduced the family physician program, which included provisions stipulating the salary and remuneration of family physicians. These provisions were later abolished by the Swedish Social Democratic Party but were still partially retained in healthcare systems of all Swedish provinces.

TABLE 11.24   Changes in Healthcare Services in Sweden From 1986 to 2003

Indicator	1986	1990	1996	2003
Annual number of visits per capita	2.7	2.8	2.9	2.8
Number of hospital beds per 1,000 people (acute diseases + psychiatric disorders)	7.4	5.8	3.6	3.1 (2002)
Number of inpatients per year at acute care hospitals	15	17	42	–
Number of healthcare practitioners per 1,000 people	52.7	52.7	39	31.9 (2002)
Share of private hospital beds (%)	6.7	7.6	22	27

In 1991, the government of Sweden issued the Maximum Waiting Time Guarantee to address long waiting times in Sweden. This guarantee stipulated that patients have the right to choose other medical institutions if the original medical institution does not provide treatment within three months of the treatment decision.

In 1992, the Ädel Reform shifted the responsibility of elderly care at healthcare institutions or care centers from the central government to municipalities.

In 1994, the Swedish government promulgated the Act on Freedom to Establish Private Practices and began encouraging the establishment of private healthcare institutions.

In 1997, the government promulgated a series of reforms, such as the Act on Supervision, Quality Systems, and Law on Priorities, to further guarantee healthcare quality throughout the country. These reform measures sought to establish a supervisory mechanism for all healthcare institutions, formulate general rules for addressing healthcare quality systems, and promote the utilization of primary and specialist care by introducing healthcare priorities.

In 1998, the government introduced the PBS to address the most pressing pharmaceutical issues in the process of health reform. In addition, county councils assumed the responsibility of covering the expenses for prescription drugs.

In 1999, the government of Sweden reformed dental care by implementing fixed subsidies for different types of services and free pricing systems for healthcare institutions.

5. Outcomes of Health Reforms   The outcomes of Swedish health reforms have not been systematically and comprehensively studied. Moreover, some notable changes in the Swedish healthcare system can be attributed to economic, political, and social factors rather than the implemented reforms. Nevertheless, some of the expected effects of these reforms on the Swedish healthcare system have been observed, including the improved efficiency of hospital services, reduced patient waiting times for hospitalization and surgeries, and improved health outcome indicators (Table 11.24).

However, despite the improved efficiency of healthcare services, the reforms have had a negative impact on healthcare equality to some extent. Some studies illustrated a clear increase in inequality for out-of-hospital services – for instance, the length of hospital stay for the elderly and disabled individuals has considerably reduced because of tighter hospital budgets; most of these individuals are now transferred from hospitals to primary care institutions or home-based care. The Swedish government has also noted that there is no guarantee of the quality of healthcare services for the elderly and disabled individuals.

Some reform measures have increased the share of out-of-pocket expenses for healthcare services. For instance, there was a significant increase in private payments as a share of total healthcare expenditure from 9.7% in 1990 to 15.7% in 1996 and 14.7% in 2002. Private healthcare services have also become increasingly active following the introduction of the competitive market mechanism in the reforms. Some public healthcare institutions have chosen to close or privatize because of the tightening of government budgets. Table 11.24 shows that the share of private hospital beds has increased continuously over the years. Public funding for healthcare is also expected to gradually decline, as the Swedish tax rate is expected to decrease in the long run. Additionally, there is a limit to which the share of out-of-pocket expenses can be increased before it starts to influence the accessibility of healthcare services. Therefore, there is an urgent need to establish a new nongovernmental fundraising mechanism that can also benefit the status of private healthcare services. As a result, Sweden is facing an unprecedented challenge in the dominance of public funding for healthcare services.

6. The Path of Swedish Health System Reforms in the Twenty-First Century

The Swedish health reforms in the twenty-first century have primarily focused on resolving problems that have arisen as due to cost-containment measures.

In October 2002, the enforcement of the Pharmaceutical Benefit Reform Act also gave rise to a new agency: the Pharmaceutical Benefits Board, which has the power to decide whether a drug or a medical product is eligible for government subsidies, as well as negotiate with pharmaceutical companies about their prices. The eligibility of a drug for reimbursement is now determined based on the principles of cost-effectiveness rather than on particular health indicators. However, the board can make an exception by determining the eligibility of a drug for reimbursement based on certain indicators or patient groups. Furthermore, from October 2002 onwards, reimbursable prescription drugs should be replaced with their cheapest generic counterparts in pharmacies. In particular, this method has enhanced governmental control over drug expenses and the prescription behavior of healthcare providers. The new dental care program implemented in 2002 provided a high-cost payment protection plan for elderly patients aged over 65 years to help them cope with high out-of-pocket expenses for dental care and the resulting economic risks. There was no significant progress in the reforms in 2003 and 2004. The debates over the Swedish healthcare system in the early twenty-first century mainly focused on the need for healthcare coordination because of the cost-containment measures implemented by county councils. After 2003, the delivery of specialist and acute care was clustered within the geographical boundaries of their respective counties. For example, smaller counties began to cooperate with each other to implement specialist care, despite this process being slow. On the other hand, healthcare for the elderly and patients with multiple diseases was coordinated across various care levels, such as inpatient care, primary care, institutional care, and family care. In addition, the greater central government control over the distribution of responsibilities among central, county, and local governments in providing healthcare services also became a controversial issue. The Parliamentary Committee on Public Sector Responsibilities was established in 2003 to analyze the current distribution of responsibilities. The committee was scheduled to submit their reform recommendations by February 2007.

In June 2005, the Swedish Riksdag passed a law on the management of private healthcare providers. The amended version of the Health and Medical Service Act, which came into effect on January 1, 2006, stipulated that each county government must control at least one hospital within its jurisdiction, but that it can delegate its administrative authority over regional hospitals or clinics to any other party. In such circumstances, the delegation agreement must clearly specify that both parties must not act for the purpose of making a profit and that the healthcare services provided are supported solely by public funds and insurance premiums.

Future healthcare development in Sweden seems to be moving in the direction opposite to previous decentralization policies. For example, more national action plans are being developed to encourage the coordination of elderly care, mental health care, and primary care using available resources. The Parliamentary Committee on Public Sector Responsibilities has also attempted to propose reform recommendations by analyzing the strengths and weaknesses of the current organizational and service delivery systems.

CHAPTER TWELVE

Social Health Insurance Systems of Representative Countries

 ## SECTION I. THE HEALTH SYSTEM IN GERMANY

Germany is situated in the center of Europe, covering an area of 357,000 square kilometers, and it is the largest country in Central Europe. Its population is about 80.622 million (in 2013), which is the second-largest in Europe after that of Russia. The urban population accounts for 60% of Germany's total population, and the population density is 230 people per square kilometer.

After the reunification of East and West Germany, the country was divided into 16 states. The national government takes the form of a federal republic in which foreign affairs, national defense, currency, customs, railways, aviation, post, and telecommunications are under the jurisdiction of the federal government, whereas the remaining domains (including health) are jointly administered by the federal and state governments or fall under the full autonomy of each state. Germany is one of the most developed industrialized countries in the world. In 2013, its gross national product (GNP) was US$337.333 billion, which ranked fourth in the world after the US, China, and Japan. It has the highest foreign trade volume in the world and is known as the "world champion in exports."

The health indicators of German residents have reached the level of those in advanced and developed countries. In 2012, the average life expectancy for men was 78.6 years, and that for women was 83.3 years. Due to a declining birth rate and prolonged life expectancy, the rate of population aging is accelerating, and individuals over 65 years old account for 21.1% of the total population. The main causes of death in the population have shifted from infectious diseases and nutritional deficiency in the past to cardiovascular diseases, cancer, and psychiatric disorders. The mortality rate from infectious diseases accounts for 4% of the total. In 2013, the infant mortality rate was 3.2 per 1,000 live births, and the maternal mortality ratio was 7/100,000.

The administration of the German health system is divided into three levels: the federal, state, and grassroots (community) levels. The federal and state governments both have legislative powers relating to health. In addition to performing management and guidance functions, the Federal Ministry of Health has a cooperative relationship with the state governments in terms of implementing health services. In general, the Federal Ministry of Health is responsible for formulating macroeconomic policy or policy framework, whereas each state is responsible for the specific implementation of policy. The Federal Ministry of Health does not directly determine the specific health affairs of each state.

In 1881, Germany was the first country in the world to establish social health insurance, and it was the birthplace of health insurance. More than 95% of German residents have social health insurance. The health insurance system requires residents to first consult community general practitioners (GPs). However, the doctor-patient relationship in community services is not fixed, and patients are free to choose their own physicians. GPs in the community mainly engage in independent private practice and also establish contractual relationships with hospitals that include referrals and other services. Hospitals generally do not have outpatient clinics and only provide inpatient services. The definition of the health service level set by the health insurance system can facilitate the role of community health services and the rational use of health resources.

The cost of the use of health services by German residents is mainly covered through third-party payments. Both patients and physicians lack cost consciousness, and there are virtually no economic measures for physicians to reduce patient demand. Hence, competition among healthcare institutions primarily manifests as competition on the quantity and quality of services rather than on the reduction of costs. Nevertheless, Germany's total health spending as a percentage of GDP shrank by 0.1% from 1985 to 1993 and was 8.6% in 1993. However, this spending began to increase thereafter. In 2000, health spending was 10.3% of GDP, and by 2012 it was 11.3% of GDP. It is generally believed that Germany's relatively slow growth in health spending as a share of GDP has an important relationship with the clear hierarchy of health services. That is, the health insurance system limits patients with common diseases to medical treatment from community health service institutions in order to avoid the unnecessary use of hospital services, thereby effectively controlling healthcare expenditure.

Following the energy crisis, Germany was the first country to undertake major reforms of its previous health security system. In 1976, Germany began implementing healthcare cost-containment policies that were further expanded and reinforced after 1981 and that also influenced France and many other countries. Starting in 1985, Germany undertook the reform of the healthcare provision system and the health insurance structure, including the reconstruction of the hospital financing and payment system. After 2003, Germany performed another major reform of hospitals. This reform was based on diagnosis-related groups (DRGs) and involved the quality management and cost containment of healthcare institutions. In addition, the reform also introduced a completely new approach to providing healthcare services and proposed the concept of "holistic healthcare" in order to address the fragmentation of health services in Germany.

1. Health Service System

(1) Establishment of Health Service System

In the early 1880s, Germany had already established a health service system based on insurance. The basic structure of the health service system at that time has been preserved to this day. Currently, all employees earning less than the annually adjusted minimum income threshold must enroll in the sickness funds of this social health insurance. Both the employer and employee jointly contribute to the fund at a fixed ratio (at an average of about 13.5%). In the late 1990s, about 75% of residents in Germany were covered by mandatory health insurance, another 13% enrolled voluntarily in the national sickness funds, and the remaining 12% (mainly including civil servants, high-income earners, and self-employed individuals) purchased private health insurance.

Individuals with health insurance and their dependents can receive full health coverage. They have almost unlimited access to outpatient healthcare services. Prior to 1996, outpatient services were completely free. As of 1996, only a few services (e.g., dental care) require copayments. Inpatient services are also largely free, and patients only need to pay part of the expenses for the first two weeks of a hospital stay.

One of the basic features of the health service system in Germany is the joint decisions made by the federal and local governments. Nongovernmental organizations, such as the sickness funds and the Germany Medical Association, also have an influence on decision-making. This relationship implies that a primary feature of Germany's health service system is that it is the product of coordination between the buyers and suppliers.

The federal government formulates the regulatory framework for health services, whereas the local governments provide the funds for hospital construction. The Ministry of Health is responsible for formulating the rules and regulations for the management of health service financing and provision and for health insurance.

In addition, the health service system in Germany is also characterized by self-administration. In terms of the buyers, the sickness funds occupy a central position in the national statutory health insurance and negotiate service price and quality assurance measures with healthcare institutions on behalf of insured persons. As the representatives of the suppliers, the State Chambers of Physicians (jointly forming the German Medical Association) are self-administering entities that are present in each region. Certain regions even have several such entities. Furthermore, the German National Associations of Statutory Health Insurance Physicians also represent the suppliers. Physicians providing outpatient services to persons insured by the sickness funds must be members of the local State Association of Statutory Health Insurance Physicians. The main task of this organization is to conduct negotiations with the sickness funds and other insurance agencies regarding issues such as payment methods and outpatient service payment contracts. In addition, this organization must also distribute the funding obtained from the sickness funds among its members.

Local hospitals also have a representative for their interests, that is, the German Hospital Federation (DKG). The law specifically stipulates the rights of local hospitals and also emphasizes their corresponding obligations. At the national level, the DKG conducts negotiations with the Association of Statutory Health Insurance Funds regarding the terms and conditions of the service contracts (and also with the German Medical Association under specific circumstances), such as hospital services, the composition of hospital human resources, service efficiency standards, quality control, and so on. Since 2000, the DKG has been responsible for establishing and implementing the DRG-based payment system for inpatient services, planning the form and content of holistic healthcare, applying the requirements of evidence-based medicine to evaluate the diagnosis and treatment process in hospitals, and formulating suitable and effective standards for health service provision.

(2) Status of Healthcare Institutions and Practitioners

1. Healthcare-Related Facilities

1. *Hospitals.* Hospitals in Germany refer to institutions and maternity hospitals (with more than 10 beds) that receive and care for patients and rely on physicians for the diagnosis and treatment of diseases in order to alleviate the suffering caused by diseases and promote the rehabilitation of the body. In other words, hospitals provide what is usually known as inpatient care. Hospitals can be roughly divided based on their nature into public, nonprofit, and private hospitals. Public hospitals are run by the federal government, states, state federations, municipalities, municipality federations, and insurers of social insurance (state insurance offices, professional associations, and so on). Nonprofit hospitals are run by financial groups, religious groups, or charitable organizations. The basic mode of operation is similar to that of public hospitals, and the main difference is the model for the relationship with the government. Public and nonprofit hospitals do not need to be accredited upon establishment.

   Private hospitals are those accredited under Article 30 of the German Industry Regulations. The permit for private hospitals considers whether the founder has full capacity for the guidance and operation of the hospital as a hospital operator, whether the building fulfills the criteria for a hospital, and whether other aspects are satisfactory. Unlike the model of private hospitals in China, the German government also invests in private hospitals. In general, public and nonprofit hospitals are mostly general hospitals, whereas private hospitals are specialist hospitals. Many public hospitals are state university hospitals. University hospitals and designated hospitals (e.g., municipal hospitals in metropolitan regions) are also training and teaching hospitals for physicians. In addition, public hospitals also play an important role in public health activities.

   In general, the trend in German hospitals is that the total number of hospitals and number of beds have been gradually decreasing, the proportion of private hospitals has been increasing, and the average length of a hospital stay has been decreasing. In 2000, Germany had a total of 2,258 hospitals and 568,822 beds and an average hospital stay of 11.4 days. In 2004, there was a total of 2,139 hospitals and 523,824 beds and an average hospital stay of 10.4 days. However, by 2009, the number of German hospitals once again reached 3,324 with 674,830 beds. Among the different types of hospitals, public hospitals account for one-third of hospitals and 54% of the total number of beds in the country; nonprofit hospitals account for one-third of hospitals and 38% of the total number of beds; and private hospitals account for one-third of hospitals and 8% of the total number of beds.

2. *Pharmacies.* The establishment of pharmacies is based on the German Pharmacies Act of 1960, but the standards of establishments vary slightly from state to state. Pharmacies must be run by a pharmacist with a certain number of years of experience. Germany has long implemented the separation of prescribing and dispensing. After seeking medical treatment from private clinics or hospital outpatient clinics, patients can only use their prescriptions to obtain drugs from community pharmacies. According to statistics from the German government, by the end of 2004 Germany had a total of 21,392 community pharmacies, which implied an average of one pharmacy per 3,858 residents. This ratio greatly helped the public, as patients could obtain drugs from the nearest community pharmacist after seeking medical help. Before 2004, the German government stipulated that a pharmacist could only operate one community pharmacy, and, hence, there were no chain pharmacies

in Germany. Since January 1, 2004, the government has permitted a pharmacist to operate up to three community pharmacies. As of 2004, there were 632 chain community pharmacies in Germany.

2. Healthcare-Related Practitioners

1. *Physicians.* According to the Federal Medical Practitioners' Act of 1961, physicians must have a license to practice. Physicians can only obtain their license after six years of medical education in national or state university hospitals and passing a medical examination. After October 1970, the requirement for medical students to work for one to two years as medical assistants was repealed. This repeal was due to the fundamental reform of physician training, since medical students receive practical clinical training during their university education. Based on statistics from January 2005, Germany had 394,432 physicians, of whom 42% (133,365) were family physicians, 48% (146,357) were hospital physicians, 3% worked in public health institutions, 2% were private practitioners, and 5% were other healthcare practitioners. In 2006–2013, the number of physicians per 10,000 people was 38.1.

   Upon obtaining a license to practice medicine, a physician may receive another two to five years of specialty training under the guidance of qualified specialists at hospitals designated by the specialist association of each state (a different organization from the general State Chamber of Physicians; the former is a legal entity for the assessment of specialists in accordance with the Federal Medical Practitioners' Act). The specialist association of the state in which the prospective specialist intends to practice then assesses the evidence for the successful completion of specialty training before awarding the qualification. The specialist qualification obtained in each state can be used throughout all states in Germany. Only those with specialist qualifications are able to use the title of specialist.

2. *Dentist.* According to the German Dentistry Act of 1952, all dentists must have a license to practice. As in the case of physicians, dental specialists (orthognathic surgery) have an assessment system. In 2004, the number of dentists employed was 65,000. In 2006–2013, the number of dentists per 10,000 people was eight.

3. *Office-based physicians.* A dual-track system is implemented for healthcare services in Germany, which are divided into outpatient and inpatient services. Hospitals only provide inpatient treatments and generally do not carry out outpatient services. The majority of outpatient services are provided by physicians with independent practices. Office-based physicians are divided into office-based GPs, office-based specialists, and office-based dentists. More than 98% of office-based physicians sign service contracts with health insurance agencies, and some of them specialize in providing services to patients covered by private insurance companies. In the past, only a license to practice medicine was required to become an office-based physician. However, at present, office-based physicians are not able to secure an income without also becoming statutory health insurance (SHI) physicians. Therefore, in practice, becoming an SHI physician or joining an association of SHI physicians is a key condition for starting a practice.

   Within one year of obtaining a license to practice medicine, SHI physicians must serve as assistant physicians at designated hospitals; after they have done so, an approvals committee set up within the association of SHI physicians reviews and issues permits to applicants who comply with certain conditions, such as having never previously been penalized, in accordance with the applicant's wishes (intention to be listed in the physicians' register created by the association of SHI physicians).

SHI physicians can obtain permission to practice within a specific area. Office-based specialists must possess specialist qualifications. There are 16 specialty areas. In Germany, physicians are prohibited from specializing in two or more areas or becoming both a GP and specialist.

By the end of December 2000, the ratio of office-based to hospital-based physicians was 9:11 (hospital physicians showed an increasing trend). The number of office-based physicians was 97,524 (the average number of residents served by each office-based physician was 2,294). About 98% of office-based physicians were SHI physicians. The number of dentists was 35,863, of whom 95% were office-based dentists, and about 90% were SHI physicians. The majority of income earned by office-based physicians and dentists came from the treatment fees paid by the sickness funds.

4. *Pharmacists.* According to the German Pharmacists Act, pharmacists must have a license to practice pharmacy. The training and licensing of pharmacists are specified in the Federal Pharmacists Act of June 1968 and the Pharmacy Licensing Act of October 1971. By the end of December 1998, the number of pharmacists serving in pharmacies was 28,216. In 2006–2013, the number of pharmacists per 10,000 people was 6.2.

5. *Nurses.* After three years of professional education in a nursing school, nurses can achieve the qualification for nursing only after passing a state examination. Two-thirds of nurses work in hospitals. By the end of December 2000, the number of employed nurses was 478,012. In 2006–2013, the number of nurses and midwives per 10,000 people was 114.9.

6. *Other healthcare practitioners.* Midwives, massage therapists, spa therapists, X-ray technicians, laboratory technicians, monthly nurses, and various physiotherapists must receive one to two years of education from the relevant training institutions and pass national examinations before they can obtain a license. In addition, according to the Medical Technical Assistant Act of 1971, technical assistants in the physiotherapy and radiotherapy departments are also required to undertake training within two years. By the end of December 2000, the number of employed midwives was 4,926; the total number of massage therapists, exercise therapists, and spa therapists was 11,563; and the number of medical technical assistants was 42,511.

(3) Costs of Healthcare and Hospital Services

1. Status of Healthcare Expenditure　　Although we have discussed previously that the growth of healthcare expenditure as a share of GDP in Germany is relatively slow, this share is still relatively high compared to those of other European countries. In 2003, Germany's total health spending was 10.7% of GDP, whereas the total health spending of most other European countries was much lower during the same period of time. In 2008, as shown in Figure 12.1, Germany's total health spending was 10.5% of GDP, which was still higher than the average level across major European countries.

The causes leading to this situation are fairly complex. However, one thing is clear: hospital services do not have a direct relationship with high costs. In fact, the opposite is true; Germany's spending on nonhospital services and drugs was the highest among European countries, whereas its expenditure on hospital services was not very high. Compared to those of other European countries, the costs of hospital services in Germany are moderate.

Prior to 1990, the growth of health expenditure was basically consistent with the growth of the national economy. However, since 1990s, the growth of health expenditure has surpassed the rate of economic growth. Although the cost of hospital services has increased substantially, its upward trend has been effectively controlled since 1993. The rate

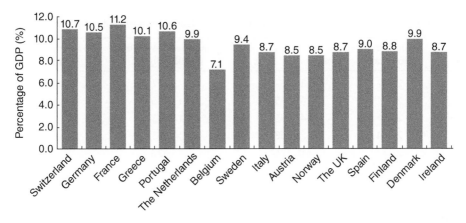

FIGURE 12.1   Total health spending as a percentage of GDP in major European countries in 2008. *Source:* World Health Statistics, 2011.

of increase is essentially consistent with economic development, and health expenditure as a share of GDP has basically been maintained at a stable level.

2. Additional Charges for Single or Double Rooms in Hospital Services   In Germany, patients who opt for single or double rooms in hospitals must pay additional charges. For single rooms, private for-profit hospitals have the highest additional charges at €61.8, followed by public hospitals at €56.7 and private nonprofit hospitals at €53.1, with an average charge of €58. As for the additional charges for double rooms, private for-profit hospitals also charge the highest amount at €40.9, followed by private nonprofit hospitals at €39.8 and public hospitals at €30.1, with an average of €34.7.

In Germany and other developed European countries, the desire for single rooms when patients are hospitalized has rapidly increased. This increase is mainly because in Nordic countries such as Denmark and Sweden, elderly care institutions beyond hospitals have been actively working towards providing single rooms (including single rooms for married couples). In keeping with this trend, the demand for single (or double) rooms in hospitals has also significantly increased, as such rooms provide patients with privacy, and it is expected that this demand will continue to rise.

In Germany, the costs of single or double rooms are generally covered by the additional charges paid by the patients (not included in the health insurance payouts). However, in practice, nearly all of these additional charges are covered by the private health insurance in which the patient has enrolled.

(4) Hospital Service Provision and Output Levels

Since 1993, hospitals have been facing a rapidly changing environment, including the introduction of the global budget system, the risk of operating losses, the promotion of outpatient surgery, and the prospective payment system introduced in 1996. These changes have dramatically altered the utilization of hospital services. As shown in Table 12.1, the average length of a hospital stay has decreased from 15.2 days in 1990 to 9.8 days in 2009. The total number of hospital beds during the same period decreased from 686,000 to 674,830. Overall, efficiency indicators, such as the volume of hospital services and the average length of a hospital stay, increased significantly. However, compared with the rest

TABLE 12.1 Changes in Germany's Hospital Service Capacity and Output in 1990–2009

Year	Number of Hospitals	Number of Beds	Annual Service Volume (1,000 people)	Average Hospital Stays (Days)
1990	2,447	685,957	13,777	15.2
1991	2,411	665,565	13,925	14.6
1992	2,381	646,995	14,233	13.9
1993	2,354	628,658	14,385	13.2
1994	2,337	618,176	14,627	12.7
1995	2,325	609,123	15,002	12.1
1996	2,269	593,743	15,232	11.4
1997	2,258	580,425	15,511	11.0
1998	2,263	571,829	15,952	10.7
2000	2,258	568,822	—	11.4
2004	2,139	523,824	—	10.4
2009	3,324	674,830	—	9.8

of the EU, Germany's number of hospital beds per 1,000 people, total number of hospital beds, and average length of a hospital stay were still above average.

1. Number of Hospitals and Beds Unlike Japan, Germany does not define hospitals based on the number of beds, but, in terms of statistics, Germany regards healthcare institutions with more than 10 beds as hospitals. In 2000, Germany had approximately 2,258 hospitals, a total of about 568,822 beds, an average of seven beds per 1,000 inhabitants, and a bed utilization rate of 86%. Among these hospitals, 890 were public hospitals, 942 were private nonprofit hospitals, and 426 were private for-profit hospitals. The distribution of beds across these three categories of hospitals was 55%, 38%, and 7%, respectively. In terms of trends, the market share of public hospitals has been shrinking, whereas that of private hospitals has been increasing. Based on the distribution of hospital sizes in 2000, more than half (1,236 hospitals or 54.7%) were small hospitals with fewer than 150 beds, and only 234 hospitals were large hospitals with more than 500 beds (see Table 12.2).

By 2009, there were 3,324 hospitals in Germany, including 872 public hospitals, 1,093 private nonprofit hospitals, and 1,359 private for-profit hospitals (40.88%), with a total of 674,830 hospital beds. The number of hospitals in Germany and the number of beds in public and private hospitals in 1970–2009 are shown in Table 12.3.

With regard to the regional distribution of hospitals, we can see from the high hospital concentration in Bavaria (accounting for about one-fourth or 23% of all hospitals) and the low concentration in Bremen (only 17 hospitals) that there is considerable unevenness in the distribution between regions.

In terms of the number of hospital beds per 100,000 people, Berlin has an especially high density of hospital beds at 1,768. There is substantial hospitalization of elderly people in Berlin. Moreover, although the number of physicians exceeds demand, many hospitals are facing an increasingly severe shortage in nursing staff.

People have a strong demand for a balanced structure of hospital beds and the number of healthcare practitioners. Figure 12.2 normalizes the data from 1975 at 100 and uses an index to track the evolution in the number of physicians and beds in hospital services. We

TABLE 12.2 Number of Hospitals with Different Numbers of Hospital Beds in Germany in 2000

Number of Beds	Number of Hospitals	Percentage (%)
Below 50	394	17.4
50–100	422	18.7
100–150	420	18.6
150–200	381	16.9
200–300	466	20.7
300–400	234	10.4
400–500	132	5.8
500–600	75	3.3
600–800	88	4.0
800–1,000	24	1.1
Above 1,000	47	2.1
Total	2,258	100.0

TABLE 12.3 Number of Hospitals, Number of Hospital Beds, and Bed Utilization Rate in Germany in 1970–2009

Item	Year (End of Year)	Total	Of Which Public	Of Which Private Nonprofit	Of Which Private for-Profit	Of Which, General Hospitals
Number of hospitals	1970	3,347	1,228	1,139	980	2,135
	1980	3,234	1,190	1,097	947	1,991
	1990	2,447	928	1,042	477	1,638
	2000	2,258	890	942	426	1,526
	2009	3,324	872	1,093	1,359	1,780
Number of beds	1970	714,879	373,675	253,239	87,965	484,776
	1980	707,713	370,717	248,717	88,279	476,652
	1990	665,957	338,825	235,284	91,848	461,555
	2000	568,822	278,041	218,457	72,324	350,128
	2009	674,830	—	—	—	—

can see from this figure that despite the sustained and stable decrease in hospital beds, the number of hospital physicians continued to increase significantly. This increase means that even with the reduction in the number of hospital beds, the excessive growth in healthcare expenditure cannot be curbed if the number of physicians is not controlled.

The reduction in the number of hospitals and beds was carried out in accordance with the Hospital Cost Containment Act of 1981 (a comprehensive amendment of the Hospital Financial Stability Act of 1972, which aimed to limit the building of hospitals and the introduction of costly medical devices) and was the result of cost containment implemented according to the need planning of public and private hospitals. Hospitals not included in

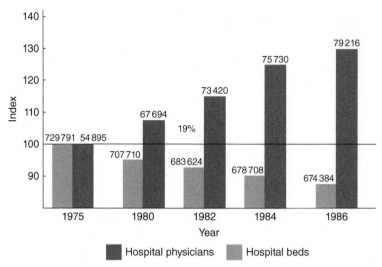

FIGURE 12.2 Number of hospital physicians and hospital beds in Germany in 1975–1986. *Source:* Statistisches Bundesamt, Statistik BAK, Statistisches Jahrbuch 1988.

the hospital need planning were unable to receive federal or state financial subsidies for construction funds.

Compared to 1960, the number of physicians increased by about 2.7-fold, and the number of residents served by each physician was reduced by half. The number of dentists was 63,485, and that of pharmacists was 49,904. This data indicate that even after considering natural changes in demographic factors, the number of physicians has been increasing significantly in real terms during this period, and this trend is expected to continue in the future (Table 12.4).

With regard to the male-to-female ratio of physicians, there were approximately 123,000 male physicians (75%) and 42,000 female physicians (25%), implying a ratio of

TABLE 12.4 Number of Physicians, Dentists, and Pharmacists in Germany in 1960–2010

Year	Number of Physicians Engaged in Healthcare	Number of Dentists	Number of Pharmacists
1960	79,350	32,509	15,776
1965	85,801	31,660	17,725
1970	99,654	31,175	20,866
1975	118,726	31,774	25,597
1980	139,431	33,240	29,674
1985	160,902	36,853	32,234
1990	177,158	38,184	33,144
2000	216,720	53,863	34,251
2005	277,885	64,609	47,956
2010	292,129	63,485	49,904

about 3:1. Hence, male physicians accounted for an overwhelming majority. Among female physicians, approximately 24,200 did not indicate a specialty (i.e., GPs), which accounted for 58% of the total, and about 17,600 did indicate a specialty, accounting for 42% of the total. Among female specialists, those specializing in general medicine, internal medicine, anesthesiology, obstetrics and gynecology, ophthalmology, and otolaryngology represent about 60% of the total (approximately 10,300 physicians).

In terms of employment patterns, the percent of physicians who were office-based and hospital-based in 1970 were 57% and 43%, respectively. These percentages began to reverse in the latter half of 1975 and were 45% and 55%, respectively, by the end of 2000, implying that the latter accounted for a higher percentage of physicians. As the total number of physicians has increased, physicians have begun to show an increasingly significant trend of specialization.

Although the number of dentists has grown at a slower rate than the number of physicians has, by 2000, the average number of German residents served by one dentist was 1,126, which was 590 fewer than that in 1960. As for the number of dentists per 100,000 people, the national average was 62.2 dentists in 2000 (an increase of 1.8 from 1999), which increased to 77 dentists by 2010. The growth of dentists in Germany was rapid during the 1990s, increasing from 38,184 in 1990 to 53,863 in 2000 and further to 63,485 in 2010. The German Dental Association is also concerned about the surplus of dentists amidst a shrinking population. The regional distribution of dentists has shown similar tendencies to that of physicians. That is, the regions where the supply of dentists has exceeded the national average are, in ascending order, Hamburg (89.3), Berlin (84.6), Essen (68.3), Bavaria (68.0), Schleswig–Holstein (65.3), Baden–Württemberg (65.2), and Bremen (63.3). Regions where the number of dentists is below average include Saarland (49.1), Rhineland–Palatinate (53.3), Lower Saxony (54.3), and North Rhine–Westphalia (55.3) (all based on states as units).

With regard to the number of pharmacists, the total number in 2000 was 34,251, and by 2010 the total number of pharmacists was 49,904, of whom 70% were female. In recent years, women have been joining this industry far more actively than they did previously. Based on the ratio of men and women in the previous year (2009), the number of men increased merely by 28, whereas that of women increased by 763.

Aside from the occupational groups above (physicians, dentists, and pharmacists), there are also other full-time staff engaged in various healthcare professions, including assistant practitioners, male and female nurses, nursing staff, midwives, physiotherapists, occupational therapists, laboratory technicians, pharmacologists, dental technicians, optometrists, spa therapists, and business and operations staff, who make up a total of 2.1 million people. Among them, nursing staff accounted for the highest number, reaching a total of 478,000 (40%), followed by nonclinical physicians (13.6%), physician assistants (12.6%), dental assistants (7.1%), nonclinical dentists (3.2%), pharmacy assistants (3.1%), dental technicians (2.8%), and nonclinical pharmacists (2.7%).

2. Introduction of High-Priced Medical Equipment   From an international perspective, Germany is also well known for taking the lead in introducing high-precision, large-scale medical devices (commonly known as "high-priced medical equipment"). The allocation of high-priced medical equipment within the European Community is shown in Table 12.5. We can see from the table that the allocation of high-priced medical equipment relative to the population density is far higher in Germany than in the other countries. Furthermore, Germany's healthcare expenditure as a share of GNP is also far higher than that of the other countries.

TABLE 12.5 Allocation of Valuable Medical Equipment and Implementation of Major Surgeries in European Countries in 1997

Country	Population (1 Million People)	No. of CT Scanners Installed	No. of Uses Per 1 Million Residents	No. of Open-Heart Surgeries	No. of Uses Per 1 Million Residents	Electro-Magnetic Wave Machines	No. of Units Per 1 Million Residents	No. of Dialysis Patients	No. of Patients Per 1 Million Residents	No. of Kidney Transplant Patients	No. of Patients Per 1 Million Residents	Magnetic Resonance Imaging (MRI)
Belgium	10	64	6.4	3,500	350.00	43	4.3	2,700	270.00	200 (1982)	20.00	7
Denmark	5	22	4.4	414	82.80	20	4.0	900	180.00	195	39.00	4
Germany	61	423	6.9	21,500	352.00	300	4.9	18,000	278.00	1,274 (1984)	20.50	30
France	53	139	2.6	8,500 (1982)	160.40	208	3.9	8,269 (1981)	156.00	800 (1981)	15.10	26
Greece	10	17	1.7	1,200 (1985)	120.00	32	3.2	1,207*	120.70	36	3.60	5
Ireland	3	5	1.7	—	—	5	1.7	—	—	—	—	2
Italy	57	201	3.5	11,000	193.00	163	2.9	12,759	222.84	104 (1981)	1.80	17
Luxembourg	0.4	2	5.0	61	153.00	1	2.5	105	262.50	5	12.50	2
The Netherlands	14	45	3.2	8,289	592.00	79	5.6	2,274	162.43	376	26.80	14
The UK	56	123	2.2	6,008	107.00	177	3.2	9,678	172.82	1,592	28.40	15

Note:
* includes home artificial dialysis; numbers in brackets indicate year of data collection
Source: Die Sozialversicherung, February 1998, S. 38.

The number of CT scanners introduced in, and allocated to, Germany is more than 2 times that of Italy, which comes in second; more than 3.4 times that of UK, which has implemented the NHS; and about 3 times higher than that of France. The number of CT scanners allocated per one million people for each country is, in descending order, 6.9 units in Germany, 6.4 units in Belgium, 5.0 units in Luxembourg, 4.4 units in Denmark, 3.5 units in Italy, 3.2 units in the Netherlands, 2.6 units in France, 2.2 units in the UK, and 1.7 units each in Greece and Ireland.

Internationally, Germany has largely maintained the highest standards in medical technology in the world and will most likely continue to further expand the research and development of various fields in the twenty-first century.

The areas that German manufacturers of medical equipment have focused on for research and development are as follows.

1. Development of diagnostic and therapeutic technology
   1. Medical testing technology
   2. Imaging technology for medical diagnoses (γ-ray, X-ray, light, microwave, ultrasound, and so on)
   3. Clinical treatment technology, such as the use of shockwave therapy
2. Medical materials and rehabilitation aids
   1. Aids and substitutes for biological organ functions (especially artificial kidneys)
   2. Biocompatible materials (especially artificial heart valves, artificial blood vessels, membranes for dialysis, and so on)
   3. Artificial joints and other visceral-type materials (artificial joints and artificial tooth roots)
   4. Aids for physically disabled individuals (aids for the visually and hearing impaired, wheelchairs, and so on)

As the latest membrane separation technology can also be applied to fat-soluble metabolites, significant improvements have been achieved in the dialysis method itself. In addition, its application has also been expanded to other fields and has given hope for the provision of better treatment for patients with chronic liver disease. These achievements are the crystallization of German medical technology, and Germany prides itself on having the best medical technology in the world.

With regard to the rapid introduction of high-priced medical equipment, many experts, including economists, have all expressed that this move would bring about a crisis with respect to the rapid rise in healthcare expenditure and have raised their concerns. It is not difficult to imagine that various high-precision, large-scale types of medical equipment will be further developed in the future. Furthermore, with the support of highly developed technological capabilities, German hospitals will continue to provide high-tech services, thereby promoting global medical development. However, when considered from the perspective of balancing insurance funds, as well as the issue of funding efficiency, it is necessary to ensure the balance and efficiency of funding utilization. Thus, it is imperative that the government adopt a more cautious attitude toward the supply and allocation of high-priced medical equipment while also actively introducing new policies to control the situation. Currently, Germany has implemented an access system for large-scale, high-priced medical equipment that is subject to strict limitations in health planning.

(5) Hospital Planning and Investment

Local governments are responsible for formulating hospital development plans. According to the Federal Hospital Financing Act, all regions throughout the country must formulate local hospital development plans and prioritize the development of hospital services. Thus, the hospitals in each region were incorporated into their local development plans according to the local demand for healthcare services and political will. Furthermore, planning according to demand also involves listing the development plans for specialties, which even include the specific numbers of beds for different specialties. Due to differences in political goals, the hospital development plans of each region also have different requirements for hospital service capacities and investment in hospital development.

For a hospital, being incorporated into the local hospital development plan has two implications. First, the hospital's capital investment (buildings and large-scale medical equipment) can be subsidized by the local government. Although local governments have their own priorities in hospital development, developmental investment in hospitals is still determined by local governments. However, hospitals do not have the legal right to require their local governments to invest in or subsidize their development. Furthermore, government subsidies and hospital ownership are not necessarily related, and subsidies are only determined by the priority level in the development plans of the local government.

The second implication is that generally only hospitals incorporated in the local hospital development plan can receive compensation from sickness funds. Therefore, whether a hospital can provide services to individuals insured under sickness funds and receive compensation is ultimately determined by the local government. Naturally, according to the Health Care Reform Act of 1989, sickness funds also have the right to enter into contracts with hospitals. However, the procedures involved are relatively complicated and require the approval of the local government.

(6) Compensation of Hospital Operating Costs

For a long time, hospitals in Germany have been implementing the principle of full cost compensation. This principle implies that sickness funds must pay for everything that hospitals carry out. In practice, payments are made through per diem reimbursement, and the per diem rate of each hospital was determined by the state government. The Health Care Structure Act of 1992 was the first major law that had a true impact on this principle. Since then, increases in sickness funds' payments of hospital services have been linked to the income from the financing activities of the funds. Since 1993, the principle of full cost compensation was also abandoned, and a global budget system was implemented in hospitals. This change meant that hospitals could face the risk of an operating deficit. In 1996, the prospective case fees and procedure fees were introduced for some hospital services. Case fees were based comprehensively on specific disease diagnoses and the corresponding therapeutic interventions, whereas procedure fees were only the fees for specific therapeutic interventions. A case fee could include multiple procedure fees. In practice, the number of patients paid by "case fees" was less than one quarter of the total, and payment standards varied significantly among different regions and different specialties.

The services for most other patients were paid for using a two-tier per diem reimbursement rate, which included the non-healthcare-related compensation rates among different hospitals and the treatment-, nursing-, and medication-related compensation rates among different specialties. Case fees, procedure fees, and per diem reimbursement have already become a part of the hospital budget. This kind of budget cannot be considered a budget in a certain sense because it is not positively correlated to the services actually provided by the hospital. Instead, it is the result of specific negotiations between the insurance funds and each hospital. Naturally, the budget still stipulates the target service volume of the hospital, and if the hospital completes this service volume, then the budget does not need to be adjusted. However, if the hospital exceeds this target service volume, then the excess will only be partially compensated. For organ transplants, only 50% of the case fees for the excess service volume are compensated. For other service items, only 25% of the case fees or procedure fees for the excess services are compensated. If the hospital does not meet its service volume, then only 40% (50% in 1999) of the incomplete portion is compensated.

2. Health Insurance System

(1) Establishment of the Health Insurance System

Germany was the first country in the world to establish a health insurance system through social legislation. In 1883, 1884, and 1889, it enacted the Health Insurance Bill, Accident Insurance Bill, and Old Age and Disability Insurance Bill, respectively. The health insurance system is centered on hospitals and SHI physicians. The German health insurance system fulfills a crucial task, function, and position in the social security (safety) system. With regard to the scope of application, level of security, and scale of financial investment, the health insurance system occupies a substantial proportion of the social security system. The health insurance system targets about 90% of the population and, together with the pension insurance, accident insurance, and unemployment insurance, constitutes the social insurance system. As enrollment in statutory health insurance is not mandatory for employees (white-collar workers) and self-employed individuals whose personal income exceeds a certain standard, such individuals may choose to enroll in private health insurance. Private health insurance covers about 10% of the population. Hospitals and health insurance physicians form the core of the healthcare provision system, providing medical benefits and public health services in terms of health insurance, accident insurance, social benefits, and other benefits and relief. The majority of hospitals are public hospitals, and the majority of office-based physicians are SHI physicians.

Historically speaking, in the late nineteenth century, a system of healthcare institutions and healthcare practitioners already existed prior to the establishment of health insurance. The system of SHI physicians was established between the latter half of the 1950s and the early 1960s after World War II. The expansion of the hospital system only officially commenced in the 1970s. On the other hand, the health insurance system was created in the late nineteenth century (1881), but the extension of its scope of application and the improvements in the benefits implemented were carried out during the early 1960s to the mid-1970s. Although the German health system and health insurance have a long history, their major developments took place after World War II. In particular, after the main sector of the social security system was established, further improvements only began in the mid-1970s. These improvements were based on the rapid economic development after World War II.

Since then, during the significant economic recession after the energy crisis, Germany had no choice but to re-evaluate and adjust its health insurance system to control the rapid rise in total healthcare expenditure. Since the implementation of the Health Insurance Cost Containment Act (1977), Germany adopted various regulatory policies not only in health insurance but also in different areas of the health system, thus resulting in major reforms of the German health insurance system.

(2) Physician System and Health Insurance

The vast majority of the physician system in the nineteenth century was dominated by independent practice and family physicians. Medical fees were paid by individuals themselves or by their employers. This system was regarded as one of the most ideal systems and, hence, existed for a long time. Prior to the establishment of health insurance, healthcare was almost always provided under such health systems. However, only about one-third of residents had access to such healthcare. Since around the mid-nineteenth century, the Prussian government and the German Reich government successively established relief funds for miners and workers (the precursors of health insurance). However, healthcare was mainly implemented under the abovementioned physician system, which completely failed to overcome the difficulties faced by the health needs brought about by rapid socioeconomic development. On the other hand, the physician class was not concerned with the working class, and the former did not contribute to the creation of health insurance, which mainly aimed to compensate physicians for medical treatment. At that time, although the relief fund system only covered about 10% of residents, a form of health insurance that targeted workers began to emerge, and various sickness funds, which were the operating agencies of health insurance, began to implement the compensation of medical benefits to insured persons according to contracts signed with physicians.

After this implementation, as the content and coverage of health insurance continued to expand, physicians began to play public and important roles in the health insurance system, and restrictions were also imposed on the private practices of physicians to a certain extent. Thus, the socioeconomic status, social standing, and social role of physicians underwent changes and gradually formed the foundation for sickness fund physicians (SHI physicians). Then, in accordance with the emergency laws of 1923 and 1931, the rules governing the contractual relationship between sickness funds and physicians were formulated. After the Second World War, the SHI physician system was established through the enactment of the 1955 Laws on the Legal Rights of Statutory Health Insurance Physicians, the 1957 Licensing of Statutory Health Insurance Physicians and Dentists, and the 1962 Federal Contract for Physicians and Dentists. After undergoing the above process, a new social relationship emerged between the health system and health insurance. Today, nearly all physicians and dentists have become SHI physicians or SHI dentists.

Health insurance is based on contracts, and the reimbursement of healthcare services is determined by the contract between each State Association of SHI Physicians and the Federal Association of Sickness Funds. There are medical treatment contracts between hospitals and sickness funds. Midwifery clinics, pharmacies, and other healthcare institutions also have contracts with the sickness funds.

The relationship between SHI physicians (including dentists) and sickness funds is intended to facilitate their cooperation to guarantee the healthcare of insured persons and their families. The specific method involves establishing treatment contracts between the state associations of SHI physicians and the associations of sickness funds (they include eight types of sickness funds: regional sickness funds, company-based sickness funds, guild-based sickness funds, sailors' sickness funds, federal miners' funds, employees' substitute funds, workers' substitute funds, and farmers' sickness funds, consisting of about 1,300 funds) in order to implement medical insurance. The associations of SHI physicians are self-administered professional associations with public authority (legal entities under public law). Any physician who has completed a year and a half of training in a hospital and has worked under the supervision of an SHI physician can register with an association of SHI physicians and become an SHI physician as long as certain conditions are met. In other words, SHI physicians follow a permit system. Based on an application made to the health insurance, a permit is issued for a specific region if a physician meets certain conditions. The permits are issued by an approvals committee consisting of an equal number of representatives from the Federal Association of Sickness Funds and the physicians' association of each state.

The regulations for health insurance are mainly based on the 368 articles in the Reich Insurance Code (RVO), and health insurance is implemented based on these provisions. Reimbursements for health insurance are based on the remuneration regulations for physicians. In accordance with the contractual remuneration decided by the Federal Association of Sickness Funds and the associations of SHI physicians, the Federal Association of Sickness Funds first pays the total sum to the associations of SHI physicians, which in turn distribute the funds to each SHI physician according to a given allocation criteria.

(3) Hospital System and Health Insurance

The hospital system began with the documents of the third meeting on the law on the standardization of the healthcare system in 1935. However, the establishment of the modern hospital system was gradually developed based on the Law on the Economic Security and Health Care Costs of Hospitals (Hospital Financial Stability Act) of 1972. This law provided the economic security needed for the construction and operation of hospitals, thus enabling the rapid development of hospital modernization, which was advocated by various parties after World War II.

In the relationship between hospitals and sickness funds, aside from the treatment contracts signed between the two parties for the implementation of health insurance, health insurance may also be implemented in hospitals without contracts in the event of emergencies. Apart from emergency situations, hospital treatments should, in theory, only be carried out with referrals from office-based physicians. Moreover, inpatient treatments in hospitals must first be approved by the sickness funds before they can be carried out. Patients are free to choose their SHI office-based GPs. However, unless they have a major reason, patients are not allowed to change their physicians at will within the three months during the validity period of the medical certificate (delivered by the sickness funds).

The reimbursement of hospital treatment is determined by the treatment contract between the sickness funds and the hospitals. Hospital-based specialists can also become SHI physicians and provide insurance treatments to individuals in hospitals. Some office-based GPs are also commissioned by the hospitals to provide inpatient treatment within the hospitals. Furthermore, there are approximately 2,500 chief physicians in hospitals who serve as individual SHI medical practitioners in their capacity as SHI physicians.

Other healthcare-related institutions have a collaborative relationship with the sickness funds. For example, when the Federal Minister of Labor decides the expenditure for midwifery clinics, all associations of sickness funds, substitute funds, and midwifery clinics must lend their cooperation. The expenditures of midwifery clinics are paid directly by the sickness funds. As for the payment of drugs, sickness funds can sign a special agreement with pharmacies.

3. Health Insurance Operations

Germany is the birthplace of the social health insurance system. In 1883, Bismarck, the "Iron Chancellor," attempted to ease the class conflicts at that time by establishing a social health insurance system in a legislative form. This system lasted for more than 120 years and is the world's oldest health insurance system. To date, Germany's health insurance has had a major impact on health insurance in countries throughout the world. Although Germany's health insurance has a long history and tradition, innovations have frequently been attempted within the system. The healthcare cost-containment policies that have been adopted to cope with changes in economic conditions after the energy crisis have also had major impacts on many countries, including neighboring France. It is expected that German health security policies will continue to have substantial impacts on all countries in the future.

(1) The Institutional System and Its Applicable Targets

The health insurance system is a branch of the social insurance system that continues to improve as society progresses. The health insurance system is composed of 292 social insurance funds, covering nearly 90% of the population, while about 10% is covered by private health insurance. Individuals with monthly incomes exceeding €3,937 (mostly freelancers or high-income earners) can choose to enroll in private health insurance. Everyone who enrolls in social insurance can also purchase private health insurance and enjoy special services, such as single-room wards and dental services.

Individuals enrolled in health insurance are further divided into compulsorily insured persons (*pflichtversicherter*) and voluntarily insured persons (*freiwillig versichert*). The compulsorily insured refers to employed persons whose monthly incomes do not exceed the statutory threshold (incomes of less than €3,750/month in 2010), unemployed persons, retirees receiving pensions, university students, and pre-employment interns. These individuals must enroll in statutory health insurance. The voluntarily insured refers to employed persons whose monthly incomes exceed the statutory threshold (incomes of more than €45,000/year in 2010), civil servants, freelancers, employers, lawyers, and military personnel. These individuals can choose between social and private health insurance companies. The voluntarily insured who have opted for private insurance companies are not free to withdraw and transfer to statutory health insurance agencies.

A comparison between the two types of insurance reveals that private health insurance pursues a balance between premiums and risks, and, hence, premiums vary with age, gender, illness, and the scope and proportion of reimbursement. The premiums of young and healthy individuals are relatively low, whereas the premiums for elderly and chronic patients are much higher than those charged by statutory health insurance companies. Therefore, it may be much cheaper for single, young adults with high incomes to purchase private health insurance than to purchase statutory health insurance. However, private health insurance companies provide coverage for a limited period, and premiums continue to rise after twelve months of enrollment. In addition, when individuals enroll in statutory insurance and meet certain conditions, their spouses and children can also receive the benefits of their health insurance. In contrast, private health insurance only provides personal coverage. Individuals covered by statutory insurance companies must contribute taxes based on a percentage of their salaries. Since January 2011, contributions are collected at 15.5% of an employee's salary, of which the employee pays 7.3% and the employer pays 8.2%. Private insurance offers many advantages over statutory insurance, such as the ability to request single rooms during hospitalization, appoint specific physicians, and avoid long waiting times during appointments. Individuals covered by statutory health insurance who wish to enjoy these benefits must purchase supplementary insurance. Currently, statutory health insurance companies cover nearly 90% of the German public, whereas private health insurance companies cover only about 10% of the German public. According to statistics from 2009, 51.4 million people in Germany contribute premiums, and, together with their family members, about 70 million people are enrolled in health insurance. Thus, we can see that the German health insurance system benefits all citizens. This system mainly uses statutory health insurance to protect the majority of the public but also satisfies the rights of employees to have the freedom of choice.

University students are given many preferential benefits under compulsory insurance. Students under the age of 30 years who have studied at university for at most 14 semesters are offered special benefits by statutory health insurance companies and only need to pay €64.77 per month in premiums. Students above the age of 30 years or who have studied more than 14 semesters (not including semesters of academic leave) can choose whether to continue their insurance coverage. Choosing to continue their insurance coverage with statutory health insurance companies leads to a substantial increase in premiums. It should be pointed out here that only students studying in public German universities or nationally recognized private colleges have access to compulsory insurance benefits. Students in language schools or private colleges not recognized by the country do not have access to compulsory insurance. Applying for insurance is a very simple process for foreign students. When applying for university admission, applicants can use the acceptance letter issued by the university's office of international affairs to apply for student insurance at the office of the statutory insurance company located in the university. Without a health insurance certificate, students are not allowed to register at the university, and foreign students are unable to renew their visas.

(2) Health Insurance Financing and Operations

Although the premiums of the general insurance system vary according to the sickness funds, all of them follow the principle of employees and employers each contributing half. The average premium rate on August 1, 1988, was 12.9%. The average premium rate of company-based sickness funds, which have relatively low rates, was 11.4%, whereas that of regional sickness funds, which have relatively high rates, was 13.5%. Premium rates have gradually been increasing. Since July 2009, a uniform premium rate based on the employee's salary was applied for statutory health insurance funds. The current premium rate is 14.9% of income, of which 7.9% is paid by the employee and 7% is paid by the employer.

The premiums of low-income (monthly income of DM 600 since January 1988) workers are paid fully by their employers. For high-income employees who choose to enroll in private health insurance instead of social health insurance, employers are required to subsidize the equivalent of one-half of social health insurance premiums.

Most of the premiums for the unemployed are paid by the employment agencies, and the difference is paid by the national sickness fund. Although miners' health insurance, students' health insurance, and disabled persons' health insurance are subsidized by government finance, these insurance types only account for about 3% of the total health insurance funds.

The premiums of pensioners are paid jointly by the insurers of pension insurance, the insured persons under the general health insurance system, and the pensioners themselves. Pension insurance bears 11.8% of the pension as a premium subsidy; the joint premium rate paid by insured persons under the general regime is 3.4%; and the actual premium paid by pensioners is 3% of their pension. Among pensioners, individuals who did not enroll in health insurance for more than half of their working life before retirement (i.e., those who became voluntary contributors) must pay separate premiums. Fund adjustments can be made among all sickness funds for the joint contributions from general insured persons to the health insurance premiums of pensioners.

The method of fund adjustment involves estimating the expenses for all pensioners within a certain period and calculating the equivalent percentage of the total basic salary of all insured persons covered by the sickness funds. For example, assuming that the rate is 3.4%, we can calculate the amount that is 3.4% of the total basic salary of insured persons covered by each sickness fund. At the end of a given period, the actual expenditure on pensioners' health insurance borne by each sickness fund can be calculated. Funds that spent less than 3.4% of the total basic salary make up the difference, whereas funds that spent more than 3.4% absorb the difference. This method is used to eliminate differences in burdens and funds among sickness funds caused by differences in the number of pensioners. In contrast, the majority of funds for farmers' health insurance comes from premiums paid personally by farmers (including premiums partially transferred from pensioners). It has been specified that premiums cannot exceed the average maximum premium of regional sickness funds in the same area. Pensioners covered by farmers' health insurance do not need to contribute premiums, and the full amount of the required costs is borne by the government.

(3) Health Insurance Benefits

The health insurance benefits in Germany include medical benefits, prevention benefits, sickness allowances, long-term care allowances, hospital benefits, maternity benefits (childbirth and pregnancy-related midwifery and medical benefits, childbirth allowance, maternity allowance, and childcare allowance), home care benefits, family benefits, rehabilitation benefits, and funeral expenses.

Some copayments are required among health insurance benefits. For example, the average cost of each drug prescription is €1.02 (the drugs for four specific minor illnesses are fully self-funded, but the costs are waived for children below the age of 16), and an average copayment of €2.5 per day is charged for 14 days of hospital benefits. However, health insurance provides a high payout rate to insured persons and their dependents. Aside from the sickness allowance, which pays full wages for the first six weeks and pays at a rate of 80% from the seventh week onwards, the remaining benefits are paid at a rate of 100%.

The benefits of farmers' health insurance have certain additional special features. Specifically, if the owner has a long-term illness or if his coworking family members are unable to work, labor is provided to replace the sickness allowance or the cost of labor is paid.

(4) Health Insurance Agencies

German health insurance is implemented by various sickness funds. Sickness funds are administered by legal entities under public law, and all positions are honorary.

On average, the number of people enrolled in a regional sickness fund is about 60,000 (about 90,000 if dependents are included), the number enrolled in a company-based sickness fund is 5,500 (about 9,400 if dependents are included), and the number enrolled in a guild-based sickness fund is 12,000 (about 20,500 if dependents are included).

Regional sickness funds are sickness funds administered according to region, characterized by their large scales and high numbers of pensioners. The percentage of pensioners enrolled in regional sickness funds is 33.6% (accounting for 29.2% of the total population). This enrollment is because, in principle, retired individuals should remain with the sickness funds in which they enrolled before retirement. However, due to migration or personal intentions, pensioners can also enroll in the regional sickness fund of their place of residence. As a result, the premiums of regional sickness funds have increased. In order to adjust the risk of such insurance funds, fund adjustments are implemented among all sickness funds for the health insurance premiums of pensioners. The management of pensioners' health insurance is implemented separately by each sickness fund.

The management system of sickness funds is based on the principle of self-administration (*Selbstverwaltung*) of social insurance. Its operation is managed by representatives selected (via election) by employers and employees and minimizes government intervention. In other words, the government implements legislation, administrative guidance, and supervision. Apart from providing subsidies for the elderly, disabled, students, and mothers, in principle the government does not bear any financial burden. In addition, excessive restrictions are avoided in the implementation of administrative guidance and supervision. Although the healthcare cost-containment policies implemented after 1976 were based on the enactment of extensive laws and the adoption of powerful measures, these policies fully respected the autonomy of the sickness funds and healthcare providers.

(5) Payment Methods of Health Insurance Premiums

Health insurance benefits are given directly to the patients by SHI physicians and hospitals according to the agreements signed between each SHI physician and hospital with each sickness fund association. The remuneration of SHI physicians (and SHI dentists) is based on the remuneration regulations for physicians (and dentists). The agreed remuneration decided between the SHI physician (or SHI dentist) association and various sickness fund associations is first paid in full by the sickness fund association to the SHI physician (or SHI dentist) association. Following this payment, the latter association pays each SHI physician (or SHI dentist) according to specific criteria. In accordance with the health insurance regulations (Social Code) amended in March 1987, the Uniform Evaluation Standard (EBM) for Insurance Healthcare came into effect in January 1988 and sought to achieve the rationalization of healthcare remuneration.

Calculation of the total remuneration is based on the number of cases, number of services, fixed amounts, and other methods. The payment standard is determined by the agreement between each state association of SHI physicians (or SHI dentists) and the sickness fund associations.

The increase in total remuneration is implemented according to the Health Insurance Cost Containment Act of 1977, which is based on the opinions formed during the Concerted Action for Health Affairs (composed of employers, employees, government, SHI physicians, SHI dentists, hospitals, sickness funds, operators of private health insurance, and pharmaceutical representatives) held twice a year during spring and fall. The rate of increase in remuneration proposed in the opinions should be within the range of the expected rate of increase in wages. However, in some specific years, the rate of increase was frozen as part of the healthcare cost-containment policy.

The payment mechanism of German social health insurance is composed of two major elements: payment method and payment level. The payment method controls supplier-induced demand. As there is information asymmetry between physicians and patients in the health market, it is difficult for consumers to protect their own interests once healthcare providers provide them with unnecessary healthcare services and drugs. To this end, the German social health insurance funds are well placed to play the role of third-party purchasers. A points system for services (*Punktesystem*) and a DRG-based system were established as the health insurance payment methods for outpatient and inpatient services, respectively. The levels of health insurance payments – that is, how much the insured (health service consumers) can be compensated and how much they have to pay relative to the healthcare expenses incurred – guide consumers to make rational choices. Payment levels are jointly determined by three variables: the deductible, cost sharing, and the ceiling. This design not only helps to control moral hazard on the demand side but also guarantees that reasonable healthcare demands can be met.

(6) Private Health Insurance

About 10% of the total population in Germany is enrolled in private health insurance, the majority of whom are high-income earners. In 1972, during the expansion in the coverage of social health insurance, the number of enrollees decreased to 4.6 million (about 6.6 million in 1965) and gradually increased thereafter.

The federal government has adopted a policy of coexistence between social and private health insurance and intends to continue maintaining this policy in the future. The purpose of this policy is to ensure competition between social and private health insurance. As mentioned above, the employers of individuals who earn above the upper threshold and enroll in private health insurance are obliged to subsidize the equivalent of half of social health insurance premiums. In addition, the policy also stipulates that the benefits of private health insurance must exceed those of social health insurance. Certain individuals covered by private health insurance are also enrolled in social health insurance, which involves insurance agreements for specific benefits, thus causing these individuals to be double insured. Private health insurance provides these enrollees with more choices that can adapt to diversified needs.

The rise in healthcare expenditure is also unavoidable for private health insurance and has caused private health insurance to adopt more rigorous healthcare cost-containment policies than social health insurance has. The stakeholders in social and private health insurance hold policy roundtables once or twice a year to discuss issues on healthcare expenditure and propose opinions and suggestions. In particular, at the beginning of 1988, the association of private health insurance put forward the following requests to the Health Insurance Structural Reform Committee of the Federal Council.

1. Individuals eligible for social health insurance should be limited to those earning an annual income less than the threshold (i.e., the current system, in which those earning above the income threshold can voluntarily choose to enroll in social health insurance, should be modified).
2. The income threshold of compulsory enrollment for workers should not be linked to the increase in the annual remuneration threshold for employees.
3. Civil servants should also be eligible to enroll in social health insurance.
4. Agricultural operators whose main income is not from agriculture should not be eligible for farmers' health insurance.
5. Individuals obliged to enroll in social health insurance whose spouses earn above the annual income threshold should not be eligible for private health insurance.
6. When reforming the regulations for physicians' remuneration, the emphasis should first be placed on the physician–patient relationship, and physicians' technical fees should be rigorously evaluated. The remuneration regulations for dentists should be the same as those for physicians in order to improve transparency.

7. To contain healthcare expenditure, patients' copayments should be a fixed rate instead of a fixed amount.
8. A reimbursement method should be adopted for individuals who voluntarily choose to enroll in private health insurance, and the maximum amount should be specified in the regulations of the fund.
9. Pensioners obliged to enroll in social health insurance should be limited to those who were members of social health insurance for half of their working years.

In summary, in order to coexist with social health insurance, private health insurance has advocated structural policy reforms that limit the scope of compulsory enrollment in social health insurance.

4. Current Status and Future Trends of Health Insurance Policy

(1) Health Insurance Cost-Containment Policies and Structural Reform

The health insurance cost-containment policy in Germany began with the Health Insurance Cost Containment Act of June 1977. This law especially reflects the extensive reform of health insurance coverage and benefits within the context of high economic growth in 1971–1972, which aimed to curb health insurance costs and prevent an increase in the burden of premiums. Due to this law, German health insurance policies underwent a major shift from expansion to containment. As a result, German health insurance has maintained a steady pace of development.

In accordance with the Health Insurance Cost Containment Act, Germany imposed restrictions on the increase in the remuneration of SHI physicians, increased patients' copayments, and performed bonus adjustments among sickness funds. In December 1981, a second Health Insurance Cost Containment Act was enacted. In accordance with this law, Germany implemented the exclusion of drugs for minor illnesses from insured drugs, a reduction in payout rates for dentures, a transparency list of imported drugs, increase of copayment ratios for drugs and treatment supplies, limitations on the rise of hospitalization costs, and so on. In addition, hospital cost-containment acts were also formulated in an attempt to curb hospital costs on the supply side. Following these acts, in 1982–1983, Germany reinforced its policies on healthcare cost containment, which involved a further increase in the copayment ratios for drugs, hospitalization, and rehabilitation and setting up home care benefits. Due to this series of legislative measures, the growth rate of health insurance premiums began declining each year. In 1971, the growth rate was 19.2%, whereas in 1988, it was only 12.9%. On the other hand, although Germany had adopted spending policies that matched its income in order to balance the income and expenditure of premiums, it was difficult to resolve the contradiction between the long-term stable balance of health insurance funds and effective coverage by depending solely on the reinforcement and maintenance of previous healthcare cost-containment policies. Therefore, a reform of the health insurance structure was carried out once again.

In May 1988, the federal government proposed a Health Care Reform Act to the Bundestag. The health insurance structural reform investigation committee of the Federal Council reviewed the reform of the health insurance structure and summarized the results in September 1988. This Act was officially enacted in December of the same year and came into effect in January 1989.

The Health Care Reform Act (Health Care Structural Reform Act) comprehensively assessed the German health insurance system. With the aim of implementing a unified structural reform, and with the basic spirit of joint relationships and self-responsibility among all health insurance funds, the following reforms were carried out.

1. Focus was placed on reimbursements for items with high demand, and benefits such as funeral expenses, drugs with low medical demand, and minor treatment supplies were abolished.
2. Reimbursements were limited to indispensable medical supplies, and fixed reimbursement levels were stipulated for one-third of semi-insured drugs, eyeglasses, hearing aids, treatment supplies, and spa therapy.
3. To strengthen self-responsibility and health management, sickness funds expanded and strengthened policies related to health education, health maintenance, and health promotion. The specific measures include (1) conducting health checks for the heart, circulatory system, kidneys, liver, and diabetes every two years for individuals aged 35 and above; (2) implementing dental preventive measures for individuals above the age of 14 years; (3) conducting group dental examinations in kindergartens and schools; (4) expanding the age range for routine physical examinations from children below the age of four years to those below the age of six years; and (5) the provision of health education in schools and kindergartens by physicians.
4. To effectively overcome common and frequently occurring diseases that endanger the health of people (cancers, heart diseases, circulatory disorders, rheumatism, allergies, psychiatric disorders, AIDS, and so on), the support for research on healthcare prevention programs, experimental treatments, and early detection should be strengthened.
5. The reimbursement for dentures should, in principle, be 50% of the necessary expenses. However, those who regularly receive preventive dental examinations were given an additional 15% reimbursement, thus receiving a total reimbursement of 65% (all sickness funds may reimburse 40–60% of the necessary expenses according to the regulation, up to a maximum of 75%).
6. The copayment ratio of drug costs was increased (the average cost of each prescription was increased from €1 to €1.5).
7. Low-income individuals under 18 years of age were exempted from paying certain patient copayments.
8. In order to support home care, since 1989 employees providing special care services are given four weeks of leave per year (substitute nursing staff are dispatched, and in 1991 substitutes were dispatched at least 25 times a month for one hour each time) or a care allowance of €204.5 per month is paid (the funding source for these expenditures comes from about €3.3 billion of the €7.2 billion saved).
9. The economic efficiency of hospitals was increased, and excess beds were reduced. The specific measures include (1) strengthening the extent to which sickness funds participate in state hospital planning and recognizing the rights of funds to terminate contracts in the case of low demand and inefficient hospitals; (2) distinguishing previous healthcare and special institutions from hospitals and reclassifying them as "prevention and rehabilitation institutions," incorporating them into the same contractual system as hospitals, and requiring nursing homes with inpatient treatment among the contracted institutions to be effective and relatively inexpensive; (3) further limiting the reimbursements for spa therapy and the use of special facilities in the contracts between hospitals and sickness funds; (4) requiring SHI physicians to guide patients to cheaper community hospitals according to their medical requirements and creating

hospital cost comparison tables as references for SHI physicians and sickness funds; and (5) ensuring the implementation of prehospitalization diagnoses and post-discharge treatments in order to strengthen the coordination of outpatient and inpatient benefits and reduce the length of a hospital stay.

10. State governments can modify the number of medical students to control the number of physicians.

11. Modifying the remuneration of SHI physicians should be based on the balance of income and expenditure in premiums, as with other reimbursements.

12. Reimbursements for prescriptions by SHI physicians (drugs, hospitalization, spa therapy, and so on) must be made according to the standard content stipulated, and those that exceed this scope must be reviewed.

13. Insured persons have the legal right to request that sickness funds provide information related to their own healthcare expenses and healthcare content.

14. The previous system of consulting physicians was revised such that all SHI physicians must implement the medical consultation services of the sickness funds.

15. The system in which hospital-based physicians are automatically SHI physicians was repealed, the requirement for physicians to pass national medical examinations to become SHI physicians was preserved, and the special treatment of physicians was abolished in order to improve the quality of physicians.

16. The mark-up percentages of pharmacies were divided into three levels, 3%, 5%, and 7%, according to sales volume.

17. If cheaper drugs of similar efficacy are available in pharmacies, then reimbursements for those drugs are given priority.

18. In the case of a surplus, all sickness funds must reimburse the premiums as stated in the agreement; in the case of a deficit, reimbursement can be suspended.

19. The structural modernization of the health insurance system was promoted. The specific measures include (1) unifying the regulations for the collection, reimbursement, and management of premiums among all sickness funds; (2) stipulating the obligation for fund adjustments among the same type of sickness funds to eliminate the disparities in premiums; (3) adjusting the burden of health insurance borne by pensioners and increasing the level of concern of all sickness funds towards pensioners; (4) applying the same premium rates to pensioners as to other general insured persons; and (5) introducing an income threshold system for workers who are obliged to enroll in insurance.

20. A review system was established for the Concerted Action for Health Affairs that aimed to balance the income and expenditure of premiums.

21. The laws and regulations related to health insurance were re-consolidated and incorporated into the Social Code to facilitate inspection and supervision by the public.

The problem of overly rapid growth in Germany's health insurance costs was resolved through the effectiveness of the Health Insurance Cost Containment Act. The growth rate of health insurance costs was 4.9% in 1977, 10.9% in 1980, 7.5% in 1990, and 8.2% in 2000. There was a significant decrease compared to the period before the Act was enacted (the average annual growth rate was 19.2% in 1971–1975), and the average premium rate showed almost no increase since 1976 (11.3% in 1976, 11.4% in 1980, 11.6% in 1990, and 11.8% in 2000). Therefore, the issue of balancing health insurance funds has been relatively stable the past few years.

However, the growth rate of health insurance costs has still been rising each year and is accompanied by a gradual increase in premium rates. In particular, the healthcare expenses incurred by pensioners have been accounting for a higher share of health insurance cost, and the growth rate of payouts per capita is 16.4%, which is far higher than the 10.8% of general insured persons. The growth rate of pensioners' premium rates in 1990–2000 was 7.8%, whereas that of general insured persons was 4.5%. Therefore, the growth rate of payouts for regional sickness funds, which have a higher number of pensioners, surpassed that of all sickness funds at 13.2% in 2000.

In summary, reforms of the health security system were undertaken at an unprecedented scale. These reforms were characterized by the proposal of the following new policies: (1) Regarding the stable balance of health insurance funds as the top priority by abolishing certain benefits, reducing reimbursement rates, improving patient copayments, strengthening healthcare efficiency and cost-effectiveness, and so on. (2) Reinforcing savings on expenditure and using the savings to expand and strengthen disease prevention, health management and promotion, and the development of home care programs.

(2) Containment Policies of Healthcare Provision

Although the total number of hospitals has decreased since 1970, the total number of beds and the number of beds per 100,000 residents have not changed significantly. However, hospital healthcare expenditure has continued to rise due to heightened hospital functions (increase in high-priced medical equipment, facilities, healthcare practitioners, and so on) and a larger elderly population. The Hospital Finance Amendment Act enacted in December 1981 emphasized the rationalization of hospital operations and stipulated the following items: (1) the improvement of concepts for hospital operations, (2) the rationalization of calculation methods for nursing and other fees, (3) assurances that health insurance funds have a say in hospital operations, and (4) the reduction of investments in hospital funding (investment from insurance funds). These measures were applied to further improve the efficiency and cost-effectiveness of hospital operations to curb the excessive growth in hospital healthcare expenditure as much as possible. On the other hand, the total number of physicians has been increasing each year, along with the number of SHI physicians. Not only is the rapid increase in SHI physicians related to the rise in healthcare expenditure, but it also leads to increased competition among SHI physicians and a decrease in income. The Need Planning Law of Statutory Health Insurance Physicians enacted in December 1986 controlled one of the causes for the rise in healthcare expenditure, namely, the increase in SHI physicians. Licenses for SHI physicians were restricted in areas with surplus SHI physicians (areas below 50% nationwide) in order to achieve the appropriate distribution of SHI physicians and healthcare cost containment. This law was an amendment based on the Health Insurance Promotion Act enacted in 1976 to address the lack of physicians, which revised the need planning of SHI physicians in order to prevent the over-concentration of SHI physicians in specific areas, thereby avoiding the resulting surplus in local supply. However, this law does not impose restrictions on the overall scope of SHI physicians and only limits the new addition of licenses for SHI physicians in oversupplied areas within a certain period of time or in each medical field. In December 1983, the decree on licenses for SHI physicians was amended and extended the approval process for SHI physicians from six months to eight months. The Federal Medical Practitioners' Act was amended in December 1985, which means that, since 1986, all medical students who have completed their university education must receive two years of training as clinical physicians to obtain their licenses to practice medicine. The purpose of these measures regarding the supply of physicians was to maintain the current quota of medical graduates, provide physicians who have received adequate training, extend the duration of education and training, and ensure the rational supply of physicians.

Such containment policies for healthcare provision seek to rationalize the healthcare providers, thus promoting the efficiency and cost-effectiveness of insurance healthcare. Their purpose is to work together with health insurance containment policies to achieve the stability and balance of health insurance funds. These policies were established from a long-term perspective, and bolder policies have continuously been proposed based on their outcomes. Since January 1985, Germany has implemented the New Hospital Financial Stability Act and has striven to adopt measures to curb the soaring healthcare expenditure of hospitals. Unfortunately, during the evaluation of these reforms in the late 1990s, the reforms were generally considered effective but not ideal. Furthermore, the most significant factor in the rising healthcare expenditure of hospitals was due to the continued increase in the number of healthcare practitioners. Thus, the issue of healthcare provision is a deep-rooted and intractable problem.

(3) Issue of Funding Balance in Health Insurance

Germany experienced rapid economic growth from the latter half of the 1960s to the early half of the 1970s. During this period, the income of health insurance had a stable growth rate that was sufficient to cope with the rise in spending required by the expansion of health insurance and the expansion of the health system, including hospitals and medical practitioners. Apart from deficits in 1955 and 1969, health insurance maintained a balance between income and expenditure from 1950 until 1973.

Due to the significant increase in spending after the latter half of the 1970s, it became more challenging to maintain the balance between the income and expenditure of premiums. The considerable increases in spending in 1974 and 1975 led to the loss of balance between income and expenditure, resulting in deficits in 1975 and 1979. It was expected that if the situation could not be rectified, it would lead to continuous and substantial deficits. At that time, the increasing premium rate was about 11.3%. Coincidentally, the occurrence of the oil crisis led to a rapid decrease in economic growth, which meant that large increases in wages were impossible. Moreover, the premium rates were also relatively high, and the contributions of employers and employees could not be increased further. Consequently, the government could only adopt an income-oriented expenditure policy to achieve the balance and stability of health insurance funds.

Therefore, since 1976, policies to contain health insurance expenditure have been vigorously implemented. As a result, the growth rate of health insurance expenditure decreased significantly after 1976 and showed a surplus instead in 1976–1978. However, the growth rate of health insurance expenditures showed a subsequent trend of increase and reached a considerable deficit in 1979.

As the previous health insurance cost-containment policies were also flawed, they became ineffective. Hence, it was expected that without remedying the situation, the funding deficit of health insurance would become more serious in the future. In view of the need to further pursue health insurance cost-containment polices in 1982, the federal government proposed a second Health Insurance Cost Containment Act in the fall Parliamentary session of 1981. This act was formally enacted in December 1981 in conjunction with the amendment of the Hospital Financial Stability Act (Hospital Cost Containment Act) proposed to Parliament in April 1981. The amendment of the Hospital Financial Stability Act mainly involved controlling hospital construction and the introduction of medical devices and limiting the increase in daily hospital healthcare expenditure. Hospital cost containment was enforced on targets that were not previously incorporated in the law.

5. Health Reforms in the Twenty-First Century

On January 1, 2000, Germany officially implemented the Health Care Reform Act of 2000. This campaign was initiated by the German government to restructure the health service system. This reform had a major and far-reaching impact on all aspects of hospitals. The main contents of the reform and its impacts are described next.

(1) Strengthened Budgetary Control

In recent years, the German government has been striving to find solutions to the lack of strict cost-containment measures in social health insurance. For example, recent reforms restricted the rise in the cost of hospital services to within the range of the growth rate for insurance funds. Additional costs are only permitted under certain circumstances, such as when the number of patients increases or when the composition of health services changes. This type of budgetary restriction measure was expected to maintain the current level of health services without requiring additional capital investment. However, such measures may instead unleash the potential to promote the overall efficiency of the health service system.

(2) Hospital Payment System

The goal of the Health Care Reform Act of 2000 was to change the existing hospital service payment system and establish a comprehensive payment system based on DRGs before 2003. The National Associations of Sickness Funds and the hospitals were the main departments and institutions responsible for implementing these reforms. The decisions of these institutions and departments had to be based on the principles of the new payment system, such as the basic structure of the system, the method of calculating cost weights, and the classification standards for disease diagnosis.

By the end of June 2000, the German sickness funds and the Hospital Federation decided to reform the hospital compensation system by referring to the Australian refined DRG (AR-DRG) system. The AR-DRG system consists of 409 basic DRGs, each of which represents a patient group with similar clinical conditions that require similar treatment methods. Each group can further be divided according to disease severity and complexity. At present, the AR-DRG system has a total of 661 DRGs. The outcome of the negotiations between the German sickness funds and the Hospital Federation was to increase the number of DRGs from 661 to more than 800 according to the actual payment needs of German hospitals.

Several issues had to be resolved before the implementation of the DRG system in 2003.

1. The sickness funds and the German Hospital Federation had to establish a supplementary payment system to cover aspects that could not be compensated through DRGs, such as emergency care, the training of nursing staff, the depreciation of hospital infrastructure, and so on. Due to the varying interests of different sickness funds, negotiations in this regard progressed slowly.
2. An agreement had to be reached regarding the financial system, principles, and content.
3. The coding of the basic AR-DRG system and the related diagnostic and treatment groups had to be completed.
4. An agreement had to be reached regarding costs and pricing before December 31, 2001.

However, the legislative and economic framework of the new hospital payment system has not yet been formulated. It is still doubtful as to whether the expectations of the policymakers are too high concerning the ability of the reforms to improve hospital service efficiency. At present, it is still difficult to determine whether the payment system can reflect the specific characteristics of different hospitals. For example, some hospitals have high service levels, others provide more emergency services, and some are teaching hospitals. In legal terms, improving the service pricing of these hospitals is not a good solution, as such improvements will cause these hospitals to have more expensive service prices than their competitors have, which will discourage patients from choosing these hospitals.

In future DRG-based payment methods, prices will be set according to the average cost nationwide. This pricing is unfavorable to hospitals with higher costs than the social average, especially public and nonprofit hospitals, as the labor costs of these hospitals are difficult to reduce due to the influence of labor unions. As a result, hospitals will face greater financial risks than they do currently. As of now, DRGs have mainly achieved the following outcomes. (1) They established a new set of hospital cost management methods. The DRG-based payment system has changed the income strategies of hospitals, altered their organizational structures, helped to optimize medical procedures, and facilitated hospital cost accounting and management. (2) They have created a new language for communication among all involved parties. The implementation of the DRG-based payment system has alleviated the difference in perspective between physicians and managers. Thus, the communication gap between the two has been eliminated to a certain extent and has facilitated their coordination and communication. (3) They have achieved preliminary results in shortening the length of hospital stays.

(3) Guarantee of Service Quality

Prior to the Health Care Reform Act of 2000, legislators mainly focused on quality control of health services, as the public believed that hospitals need to strengthen quality management and safeguard the interests of patients. Various political parties have also proposed a number of policies to guarantee the quality of healthcare services. Hospitals took the lead in the establishment of quality control measures for the overall health service system. However, when drafting the Health Care Reform Act of 2000, legislators were no longer conservative. Hence, quality assurance and quality management became mandatory regulations, and providers who do not comply with the national quality management regulations are severely punished.

The Health Care Reform Act of 2000 also stipulated the responsibilities of health service agencies and societies to evaluate health services. The evaluation committee assesses the quantity, efficiency, and suitability of various diagnoses and treatments provided by hospital services. If a treatment method fails to meet the criteria during evaluation, insurance funds decline to pay the expenses. In addition, a newly formed coordination committee was made responsible for formulating the standards for evaluating the suitability and efficiency of diagnoses and treatments provided under hospital services. The evaluation process follows the principle of "evidence-based medicine," and 10 types of treatment regimens with suspected problems are evaluated each year.

(4) Promotion of Integrated Healthcare

A major problem with the German health service system is the lack of coordination between outpatient and inpatient services. "Integrated healthcare" was introduced in the

Health Care Reform Act of 2000 and aimed to eliminate the gap between the two services. Integrated healthcare may ensure that health services are more patient-oriented. At the same time, legislators also hoped that integrated healthcare could reduce the cost of health services. The law permitted the creation of contracts or agreements among various insurance funds, among healthcare institutions, and between insurance funds and healthcare institutions to implement different forms of integrated healthcare.

(5) Alternatives to Inpatient Treatment

In the German health service system, the differences in the services provided by office-based physicians and hospitals are stipulated in the law. Office-based physicians provide outpatient services, whereas hospitals are responsible for providing inpatient services. In 1993, policymakers began to downplay the division of labor between the two and allowed hospitals to conduct ambulatory outpatient surgery. However, the types of such surgeries are regulated by the National Ambulatory Surgery Directory. The introduction of the "alternative measures to inpatient treatment" in the Health Care Reform Act of 2000 further expanded the types of ambulatory surgery. The implementation of this change was accomplished through agreements between suppliers, purchasers, and other relevant parties. In addition, the law advocated the establishment of a single-payer system that specifically covers the service costs of ambulatory surgeries and other "alternative measures to inpatient treatment" provided by clinics and hospitals.

6. Health Insurance System Reforms by the Grand Coalition Government

(1) Introduction of Universal Health Insurance

On New Year's Day in 2009, Germany achieved universal health insurance for the first time in history. Any German resident who does not have other adequate health security measures is obliged to enroll in the sickness funds. That is, according to the relevant rules and conditions, individuals have to enroll in either statutory health insurance or private health insurance. As a transitional measure, individuals who were previously covered by the statutory health insurance system and currently do not have health insurance must meet the following requirements.

1. From April 1, 2007, onwards, all individuals are obliged to re-enroll in statutory health insurance; as of July 1, 2007, those who were previously covered by the private health insurance system and currently do not have health insurance can choose to enroll in private health insurance again. (2) Individuals first received health insurance coverage under the framework of the standard tariff and switched to the basic tariff on January 1, 2009.

(2) Improvement of Health Service Provision

The main measures to improve health service provision are as follows. (1) The scope of health services was expanded. Hospitals were allowed to provide outpatient services that were originally not permitted to critically ill patients; pain relief could be provided to terminally and critically ill patients; the sickness insurance agency was required to pay for the cost of rehabilitation, vaccination, and childcare costs for parents; and eligible individuals could receive home care services instead of moving to a nursing home. (2) Greater emphasis was placed on safety and cost-effectiveness in drug supply. The cost-efficacy-evaluation mechanism was introduced. Under this mechanism, when a new drug is prescribed, another physician should be consulted to fully evaluate the cost-effectiveness and safety of the drug. Sickness insurance agencies should negotiate discount contracts with drug manufacturers to compete for lower drug prices.

(3) Promotion of the Modernization of Statutory and Private Health Insurance Agencies

1. Statutory health insurance agencies may formulate different fee standards and contracts according to the preferences of insured persons; thus, insured persons enjoy greater freedom of choice, and more mechanisms for competition among the statutory health insurance agencies are introduced. Insured persons are encouraged through relevant measures to strengthen their awareness of self-care responsibilities (e.g., receiving preventive checks). Various health insurance agencies provide more forms of services and fee plans for selection. To reduce bureaucracy and streamline the institutions, the highest-level associations for each of the seven health insurance agencies were merged into one to uniformly represent the negotiations of all statutory health insurance agencies. All insurance agencies (including cross-category agencies) are permitted to merge freely.

2. Private health insurance agencies, since the beginning of 2009, must provide basic insurance coverage similar to that of statutory health insurance, with premiums that should not exceed the standards of the latter. For individuals intending to be insured, companies have the mandatory obligation to contract (*Kontrahierungszwang*) and are not permitted to charge additional risk premiums (*Risikozuschläge*). Insured persons are allowed to change insurance companies; old-age provisions (*Alterungsrückstellungen*), which were previously barred from switching companies and competition, can now be transferred among different insurance policies within the same insurance company or between different insurance companies.

(4) Financial Reform of the Health Security System

Reforms were undertaken on the health fund financing and claims-payment financing methods. In the beginning of 2009, a health fund model (*Gesundheitsfonds*) was introduced for the financing of the statutory health insurance funds. The health fund model incorporated a design involving contributions from both parties (Figure 12.3).

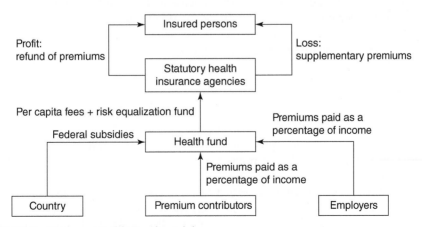

FIGURE 12.3 German Health Fund model.

The sources of funding included the country, premium contributors, and employers. However, the sickness insurance agency requires the insured to pay additional premiums when it earns a loss, and it refunds part of the premiums to the insured when it earns a profit. After the fund was established, it was responsible for financing more than 95% of health expenditures.

SECTION II. THE HEALTH SYSTEM IN FRANCE

France is situated in Western Europe, where it has the largest land area, covering approximately 551,000 square kilometers. In 2013, the total population was 66.028 million, of which 78% live in cities, and 8% are engaged in agricultural production. The capital, Paris, has a population of 2.21 million, accounting for about 3.5% of the total population, and it is the political, economic, and cultural center of the country. France is a relatively industrialized country with an economically open system. Its GDP per capita in 2013 was US$42,503.30.

France implements a constitutional presidential system, in which the president appoints a prime minister to form a cabinet. The country is divided into 22 administrative regions and 95 counties (or departments). The national health administration is mainly led by three bureaus within the Ministry of Social Affairs and National Solidarity: the General Directorate of Health, the Hospital Directorate, and the Medical Devices Directorate. The 22 administrative regions and 95 counties (or departments) each have their own health and social affairs agencies. In addition, the Directorate of Labor Relations (equivalent to the Ministry of Labor) has a director of labor and occupational health affairs who is responsible for the management of occupational health.

France's healthcare spending in 2012 was 11.7% of GDP. Healthcare financing in France mainly depends on government funding allocations, sponsorships, and the social insurance system, which covers all residents. French residents have a good health status. In 2012, the population had a birth rate of 12.6%, a mortality rate of 8.7%, an infant mortality rate of 3.5 per 1,000 live births, and average life expectancies of 86.1 years for women and 79.2 years for men. However, the age structure of the French population has shown trends of aging. In 2013, individuals over 65 years old accounted for 17.9% of the population. In 2006–2013, the number of physicians per 10,000 people was 31.8, the number of nurses and midwives per 10,000 people was 93, and the number of hospital beds per 10,000 people was 64. To alter its population structure and achieve the goal of maintaining national fertility, the French government adopted policies to encourage fertility and strengthened healthcare for women and children.

1. Health Service System

(1) Healthcare Provision System

Physicians and other healthcare practitioners have their own professional organizations. Physicians belong to two types of professional organizations: the Order of Physicians (*L'Ordre des Médecins*) and the medical unions (*les syndicats médicaux*).

The Order of Physicians was created in 1945. The Order of Oral Surgeons and Order of Midwives were also established in the same year. The Order of Physicians requires all physicians (except for nonexecutive positions) to join the French Medical Council (mandatory participation). The French Medical Council monitors the ethics, quality, and quantity of physicians according to the Code of Medical Ethics (decree of November 28, 1955). The Order of Physicians is a three-tier organization divided into the county, regional, and national levels. The counselors for each Order of Physicians are selected from among the Orders in the level below.

The medical unions were established in 1881 (officially recognized in 1882), which was 60 years earlier than the creation of the Order of Physicians. The medical unions were formed for the purpose of seeking economic and social progress among fellow practitioners. The unions differ depending on the type of occupation or political opinions. The largest and most representative of the national medical unions is the Confederation of French Medical Unions (*La Confédération des Syndicats Médicaux Français*, CSMF), which is said to include 67% of private practitioners as members. Another nationally representative medical union is the Federation of French Physicians (Fédération des Médecins de France, FMF), which claims to have 13,000 members. However, this figure seems to be an exaggeration.

The CSMF was established in 1928 and has been responsible for negotiating with health insurers since 1945. However, the "standard agreement" (convention type) adopted according to the decree of May 12, 1960, led to fierce internal conflict within the CSMF, which caused the opposing parties to splinter and form their own organizations, which eventually merged in 1968 to officially form the FMF. In addition to the CSMF and FMF, which were the nationally representative organizations of physicians, the participants in national agreements also included the national federation of resident physicians, contract physicians and civil service physicians, and the union of university hospital physicians.

Legislation concerning healthcare practitioners mainly includes the 1927 Medical Charter (*Charte Médicale*); the 1945 Ordinance Related to the Practice and Organization of Physicians, Dentists, and Midwives; the 1955 Code of Medical Ethics; the 1953 Public Health Law; the 1967 Code of Ethics for Dentists; the 1971 Code of Ethics for Midwives; and the 1971 Amendment to the Social Insurance Code (coordinated amendments were made to the Code of Medical Ethics and Social Insurance Code). Currently, the activities of healthcare practitioners are protected and bound by these laws. Hospitals in France began as shelters for the poor owing to religious charitable activities. Prior to the French Revolution, hospitals were maintained through donations and farm income and, hence, did not charge fees. After the outbreak of the French Revolution, these facilities were used as "Citizens' Hospitals" and were charitable facilities that were basically free. After the promulgation of hospitals laws on August 7, 1951, although hospitals inherited some of their previous practices, they began to transition from hospitals run by religious groups to public hospitals. Thereafter, hospitals were run by cities, towns, and villages. In addition to income from donations, hospitals also relied on financial assistance from their cities, towns, and villages.

As hospitals were not fully staffed with physicians at that time, they did not require much money, and the contradictions in funding were not prominent. However, with the medical advancements of the nineteenth and twentieth centuries, excellent physicians began gathering in hospitals, and, in turn, hospitals needed to find new funding sources. In addition, with the development of social insurance, the service targets of hospitals were not just the poor population but also included general patients, who wished to be treated by good physicians. Hence, "pay-per-diem" was adopted as the new payment method for hospital fees. The law of December 21, 1941, stipulated that fee-paying patients shall be individuals who qualify for per diem hospital fees. The law also determined the remuneration for physicians and recognized the creation of open clinics.

During the nineteenth and twentieth centuries, private hospitals gradually developed into two types. The first type was hospitals built by physicians that targeted fee-paying patients, where the remuneration of physicians (including surgeons and gynecologists), costs of medical assistants, and accommodation fees were paid per diem (i.e., for-profit hospitals). On the other hand, state-owned railway and mining companies constructed general hospitals that provided free healthcare (hospital remuneration paid by the companies). The operating agencies of the social insurance system and some mutual aid societies also constructed hospitals of a similar nature. There were also special hospitals for tuberculosis and psychiatric disorders. These hospitals are known as nonprofit hospitals.

In order to accommodate the changes in the functions of these hospitals, the ordinance of December 11, 1958, sought to modernize hospital organization and interior structure and to implement the restructuring of hospitals. In other words, it divided public general hospitals according to importance into regional, local, and general hospitals. Specialized hospitals included mother-baby units and elderly care centers. Previous public special hospitals continued to exist in their original forms. In addition, general hospitals began to implement emergency care, ambulatory care, day hospitals, in-home medical care systems, and so on.

However, not only are public and private hospitals differentiated in the law, but the treatment provided by them under health insurance differs significantly, as well. To eliminate this difference between public and private hospitals, France enacted the hospital reform law on December 31, 1970, which made the concept of "public hospital service" applicable to private hospitals such that private hospitals are also imbued with a public social mission. The hospital reform of 1970 divided hospitals into the following four categories: (1) general hospitals, which aim to provide diagnoses and short-term hospital treatments; (2) local hospitals, which aim to provide nursing care, convalescence, or functional rehabilitation; (3) specialist hospitals, which aim to provide treatment for specific diseases; and (4) specialized hospitals, which include mother-baby units and elderly care centers. The main contents of the hospital reform law are as follows: the establishment of a national public hospital system, the establishment of rules to regulate the practice of public and private hospitals, and the reform of public hospital operations.

(2) Hospital Services

Healthcare institutions in France can be divided into three types: public hospitals, private nonprofit hospitals, and private for-profit hospitals. There are various forms of hospital ownership, including public hospitals, church-run hospitals, union clinics, and private clinics, as well as charity-run hospitals and hospitals affiliated with certain large companies and financial groups. Public hospitals provide nearly two-thirds of all inpatient treatment. One characteristic of French hospitals is that the number of private hospitals exceeds that of public hospitals, but the former tend to be smaller than the latter. In fact, the healthcare institutions that provide high-tech medical services are public hospitals centered on universities (*centre hospitalier universitaire*, CHU).

Before the twentieth century, French physicians were mainly individual private practitioners, and since the Middle Ages hospitals had mainly been institutions for poverty relief or charity rather than healthcare institutions. By the twentieth century, the continuous advancement of healthcare standards, together with the enrichment and improvement of the social security system, meant that not only low-income groups but also high-income groups began to take notice of hospitals. Hospitals only began to take the form of modern healthcare institutions at this point in time. The new management introduced in the hospital reform plan "Hospital 2007" (and its extension "Hospital 2012") led to the establishment of a new hospital financing model: T2A. This model determines the allocation of funds according to outpatient and inpatient DRGs (each disease code corresponds to each specific medical price in the *groupes homogènes de séjours*, or GHS) so as to achieve a balanced budget.

Although the legal system for hospitals has existed for a long time, it was not until 1941 that the hospitals' legal status was clarified. The hospital system was reformed in 1958 and 1968, followed by the 1970 Law on Hospital Reform (Law No. 70-1318, hereinafter referred to as the Hospital Reform Law), which ultimately formed the basis for the current hospital system.

1. Public and Private Hospitals   Table 12.6 shows the number of hospitals and beds in 2000 in France. Specifically, there were 1,849 public hospitals (41.2%) with 509,936 beds (70.6%) and 2,637 private hospitals (58.8%) with 212,442 beds (29.4%). Thus, although the number of public hospitals is smaller, they are usually of larger size and, hence, account for a greater number of beds.

TABLE 12.6   Composition of Hospitals and Beds in France in 2000

Item	Number of Legal Subjects	Number of Institutions	Number of Beds
[Public]			
Regional hospital centers (*centre hospitaliers*)	29	239	114,036
Hospital centers (*centres*)	202	344	148,451
Hospitals (*hôpitaux*)	301	396	104,833
Local hospitals (*hôpitaux locaux*)	342	368	52,908
Medium-stay centers	81	135	14,304
Other subjects (*autres*)	4		819
Specialist psychiatric hospital centers	98	210	74,585
Other public institutions		157	
Total	1,057	1,849 (41.2%)	509,936 (70.6%)
[Private]			
For-profit hospitals		1,523	104,167
Nonprofit hospitals		1,092	90,364
Of which:	Hospitals not participating in public hospital service	665	39,301
	Hospitals participating in public hospital service	427	51,063
Private psychiatric hospitals		22	17,911
Total		2,637 (58.8%)	212,442 (29.4%)
Total of public and private hospitals		4,486 (100.0%)	722,378(100.0%)

Notes:
(1) The difference in the number of legal subjects and institutions is because, for example, the Assistance Publique-Hôpitaux de Paris (a healthcare trust) is considered one legal subject but consists of 42 independently operating hospital institutions.
(2) Private hospitals also include cases such as the French Red Cross hospitals, but only the number of hospital institutions was counted.
(3) According to the Hospital Reform Law, public hospitals refer to five types of hospitals: municipal, inter-municipal, regional, inter-regional, and national hospitals.

The separation of ownership and management rights in French public hospitals implies that all major issues concerning hospital construction and development are handled by the management committee, whereas routine operations are handled by the hospital director. Public hospitals come under the responsibility of a board of directors. The directors may vary according to the hospital in question. However, due to considerations for the opinions of the management and service targets, the board must include representatives of social insurance funds and local public bodies. Although the board of directors is the highest decision-making body, the specialization of healthcare and the increasing share of social security in the hospital budget imply that the hospital director (*directeur d'hôpital*) is usually in charge of the routine operations of current hospitals. Therefore, the hospital director occupies a relatively high position in a French public hospital.

As for private hospitals, the ordinance of April 24, 1959, defines private hospitals as "all healthcare institutions that are not public in nature, and are not run by national, municipal, and public institutions" (Article 13). However, unlike public hospitals, a private hospital is not necessarily run by a single legal subject, and the involvement of two or more companies is not uncommon. Private hospitals can be categorized according to the operating entity as follows (Figure 12.4).

1. The operating entities of for-profit hospitals include (1) individuals (*propriétaire exploitant*) and (2) companies (*société*).
2. The operating entities of nonprofit hospitals include (1) associations, (2) foundations (*fondation*), (3) religious corporations (congregation), (4) social security funds (*caisse de sécurité sociale*), and (5) mutual insurance associations (*sécurité mutualiste*).

A considerable proportion of for-profit hospitals consists of joint-stock and limited companies. On the other hand, the majority of nonprofit hospitals exist as associations, which are established according to the Law of July 1, 1901, Relating to the Contract of

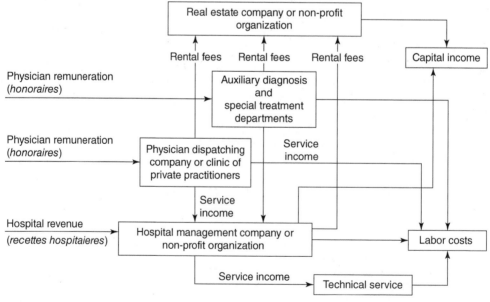

FIGURE 12.4 Concept of French private hospitals.

Associations. This distinction is because dues may only be returned upon the dissolution of the association, but associations can enjoy value-added tax, gift tax, and other concessions. Hospitals taking the form of foundations are mostly cancer and psychiatric hospitals.

2. Public Hospital Service In France, both public and private hospitals occupy important positions. At the beginning of the twentieth century, the numbers of various types of private hospitals began to increase, and the compensation system for healthcare expenses established in the social security system strengthened this development. However, the fierce competition caused by the increase in the number of private hospitals led to the prioritization of interests, which caused the gradual emergence of vicious competition in healthcare. Along with the occurrence of this phenomenon, public hospital service (service public *hospitalier*) emerged to play a coordinating role in healthy competition and social welfare. Hence, Article 2 of the Hospital Reform Law defines public hospital service as follows: "Public hospitals provide security for the diagnosis, examination, and treatment (emergency treatment in some cases) of patients and pregnant women who were sent or have come to the hospitals and provides security for hospitalization as necessary." Public hospital services mainly include (1) cooperating with the university and graduate education of physicians and pharmacists and the training of medical personnel; (2) cooperating with preventive medical services and implementing their adjustment policies; and (3) participating in medicine, medical research, and health education. Physicians in private practice may be required to participate in public hospital service. Hospitals that were incorporated into public hospital service became the core of regional healthcare and were obliged to provide residents with the same basic medical and emergency services.

The participation of private nonprofit hospitals in public hospital service must be approved by the relevant authorities. On the one hand, these hospitals have the same obligations as public hospitals do, but, on the other hand, they can enjoy the same treatment, including receiving payments of medical fees and subsidies for healthcare institutions from the state and social security funds. Private hospitals other than those described above (i.e., for-profit and nonprofit hospitals not involved in public hospital service) adopt third-party payment methods (direct payments of costs borne by insurers to healthcare institutions) according to the agreements signed with the social security funds.

The operation of French public hospitals mainly relies on the support of state funding, and a strict budget is implemented for all expenditures. The government has passed legislation to implement a tiered management system for hospitals that is administered jointly by the Ministry of Health, local governments, and health administrations. Although the government gives public hospitals considerable autonomy in operation and management, investment and development are strictly conducted according to plan, which enables a high level of transparency and facilitates supervision. Hospital revenues are mainly from health insurance reimbursements, and reimbursement standards are negotiated annually between the state and healthcare industry organizations. The government promotes the improvement of health service quality by reviewing and certifying the quality of healthcare institutions and assessing the quality and safety factors of their medical care.

3. Hospital Classification Based on Public Hospital Service The Hospital Reform Law placed a greater emphasis on hospital classification according to hospital technology and equipment compared to previous laws. Following this classification, new classifications based on hospital conditions and regional service functions were gradually introduced.

After undergoing three revisions, the current classification of French hospitals is as follows.

1. *Hospital centers (*les centres hospitaliers*).* These mainly include regional hospital centers (*les centres hospitaliers régionaux*), specialized hospital centers (*les centres hospitaliers spéciaux*), general hospital centers (*les centres hospitaliers generaux*), and sector hospital centers (*les centres hospitaliers de secteur*).
2. *Convalescence, treatment, rehabilitation, or psychiatric medium-stay centers.* These mainly include convalescence centers (*les centres de convalescence*); medical cure centers (*les centres de cure medicale*); rehabilitation centers (*les centres de réadaptation*); convalescence and cure centers (*les centres de convalescence et de cure*); convalescence and rehabilitation centers (*les centres de convalescence et de réadaptation*); cure and rehabilitation centers (*les centres de cure et de réadaptation*); convalescence, cure, and rehabilitation centers (*les centres de convalescence, de cure et réadaptation*); and post-cure centers (*les centres de postcure*).
3. Long-stay centers (*les centres de long séjour*).
4. Local hospitals (rural hospitals).

Among these hospitals, (1) are for acute, short-term inpatient treatments; (2) are inpatient institutions providing treatment during convalescence for chronic diseases and training for functional rehabilitation; (3) are institutions providing medical care for elderly people who have lost the ability to care for themselves; and (4) are hospitals in rural villages, mountain villages, and other remote areas. However, (2) and (3) are not necessarily separate from (1) and mostly use affiliated buildings of the same institution as wards.

The difference among hospital centers classified under (1) is that regional hospital centers are the largest and have the most equipment and medical departments; they mainly provide high-tech specialized healthcare and serve as regional healthcare centers. In contrast, general and sector hospital centers (in descending order) have fewer approved medical departments and less equipment, and they serve as supplementary healthcare institutions in a given region. Specialized hospital centers are institutions for the treatment of specific diseases and are almost entirely devoted to psychiatry.

4. Classification Based on the Tasks of Various Hospital Institutions   Based on the distribution of tasks, the hospital institutions in France can roughly be divided into hospital centers, convalescence and rehabilitation centers, and inpatient units. Hospital centers can further be categorized according to size and specialization into regional hospital centers, general hospital centers, and specialist hospital centers. Regional hospital centers are located in the major cities of the 21 regions. They provide advanced medical care and conduct medical education and research. They are hospitals that serve central tasks in the regions. General hospital centers are established in areas with populations of 100,000–200,000 and must include medicine, surgery, obstetrics, and pediatrics departments. Specialist hospital centers refer to tuberculosis hospitals, psychiatric hospitals, and so on. Convalescence and rehabilitation centers are healthcare institutions for the convalescence of patients with chronic diseases and those requiring rehabilitation. Inpatient units are healthcare institutions that are situated in remote areas and have the minimum level of medical equipment.

Table 12.7 shows the number of beds in French healthcare institutions over time. The number of beds in public general hospitals (regional hospital centers, general hospital centers, and inpatient units) is more than twice that in private healthcare institutions (e.g., hospitals, convalescence, and rehabilitation centers), but the difference in the number of

TABLE 12.7 Number of Beds in French Healthcare Institutions over the Years

Year	Public General Hospitals	Private Healthcare Institutions	Public Elderly Care Homes	Private Elderly Care Institutions
1970	412,520	170,000	80,329	75,800
1980	489,159	191,630	122,840	132,715
1990	512,520	238,418	180,329	198,452
2000	520,866	271,212	273,896	257,039

Source: French National Institute of Health and Medical Research, Statistical Yearbook of France, 2001.

beds on the regional level has not yet been eliminated. In recent years, hospital reform has sought to establish a public hospital service system for private hospitals that have signed agreements with public hospitals (a system that gives private hospitals a public service mission). Although, in accordance with the Hospital Reform Law, the authorities have formulated a plan for the allocation of beds based on the "health map" (*carte sanitaire*) of all healthcare institutions and their utilization efficiencies, the expected results have yet to be achieved.

(3) Health Map

The health map (*carte sanitaire*), which is an important part of regional health planning, has been used to achieve the planned provision of healthcare. France first proposed the health map in 1969. After discussions, the health map was explicitly written into the Hospital Reform Law.

1. Role of the Health Map The health map can be used as a guideline to guide the establishment of healthcare institutions and is the earliest pioneer of regional health planning. It is not merely a means of restricting health resources, and its purpose covers the following aspects:

1. Providing the basic healthcare needs of residents under the most optimal conditions.
2. Adjusting and supplementing public and private hospitals to ensure the most rational operation of healthcare institutions.
3. Achieving the most rational layout, allocation, and utilization of healthcare resources.

2 .Content of the Health Map The health map divides the country into 284 health sectors (*secteurs sanitaires*) and 21 health regions (*régions sanitaires*). The purpose of health sectors is to provide residents with general healthcare. The standard for delineating health sectors is usually a range that can be reached within 30 minutes by transportation and is generally based on one or several municipalities as units. Health regions aim to provide residents with high-tech and specialized healthcare, and their ranges are based on the administrative regions (*région*) with the core area as the allocation unit. At least one regional hospital center is established within each region.

Secondly, the healthcare needs of each health sector are determined based on the demand index for hospital beds and equipment. This demand is determined by the Ministry of Health and Welfare based on the number of inpatients, the total number of bed days, the average length of a hospital stay, and bed utilization rates in each health sector followed by considerations for the specificities of each area (large cities, remote areas, and so on).

The supply and demand relationship of beds and equipment in each health sector and health region is objectively determined based on the relationship between demand and existing beds and equipment. The procedure for the creation of the health map is shown in Figure 12.5.

3. Limitations Based on the Health Map   The health map focuses on the following two aspects: (1) the set-up, expansion, and modification of hospital beds; and (2) the installation of large-scale, high-priced medical equipment. The application of (2) is based on Articles 84 to 247 of the decree of April 5, 1984. Computed tomography (CT) scanners, nuclear magnetic resonance (NMR) CT, and other large-scale medical equipment have been listed as requiring the approval of the Director-General of Health and the county prefect prior to

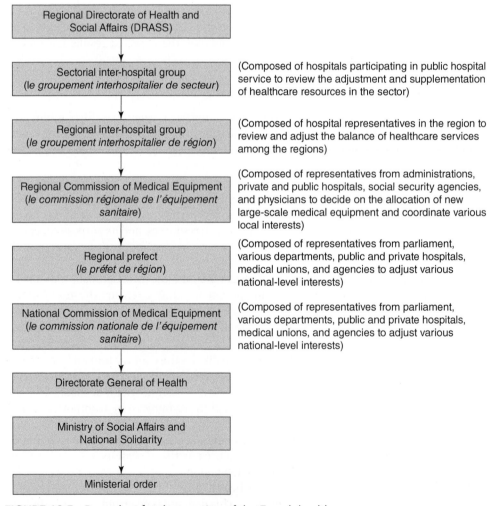

FIGURE 12.5 Procedure for the creation of the French health map.

acquisition. With regard to (1), approval for setting up and adding hospital beds has become more stringent.

4. Evaluation of the Health Map   In 1996, the French government invited domestic and foreign experts to evaluate the policies and implementation of the French health map, and the conclusions are as follows.

The advantages of the health map include the following: (1) the establishment of hospitals and the installation of equipment are restricted by regulations, thereby achieving planned allocations; (2) limited national adjustments are made to the allocation of hospital resources; and (3) the increase in beds is under control.

The relative disadvantages are as follows: (1) a long period of time is needed to research and formulate the health map; (2) although the health map can control the set-up of hospitals and beds, it does not have significant control over the existing oversupply of current inventory; and (3) it is not an effective approach to reduce the inter-regional gap in healthcare resources.

2. Healthcare Practitioners and Mobility

(1) Basic Status of Practitioners

Due to the specialization of medicine and healthcare, in addition to traditional healthcare practitioners, such as physicians, pharmacists, and nurses, a variety of other healthcare practitioners have emerged who can be roughly divided into the following categories.

1. In accordance with public health regulations, professional healthcare practitioners with a prefectural entrance system, a monopoly of practice, and mandatory registration required by professional bodies include physicians, dentists, midwives, and pharmacists.
2. In accordance with public health regulations, professions with a prefectural entrance system and a monopoly of practice but without mandatory registration with professional bodies include nurses, massage therapists, physiotherapists, podiatrists and orthotists, speech therapists, and vision therapists.
3. In accordance with public health regulations, professions with a prefectural health directorate registration system and a monopoly of practice but without professional bodies include opticians (optometrists) and hearing aid practitioners.
4. Professions without provisions in public health law but that are awarded national qualifications and have a customary system include occupational therapists, clinical laboratory technicians, and radiographers.
5. Professions without a qualification system include female orderlies and caregivers.

In addition, other healthcare-related occupations include nutritionists, clinical psychologists, and hospital administrators.

After receiving the required education for a certain period of time, all healthcare practitioners must obtain a license before they can begin practicing. Physicians must obtain the national physician's license after completing seven years of education in a university medical faculty. Dentists must obtain the national dentist's license after completing five years of education in the dental faculty of a university medical school. Midwives and nurses must obtain the national midwife's and nurse's licenses after three and two years of education, respectively. In addition, physiotherapists who have completed three years and podiatrists who have completed two years of education must also obtain national licenses.

TABLE 12.8 Number of Healthcare Practitioners (Main Occupational Categories) in France over the Years

Year	General Practitioners	Specialists	Dentists	Pharmacists	Midwives	Nurses
1960	33,109	20,348	16,410	15,293	8,500	96,876
1970	43,550	21,641	20,571	17,533	8,749	148,601
1980	57,715	33,727	27,683	19,900	8,899	219,032
1990	64,985	38,726	31,101	27,078	9,195	273,934
2000	76,195	42,357	35,822	29,470	8,874	382,666

Source: INSE, Annuaire statistique de la France, 2001.

The specialist system was introduced in 1949. Physicians who wish to become specialists must undertake further education for a certain number of years (the length of study is determined by the specialist qualification review committee established by each specialty and is usually three years) and pass the examinations run by the university medical faculty before they can obtain specialist diplomas awarded by the Ministry of Education. The changes in the number of healthcare practitioners over time are shown in Table 12.8. The numbers for each type of profession have been increasing each year, especially those of physicians and nurses.

(2) Physicians

1. Characteristics of the French Physician System Historically, the French physician system was separate from hospitals, as the latter originated from poverty-relief and charitable organizations for the poor, whereas the former developed from providing diagnoses and treatments to the rich. Therefore, even with the establishment of social security and the strict limitations of modern-day public health regulations, physicians' concept of healthcare service is still strongly influenced by the principle of "liberal medicine" (*médecine libérale*). This principle incorporates the free choice of physicians, the freedom to prescribe, and the freedom of private practice. This concept has also influenced the social security system and public health regulations.

The characteristics of the French physician system can be summarized by the following four points.

1. There is no national physician examination, and only the university graduate qualification, the State Diploma of Doctor of Medicine (*diplôme d'État de docteur*), is needed to become a physician.
2. Physicians are divided into two types: general practitioners (*généraliste*), who serve as family doctors, and specialists (*spécialiste*).
3. Prescribing and dispensing are separate responsibilities, and physicians are prohibited from dispensing drugs unless they are given special permission in remote areas without pharmacies.
4. Private practitioners do not own hospital beds and do not have large or expensive equipment other than simple medical tools.

2. Physician Training Methods Physician training is carried out by university medical faculty, and the training units are the university hospitals (*centre hospitalier universitaire*, CHU) in which medical faculties and regional hospital centers are integrated (after 1958).

At least one CHU has been established in each region. There are currently 11 CHUs in Paris and 25 CHUs outside of Paris.

Since 1985, medical students have been required to undertake at least eight years of medical studies. The outline of the training process for physicians is shown in Figure 12.7. The medical faculty shares the same course as the dental faculty in the first year, and the two faculties are separated at the final entrance examination at the end of the first year. To become a specialist, a physician must pass the internship examinations (commonly known as the "C exams"). According to regulations, the qualification for taking the internship examinations is only granted in the fourth year of the second cycle of medical studies. Among the 2,568 qualified specialists in 1984, about 69% (1,760 candidates) passed the C exams directly, whereas the rest were candidates from the general practitioner course or transferred from other specialist courses. The pass rate of the internship examinations is low, with only 46% of the candidates passing the examinations.

Thus, there are no special national examinations for specialists. To become a specialist, a physician only needs to complete the specialist course to obtain the Certificate of Specialist Studies in Medicine (*certificat d'études spécialisées de médecine*, CES) and receive individual accreditation by the Regional Order of Physicians according to the eligibility criteria set by the National Order of Physicians. Therefore, even graduates of the specialist course can still choose to practice as general practitioners. However, once a physician has accepted a specialist accreditation, he is obliged to only perform the healthcare services stipulated within his medical specialty.

Although specialists have the obligations described earlier, they also enjoy the following privileges. (1) They receive the title of specialist in prescriptions and personal directories. (2) They can enjoy the benefits of medical remuneration paid by health insurance.

3. Problems The problems encountered in the French physician system can be summarized according to the following three aspects.

1. *Excessive number of physicians.* The average age of French physicians is 42.4 years, and the age structure is such that half of physicians are under 40 years old because, in the past 10 years, the number of medical students has increased from 105,000 to 145,000.

   In other words, the number of medical students has increased drastically over the past 20 years. In 2002, the number of physicians per 100,000 people was 256.4. In overall terms, there was already a tendency towards the oversupply of physicians. In 2003, the total number of physicians reached 179,574, of whom 118,518 were private practitioners and 61,056 were salaried physicians. The specific categories are shown in Figure 12.6. Planned physician training has long been a major issue in France (Figure 12.7). Therefore, since the 1990s, the number of students who qualify for the second cycle of medical studies has been capped in an attempt to begin reducing this number. The number of physicians is expected to continue to rise in the future. By 2010, the number of physicians in France was 213,821, and the number of physicians per 100,000 people reached 350 (Table 12.9).

2. *Inter-regional differences in the number of physicians.* Figure 12.8 shows the sex and age structure of French physicians (including salaried physicians and private practitioners). Physicians in the age group of 30–45 years accounted for a relatively large proportion of the total, and there were more male than female physicians. Although there is an overall surplus of physicians, there are significant disparities between the north and south and between urban and rural areas. Hence, areas with inadequate healthcare services still exist, which also causes an imbalance in the incomes of physicians.

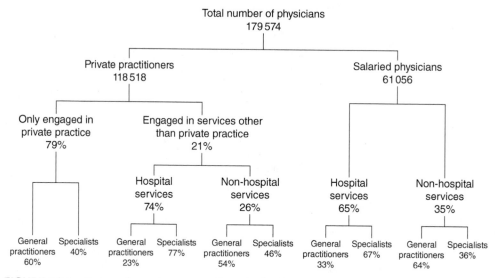

FIGURE 12.6 Types of practice among French physicians in 2003.

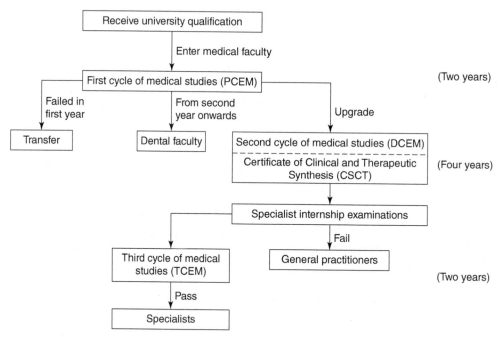

FIGURE 12.7 Training process for physicians in France.

3. *Differences between general practitioners and specialists.* In general, although specialists have 30% fewer working hours than general practitioners have, their incomes are 30% higher. Thus, the number of medical students who wish to become specialists has increased. Therefore, general practitioners are often considered to be specialist interns who failed and are not appraised in terms of their roles as family doctors. Furthermore, the structure of the medical community is such that the highest level of medical consultant (patron) is a university professor. Thus, the structure of physicians who provide healthcare services in France has become seriously distorted.

TABLE 12.9 Number of Physicians in France in 1986–2010 (Unit: Person)

Item		1986	1991	1996	2001	2010
Total number of physicians	Number of physicians	126,526	152,229	169,970	178,396	213,821
	Number per 100,000 people	229.8	270.4	296.7	307.4	350
Private practitioners	Number of physicians	85,448	102,507	114,346	119,958	—
	Number per 100,000 people	155.2	182.1	199.6	206.7	—

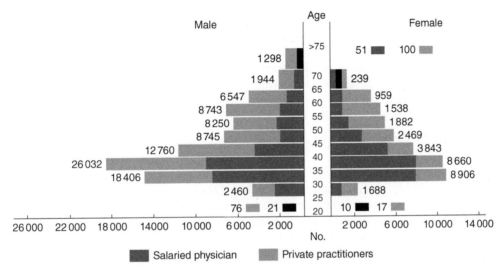

FIGURE 12.8 Sex and age structure of French physicians. *Source:* Ministry of Social Affairs and Employment, Statistical Yearbook of Social Health.

(3) Pharmacists

In 1985, France fully implemented the separation of prescribing and dispensing and adopted measures giving preferential treatment to pharmacists, which has become a feature of the French pharmacist system.

1. Pharmacists have a monopoly of practice not only for drugs but also for items such as bandages for medical use, medicinal plants stored in pharmacies, insecticides, contact lens solution, and a wide range of other products.
2. The scope of business in which pharmacists are obliged to participate is not limited to pharmacies but also includes drug wholesalers and the pharmaceutical industry.
3. When physicians' prescriptions are not suitable, pharmacists have the right to express their opinions to the physicians and request corrections.

As of 2010, there were 75,432 pharmacists in France serving in various fields, with an average of about 121 pharmacists per 100,000 people. The training method for pharmacists is similar to that for physicians. Restrictive measures are imposed on the number of students who pass the final examinations at the end of the first year in order to implement planned training. As for the length of study, the first cycle is one year, and the second cycle is four years. The pharmacist internship examinations are conducted in the fourth year of the second cycle. Those who pass must undertake one year of internship before they can graduate with a State Diploma of the Doctorate of Pharmacy (*diplôme d'état docteur pharmacie*). Outstanding students can directly enter the third cycle before the internship and develop at a higher level. This route is mainly for the training of teachers and senior researchers and involves another four years of education.

(4) Other Healthcare Practitioners

The training of other healthcare practitioners is carried out by professional training institutions beyond universities. However, due to the requirements of the technical operations in internships, these institutions are mostly attached to hospitals. There are currently about 660 training institutions, of which 79% (or 514) are public, thus indicating that public institutions account for a higher percentage of the total.

The number of students attending these training institutions is about 60,000. Among them, quotas for the training of state-accredited nurses, midwives, massage and physical therapists, and psychotherapists are determined annually by the ministerial order in order to implement planned training.

3. Health System Reforms

(1) Reform Background

Under the background of medical specialization and the reliance of full health insurance on social security, the surge in healthcare costs has not only gradually become an operational difficulty in balancing health insurance funds but has also become a limiting condition of socioeconomic development. This trend is relatively significant in France as well. Since the 1980s, France has introduced concepts of healthcare cost containment, such as the global budget, and has actively undertaken reforms. In addition, the most recent trend is to re-evaluate the healthcare provision system from the perspectives of mid- to long-term development and structural adjustment. The specific methods involve reducing hospital beds for psychiatry or changing their use and actively introducing new methods and forms of healthcare provision to replace hospitalization. According to current law, French health system reforms aim to achieve four goals: the modernization of healthcare institutions, residents' access to high-quality medical care, the centralization of preventive healthcare, and the regionalization of health policies.

(2) Day Hospitalization

Day hospitalization mainly provides day care services and evolved about 20 years ago into a type of healthcare service that mainly targets psychiatric treatment. It has now been extended to other areas, including the diagnosis and treatment of cancer, diabetes, and hypertension. Currently, there are 1,550 beds in public institutions and 1,268 beds in private institutions for day hospitalization (not including psychiatric disorders), giving a total of 2,818 beds, and the total number of hospitalization days is 302,000 days. Day hospitalization in the Assistance Publique – Hôpitaux de Paris accounts for 1% of its hospital beds and 0.4% of hospitalization days.

The costs for this service are paid from the global health insurance budget. Opinions differ as to whether day hospitalization should be continued in the future. However, proponents of this service list the following benefits. (1) It avoids the isolation of patients from their families. (2) It saves on the cost of nighttime hospitalization.

(3) Home Healthcare

Although the home-based therapy system, also referred to as "home care," is explicitly stipulated in the Hospital Reform Act (Article 4), due to the negative attitude held by health insurance funds towards the popularization of home-based therapy in the past, the only explicit administrative proposal for the promotion of this system appeared on March 12, 1968.

A primary feature of home healthcare in France is that the attending physician cooperates with hospital physicians and nurses to provide discharged patients with home rehabilitation, maintenance therapy, or palliative treatment in hospice care in accordance with the treatment provided by hospital physicians.

In total, 32 healthcare institutions provide home-based therapy service; 10 of them are public hospitals (including Assistance Publique – Hôpitaux de Paris), and 22 are nonprofit associations. The average age of users is 63 years, 45.6% of users are over 70 years old, and the main service targets are elderly persons with chronic diseases. In 1982, the specific diseases addressed were, in descending order of frequency, cancers (47.6%), circulatory system diseases (14.7%), sports injuries including fractures (8.8%), neurological and sense organ disorders (8.1%), and other conditions (20.8%).

Reimbursements from health insurance were previously based on fixed contractual fees (per diem units) with the Regional Health Insurance Fund (*Caisse régionale d'assurance maladie*, CRAM). However, in 1985, public hospitals started to have the same healthcare expenditures as general hospitals, and expenditures were paid from a global budget.

The reasons for promoting the home-based therapy system in the future are as follows.

1. Providing therapy in a patient's daily living environment may promote early recovery.
2. Terminal care can be provided at home even for incurable diseases.
3. It is cheaper than hospitalization.

(4) Home Care

The point at which home care first appeared in the law was in Law No. 78-11 on January 4, 1978, which was an amendment to the law relating to social and medical institutions (Law No. 75-535 on June 30, 1975). Based on this amendment, home care was incorporated into Clause 3 of Article 27, which stipulates that home care can be reimbursed by health insurance.

Home care is equivalent to a system of visiting nurses in which nurses provide care for the elderly according to physicians' prescriptions and coordinate with massage therapists and physiotherapists when necessary. Home care is now considered a vital component of home assistance services for the elderly.

Among the main bodies implementing home care, public institutions account for 31%, associations account for 57%, social insurance funds account for 9%, and other institutions account for 3%. Thus, associations play a central role in home care.

In terms of costs, insured persons are covered by health insurance funds, whereas uninsured persons are covered by their respective counties. Thus, the beneficiaries bear no cost. The costs borne by health insurance in 2003 reached €1.9 billion, 70% of which was covered by the general regime.

Home care has been actively promoted for the following reasons.

1. Hospitalization can be avoided within the permissible scope of medical and social conditions.
2. Patients are able to return quickly to their homes upon discharge.
3. Patients' health statuses can still be monitored, and deteriorations in their conditions can be alleviated.
4. Patients can be prevented from entering social welfare institutions, reducing the social burden.

(5) Financing of Healthcare Institutions

In France, there is fierce competition not only between private and public hospitals but also among public hospitals. However, such competition cannot be regulated by relying solely on market laws. Regulation also requires the intervention of government departments to guarantee that everyone has access to equal healthcare. In 2007, the healthcare reform plan established a new model of hospital financing (T2A) to determine the allocation of funds and thereby achieve a balanced budget. The state formulated specific healthcare prices based on experiments conducted in pilot hospitals, and healthcare institutions were reimbursed by health insurance according to this price list. The government finances healthcare activities through the Missions of General Interest and Contracting Support (MIGAC), which does not include GHS prices. For public hospitals, this reform has profoundly affected the routine practices, actions, and organizational structures of hospitals.

Public hospitals will eventually adapt to the reforms by increasing their total outputs and/or reducing unit healthcare costs. Regardless of whether hospitals have financial difficulties, they should all seek to balance their own accounts. That is, they should ensure the profitability of healthcare activities by reducing fixed unit costs. The T2A model that was implemented under the reform can also be regarded as rewarding the output of hospitals. This concept, which originates from the commercial private sector, poses a challenge to the values of public hospitals and the meaning of the work performed by healthcare workers. Many problems and difficulties were encountered in the process of implementing the T2A model, leading to numerous disputes and ultimately causing the government to postpone the original deadline of 2012 for the formation of public-private partnerships. In January 2006, a report published by the General Inspectorate of Social Affairs (*Inspection Générale des Affaires Sociales*, IGAS) indicated that the GHS prices of public hospitals were 1.81 times those of private hospitals. Although this gap does not seem significant, this figure does not take into account the constraints of public hospitals. In addition to several complex technical factors, two points require special attention: the full manifestation of the mission of the public healthcare industry and its impact on employment in this industry. Under these circumstances, public hospitals should assume responsibility for treating major illnesses and serving the poor. If the T2A model did not exacerbate the inequality of healthcare for citizens, then why does the issue of unequal resource distribution among healthcare professionals persist? This point warrants further reflection.

4. Health Insurance System

French social security (*sécurité sociale*) mainly refers to health insurance, pension insurance, and family benefits. Insurance for work-related injuries is occasionally covered by the sickness funds (general regime) and, hence, is included in social security.

Each of the three areas of social security has its own history. Of these areas, health insurance is combined with the state of the health service provision system, which includes healthcare institutions, physicians, and nurses. It is also closely related to the culture and national conditions of France.

(1) The History and Development of the Health Insurance System

1. History of the Health Insurance System

1. *Rudimentary stage before World War II.* Compared to France, neighboring Germany began the establishment of its social security system at a much earlier time. France can be said to have implemented its current social security system only after World War II. Naturally, there were several rudimentary stages before this point that can roughly be summarized as follows.

   Firstly, in accordance with the law of April 9, 1898, the employer-covered employee compensation system for industrial accidents, which constitutes a part of the current social security system, was created.

   In accordance with the law promulgated on April 5, 1910, an "Old-Age Pension" was created for employees. This pension was followed by the creation of the employer-covered family allowance system in November 1916 by regional enterprises in Grenoble.

   As for health insurance, a social security system had already been implemented in the Alsace-Lorraine territory, which Germany returned to France after World War I. In order to popularize this system, the French government began to enact relevant laws and established separate systems for health insurance and pension insurance in accordance with the laws enacted between 1928 and 1930. Although the enrollment conditions and benefit standards of this system were neither reasonable nor adequate, the compulsory social security system that targets workers became a solid foundation for today's health insurance system.

2. *Establishment of the general regime after World War II.* In accordance with the ordinances of October 4, 1945, and October 19, 1945, a "general regime" (*régime général*) was established and implemented, and its scope of application was gradually expanded.

   The general regime, as suggested by the name "general," did not differentiate between employees and the self-employed. This bold reform was intended to create a security system that covers all areas, including pensions, healthcare, and family benefits. France made this choice after a long period of deliberation over whether to adopt the British national security system or the German social insurance system.

   The French general regime covered 53% of the country's population in 1946. However, it soon resulted in conflicts between ideals and reality. The first conflict was the refusal of employee groups that existed before the creation of the general regime to merge with the general regime and the independence of self-employed and agricultural groups. The second conflict was the separation of the pension insurance, health insurance, and family benefit systems in 1967 and the introduction of independent calculation methods for income and expenditure. After encountering these conflicts and difficulties in practice, the broad and consistent policies implied by the name "general regime" did not seem to fit with reality.

   In 1975, the principle of universal insurance was proposed. Employees and workers who were previously uninsured were gradually incorporated into the social security system, especially the general regime. In 1978, universal insurance was nearly entirely achieved, and the population not covered by public social security was only 0.4%. In 1996, the French Parliament passed four bills, which stipulated that (1) major reforms of the French health insurance system must be deliberated and passed by Parliament, (2) the contribution base must be determined by the national income, (3) a global budget shall be implemented, and (4) a lump-sum system shall be implemented for the payment of inpatient healthcare expenditure. These laws and regulations gradually clarified the role and content of social insurance for diseases, promoted the establishment and improvement of the French health insurance system, and hence further encouraged the development of the medical and health industry.

Overall, the French social security system, which is thought to have originated from guilds in the Middle Ages, developed at an early stage, but it was burdened by historical baggage, and thus the completion of the system occurred much later than expected. Thus, the French social security system has significant links to French culture, customs, and social relations.

2. Development of the Health Insurance System   The history of health insurance in France began with the enactment of the Social Insurance Law between 1928 and 1930. Before this law, the compensation system for healthcare benefits implemented by cooperatives, which was a form of rudimentary insurance, already existed as of the late nineteenth century (e.g., the law enacted on April 1, 1898, that recognized mutual societies for sickness and the elderly). In particular, the mutual societies for miners, railway workers, and other employees continue to exist to this day and have become special regimes within the social insurance system.

As with old-age insurance, the historical development of health insurance varied according to occupation type and social status. The first step was the Social Insurance Law in 1930, which mainly benefited employees, whereas self-employed individuals and farmers only had access to health insurance long after the Second World War. The universal access of all residents to health insurance was only achieved with the General Social Insurance Law of 1974.

After World War I, France recovered the Alsace-Lorraine territory (including Bas-Rhin, Haut-Rhin, and Moselle), where German-style social insurance had been implemented, from Germany. This recovery triggered France's drafting and enactment of the Social Insurance Law of 1930, which resulted in the establishment of the earliest mandatory health insurance. Under the commission of the senior administrator for Alsace-Lorraine, Fernand Merlin, the Parliamentary member elected by Alsace, Anselme Patureau-Mirand, formed a special committee in 1920 that drafted the Social Insurance Law. The Minister of Labor of Aristide Briand's cabinet, Charles Daniel-Vincent, proposed the bill to the National Assembly in 1921. After major revisions, the bill was passed in the National Assembly in 1924 and was referred to the Senate for deliberation, where further revisions were made. Finally, after seven years, the bill was passed by the Senate on March 14, 1928. However, due to imminent elections and strong opposition from farmers and physicians, the government had no choice but to postpone its implementation. After further revisions, the government enacted and implemented the Social Insurance Law on April 30, 1930. In the aftermath of World War II in 1945, within the context of demands for the establishment of a new post-war order, France promulgated the presidential decree of October 4, 1945, on the organization of social security. This decree became the foundation for the provision of social insurance to all residents (Table 12.10).

TABLE 12.10 Starting Year of Health Insurance for Occupational Categories in France

Occupational Categories	Starting Year
National and regional civil servants	1928–1930
Miners and railway workers	Nineteenth century
Industrial and commercial workers	1928–1930
Agricultural operators	1928–1930
Students	1961
Self-employed, nonfarm workers	1948
Disabled war veterans	1954
Pension beneficiaries	1964
Others	1974

Nevertheless, due to the social industry structure at that time, social insurance schemes continued to exist as separate systems divided according to occupational type and social class. At the same time, the general regime, which was centered on industrial and commercial workers, became the foundation for the establishment of the social insurance system. Those who were eligible for the general regime accounted for about 70% of the population.

Furthermore, the outline of health insurance, which was based on the provisions for social insurance centered on the presidential decree of 1945, later became the Social Security Code in 1956. Its contents are as follows.

1. The medical fee schedule shall be formulated and proposed by the medical unions of each county.
2. The medical fee schedule shall be recorded in the agreements signed between the local social insurance funds and medical unions.
3. The medical fee schedule must be approved by a national tripartite commission composed of representatives for physicians, social insurance agencies, and the government.
4. The national tripartite commission (National Commission of Medical Fees) has the power to reject fee schedules or request their revision. If it is not possible to produce a medical fee schedule that meets the commission's approval, the commission itself can formulate an applicable fee schedule (tariff applicable).
5. The medical fee schedule is applicable to the medical procedure groups (nomenclature) prescribed by each region. The fee schedules only determine a certain number of medical procedures. The amount of healthcare reimbursement is calculated by multiplying the fees for basic acts by the coefficients of medical procedures for each group.
6. When seeking to charge fees higher than those listed in the fee schedule, the county mediation committee shall consult with physicians regarding the reasons for overcharging based on the needs of the patients or the social insurance agencies and reach a decision as to whether the higher fees are appropriate.

According to the provisions of the fee schedule, the insurance funds reimbursed 80% of the fees paid by the insured to the physicians, and the remaining 20% were paid by patients. In 1956, A. Gazier believed that these provisions would cause social problems, and, hence, proposed the Gazier plan, which sought to implement further reforms of the health insurance system. The key points are as follows: (1) the determination of the medical fee schedule according to economic principles; that is, a patient's ability to pay must be considered when determining the fee schedule, which is then determined by an agreement reached between physicians and funds; (2) the implementation of third-party payments; (3) the right to overcharge is limited to at most 15% of physicians in each county; and (4) in counties where no agreement has been reached, funds can set up clinics similar to those operated by cooperatives to provide free medical treatments (benefits in kind) as a form of sanction.

This last item, in particular, was a major threat to physicians. Therefore, until 1960, France's social health insurance remained in a state of controversy and confusion that revolved around the Gazier plan. Ultimately, physicians adopted a strong stance by abandoning the agreement and going on strike, which prompted the government to issue the decree of May 12, 1960, which focused on the use of the "standard agreement (convention type)," to resolve the chaos. The reform of 1960 was one of the most important measures adopted, but physicians were still strongly opposed to it. Nonetheless, the major amendments to the "medical procedure groups (nomenclature)" formulated in 1945 led to the establishment of contracting agencies by counties and cities. The first signs that the French social security system was heading towards true maturity were the laws of January 21, 1961, and January 2, 1978, relating to social security. By the end of January 1961, 78 of the 90 counties had entered into agreements, and 8.7 million of the 13 million people who qualified for the agreement were insured.

The agreement of 1960 was as follows. Physicians were obliged to charge fees according to the agreement, and patients could be reimbursed for 80–100% of the funds based on these fees. The exception was that, depending on a patient's financial situation, if that patient had special service needs, then only physicians with the right to overcharge could charge more than the amount stipulated in the agreement. A coordinating committee composed of representatives for physicians and social insurance agencies was established in each county and was responsible for settling overcharging issues and disputes between physicians and social insurance funds. Based on this "standard agreement" method, the majority of French people became eligible for health insurance, but this agreement also resulted in a 29% increase in the number of visits per year and an 11% increase in healthcare expenditure per capita.

Thereafter, in 1966, France expanded the coverage of its four systems to accommodate self-employed professionals. In 1971, civil servants, agricultural workers, and railway workers were given medical compensation under the general regime. In the meantime, in 1967, France implemented reforms of health insurance operations and management organizations. Following these reforms, in 1974, the law on the universalization of social insurance was established to guarantee common basic benefits to all residents. Then, in December 1974, the Insurance Fund Adjustment Act was enacted to implement fund adjustments among the systems. After the energy crisis of 1973, the status of health insurance funds deteriorated rapidly. To cope with this situation, the legislative measures adopted after 1976 all focused on fund strategies and healthcare cost-containment policies.

(2) Types of Health Insurance Systems

In general, the French social security system can be divided into three groups according to occupational categories: employee groups, self-employed and liberal profession groups, and agricultural groups. France does not have a regional insurance system, like Japan's National Health Insurance, or a special cross-sectional system targeting the elderly, like Medicare in the US. Retirees in France continue to participate in the preretirement health insurance system. The numbers of people covered by the various health insurance systems

TABLE 12.11 Number of People Eligible for Different Health Insurance Systems in France

System	Eligible Persons (1,000 People)
(1) Employee system	
(A) General regime	45,792
(B) Systems targeted by fiscal adjustment	5,474
Sailors	350
Agricultural workers	1,774
Notary clerks	89
Employees of the Autonomous Operator of Parisian Transports (RAPT)	128
State-owned railway workers	1,233
Miners	552
Military	1,223
Employees of Banque Nationale de Paris (BNP)	48
Clergy	77
(A+B)	51,266
(C) Employee system excluding A and B	78
Employees of the state-owned water company	7
Employees of the Paris Chamber of Commerce	7
Nonresident French nationals	64
(A+B+C)	51,344
(2) (D) Nonemployee System	6,952
Agricultural operators	3,538
Self-employed and liberal professions (nonagricultural)	3,414
(E) (Other agricultural workers)	10
Total (A+B+C+D+E)	58,306

Note:
(1) The total population of France does not match the total population eligible for health insurance because some people enroll in more than one system.
(2) The total number of 58.306 million includes insured persons (23.504 million), those covered by old-age insurance (10.165 million), and dependents (24.637 million).
(3) In addition to private commercial and industrial employees, A (the general regime) also includes national and regional civil servants (4.561 million people) and students (76,000 people).

in France are shown in Table 12.11 and are grouped into two categories: the employee and nonemployee systems.

1. Employee Groups Such groups include national and regional civil servants, state-owned railway workers, military personnel, sailors, miners, and other employees with special identities, as well as private industrial and commercial employees. These employee groups have their own health insurance system and management organizations (for civil servants, however, reimbursements for healthcare services are performed through the general regime). Although the systems targeting civil servants, miners, sailors, and state-owned railway workers have had a longer history of establishment, the "general regime" targeting private industrial and commercial employees now occupies a dominant position in health insurance. Individuals who enroll in the general regime (insured individuals and their dependents) account for 80% of the total population, and their healthcare expenses also account for 80% of the total. The significant share of the general regime is the result of socioeconomic changes, the development of the salaried class, and the gradual decline of agriculture. In 1954, the salaried class only accounted for 60% of all workers, but in 2003, it accounted for 87%.

2. Self-Employed and Liberal Profession Groups (Nonagricultural)　This group consists of merchants, artisans (nonsalaried persons who possess their own technology and create their own crafts), sole proprietors, and other self-employed persons, as well as physicians, lawyers, and other liberal professions. The health insurance system for this group is implemented by a single fund known as the National Health Insurance Fund for Self-Employed Persons (*Caisse National d'Assurance Maladie des Professions Indépendantes*, CANAM). However, the vast majority of physicians enter into health insurance agreements, and most of them join the general regime.

It took a relatively short time to establish the health insurance system for the self-employed and liberal profession groups. This system was created according to the laws of 1966 and began operation in 1969. It provides lower levels of healthcare benefits than other systems provide. Hospitalization costs (including technical fees, drug costs, and living costs) are basically the same as those of the other systems, with a copayment rate of 20%. However, the copayment rate for healthcare costs other than hospitalization is 50%. In addition, injury and disability and maternity allowances are not included in the healthcare benefits. The reimbursement standard of this system is used as a reference standard for the adjustment of compensation between the systems for the employee group and other groups.

3. Agricultural Groups　France is a relatively agricultural country that has retained the traditions of agricultural prosperity and the features of agricultural countries, such as the substantial impact of good or bad harvests on farmers' incomes. Therefore, the agricultural health insurance system exists as an independent domain in the French social security system. However, the population covered by the agricultural health insurance system is only 7% of the working population. Moreover, the government and other national systems (especially the general regime) require substantial financial assistance to provide this system. The eligible population for the agricultural health system is mainly agricultural workers (tenants). The general regime has been providing financial assistance to this system for agricultural workers since 1963.

(3) Health Insurance Premiums and Benefits

1. Premiums (Cotisation)　In principle, premiums are calculated based on a fixed percentage of income. According to the premium rate stipulated by the country's health insurance system, an insured person pays 6.8% of his salary, and his employer pays 12.8%. Employees' premiums are deducted uniformly from their salaries by their employers. Pension beneficiaries and unemployed persons are also required to contribute to health insurance premiums. Pensioners contribute 1.4% of their pensions. Those who receive private pensions contribute 2.4% of their pensions. Unemployed persons contribute 2% of their minimum guaranteed incomes and 1% of their unemployment benefits and training allowances. The high premium rates in France are due to the wide range of healthcare benefits (including compensation for reduced income due to illness), the trajectory of population aging, the absence of state treasury burdens in principle, and so on. High premium rates, especially the heavy burden on employers, have had a significant impact on French economic activity and have caused heated debate within the country.

2. Fiscal Adjustment Fiscal adjustment refers to changes in the distribution of various occupations together with socioeconomic development and changes in the income levels of the working population. Correspondingly, fiscal adjustments in health insurance and pension funds refer to transfers and adjustments made in the insurance funds according to the population balance and the ability to levy (that is, transfers and adjustments only between incomes and the employee system). Another form of fiscal adjustment takes place within the general regime, in which funds are transferred among health insurance, old-age pensions, and family benefits. Broadly speaking, in the case of health insurance (with comparable deficits and surpluses), old-age pensions (with large deficits), and family benefits (with surpluses), funds are generally transferred from family benefits to old-age pensions (Table 12.12).

TABLE 12.12 Current Status of Fiscal Adjustments in French Health Insurance

System	Number of Contributors Per Beneficiary (Premium Contributors/ Beneficiaries) (Number of Eligible Persons)	Transfer Amount (Million €)	Share of Transfer Amount (Transfer Amount/Total Healthcare Benefits For Each System)
General regime	0.37	+1,382.2	3.7%
Agricultural workers	0.36	+15	0.8%
Military	0.28	−111.4	14.7%
Miners	0.13	−387.7	52.8%
State-owned railway	0.20	−392.8	30.1%
RAPT	0.30	−3.8	2.5%
Sailors	0.18	−52.4	21.0%
Notary clerks	0.39	+7.3	10.0%
BNP	0.35	+40.1	60.0%
Agricultural operators	0.27	−520.3	16.8%
Self-employed and liberal professions	0.36	+38.5	1.8%
Overall employee system	0.36	Total transfer amount	
Overall health insurance system	0.36	≈ 1,468	

Note:
For transfer amounts, "−" indicates the receipt of a transfer and "+" indicates the provision of a transfer.

3. Insurance Benefits (Prestations) In terms of health insurance, healthcare benefits can be divided into "medical service benefits" (actual coverage for medical expenses) and "income-loss benefits" (compensation for the loss of income due to illness).

1. Healthcare Benefits
   1. *Medical service benefits.* Although residents can seek outpatient treatment directly from hospitals, they generally do not go directly to major hospitals or university hospitals for minor ailments such as a cold or abdominal pain. Most patients first visit general practitioners according to their own choice and, if necessary, are referred to major hospitals by the general practitioners.

      General practitioners in private practice do not have large-scale medical devices or high-priced medical equipment such as CT scanners. These small clinics are usually equipped with a weighing scale, an examination table, a sphygmomanometer, and a stethoscope; the drugs price list, commonly known as VIDAL, is also displayed on the desk.

      For outpatient visits, the patient first pays the full amount of the medical fee to the physician and then receives a 75% reimbursement from the regional sickness fund. As for pharmacies, patients must pay the full drug cost to pharmacies and claim either a 70% or 40% reimbursement from the regional sickness fund depending on the drug costs (the copayments for certain drugs could be zero or the full price). Patients only need to pay 20% of the total cost of hospitalization, including technical fees, drug costs, nursing fees, and bed fees. In addition, there is a partial fixed copayment (€5.3 per day in 2003), and the reimbursement rates are shown in Tables 12.13 and 12.14.
   2. *Income-loss benefits.* In order to compensate for the loss of income caused by the inability to work due to illness, beneficiaries are paid an average of half of their daily income (this per diem rate is subject to a maximum) as a sickness benefit. The maximum duration of payment is three years. The CANAM system does not provide income-loss benefits.
2. *Maternity benefits.* For healthcare services related to childbirth, including childbirth fees, healthcare fees, drug costs, and hospitalization, a 100% reimbursement is given, and no copayment is charged. In order to receive income-loss benefits, social security registration must be completed at least 10 months before the birth, and pregnancy registration must be completed with the regional sickness fund before the fourth month of pregnancy. Beneficiaries must also receive at least four regular checkups before giving birth. Maternity benefits are 84% of standard income (used to calculate the income standard of old-age pensions). In addition to maternity benefits, post-childbirth recuperation benefits are also paid limited only to the beneficiary). The CANAM system also provides these benefits.

   The reason that France has adopted these incentives for childbirth is its population policy of encouraging childbirth in order to increase the low birth rate.
3. *Global budget system for healthcare.* Inpatient services in France are mainly provided by hospitals. The annual budget allocated to each hospital is determined by multiplying the number of patients by the average daily expenses in the past year. However, this method of budget preparation has been carried out crudely and unsystematically in the past, and strict management has been absent in budget implementation.

TABLE 12.13 Healthcare Reimbursement Rates for Different Health Insurance Systems in France

Item	Farmers, Military, and Sailors in the General Regime	Notary Clerks	State-Owned Railway Workers	BNP	Nonresident French Nationals	Self-Employed and Liberal Professions
Outpatient services						
Technical fees						
Physicians	75	90	80	80	75	50
Healthcare-related workers (healthcare workers)	60	90	80	80	75	50
Pharmaceutical costs						
High-priced drugs without substitutes	100	10	80	100	100	50
Drugs with limited clinical efficacy	40	50	80	100	100	50
Other general drugs	70	90	80	100	100	50
Examinations	65	90	80	75	65	50
Inpatient services	80	90	10	80	80	80
Transfer fees	70	10	10	100	70	80

The "global budget system," which aims to control healthcare expenditure, has been implemented since 1984. Hospital outpatient services were also included in 1985. The new budgeting system stipulates the following. (1) Strict budget preparation should be implemented for the following year, and the deficits of the previous year should not be transferred to the budget. (2) The rationalization of hospital management, on which rationalized decisions regarding the hospital budget can be based, is required. (3) The annual budget is divided into 12 months and allocated on a monthly basis, regardless of variations in expenditure across different months. (4) In order to address the issue of arbitrariness, irresponsibility, and inefficiency across all hospital departments, the overall hospital budget is used to control each department. A hospital director (nonphysician) is appointed, is given the authority over the hospital budget, and assumes the responsibility for hospital operations. This global budget system has gradually taken effect and has shown signs of alleviating the rise in inpatient costs.

TABLE 12.14 Benefits for Different Health Insurance Systems in France

| Type of system | Healthcare Benefits | | Maternity Benefits | | Work Injury and Occupational Diseases | | | Disability Pension | Temporary Death Benefits |
| | | | | | Temporary Disability | | Permanent Disability | | |
	Medical Service Benefits	Income-Loss Benefits	Medical Service Benefits	Income-Loss Benefits	Medical Service Benefits	Income-Loss Benefits	Lifelong Pension		
General regime (private industrial and commercial employees)	*	*	*	*	*	*	*	*	*
Systems related to the general regime (national and regional civil servants and employees of state-owned gas and electric companies)	*		*						
Sailors	*	*	*	*	*	*	*	*	*
Military	*		*						
Notary clerks	*	*	*	*					
RAPT	*	*	*	*	*				*
State-owned railway workers	*	*	*		*				*
Mining	*	*	*	*	*	*	*	*	*
BNP	*		*						
State-owned water company workers	*		*						
Chamber of Commerce	*	*	*	*				*	*
Church clergy	*		*						
Nonresident French nationals	*	*	*		*	*	*	*	
Agriculture Workers	*	*	*	*	*	*	*	*	*
Operators	*		*	*				*	
Others	*		*						
Self-employed and liberal professions (nonagricultural)	*		*	*					*

Note:
* indicates this benefit is available.

4. Collection and Reimbursement System   The eligible targets of the French health insurance system can roughly be divided into three types: employee groups, self-employed and liberal profession groups, and agricultural groups. However, the general regime targeting employee groups is the most predominant in terms of the number of systems, as it consists of more than 20 types of systems. Each system does not necessarily have its own mode of operation (reimbursement and collection). For example, the system for national or regional civil servants uses the structure of the general regime to provide health service benefits. The operational management and organization of the general regime are shown in Figure 12.9.

5. Status of Insurance Fund Operations   The content of healthcare expenses varies according to their definition. In general, the concept of healthcare expenditure (*consummation médicale totale*) in France is relatively broad. For example, it includes disease prevention funds (school healthcare, family planning, maternal and child healthcare, and so on). Fertility, eyeglasses, and spa therapy are regarded as insurance benefits, and disability pensions and work injury expenses are sometimes included in health insurance as well.

In 2010, the budget for health insurance costs passed by the French Parliament was €162.4 billion. Of this total, hospital costs amounted to €71.2 billion, accounting for 44% of health insurance costs. Health insurance costs include benefits for healthcare services and devices (eyeglasses, assistive devices) as well as for preventive services. Total health insurance expenditure includes not only healthcare but also benefits, such as income allowances for ceasing work due to a work-related injury or pregnancy and disability pensions (Figure 12.10). The cost of paying for the risks (including sickness, childbirth, disability, and work-related injury) to the beneficiaries of the insurance system also includes a copayment.

(4) Health Insurance Agreement and Medical Fee System

1. Health Insurance Agreement

1. *Conclusion of agreements.* The purchase and sale of healthcare services (method of health service provision, payment of healthcare expenditure, prices and review methods, and so on) are based on the "agreement" reached between the healthcare provider and the payer. Any prior agreement reached between the relevant parties is not questioned by the government. When concluding the agreement, the healthcare providers are the medical unions, negotiating from the position of trade unions to pursue their own best interests. In specific terms, the national medical unions centered on private practitioners and salaried physicians represent all healthcare practitioners. The payers are the representatives from the National Sickness Insurance Fund for Employees (the general regime with private employees as members), the Central Fund for the Agricultural Mutuality (targeting farmers), and the National Sickness Insurance Fund for Self-Employed Persons (targeting self-employed persons).

   Both parties must reach a consensus on all matters related to the revision of healthcare prices, and the agreement can be concluded after obtaining the approval of the central government. The content of the agreement is announced by the central government. In practice, prior to concluding the agreement, the parties concerned understand the intentions of the central government, and the central government coordinates the negotiations by prompting both parties and persuading them to reach an agreement. If an agreement cannot be reached, the central government intervenes.

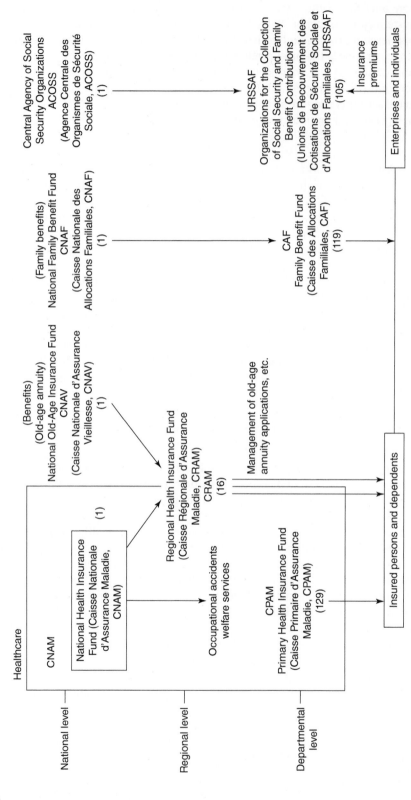

FIGURE 12.9 Management organizations of the General Health Insurance regime in France (numbers in brackets indicate the number of institutions).

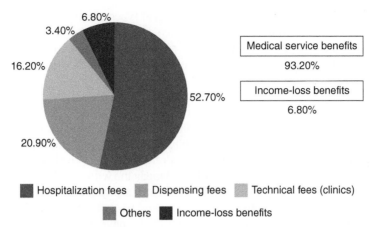

FIGURE 12.10 Content of healthcare benefits for the general regime in French health insurance

2. *Difference between contracted and noncontracted physicians.* Physicians are free to choose whether to enter the "agreement." However, as of December 31, 2003, only 593 (0.3%) out of a total of 179,574 physicians were noncontracted. Therefore, virtually all healthcare is provided by contracted physicians. The difference between contracted and noncontracted physicians lies in the remuneration paid by the sickness funds. More precisely, there is a significant difference in the prices for physician consultation (technical fees) that patients can claim for reimbursement from the sickness funds. For example, for the same "consultation," the difference between a contracted and a non-contracted general practitioner is nearly 20-fold (in the case of Paris, this difference is €11.4 vs. €0.6).

3. *Three types of contracted physicians.* Contracted physicians can be divided into the following three types. (1) General contracted physicians: These physicians provide medical treatment according to the agreed prices. About 70% of all contracted physicians belong to this type. (2) Contracted physicians with surcharges (*dépassement d'honoraires*): These physicians are able charge patients more than the agreed prices. Physicians of this type have received exceptional individual recognition due to superior technical qualifications, experience, or reputation. Currently, such physicians are holders of previously acquired rights and account for only 6–7% of all contracted physicians. (3) Liberal contracted physicians: These physicians are also known as "Sector 2 contracted physicians" and are free to choose the amount to charge for medical treatment. Such physicians currently account for 20% of all contracted physicians. There are more Sector 2 physicians in large cities, such as Paris and Lyon, as well as more specialists than general practitioners.

   The sickness funds provide tax benefits and reduced social insurance premiums to the first two types of contracted physicians but impose partial restrictions on liberal contracted physicians. The purpose of having different treatments among contracted physicians is to encourage more physicians (especially high-quality physicians) to become contracted physicians.

   Although these contracted physicians vary in terms of patient costs, their relationships with the sickness funds depend on a single, uniform agreement of fees, and reimbursements are also made according to these uniform fees. Expenses exceeding the agreed prices are fully borne by patients for both surcharges and liberal charges.

2. French Medical Fee System   There are several types of payment methods for medical fees under social health insurance. In France, the payment of medical fees is known as the reimbursement method. That is, upon consulting a physician, a patient pays the medical fees directly to the physician, and the sickness fund fully or partially reimburses the patient.

Why has this method been adopted by French social health insurance? One of the main reasons is the demand for the principle of liberal medicine to be fully implemented in French healthcare. This principle includes the freedom of private practice, patients' freedom to choose a physician, and the freedom to prescribe. However, more importantly, the physician is free to decide the medical fees. Therefore, this reimbursement method is the product of combining France's traditional principle of liberal medicine with social health insurance. In particular, in traditional liberal medicine, the freedom of physicians to decide medical fees stems from direct negotiations between physicians and patients (known as *l'entente directe*). To put it in plain terms, the historical evolution of the payment method for medical fees in France can be seen as the integration of this principle of direct negotiations into social health insurance. The various incompatibilities between physicians and the social insurance system have all originated from the contradictions between the principle of direct agreement and social health insurance.

The principle of direct negotiation advocated by physicians is also known as individualistic healthcare. It is suitable for the social system of various occupational and social class stratifications, but it is not suitable for a collectivistic social system. Although the social health insurance systems of other Western developed countries exist within capitalist economies, most of them have been socialized and even have completely abandoned the principle of direct negotiation. Nevertheless, the health services and health insurance (reimbursement method) of France still retain a trace of individualism.

However, since 1992, the direction of reform has turned toward the socialization of social insurance, which seems to hint at the fact that changes have begun to occur in the individualism of occupational categories and social classes that underlie the formation of social tendencies in France. Hence, the individualistic reimbursement method for the payment of healthcare expenses in France has also been influenced to adapt to these changes.

1. *National agreement* (Convention nationale). The agreement of medical fees underwent major changes in 1993. In the past, decisions on medical fees were entrusted to agreements reached by each county. However, in accordance with the law of July 3, 1993, the county-level agreement method was abolished in favor of a national, unified standard agreement. As healthcare expenditure continued to increase rapidly, the government authorities believed that it was necessary to seek a thorough countermeasure when formulating the eighth economic and social development plan. Hence, it explicitly proposed the abolishment of the existing fee-for-service system for medical acts.

   Physicians responded quickly and dynamically to this proposal and advocated a more binding method of determining medical fees based on a unified national standard agreement. After a year-long discussion with the National Health Insurance Funds, the current national unified standard agreement between the national medical unions and the National Health Insurance Funds was reached on October 28, 1994. Prior to the conclusion of the National Agreement, the government confirmed its compliance with the principles of liberal medicine and issued a statement declaring the preservation of the fee-for-service system.

Furthermore, a coordinating committee composed of physicians and health insurance agencies was established. This committee was responsible for resolving disputes related to the implementation of the agreement in each county, and a medical statistic known as the summary of medical fees, which aimed to reflect the number of consultations, the trend in healthcare expenses, and the appropriateness of medical fees for each physician, was specially created. Although this statistic is not legally binding, relevant physicians may be excluded from the agreement in the event of major adverse incidents, and the statistic constrains medical malpractice to a certain extent.

The national standard agreement can be regarded as a major achievement resulting from the accumulation of experience in the socialization of traditional liberal medicine over a quarter of a century since 1970. Therefore, on the one hand, physicians have retained (1) the fee-for service system and (2) the right to overcharge. On the other hand, insurers have won a national fee schedule that has binding power over all physicians. In summary, physicians mainly possess the right to implement the fee-for-service system, whereas, to insurers, this right is a distortion of social health insurance.

According to the national standard agreement, the principle of direct negotiation was replaced by the principle of collective agreement (*l'entente collective*). Thus, insurers achieved their goal of many years, but physicians also retained the right to make direct remuneration decisions in the form of the fee-for-service system. Furthermore, since the right to overcharge partially retains the principle of direct negotiation, the number of physicians exercising this right began to increase and accounted for 20% of all private practitioners by 1996, implying that nearly 10,000 physicians enjoyed this privilege. Although most of them were hospital physicians, who automatically have the right to overcharge, this figure indicates that there were significant limitations in achieving the policy objectives of the national standard agreement.

The drafting of the Fifth National Standard Agreement began in early April 1997. This agreement also incorporated healthcare containment policies (improvement of economic responsibility, improvement of healthcare quality, and so on) under the principle of freezing the increase in medical fees and controlling the growth rate of healthcare expenditure to within the range of GDP growth. This principle led to resistance from physicians. By 1998, the new agreement had even resulted in general confusion caused by local strikes and a unilateral increase in medical fees by medical unions. Subsequently, the negotiations between the National Health Insurance Funds and the Federation of French Physicians were successful and led to the signing of the Fifth National Standard Agreement on May 29, 1999. However, the Confederation of French Medical Unions, which represented the majority of physicians, strongly opposed this agreement and called on physicians to boycott the agreement or launch counterpropaganda. By January 2000, the Confederation of French Medical Unions finally decided to sign the new agreement, and the agreement, which incorporated healthcare cost-containment policies, was finally accepted by the physicians.

The contracting parties for the insurers were the National Sickness Insurance Fund for Employees, the Central Fund for Agricultural Mutuality, and the National Sickness Insurance Fund for Self-Employed Persons.

2. *Fee schedule and medical procedure groups.* As specified in Articles 8 to 10 of the Fifth National Standard Agreement, the medical fees of physicians shall be calculated according to the agreed fee schedule for medical procedure groups; that is, the agreed

fee schedule only makes provisions for the key-letters (*lettres-clé*) of medical procedure groups stipulated in Article 2. Physicians can calculate the remuneration for procedures using the key-letter of the medical procedure group and the coefficient attached to it.

Thus, the French medical industry groups adopted the following dual structure:

$$\text{Medical procedure group} = key\text{-letter}$$
$$\text{Relative importance of medical procedure} = \text{coefficient}$$

The content represented by the key-letters is shown in Table 12.15.

Medical fees are calculated by multiplying the price of the key-letter for the medical procedure by its coefficient. For example, the key-letter for an appendectomy is listed as K50. Hence, the cost of K, €1.03, multiplied by 50 gives $50 \times 1.03 = €51.83$.

3. *Medical and hospitalization fees for hospitals.* Hospitalization fees (*prix de jour/dépenses d'hospitalisation*) are not consistent but rather vary across different hospitals. In fact, hospitalization fees may even vary across different wards and departments in the same hospital.

This variation arises because hospitalization fees are calculated based on the original prices charged by each hospital or each medical department. In public hospitals, the original prices of each department are calculated each year and reported to the hospital management committee. The county prefect then stipulates the hospitalization fees based on this report. The average daily hospitalization fee is calculated by dividing the expenditure budget of the previous year by the average number of days of a hospital stay in the past three years. The basis of calculation includes costs for meals, heating, electricity and gas fuel, labor, drugs, medical devices, loan repayments, repairs, depreciation, and deficits from previous years. It is worth noting that drug costs are included in hospitalization fees. Due to the large share of costs accounted for by drugs and medical devices, the amount used has a significant impact on hospitalization fees.

TABLE 12.15 Content of Key-Letters for the Calculation of Medical Fees in French Health Insurance

Key Letter	Content	Key Letter	Content
C	Consultation by general practitioner, dentist, or midwife	D	Services by dental specialist
Cs	Consultation by specialist	SF	Special services by midwife
CNpsy	Consultation with neurologist, psychiatrist, or other specialists	SFI	Nursing care by midwife
V	Visit by general practitioner, dentist, or midwife	AMM	Services by massage therapist or physiotherapist
Vs	Visit by specialist	AMI	Services by nurse or male nurse
VNpsy	Visit by neurologist or psychiatrist	AMP	Services by podiatrist
K	Surgical procedures and specialist services	AMO	Services by speech therapist
Z	Services by physician or dentist using scientific instruments	AMY	Services by orthoptist

In the case of private hospitals, fee agreements are signed directly with sickness insurance funds, and the healthcare expenditures of insured persons are reimbursed according to this fee schedule. The costs covered by the insurance funds do not exceed the hospitalization fees for public hospitals of a similar nature. Moreover, the costs for examinations, pathological diagnoses, blood transfusions, and so on are not included in the agreement.

In general, there are two types of medical treatments in hospitals. The first is free medical services for the military, recipients of social assistance, and so on. The second is services covered by health insurance and other fee-based medical services. The latter case is similar to that of private practitioners, as physicians are paid by hospitals according to the medical fees calculated based on the medical procedure groups. However, physicians do not receive the full amount of the medical fees but rather the balance after the hospital deducts a certain percentage as a management fee. Using the radiology department as an example, the percentage of deduction is up to 50% plus another 5% for administrative fees.

(5) Health Insurance Management Systems

The model adopted by the French health insurance system involves "government decision-making, private operations, and vertical management." Health insurance decisions are submitted by the central government to the Parliament for approval and are implemented after a decree is enacted. The government entrusts the central and regional health insurance agencies to implement specific policy requirements according to the agreement signed with the government and to administer social insurance affairs. The management system is mainly divided into three major systems.

1. *Fund collection system.* The basic social insurance in France has a hybrid financing system whereby the separation of income and expenditure is implemented within a vertical management model of social insurance funds (includes sickness insurance, work injury insurance, pension insurance, and family benefits). Funds are collected uniformly by the Central Agency of Social Security Organizations (ACOSS) and its subordinate local Organizations for the Collection of Social Security and Family Benefit Contributions (URSSAF). The collection of social insurance premiums, also known as social insurance contributions (*contribution sociale généralisée*, CSG), includes individual social insurance contributions based on income levels and social insurance contributions paid by employers.
2. *Health insurance management system.* This system is composed of the National Settlement Center for Health Insurance Management and its subordinate Regional Health Insurance Management Offices. These are the leading and core departments of health insurance management in France, and they play an important role in France's health insurance.
3. *Health insurance payment system.* This system is composed of the national and regional health (pension) insurance settlement centers and mainly undertakes direct payments of approved health insurance fees. Basic health insurance pays for 77% of healthcare expenditure in France, and, of the remainder, 12.5% is paid by supplementary health insurance, 1.5% is subsidized by national assistance programs, and 9% is funded by families and individuals. In 2006, basic social insurance expenditure in France was €526.2 billion, accounting for 29.4% of GDP, of which, health insurance expenditure accounted for 11.7%.

(6) Basic Characteristics of the Health Insurance System

The health insurance system in France has the following characteristics.

1. The insurance system exists as national cross-sections of occupational groups, and its operation is carried out by representatives of employees and employers.
2. There is no regional insurance.
3. There is no health insurance system specifically targeting the elderly, who remain in their previous health insurance system after retirement.
4. Apart from agriculture, mining, and other special sectors, there are virtually no subsidies from the state treasury.
5. Benefits covered by insurance include maternity benefits, eyeglasses, and assistive devices.
6. Inpatient services are paid according to a fee-for-service system, and outpatient services are paid using the reimbursement system. The reimbursement rate (copayment rate) varies according to the system and type of benefit. Physicians' remuneration for consultation is paid on a per-case basis.
7. The premium rate is high (19.6%), and contributions by employers are about twice those of employees (12.8% for employers, 6.8% for employees).
8. There is no difference between the healthcare benefits received by employees and their dependents.

5. Health Insurance Issues and Reforms

(1) Main Existing Issues

1. Insurance Fund Deficits Caused by Excessive Growth in Healthcare Expenditure   Due to its focus on a high level of security and welfare, French health insurance has placed a greater emphasis on the provision of healthcare services and less on people's ability to pay. As a result, some patients have abused insurance claims, drugs, and examinations and have exaggerated minor illnesses. The emphasis on the provision of services has also led some to believe that health insurance should cover a greater proportion of healthcare expenditure, which has resulted in a drastic increase in health insurance costs. At present, health insurance accounts for 34.6% of overall social welfare spending, second only to pensions (44.1%). This level of spending has especially been the case in recent decades. Due to the economic downturn, increased unemployment, population aging, and lower statutory working hours in France, the growth rate of annual health insurance contributions is far lower than that of health insurance expenditures. France's health insurance expenditure has long exceeded its income, which has continued to exacerbate this deficit. Thus, this issue has now come under the scrutiny of all sectors in French society.

According to statistical analysis, healthcare expenditure in France as a share of GDP was 3.4% in 1950 and increased to 4.7% in 1960, 6.4% in 1970, 7.6% in 1980, 8.8% in 1990, 10.1% in 2000, and 11.2% in 2008. In 1975–1990, the elasticity of healthcare spending to GDP reached 1.79. Health insurance expenditure in France was €83.3 billion in 1995 and €85.3 billion in 1996. Healthcare spending per capita was €148.5 in 1950 and increased sharply to €274.4 in 1975, €1,753.1 in 1995, €2,617.5 in 2000, and €2,945.1 in 2008.

The coverage of healthcare expenditure is extremely broad in France, as it includes disease prevention, maternity benefits, eyeglasses, assistive devices, and spa therapy.

The increase in this healthcare expenditure far exceeds that of GDP and household expenditure and, thus, has become the most prominent issue in France. In 2008, healthcare expenditure (the broad concept of healthcare expenditure mentioned above) accounted for 11.2% of GDP. Population aging in France is similar to that of Japan, and France is one of the oldest countries in the world. Despite differences in the scope of healthcare expenditure, its rapid growth as a share of GDP is a phenomenon that can no longer be ignored.

As the expenditures of health insurance funds in France have long exceeded their incomes, these funds are now facing serious deficits. Despite undertaking more than 10 major and minor reforms since 1975, France's health insurance funds have continued to produce yearly deficits and are currently facing serious difficulties. According to statistics, the health insurance deficit in 1993 was €4.2 billion and increased to €31.6 billion in 1994, €5.5 billion in 1995, €5.2 billion in 1996, and €12.3 billion in 2004.

This situation is undoubtedly related to the slow economic development, market decline, increased unemployment rate, and reduced purchasing power that France has experienced in recent years. However, another important cause for this situation is the flaws and imperfections that exist in the health insurance system and health insurance policies. Given these circumstances, the issues that have been of great concern to successive French governments and all levels of society include further implementing reforms of the health insurance system, improving and reforming the social security system, rationally allocating and utilizing healthcare resources, increasing the efficiency of healthcare services, and controlling the rise in healthcare expenditure.

On November 16, 1995, the prime minister of the French government, Alain Juppé, proposed a reform plan of the social security system to the National Assembly. The purpose of this reform was to increase the assigned taxes of the whole society and revise the financing of health insurance, thereby gradually shifting from social health insurance contributions to an income tax. Its aim was to establish a new, unified, efficient, and universal health security system, thus fundamentally altering the passive situation in which health insurance expenditure exceeds its income.

2. Imperfect Health Insurance System that Lacks Competition and Interest Constraints   The French health system is still imperfect, and its health insurance lacks uniformity. In addition to the common system that covers the main population, the French health insurance system also includes smaller systems for several industries that are difficult to incorporate into the common system. The various systems established by individual industries cover small populations, provide limited mutual aid, and often encounter problems as the industries decline. For example, there is a large deficit gap for coal miners due to the decline of the industry, the large number of old workers, and the small number of new workers. The coexistence of multiple systems has led to difficulties in unifying health insurance payment standards, which is unfavorable for the government's unified management of health insurance overall. In France, the specific work involved in health insurance is mainly undertaken by the various health insurance fund organizations. Insurance fund organizations reimburse healthcare institutions based mainly on the content, quantity, and price of the healthcare services provided. Due to the lack of effective incentive measures to control the use of healthcare resources, providers, consumers, and third parties have yet to establish comprehensive constraint mechanisms for healthcare cost containment. Moreover, there are no mutual restrictions in the interest relationships among the three parties in the payment of healthcare expenditure, and both providers and consumers lack cost awareness. These factors have resulted in the waste of healthcare resources. For instance, the fee-for-service system for physicians often motivates them to provide unnecessary services to receive compensation. Furthermore, some patients often request their physicians to provide certain unnecessary and costly healthcare examinations and services that are not based on the needs of their conditions. This excess service provision has also led to a continuous increase in healthcare needs and health insurance costs.

3. Misallocation of Health Resources and Low Utilization Efficiency   At present, there is a misallocation of health resources among the French population and an unreasonable geographical distribution. There are too many physicians in large cities and shortages in rural and remote areas. The number of physicians in areas south of Paris is too high, whereas it is relatively low in areas north of Paris. For example, the number of physicians in greater Paris is six times higher than that in Haute-Saône, and the number of specialists in greater Paris is 15 times higher than that in Corrèze. The current number of healthcare workers in France is double that of 20 years ago. The number of physicians per 1,000 people is 2.7, which is second only to Germany and is higher than those of the US (2.3), Japan (1.6), and the UK (1.4). The number of beds per 1,000 people in France is also the highest in Europe, but the utilization efficiency of beds is relatively low. This misallocation of health resources has become a serious issue for France's health insurance and has led to differences in the health statuses of populations between urban and rural areas and across different regions. In concrete terms, these differences are reflected in the differences in the morbidity and mortality rates between urban and rural areas.

(2) Measures and Effects of Health Insurance Reform

1. Increase in Income and Expansion of Funding Sources   Since the late 1970s, the French government has repeatedly raised the contribution rates of all health insurance funds. In the most recent instance, the individual health insurance contribution was increased from 4.5% to 6.8% of the total salary, whereas the contributions of employers increased from 8% to 12.8% of the employees' salary.

The contribution base for health insurance was further expanded from salaried income to all income. That is, in addition to individual salaries, the contribution base also included stocks, bonds, deposit interest, real estate rental income, and other capital income. The premiums paid by insured persons are mainly determined by their levels of economic income, whereas the health insurance services enjoyed by the public are not differentiated based on the level of premiums contributed. Thus, mutual aid is achieved between high-income and low-income earners and between high-premium and low-premium insurance fund organizations, thereby reflecting the country's level of social health insurance.

2. Encouraging Diverse Competition and Reform Payment Methods   The health insurance fund organizations in France place great emphasis on diverse competition and self-administration. The former concerns the external conditions of the operating system, whereas the latter emphasizes the internal environment of the operating system. The government only undertakes administrative interventions when unacceptable consequences are brought about by market mechanisms. The government's emphasis on the self-administration of health insurance fund organizations aims to maximize the service functions of health insurance fund organizations and to take into account the interests of all parties concerned.

The government has strengthened the management and supervision of health insurance expenditures and has strictly controlled the payment standards for health insurance premiums. The government has reviewed and assessed various new medical technologies and has clearly stated the opinion that health insurance should not pay for ineffective and costly new medical technologies. The government has repeatedly reduced the reimbursement rates for healthcare and drugs. In 1993, the reimbursement rate of medical fees was reduced from 75% to 70%, that of general drugs was reduced from 70% to 65%, and that of drugs with minimal efficacy was reduced from 70% to 40%. Apart from vitamins D and B, vitamins were excluded from health insurance reimbursements. The reimbursement rate of nutritional supplements was reduced from 40% to 35%. Furthermore, patients' copayment ratios for medical expenses and drug costs were increased.

Cost accounting was strengthened to achieve economic efficiency, thus encouraging patients to adopt appropriate attitudes towards healthcare services. Patients' copayment ratios for healthcare expenditure were increased moderately, and their cost awareness was enhanced by adjusting their economic benefits, thereby achieving healthcare cost containment. In accordance with the Social Security Fund Law passed in 1997, the government imposes deficit restrictions on health insurance funds and proposed income-oriented expenditures of health insurance funds. In addition, the National Assembly is required to review and approve the annual budget resolutions, stipulate the annual increase in health insurance expenditure, and strictly control the growth ratio of health insurance expenditure during its implementation at each level.

A DRG-based payment system was implemented, and reforms have been undertaken since 2003 on the reimbursement allocation system for healthcare institutions. Instead of a simple budgeting system, a fund allocation system that combines a budgeting system, a measurement system, and a DRG-based payment system was implemented. The public welfare components of public healthcare institutions (e.g., public health services, physician and nurse training, psychiatric hospitals, drug rehabilitation and prevention, the construction and operation of blood and organ banks, and other costs) are managed based on a budget. Budget-based allocation is implemented for the fixed costs of hospital operation (personnel and equipment costs), whereas per-case and DRG-based payment systems are implemented for outpatient and inpatient services. Different costs are charged for patients with the same disease in different age groups, and the cost standards for those aged 60 years and above are especially high. Different costs are also paid for the same disease across different regions. To accurately measure the quantity of medical activities, the French-style Program for Medicalization of Information Systems (*Programme de Médicalisation des Systèmes d'Information*, PMSI) was established to determine the caseload and cost payment standards for the treatment of various diseases according to the International Classification of Diseases. Currently, France has identified more than 2,300 DRGs (or *groupes homogènes de malades*, GHM) for the calculation of payment costs.

3. Optimization of Health Resource Allocation and Utilization and Control of Health Insurance Expenditure   The French government has implemented a "global budget" on its health system, which is a new method of hospital investment and financial management. Under the premise of achieving healthcare goals and guaranteeing national health, the government has strengthened the planning of healthcare expenditure, optimized the allocation and utilization of health resources, and eliminated waste to reduce and control healthcare expenditures. In addition, the government has also restricted the expansion and growth of healthcare institutions, controlled the continuous increase in the healthcare workforce, limited unnecessary medical tests and examinations, reinforced the supervision and management of healthcare expenditure, and contained the overuse of health insurance services.

After President Jacques Chirac took power, the government once again implemented austerity policies that reduced fiscal expenditure and expanded economic development. Thus, on the one hand, tax collection was expanded, and, on the other hand, social security expenditure was reduced (including health insurance expenditure) in an attempt to fundamentally alter the passive situation of continuous yearly deficits in social security caused by expenditure greater than income.

This reform was promulgated and implemented nationally on January 1, 1996. Its main contents include (1) levying a 0.5% social insurance amortization tax (*caisse d'amortissement de la dette sociale*, CADES) on all persons, including those receiving pensions and unemployment benefits; (2) increasing the daily hospitalization fees paid by patients, separating hospital insurance, and establishing a special hospital management institution to strengthen management; and (3) implementing and promoting a national "global budget method" to strengthen the planning and management of healthcare expenditure, thereby effectively controlling health insurance expenditures.

These measures have produced preliminary results. The first measure increased the national taxes collected each year by €3.7 billion. The second measure has increased the hospitalization fees paid by patients, that is, patients' hospitalization fee copayments increased from €8.4 to €10.7. This measure, to a certain extent, has constrained the growth of demand for inpatient services and controlled expenditure on these services, which account for nearly 60% of total health insurance costs. The third measure has strengthened the government's macro-control over the budget for healthcare services. The implementation and promotion of the global budget method has further encouraged the control of healthcare expenditure by healthcare institutions and has optimized healthcare services. Thus, it is one of the key measures to promote the reform of the health insurance system and reduce the fiscal deficit of social security.

In 2004, the French minister of health, Philippe Douste-Blazy, announced recommendations for the reform of the health insurance system. He called on government departments, all sectors of society, and all citizens to share in the responsibility of eliminating the long-standing debt of the French health insurance system and reducing the country's financial burden. This reform measure has slowed the upward trend of costs. In 2007, health insurance returned to a deficit of €4.6 billion, rather than the prereform projection of €9 billion, thus restoring the balance of finances. The National Objective for Health Insurance Spending (*Objectif National des Dépenses d'Assurance Maladie*, ONDAM) was achieved, and the upward trend of prescription costs was effectively curbed.

The reform of the health insurance system is a complex social project. As this reform involves multiple aspects and an extensive scope with varying degrees of adjustment for the interests of different social classes, it has also faced resistance from society, the public, and the healthcare sector. Under the premise of guaranteeing the operation and development of the healthcare industry, the French government has adopted such measures as controlling total health investment, reducing healthcare expenditure, increasing the efficiency of healthcare services, and reforming payment methods to ensure social stability and economic development in France. Within the scope permitted by socioeconomic levels, this reform aims to improve the service content of health insurance, strengthen the management of health insurance funds, and deepen the reform of the health industry.

4. Reforms of the Hospital Management System and Operational Mechanisms The first management system reform involved continuing the promotion of regional health planning. In 2003, the regional health planning system focused on classifying the grades of hospitals based on their technological capabilities in certain fields, thereby maintaining mutual cooperation among hospitals. From 2005 to the present, regional health planning has focused on promoting the formation of an intra-regional hospital network. Each hospital shall strive to achieve full cooperation to ensure that the hospital network provides more comprehensive healthcare services. The second reform involved signing hospital development contracts. Contracts were signed between regional hospital agencies (*agences régionales de l'hospitalisation*, ARH) and public hospitals to set three- to five-year development goals and tasks for hospitals, including health service provision, healthcare quality, information system and management efficiency, and so on. The contract determines the funding method for hospital projects. If the hospital is considered to be inefficient, it can only obtain resources by improving its own efficiency; if the hospital is very efficient, then it can receive additional funding through the ARH. The third reform involved strengthening hospital cooperation. Agreements were signed between hospitals to strengthen cooperation, for example, by transferring emergency staff from less busy hospitals. Cancer treatment involves cooperation between public and private hospitals to ensure that patients can receive comprehensive healthcare services. The fourth reform involved a downward shift in the focus of management. By strengthening the management authority of ARHs, the focus of management was shifted from the central to the regional level. The demographic and epidemiological characteristics of each region were taken as primary indicators in the formulation of hospital planning in regional health planning.

As for reforms of hospital operational mechanisms, the first involved implementing the management of major departments. Promoting the system of "major department management" has enabled the rationalization of hospital organizational structures. There are no unified standards and requirements for major departments. Each hospital can establish major departments based on its departmental features and actual conditions. The heads of departments are jointly appointed by the hospital director and the management committee. Major departments also have management committees that meet three to four times every year to discuss and decide on daily affairs. The second reform involved simplifying management. By promoting hospital development and simplifying hospital management, hospitals were provided with more room for reform and adjustment, which gave healthcare workers more autonomy in management decisions. Physicians were placed in charge of major departments and have autonomy in their organization and management. However, hospitals are still subjected to strict limitations in other aspects. The management committees are still under the management of the Ministry of Health and ARHs. Management systems, such as employee recruitment, investment, and the use of new technologies, still require the approval of the relevant management authorities.

6. Healthcare Cost-Containment Policies

(1) Preliminary Policies for Healthcare Cost Containment

As France has universal health insurance, most of its healthcare expenditure is covered by social health insurance (the average compensation rate of the general regime is 90%). The growth rate of healthcare expenditure in France far exceeds that of its GDP. The total healthcare cost in 2003 was 10.1% of GDP and reached 11% in 2007 and 11.2% in 2008; this figure was 7.0% in 1980. In 2007, the government's total health spending as a share of total healthcare expenditure was 79.0%, total private health spending as a share of total healthcare expenditure was 21.0%, the government's total health spending as a share of total government spending was 16.6%, and social security health expenditure as a share of total government health spending was 93.4%.

Therefore, the control of total healthcare expenditure is equivalent to the control of health insurance expenditure. On the other hand, about half of health insurance benefits are used for inpatient services in hospitals. Thus, at this stage, healthcare cost-containment policies are equivalent to containment policies for inpatient healthcare expenditure. Since 1975, France has been implementing inter-regime fund adjustments, funding measures (e.g., increasing premiums), and various healthcare cost-containment policies to address the increase in health insurance expenditures and the consequent financial issues.

First, in accordance with the Fiscal Adjustment Law of 1974, fiscal adjustment has been implemented among all social insurance sectors and regimes since 1975 in the hope of eliminating the considerable deficit of the social insurance sector. However, the deficit continued to increase. Therefore, after 1976, France implemented drug reimbursement controls (reduction of drug prices; reduced reimbursement rates for certain drugs, such as nutritional supplements; etc.) and a continued increase in premium rates (16.95% in 1976, 17.95% in 1977, and 18.95% in 1979). In particular, after 1979, strong healthcare cost-containment policies were implemented, and new sources of insurance funds were added as countermeasures to reduce expenditure and increase income.

The healthcare cost-containment policies mainly included (1) controlling hospital healthcare expenses; (2) limiting the number of medical students; (3) establishing social insurance management and supervisory committees to strengthen supervision and management; (4) increasing the personal copayment ratio; (5) cutting administrative expenses for social security and similar funds; (6) strengthening the prevention of smoking, alcohol poisoning, and accidents; (7) reducing the costs of tests; (8) strengthening the medical supervision of insured persons on sick leave by consulting physicians; (9) enhancing the sense of responsibility among physicians and insured persons; and (10) adopting a ratio system in the agreement between insurers and pharmacist groups, pharmaceutical company groups, and inspection agency groups.

Measures to add new sources of insurance funds included (1) increasing insurance premiums, (2) collecting health insurance premiums from retirees (1% of basic pensions and 2% of supplementary pensions), (3) abolishing the special tax for car insurance and creating compulsory insurance for motorists to raise funds for the healthcare expenses of injuries caused by car accidents, (4) increasing taxes on tobacco and alcohol, (5) levying a special sales tax on pharmacists equivalent to 1.5% of net income (limited to once a year), (6) levying a special tax of 2.5% on the publicity expenses of pharmaceutical companies (limited to one time), and (7) reducing special government expenditures.

In the late 1980s, France adopted new drug price regulations and limitations. In addition, the presidential decree of 1945 abolished the long-standing drug price system and replaced it with a system in which pharmaceutical companies attached suggested retail prices and applied for the registration of new drugs with the Ministry of Health. For existing drugs, the method of repricing each product was abolished, and instead the rate of price increase was determined at regular intervals according to economic conditions. At that point, pharmaceutical companies could set different price increase rates for each product. Furthermore, the committee for determining the prices of reimbursable drugs became a neutral committee that was responsible for comparing new and existing drugs and expressing its opinions on the prices of reimbursable drugs. Private practitioners can now select cheaper drugs with the same efficacy from this price list.

In the 1990s, the above healthcare cost-containment measures complemented the measures to increase the sources of insurance funds by raising health insurance premiums, thus alleviating the severe funding deficit of healthcare expenditures. Nevertheless, the social insurance funds were still mired in chronic deficits. For example, from 1993 to 1996, the annual deficits were €8.6 billion, €8.5 billion, €9.4 billion, and €9.6 billion, respectively; the deficits of the sickness funds were €4.2 billion, €4.8 billion, €5.5 billion, and €5.2 billion, respectively.

(2) Further Policies for Healthcare Cost Containment

Although the above measures have achieved certain results, there are still doubts over the true extent of their effects. Thus, controlling the rapid growth of healthcare expenditure is still fraught with difficulties and requires further reform. In the 1990s, France began a new round of social security reforms, ultimately leading to the enactment of the new Social Security Act on April 24, 1996, which also forms the basic legal framework of the current French social security system. In 2000, the healthcare cost-containment plan explicitly stipulated (1) the unification of the health insurance system and greater control of healthcare expenditure, (2) the reform of healthcare provision institutions (regional health planning, community orientation, informatization, introduction of healthcare evaluation indicators, and quality management), (3) a special system for balancing old-age pension finances and the construction of a supplementary health insurance system (care insurance system), (4) the reform of the family healthcare fund system, (5) further clarifications of the responsibilities of relevant organizations in the social security system, and (6) management system reforms to balance social security finances.

1. Unification of Health Insurance System and Healthcare Cost Containment   In the past, deficits in specific sickness insurance funds were usually covered through transfers from other funds and regimes. These transfers mainly occurred in the form of supplements from the family healthcare fund to other sectors or from the general regime to other sectors, especially to the agricultural sector, to ensure the unification of the health insurance system. Further healthcare cost-containment policies required all sectors to formulate premium rates and collect them rationally under an equitable system. Thus, based on existing industrial and regional insurance organizations, the family healthcare fund was developed, and sickness insurance affairs were further expanded. To maintain the balance of funds by supplementing social security deficits, the social security amortization tax introduced on January 1, 1996, was further increased. The French health insurance industry was once described as having brain-wracking difficulties at every step.

2. Global Budget Planning and Regionalization of Healthcare Expenditure   The introduction of the global budget planning system for healthcare expenditure is one of the most decisive measures in France's healthcare expenditure reform. The global budget system of healthcare expenditure refers to the sum of healthcare expenditure across four sectors, public hospitals, private hospitals, liberal healthcare, and social healthcare, and is determined by Parliament.

1. *Public hospitals.* The budget for healthcare activities for the current year is based on the hospital plan of the current year and the quantity of healthcare services provided in the previous year, and it is implemented according to the global budget payment system. The final accounts are examined by the regional accounting inspectorate and regional hospital agency, and the results are submitted to the central accounting inspectorate, which in turn reports to Parliament after its investigations. Based on this report and the opinions of the National Health Conference on health service priorities, Parliament reviews the national and sickness fund budgets and reaches a resolution. The confirmed

national budget is then allocated according to the actual hospital services provided by each region and the status of healthcare services. The budget allocated to each region is then distributed by the regional hospital agency to hospitals in the region.

2. *Private hospitals.* In the past, inpatient healthcare expenditure was decided by negotiations between insurance funds and hospitals. Further healthcare cost-containment policies require state, insurance fund, and hospital representatives to conduct negotiations on the national global budget to determine the National Quantified Objective (*Objectif Quantifié National*, OQN). As with public hospitals, this amount is allocated to each region and then distributed to institutions within the region by regional hospital agencies.

3. *Liberal healthcare.* The global budget is determined by the state and funds according to healthcare cost analysis results from the previous year. The budget determination is followed by the signing of agreements between the insurance funds and medical unions in which the targets for healthcare costs and remunerations for medical treatment are determined according to the global budget. If healthcare expenditure exceeds the target amount due to the provision of medical procedures without justifiable reasons, the physicians bear full responsibility and return the excess healthcare expenditure to the insurance funds. With regard to quality assurance, a binding healthcare evaluation indicator (*Références Médicales Opposables*, RMO) was introduced in 1994 to enable physicians to consciously contribute to healthcare cost containment. This indicator was developed by the National Agency for the Development of Medical Evaluation (ANDEM; now restructured to form the National Agency for Accreditation and Evaluation in Health, ANAES) based on unanimous agreements among foreign and domestic experts. Physicians must issue receipts to patients after providing medical consultations according to this indicator. Physicians who do not comply with this indicator are penalized according to the severity of the violation, and punishments may involve the termination of payments from sickness funds and the removal of qualifications as contracted physicians.

4. *Social healthcare sector.* This sector is mainly responsible for the healthcare of disabled persons and patients with opioid poisoning. The procedures for this sector are similar to those for the public hospital sector. After the share of the national global budget allocated to each region is determined, the regional government decides the amount allocated to each institution.

3. Regional Hospital Agency (ARH)   Hospital services are jointly managed by the Regional Directorate of Health and Social Affairs (*Direction Régionale des Affaires Sanitaires et Sociales*, DRASS) and the Regional Health Insurance Fund (*Caisse Régionale d'Assurance Maladie*, CRAM). First, hospitals set the number of beds for internal medicine, surgery, gynecology, and other departments according to the Regional Health Organization Plan (*Schéma Régional d'Organisation Sanitaire*, SROS) and specify the number of high-value medical devices. When making adjustments to hospital beds and departments or adding new high-value medical devices, healthcare institutions need to submit annual plans to the DRASS, which reviews the rationality of the quantity and the reasons for the additions. The DRASS officials for public health and social issues also conduct comprehensive inspections of the medical, financial, and legal aspects of the plan. After inspection and approval, public hospitals providing insured services operate according to the hospital plan, and a global budget is paid by the CRAM; private hospitals providing insured services are contracted with the CRAM, and the costs are covered by the funds for insured services. Public and private hospitals that join this system are both managed by the regional health plan, and the difference in the payment method lies in whether the global budget or agreement method is adopted.

As the target value for the annual rate of increase in hospital healthcare expenditure is set by the state, public hospitals usually exceed the target value to a larger extent than private hospitals do. Thus, attention should be paid to the operational efficiency of the former hospital type. However, private hospitals have also been accused of providing low-cost healthcare services, such as ambulatory surgery, dialysis, and childbirth delivery, to wealthy groups in middle class or above, whereas public hospitals are more focused on treating poorer patients and complicated cases. Thus, it is necessary to evaluate common costs to ensure the equal and rational distribution of healthcare expenses and resources. As a result, the government has established ARHs, which are headed by executive committees consisting of representatives from the DRASS and the CRAM, in 24 regions. Their task is to determine the amount of hospital healthcare expenditure (public and private) allocated to each hospital; certify the beds, departments, and high-value medical devices of hospitals in the region; and formulate the regional healthcare plan. In order to further enhance healthcare quality, all hospitals are required to submit quality assessment reports within the next five years. The ARHs then analyze the unit costs of DRGs and assess the overall service quality of hospitals. Based on this analysis, unified adjustments are made to the budget allocation and regional healthcare planning agencies. Initially, uniform national standards for quality assessment were absent. Each healthcare institution performed its own independent assessment until 1998, when the ANAES national quality assessment method was adopted.

4. Promotion of Information-Based Management   The healthcare behaviors of physicians in the past were performed under the principles of freedom. Only the codes and scores of medical procedures were sent to the sickness funds, which did not receive information about the specific contents of the medical procedures provided. For instance, KC-50 represents 50 points for surgical treatment, which is equivalent to a surgery such as an appendectomy. The Hospital Reform Law of 1991 stipulated the implementation of reporting obligations for hospital information planning, which required the content of medical procedures and their corresponding costs to be reported to the management accounting fund and the state. Since 1997, all hospitals nationwide, both public and private, have adopted the DRG method when reporting to an ARH. Thus, the healthcare content provided by hospitals has become more transparent, enabling the state to formulate a more rational budget. In addition, this information has also become a specific countermeasure to eliminate regional differences in healthcare expenditure by facilitating its distribution from high to low areas.

As for private practitioners, insurance funds formulated medical fee schedules for each physician in the past and were responsible for inspecting physicians charging higher-than-average fees for the same specialty within a given region. As the specific contents of medical procedures were unclear, these inspections were ineffective. In 1993, the government required all private practitioners to record the diagnosis, medical procedure, and the pathology and diagnosis code (CPD) on a receipt. As this method could not adequately protect the personal privacy of patients, it was strongly opposed by physicians and was not implemented. In 1994, the RMO, which specified the obligation to issue a receipt when providing a medical consultation, was introduced. In the year the RMO was introduced, it was expected to reduce healthcare expenditure by €51.4 million. In both the attempt to improve the transparency of healthcare content and to rationalize the negotiations between medical unions and sickness funds, the failure to introduce the CPD has demonstrated that the road to achieving the informatization of private practice is not smooth.

In the late 1990s, the government adopted the medical management records and health records system, which aimed to manage the records of examinations, medications, and other healthcare services. This system was intended to facilitate the management of overutilization by patients, the control of unnecessary healthcare services (especially repeated hospital visits and unrealistic hospitalizations), and the provision of medical information in emergencies. A future goal is to establish an IC-card medical information system in which an IC-card computer terminal is installed in the clinics of private practitioners and a patient's information is displayed when the physician's and patient's IC-cards are inserted. Physicians can refer to the patient's medical records (including records from other physicians) during a consultation, and the contents of the consultation are then recorded on the electronic medical records card. All information is then transferred via the network system to the sickness funds. This system will play an important role in information selection, the analysis of healthcare expenditure, information utilization, ensuring authenticity of patient information, and protecting patients' personal privacy.

The acceleration of population aging and the advancement of medical technology have led to the rapid rise in healthcare expenditure. In the meantime, France's socioeconomic growth has been relatively slow. In 1999, the deficit of health insurance funds was €700 million, and it increased drastically after 2000 and reached €11.6 billion in 2004. The immense deficit in healthcare expenditure indicates that previous cost-containment measures have been relatively ineffective. This outcome is manifested as follows. Due to the high reimbursement rate for outpatient expenses, patients often make multiple visits for one illness. Due to the high reimbursement rate for drugs and the inadequate management of drug reimbursement types, the drug consumption per capita of French residents is much higher than that of other European countries. The declining efficiency of public hospitals has reduced the utilization efficiency of state-owned healthcare resources. Against this backdrop, the French government launched the health system reform plan in early 2004. The content of the French reform plan related to the payment of healthcare expenditure mainly includes the following measures.

1. *Primary-care physician (*médecin traitant*) system.* The newly enacted Health Insurance Law stipulates that every resident must declare his or her own primary-care physician (private practitioner) who is responsible for the first consultation. If the patient directly seeks medical treatment from other healthcare institutions without going through a primary-care physician, the compensation rate of the health insurance fund is greatly reduced. Primary-care physicians reduce the number of outpatient visits by regulating the health-seeking behaviors of patients, thereby controlling outpatient healthcare expenditure.

2. *Reduction of patients' reimbursement rates for outpatient fees.* The French healthcare reform in 2004 increased patients' copayment rates for each outpatient visit by €1. It also stipulated that health insurance agencies had the right to determine the reimbursement rate for drugs based on the economic growth rate of the current year. Thus, a dynamic link was established between health insurance reimbursement and health insurance financing, which enabled a compensation mechanism with income-oriented expenditure, thereby ensuring the safety of health insurance funds.

3. *Controlling the scope of drug use.* Special drug review agencies were established to strictly screen the types of drugs included in the health insurance reimbursement list and to eliminate duplicated, ineffective drugs that have low cost-effectiveness. Economic incentives were given to physicians who use generic drugs in the form of agreements to achieve the aim of reducing the share of drug costs in healthcare expenses.

4. *Promotion of patient electronic medical records.* A common system of patient electronic medical records, which enables the use of patient medical information by different institutions, was promoted among healthcare institutions, thereby preventing duplicate examinations and reducing the waste of healthcare resources.

5. *Changing the budgeting method of public hospitals.* To improve the efficiency of public hospitals, France has implemented reforms for the payment of healthcare expenditure in public hospitals based on medical informatization (PMSI). Given the premise that adequate funds were available to protect public welfare projects, including teaching in public hospitals, the construction of key disciplines, and emergency care, a payment method based on service units (T2A), which is similar to that in private hospitals, was applied to the healthcare services of public hospitals. The specific method is as follows. Inpatient healthcare services are broken down into a number of equivalent service units, and the total number of service units completed by all hospitals in a given region and year is counted. After subtracting the budget for public service expenditure from the budget for inpatient healthcare services in the entire region, the remainder is divided by the total number of service units to calculate the reimbursement rate for each service unit. Finally, the reimbursement rate for each service unit is multiplied by the number of service units provided by each hospital in the current year to obtain the total amount of health insurance payment for a given institution. The purpose of this reform is to improve the working efficiency of public hospitals. It can be seen that France has always adopted a management approach to public hospitals through which providers invest in infrastructure construction, and health insurance funds pay for hospital service provision. Since 2004, the French government has further reformed the provider payment mechanism. Given the control of the overall amount, the basic health insurance fund payments were redistributed according to the service volume provided by public hospitals, thereby improving the working efficiency of public hospitals.

As of today, the above reforms have achieved positive results. The growing deficit in France's healthcare expenditure has been effectively controlled. In 2006, the deficit in healthcare expenditure was reduced to €6.5 billion. Based on the original growth rate of €2.5 billion per year, the deficit was projected to reach €16.5 billion by 2006, which implies that the new policy reduced the deficit by €10 billion. However, a report by the French Parliament also pointed out that the decline in the deficit of healthcare expenditure should also partly be attributed to the financing of healthcare expenditure. For example, the financing of healthcare expenditure in 2006 and 2007 added €2 billion and €4 billion, respectively. The report also states that, among the healthcare reform policies, those that had a direct effect on cost containment included linking the healthcare reimbursement rate with national economic growth and encouraging the use of generic drugs. Although other policies, such as the primary-care physician system, the promotion of electronic medical records, and changes in the public hospital payment system, have standardized the framework of healthcare services, their immediate effect on healthcare cost containment is not clear in the short term.

 ## SECTION III. THE HEALTH SYSTEM IN JAPAN

Japan is an archipelago nation in East Asia. It consists of four main islands, Hokkaido, Honshu, Shikoku, and Kyushu, and several smaller islands. Its total land area is 377,000 square kilometers, of which 76.0% are mountainous areas and 14.8% are cultivated land.

In 2013, its population was 121.339 million, of which the population aged over 65 years accounted for 25.1%, and 92.5% of the population lived in urban areas, making it the third most urbanized nation in the world.

The constant improvement in Japan's healthcare system, the development of medical science and technology, and the improvement in people's living conditions have promoted the continuous enhancement of residents' healthcare levels. The average life expectancy in Japan has continued to increase. In 1920, the average life expectancy of the Japanese was only around 45 years. By 1985, the average life expectancy of men was 74.8 years and that of women was 80.4 years. Japan has a rapid rate of population aging. In 1990, the percentage of the population aged over 65 years reached 12%. Thus, Japan took the lead in becoming an aging society and had the highest life expectancy in the world. In 2000, the life expectancy at birth in Japan was 81 years: 78 years for men and 85 years for women. In 2012, the life expectancy at birth was 83.1 years: 79.9 years for men and 86.4 years for women. In order to cope with this unprecedented level of population aging in the history of mankind, Japan has adopted numerous measures and attempts in healthcare and welfare, including the development of community health services. The emphasis on elderly care is a distinctive feature in Japan's community health services.

The Cabinet is the core leadership of the central government. Institutions led by the Cabinet include the Cabinet Office, the Prime Minister's Office, and the 12 administrative ministries. The Ministry of Health, Labour and Welfare (MHLW) is the national-level health administration department. The administrative divisions of the country include one metropolis (Tokyo), one circuit (Hokkaido), two urban prefectures (Osaka and Kyoto), and 43 prefectures (including Okinawa). This level of administrative division lies between the central and municipal levels. At this level, there are 47 health-related departments and bureaus in the country with different names, such as the Health Bureau, the Environment and Healthcare Department, and the Health and Environment Department. Subordinate to these health-related bureaus and departments are public health centers, which serve both administrative and institutional functions. These centers implement health-related administrative work within their jurisdiction, while also serving as central institutions for public health activities such as disease prevention, healthcare promotion, and environmental health improvement. The administrative divisions below the prefecture level include city, town, and village, which are municipal autonomous organizations. In terms of health administration, large cities with a population greater than 1 million generally have health and public cleaning bureaus; medium cities with a population of 100,000 to 1 million have health bureaus (or departments); cities with a population smaller than 100,000 or towns have health divisions that are sometimes combined with national health insurance affairs and are known as the healthcare divisions. Villages often have health sections (units) or resident sections (units) that undertake health affairs. Municipalities have public health centers where residents can engage in various health promotion activities.

In 1961, Japan implemented the National Health Insurance (NHI) system, and all residents of Japan are required by law to enroll in health insurance. Insured residents are free to choose any healthcare institution for treatment, and individuals only need to pay a small portion of the costs. Japan's health insurance is a relatively successful health security system that has had a certain extent of international influence.

After the formation of the universal health insurance system, Japan continued to make adjustments according to the actual conditions of its economy and healthcare needs.

In 1973, free healthcare was provided to the elderly, tuberculosis patients, and patients with psychiatric disorders. Since the 1980s, the acceleration of population aging, the continuous improvement of medical science and technology, and the diversification of people's demand for health services led to a rise in healthcare expenditures. In particular, healthcare expenditure for the elderly accounted for an increasing proportion of total costs, which led to increasingly prominent financial problems for health insurance. On top of these problems, a slump in the national economy weakened the government's ability to compensate the health insurance system, which further exacerbated its health insurance's financial difficulties. Therefore, based on its original universal insurance system, Japan undertook a series of adjustments to its health insurance and to the healthcare and welfare system for the elderly to ensure that citizens have equal access to, and free choice in, the health services they receive. In addition, Japan has also strengthened its healthcare cost-containment efforts, including exerting control over supply and demand, by, for example, increasing the copayment ratios of individuals.

At the turn of the twenty-first century, under the pressure of population aging, Japan began to focus on developing community-based care for the elderly as an important measure to ease the financial burden on health insurance. To further clarify the copayment ratios of healthcare costs, the piece-rate system was replaced by a fixed-amount system for the implementation of managed health insurance. In terms of health insurance for the elderly, long-term care insurance that aimed to transfer the long-term care of elderly patients from the hospital to the community (i.e., at home, elderly welfare homes, and elderly healthcare facilities) was introduced.

Japan's health insurance can be roughly divided into two categories: employee insurance and community (regional) insurance. Employee insurance includes government-managed health insurance (mainly for small- to medium-sized enterprises), industry-managed health insurance (mainly for large enterprises), mutual aid insurance (for national civil servants, local civil servants, and private school personnel), and seaman's insurance. Japan's health insurance belongs to the category of social health insurance. It is mandatory, and individuals cannot choose the type of insurance in which they enroll, which is determined by their occupations.

The funding sources for the various health insurance organizations are mainly the insurance premiums paid by employers and employees, and the national and local governments provide certain subsidies based on the composition of insured persons in each health insurance organization. As the composition and health levels of insured persons differ across insurance organizations, there are also variations in the premium amounts paid.

The health insurance service providers (hospitals, clinics, and pharmacies) and staff (physicians and pharmacists) have all signed contracts with health insurance organizations specifying the health insurance term limit and the range of the area covered. The contracts are jointly approved by insurance organizations and local governments. As all healthcare institutions have signed contracts to provide insured services, insured persons can seek medical treatment from any hospital or clinic.

Japan established health insurance systems for the elderly and retirees in 1983 and 1984, respectively. The purpose of implementing a health insurance system for the elderly is to provide the elderly with a comprehensive range of healthcare services, including disease prevention, treatment, and rehabilitation. In addition, it allows the uneven burden among health insurance systems caused by differences in the proportion of elderly persons to be adjusted, thus ensuring equality of health insurance to a wider extent.

The national healthcare cost in Japan is increasing at a rate of about 6% per year, reaching ¥34 trillion in 2002. Of this cost, healthcare expenditure for the elderly has been increasing at a rate of 8% per year. The healthcare cost per capita for the elderly is five times that for other groups, and the healthcare expenditure of individuals over 70 years old accounts for one third of the national healthcare expenditure.

1.Health System

In terms of function, the Japanese health system is mainly composed of the service provision system (healthcare institutions and healthcare workers) and the management system (medical and healthcare management system).

(1) Status of Healthcare Institutions

Healthcare institutions with at least 20 beds are known as hospitals, and those without beds or with fewer than 19 beds are known as clinics. According to the provisions of the Medical Care Act, hospitals must provide scientific and reasonable treatment to injured or sick persons and should possess excellent facilities and equipment. However, there are no strict requirements for clinic facilities. The Hospital Medical Care Act differentiates between general hospitals and other hospitals in terms of staffing standards, facility standards, and management-level responsibilities.

The classification of hospitals in Japan based on ownership could yield as many as 25 types. However, hospitals are customarily divided into national hospitals (run by central government departments such as the Ministry of Health, Ministry of Culture, and Ministry of Labor), public hospitals (run by local governments), and private hospitals. Hospitals can also be classified according to healthcare function into general hospitals, specialist hospitals, regional healthcare auxiliary hospitals, psychiatric hospitals, and tuberculosis hospitals. General hospitals are those with more than 100 beds, complete medical departments (i.e., they must include internal medicine, surgery, obstetrics and gynecology, pediatrics, ophthalmology, otorhinolaryngology, and so on), and equipment and facilities that meet certain standards (i.e., they must contain chemical, microbiological, and pathological testing equipment; an autopsy room; research laboratories; classrooms; a library; and other facilities stipulated by the central Ministry of Health).

According to the "Dynamic Survey of Medical Institutions" by the MHLW, as of the end of March 2008, Japan had 176,215 healthcare institutions of various types (Table 12.16), which included 8,832 hospitals (5%), 99,455 general clinics (56.4%), and 67,928 dental clinics (38.5%). The total number of healthcare institutions showed an increasing trend from 2000 to 2008. Among these institutions, the number of hospitals has tended to decrease, whereas the number of clinics has tended to increase. According to the types of

TABLE 12.16   Number of Different Healthcare Institutions in Japan in 2000–2008
(Unit: Institutions)

Healthcare Institutions	2000	2002	2004	2006	2008
Hospitals	9,266	9,187	9,077	8,943	8,832
Of which: Psychiatric hospitals	1,058	1,069	1,076	1,072	1,077
Tuberculosis sanatoriums	3	2	2	1	1
General hospitals	8,205	8,116	7,999	7,870	7,754
General clinics	92,824	94,819	97,051	98,609	99,455
Dental clinics	63,361	65,073	82,286	67,392	67,928
Total	165,451	169,079	172,685	174,944	176,215

Source: Dynamic Survey of Medical Institutions by the Ministry of Health, Labour and Welfare (conducted annually on October 1; data from end of March 2008).

services provided, there are currently 7,754 general hospitals, 1,077 psychiatric hospitals, and 1 tuberculosis hospital in Japan.

Government-run hospitals include national hospitals, various public hospitals, and hospitals run by social insurance and other related groups. Such hospitals can obtain certain financial subsidies and enjoy tax-exemption policies. Private hospitals refer to civilian-run and privately run hospitals, which must pay taxes according to regulations. As of 2008, private hospitals accounted for 80.6% of hospitals in Japan, whereas government-run hospitals accounted for only 19.4% of hospitals, and the number of beds owned by the latter accounted for 30.6% of the national total. In 2002, the average number of beds per 10,000 people was 133.4, ranking second in the world, which was higher than that in many other developed countries, including the US. By 2009, Japan had an average of 139 beds per 10,000 people.

Since 1960, Japan has gradually established several high-level medical centers for special diseases, including the National Cerebral and Cardiovascular Center and the National Cancer Center. Many prefectures have also established prefectural cancer prevention and treatment centers and adult disease centers. A few large cities have also established children's medical centers and maternal and child health centers. Furthermore, dedicated healthcare facilities for individuals over the age of 65 have also been set up.

There are 104 teaching hospitals in medical schools, of which 44 are state-owned, 11 are public, and 49 are private; there are also 6 hospitals affiliated with university research institutes. Teaching hospitals are generally equipped with a large number of advanced medical instruments and have an average of 486 beds per teaching hospital. The main purpose of teaching hospitals is to teach and train medical undergraduates and graduate students. The state has also designated 179 teaching hospitals for post-graduate medical residency training.

National hospitals are invested in and built by the state. Their funds mainly come from the central government, followed by funding from social health insurance programs and payments by patients. The main sources of funding for public hospitals are local governments, and the remaining sources are the same as those for national hospitals. National and public hospitals can obtain various annual subsidies from the state and local governments to pay for labor, infrastructure, equipment, and so on. The law stipulates the "self-funding principle" for hospitals; that is, hospitals should cover recurring expenses using income from providing inpatient healthcare services. In addition to undertaking healthcare work, hospitals and outpatient institutions are also required to actively undertake public health work, which is self-funded by the healthcare sector. Most private hospitals have private capital, but they may also receive government loans. The pension welfare service public mutual aid association of the medical care fundraising association may also provide long-term, low-interest loans to private hospitals. The responsibility for fundraising, payment collection, and debt repayment of private hospitals rests with private individuals. One of the main financing avenues is through healthcare income. Medical funds are fully financed by the government and form medical fund institutions (corporate bodies) to provide long-term, low-interest loans to private hospitals, clinics, and so on for the acquisition of equipment and the improvement of service levels. It is difficult for other financial institutions to provide such low-interest loans.

The vast majority of hospitals in Japan are nonprofit and are built with investments from state or local governments. Individual contributions to health insurance comprise 70% of investment in hospitals, and government subsidies comprise 30%. These subsidies are mainly used for the acquisition of large-scale medical devices and equipment, building repairs, and covering hospital operating deficits. The current level of healthcare services in Japan is relatively high. However, there is also an uneven distribution of healthcare institutions, leading to the overconcentration of institutions and, thus, the over-provision of healthcare services in certain areas. In contrast, certain mountainous areas, smaller islands, and peripheral regions have too few healthcare institutions, which are insufficient to meet the healthcare needs of these areas.

(2) Status of Healthcare Workers

1. Composition of Healthcare Workers

1. *Clinical physicians.* In 2002, the number of registered physicians in Japan was 261,806, the number of physicians per 100,000 people was 192.5, and the average number of people served per physician was 520. Physicians practicing in healthcare institutions accounted for 95.6% of the total, of whom 30.1% were founders or legal representatives of hospitals and clinics and 65.5% were employees of healthcare institutions. Physicians working in education and research institutions accounted for 2.1% (4,857) of all physicians. In 2008, there were 286,699 registered physicians in Japan, and the number of physicians per 100,000 people was 224.5 (Table 12.17).

2. *Dentists.* At the end of 2002, there were 87,624 registered dentists in Japan, with 97.5% practicing at dental healthcare institutions. Of them, 62.9% were founders or legal representative of dental institutions, and 201 were engaged in administrative and public health work. By 2008, Japan had a total of 99,426 registered dentists, and the number of dentists per 100,000 people was 77.9, as shown in Table 12.17.

3. *Pharmacists.* At the end of 2002, there were 202,400 registered pharmacists in Japan; the number of pharmacists per 100,000 people was 155.6; and the number of people served per pharmacist was 645. Of this total, 74.4% practiced in pharmacies, 24.3% practiced in hospitals and clinics, and another 1.3% were engaged in research. By 2008, Japan had a total of 267,751 registered pharmacists, and the number of pharmacists per 100,000 people was 209.7, as shown in Table 12.17.

4. *Public health nurses, midwives, and nurses.* As of the end of 2002, there were 28,841 public health nurses in Japan, of whom 28.1% practiced in public health centers, 49.5% practiced in street and village health centers, 5.1% practiced in hospitals, and 4.3% practiced in clinics.

TABLE 12.17   Changes in the Number of Clinical Physicians, Dentists, and Pharmacists in 1960–2000 in Japan (Unit: persons)

Type of Physician	Indicators	1960	1970	1980	1990	2000	2008
Clinical physician	Total number	103,131	118,990	156,235	211,797	255,792	286,699
	Number per 100,000 people	110.4	114.7	133.5	171.3	201.5	224.5
Dentist	Total number	33,177	37,859	53,602	74,028	90,857	99,426
	Number per 100,000 people	35.5	36.5	45.8	59.9	71.6	77.9
Pharmacist	Total number	60,257	79,393	116,056	150,627	217,477	267,751
	Number per 100,000 people	64.5	76.5	99.1	121.9	171.3	209.7

Source: "Survey of Physicians, Dentists, and Pharmacists," Statistics and Information Section, Minister's Secretariat, Ministry of Health, Labour and Welfare, 2009.

The number of practicing midwives in the country was 24,683, of whom 10.8% practiced in midwifery homes, 71.8% practiced in hospitals, and 10.8% practiced in clinics.

As of the end of 2002, there were 1,108,463 practicing nurses in Japan, and the ratio of physicians to nurses was 1:4. Among them, 74.9% practiced in hospitals and 18.4% practiced in clinics.

2. Training and Education of Healthcare Workers

1. *Residency training system.* (1) *Medical education and residency training.* According to the Medical Practitioners' Act, physicians seeking to engage in clinical work must undertake at least two years of residency training in a university hospital with a medical training course or a hospital designated by the MHLW. (2) *Basic concept of residency training.* Residency training must enable physicians to develop good clinical work attitudes and to acquire basic diagnostic and treatment skills. (3) *Implementation status.* As of April 1, 2009, a total of 2,372 specialized residency training hospitals and 135 university hospitals have participated in the resident training system.
2. *Physician training, licensing, and further education.* Japan currently has 80 medical colleges (including medical schools in general universities), of which 43 are national medical colleges, 8 are public, and 29 are private. Table 12.18 shows the supply and demand of Japanese physicians from 2000 to 2025. In the future, the supply of physicians in Japan will exceed its demand; that is, Japan's local medical education is able to meet the demands of its domestic health services for physicians. By 2025, the median difference between the supply and demand of physicians will be 16,000.

   Medical education in Japan involves a six-year system for medicine and dentistry followed by four years of specialty education after graduation. In 1964, the internship and national medical examination systems were introduced from the US. High school graduates are required to pass an examination to enter medical schools, where they receive two years of preclinical education followed by four years of clinical education. After graduation, they must pass the National Examination for Physicians and be approved by the relevant department to obtain a medical license. In 1968, the internship system was abolished, and the Medical Practitioners' Act was amended to require medical graduates who have obtained medical licenses to undertake another two or more years of specialist residency training. Specialist residents must practice in teaching hospitals or hospitals designated by the MHLW. In accordance with Article 5 of the Medical Practitioners' Act, physicians must pass the National Examination for Physicians and be granted a medical license by the Minister of Health in order to obtain their medical qualifications.

TABLE 12.18 Supply and Demand of Japanese Physicians in 2000–2025 (Unit: 1,000 people)

Year	Demand			Supply		
	Lower Quartile	Median	Upper Quartile	Lower Quartile	Median	Upper Quartile
2000	244	249	280	258	263	267
2005	247	260	290	266	276	285
2010	247	270	295	275	289	302
2015	244	278	297	292	301	318
2025	233	291	348	305	305	344

Private practitioners have always played a major role in Japan. The implementation of the universal health insurance system relies heavily on private practitioners to provide healthcare services. Private practitioners are generally graduates of medical school who have also obtained a "Doctor of Medicine" degree after studying for four or more years. Private practitioners have a high level of prestige in the community, and the country's health policies are also adapted to private practice. The vast majority of private practitioners form the backbone of the regional medical associations and the Japan Medical Association. The Japan Medical Association is an authoritative medical group in Japan. All regions have also established voluntary unions of professional institutions that have played major roles in professional and academic development.

The clinical training of physicians is divided into three stages: undergraduate studies, postgraduate training, and lifelong learning (continuing education). Article 16 of the Medical Practitioners' Act stipulates that physicians shall strive to undertake two years of advanced clinical training, which shall take place at a university hospital designated by the MHLW, after obtaining their medical licenses. The state provides training subsidies to the university hospitals and designated hospitals that provide advanced training. Furthermore, in order to cultivate excellent general practitioners, more funding is provided to trainees studying multiple disciplines. In 1998, the MHLW established regional medical training centers in 15 national healthcare institutions, 11 public healthcare institutions, and two public-welfare corporations as sites for the lifelong learning of physicians.

3. *Dentist training, examination, and further education.* In 1998, there was a total of 29 dental colleges and medical schools in Japan, of which 11 were national, 1 was public, and 17 were private. The number of current students was 3,005. In accordance with Japan's "Dental Practitioners' Act," after passing the national examination and receiving a dental license, dentists generally must undertake one year of clinical training. The training sites are university hospitals and dental hospitals designated by the MHLW.

3. Physician Wage Management   Physician wages in Japan are controlled by the government's macroeconomic policies. According to the Hospital Act, groups, legal persons, and individuals applying to set up hospitals and clinics must list the wage level standards for all healthcare workers in the application, which is then submitted to the local governor (or mayor) for review and approval.

Physician wages in Japan are characterized by the following features. Physician wages are higher than those of other industries. The wages of physicians in private hospitals are higher than those of physicians in national and public hospitals. The wages of physicians with mobile professions are higher than those of fixed, salaried physicians.

(3) Healthcare Management System

1. National Health Administration System   The national-level health administration department is known as the MHLW. The management of healthcare by the MHLW is mainly through the formulation of relevant rules and regulations, health policies, and proposals for the amendment of relevant laws. Its main tasks are as follows. (1) *Health and medical services.* This task involves formulating disease prevention measures, improving environmental health, providing adequate facilities for healthcare services, training healthcare workers, controlling the quality of pharmaceutical preparations, controlling narcotics, and carrying out other administrative affairs. (2) *Social welfare services.* Various methods are used to provide the poor with services to maintain a minimum standard of living; to provide financial assistance to the disabled and widowed families, thus enabling them to be self-reliant; to provide children with adequate healthcare services and preventive measures; and to resolve the growing problem of elderly care. (3) *Social health insurance*. This task involves the management and implementation of various health insurance and pension plans to reduce the personal economic burden caused by diseases, old age, and disability.

The MHLW is responsible for managing national hospitals, sanatoriums, and various medical research institutions (e.g., the National Cancer Center and the National Cerebral and Cardiovascular Center).

Aside from the MHLW, the Sports Bureau of the Ministry of Education, Science, and Culture; the Labor Standards Bureau of the MHLW; and the Environment Agency also participate in health-related administrative work. Among them, the Sports Bureau of the Ministry of Education, Science, and Culture is responsible for the health administrative affairs of schools; the Labor Standards Bureau of the MHLW is responsible for the administrative affairs of labor health; and the Environment Agency is responsible for the administration of natural and man-made environmental hazards.

2. Local Health Administrations   In general, large cities with populations above one million have health and public cleaning bureaus; cities with populations above 100,000 have health bureaus (or departments); towns with populations below 100,000 have health divisions; and villages have health units.

There are 47 health-related departments and bureaus below the national level, but they have different names (including 19 Health Bureaus, 10 Environment and Healthcare Departments, 3 Health and Environment Departments, 5 Healthcare and Environment Departments, 2 Healthcare Departments, 1 Healthcare and Health Department, and 7 Health and Welfare or Welfare and Healthcare Departments). The local health departments and bureaus manage the health administrative affairs within their regions. They are responsible for the administration of healthcare, drug administration, preventive care, environmental hygiene, and food hygiene as well as running the national health insurance, reviewing applications for opening hospitals in the region, and so on. Furthermore, they are responsible for the direct management of public health centers, health research institutions, mental health centers, and other public research institutions and hospitals.

Public health centers are subordinate to the local health departments and bureaus. There are more than 850 public health centers in Japan. They serve both administrative and institutional functions, implementing health-related administrative work within their jurisdictions while also performing preventive healthcare. Public health centers are central institutions for public health activities such as disease prevention, health promotion, and environmental improvement. Their work is linked directly to the physical and mental health of residents within a specific area. The sizes of public health centers vary regionally, with public health centers under the direct jurisdiction of 31 major cities in the country and 23 special wards in Tokyo. As for other regions, it has been stipulated that, in principle, there should be one public health center for every 100,000 people. School health and meal management divisions (units) are established in the Board of Education of public schools. In private schools, this task is assumed by the executive divisions of governmental departments and bureaus. The prefectural and municipal Labor Standards Bureaus are directly under the leadership of the MHLW. Subordinate to these bureaus are the Labor Standards Inspection Offices, which are the first-line agencies for administering labor standards. Normally, these offices perform supervision and guidance in accordance with the Labor Standards Act, the Industrial Safety and Health Act, the Pneumoconiosis Act and so on, and they also handle the payment of workers' accident compensation insurance and other tasks. Cities with populations smaller than 100,000 and towns have health divisions that are sometimes combined with national health insurance affairs and are known as healthcare divisions. Villages mostly have health sections (units) or resident sections (units). In accordance with the requirements of the MHLW, health centers have been successively established in all municipalities. Health centers are not administrative institutions but venues to effectively implement various health promotion activities at the municipal level. The mission of health centers is to promote the development of the National Health Movement and provide local residents with services such as vaccination, health consultation, health education, and health checkups for areas including maternal and child health, mental health, occupational health, environmental hygiene, food hygiene, school health, and elderly healthcare.

3. Health Policy and Legislation   The Constitution of Japan states that "the State shall use its endeavors for the promotion and extension of social welfare and security and of public health." In accordance with its Constitution, the Japanese government has gradually formulated various health laws, regulations, and policies. There are currently more than 110 health laws and regulations, most of which were enacted after World War II. These laws have had a significant impact on the management of healthcare, and all levels of health administrative departments are managed according to the law. Thus far, Japan's existing laws include 9 on disease prevention; 25 on environmental hygiene; 11 on public health, health management, and health statistics; 14 on healthcare services and healthcare workers; and 9 on drugs. There is also other health legislation related to social welfare, social health insurance, and so on. In order to comprehensively implement these acts, numerous regulations and detailed rules were also formulated. In addition to the national legislation above, local governments have also formulated various regional health acts and policies in accordance with the Local Autonomy Act. The government has also established special supervision and inspection agencies.

4. Government Management of Hospitals
  1. *Legal constraints.* The law stipulates that the administrators of healthcare institutions must be physicians, the administrators of general healthcare institutions must be clinical physicians, the administrators of dental institutions must be dentists, and the administrators of midwifery homes must be obstetricians or gynecologists. The founder of a healthcare institution must personally undertake its management if he meets the criteria for an administrator. However, the founder can also to entrust its management to others given the approval of the local governor. Unless approved by the local governor, the medical staff of a healthcare institution shall not assume the role of administrator for other healthcare institutions. The Medical Care Act stipulates that the minister and local governors can, if necessary, order the health workers of healthcare institutions to submit medical records, accounting books, and other articles. Healthcare institutions must be equipped with medical personnel and facilities in accordance with the regulations of the central health authority (the MHLW).
  2. *Adjustment of distribution.* Japan's central health administration authority (the MHLW) has the power to implement large-scale system reforms to national healthcare institutions. Its basic policies include mergers, closures, and transfers, which aim to achieve the rational distribution of various healthcare institutions. Specifically, national institutions that struggle to perform due to the presence of public or private institutions of similar sizes within the same area are targets of closure. Similar national institutions within a short distance of each other are merged. National institutions that have a certain impact on the healthcare activities of local residents but could be more effectively

managed if they were transferred to local governments or private groups are subjected to the transfer of management and operation rights.

3. *Rational division of labor.* The MHLW has ordered the progressive transfer of primary and general healthcare services to public and private healthcare institutions, thus shifting the primary role of national healthcare institutions to the following objectives: (1) to perform policy-level healthcare activities, that is, to overcome diseases that pose a significant threat to the health of residents, such as cancers, cardiovascular diseases, neurological diseases, and other intractable diseases; (2) to play a leading role in the treatment of tuberculosis, severe physical and mental disorders, nutritional disorders, and leprosy and to conduct various clinical studies; (3) to provide other public and private healthcare institutions with high-precision equipment, laboratories, and technical support for healthcare and scientific research; (4) to undertake the training of clinical physicians and specialists for all levels of hospitals and the education and training of hospital administrators; and (5) to collect medical information and promote the results of medical research.

4. *Functional evaluation.* The government's functional evaluation of healthcare institutions is also a key component in its management of healthcare institutions. The evaluation criteria relate to hospitals' organizational structures, the status of facilities and equipment, the basic state and rationality of operations, the level of regional demand, the comfort of patient services and patient satisfaction, the level of medical technology, and healthcare quality.

2. Health System Issues and Reforms

(1) Issues Faced by the Health System

The ideal model of a health system is one where "everyone can receive the best treatment anytime and anywhere." However, due to limited health resources, this ideal is difficult to achieve. Nevertheless, providing the most effective healthcare possible with limited resources is an ultimate goal that every health system can achieve.

Japan's health system occupies an important position in its social security system. Following its post-war development, Japan has now achieved the highest life expectancy in the world and a high level of healthcare, and its health system has played an undeniable role in this achievement. However, after decades of development, especially since the 1990s, significant changes have taken place in the healthcare environment, including a low birth rate, rapid population aging, an economic downturn, advancements in medical technology, and changes in people's health awareness. These factors have led to urgent problems in Japan's health system (Figure 12.11).

1. Increased Healthcare Expenditure and Overburdened Health Insurance   From 1960 to 1978, the annual growth rate of Japan's national healthcare expenditure has remained above 10%, and the increase was especially large during the latter half of the 1960s to the 1970s. The reasons for the high healthcare expenditure in Japan are, first, that the implementation of universal social health insurance increased the avenues for seeking medical treatment and, second, that the costs of drugs, examinations, and other healthcare services have increased with the increase in prices and wages. Japan's excessively high drug prices are well known. Among developed countries, drug prices in Japan are 1.1 times those of the US, 1.4 times those of Germany, 2.7 times those of France, and 2.7 times those of the UK. The extensive use of expensive medical devices and equipment by Japanese hospitals is also

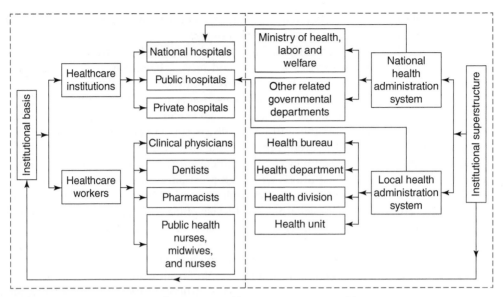

FIGURE 12.11 Framework of Japan's health system institutional basis.

another factor leading to the rise in healthcare expenditure. With the increase in the elderly population, the healthcare expenditure of the elderly accounts for a substantial proportion of overall healthcare expenditure. According to statistics by the MHLW, the average healthcare expenditure of those over 70 years old has risen by 2.5-fold, from ¥254,000 in 1977 to ¥636,000 in 1993.

The healthcare expenditure of individuals aged 0–69 years increased by 2.1-fold from ¥58,000 to ¥123,000. In 2000, Japan's national healthcare cost was approximately ¥30 trillion, one-third of which was spent on elderly healthcare. By 2008, Japan's healthcare cost had reached 8.3% of national income. According to statistics by the MHLW, total healthcare expenditure paid to healthcare institutions (national healthcare expenditure) in 2009 was ¥36.0067 trillion (about RMB 3 trillion), which represented an increase of ¥1.1983 trillion (or 3.4%).

"Social hospitalization" is also a long-standing problem of the Japanese health system. It is caused by certain elderly persons who should receive care in special nursing homes or at their own homes but who refuse to be discharged from long-term hospitalization. This issue, on the one hand, affects patients who need to be hospitalized for treatment and, on the other hand, results in idle and wasted healthcare resources. The most significant problem is that "social hospitalization" has led to a rise in health insurance costs. Based on 1996 prices, the monthly cost of elderly persons living in special nursing homes was ¥260,000, whereas the monthly cost of hospitalization was ¥430,000. Officially, these costs were paid for by health insurance but, in practice, they increased the burden on a generation of the working population. The incompleteness of the hospice care system was also a major cause for the high levels of average healthcare expenditure. The role of hospice care is to alleviate a patient's suffering, reduce the fear of death, and allow the patient to gradually accept the idea of death. However, according to a relevant report, 60% of a patient's suffering is caused by psychological factors, and the provision of careful and considerate psychological comfort can reduce 60% of a patient's suffering. This item alone can reduce the burden of drug costs. In Japan, the primary goal of hospice care is to extend life. Hence, substantial investments have been made in technology, equipment, and drugs to preserve patients' lives. The closer a patient is to death, the higher these healthcare expenditures become. Thus, this issue is also one of the major causes of the high level of hospital healthcare expenditure.

2. Low Healthcare Quality and Decline in Residents' Satisfaction Along with the increase in healthcare expenditure, the degree of trust that Japanese residents have towards the health system has also been decreasing. The incompleteness of the "three-hour waiting time, three-minute consultation" healthcare provision system, the inadequate explanations and levels of understanding provided to patients, the information asymmetry between hospitals and patients, medical accidents, and other issues have triggered people's dissatisfaction towards the quality of healthcare. According to a survey by Harvard University on Japan, Canada, Germany, the UK, and the US (Liu JX, 2002), Japan's overall satisfaction with healthcare was the lowest (at 67%), which was 20 percentage points lower than that of the second-lowest country, the UK (at 87%). Japan's low quality of hospital service is also reflected in the number of healthcare workers. In Japan, the average number of healthcare workers (including physicians, nurses, administrative staff, and technicians) serving one inpatient is 1.0, and the average length of a hospital stay for each inpatient is 30 days. In contrast, the average number of healthcare workers (excluding physicians) serving one inpatient in the US is 4.5, and the average length of a hospital stay is only 5.5–5.6 days. Thus, although the number of healthcare workers in the US is 4.5 times higher than that in Japan, the average length of a hospital stay is only one-sixth that of Japan. The average number of healthcare workers serving 1 inpatient in the UK is 3.0, and the average length of a hospital stay is about 10 days. Germany and France both have 2.5 healthcare workers serving 1 inpatient, and the length of a hospital stay is 12–13 days. Thus, it can be seen that the average number of healthcare workers serving one inpatient is inversely proportional to the length of a hospital stay.

Among developed countries, Japan is the only country where the average number of physicians and nurses serving one patient has remained unchanged compared to 30 years ago. This figure has nearly tripled in the US, France, Germany, and the UK compared to 30 years ago. This outcome is because Japan has continued to increase the number of beds, and the rate of increase in Japan is two to five times higher than those of other countries. Increasing the number of healthcare workers can reduce the length of a hospital stay and improve the efficiency of healthcare provision. Although an increase in healthcare workers would increase the unit price of healthcare expenditure, the overall costs would not increase due to the shorter hospital stay length. In recent decades, other developed countries have reduced the number of beds and the length of a hospital stay while also increasing the number of nurses and improving healthcare quality. In contrast, Japan has spent a considerable amount on the introduction of various medical devices. Currently, the numbers of CT scanners and other costly examination devices are three to seven times those of the UK and the US, and Japan accounts for nearly half of this type of equipment across OECD countries.

Japan's economy is unlikely to experience rapid development in the short term. Thus, during the process of its declining birth rate and population aging, a continuous increase in healthcare expenditure will certainly increase the burden of its citizens, which will further decrease their trust in the health system. Therefore, Japan's health system is faced with the urgent task of reform.

(2) Health System Reform

In summary, in order to adapt to these changes and provide healthcare that can meet the needs of its people, Japan has begun to undertake major reforms to its health system, which include the healthcare system, the medical pricing system, and health insurance system.

1. Basic Direction of Reform   The specific direction of Japan's health system reform is to carry out comprehensive, phased reforms of the health system; control the rise in healthcare expenditure; clearly specify the functions of healthcare institutions; improve the efficiency of healthcare institutions; and ensure the provision of healthcare to patients. With regard to the healthcare system, health management and disease prevention have been actively implemented, and information disclosure has been applied to expand patients' choices. In addition, health service functions have been subjected to differentiation and intensification to provide citizens with high-quality and efficient healthcare services. In terms of the medical payment system, a medical pricing system was established that accurately reflects advancements in medical technology and the operating costs of healthcare institutions. As for the health insurance system, the equal distribution of benefits and burdens has been achieved among various systems and generations (e.g., the retired elderly population vs. the younger working population) based on the principle of "national insurance." The integration, optimization, and expansion of insured persons was performed to establish a sustainable and stable system. In terms of the elderly healthcare system, more importance has been attached to healthcare for the elderly due to the growth of population aging. When responding to the rapid growth in healthcare expenditure for the elderly, attention was also given to the equal distribution of the burden between the generations, the focus of public funding policy shifted to latter-stage elderly persons, and insurance premiums, which have become a major pressure on insured persons, were reduced. There are three key points regarding the basic reforms of the health insurance system. (1) The scope of national security is limited to the minimum national standard of living, which combines self-responsibility with self-help. (2) The concerns of the elderly regarding their care in old age should be addressed, but the growing intergenerational inequalities should also be rectified. To this end, reforms must be implemented to the existing elderly health system to ensure an independent and stable system. (3) Market mechanisms should be introduced to improve the efficiency and quality of healthcare services through a suitable assessment of healthcare institutions and competition in service provision.

2. Specific Reform Measures   In November 1996, several Japanese councils related to social security discussed the future direction of development for the social security system. The discussion led to the conclusion that the health system should follow the following three basic principles: further improvements in the quality of healthcare services, coverage of all citizens, and effective provision of healthcare services.

Measures to improve the quality of healthcare services were as follows. (1) *The classification of healthcare institutions.* In order to better provide healthcare services and guide patients to the appropriate healthcare institutions, the functions of healthcare institutions should be explicitly stipulated, with clear divisions into general hospitals, specialist hospitals, and clinics. In addition, an appropriate pricing and payment system for healthcare expenditure should be established based on the functions of each healthcare institution. (2) *The improvement of healthcare services.* This reform was especially needed in the case of healthcare services for acute diseases. After the implementation of long-term care insurance, the coverage of care services (originally covered by health insurance) was switched to long-term care insurance. Hence, under the health insurance system, the quality of health-care services had to be improved, especially in the treatment of acute diseases, to ensure that the healthcare environment could meet its requirements. Furthermore, patients were also encouraged to receive follow-up services after treatment. (3) *The reform of the drug provision system.* (4) *Information provision.* To ensure that patients can make choices with full knowledge of the available information, a comprehensive information system must be established and provided.

In 1997, the MHLW proposed the following reforms. (1) *Revision of the payment system for healthcare expenditures.* The new payment system would merge the existing fee-for-service and DRG-based systems. The specific methods for merging would be determined according to the hospital and disease types. For example, a DRG-based payment system would be implemented for the treatment of chronic diseases, whereas a fee-for-service system would be applied to the treatment of acute diseases. (2) *Drug pricing system.* Under the current system, drug prices are based on a list approved by the MHLW. Under the new system, the ceiling price is determined based on the market price. (3) *The reform of the healthcare provision system.* To clarify the responsibilities of each healthcare institution, major hospitals will mainly provide inpatient treatment in the future. Outpatient services provided by major hospitals will have higher copayment rates. In addition, general practitioner services must be developed to control the number of beds and physicians. (4) *Revision of health insurance methods.* Currently, health insurance is based on occupations and regions, with differences in contributions and insurance premiums. This system will be reformed in the future to achieve a balance. (5) *A new elderly health insurance program will be established that will separate health insurance for the elderly from that for other groups in the future.* Under the new program, elderly persons will be required to pay premiums, but consideration will still be given to the difficulties of elderly persons with low incomes, who can still receive subsidies from the government and other health insurance. Urgent reforms are needed for elderly healthcare in Japan and the health insurance that supports it.

On November 1, 2000, due to the majority approval of the ruling coalition (consisting of the Liberal Democratic Party, Komeito, and the New Conservative Party) and the 21st-Century Club, the Health and Welfare Committee of the House of Representatives passed the Health Insurance Act and other related amendments by a forced vote. One of the key components was to change the copayments for hospital outpatient services by patients aged over 70 years from a "fixed-amount system" to a 10% "fixed-rate system." The MHLW called this measure "the first step towards reform." As for the sharp rise in healthcare expenditure, a series of policies was adopted in 2000, including the curbing of healthcare provision, the expansion of elderly care facilities, the promotion of self-care efforts, and the encouragement of the proactiveness of the private sector. To solve the problem of long-term hospitalization among the elderly, new elderly care facilities were built to meet their long-term care needs through family and community care. Healthcare expenditure is calculated by adding the number of treatments in different age groups and the number of items per treatment for different age groups. Hence, in order to achieve healthcare cost containment, one must either reduce the number of treatments or control the number of items per treatment. Because the number of treatments increases as the population ages, it would be impossible to reduce healthcare expenditure without formulating strong measures for elderly healthcare. These measures included repealing free healthcare for the elderly, introducing small copayments for insured persons, improving elderly healthcare facilities, and promoting home healthcare and home care. In order to improve healthcare quality, physicians must undertake more than two years of clinical training, and dentists must undertake more than one year. Since 2004 for physicians and 2006 for dentists, those who do not undertake training are not able to register for private practice. Furthermore, the standards for nurses allocated to general hospital beds were improved, which decreased the number of patients served by one nurse from four to three.

The MHLW announced the draft healthcare reform in September 2001. Its specific contents were as follows. (1) The individual copayment rate of health insurance was increased. Starting in 2002, persons enrolled in health insurance who seek medical treatment from healthcare institutions must pay 20% of the costs. In addition, this percentage increased to 30% in 2003. (2) "Elderly healthcare" was postponed until the age of 75 years. The recipients of Japan's existing elderly healthcare system were persons over 70 years old. After the reform, this age was raised to 75 years within 5 years. Patients over 75 years old were required to pay 10%, whereas those above a certain income level and those aged 70–74 years were required to pay 20%. (3) Residents of "special nursing homes" were required to pay for their own room rates and utility bills. In the existing long-term care insurance system, the utility bills of residents in "special nursing homes" were included in the benefits for long-term care and were paid directly by insurance. After the reform, the room rates and utility bills of residents could be borne by individuals as "hotel costs."

3. Health Insurance System

(1) Historical Evolution of the Health Insurance System

Japan was one of the first countries in the world to establish a health insurance system. Its management framework was introduced from Germany in its early stages, and certain American practices were also adopted after the Second World War. After that, a series of health laws and policies were formulated, thus forming a health insurance system that is unique to Japan.

The Japanese government formulated the first set of health insurance laws, the Health Insurance Act, in 1922. This Act covers private enterprises with more than 10 employees and marked the establishment of Japan's health insurance system. Due to the impact of natural disasters, this Act was only formally implemented in 1927. Since then, Japan's health insurance system has undergone a process of continuous practice and improvement.

In 1934, in order to expand the scope of health insurance, this Act expanded its coverage to private enterprises with more than five employees. At this point, Japan's health insurance system covered only industrial workers. In 1932, the agricultural crisis in Japan created a large demand for farmers' insurance. Hence, in 1938, Japan formulated the National Health Insurance Act, which expanded the coverage of health insurance to general citizens. In the same year, the Japanese government established the Ministry of Health and Welfare. In 1939, the Seaman's Insurance Act and Employees' Health Insurance Act were promulgated. The introduction of the four laws above expanded the coverage of health insurance from industrial workers to seamen, government employees, and so on.

Between 1948 and 1956, Japan successively enacted the National Public Servants' Mutual Aid Association Act and the Private School Personnel Mutual Aid Association Act, which covered national public servants, local public servants, and private school personnel, thus including employees of public enterprises under the coverage of health insurance. In 1958, the National Health Insurance Act was fully amended to include farmers and other self-employed persons who were still outside the scope of health insurance. In 1961, the National Health Insurance Act was amended to impose mandatory health insurance for all Japanese people; that is, all citizens were covered by the health insurance system.

This explanation describes the development process of the initial establishment of Japan's health insurance system. The composition of this system was subsequently divided into two major components: Employees' Health Insurance and National Health Insurance. These two major components each had their own development trajectories.

1. In 1942, in order to eliminate cases of duplicate insurance, the Employees' Health Insurance was unified, and healthcare payments for the dependents of employees were legalized (the ratio of insurance payments was 50%). In 1947, the Health Insurance Act abolished health insurance payments for work-related accidents. In 1953, as part of the Employees' Health Insurance, the "Day Laborers' Health Insurance Act" was introduced. In 1954, treasury support mechanisms began to be introduced to the government-administered Employees' Health Insurance. Thereafter, from 1956 to 1973, the Japanese economy entered a period of rapid growth, and the government began to implement its health insurance goals, which were centered on National Health Insurance; hence, there were minimal changes to the Employees' Health Insurance during this period. In 1971, the government proposed to "improve national welfare and rectify the mistake of neglecting to enhance the lives of citizens in high-growth policies." Under the guidance of these ideas, the government made epochal amendments to the Employees' Health Insurance. The treasury burden of the government-administered Employees' Health Insurance was fixed (at 10% or more), the insurance payment for dependents was increased to 70%, and a system for high-cost medical care was introduced. In 1984, due to ever-increasing healthcare expenditures, another round of major amendments was made to the Employees' Health Insurance to equalize the payments and contributions of the health insurance system. The contribution rate by insured persons was increased to 10%, and the standards for the Day Laborers' Health Insurance were unified. In 1992, the government-administered Employees' Health Insurance adopted medium-term financial operations. The Employees' Health Insurance was gradually refined through these major amendments.

2. The National Health Insurance was implemented in July 1938. The main implementation bodies were the municipal governments and the mutual aid associations voluntarily established by occupational units. In 1948, in response to the difficulties in health insurance caused by post-war economic chaos, the National Health Insurance underwent a major revision whereby mutual aid associations were replaced by municipal public administrations to implement the mandatory enrollment of insured persons. The Social Insurance Medical Fee Payment Fund, which integrated the insurance review and payment of medical fees, was created. In addition, the copayment system was restored, and premium rates were increased. In 1958, the National Health Insurance Act was fully amended to promote social health insurance, and the payment rate of social health insurance was fixed at 50%. In 1961, the National Health Insurance was promoted nationwide. In 1963, the payment rate for persons insured by the National Health Insurance was increased to 70%. In 1968, the same benefits were given to the dependents of insured persons. In 1988, the basic insurance stabilization system was established. In 1990, the treasury expanded its subsidies for the National Health Insurance and strengthened its regulatory functions. Japan's social health insurance system, which covered all citizens, improved day by day and eventually became a reliable health security system for Japanese citizens.

(2) Development of the Health Security Act

Japan first became an aging society in 1970, and the number of people over 65 years old reached 10.65 million in 1980. In response to the challenges of population aging and the low birth rate, Japan's health security legislation has undergone major adjustments surrounding these issues. In 1972, the Japanese government fully amended the Elderly Welfare Act and implemented a free healthcare system for the elderly. In 1973, the Health Insurance Act was further amended to increase dependents' payments of medical expenses to 70%, and a high-cost medical fee payment system was established. In addition, the ad hoc treasury subsidies to the government-administered health insurance fund were designated as treasury subsidies to the permanent budget for the first time, and the subsidy rate was above 10%.

Since the 1980s, the Health Insurance Act and the National Health Insurance Act underwent multiple revisions to address this problem. In 1980, the Health Insurance Act increased dependents' medical payments for hospitalization to 80%, revised the floating range for the upper limit of the standard remuneration scale, and amended the cap on insurance premiums. In addition, the "Special System for Retired Insured Persons," the "National Health Insurance System for Retired Persons," and the "Health Insurance System for Specific Industries" were created in succession. In 1982, the Japanese government enacted the Elderly Healthcare Act, which separated bedridden persons over 65 years old and elderly persons over 70 years old from the National Health Insurance and incorporated them within the scope of this Act. In 1984, the Health Insurance Act made significant changes to health insurances that provided greater medical benefits than the National Health Insurance. The health insurance benefits for employees were reduced from 100% of incurred expenses to 80%; copayments borne by retirees for outpatient and hospitalization expenses were 20%; and copayments borne by dependents of employees were 30% for outpatient expenses and 20% for hospitalization expenses. However, the rate of population aging had far exceeded the expected level in the initial design of the system. Hence, to ease the pressure on the elderly health and medical services fund, in 1986 the Japanese government had no choice but to revise the free healthcare system stipulated in the Elderly Healthcare Act, which increased the copayments and raised the percentage of costs paid by the insured. In 1988, Japan amended the National Health Insurance Act to create the "insurance fiscal adjustment system" and "special adjustment system." The insurance fiscal adjustment system refers to contributions by municipalities equivalent to 10% of medical expenses to establish an adjustment fund, which is used to balance the actual burden among regions. The special adjustment system provides for reductions of health insurance premiums for low-income groups.

In the 1990 amendment of the National Health Insurance Act, provisions relating to the expansion of treasury support, the strengthening of fiscal adjustment functions, and the rational adjustment of the treasury burden in the elderly healthcare fund were added. In 1991, Japan amended the Elderly Healthcare Act to reduce copayments and introduce price-floating mechanisms, increase the proportion of nursing care in public spending, and establish a visiting nursing system for the elderly.

In 1994, corresponding amendments were also made to the Health Insurance Act. These amendments involved reforming health insurance benefits related to accompanying care and nursing and promoting home healthcare. In addition, the Council of Elderly Healthcare and Social Welfare was established.

In 2000, the Long-Term Care Insurance Act was implemented to provide long-term care exclusively for the elderly. In 2002, the Elderly Healthcare Act and its implementation order were amended once again. These amendments involved increasing the copayments for elderly healthcare, raising the age for insurance beneficiaries to 75 years, adjusting out-of-pocket expenses, abolishing the fixed-amount selection system, adjusting the limits for copayments, and abolishing the upper limit and adjusting the lower limit for elderly enrollment rates related to the estimation of elderly healthcare financing. The most recent revision to Japan's Health Insurance Act was the "Outline of Health System Reforms" promulgated by the government in June 2006. This outline mainly involved three types of amendments to the Health Insurance Act: the rationalization of healthcare expenditures, the establishment of a new healthcare system for the elderly, and the reorganization and integration of insurers.

(3) Current Status of the Health Insurance System

1. Basic Health Insurance System   After nearly 50 years of development, Japan's health insurance system has become self-contained. It consists of two independent health insurance systems: industrial insurance for salaried employees and regional insurance for farmers and individual industrial and commercial households. The Employees' Health Insurance, which covers the majority of the population, can be divided into seven categories. It includes the Union Managed Health Insurance for large enterprises with more than 700 employees (equivalent to a trade union); the Government Managed Health Insurance for small- to medium-sized enterprises with fewer than 700 employees; and separate health insurance systems for temporary workers, seamen, national public servants, local public servants, and private school personnel.

According to statistics by the MHLW from July 2008, a total of 128.81 million people in the country have enrolled in various health insurance programs. Among them, the National Health Insurance covers the largest number of people (about 51.27 million), followed by the Government Managed Health Insurance (about 35.94 million), and the Union Managed Health Insurance (about 30.47 million). Another 9.44 million people are enrolled in mutual aid association insurance, and about 13 million are enrolled in the Senior Citizens' Health Insurance. In addition, about 160,000 people are enrolled in the Seaman's Insurance, and 1.53 million are enrolled in other livelihood protection systems.

1. *Government Managed Health Insurance.* The number of people covered by the Government Managed Health Insurance is second only to the National Health Insurance, and it is the second-largest health insurance system in Japan. Its main targets are the employees of small- to medium-sized enterprises, and it has only one insurer in the country, the Social Insurance Agency.

The out-of-pocket healthcare expenses of those insured by the Government Managed Health Insurance was originally 20%, but it was revised to 30% in April 2003. The statutory general premium rate is 8.2% (half each paid by the company and the employee) of the average wage grade (including bonuses), but it can be adjusted by the MHLW to between 6.6% and 9.1%, subject to a review by the Social Insurance Council.

The income of the Government Managed Health Insurance includes premium revenues, treasury subsidies, and other sources. In 2006, the total income of the Government Managed Health Insurance was ¥6.9487 trillion, the total expenditure was ¥6.837 trillion, and the surplus for that year was ¥111.7 billion. As of the end of 2006, the Government Managed Health Insurance Fund had accumulated a surplus of ¥498.3 billion. From 1993 to 2003, the Government Managed Health Insurance had an annual deficit for 10 consecutive years. In 2008, the budget for the Government Managed Health Insurance system was ¥825.4 billion.

2. *National Health Insurance.* The National Health Insurance is the health insurance system that covers the largest population in Japan's health security system. It mainly targets farmers, individual industrial and commercial households, and unemployed persons. Health insurance services are provided by the municipalities in which the insured persons reside.

   Although the National Health Insurance Act was enacted in 1938, the national treasury only began to subsidize this system in 1955. After the Act was amended in 1958, the out-of-pocket medical expenses of the insured were limited to 50%, and were further limited to 30% after 1963. In 1968, the dependents of the insured also began to enjoy the benefits of having their out-of-pocket expenses limited to 30%.

   The National Health Insurance generally takes two forms: the National Health Insurance Union for unions of self-employed persons in a given industry (e.g., physicians, dentists, pharmacists, and so on) and municipal National Health Insurance. Of these two forms, the municipal National Health Insurance forms the main body of the National Health Insurance. As of July 2008, the number of insurers under municipal National Health Insurance was 1,818 and the number of people insured was 51.27 million, accounting for 36.8% of the total number of people enrolled in health insurance. The number of people enrolled in the National Health Insurance Union during the same period was only 3.89 million.

3. *Union Managed Health Insurance.* Since April 2003, the out-of-pocket expenses of those covered by Union Managed Health Insurance have been 30% of their total healthcare expenses, and that of their dependents has also been 30%. As of the end of 2006, the average premium rate for all health insurance unions was 7.484%, with employers and individuals bearing rates of 4.149% and 3.335%, respectively. In 2006, the total income of Union Managed Health Insurance was ¥6.0077 trillion, the total expenditure was ¥5.7708 trillion, and the surplus of that year was ¥236.8 billion. In 2008, the subsidy budget given by the national treasury to Union Managed Health Insurance was ¥500 million.

   Union Managed Health Insurance mainly targets large enterprises with more than 700 employees, and the insurers are the individual health insurance unions. As of December 2008, there were 1,497 insurers within Union Managed Health Insurance, 272 of which were comprehensive health insurance unions.

4. *Mutual Aid Association Insurance.* The mutual aid association insurance system can be divided into seaman's mutual aid association insurance, national public servants mutual aid association insurance, local public servants mutual aid association insurance, and private school personnel mutual aid association insurance.

   1. The seaman's mutual aid insurance system was established in 1939 according to the Seaman's Insurance Act, with the state serving as the insurer. In July 2008, the total number of insured seamen in the country was about 160,000. In 2006, the premium rate for seamen was 9.1% of the standard monthly wage (half of which was by the seaman and half by the ship owner).

   2. The national public servants' mutual aid insurance system was established in 1948 according to the National Public Servants Mutual Aid Association Act, with the mutual aid associations of each central government agency serving as the insurers. As of the end of 2006, there was a total of 21 mutual aid associations in the country. The number of insured persons was 1.11 million people, the number of dependents was 1.42 million people, and the average number of dependents per insured person was 1.27. The premium rate is adjusted by each mutual aid association according to the state of income and expenditure, and, hence, varies across government agencies. In 2006, the lowest premium rate was 5.51%, and the highest was 8.60%.

3. The local public servants' mutual aid insurance system was established in 1962 according to the Local Public Servants Mutual Aid Association Act, with the mutual aid associations of each local public organization serving as the insurers. As of the end of 2006, there were a total of 54 mutual aid associations in the country. The number of insured persons was 2.87 million people, the number of dependents was 3.47 million people, and the average number of dependents per insured person was 1.21. The Local Public Servants Mutual Aid Association Insurance is the same as the National Public Servants Mutual Aid Association Insurance in that the premium rate is adjusted by each mutual aid association according to the income and expenditure for that year.

The premium rate in 2006 was 8.72%.

4. The private school personnel's mutual aid insurance system was established in 1953 according to the Private School Personnel Mutual Aid Association Act, with the unified Japan Private School Revitalization Mutual Aid Association serving as the insurer. As of the end of 2006, the number of insured persons was 470,000 people, the number of dependents was 370,000 people, and the average number of dependents per insured person was 0.79. The premium rate is currently 7.37%.

5. *Elderly Healthcare System.* The elderly healthcare system is a new health security system established in 1983 to cope with the challenges of population aging and to achieve a balance among various systems, especially given the difference in the payment levels for elderly healthcare expenses in the National Pension System. This system mainly targets persons over 70 years of age (in exceptional circumstances, such as in the case of being bedridden, individuals can also use this system from the age of 65 years).

Of the total expenses (apart from those borne by the patient), 42% are paid by subsidies from the central treasury and local governments, and the remaining 58% are shared among various health insurance systems. The elderly healthcare system has significantly evened out the differences in payment levels among various systems.

2. *Comparison of Municipal National Health Insurance, Government Managed Health Insurance, and Union Managed Health Insurance* The region-based municipal National Health Insurance and the employment-based Government Managed Health Insurance and Union Managed Health Insurance currently form the main body of Japan's health security system. The total number of people covered by these three insurance systems is 117.68 million, accounting for 88.47% of the total population. They are also the three largest systems in the "universal insurance" system. Table 12.19 shows the comparison of the municipal National Health Insurance, Government Managed Health Insurance, and Union Managed Health Insurance with regard to the number of insurers; the types, number, and average age of insured persons; the adjusted premiums per household; the national treasury burden; and healthcare expenditure per capita.

(4) Reforms of the Health Insurance System

1. Background of Health Insurance Reforms

1. *Changes in population structure.* According to the 1997 population statistics and projections for Japan published by the National Institute of Population and Social Security, by 2050 Japan's average life expectancy will be 79.43 years for men and 86.47 years for women. The population birth rate is expected to decline from 1.42 in 1995 to 1.38 in 2000 and then gradually increase until 2030 and stabilize at 1.61. Therefore, the elderly population will increase, and the working population will decrease. According to the projections, the population over 65 years old will increase

TABLE 12.19 Comparison of Municipal National Health Insurance, Government Managed Health Insurance, and Union Managed Health Insurance

Item	Municipal National Health Insurance	Government Managed Health Insurance	Union Managed Health Insurance
Number of insurers (end of March 2007)	1,818	1	1,541
Insured persons	Self-employed, farmers, and so on	Mainly employees of SMEs	Mainly employees of large enterprises
Number of insured persons (end of March 2007)	47.38 million	35.94 million (19.50 insured persons and 16.44 dependents)	30.47 million (15.46 insured persons and 15.02 dependents)
Average age of insured persons[1] (2006)	55.2 years (44.6 years)	37.4 years (35.0 years)	34.3 years (33.1 years)
Percentage of elderly insured persons[2] (end of March 2007)	22.5%	3.9%	1.80%
Adjusted premiums per household[3] (2006)	¥155,000	¥170,000 (¥341,000)	¥187,000 (¥415,000)
Treasury burden (healthcare)	43% of payment amount, and so on	13% of payment amount (16.4% of elderly healthcare premiums)	Fixed amount (budget subsidy)
Healthcare expenses per capita[4] (2005)	¥174,000	¥117,000	¥101,000

Note:
(1) The figures in parentheses do not include the data of insured persons over 70 years old.
(2) Includes bedridden individuals over 65 years old.
(3) The figures in brackets are the contributions paid by the employer.
(4) Excludes the values for recipients of elderly healthcare.
Source: Ministry of Health, Labour and Welfare, The "Overview of the Health Insurance System in Japan" published on July 4, 2008.

from 18 million in 1995 to 32 million in 2050, the working population aged 15–64 years will decrease from 87 million in 1995 to 55 million in 2050, and the proportion of the population over 65 years in the total population will increase from 14.5% in 1995 to 27.4% in 2025 and 32.3% in 2050. The acceleration of population aging and the decreasing proportion of children in the population have had a profound impact on Japan's social security. By 2025, the burden of social security contributions as a share of national income is expected to increase from 29% to 35.5%.

2. *Deterioration of health insurance income and expenditure.* In 1995, national healthcare expenditure had reached ¥27.2 trillion, accounting for more than 7% of the national income, and it continued to increase at an annual rate of 6%. The healthcare expenditure of the elderly population was about ¥8.9 trillion, accounting for one-third of the total healthcare expenditure, and it continued to increase at an annual rate of 8% after 1995. Due to the slow growth in national income (annual growth rate of about 1%) and the inability to drastically increase income from contributions, deficits began to appear in the health insurance programs. For example, the deficit of the Government Managed Employees' Health Insurance program in 1996 was more than ¥5 trillion. As for the Union Managed Employees' Health Insurance program,

1,137 health insurance agencies (more than 60% of the total) had deficits in 1995. The government-managed health insurance had accumulated a deficit of ¥1.5 trillion in 1996, which was reduced to ¥300 billion by the end of the year. In addition, among the National Health Insurance programs managed by local governments, more than 60% of municipalities were in deficit.

The fundamental cause for the deficit in health insurance is the unbalanced development between healthcare expenditure and the national economy. In 1995, healthcare expenditure reached ¥27 trillion, and the amount per capita was ¥220,000. The annual growth rate was 5–6%. In the meantime, the economy remained in a sluggish state. Since 1992, the growth rate of national income has fluctuated around a low level of 1%, which inevitably led to the slow growth of income-based health insurance premiums. Thus, in the face of increasing healthcare expenditure, the deterioration of health insurance deficits was unavoidable.

Of the rise in healthcare expenditure, the increase in that of the elderly population is the most prominent, as it is growing at an annual rate of 8%. In 2004, the healthcare expenditure of the elderly population (aged over 70 years) accounted for one-third of the national healthcare expenditure. With the continued exacerbation of population aging, the increase in elderly healthcare expenditure will inevitably persist. It has been estimated that health insurance premiums will increase from 8.2% of national income in 2004 to 20% in 2025. Thus, we can see that the rapid rise in elderly healthcare expenditure is the main cause of increase in overall healthcare expenditure, which in turn has led to financial deficits and operational crises among insurers. Furthermore, the intensification of population aging, advancements in medical technology, and the increasing demand by patients for quality healthcare services have gradually exposed the problems in healthcare service provision, healthcare service fee standards, and the health insurance system.

2. Framework of Health Insurance Reforms   In the "National Healthcare and Health Insurance Reform Plan for the Future" (Second Report) published in July 1996 by Japan's Central Social Insurance Medical Council, future health insurance reforms were divided into three phases (Table 12.20). The first phase was until 2000, the second phase was until 2005, and the third phase was until 2010. The first phase focused on reforms of benefits and burdens. The second phase used health system reforms as the breakthrough to establish a rational system of medical fee standards. The third phase emphasized the comprehensive reform of the health insurance system and the control of overall healthcare expenditure. Health insurance reforms were divided into five types: (1) reforms of benefits and burdens, (2) structural reforms of the health insurance system, (3) reforms of fee standards, (4) reforms of the healthcare provision system, and (5) informatization and other aspects.

With the acceleration in population aging, Japan's national healthcare expenditure has recently been growing at an annual rate of 3–4%. To ensure the sustainability of the health security system, the MHLW announced the Trial Reform of Health System Structure in December 2005, which laid out the basic direction for the structural reform of the health system. The discussions between the government and the Health Care Reform Committee of the ruling party led to the conclusion of the Outline of Health System Reforms. After deliberations by the House of Representatives and the House of Councilors, it was passed on June 21, 2006. The "Outline of Health System Reforms" mainly involved three types of amendments to the Health Insurance Act: the rationalization of healthcare expenditure, the establishment of a new healthcare system for the elderly, and the reorganization and integration of insurers.

TABLE 12.20 Three-Phased Framework of Japan's Health Insurance Reforms

Item	First Phase (1997–2000)	Second Phase (2001–2005)	Third Phase (2006–2010)
Focus	The focus was on healthcare benefits, ensuring the equality of benefits and burdens, and embarking on reforms of the healthcare provision system.	The focus was on the complete reform of the healthcare provision system and the standardization of insurers' actions.	The focus was on completing the restructuring of the health insurance system and controlling the rise in overall healthcare expenditure.
Reforms of benefits and burdens	■ Emphasis on reforms of benefits ■ Reform of patients' copayments and benefits for drug costs ■ Increase in health insurance premiums	■ Deepening reforms of benefits and burdens	■ Completing the restructuring of the health insurance system ■ Controlling the rise in overall healthcare expenditure ■ Ensuring the rationalization of drug use
Reforms of the institutional structure	■ Reform of the elderly healthcare system ■ Reform of the insurance system ■ Reform of the National Health Insurance system	■ Balancing the relationship between insurers and healthcare institutions ■ Undertaking the restructuring of various health insurance systems	■ Enhancing the stability of the elderly health insurance system ■ Expanding patients' freedom of choice while also enhancing personal responsibility
Reforms of medical fee schedules	■ Reform of medical fee schedules to promote the reform of the healthcare provision system	■ Establishing medical fee payment systems that are suitable for the new healthcare provision system	■ Stabilizing the growth rate of healthcare expenditure
Reforms of the healthcare provision system	■ Elimination of social hospitalization ■ Adjustments to the number of beds and physicians ■ Functional differentiation and cooperation of healthcare institutions	■ Complete reform of the healthcare provision system, including adjustments to the number of beds	■ Reducing the average length of a hospital stay ■ Improving the overconcentration of patients in major hospitals
Informatization and other aspects	■ Use of insurance cards for health insurance identification ■ Improvement of medical information	■ Fully implementing the computerization of health insurance invoices	■ Direct signing of contracts by insurers with healthcare institutions to strengthen their supervisory functions

3. Specific Content of Reforms to the Health Insurance System   After the promulgation of the Outline of Health System Reforms in Japan, reforms were mainly implemented to address seven issues, as follows:

1. *Measures to control the growth of elderly healthcare expenditure.* In the first phase, the first measure was to establish a new elderly health insurance system, which eventually joined the Employees' Health Insurance, the National Health Insurance, and

other systems, and to reform the unified national health insurance system. The second measure was to reform the existing elderly healthcare system and to reform the transfer fund and patient copayment systems. The second phase involved the implementation of the Long-Term Care Insurance Act to improve the elderly health insurance system. The third phase aimed to ensure greater stability in the elderly health insurance system.

2. *Health insurance measures after the establishment of the long-term care insurance system.* In the first phase, the first measure was to eliminate social hospitalization, improve long-term care services, strengthen hospital consultation and guidance, adjust the number of beds, and eliminate excess beds. The second measure was to enhance the capacity for acute-phase medical treatment, adjust the standards for staff allocation, and promote the construction of single-room wards. The second phase involved the further elimination of social hospitalization. The third phase involved shortening the average length of a hospital stay.

3. *Provision of high-quality and efficient healthcare services.* The first phase involved enhancing the construction of beds in private homes, establishing community-based healthcare mutual aid networks, strengthening the functions of primary clinics, and adjusting the numbers of beds and physicians. The second phase involved the further promotion of networks among healthcare institutions and rationalizing the number of physicians. The third phase involved eliminating the "three-hour waiting time, three-minute consultation" phenomenon and improving the over-concentration of patients in major hospitals.

4. *Reforms of medical fee schedules.* The first phase involved reforming medical fees, establishing fee standards for hospitals with different functions, and switching from the existing fee-for-service system to a fixed payment system. The second phase involved stabilizing the growth rate of healthcare expenditure.

5. *Reforms of the drug pricing system.* The first phase mainly involved establishing a drug pricing system based on market prices to reduce price differences in drugs and ensure transparency in setting drug prices. In the second phase, the new drug pricing system was implemented. The third phase involved the rationalization of drug use.

6. *Reforms of the health insurance system.* In the first phase, the government managed and balanced the financial income and expenditure of health insurance and gradually adjusted the premium rates and patients' shares of out-of-pocket costs. The second phase involved implementing measures for health insurance, unifying reimbursement rates, researching measures to meet the diverse needs of patients, and undertaking reforms of premium payment methods and cash reimbursements. The third phase involved balancing the income and expenditure of health insurance, ensuring the equality of benefits and burdens, and enhancing personal responsibility while also expanding patients' freedom of choice.

7. *Promoting informatization and enhancing insurers' supervisory functions.* The first phase involved providing patients with more information, building a comprehensive medical information system, and providing insured persons with more medical information from insurers. The second phase involved the construction of a comprehensive medical information system and the establishment of an evaluation system for healthcare institutions by insurers. The third phase involved improving the quality of healthcare, strengthening the responsibility of insurers, the direct signing of contracts between insurers and healthcare institutions, and reinforcing insurers' supervisory functions.

The reform measures proposed in the Outline of Health System Reforms that have been implemented since 2006 include increasing the out-of-pocket medical expenses of elderly persons with incomes equivalent to those of employed persons from 20% to 30%, increasing the share of out-of-pocket meal and accommodation expenses for convalescent and hospitalized elderly persons, increasing copayments for high-cost medical care to a level equivalent to the total remuneration (including bonuses) while also taking low-income earners into account, and reconstructing the combined use of insured and uninsured medical treatments.

The reform measures proposed in the Outline of Health System Reforms that have been implemented since 2008 include increasing the out-of-pocket expenses of patients aged 70–74 years from 10% to 20%; reducing the percentage of out-of-pocket expenses for infant and child patients, as this percentage was previously only applicable to infants under the age of three but was since adjusted in April 2008 to include all precompulsory education infants and children; creating a new elderly healthcare system and reforming the original system, which includes establishing a later-stage elderly healthcare system targeting those over 75 years old and implementing the financial adjustment of various systems based on the number of insured persons to address the healthcare expenditures of early stage elderly persons aged 65–74 years; the corporatization of the Government Managed Health Insurance, which involves separating the insurance from the government, establishing a National Health Insurance Association, and allowing premiums to be set by prefectures based on local healthcare expenditure conditions; the reorganization of long-term care beds according to medical necessity so that they are limited only to patients with high medical needs and patients with low medical needs are transferred to residential services (e.g., nursing care apartments) or elderly healthcare facilities.

(5) Unified Reform of the Health Insurance System

Japan's current health insurance system is complex, and its operating bodies are complicated, involving different levels of contributions and benefits, which has weakened the equality of social insurance systems (e.g., of health insurance). In view of this, several experts and scholars have advocated for the unification of the various systems into a single health insurance system that will facilitate the elimination of differences in financing and benefits while also achieving risk dispersion and guaranteeing fund security.

However, the various systems have their own development characteristics, vested interest groups, accumulated assets, and self-contained management methods. Furthermore, each insurance system has also formed intricate links with the ministries, agencies, and enterprises under its jurisdiction. Hence, the unification of these systems may also affect the operational efficiency of insurance due to the increased number of insured persons and the expansion in coverage. As pointed out in the "Final Report of the Special Commission for the Unification Prevention of Fiscal Adjustment" published on December 4, 2008, by the Japan Federation of Health Insurance Organizations, it is currently unreasonable and unrealistic to achieve the unification of Japan's health insurance system.

4. Framework of the Long-Term Care Insurance System

After three years of preparation, the Japanese government formally began implementing the long-term care insurance system on April 1, 2000. The implementation of this new health security system brought about a "major revolution in the concept of long-term care" to Japanese society and citizens. The basis for the creation of this system was the severity of "low birth rate and population aging," whereas the practical cause of its creation was the accelerated increase in elderly bedridden and dementia patients.

The long-term care insurance system has gradually matured after eight years of development and improvement. As of April 2008, the number of people receiving long-term care insurance services had reached 43.8278 million, including 8.7923 million recipients of preventive care services and 35.0572 million recipients of long-term care services. The basic framework of the current long-term care insurance system consists of 10 aspects.

(1) Main Body of Long-Term Care Insurance

Currently, Japan's laws and regulations on long-term care insurance mainly include the Long-Term Care Insurance Act, the Implementation Order for the Long-Term Care Insurance Act, and the Implementation Rules for the Long-Term Care Insurance Act. The insurers of long-term care insurance mainly include municipalities. In addition, the system is also supported by the state, prefectures, health insurers, and pension insurers. The insured persons are grouped into Category 1 and Category 2. "Category 1 insured persons" refers to individuals over 65 years old. Specifically, the beneficiaries include insured persons requiring long-term care due to their bedridden state or dementia, insured persons who require special care to alleviate or prevent the deterioration of their frail state, and insured persons who require support for routine tasks such as housework and self-care. "Category 2 insured persons" refers to persons aged 40–64 years who have enrolled in health insurance. Specifically, the beneficiaries include insured persons who require long-term care and support due to 16 specific age-related diseases. These 16 specific diseases include advanced cancer, rheumatoid arthritis, amyotrophic lateral sclerosis, ossification of posterior longitudinal ligaments, fracture-induced osteoporosis, presenile dementia (dementia), Parkinson's disease and related disorders, spinocerebellar degeneration, spinal canal stenosis, progeria, multiple system atrophy, diabetic neuropathy, diabetic nephropathy, diabetic retinopathy, cerebrovascular disease, chronic obstructive pulmonary disease, and osteoarthritis with significant deformation in bilateral knee joints or hip joints.

(2) Financing and Benefits of Long-Term Care Insurance

The collection of long-term care premiums in Japan is based on the status of the insured persons. Specifically, the premiums of Category 1 insured persons are deducted before the payment of pensions. The premiums of those who cannot have them deducted directly from their pensions are collected by their respective municipalities. The premiums of Category 2 insured persons are collected through the various health insurance systems. The various municipalities entrust the review and payment of long-term care costs to the prefectural Federation of National Health Insurance Organizations (FNHIO). Care service providers are paid 90% of the costs incurred by the services provided.

The contribution standard for long-term care insurance premiums is obtained by multiplying the basic amount by the coefficient. That is, insured persons are divided into five levels based on their incomes. Levels 1–3 include insured persons or households exempt from residence taxes, and their coefficients are 0.5–1. Level 4 includes insured persons with annual incomes below ¥2.5 million, and its coefficient is 1.25. Level 5 includes insured persons with annual incomes above ¥2.5 million, and its coefficient is 1.5.

According to the statistics and projections of the MHLW, the average premium for long-term care insurance was ¥2,400 in 2000, ¥2900 in 2005, and ¥3600 in 2010.

In principle, beneficiaries of long-term care services only need to pay 10% of total care service expenses, whereas the rest is shared among the central (25%), prefectural (12.5%), and municipal (12.5%) governments, and the premium income is paid by long-term care insured persons (17% is borne by premium income from Category 1 insured persons, and 33% is borne by Category 2 insured persons). In addition, care service beneficiaries also need to pay accommodation and meal expenses to their care service providers.

(3) Services and Management of Long-Term Care Insurance

1. Daily Management of Japan's Long-Term Care Insurance Japan's long-term care insurance is a system in which the central government uniformly formulates the policies to standardize service items and benchmarks, and its operation involves the joint participation of individuals, families, communities, and local and central governments. The service recipients of long-term care insurance are elderly patients who are bedridden or have dementia. This model is a major departure from the traditional family care model for the elderly and helped to realize the socialization of family care. In addition, the services are provided by the local governments of municipalities and by civil society organizations. This provision not only helps the country play a guiding role in care services but also promotes the enthusiasm of local governments and civil society organizations in providing better care services for the elderly. However, it should also be noted that the long-term care insurance system is a product of low birth rate and population aging and the inadequate provision of social security. Hence, it still has many deficiencies. Of these issues, the most controversial are whether the transition from the original social welfare approach to the social insurance approach for the elderly is a historical regression and whether the provision of high-quality, affordable and accessible care for the elderly can be sustained. More investigation is needed to explore these issues, and further observations should be made over a longer period of time.

The formulation of the daily long-term care insurance plan is carried out by the municipalities and prefectures according to the basic guidelines for long-term care insurance stipulated by the state whereby municipal long-term care insurance plans and prefectural long-term care insurance support plans are formulated to implement the preparation of infrastructure for long-term care services.

2. Application Procedures for Basic Long-Term Care Services The application procedures for basic long-term care services are as follows. When applying for care services, applicants must first apply for a long-term care requirement certification from the municipality in which they reside. This procedure can be performed by the applicants or their family members. Applicants may also entrust their applications to local integrated support centers, home care support units (care plan development units), long-term care insurance facilities, or community-based care and welfare facilities for the elderly.

Following this step, the municipality must provide a certification of long-term care (support) requirements. The municipal Long-Term Care Certification Review Committee base their review and decision on the results of the certification investigation and the opinions of the treating physician. The results of the decision are divided into three groups: no support required, support levels 1–2 required, and care levels 1–5 required. Elderly persons who are determined as not needing care or support can use local support services, including preventive care services; integrated support services; and any other services provided by community-based integrated support centers. Elderly persons requiring support levels 1–2 can use 13 types of home preventive care services and three types of community-based preventive care services. Elderly persons requiring care levels 1-5 can use 13 types of long-term care services, 6 types of community-based care services, and 3 types of facility services.

Next, the applicant enters the formulation stage for long-term care plans. If preventive care services are required, the insured persons may entrust the planning to the local integrated support center. If in-home care services are required, they may entrust the plan to the in-home care support unit or develop a plan themselves and submit it directly to the municipality. If facility services are required, they may apply directly to the care service provider or be referred by the care manager.

Finally, the applicant enters the stage of care service utilization. The insured person may sign a contract with the care service provider after a full consultation regarding the specific service content and date, time, and expenses of utilization. If the insured person wishes to change his service content, he may negotiate directly with the care manager, local integrated support center, or service provider.

3. Payment Coverage of Long-Term Care Insurance After long-term care insurance is purchased, it can provide insured persons with two major types of services: in-home and facility long-term care services. In-home care services involve users living in their homes and receiving long-term care by visiting elderly care facilities at regular or irregular intervals or home visits by home care workers. These care services are provided on a 24-hour basis. Specifically, in-home care services include home-visit long-term care; home-visit bathing; home-visit nursing care; home-visit and facility rehabilitation training; home-visit medical care management and counseling by physicians, dentists, and pharmacists; day home care; short-stay care; care service with mutual support for elderly individuals with dementia; care service in for-profit homes; payment for the rental of welfare devices and the purchase of special equipment (e.g., special urine collection devices); payment for home renovations and modifications; and in-home support services. Facility care services include long-term stays in special elderly rehabilitation facilities, long-term stays in elderly healthcare facilities and sanatorium-type wards, sanatorium-type wards for elderly patients with dementia, and other inpatient services in long-term care facilities. In addition to the benefits above, each municipality can also provide the following services to Category 1 insured persons according to their respective financial resources and regional needs: washing and drying of bedding required for long-term care, long-term care education, home care exchanges, and meal delivery for single insured persons.

In addition to the central government's transfer payments and funding for half of the insurers' service expenses, the prefectures also have financial stabilization funds for long-term care insurance to ensure the financial stability of the municipal long-term care insurance systems and the normal operation of insurers' affairs. In the event of crises within the municipal long-term care insurance funds, apart from adjusting the insurance premiums, the municipalities may also request the prefectures to allocate funds from the financial stability fund for assistance.

5. Healthcare Cost-Containment Policies

(1) Growth Characteristics of Healthcare Expenditure

1. Population Aging and Continuous Expansion of Elderly Healthcare Are the Main Causes for the Surge in Healthcare Expenditure In 1973, Japan became an aging society, and the government established free healthcare for individuals over 70 years old.

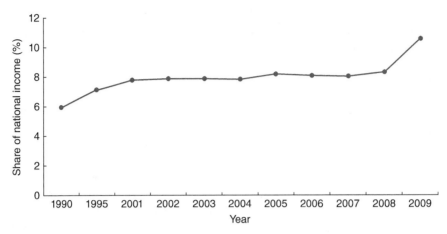

FIGURE 12.12   Healthcare expenditure as a share of national income in 1990–2009.

This year was known as the "first year of welfare." Due to the sharp increase in elderly healthcare expenditure, spreading the healthcare risks of the elderly has become a main component of Japan's health insurance system reforms. The growth rate of healthcare expenditure was 4.5% in 1990, 5.9% in 1991, 7.6% in 1992, 3.8% in 1993, 5.9% in 1994, 4.5% in 1995, 5.8% in 1996, 1.9% in 1997, 2.6% in 1998, and 3.7% in 1999. Healthcare expenditure per capita has consistently shown an upward trend, reaching ¥240,000 in 1999, an increase of 3.7% compared to 1998 (¥236,000). Healthcare expenditure as a share of national income was 3.42% in 1955, increased to 5.22% in 1975, and has been increasing annually since the 1990s. It was 5.87% in 1990, 7.12% in 1995, 7.8% in 2001, 8.2% in 2005, and 8.3% in 2008. In 2009, this figure increased to 10.61%, which was the first time since the survey began in 1954 that it exceeded 10% (Figure 12.12).

In 1999, before the implementation of the system reforms, healthcare expenditure exceeded ¥30 trillion for the first time and increased by 3.7% compared to the previous year; healthcare expenditure as a share of national income also increased by 0.28 percentage points from 7.8% in the previous year to 8.08% in that year. According to the official statistics of the MHLW, among the factors leading to this rate of increase, the population increase accounted for 0.2%, population aging accounted for 1.6%, while other factors due to increased healthcare capacity and changes in the disease structure accounted for 1.9%. In terms of different age groups, the healthcare expenditure for each elderly person was five times that for each young person, with an annual growth rate of 9.1% (the annual growth rate of total national healthcare expenditure was only 5.8%). This comparison is only based on data from 1996. Based on data from subsequent years, the growth rate was 5.7% (1.9%) in 1997, 6% (2.6%) in 1998, and 8.4% (3.7%) in 1999. In 1999, Japan's healthcare expenditure for the elderly was ¥11.8040 trillion, which was an increase of ¥917 billion from the previous year, and this figure is still showing an upward trend. Elderly healthcare expenditure as a share of the national total was only 10.9% in 1983 but increased to 38.2% in 1999. As a share of national income, it has increased nearly sevenfold from 0.45% in 1983 to 3.08% in 1999.

2. Fastest Growth in Drug and Elderly Care Expenses   Japan's health insurance can be examined in terms of treatment types. In 1999, general medical expenses amounted to ¥24.1320 trillion, accounting for 77.6% of overall national health insurance expenditure;

dental medical expenses amounted to ¥254.4 billion, accounting for 8.2% of overall expenditure; drug costs amounted to ¥2.4251 trillion, accounting for 7.8% of overall expenditure; and other expenses accounted for 6.4% of overall expenditure. Among general medical expenses, inpatient medical expenses amounted to ¥11.399 trillion, accounting for 36.8% of expenses, and outpatient medical expenses amounted to ¥12.6142 trillion, accounting for 40.8% of expenses. Of the latter, expenses for medical treatment in general community clinics and hospital outpatient services accounted for 23.1% and 7.7% of expenses.

In terms of the growth rate, in 1999, general medical expenses increased by 2.3% compared to the previous year and dental expenses increased by 1.0%. In contrast, drug expenses increased by 21.1% (¥423.3 billion), long-term care expenses of elderly healthcare institutions increased by 15.2%, and in-home elderly care expenses increased by 29.5%. Moreover, these expenses continued to increase as continuous improvements were made to elderly healthcare institutions. In 2000, medical expenses were ¥24.3 trillion, which was an increase of 0.70% compared to 1999. Pharmaceutical expenses had always experienced negative growth in previous years. However, with the progress in reforms separating prescribing and dispensing, pharmaceutical expenses instead increased by 15.6% in 2000, surpassing dental fees for the first time, which had only grown by 0.4% compared to the previous year.

3. Healthcare Expenditure of Persons Over 65 Years Old Accounts for More than Half of All Healthcare Expenditures As for different age groups in Japan, the national health insurance expenditure of individuals over 65 years old was ¥15.4797 trillion in 1999, accounting for 50% of overall health insurance expenditure. Given a more detailed classification of age groups, both the volume and rate of growth of the healthcare expenditures of individuals under 65 years old was positively related to the increase in age. As for those over 65 years old, the percent of healthcare expenditure for those aged 70–75 years was nearly twice that of those over 75 years old, and the former group also had the highest rate of expenditure growth. According to a report released by Japan's Social Insurance Bureau in 2005, the lifetime healthcare expenditure per capita of Japanese people was about ¥23 million, with individuals under 70 accounting for 51% and individuals over 70 accounting for 49%; the healthcare expenditures of individuals over 75 account for one-third of the total. The age distribution of healthcare expenditure per capita in 2005 was as follows: ¥819,000 for persons over 75, ¥521,000 for persons aged 65–74, ¥174,000 for persons aged 20–64, and ¥112,000 for persons aged 0–19.

The general medical expenses of individuals over 65 accounted for 50.5% of the total in 1999, which exceeded that of individuals under 65 for the first time. The general medical expenses of persons under 65 increased continuously with age. For both national and general health insurance, the composition ratio and growth in healthcare expenditure per capita showed upward trends with increasing age. However, among individuals over 65, the ratio of general medical expenses for those aged 70–75 years was 39.4%, and the ratio of those over 75 years old was 27.0%.

By classifying general medical expenses according to different disease types, it was found that, in 1999, the healthcare expenditures of patients with kidney, heart, and other circulatory system diseases accounted for 22.9% of the total, followed by cancer, which accounted for 11%. The expenditures of patients with respiratory diseases accounted for 8.6% of the total, and orthopedics accounted for 7.7% of the total. In terms of different age groups, among those under 65, healthcare expenditure was highest for circulatory system diseases, followed by respiratory diseases. Circulatory system diseases also ranked first among those over 65 years old, but the healthcare expenditure for cancer was higher than that for respiratory diseases.

In 2000, the total healthcare expenditure of those under 65 years old was ¥15.4539 trillion, whereas that of those over 65 years old had increased sharply and reached ¥15.4890 trillion. The healthcare expenditure per capita for those under 65 years was ¥146,500, whereas that of those over 65 years old was ¥730,300. Looking at national healthcare expenditure for 2009, the healthcare expenditure of individuals over 65 years old was ¥19.9479 trillion, which accounted for 55.4% of the total. The healthcare expenditure of those over 75 years old was ¥11.7335 trillion, which accounted for 32.6% of the total. The healthcare expenditure per capita of persons over 65 was ¥687,700, whereas that of persons under 65 was ¥163,000. The proportion of patients' out-of-pocket medical expenses was 13.9%, and the proportion covered by insurance was 48.6%, which both decreased by 0.2 percentage points compared to the previous year. The proportion covered by public funds from the central and local governments increased by 0.4 percentage points to 37.5%.

(2) Healthcare Cost-Containment Policies

The drastic increase in Japan's healthcare expenditure is mainly due to population aging and its corresponding rise in elderly healthcare and medical costs. This increase has exposed the problems related to elderly medical and healthcare in Japan's health system. The first is the problem of "social hospitalization." This problem is caused by certain elderly persons who should receive care in special nursing homes or at their own homes but who refuse to be discharged from long-term hospitalization. This situation, on the one hand, affects patients who do need to be hospitalized for treatment, and, on the other hand, also results in wasted healthcare resources. The rise in health insurance expenditure caused by social hospitalization, in effect, leads to an increase in the burden borne by the next generation of the working population. The second problem is the incompleteness of the "hospice care system," which was another major cause for the high average levels of healthcare expenditure. The role of end-of-life treatment is to alleviate a patient's suffering, reduce the fear of death, and make it possible to gradually accept the idea of death. However, according to a relevant report, 60% of a patient's suffering is caused by psychological factors, and the provision of careful and considerate psychological comfort can reduce 60% of suffering. This item alone can reduce the burden of drug costs. In Japan, the primary goal of end-of-life treatment is to extend life. Hence, substantial investments have been made in technology, equipment, and drugs to preserve patients' lives. The closer a patient comes to death, the higher the healthcare expenditure becomes.

Thus, the main direction of healthcare cost-containment policies for the elderly lies in controlling the provision of healthcare, expanding healthcare facilities for the elderly, promoting self-care efforts, and utilizing the proactiveness of the people. To solve the problem of long-term hospitalization among the elderly, new elderly care facilities were built to meet their long-term care needs through family and community care. Healthcare expenditure is calculated by adding the number of treatments in different age groups and the number of items per treatment for different age groups. Hence, in order to control healthcare costs, both the number of treatments must be reduced, and the number of items per treatment must be controlled. Since the number of treatments increases as the population ages, it is impossible to reduce healthcare expenditure without formulating strong measures for elderly healthcare. These measures include repealing free healthcare for the elderly, introducing small copayments for insured persons, improving elderly healthcare facilities, and promoting home medical care and home care as replacements for hospital care.

(3) Specific Measures

On November 1, 2000, the Health Insurance Act and other related amendments were passed by a forced vote in the Health and Welfare Committee of the House of Representatives due to the majority approval of the ruling coalition (consisting of the Liberal Democratic Party, Komeito, and New Conservative Party) and the 21st-Century Club. One of the key components was to change the copayments for hospital outpatient services for patients over 70 years old from a fixed-amount system to a 10% fixed-rate system. The MHLW called this measure "the first step towards reform."

According to the draft healthcare reform announced by the MHLW in September 2001, its specific contents were as follows. (1) The individual copayment rate of health insurance was further increased. At that time, persons enrolled in health insurance seeking medical treatment from healthcare institutions had to pay 20% of the costs. From 2003 onward, this percentage was increased to 30%. (2) Elderly healthcare was postponed until the age of 75 years. The recipients of Japan's existing elderly healthcare system were individuals over 70 years old. After the reform, this age was increased to 75 years within five years. Patients aged over 75 years would pay 10%, whereas those above a certain income level and those aged 70–74 years would have to pay 20%. (3) Residents of "special nursing homes" were required to pay their own room rates and utility bills. In the previous long-term care insurance system, the utility bills of residents in special nursing homes were included in the benefits for long-term care and were paid directly by the insurance. After the reform, the room rates and utility bills of residents were borne by the individuals as "hotel costs."

(4) Prospects for the Effectiveness of Cost-Containment Policies

Japan's healthcare cost-containment policies above mainly involved increasing patients' out-of-pocket expenses and optimizing healthcare institutions. These measures will have a negative impact on Japan's economic development in the short term. However, from a medium- to long-term perspective, these reforms will be able to control the excessive and persistent growth in healthcare expenditure, increase citizens' trust in the health insurance system, and eliminate people's healthcare insecurities, which will all contribute to economic development. According to the calculations of the Japan Research Institute, in the absence of reforms, by the height of population aging in 2025, Japan's national healthcare expenditure will reach ¥60.1 trillion, and its share of national burden (share of GDP) will increase to 7.5%. In contrast, if reforms are carried out, the national healthcare expenditure will remain at ¥46.3 trillion in 2025 (reduction of 23%), and its share of national burden will be controlled at 5.8%, which is lower than the current level.

In recent years, the long-term economic downturn and the continuous increase in the elderly population has led to a substantial increase in Japan's healthcare expenditure, which now ranks quite high in the international community. These crises have placed a heavy financial burden on the out-of-pocket expenses of Japanese residents, insurance payers, and healthcare institutions. In April 2003, the Japanese government implemented the innovative diagnosis procedure combination (DPC) payment system to replace the traditional fee-for-service system. DPC was developed by Japanese experts over four months from June to October 2002 and was based on the relevant data of 267,000 discharged patients. This new payment system includes two parts: a per-diem prospective payment and a fee-for-service payment. Based on the ratio between the average length of a hospital stay for a given DRG and the average length of a hospital stay for a given hospital, the standard for the per-diem prospective payment of healthcare expenses can be divided into three stages.

This adjustment ensures that each hospital can obtain the remuneration for the previous year. The fee-for-service payments to physicians are still based on the fee schedule formulated by the government.

Although this new payment method has reduced the average length of a hospital stay for inpatients, it did not reduce the growing healthcare expenditures of inpatients and outpatients. In April 2004, the DPC payment system and the DPC DRG-based classification were implemented at the same time. This system more clearly reflects the use of healthcare expenses for expensive drugs and consumables, serious diseases, and complications. A new two-year plan has been piloted in 51 general hospitals. This new payment system will be implemented in all hospitals in the future.

 SECTION IV. THE HEALTH SYSTEM IN POLAND

Poland is one of the oldest countries in Europe. It is situated in Central Europe, bordering Lithuania, Belarus, and Ukraine to the east; the Czech Republic and Slovakia to the south; Germany to the west; the Baltic Sea to the north; and the Russian enclave Kaliningrad to the northeast. It is the most populous country (38.531 million in 2013) with the largest land area (312,685 square kilometers) in Central and Eastern Europe.

From the 1970s to the 1980s, the health status of the Polish population was relatively poor and was lower than the average level of countries in the European Union (EU). By the 1990s, the parallel development of reforms to its health system and to its national economic system led to the improvement of the health status of its population. The health system reforms in Poland share some similarities with those of many national economic systems. Hence, conducting an analysis and review of Poland's health system reforms can provide a reference for health reforms in transitional countries.

1. Overview of Socioeconomic Development

(1) Political and Economic System

The Republic of Poland was established in 1989, and there were changes in the political regime. The Polish political system has also experienced repeated upheavals due to major reforms. At present, it is primarily divided into four levels. The topmost administrative body is the Parliament, which consists of the lower house (the *Sejm*) and the upper house (the Senate). The president is elected through national elections to serve a five-year term and can only be reelected once. With the approval of the *Sejm*, the president is able to appoint the prime minister. The cabinet is composed of the Council of Ministers. Its members are nominated by the prime minister, appointed by the president, and approved by the *Sejm*. The president has the right to veto any legislative proposal and decision, and the vetoed proposal can only be passed with a three-fifths-majority vote with at least half of the assembly present. The second level of administrative bodies is the "voivodeships" (provinces). In 1999, the Republic of Poland was divided into 49 voivodeships, which were later replaced by 16 new voivodeships. Each voivodeship is managed by a "voivode" (provincial governor) who is directly appointed by the central government. The third level of administrative bodies is the "*powiats*" (counties), which was repealed in 1975 but was later reinstated by Parliamentary vote in October 1998. The fourth level of administrative bodies is the "*gminy*" (municipalities) and is led by local municipal councils, which have independent legal personhood. Townships (*osiedle, dzielnica,* or *sołectwo*) are committees that represent the population of a certain area.

Traditionally, the Polish economy is based on industry and agriculture. Since the transition from a planned economy to a market economy in 1989, the Polish economy gradually began showing signs of recovery from the economic downturn of the late 1980s and early 1990s. Since the mid-1990s, the majority of its economic indicators began to show stable growth. In the early 1990s, there was a significant decline in Poland's GDP, but, by the mid-1990s, the GDP growth rate was nearly 7%. After 2000, its GDP growth slowed down, and it was 1.7% in 2013. Although during the initial period of transition from a centrally planned economy to a market-based economy, the inflation rate was extremely high, reaching up to 76.71% in 1991, it declined steadily over a 10-year period and fell to 0.79% in 2003, which was comparable to that of Western European countries. In 2010, the inflation rate was 2.71% (Table 12.21). Overall, the Polish economy developed relatively quickly. Based on current prices, its GDP in 2013 was about US$525.8 billion, and its GDP per capita was US$13,648. Poland joined the EU in May 2004 and has the largest market and growth potential among new EU member states. Currently, the major problems in the Polish economy are a high unemployment rate and severe fiscal and trade deficits. The high unemployment rate was prominently exposed after the transformation of its economic system and mainly manifested in the early 1990s. The annual registered unemployment (which is less than the real unemployment rate) increased at a three-fold rate and reached 19.6% in 2003 (Table 12.22). In addition, Poland's fiscal deficit in 2005 was about US$9.5 billion, and its trade deficit was about US$11.5 billion. In 2010, its fiscal deficit was about US$26 billion, and its trade deficit was about US$5.7 billion. Despite the presence of various problems and difficulties, Poland's Human Development Index (HDI) has improved and was 0.813 in 2011, ranking 39th in the world.

(2) Current Status of Population and Health Development

Poles account for 97.5% of the national population, and the remainder includes other ethnic minorities such as Belarusians, Germans, Lithuanians, and Ukrainians. The population is 95% Catholic. Poland has greater uniformity in terms of race, language, and religion compared to other European countries.

During World War II, the country suffered heavy losses, and one-fifth of its population perished, including nearly all of the Polish Jews. In 2010, Poland's total population was 38.184 million, of which 61.2% resided in cities. As with many EU countries, Poland's birth and death rates have essentially remained unchanged in recent years, and has even shown negative population growth (Figure 12.13). Studies have estimated that, by 2050, the

TABLE 12.21 Macroeconomic Indicators of Poland in 1991–2013

Indicator	1991	1995	2000	2003	2006	2009	2013
GDP growth rate	−7.02	6.95	4.26	3.87	6.23	1.61	1.7
Per capita gross national income, GNI (US$)	5,530	7,320	10,480	11,870	14,690	18,250	13,240
Registered unemployment rate (%)	—	13.30	16.10	19.60	13.80	8.20	10.4
Annual inflation rate (%)	76.71	28.07	10.06	0.79	1.11	3.83	—
Human Development Index (HDI)	—	0.727	0.77	0.791	0.795	0.807	0.834

Source: World Bank, 2014.

TABLE 12.22 Demographics and Health Indicators in Poland in 1991–2012

Indicator	1991	1995	2000	2003	2006	2009	2012
Total population (10,000)	3,824.62	3,859.50	3,845.38	3,820.46	3,814.13	3,815.16	3,853.60
Percentage of population over 65 years old (%)	10.29	11.14	12.27	12.92	13.31	13.48	14.00
Percentage of urban population (%)	61.34	61.50	61.70	61.58	61.44	61.26	60.70
Crude birth rate (%)	14.3	11.2	9.8	9.2	9.8	10.9	10.0
Crude death rate (%)	10.6	10	9.5	9.6	9.7	10.1	10.0
Average life expectancy	70.59	71.89	73.75	74.60	75.14	75.70	76.80
Infant mortality rate (per 1,000 live births)	14.7	12.1	8.3	7	6.2	5.4	4.5
Maternal mortality rate (1/100,000)	—	—	—	4	2.9	2	—

Source: World Bank Database, 2014.

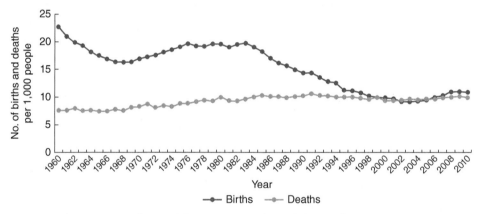

FIGURE 12.13 Patterns of natural fluctuations in the Polish population in 1960–2010.

resident population in Poland will drop to 31.9 million, which is a decrease of 6.28 million compared to 2010. It was expected that, by 2025, the percentage of persons over 65 in the total population will increase to 37.9% (Table 12.22).

It was not until the 1990s that the health indicators of the Polish population made comprehensive progress. As shown in Table 12.22, the average life expectancy of the Polish population increased from 70.59 years in 1991 to 76.8 years in 2012. The infant mortality rate also showed a significant decline from 14.7 per 1,000 live births in 1991 to 4.5% in 2012. The decline in birth and mortality rates and the extension of life expectancy will inevitably lead to the problem of population aging. The percentage of people over 65 years old increased from 10.29% in 1991 to 14% in 2012.

Due to the significant increase in the demand for health services, the financing of the health system will also be further influenced. Population aging and the continuous shrinking of the total population will disproportionately increase the tax burden on the working population. Healthcare expenses will be borne by a small group of people, which will increase the cost of healthcare. This increase will ultimately lead to the formation of a new consumption structure. With regard to causes of death, as in other industrialized countries, cardiovascular disease ranked first (accounting for about 50% of deaths), followed by cancer (about 24%), with poisoning and injuries ranking third.

2. Health Service System

(1) Structure and Management of Health Organizations

After World War II, Poland established the Ministry of Health to implement centralized health management within the context of a planned economy, emphasizing that healthcare is a public responsibility. Although it almost completely imitated the Soviet model, Poland retained a few of its own characteristics. For example, some of its individual clinics were preserved. In the 1990s, health financing in Poland was still based mainly on national taxes, but Poland had begun to implement policies of decentralization in the public health sector, including the reorganization of the hierarchical healthcare system. The first step involved strengthening the health management authority of provincial governments. In 1991, the management authority for the majority of health services was transferred from the Ministry of Health and Welfare to the provinces, and management for a small proportion of services was transferred to townships. The second step began in 1993 and involved devolving the ownership rights for the majority of public healthcare institutions to provinces and townships; prior to this, townships rarely participated in healthcare services. The third step occurred in 1998 and involved the reinstatement of counties, which were responsible for county-level hospitals.

1. Structural Framework of Health Organizations　Since 1999, the Polish healthcare system has undergone major structural reforms, the most prominent of which was the establishment of 16 regional sickness funds and a separate sickness fund for public servants (e.g., the military and railway workers). These funds were merged in 2003 to form a single National Health Fund (NHF). In 2005, the management and financing functions of the healthcare system were distributed among three types of institutions: the Ministry of Health, the NHF, and territorial self-governments, as shown in Figure 12.14.

1. *Ministry of Health.* Since 1989, the Ministry of Health gradually evolved from its role as a healthcare financer and provider to that of a policymaker and regulator. In general, the Ministry of Health is mainly responsible for the formulation of national health policies and major investments. First, the overall Ministry of Health is responsible for health services, their organization and management, and the adjustment of specific health policy projects in accordance with the cost-benefit principle. Certain areas come under the direct management of the Ministry of Health, such as national emergency medical services, convalescence, and rules and regulations for the medical professions. Second, the Ministry of Health engages in management of medical research and medical education. However, its management functions are limited to only government-funded health service institutions, including the National Medical Center of Post-Graduate Education, the National Center of Child and Maternal Health, and the National Institute of Cardiology. The institutes of medicine, university hospitals, and research institutes are semi-autonomous, but the final decision-making power still lies with the Ministry of Health. Third, the Ministry of Health is responsible for implementing national public health programs, training healthcare workers, partially funding medical equipment, and formulating and monitoring healthcare standards. In addition, the Ministry of Health also assumes

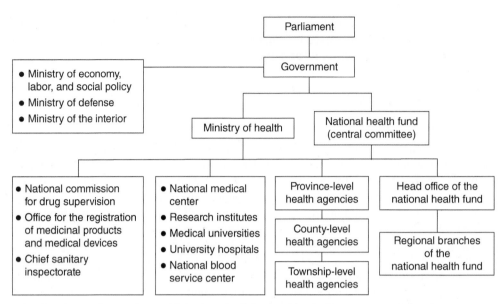

FIGURE 12.14 Organizational framework of the health service system in Poland

several supervisory and management functions, including monitoring the safety of drugs, medical devices, biological products, and cosmetics, and controlling the market access of drugs and foods using genetically modified microorganisms. In addition, it is also responsible for health inspections, including the evaluation of food safety and food quality during production and sales, and the supervision of food raw materials and finished goods design.

2. *National Health Fund (NHF).* The NHF began its operations in 2003 and is mainly responsible for the financing of healthcare services. In its role as a fund holder, the NHF signs service provision contracts with service providers after the competition for public funds or negotiations. The NHF funds health service institutions according its available financial resources. As a holder of public funds, the NHF is prohibited from engaging in for-profit activities. It cannot operate or own healthcare institutions or pharmaceutical companies, nor can it be a shareholder of health service provision and pharmaceutical trading companies. The NHF is supervised by the NHF Council. The Council is composed of nine members appointed by the prime minister, who serve a five-year term. An NHF department had been established prior to October 2004, but it was later repealed by the Act on the Public Funding of Healthcare Services. The NHF implements a director responsibility system, and the directors are appointed by the NHF Council. The deputy director of medical affairs must be a physician. The deputy director is nominated by the director and is subject to approval or rejection by the NHF Council.

3. *Local self-governments.* On January 1, 1999, Poland introduced a three-tier government administrative structure (i.e., province, county, and township). The health management agencies at each level of self-government are responsible for the following three aspects: the formulation of strategies and plans based on regional health needs, health promotion, and the management of healthcare institutions.

4. *Healthcare units.* The establishment and management of healthcare units may take any form prescribed by the relevant laws. Moreover, the law also stipulates that healthcare

units are autonomous institutions in terms of their organization, personnel, assets, and finances. Their main responsibilities are to provide health services and promote health. Healthcare units include (1) hospitals, chronic medical care homes, private nursing homes, nursing homes, convalescent homes, or other institutions that can provide healthcare services on a 24-hour basis or during regular working hours; (2) outpatient departments, health centers, or outpatient clinics; (3) institutions that can provide emergency care services; (4) diagnostic laboratories; (5) dental restoration or orthodontic clinics; (6) rehabilitation centers; (7) nurseries; and (8) other institutions that can meet the requirements of the Act.

2. Implementation of Management Functions

1. *Planning.* Poland's Ministry of Health regularly drafts a national health plan. Each province must also draft its own health plan based on the number and scope of health services that are required to meet the health demands of the residents in the province. Specifically, these plans include (1) the health status of the population in the province and the status of their health service needs and (2) a summary of policies and commitments to meet the health service needs of the population and thereby improve their health status that also specifies issues that should be prioritized. Once these plans are drafted, the NHF will formulate a health service provision plan according to these health plans. The health service provision plan details the basic health service needs and the health service volume required to satisfy these needs. It also proposes solutions to potential problems that may emerge in the future. The planning for and meeting of the population's health service needs are implemented based on temporal (short-term, annual, or long-term planning) and geographical/regional conditions.

   The formulation of a plan with clear goals and the monitoring of evaluable indicators both play crucial roles in achieving the better regulation of health service behaviors and implementing the functions of the health service system. Poland currently formulates a National Health Program (NHP) once every 10 years. Using the NHP for 1996–2005 as an example, its strategic goal was to enhance the health status of the population and improve the health-related quality of life in a multi-sectoral program in accordance with the WHO's concept of "achieving health for all." The plan focused on health and health determinants, health promotion, and public health policies. The three key areas of activities that aimed to achieve this strategic goal are as follows: (1) creating the conditions, cultivating awareness, increasing knowledge, and improving the skills for individuals to choose a healthy lifestyle and take actions to improve their own health statuses or those of others; (2) creating a supportive environment for health, work, and education; and (3) improving health equality to ensure that everyone can have equal access to health services.

   Since 1998, actionable goals with reasonable indicators have been monitored. A detailed NHP monitoring report is prepared every year and submitted to the Ministry of Health. This report is prepared based on the data provided by national institutions and related organizations (National Institute of Cardiology, Maria Skłodowska Curie Memorial Cancer Centre and Institute of Oncology, National Institute of Health, and National Food and Nutrition Institute). Based on the NHP monitoring report, it is possible to know whether the expected goals and health benefits have been accomplished on time and to predict the probability of completing the entire plan by the final year. If these goals are not completed on time, the relevant departments will adopt more effective measures. These unfinished goals are also taken into account when designing the NHP for the next ten years.

2. *Legislation.* The regulation of the Polish health system is mainly achieved through numerous laws and regulations. The first of these laws is the "Constitution of the Republic of Poland," which has the highest authority. Article 68 of the Constitution stipulates that all citizens shall have equal access to healthcare service irrespective of their ability to pay. This article implies that it is the responsibility of the state to protect the health of its citizens and to guarantee equal access to and service quality of healthcare services. The Constitution also specifically points out that public authorities shall ensure special healthcare to children, pregnant women, disabled people, and elderly persons and shall combat epidemic illnesses and prevent the negative health consequences of environmental degradation.

Under the guidance of the Constitution and combined with the actual needs of the management of the health service system, as of 2005 the Polish government has successively issued 13 laws related to healthcare services. Specifically, these laws are the State Sanitary Inspection Act, the Health Care Institutions Act, the Medical Profession Act, the Nurses and Midwives Act, the Physicians' Profession Act, the Universal Health Insurance Act, the Medicinal Products Act, the Pharmaceutical Act, the Medical Devices Act, the Act on the Registration of Medicinal Products, Medical Devices, and Biocidal Products, the Act on Universal Health Insurance and National Health Fund, the Act on the Public Funding of Healthcare Services, and the Act on Public Aid and Restructuring of Public Health Care Institutions. The successive introduction of these laws produced good results in regulating the processes, institutions, personnel, and equipment used in health service provision. The Medical Profession Act, for example, specified the form that shall be taken by a private practice (outside of healthcare institutions), for example, as an individual or group practice. Only those with both a physicians' license and a license for individual practice can establish an individual practice. In addition, individual practice also requires registration with the designated regional chamber of physicians and dentists. Establishing a specialist practice requires the practitioner to possess the corresponding specialist medical skills. Both forms of individual practices can only provide healthcare services at their place of registration. The healthcare services provided by physicians within the designated area are also governed by this Act.

It is also worth noting that the adjustment of these laws was performed in a timely manner. For example, in 2003, the Constitutional Tribunal ruled that the Act on Universal Health Insurance and National Health Fund was unconstitutional and gave the government one year (by the end of 2004) to revise this Act to align with the Constitution. Subsequently, the government issued a new bill, the Act on the Public Funding of Healthcare Services, which was passed in the *Sejm* on August 27, 2004. In this new Act, the list of healthcare services funded by the NHF was very much in line with the requirements of the Constitutional Tribunal. In addition, this new Act explicitly regulates the management of waiting lists for adjunctive therapy and hospital treatment. Furthermore, the issues concerning the burden of healthcare services for the homeless and uninsured population were also explicitly regulated.

3. *Management.* In accordance with the many laws related to healthcare services, the relevant institutions must elaborate in detail the relevant management responsibilities and specific management procedures. For example, in accordance with the Universal Health Insurance Act, the social health insurance system must be established based on the signing of contracts between payers and providers. Hence, the procedures for contract signing need to be clarified. The NHF published an announcement that included the relevant provisions of the Decree of March 25, 2003, issued by the Ministry of Health,

which was used to explain the procedures for signing healthcare service contracts with the NHF. Its contents included inviting interested persons and organizations to participate in negotiations, calling for tenders to provide healthcare services, appointing and dismissing the tender committee, and clarifying the responsibilities of the tender committee (classification regulations Article 55, Paragraph 493) and the NHF (Article 78, Paragraph 5).

According to the provisions of the Act on the Public Funding of Healthcare Services, the NHF signs healthcare service contracts based on the results of negotiations. The NHF must send invitations in order to open negotiations and issue announcements.

A social affairs committee is set up in each provincial branch by the president of the NHF. This committee consists of 14 members, including invited local health authorities and union representatives. The objective of the social affairs committee is to provide policy recommendations for provincial health planning and province-related national healthcare service planning as well as to regularly analyze the complaints and suggestions of insured persons (excluding affairs involving healthcare supervision).

4. *Supervision.* The Healthcare Institutions Act (1991) clearly stipulates the requirements for practitioners in healthcare institutions, specifically that healthcare services can only be provided by individuals with a license to practice medicine. In addition, this Act also clearly stipulates the scope of management for all levels of government authorities and the management authority of entrusted agencies or individuals. Healthcare institutions and their founders are managed uniformly by the Ministry of Health. The Ministry of Health authorizes local government officials (provincial-level) to supervise public and nonpublic healthcare institutions within their jurisdiction.

For this purpose, the state has also established a special supervision agency. This agency is composed of national consultants appointed by the Ministry of Health. Provincial consultants for provincial units are appointed after discussions between the provincial governor and the relevant national consultants.

Another form of supervision specified in the Act is implemented by the founder of the healthcare institution. This form of supervision includes medical supervision and is also known as supervision of "the implementation of statutory tasks, accessibility of healthcare services, and quality assurance of services."

The main goal of self-governments (including professional self-governments) is to implement statutory tasks. Article 17, Paragraph 1, of the Constitution of the Republic of Poland stipulates, "By means of a statute, self-governments may be created within a profession in which the public repose confidence and such self-governments shall concern themselves with the proper practice of such professions in accordance with, and for the purpose of protecting, the public interest." At present, there are more than 12 such self-governments in Poland, including self-governments for physicians, dentists, laboratory diagnosticians (medical biologists), pharmacists, nurses, and midwives.

(2) Healthcare Service Delivery System

According to Poland's Health Care Institutions Act, healthcare institutions include hospitals, chronic medical care homes, nursing homes, health centers, emergency services, diagnostic laboratories, dental clinics, rehabilitation centers, and child care institutions. These healthcare institutions are autonomous bodies in terms of their organization, personnel, assets, and finances. Hospitals in Poland are divided into three levels. Primary hospitals are run by county governments and generally include four basic departments: internal medicine, surgery, obstetrics and gynecology, and pediatrics. Secondary hospitals are run by provincial governments and provide more detailed specialized services, including cardiovascular medicine, dermatology, oncology, and urology. Tertiary hospitals are run by national ministries or universities and provide highly specialized healthcare services.

1. Primary Healthcare   Until 1991, the concept of family doctors or general practitioners had not yet emerged in Poland. Primary care physicians were mainly internal medicine physicians, gynecologists, and pediatricians providing care in general hospitals. Historically, little emphasis has been placed on primary healthcare. The education system had been dominated by narrow specialist education, and undergraduate medical education did not offer courses on primary care. Primary care physicians referred patients to specialists based on their conditions, which is a task that usually falls to general practitioners in western European countries. Some people also bypassed primary care physicians and directly sought medical treatment from specialists with better medical equipment. Primary care physicians lacked training, and their clinics were poorly equipped. Thus, primary care physicians had low status in the field of medicine, which was also reflected in the attitudes of patients to a certain extent.

In 1991, a "family medicine" strategy was developed to enhance the status and service quality of primary care physicians. In 1992, the School of Family Medicine was established in Warsaw to support this model. In addition, training in general medicine was given to specialists after graduation. As of 2004, 7,000 physicians had obtained degrees in family medicine. However, this number is far lower than the 150,000 family physicians needed according to estimates by the Ministry of Health. This shortage is compensated by the original primary care physicians, most of whom have degrees in internal medicine. Furthermore, another 5,000 pediatricians and 3,000 gynecologists also provide primary care services within their respective specialties.

The development of the so-called family beds also received strong support. In this program, hospital services in the traditional sense can be provided by a family physician in a patient's home. This type of service not only reduces the economic burden but also avoids the psychological stress caused by hospitalization and is more conducive to services for chronic and pediatric patients.

Polish physicians, who previously tended to work in hospitals, are now more inclined to work in primary care institutions. When emergency services are not needed, primary care physicians should provide healthcare services in the patient's home. In 2002, the number of outpatient visits per capita was 5.6, which was lower than the 6.3 visits of the original EU member states (joined before May 2004) and the 8.4 visits of new EU member states. It can be foreseen that the hospital certification and registration system will lead to the closure of many small hospitals, and the number of beds will shrink by at least 10%. The beds for pediatrics and infectious diseases, which have the lowest utilization rates, will be the first reduction targets. Acute beds for psychiatry, pediatric emergency surgery, and other specialties (e.g., oncology) will also be reduced. Certain acute wards will be changed to rehabilitation, long-term care, or hospice care wards.

2. Secondary and Tertiary Healthcare
   1. *Specialist outpatient healthcare.* Specialist outpatient care is strictly separated from inpatient healthcare. Specialist outpatient services are based in individual healthcare institutions with the exception of those in major cities. The specialist outpatient services of

major cities developed on the basis of former specialist healthcare centers, which have now become independently operating healthcare institutions.

2. *Management of Hospitals and Inpatient Services.* The organization, operation, administration, management, establishment, reform, financing, and closure of hospitals are all regulated by the Health Care Institutions Act of 1991 and its enforcement clauses. Hospitals established by territorial self-governments are usually known as county-level (powiat-level) hospitals. In 2004, 90% of public health and healthcare institutions were established by territorial self-governments. Healthcare institutions established by national ministries are known as ministerial hospitals, such as the Ministry of Health Hospital Units, Ministry of the Interior Hospital Units, or Ministry of Defense Hospital Units. The Health Care Institutions Act stipulates that the names of specialist healthcare institutions may reflect the scope of services provided by the institution.

Hospitals that are established by medical schools and participate in scientific research, education, healthcare services, and health promotion are known as clinical hospitals or university hospitals. There are no formal requirements for the referral level of such hospitals.

In brief, hospitals provide healthcare services in four basic departments: internal medicine, surgery, obstetrics and gynecology, and pediatrics. Hospitals are divided into different levels based on the conditions of the departments. Hospitals with only these four departments are known as primary hospitals and are mainly established by self-governments. Most secondary hospitals are established by provincial self-governments and also provide other specialist departments, such as cardiovascular medicine, dermatology, oncology, urology, or neurology. These hospitals are known as provincial-level (voivodeship-level) hospitals. Tertiary hospitals are mainly university or ministerial hospitals with highly specialized services provided by top medical experts. The National Institute of Cardiology, the Maria Skłodowska Curie Memorial Cancer Centre and Institute of Oncology, and the National Institute of Maternal and Child Health are all tertiary hospitals. This classification was implemented when sickness funds were still in existence, and, although it is currently not implemented, these names are still in use. There are very few private, church, or NGO hospitals in Poland. In 2003, there were 732 public hospitals and only 72 nonpublic hospitals.

In 2002, the number of emergency hospital beds in Poland was 4.7 beds/1,000 people, which was lower than the average level of new EU member states (5.2 beds/1,000 people) but higher than the EU average of 4.1 beds/1,000 people. The longitudinal analysis only considered the total number of beds in Poland. As major changes occurred during the 1990s in the definition of emergency hospital beds, the longitudinal analysis of emergency hospital beds is misleading.

As in many other European countries, the number of beds in Poland had decreased sharply over the past decade from 6.3 beds/1,000 people in 1990. The average length of a stay in a general hospital decreased from 9.3 days in 1999 to 7.9 days in 2002. The indicator describing the number of patients served per bed per year increased from 34.7 patients in 1999 to 38.8 patients in 2001. In 2001, the utilization rate of hospital beds was 74.5%, which was similar to that of other European countries. Since 1999, the utilization rate of hospital beds increased significantly together with the decrease in the number of beds.

Changes in the Polish health service market and its population structure, as well as the reforms to national management mechanisms, have led to a relatively small reduction in the number of hospitals but have resulted in major changes in their internal structure. The number of beds for pediatrics and infectious diseases, which have the lowest utilization rate, has decreased. Other beds have been adapted for chronic patients, rehabilitation patients, long-term care recipients who cannot engage in self-care, palliative treatment patients, hospice care patients, and psychiatric patients. The few new private hospitals generally provide general medical services and surgical services, and some of them have also signed contracts with the NHF.

3. *Emergency Services and Emergency Medicine.* Poland's emergency services have been in existence for more than 100 years. These services are usually independent departments known as emergency medical services. They are established based on geographical areas (province, county, and township) and are provided free of charge by the government. Critically ill patients and all patients after 10 p.m. can use the ambulance service free of charge. Currently, a new system of emergency service is being created through the establishment of hospital emergency departments. The main goal of the new system is to improve life-saving facilities, primarily by shortening the time interval from an emergency call to a hospital arrival by 75% (shortened to 8 minutes in cities and 15 minutes outside cities) and by cooperating closely with the fire department and the police.

To accomplish this goal, improvements are still needed to the system, such as increasing the number of dispatch centers and improving their distribution, increasing the number of ambulances, constructing and equipping hospitals with emergency departments, and determining the standards of emergency calls to ensure the availability of ambulances within the scope of physician supervision and coordination.

The government planned to build a national network of 270 hospital emergency departments by the end of 2005. In May 2004, 110 emergency departments were in operation, and 208 were being restructured.

The new emergency system that is currently being planned is shown in Figure 12.15.

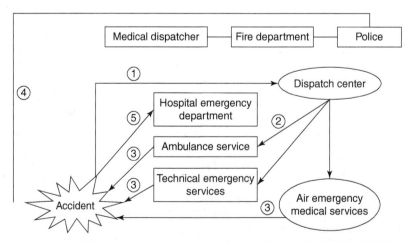

FIGURE 12.15 The organizational structure of Poland's emergency service system.

(3) Healthcare Human Resources and Training

Medical practitioners can be divided into two categories: practitioners certified by the EU sectoral system and practitioners certified by the EU general system. The first category involves five types of practitioners: physicians, dentists, nurses, midwives, and pharmacists. The second category involves the following allied practitioners: laboratory diagnosticians (medical or clinical biologists), speech therapists, physiotherapists, dental assistants, nutritionists, opticians, hearing therapists, dental hygienists, school health workers, orthopedic surgeons, child health workers, medical rescuers, occupational therapists, medical laboratory technicians, dental technicians, pharmacist assistants, medical imaging technicians, medical massage therapists, orthopedic surgical technicians, and radiation protection officers.

1. Physicians and Dentists   The numbers of physicians, nurses, and other healthcare workers per capita in Poland are all lower than in most western European countries. In 2002, the number of physicians in Poland was 2.3 physicians/1,000 people, which is lower by one-third than the average level of countries that joined the EU before 2004 (3.6 physicians/1,000 people). It is also lower than in the majority of central and southeastern European countries, new EU member states (2.8 physicians/1,000 people), and Commonwealth of Independent States (CIS) countries. Despite the new developments in family medicine in Poland, the number of specialists is still high, and the ratio of specialists to primary care physicians is greater than 3:1.

1. Medical and dental education
    1. *Basic medical education/* There are 11 medical colleges in Poland. In 2002, 2,473 physicians and 901 dentists graduated from these colleges. Thereafter, the number of graduates decreased continuously, with only 2,387 physicians and 753 dentists graduating in 2004. All graduates of medical colleges must complete postgraduate education. This requirement is imposed by the "Act on the Professions of Physician and Dentist" enacted on December 5, 1996. According to this Act, the postgraduate education of physicians and dentists must comply with two new regulations: the completion of a one-year postgraduate internship followed by national examinations and the independent choice of a medical or dental specialty.
    2. *One-year compulsory postgraduate internship.* The one-year compulsory postgraduate internship specifically targets newly graduated physicians, and their hospital work is intended as additional training in the learning stage. The internship is conducted based on the following principles. The internship hospital shall be designated by the provincial government. Hospital interns have the same status as formal employees, and expenses during the internship are covered by the government budget through the provincial government. There are two starting times for internships, namely, October 1 and March 1 of every year. The length of the internship is 13 months for physicians and 12 months for dentists. To complete this internship, interns must be approved by the internship coordinator and pass the national examination. If these two conditions are met, interns can obtain the medical practitioner certificate.
        The scope of the national examination does not exceed that of internship activities. Hence, the examination can be used to evaluate the quality of training in designated hospitals. The examination is a nationally unified multiple-choice test that is held twice a year, with different questions for physicians and dentists.

Specialist trainees can only provide specialist medical services after obtaining the license to practice medicine or dentistry in the Republic of Poland and passing the entrance examination for specialist training. Foreign physicians and dentists who have not undergone these procedures must be certified by the Ministry of Health before practicing. This new single-level specialist system is applicable to basic disciplines (internal medicine, emergency medicine, and family medicine) and other medical disciplines. In addition, physicians can only apply to study another specialty after they have completed the professional training for a basic discipline.

3. *Residency training.* Specialists in training are also known as resident physicians. The training costs are funded by the state budget and are allocated by the Ministry of Health to the healthcare institutions responsible for organizing specialty training. Physicians applying to become resident physicians must have the necessary qualifications, which mainly refer to the aforementioned entrance examination. After passing the examination, they sign a professional training contract with the hospital. Approximately 800 physicians undertake residency training each year. In 2004, more than half of resident physicians were assigned to three basic disciplines: internal medicine, emergency medicine, and family medicine. The Ministry of Health planned to expand the scale of residency training and increase the number to 2,000 resident physicians by 2005.

Specialized training can only be performed in accredited institutions. Accreditation and qualification are necessary procedures that aim to assess whether designated healthcare institutions and the education they provide are able to meet professional standards. Once qualified, these healthcare institutions are authorized to undertake specialized training. The government sets the standards for the number and training of medical workers, the organizational structure, equipment, and research foundations, and the outline and scope of health service provision. The accreditation process is also related to inclusion in the list of authorized training healthcare institutions. Once an institution is authorized, the Ministry of Health allocates a specific number of training places to the institution. The provincial public health centers are responsible for registering physicians and dentists who are undertaking specialty training in the province.

4. *Continuing education.* According to the code of medical ethics, all physicians or dentists are obliged to master new knowledge and skills and to continuously improve their professional standards. To this end, the Chamber of Physicians and Dentists adopted a resolution that laid the foundation for achieving this goal through self-learning and other forms of postgraduate education. Similarly, in accordance with the provisions of the Act on the Professions of Physician and Dentist of December 5, 1996, physicians have the right and obligation to enhance their own professional standards, which includes different forms of postgraduate training.

2. Medical license

1. *Specialty examination and EU-wide physician qualification.* Under the new system, the national specialist examination must be taken after the completion of all specialty training. Once physicians have passed this examination, they will be awarded a specialist degree certificate. The Medical Examinations Center (Centrum Egzaminów Medycznych, CEM) is responsible for organizing and implementing national-level examinations as well as other examinations related to graduate education and professional development for physicians, pharmacists, and other medical professionals. The national examination consists of three parts, including practical,

written, and oral examinations. It is held twice a year in the spring and fall. The regional self-government for physicians or dentists issues medical licenses for their respective professions to those who pass the examination.

The regional medical chamber also handles the issuing of physician's or dentist's licenses to citizens of other EU member states, provided that they meet the requirements above (with some reservations for specific regulations passed for certain EU countries). In addition, citizens of other EU member states must fulfill the following requirements: relevant proof of qualifications to conduct medical practice in their home country that has been certified by the authorities of that EU member state; a diploma proving that the applicant is qualified to practice medicine or dentistry with full legal capacity; proof of full physical and mental capacity to practice medicine or dentistry; an absence of ethical issues; and the ability to issue a written statement indicating that the applicant has good writing and speaking skills in the Polish language.

2. *Licensure and number of licenses.* Since 1970, the number of physicians per 1,000 people has been increasing gradually, as have the numbers of pharmacists, qualified nurses, midwives, and dentists. However, the decline in the number of qualified nurses after 1997 attracted widespread attention. Although the total number of healthcare professionals was sufficient, there were shortages in certain specialties that urgently required retraining. The level of wages, working conditions, and work enthusiasm were issues facing healthcare workers in Poland. The government budget crisis in 1992 led to widespread unemployment among healthcare workers, but job positions gradually stabilized again after the crisis. In all former socialist states, the wages of healthcare workers are lower than those of general workers. This phenomenon still exists in Poland. To control inflation, the government adopted measures to reduce the wages of the public sector throughout the 1990s. As a result, many Polish physicians flocked to better-paid western European countries, especial the UK and Germany. Due to the lack of a mandatory registration system, the number of physicians and nurses working abroad is difficult to estimate.

According to data provided by the Polish Chamber of Physicians and Dentists, from May 4, 2004, to April 30, 2005, 2,533 physicians obtained medical qualification certificates, and 797 dentists obtained dentistry qualification certificates. These certificates are required to practice medicine or dentistry in other EU countries. Therefore, this figure can be used to estimate the number of physicians and dentists leaving Poland to work abroad over 12 months. According to the UK General Practitioners Committee, in August 2005 alone the number of physicians registered in the UK with Polish junior doctor qualifications was 1,211.

In 2003, physicians working in the public health sector earned an average of €750 per month before tax, and nurses earned €400. Many physicians and other healthcare professionals hope to narrow the wage gap with their counterparts in western European countries. Hence, many of them increase their incomes by accepting "bonuses." In 2003, a survey conducted by the Stefan Batory Foundation found that 57% of respondents admitted to bribing healthcare workers (Kubiak, 2003). However, it should be acknowledged that although the current wages of physicians in neighboring western European countries are 5 to 10 times higher than those of Poland, their consumption levels are only 2 to 3 times higher. Hence, the only means to eliminate unofficial payments and to reduce the widespread outflow of healthcare workers is to increase the wages for practitioners in public healthcare institutions to an acceptable level.

The goal of health sector reforms is to strengthen primary healthcare and ensure a more reasonable geographical distribution of health human resources. As in many other countries, Poland's health resources are mainly concentrated in urban areas. Although less than two-thirds of the Polish population lived in cities in 2004, cities accounted for nearly three-quarters of healthcare workers (of which, physicians in cities accounted for three-quarters of the national total). Therefore, health sector reforms must include effective measures to guide healthcare professionals towards practicing primary healthcare in rural areas.

3. *Medical practice.* Engaging in medical activities implies the provision of health services, especially the following: examining the condition of a patient's physical health, diagnosing and preventing diseases, implementing the appropriate treatment and rehabilitation, providing consultation services, and providing professional advice and issuing health certificates.

The dental care services provided by dentists include the diagnosis and treatment of dental diseases, maxillofacial deformities, and other related diseases. Scientific research and teaching are another form of medical practice, but they are only involved in medical education, medication, and health promotion. Each physician's duty in the practice of medicine is to prevent, diagnose, and treat diseases using the best medical knowledge and the most feasible methods while observing the code of professional ethics and striving to achieve professional accuracy.

4. *Chamber of Physicians and Dentists.* The Polish Chamber of Physicians and Dentists and its branches form the main entity of the self-government for physicians. Currently, there are 24 regional chambers and one Military Chamber of Physicians and Dentists. All physicians and dentists must join this association. The self-government for physicians operates according to the relevant provisions of the "Act on the Chambers of Physicians and Dentists."

The Chamber and its regional branches have jurisdiction over medical responsibility and arbitration. In accordance with the relevant provisions in the "Act on the Chambers of Physicians" promulgated on May 17, 1989, members of the self-governments for physicians and dentists are obliged to be responsible for violations of medical ethics and obligations and for violations of the rules of the medical profession before the health courts.

2. Nurses and Midwives   According to existing law (the Nurses and Midwives Act of 1996), nurses and midwives are independent professions. The term "independent profession" implies that nurses and midwives are qualified to provide independent health services, especially medical services, and do not rely solely on physician orders. Thus far, nurses and midwives are still considered auxiliary healthcare workers. In accordance with the aforementioned law, the scope of the duties and capacities for nurses and midwives has greatly expanded, which has increased their knowledge and qualification requirements and also led to reforms to the healthcare system and institutions. The most dominant change is that nurses are now able to engage in independent nursing activities.

1. *Nursing and midwifery education.* Nursing and midwifery education is currently undergoing reforms. Traditional nursing schools will be closed, and a new system based on issuing licenses and awarding master's degrees will be established. Medical universities currently provide two models of nursing training: three years of degree education and supplementary education for individuals without degrees. After obtaining a

nursing degree certificate, a nurse can continue to study for another two years to obtain a master's degree. The aim of this reform is to improve the academic qualifications of nurses and midwives. At present, there are 200,000 practicing nurses and midwives in Poland, but only 4,000 have graduated from higher education institutions.

2. *Certificate to practice nursing and midwifery.* According to the relevant provisions of the aforementioned law, only nurses and midwives who have received degree certificates issued by the regional chamber of nurses and midwives can engage in medical and health services in the relevant professions. All nurses who obtained nursing school diplomas before the reform also have the same qualification to practice under the new regulations.

3. *Postgraduate education for nurses and midwives.* According to the Nurses and Midwives Act, nurses and midwives not only have the right but also the obligation to participate in different types and forms of postgraduate medicine to improve their professional standards and acquire new knowledge and skills. Postgraduate education must be provided by a specially authorized unit or an individual who is recognized by the regional chamber of nurses and midwives as being qualified to organize postgraduate education.

4. *Medical practice of nurses and midwives.* Similar to physicians, nurses and midwives have a duty to serve patients using the best medical knowledge, most feasible methods, and professional accuracy while observing the code of medical ethics. The practical activities of nurses and midwives also include teaching and research in their respective areas and the management and supervision of nurses and midwives. Nurses and midwives have a duty to maintain the confidentiality of a patient's condition and other related professional information. Nurses and midwives have the right to obtain information from physicians regarding a patient's condition, diagnosis, treatment- and rehabilitation-related procedures, and possible consequences of treatment. They are also responsible for treating patients according to physician orders.

  The self-governments for nurses and midwives represent their professions and their interests. These self-governments are established in the form of organizational entities, such as the Chamber of Nurses and Midwives and its regional chambers. Members of regional chambers are nurses and midwives practicing within that region under its jurisdiction.

  The task of the professional self-governments for nurses and midwives is to confirm the relevant documents for licensure and to handle the registration of nurses and midwives. In addition, the Chamber of Nurses and Midwives also advises on issues related to undergraduate and postgraduate education, including specialty education and healthcare, as well as the legal regulations related to the practice of nursing and midwifery. Professional self-governments also supervise the actions of nurses and midwives and are responsible for adjudicating medical liabilities and conducting arbitration.

3. Other Medical Professions Prescribed by Law

1. *Pharmacists.* In accordance with the Act on the Chambers of Pharmacists enacted on April 19, 1999, to engage in the practice of pharmacy, an individual of sound physical health and full legal capacity must receive at least five years of university-level pharmacy education, undertake at least six months of internship, and obtain a master's degree in pharmaceutical sciences or an equivalent academic qualification recognized by EU countries. Pharmacists must be certified by the relevant regional chamber of pharmacists in order to work as a pharmacist in the Republic of Poland.

For citizens of EU countries, the qualification to practice pharmacy is regulated by a special legal document that mainly includes a checklist of diplomas and certificates and other documents issued by these countries. These documents prove that the individual has the necessary qualifications to work as a pharmacist in the Republic of Poland. The list is developed in detail by the Ministry of Health and is announced to the public.

Pharmacists are not permitted to practice as physicians, dentists, or veterinarians at the same time as they practice as pharmacists. The professional goal of pharmacists is to protect the health of the people, which specifically includes the following tasks: (1) providing medicinal products and medical devices through pharmacies and drug warehouses and supervising the operation, storage, and use of drugs and medical devices; (2) drug production and distribution; (3) evaluating the quality and authenticity of pharmacy and over-the-counter drugs; (4) providing drug information and therapeutic efficacies and applying for the required medical devices according to the needs of pharmacies and drug warehouses; (5) operating pharmacies, hospital drug retail outlets, or drug warehouses; (6) participating in drug administration and supervision, especially the drug supervision of healthcare institutions; (7) participating in clinical investigation and research conducted by hospitals; and (8) participating in drug research, monitoring the adverse effects of drugs, and reporting the findings to the relevant departments.

The self-government for pharmacists is bound by the Act on the Chambers of Pharmacists of July 21, 2001. According to the relevant provisions of the law, the Chamber of Pharmacists is responsible for formulating the task list of the self-government for pharmacists. The Chamber of Pharmacists is also an advisory body responsible for providing opinions and suggestions on activities related to the pharmaceutical industry and issues related to the trading of medical devices. The Chamber also has a duty to issue expert opinions, submit proposals for undergraduate and postgraduate pharmacy education, authorize pharmacists to practice, and handle the registration of pharmacists. As with other self-governments, the self-government for pharmacists is responsible for ensuring that its members are performing their duties correctly, supervising the actions of pharmacists, and performing the adjudication of professional liabilities and arbitration.

2. *Laboratory diagnosticians (medical or clinical biologists).* Individuals working as laboratory diagnosticians must have higher education diplomas and be of sound physical and mental health. They must be sworn in as laboratory diagnosticians, and their names are included in the list of laboratory diagnosticians.

There are two routes to becoming a laboratory diagnostician. The first is to obtain a master's degree in diagnostic analysis at a medical school. The second is to graduate in another profession that can provide solid background knowledge to practice as a laboratory diagnostician. The list of other professions is determined by the National Chamber of Laboratory Diagnosticians. However, the second route still requires postgraduate studies in the field of laboratory analysis and undergoing a review.

Laboratory diagnosticians conduct medical activities in laboratories. According to the "Laboratory Diagnostics Act" passed on April 20, 2004, laboratory diagnosticians have the following duties: (1) performing laboratory tests and examinations to clarify the physical, chemical, and biological properties of the analytes and analyzing the composition of bodily fluids, secretions, excretions, and tissues for the purposes of prevention, diagnosis, treatment, and public health epidemiology; (2) performing microbiological testing of bodily fluids, secretions, excretions, and tissues for the purposes of prevention, diagnosis, treatment, and public health epidemiology;

(3) performing histocompatibility testing; and (4) evaluating the quality and effectiveness of the above tests as well as the interpretation and normative analysis of laboratory results.

Laboratory diagnosticians are responsible for scientific research and teaching in laboratory diagnostics and the management of laboratories. In addition, laboratory diagnosticians have the right to participate in procedures and activities related to the collection of patients' biological materials.

Self-governments for laboratory diagnosticians have been established. The National Chamber of Laboratory Diagnosticians is a legal organizational entity that is also a self-government. The self-governments are supervised by the Ministry of Health in accordance with the principles and scope stipulated in the Laboratory Diagnostics Act. The Chamber has the authority to supervise and evaluate the actions of laboratory diagnosticians. To this end, the Chamber has designated inspectors and assigned them with the relevant functions.

According to the legal stipulations, the practice of laboratory diagnosticians is protected by law. The Chamber of Laboratory Diagnosticians decides who can or cannot be included in the list of laboratory diagnosticians. Upon the submission of a written request, death, or a court verdict to withdraw their qualifications, a laboratory diagnostician is removed from the list. Those who do not pay their membership fees for more than 12 months are also removed.

3. *Medical rescuers and medical dispatchers.* The establishment of the emergency medical system was based on the Act on the State Emergency Medical System, and its aim was to ensure the safety of citizens. In accordance with this Act, two medical professions were created: medical rescuers and medical dispatchers. Candidate medical rescuers must pass a national examination and obtain a university degree (or an equivalent academic qualification) to receive a license to practice. These requirements ensure that medical rescuers have uniform knowledge and skills regardless of their academic backgrounds. Knowledge acquired in higher vocational schools and medical specialized secondary schools better enables graduates to perform tasks independently or under the supervision of emergency physicians.

4. *Psychologists.* The services provided by psychologists play an important role in the diagnosis and treatment of certain diseases. The Act on the Profession of the Psychologist and the Self-Government of Psychologists was formally implemented on January 1, 2006. The law stipulates that the services provided by psychologists include diagnosis, advice, and decisions concerning psychotherapy and psychological support.

Other medical professions include speech therapists, physiotherapists, dental assistants, nutritionists, opticians, hearing therapists, dental hygienists, school health workers, orthopedic surgeons, child health workers, occupational therapists, medical laboratory technicians, dental technicians, pharmacist assistants, medical imaging technicians, medical massage therapists, orthopedic surgical technicians, and radiation protection officers.

3. Health Insurance System

(1) Main Health Insurance System

In the 1990s, healthcare in Poland was mainly funded by the government through budget allocations by the Ministry of Finance. The funds were mainly allocated by the providers of healthcare services, such as central government departments and provincial-, county-, and township-level units. In the 1990s, Poland's healthcare expenditure as a share of GDP and the national budget dropped slightly from an already low level. As it was difficult for state finances to maintain reforms and the public was unable to pay sufficient insurance premiums, the restructuring of health service financing remained in a state of stagnation. The reduction in budget allocation has increased the financial pressure on the health system. The goal of the new insurance plan is to develop new sources of income, regulate the financing of the health sector, further implement the decentralization (regionalization) of healthcare services, and introduce market mechanisms to increase efficiency. According to the results of a national randomized household survey in 1994, the out-of-pocket expenses of residents have increased significantly. The hope is that in the future, informal payments, including bonuses, can be replaced by insurance costs to a large extent.

The Universal Health Insurance Act of 1997 was formally implemented in January 1999. The implementation of this Act altered the financing system. After its enactment, there were two main sources of funding. The first was insurance funds, which directly financed the healthcare expenses of patients through contracts with service providers. The second was government budgets (state, province, or township), which continued to provide financial support for public health services, the main costs of all health services, tertiary specialist services (e.g., organ transplants), and high-cost drugs (e.g., immunosuppressants).

1. Statutory Health Insurance   In 1999, Poland implemented the reform of universal health insurance in accordance with the Universal Health Insurance Act. Its basic contents are as follows:

1. Companies (employers) contribute 8.5% of their employees' total wages to the health insurance fund in the form of taxes, and the insured persons (employees and their dependents) are given access to free basic healthcare services in contracted hospitals. If employers wish to provide employees with better healthcare benefits, they can purchase special health insurance for their employees in addition to the basic health insurance. Individuals can purchase commercial health insurance. Farmers, agricultural workers, and industrial workers (a total of two million in the country) do not pay personal contributions. The social insurance agencies are responsible for keeping statistics on insured persons, and their insurance is purchased only by the state. About 7% of health insurance funds are government subsidies.

   At the end of 2004, health insurance coverage in Poland was about 98.5%. Insured persons were free to choose their healthcare institutions and had access to free healthcare services, such as family physicians, specialist outpatient services, rehabilitation treatment, and medical care. However, they were required to pay meal expenses for hospitalization and 50% of the costs for drugs on the list of medications reimbursable by health insurance.

2. The state established a health insurance fund administration that is responsible for collecting and managing insurance premiums, calling for tenders from healthcare institutions that provide services, contracting with successful tendering institutions, and paying contracted institutions the healthcare expenses of patients.

3. The Ministry of Health developed healthcare policies and formulated detailed implementation rules and regulations for the Universal Health Insurance Act. It is also responsible for supervising and managing the access, quality, and actions of healthcare institutions and supervising the income and expenditure of the national health insurance fund. In addition, the government provided subsidies for certain special disease types and major diseases and directly administered university hospitals and research institutes.

4. Healthcare institutions that have contracted with the health insurance fund administration are responsible for providing healthcare services to insured persons. Contracted hospitals are selected through a tendering process. Successful tenderers receive income for healthcare services from the health insurance fund administration, as stipulated in the contract. The prices of healthcare services are set by hospitals during the tendering process.

Poland's reforms of the health insurance system have yielded substantial results, especially in reducing the national burden and encouraging competition among healthcare institutions.

2. Scope of Health Insurance Coverage In 1952, the Polish government began to promote the widespread availability of healthcare services. The health reforms in the 1990s were also efforts to keep this commitment. The Health Care Institutions Act of 1991 and subsequent related regulations stipulated the scope of basic services that must be provided. Only a small proportion of healthcare services were excluded, such as alternative treatments and cosmetic surgery. It also did not include some services in health resorts (spas), but those who were eligible for healthcare services could still receive free dental care and treatment at these spas.

The Universal Health Insurance Act of 1997 and its subsequent amendments proposed risk-free health insurance coverage for the entire population; this topic will be discussed later. As before, some service items were excluded, such as cosmetic surgery and treatments unrelated to diseases in healthcare institutions.

The Universal Health Insurance Act and the Act on Universal Health Insurance and National Health Fund were enacted on January 23, 2003, and were only implemented at the end of 2004. These two Acts clearly define the scope of healthcare services under the insurance plan. They also point out the goals of healthcare services, which include maintaining and restoring human health, preventing diseases and injuries, early diagnosis and treatment, and preventing and reducing disability. Insured persons have the right to obtain medical examinations and consultations, diagnostic tests, preventive healthcare, outpatient services, inpatient services, emergency services, rehabilitation, nursing, a supply of drugs and medical devices, the provision of orthopedic equipment and assistance, perinatal care, childbirth and postpartum recovery, palliative treatment, and proof of temporary or permanent disability. In terms of dental services, an exact pricing system has been established for standard dental procedures and dental materials according to the provisions in the Decree issued by the Ministry of Health.

The basic services that must be provided do not include the following:

1. Services that are funded based on different regulations, including occupational healthcare and high-tech medical services that are directly funded by the state budget.
2. The issuing of drivers' health certificates and other medical certificates for in-depth treatment, rehabilitation, and non-work-related disability within the scope of statutory entitlement at the request of the insured person (unless these must be submitted to welfare agencies or to receive a nursing care allowance). These regulations cover the social insurance of employees and farmers, continuing education, children, primary school students, trainees participating in teachers' training centers, and university students participating in sports and leisure activities.
3. Healthcare services provided by institutions such as health resort hospitals or nursing homes with the aim of addressing the issues that led the insured person to visit these healthcare institutions.

4. Nonstandard dental services.
5. Nonstandard vaccinations.
6. Other nonstandard health services listed in a decree announced by the Ministry of Health.

The Decree of April 4, 2003, promulgated by the Ministry of Health was the implementation clause for the Act on Universal Health Insurance and National Health Fund (Article 47). It specifies the following nonstandard healthcare services: plastic or cosmetic surgeries unrelated to diseases and their sequelae, congenital malformations or injuries, sex reassignment surgery, and acupuncture therapy (except for pain relief). The excluded service items were very limited, and these items have not changed with the transition from sickness funds to the NHF, nor have they been affected by the Act on the Public Funding of Healthcare Services enacted on August 27, 2004.

The OECD report in 2000 recommended that the scope of excluded services be further expanded to reduce the "package of promised services" financed through health insurance funds. However, this recommendation was not implemented.

In the service contract signed between the health service provider and the NHF branch (formerly the sickness fund), the limitations imposed on the volume of health service provision is a typical feature of the current insurance system, which usually limits people's access to health services. The restrictive measures, which aimed to impose strict financial constraints on health fund holders, resulted in patients being denied timely inpatient and outpatient services (especially at the end of the year for the basic accounting period) and led to longer waiting times. As a consequence, patients were forced to visit private health clinics or purchase health services through informal channels (bonuses), which gave easier access to services. In some cases, the waiting times were very long, especially for patients undergoing cancer surgery, which was detrimental to their health.

The final conclusion was that although the scope of health services guaranteed by law was extensive, in practice the contractual terms enforced to restrict costs have limited patients' access to health services. Thus, patients had no choice but to purchase services from the private or public sector, which increased their additional out-of-pocket expenses.

3. Financial Input by the State and Local Governments   In the reformed health service system, financial input by the state and local governments accounted for a very limited proportion of health service financing. At present, these expenditures only play a complementary role. In general, public health goals, health insurance funds for special populations (e.g., unemployed persons receiving social security benefits, pension recipients, farmers, and veterans), and investments in public healthcare institutions are derived from these inputs. The majority of funds to implement health projects are transferred to the NHF. The list of highly specialized services, which were funded by the Ministry of Health budget and based on contracts signed with service providers, was repealed. The NHF and its branches are responsible for the listed items that were agreed upon in the contract.

The funds from the state budget are mainly used for healthcare services for life-threatening conditions, such as accidents or childbirth, and for uninsured persons who do not have to pay health premiums. The Ministry of Health agrees to cover the expenses for diseases that cannot be diagnosed or treated in the country and must be treated abroad.

(2) Main Health Insurance Payment Methods

In 1999, health reforms involving an internal market were carried out in the health service system. This process was achieved through the introduction of universal health insurance and the establishment of independently managed sickness funds. These reforms included greater freedom in acquiring and utilizing public resources for use in the domain of health services. Due to the implementation of these measures, the responsibility for purchasing health services was separated from the providers, thus creating two major roles: purchasers and providers of health services. These health reforms brought about a fundamental change. In less than a year, all healthcare institutions had gained independent statuses and were able to sign contracts with sickness funds. They were released from the original budget financing, budget accounts, and reporting system and began to raise funds through service activities (these service activities were based on the financial terms of economic entities).

The Universal Health Insurance Act of 1997 was established on the basis of competitive tendering for health services, which set the principle of resource distribution for sickness funds. The terms and procedures for signing contracts, including the requirements for health service providers, rules governing the tendering for health services, and other conditions have been detailed in their respective provisions. At the end of 1998, the sickness funds began reviewing tenders, conducting negotiations, and signing contracts. In the first year of the reform, sickness funds could contract with any public or private health service providers that met the requirements (qualifications of healthcare workers and infrastructure, including devices and diagnostic equipment) and had the intention to sign a contract. The terms and conditions of health fund management and the signing of health service contracts were implemented in accordance with the relevant provisions of the Universal Health Insurance Act and the recommendations from the representatives of the health reform. The 17 sickness funds could autonomously set the allocation ratio of funds for different kinds of health services, determine the services that require contracting, and negotiate the prices of individual services.

1. Payment of Hospitals   Emergency and short-term hospitalization are the major service areas for reforms to the funding system. As mentioned above, the sickness funds had undergone reforms to their financing mechanisms for several consecutive years, such as, for example, consolidating the costs of individual services, differentiating inpatient services based on the average length of a hospital stay, separate financing for the hospital admission office, and introducing the DRG-based financing system to a certain extent. In 2003, on the basis of clarifying service procedures and basic prices, a unified hospital service classification standard (more than 1,000 groups) was introduced. This standard helped to resolve the limited volume of inpatient services and increase the accessibility of services without increasing costs. However, the lack of financial resources was still a major problem; although the volume of hospital services was increasing, hospital income was still decreasing. This issue was another factor that has led to the increase in hospital debt.

1. *Payment rules.* The general rule for payment methods is to make payments at the beginning of the month and to adopt different accounting cycles (once per month, once per quarter, or once per year). Most services use a direct funding mechanism. The prices of most individual services (e.g., expert consultations or inpatient services) are fixed, and the prices of day services in hospitals and other inpatient institutions are

also mostly fixed. The global budget system may sometimes be adopted as the funding method. The capitation system is implemented for primary healthcare but does not account for differences in health risks and number of visits in the population. Under previous systems, primary care physicians served as gatekeepers and referred patients to other service providers in the public health service system. Many conclusions and recommendations have been drawn based on the review and evaluation of the operations of the funding mechanism in the first fiscal year. More accurate definitions were needed for the requirements and standards for real estate and equipment and the scope of health services delivered by providers. In addition, as the fund holders, sickness funds were responsible for fund management, and there was a need to define special services more accurately.

In order to improve the signing of hospital service agreements, some sickness funds introduced their own DRG-based systems in 2000. According to the DRG-based systems, hospitals were responsible for issuing checklists of diagnoses, diagnostic tests, and treatment procedures. By analyzing the relationship between hospital expenses and patient treatments for DRGs, the approximate costs of individual DRGs could be derived. Most sickness funds began to use new directories of service categories, such as "short-term hospital treatment" and "day surgery," and differentiated hospital treatments according to differences in procedures.

In the field of specialist consultation, basic tests and procedures were required to be defined within the scope of comprehensive consultation. These tests and procedures were more expensive than routine consultations based on diagnostic tests. With regard to hospital services, service accessibility was often considered in contract negotiations, and waiting times were the main indicator of accessibility. In terms of dental services, the definition of key indicator systems had been verified. For example, service items with poor clinical efficacy also had lower prices. In the field of rehabilitation, there were fixed prices for various treatment procedures and services. It was also common to sign for comprehensive rehabilitation service packages.

2. *Negotiation mechanisms.* In terms of price negotiations, sickness funds did not need to consider the service costs calculated by service providers. They were in a monopolistic position and, hence, could use this advantage to set price standards and limit the number of services (the number of agreements reached). From the perspective of fund holders, this approach was reasonable as the funds for signing health service contracts were limited by the available resources. However, this action caused service providers to face serious financial problems. The payment of additional services outside of service contracts became an issue of concern. Many factors can cause healthcare institutions to generate debt, the vast majority of which are due to hospitals, and this phenomenon began at the start of operations in the new system. These factors mainly included service structures that were not reflected in contracts or the limited capacities and cost burdens of health service providers. Due to fixed prices and price limitations imposed by sickness funds, dissatisfaction grew among the founders of institutions during the process of restructuring public hospitals, and the growth rate of the financial resources managed by sickness funds was also relatively low. The relevant departments strived to gradually standardize service contracts, first by introducing unified definitions of service, quality, and waiting times and also by formulating standards to resolve the differences between the number and type of services stipulated in contracts and their actual implementation. In addition, the sickness funds made efforts to improve the monitoring system with regard to the qualifications of healthcare workers, infrastructure, the accuracy of medical documents, the reliability of service data, the quality of health services, and accessibility in order to enhance the monitoring of service provision and implementation.

The proportion of private health service providers that contracted with the sickness funds continued to increase in terms of volumes and funding amounts, especially in the areas of primary healthcare and dental services. In 2000, within the primary healthcare sector, the percentage of contracts with private health service providers exceeded 90% for three sickness funds, and only five funds had percentages below 50%. A similar situation occurred in the field of dental services. Due to the limited number of private hospitals, contracts with public hospitals were very common.

The new healthcare financing system began its development at the start of its operation and is still continually improving. In 2003, the NHF established contractual terms with service providers, setting out the exact scope of the terms and the routine and final regulations. In addition, detailed requirements for various services, including primary healthcare, outpatient specialist services, inpatient services, mental health and addiction services, medical rehabilitation, long-term care, dental services, convalescent services, emergency services and health transport, disease prevention and health promotion, single-contract services, orthopedic equipment, and medical devices, were established.

2. Payment of Physicians   The capitation funding mechanism based on patient lists has been widely recognized by sickness funds and approved by the NHF. Basic prices are adopted and differentiated according to three age groups (0–6 years, 7–64 years, and over 65 years) that enjoy different benefits (provided to nurses and community midwives, school-age children, and retirees of social welfare homes or nursing homes). The basic price level is also a common problem. For example, the price in 2003 remained at the level of 2002, but physicians were required to provide additional 24-hour healthcare services. This change led to protests among primary care physicians. Through negotiations with primary care physicians who went on strike, a price agreement to increase the capitation fee was finally reached. However, there is still a lack of consistency and significant differences in prices paid across the country.

(3) Status of Healthcare Expenditure

1. Healthcare Expenditure Per Capita   In 2010, Poland's health expenditure per capita was US$917.11. After correcting for inflation (calculated based on the prices in 1997), the average annual growth rate of healthcare expenditure per capita in Poland was 2.6% from 1995 to 2010. From 1995 to 2008, healthcare expenditure per capita showed a trend of steady growth. In 2009 and 2010, expenditure decreased and stabilized, as shown in Table 12.23 and Figure 12.16.

2. Healthcare Expenditure and Economic Growth   In 2010, the total healthcare expenditure in Poland was 7.46% of GDP. In the past 15 years, regardless of Poland's GDP growth rate, total healthcare expenditure as a share of GDP has shown a trend of steady growth, which indicates the sustainability and stability of health investment in Poland (Figure 12.17).

3. Funding Sources   In 2010, the share of spending by the Polish government and government agencies (public sector) accounted for 72.62% of total healthcare expenditure, and the share of personal out-of-pocket expenses was 22.06%. Since 1995, the share of public spending in total health expenditure has remained relatively stable at around 70%, and the share of personal out-of-pocket expenses has shown a steady decline (Figure 12.18).

TABLE 12.23 Indicators Related to Healthcare Expenditure in Poland in 1995–2010

Indicator	1995	1996	1997	1998	1999	2000	2001	2002	2003	2004	2005	2006	2007	2008	2009	2010
Healthcare expenditure per capita (US$)	197.64	237.95	227.81	263.74	248.76	246.98	292.02	328.59	354.28	410.51	494.20	555.49	717.18	972.51	829.48	917.11
Healthcare expenditure per capita measured by purchasing power parity (PPP) (constant 2005 international $)	406.2	472.9	492.5	553.6	567.6	583.5	641.8	732.9	748.1	807.4	856.7	934.3	1077.8	1264.7	1390.7	1476.1
Total healthcare expenditure as a share of GDP	5.48	5.88	5.61	5.91	5.73	5.52	5.86	6.34	6.24		6.21		6.43	7.00	7.35	7.46
Personal out-of-pocket expenses as a share of total expenditure	27.11	26.61	28.04	34.62	28.87	29.97	28.10	25.44	26.43	28.11	26.12	25.59	24.23	22.42	22.30	22.06
Government health spending as a share of total expenditure	72.89	73.39	71.96	65.38	71.13	70.03	71.90	71.16	66.27	64.67	64.65	69.90	70.84	72.24	72.32	72.62

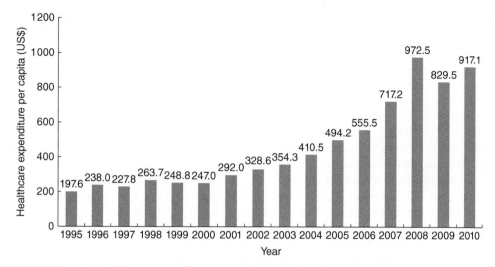

FIGURE 12.16   Healthcare expenditure per capita in Poland in 1995–2010.

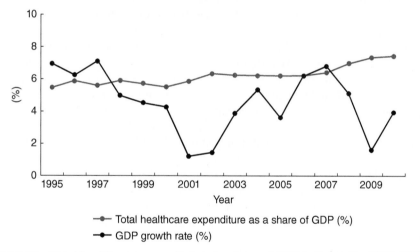

FIGURE 12.17   Total healthcare expenditure as a share of GDP in Poland in 1995–2010.

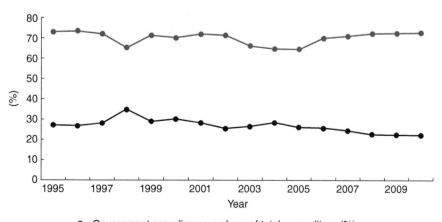

FIGURE 12.18   Composition of total healthcare expenditure in Poland in 1995–2010.

4. Reforms to the Health System and Social Security Planning

(1) Historical Course of Reform

The ongoing health reforms in Poland began in 1989. Prior to 1989, there were three relatively important healthcare reforms. The first reform took place during the early founding of the country and aimed to establish free and universal public health services. The purpose of the second reform was to provide comprehensive health and social services to all regions. In 1960, the Ministry of Health changed its name to the Ministry of Health and Welfare. In 1972, integrated healthcare units (*zakład opieki zdrowotnej*, ZOZ) were established to manage hospitals, clinics, specialists, and primary healthcare. The aim of the third reform was to achieve the decentralization of public administrative power. In 1983, the authority of the Ministry of Health and Welfare was reduced, whereas the authority of provincial and county governments and the ZOZ was enhanced. In 1989, Poland underwent reforms to its political system that also led to changes in its health system. The changes in the health system were mainly reflected as decentralization (regionalization).

The Universal Health Insurance Act was enacted on February 6, 1997, and implemented on January 1, 1999, after revisions. This law made fundamental changes to the structure and funding sources of the public health service system. The establishment of mandatory health insurance abolished the centralized health service system funded by the national budget. The purpose of mandatory health insurance was to ensure that citizens had equal access to health services. This system was administered by government departments (the Ministry of Health and provincial health departments). Health services were provided by public healthcare institutions with the status of budget entities. The new system established 16 regional sickness funds and 1 sickness fund for uniformed public servants. These organizations became the holders of public healthcare funds and mainly fundraised through health insurance. Access to health services was related to whether an individual was enrolled in mandatory health insurance and whether he or she contributed to insurance premiums. Public healthcare institutions were transformed into independent healthcare institutions that earned income through health services and were responsible for their own profits and losses. In April 2003, the sickness funds were replaced by the NHF. This measure, on the one hand, was due to the dissatisfaction of insured persons towards the new system and, on the other hand, was due to political reasons.

The reform of 1997 and its multiple amendments finally introduced two major public funding sources for health services: the NHF and fiscal budgets (including the fiscal budgets of national, provincial, county, and township government departments). Due to its dual nature, this system is known as the insurance-budget system. The specific course of its development is as follows.

1. Reforms in 1989–1998 The focus of reforms during this period was the deepening of decentralization and the strengthening of primary healthcare. Polish health services had followed a strictly centralized system. In 1989, the government began to discuss the restructuring of the health service system. In the early 1990s, Poland continued its transformation of the public sector and the reorganization of its hierarchical health service system, thus gradually transferring the majority of management rights for health services and the ownership of public facilities to provincial and local governments. In 1998, county-level governments were reinstated and were responsible for the administration of county-level hospitals. In terms of primary healthcare, the focus on family medicine led to improvements in primary healthcare. The "family medicine" strategy was formulated, and the School of Family

Medicine was established to support this strategy. In addition, post-graduate training in general medicine was also given to specialists.

2. Reforms in 1999–2002   The Polish health system underwent major structural reforms during this period. On January 1, 1999, the implementation of the Universal Health Insurance Act led to fundamental reforms to the structure and funding sources of the public health service system. This reform was predominantly manifested as the introduction of mandatory health insurance and the creation of 16 regional sickness funds and 1 separate fund for public servants (e.g., the military and railway workers). The sickness funds were the holders of public healthcare funds and signed contracts with independent healthcare institutions to purchase health services. Citizens' access to health services was determined by whether they were enrolled in mandatory health insurance and whether they contributed to insurance premiums. Another prominent feature of this period was that nearly all healthcare institutions were separated from the original budget financing, budget accounts, and reporting systems, thus becoming independent institutions that could contract with the sickness funds. The Universal Health Insurance Act ultimately shifted the funding source for health services from one predominated by the state budget to an insurance-budget system predominated by health insurance funds and supplemented by the state budget. However, the changes in funding sources did not lead to significant improvements in the public income of health services.

3. Reforms After 2003   Due to the dissatisfaction of the insured towards the reforms and various political reasons, the 17 sickness funds were ultimately replaced by the NHF. However, its functions essentially remained unchanged. The NHF manages the insurance funds and is responsible for planning and purchasing health services. To a certain extent, this reform was also a result of the lack of policy stability at the central level of the Polish health system. The Act on the Public Funding of Healthcare Services enacted in August 2004 brought about a new opportunity for healthcare reforms. This Act introduced new rules for the contracting of health services and stipulated the specific obligations of the NHF.

The results attained by the reforms since the 1990s are worthy of recognition, especially the reduction in the number of beds and the elevation in the status of family physicians. Moreover, national health planning has also ensured that prevention and health promotion received greater attention. However, its existing problems should not be ignored. The inadequacy of financial resources for public health, the reduced accessibility of health services, and increased personal health expenditures have already led to widespread public dissatisfaction towards health services and have affected the public's confidence in the reforms.

(2) Reform Characteristics

1. Establishment of a Legal System   The health reforms in Poland were supported by numerous pieces of legislation. During the process of reform, the government promulgated a series of bills, from the Universal Health Insurance Act, which had a profound impact on reform, to the most recent Act on the Public Funding of Healthcare Services. Each bill clearly stipulates the purpose of the reforms and the rights and obligations of relevant sectors, thus enabling affairs to be conducted according to law.

2. Health Service Provision   The Constitution of the Republic of Poland stipulates that all citizens shall have equal access to healthcare services, irrespective of their ability to pay, and public authorities shall ensure special healthcare to children, pregnant women, disabled persons, and elderly persons. The Act on the Public Funding of Healthcare Services included homeless persons in health insurance and stipulated that their premiums shall be paid by social healthcare institutions.

3. Formulation of Health Policies Health policies should be established by the public and should be able to target all social classes. The 1996–2005 National Health Programme (NHP), which was formulated based on this principle, significantly improved the health status of the Polish population. This measure was a major victory in Polish health reforms. The success of the 1996–2005 NHP indicates that the focus of health policies should be shifted from centralization in high-level state management to public participation.

4. Healthcare Benefits and Distribution The Universal Health Insurance Act and its subsequent amendments proposed risk-free health insurance coverage for the entire population. The Universal Health Insurance Act and the Act on Universal Health Insurance and National Health Fund enacted on January 23, 2003, clearly define the scope of healthcare services under the insurance plan. The scope of healthcare services protected by the law was relatively broad. However, in practice, the contractual terms that were enforced to limit costs led to long waiting times for patients and reduced access to health services. Thus, patients were forced to purchase health services from private institutions or the public health sector, which instead increased their additional healthcare expenditures.

5. Social Healthcare The advent of population aging necessitated the development of social healthcare and long-term care. Under the centralized "Semashko" model, which was built as a multi-tiered healthcare system with a strongly differentiated network of service providers, where each of the five levels corresponded to the severity of the disease, the development of social healthcare was less than ideal, and many patients were cared for by their families. In the 1990s, voluntary and nongovernmental organizations developed rapidly and played an important role in the provision of nursing, hospice care, rehabilitation services, long-term inpatient services, and community services. As for the government, beds with low utilization rates were adapted to beds for chronic diseases, rehabilitation, long-term treatment, palliative care, and psychiatric treatment to meet the needs of patients.

CHAPTER THIRTEEN

Commercial Health Insurance and Medical Savings Account Systems of Representative Countries

 ## SECTION I. THE COMMERCIAL HEALTH INSURANCE SYSTEM IN THE UNITED STATES

The United States (US) is located in the central part of the North American continent. It has an area of 9.37 million km² and a population of roughly 327.17 million (as of 2018). White Americans account for more than 80% of the total population, followed by African Americans accounting for about 11% and other ethnic groups accounting for about 9%. The US is a typical free market economy, whereby market regulation is the main method of resource allocation, and private enterprises are the major players in economic operations. The economic behaviors of the government mainly involve offsetting market failures, maintaining market order, and ensuring economic stability. In 2012, the life expectancies at birth for men and women in the US were 76.4 years and 81.2 years, respectively. In 2013, the infant mortality rate was 5.9 per 1,000 live births, and the maternal mortality rate was 28 per 100,000 live births. The percentage of the US population aged over 65 years was 14%. The natural population growth rate was 0.7%, and the GDP per capita was US$53,042.

The US is the largest capitalist country in the world. Although its main political parties – the Democratic Party and Republican Party – claim to have differing political views, they are both committed to safeguarding the interests of the monopolistic consortia after taking office. The impact of the political system on healthcare is reflected in nearly every presidential election. Although the promises of health reform for the public good have given rise to new reform ideas, these ideas are rarely implemented. This is a major reason for the relative stability of the healthcare system in the US.

The US government has rather weak control over the healthcare industry, which is largely predominated by commercial healthcare institutions with strong monopolistic power. The consortium of healthcare institutions and health-related businesses (e.g., health insurance agencies) has become an important aspect of various healthcare services and their management. The allocation of healthcare resources is mainly balanced via market regulation, and the government has limited ability to implement the macroprudential regulation.

The US has injected enormous capital into healthcare, which accounted for 17.9% of GDP in 2012, equivalent to US$8,895 per capita. Healthcare expenditure ranked third after defense and education. The main sources of funding were the government (41%) and individuals (59%). Hospitals made up the largest share of healthcare expenditure (59%), followed by community healthcare centers (e.g., family medicine services and nursing homes), which contributed about 28% of the total expenditure. From 2000 to 2008, the US economy grew by US$4.4 trillion, of which one-fourth was spent on healthcare. The Congressional Budget Office estimated that the total healthcare expenditure will increase from 17.9% of the GDP in 2012 to 30% in 2035. As noted above, the US is a federal country with a free-market economy. The diversification of administrative and economic systems has an important impact on the US healthcare system, which is mainly characterized by its diverse operating and delivery models.

The US healthcare system has been completely marketized and is mainly composed of private medical holdings and private hospitals. There are only a handful of public healthcare institutions. With the exception of the military and veterans' affairs healthcare systems, most public institutions are primary care institutions that are mainly distributed in rural and impoverished areas, where private healthcare institutions are reluctant to serve. Many so-called public hospitals are in fact operated by private medical holdings. However, the vast majority of private healthcare institutions are nonprofit organizations that strictly follow a nonprofit management and business model. All profits are used for the construction and development of hospitals; shareholders do not receive any return on investment.

The US is a federal republic, in which all state governments have independent legislative, executive, and judicial systems. The state governments are also endowed with the authority to establish their own healthcare service systems and formulate the corresponding policies and regulations. As the state governments hold primary responsibility for healthcare funding, the federal government only provides policy guidance and financial support for certain healthcare programs. Therefore, based on the principle of unified administrative and financial powers under this system, the healthcare systems of different states are not only permitted to differ in terms of administration, service delivery, and health protection but also tend to show substantial disparities.

The US is one of the few developed countries without a universal health insurance system. Medicare and Medicaid recipients account for only around 23% (54.10 million) of the US population, and more than half of the Americans rely solely on private insurance, while the remaining 14% have not enrolled in public or private health insurance schemes. The number and percentage of uninsured Americans from 1987 to 2008 are shown in Figure 13.1.

1. Healthcare Institutions

(1) Types and Functions of Healthcare Institutions

1. Types of Healthcare Institutions   There is considerable diversity in US healthcare facilities. For example, clinics (i.e., private practitioners) range from simple outpatient clinics to clinics equipped with advanced medical devices, outpatient surgery centers, birth centers, emergency care centers, practices that serve as the basis for home-based medical and nursing care, and hospice care centers. Hospitals have an average of 179 beds and are

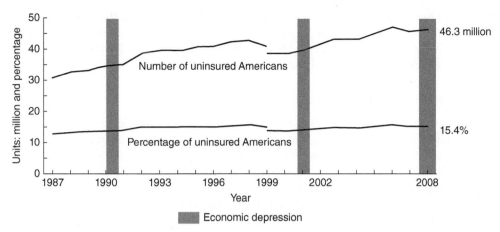

FIGURE 13.1 Number and percentage of uninsured Americans from 1987 to 2008. *Source:* US Census Bureau, Current Population Survey, 1987–2008 Annual Social and Economic Supplements.

well-stocked with medical equipment. In addition to providing healthcare services, many hospitals also serve as research and educational institutions. There are also public hospitals (e.g., hospitals run by charities) that do not target the general public.

Nursing homes are facilities for the long-term care, nursing or rehabilitative care of patients with chronic diseases. In addition to hospital services, nursing homes provide health and social welfare services for patients. Currently, the number of nursing home beds has exceeded that of hospital beds. Furthermore, nursing homes have become the largest recipient of Medicaid reimbursement.

2. Hospitals   In 2008, there were 5,815 hospitals in the US with 951,045 beds. Among these hospitals, 213 were federally owned. On average, there were 29 hospital beds per 10,000 people in the US from 2006 to 2012.

Broadly speaking, hospitals can be classified into short- and long-term inpatient hospitals, which have average lengths of hospital stay of less than and more than 25 days, respectively. Short-term inpatient hospitals include nonprofit hospitals (65%), state hospitals (18%), for-profit hospitals (10%), and federal hospitals (7%). Long-term inpatient hospitals, on the other hand, include psychiatric hospitals and tuberculosis hospitals, 90% of which (based on the number of beds) are either state or federal hospitals.

The number of hospital beds at short-term inpatient hospitals changed very slightly from 1980 to 2000, whereas among long-term inpatient hospitals, the number of psychiatric hospital beds decreased by 17% over that same period. An increasing trend was also evident in the number of for-profit hospitals for short-term inpatient care, with the proportion of their beds to the total number of hospital beds increasing from 6% in 1970 to 10% in 2000.

3. Nursing Homes   Nursing homes include both skilled nursing facilities (SNFs) and intermediate care facilities (ICFs). The latter account for about 90% of nursing homes in the US, while the former account for the remaining 10%.

Due to population aging, the number of nursing homes in 1986 with more than 25 beds was 16,033 nursing homes (70% of which are for-profit), and the total number of beds was

1,618,480 beds, which represented an increase of 25% compared to the previous decade. The number of beds per 1,000 people aged over 65 years was 56, and this figure only fluctuated slightly during this period. In the US, the total number of beds in hospitals and nursing homes was 2,912,276 beds, and the number of beds per 100,000 people is 1,200.

(2) Utilization of Healthcare Institutions

1. Clinics and Hospitals   Patients in the US tend to first seek medical attention from nearby private practitioners, who traditionally have the freedom to charge patients based on their technical capabilities. However, these medical charges are established according to the balance between free competition and self-regulation. Hence, the medical charges must not exceed the average level of that region by a significant amount. Most hospitals adopt an open system, whereby a private practitioner who has signed a contract with the hospital can refer a patient for admission to the hospital when necessary. The private practitioner might participate in the inpatient services at the hospital and conduct follow-ups or treatments after the patient has been discharged. In such circumstances, the patient must pay both the private practitioner and the hospital.

In 2000, the US recorded seven visits per capita to clinics and hospitals (12 visits per capita for elderly adults aged over 65 years), among which clinics accounted for 56%, hospitals 15%, telephone consultations 13%, and others (e.g., home visits) 16%. Furthermore, the number of visits per capita for dental care services was two visits per year. Short-term inpatient hospitals had a total of 35.48 million visits with an average length of hospital stay of 6.3 days. Compared to 1980, the number of inpatients declined by 7%, while the average length of hospital stay shortened by 11%. On the other hand, there were 272.83 million outpatient visits, which showed an increasing trend in recent years. The utilization rate of short-term inpatient beds declined from 76% in 1980 to 72% in 1995, while the utilization rate of long-term inpatient beds remained at about 87%.

In 2002, the US spent approximately US$155.3 billion on healthcare, much of which comprised hospital charges (39%), physician charges (20%), and drug expenses (7%). A total of US$1,904 per day was spent on inpatient charges incurred at short-term inpatient hospitals, which was more than twice the cost seven years prior. Hospitals and physicians both receive fee-for-service payments. However, the rapid emergence of managed healthcare programs, including health maintenance organizations (HMOs) and preferred provider organizations (PPOs), has led to the widespread application of prospective capitation models. Additionally, prospective payment systems (PPS) have been adopted for the reimbursement of inpatient services covered by Medicaid. A PPS compensates hospitals according to the fixed amounts specified for the 467 diagnosis-related groups (DRGs), irrespective of the number of service items.

Among US residents under the age of 65 years, 76% have purchased private health insurance, and 6% are Medicaid recipients. All elderly residents aged over 65 years are covered by Medicare, among whom 72% are covered by Medicare and private insurance, while 6% are covered by Medicare and Medicaid, which will reimburse 75–80% of medical expenses after the deductible has been met.

Patients must pay a considerable share of medical expenses, regardless of whether they are covered by social or private insurance. A key objective of the Medicare Amendments of 1988 was to reduce these heavy out-of-pocket expenses (including the newly established prescription drug coverage). In addition, 14% of the US population is uninsured and must pay the full amount of medical charges at their own expenses.

2. Nursing Homes   In 2000, 1.85 million individuals were admitted to nursing home, among whom those aged 65–74 years accounted for 16%, those aged 75–84 years accounted for 39%, and those aged over 85 years accounted for 45%. In terms of gender, males and females accounted for 25% and 75%, respectively, while individuals who were capable of self-care – in terms of eating, toileting, and dressing – accounted for 61%, 39%, and 25%, respectively.

The share of nursing home expenses out of the total US healthcare expenditure increased from 4.9% in 1965 to 11.7% in 2000 (when it was roughly US$78.6 billion). In addition, the shares of nursing home expenses out of the total Medicare and Medicaid expenditures were 1.4% (US$1.8 billion) and 36% (US$46.6 billion), respectively. Overall, nursing home expenses were shared among admittees (57%), Medicaid (42%), and Medicare (1%). Nursing homes imposed an average admission fee of US$1,456 per month. Admittees were still eligible for Medicare reimbursement within 150 days (100 days before the Medicare Amendments of 1988) after being discharged, during which they must only pay a fixed amount of out-of-pocket expenses (about US$20 per day). However, long-term admittees who have stayed in nursing homes for more than 150 days must bear the full cost of expenses incurred after 150 days. Therefore, some elderly Americans have no choice but to apply for Medicaid after they have exhausted their personal assets.

(3) Hospital Reforms and Development

1. Hospital Quality Assessment   The US has arguably the best healthcare quality in the world due to its strong economic and technological support. Currently, healthcare development in the US is driven by hospitals. This is in stark contrast to the past when many US hospitals were poorly equipped. However, hospital quality in the US has improved dramatically following the implementation of regional health plans and the assistance for hospital construction in accordance with the Hospital Survey and Construction Act (also known as the Hill–Burton Act), which was enacted after World War II. In addition, improvements in hospital quality can also be attributed to the efforts of the Joint Commission on Accreditation of Healthcare Organizations (JCAHO).

The JCAHO adopted the hospital standardization program established by the American Surgical Association in the 1920s. It is mainly composed of the American Hospital Association (AHA), the Association of American Physicians (AAP), the American Society of Internal Medicine (ASIM), the American Surgical Association, and some NGOs established in 1951. It has a strict accreditation system for hospitals in the training of specialists, which in turn provides hospitals with a strong motivation to improve their medical facilities. The JCAHO also imposes high accreditation standards for each renewal of accreditation. As a result, hospitals must constantly seek to improve their service quality while also competing with each other.

The functional differentiation and collaboration between hospitals and clinics facilitate the effective investment of expensive medical facilities and the qualification check of hospital-contracted physicians. Furthermore, the widespread promotion of the specialist system has improved physicians' participation in research and the expansion of equipment at hospitals. Since the 1950s, the US government has begun to inject a massive amount of capital into various medical research institutes, such as the National Institutes of Health (NIH), which has also contributed to a dramatic improvement in hospital services.

2. Changes in Hospital Industry   The US healthcare system is a public system to a certain extent, with about 40% of the total healthcare expenditure being covered by public funds. However, it is essentially a liberal system that relies on well-developed healthcare marketization; as such, it differs markedly from the Japanese system, which prohibits profits and dividends and imposes advertising restrictions. However, on the one hand, this hospital-centered healthcare industry has completed its rapid growth; on the other hand, administrative authorities have begun to implement various policies targeting hospital providers that aim to suppress rising medical expenses.

Mergers and acquisitions among hospitals in the US have given rise to highly competitive hospital clusters and franchises. Moreover, the participation of large enterprises has promoted the industrialization of healthcare services, as well as hospital rationalization and diversification. The US healthcare market has also expanded alongside the diversification of healthcare demands. Since the nineteenth century, the hospital-centered healthcare system has gradually shifted towards the replacement of inpatient facilities with outpatient surgery centers and home-based care to ensure a comfortable living environment for patients. Hospitals with reduced inpatients and bed utilization began to attract users by providing convenience, comfort, and a trustworthy and respectful environment. The rapid development of cutting-edge technology in the 1980s, along with the healthcare cost-containment policies formulated by the Reagan administration in accordance with the principles of marketization, have promoted the implementation of a development model that is compatible with the healthcare industry and has driven the reform of the physician–patient relationship.

3. Concepts for Hospital Development The US healthcare environment has undergone considerable changes in the past. Hospitals that once aimed to only treat patients have gradually changed their developmental concept, becoming comprehensive centers for counseling and health promotion that aim to improve the quality of life. The growth rate of inpatient charges has slowed down in the two decades since the introduction of the PPS, but the expenses for outpatient, physician, and other specialized services have remained high. The US federal government considered the PPS as a cornerstone of the future health security system and has continued to show a strong desire to undertake fundamental health reforms.

The economic effects of healthcare-related activities have begun to receive more positive appraisals, as they improve the health status of the labor force via the prevention and treatment of diseases and induce the productivity of healthcare-related industries, such as biotechnology. The US has to make new development choices to ensure healthcare quality while also controlling for an excessive growth of healthcare expenditure.

(4) Integrated Care Organizations

Integrated care organizations are jointly formed by hospitals and physicians that were once independent practitioners. Joint ventures and mergers are the two basic forms of such organizations. A joint venture refers to a new legal entity established by various parties via a contract, while a merger involves a change of ownership such that the transferrer loses its independent existence. The integrative process of US healthcare service organizations has followed two directions: horizontal integration among physicians, and vertical integration among physicians, hospitals, and insurance agencies.

1. Integrated Care Organizations Among Physicians
   1. *Preferred provider organizations (PPOs).* PPOs are joint ventures among physicians that usually negotiate with medical expense payers (i.e., employers and insurance companies) on the standard fees or discount rates for certain services in exchange for its members being listed as preferred providers (employers or insurance companies

provide a list of recommended providers to their employees or insured persons) to reduce medical expenses. Such organizations must be subject to quality control and utility management.

2. *Independent practice associations (IPAs).* IPAs are typical organizational entities that negotiate with employers and insurance companies on behalf of physicians and represent their interests. They differ from PPOs in that they accept prospective capitation (per member per month) and provide services that fall within the scope of the contract.

3. *Group practices.* These are medical practices comprising more than three physicians who share business operations, facilities, and management resources. Their revenues are allocated on a preagreed basis.

4. *Partially integrated medical groups (PIMGs).* These are larger legal entities consisting of physicians and can be partnerships or professional corporations, wherein members retain some degree of autonomy.

5. *Fully integrated medical groups (FIMGs).* FIMGs involve more extensive cooperation and centralized management, which has complete authority over all aspects of healthcare services, including quality and utility management.

2. Integrated Care Organizations for Physicians and Hospitals

1. *Physician-hospital organizations (PHOs).* PHOs usually consist of a hospital and its healthcare workers but can also include multiple hospitals and physicians who work outside these hospitals. Hospitals generally occupy the central position in PHOs. In addition to providing healthcare services, PHOs may also provide other services, such as management services, accreditation, utility reviews, and quality assurance reviews.

2. *Integrated delivery systems (IDSs).* IDSs are fully integrated organizations comprising physicians and hospitals (including various types of specialist hospitals) that provide a range of healthcare, management, and information services. IDSs cover a broad geographical scope in providing these services.

3. *Management service organizations (MSOs).* MSOs mainly provide administrative management and practice management services to physicians. MSO services for physicians might be limited to financial management, but can also include contract negotiations, staff management for nonhealthcare workers, and even offices with furniture and medical facilities.

4. *Health maintenance organizations (HMOs).* HMOs provide a wide range of healthcare services that have been integrated with healthcare fundraising, making it an entity that effectively combines the services of physicians, hospitals, and insurance agencies. HMOs often adopt more comprehensive measures in attempts to control costs via a reduction in unnecessary healthcare services. For example, policyholders are given lower rates of cost sharing when seeking services within the provider network than outside it.

2. Healthcare Workforce

(1) Medical Education Systems

1. Basic Medical Education   There are currently 127 medical schools in the US. Students in the US usually enroll in a four-year medical course at a medical school after completing a four-year degree at a general university. There are also a handful of medical preparatory schools that offer a two-year medical course for high-school graduates; however, these schools have strict limitations on the number of enrolled students. Determining whether a candidate fulfills the entry requirements for medical schools usually involves comprehensive consideration of their performance during the four-year course at the general university, their score on the Medical College Admission Test (MCAT) conducted by the Association of American Medical Colleges, and the results of interviews. During these interviews, applicants are asked detailed questions about their life experiences, motives for becoming physicians, specialties, hobbies, and so on.

Although the course content for medical schools is regularly audited by organizations such as the American Medical Association (AMA) and the Liaison Committee on Medical Education (LCME), major changes are still allowed in accordance with the philosophy and characteristics of the respective universities. The 112- to 175-week medical course is mostly completed within four years. Clinical internships are carried out at nearby teaching hospitals that have signed agreements with the schools.

2. Postgraduate Education　Medical students in the US must receive internship training specified by the Accreditation Council for Graduate Medical Education (ACGME). In general, interns are not only trained at their own departments but also rotate between various departments. In 1975, the general assembly of the AMA decided to further expand the one-year postgraduate internship program into the resident training system, which takes place over a few years.

The duration of resident training varies among different specialties. For example, it is about three years for internists and GPs, and five to seven years for surgeons. Physicians are recognized by various associations as qualified specialists and GPs (there are currently 22 qualifications) upon the completion of a resident training course. The vast majority of resident physicians are able to withstand such rigorous training as they enjoy a very high social status and considerable income after becoming specialists and GPs. However, specialists and GPs are still required to continue medical education and take regular examinations.

(2) Medical Training System

1. Medical License　Medical graduates who have obtained a Doctor of Medicine (MD) degree from a medical school must then obtain a medical license in accordance with the respective state medical laws before they are permitted to engage in clinical work (i.e., run a medical practice). In general, medical licenses are applicable to the respective states only. To obtain a medical license, a medical graduate must graduate from an LCME-recognized medical school, complete the required internship training, and then pass the examination set by the National Board of Medical Examiners (NBME) or the Federal Medical Licensing Examination (FLEX). Those who have passed the Foreign Medical Graduate Examination in the Medical Sciences (FMGEMS) are also eligible for medical licensure, albeit with more restricted numbers and a higher threshold. The NBME examination comprises three parts: Comprehensive Basic Science Self-Assessment (CBSSA), Comprehensive Clinical Science Self-Assessment (CCSSA), and Comprehensive Clinical Medicine Self-Assessment (CCMSA). Many students take these examinations on a step-by-step basis upon completing a two-year medical course, at graduation, and in the first year of their internship training, respectively. FLEX carries out its examinations within the same period of time. State authorities then determine whether the candidates have passed the examinations based on their examination scores and independent weighted factors. Since the 1970s, 22 states in the US have established expiration dates for medical licenses; as such, medical practitioners are obligated to receive continuing medical education (CME) for license renewal.

2. Physician Quality Control   The quality control of American physicians is further enhanced by CME and a strict qualification system. The implementation of CME is centered on the AMA, which utilizes medical schools and other resources to organize seminars, lectures, and case discussions regularly. The AMA issues CME qualification certificates and has attempted to develop various approaches to increase physicians' motivation for CME, such as collaboration between the Nationwide Health Information Network (NHIN) and Peer Review Organizations (PRO). On the other hand, the Accreditation Council for Continuing Medical Education (ACCME) is responsible for content development and quality assessment.

Thus, it can be seen that the accreditation of medical schools, admission selection process, and physician qualifying examinations in the US have all been entrusted to legal intermediary organizations, rather than to government agencies. Additionally, the administration of medical education, postgraduate internships, and CME have been entrusted to the Association of American Medical Colleges and the AMA. It is evident that the US medical education system is characterized by its diversity and specificity. Various types of accreditation and qualifications have a limited term, and each renewal requires physicians to further improve their techniques and service quality.

3. Controlling the Number of Physicians   In 2000, there were 534,800 practicing physicians in the US and 250 physicians per 100,000 people. The number of physicians per 100,000 people fluctuated at about 140 in the 1940s to the 1960s but subsequently increased rapidly to more than 200 in 1982, 235 in 1990, and 250 in 2000.

In the early 1980s, the Graduate Medical Education National Advisory Committee (GMENAC) proposed three recommendations: a 17% reduction in admissions to medical schools, stricter limits on the number of new foreign physicians (which exceeded 3,000 each year), and restricting the increase in the number of healthcare workers other than physicians. Therefore, the number of enrollees in medical schools has decreased by nearly 1% each year since 1983 and has remained stable since the beginning of the twenty-first century. The opportunities for foreign physicians to serve in the US were reduced due to the increasingly stringent examinations. In 1975, the Visa Qualifying Examination (VQE) limited the recruitment of foreign physicians. The restriction became increasingly evident following the implementation of the FMGEMS in 1984, which only allowed a handful of foreign physicians to qualify.

A 1984 AMA survey showed that only 12% of Americans believed at that time that the country has a surplus of physicians, and most citizens perceived the shortage of physicians to be a greater problem than the surplus of physicians. Another survey showed that the average number of physician visits per week had decreased from 121 in 1995 to 107 in 2000, but the average annual income of a physician had increased from US$150,000 to US$210,000. Thus, even after correcting for changes in health policies and labor practice, it is apparent that the reduction in service volume is associated with an increase in the number of physicians.

The increase in the number of physicians can be a double-edged sword. On the one hand, it can increase the accessibility of healthcare, but on the one hand, it can also increase healthcare expenditure, thereby further aggravating the government's financial burden. Furthermore, it is indisputable that the surplus of physicians will negatively affect the healthcare quality and perhaps the entire healthcare system. In early 1970, the warning of an impending healthcare expenditure crisis issued by President Nixon became a reality. The total healthcare expenditure in the US rose from US$75 billion in 1970 to US$155.3 billion in 2002. The total healthcare expenditure as a share of GDP also increased from 7.4% to 14.9%.

The rapid increase in the number of applications for specialist practices has also flipped the GP-to-specialist ratio from 8:2 in early 1930 to 2:8 in 1969; following the restrictions in 2003, however, the ratio became close to 5:5. Since the 1970s, greater importance has been attached to preventive care and the social sciences in medical education due to public demand for greater healthcare integrity and more basic healthcare services. Furthermore, the surplus of specialists was alleviated through the institutionalization of family medicine training for GPs. However, the specialization and subdivision of medical fields are still ongoing in the US, and the ingrained emphasis on technology and depersonalized healthcare services ("medical consultation without treatment") remains prevalent.

The US is proud to have the greatest number of physicians and best healthcare quality in the world. However, it also has the highest healthcare expenditure, which does not necessarily translate to better health status among Americans compared to other developed countries. In fact, in 2003, the infant mortality rate in the US was ranked eighteenth in the world, and the US did not rank among the top 10 countries in terms of average life expectancy (males: 76 years; females: 80 years) worldwide. Furthermore, 1.5 million Americans suffered from cardiovascular diseases in 2003, half of which led to deaths (0.77 million cases), accounting for 33% of the total number of deaths in the US. In addition, among youths aged 12–17 years, approximately 12% take drugs, 16% smoke tobacco, and 31% consume alcohol.

4. Healthcare Quality Peer review organizations (PROs) are agencies led by physicians that aim to control healthcare quality. This type of agency was established in 1982 to replace professional standards review organizations (PSROs). PROs consist of several senior physicians who conduct reviews on hospital discharge, the rationality of long-term inpatient charges or high-priced medical charges, and standard healthcare quality control and information provision. PROs retain extensive authority to review Medicare reimbursement. In 1983, the US government introduced the Prospective Payment System (PPS) for Medicare reimbursement as a trump card for controlling healthcare expenditure. The implementation of PPS was only made possible via specialized healthcare quality control in hospitals performed by PROs.

5. Medical Disputes Most medical disputes in the US are associated with physicians rather than with hospitals because of the country's national conditions and healthcare system. Medical disputes between patients and attending physicians are usually resolved via medical litigation. The past decade has seen an increasing trend in medical disputes. For instance, the average number of medical ligations per 100 physicians increased from 5 cases in 1975 to 18 cases in 2003. The economic harm due to medical negligence reaches upwards of millions of dollars. As a result, the medical professional liability insurance premiums have skyrocketed at greater rates than healthcare expenditure (average annual amount of US$315 in 1975, US$6,200 in 1984, and US$48,500 in 2003). Hospitals and physicians have begun to gradually practice more defensively to prevent medical disputes, leading to over-diagnoses and over-conservative treatment for patients.

3. Health Insurance System

In 2007, the US Bureau of Justice Statistics (BJS) reported that 67.9% of Americans had some form of commercial health insurance and 27.8% of Americans had government insurance; the remaining 15.3% of Americans (about 4.568 million people) were uninsured. Furthermore, the BJS reported that among those with commercial health insurance, 60% were covered by employer group insurance, and only 9% were covered by individual

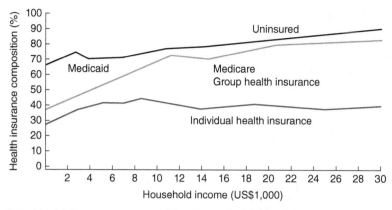

FIGURE 13.2 Health insurance status of families with different household incomes in the US.

insurance. The health insurance status of households with varying income levels in the US is shown in Figure 13.2. Families with higher household incomes tend to have greater coverage rates for various insurance schemes.

(1) Medicare

In the US, Medicare is a social health insurance program that primarily targets Americans aged over 65 years, as well as Americans aged under 65 years who require kidney transplantation or long-term hemodialysis because of chronic kidney disease. Medicare is a limited social health insurance program covering approximately 13.8% of the US population.

(2) Medicaid Scheme for Low-Income Earners

Medicaid is another US social health insurance program, funded by the federal government and administered by respective state governments. It provides noninsurance medical benefits for low-income earners, including children, pregnant women, and individuals with disabilities; it covers about 13.2% of the US population. Medicaid has been implemented in a total of 56 administrative entities, including 50 states and special districts, such as Washington, DC, and Puerto Rico.

In 2000, there were 31.04 million Medicaid recipients, incurring a total cost of US$55 billion, of which 50–80% was subsidized by the federal government based on the financial status of each state.

Medicaid mainly targets low-income families with minors (through the Aid to Families with Dependent Children program, AFDC) [AFDC was replaced by the Temporary Assistance for Needy Family (TANF) in 1996] and Americans living below the poverty line, who are elderly, visually impaired, or disabled (through Supplemental Security Income, SSI). Medicaid also targets other low-income groups as determined by the respective state governments. In 1997, there were 36 states and 4 special districts in the US that have implemented such supplemental measures.

Since 2014, most American adults aged below 65 years with an annual income of less than US$15,000 are eligible to apply for Medicaid.

The US social health insurance system also includes the health insurance system for veterans and their dependents (TRICARE) and workers' compensation.

(3) Private Medical Insurance (PMI) With a Wide Coverage

PMI has developed significantly because of the limited coverage of Medicare and Medicaid. The vast majority of Americans are covered by PMI, which implies that it occupies a more important position than public health coverage in the current US health insurance system. About three-fourths of Americans aged below 65 years are PMI policyholders. Most PMI schemes are considered corporate welfare measures, whereby insurance premiums are fully or partially covered by employers. The Centers for Medicare & Medicaid Services (CMS) reported that almost 100% of large-scale US companies purchase PMI for their employees and generally cover a large share of the premiums.

In 2008, employees in the US paid an average of 16% and 27% of the single coverage premiums and family coverage premiums, respectively. Such proportions have remained stable since 1999. Employers that provide health insurance benefits are entitled to tax incentives. The amount of health insurance premiums paid by employers has continued to rise in recent years. The premiums for family coverage have increased by 78% in 2008 compared to those in 2001, even though wages have only increased by 19% in the meantime. In 2008, the combined total of average premiums paid by employers and employees were US$4,704 for single coverage and US$12,680 for family coverage.

Even Medicare recipients aged over 65 years must pay for healthcare services that fall beyond the scope of Medicare, which has a limited scope of reimbursement. Thus, more than 70% of Medicare recipients have also purchased PMI to make up this difference.

Individual health insurance is mostly similar to group health insurance, but the former has higher deductibles and copayments. Critical illness insurance is the most commonly purchased individual health insurance. Policyholders must purchase individual health insurance at their own expense. Self-employed households can enjoy pretax deductions for the purchase of health insurance, but the majority of policyholders of individual health insurance are not entitled to such tax incentives.

(4) Children's Health Insurance Program (CHIP)

CHIP targets uninsured children from low-income families who are not eligible for Medicaid. CHIP was first created as part of the Balanced Budget Act (BBA) of 1997. The program was extended to 2013 by the Children's Health Insurance Program Reauthorization Act (CHIPRA).

In 1999–2009, the proportion of American minors under age 18 covered by PMI declined from 69% to 56%, while the coverage of medical aid for low-income earners (including CHIP) increased from 18% to 35%. The overall proportion of uninsured minors has decreased from 12% to 8% in the meantime.

(5) Other Types of Health Insurance

In addition to the aforementioned types of health insurance, the US health insurance system also includes a Pre-Existing Condition Insurance Plan (PCIP), which was created as part of the Affordable Care Act for people who have a pre-existing condition and have been uninsured for the past six months. In addition, Americans who cannot afford any type of health insurance can obtain free or low-cost care at community healthcare centers.

4. Medicare

(1) Growth and Control of Medicare Expenditure

1. Medicare Expenditure and Federal Budget Medicare was established in 1965 and implemented on July 1, 1966. Since its introduction, the US healthcare expenditure has basically increased at a slightly greater rate than the gross national product (GNP) per capita. The increasing trends in both the US total healthcare expenditure from 1995 to 2009 and the Medicare expenditure from 1967 to 2011 are shown in Table 13.1 and Table 13.2, respectively.

Medicare consists of Part A (hospital insurance), which covers inpatient care, and Part B (medical insurance), which covers healthcare services provided by physicians and outpatient care. Patients cover part of Medicare Part A expenditure while the remainder is covered by the social security tax. For Medicare Part B, as of 1988, part of the expenditure is covered by patients, while 25% and 75% of the remaining balance are covered by insurance premiums and the general federal budget, respectively. Since Medicare expenditure is almost entirely covered by the federal budget, the increase in Medicare expenses has been associated with an increase in the federal budget (including special accounts). As shown in Table 13.2, Part A accounts for a slightly greater share of Medicare expenditure than Part B.

2. Medicare Cost-Containment Policies Population aging has increased the expenditure on social security, such as healthcare and pensions, leading to an increase in the federal budget. Pensions and healthcare issues are also considered the greatest domestic challenges facing the US. Over the past two decades since 1980, the US Congress has proposed numerous healthcare-related laws, among which nearly 140 were passed and signed by the president. Many of these laws are related to Medicare, which is based on the social health insurance system, of which seven were established specifically to control the healthcare expenditure of Medicare.

For example, the DRG/PPS system (prospective capitation system) was introduced through the Social Security Amendments of 1983. Prior to the introduction of this payment system, several reforms had already been introduced under the Tax Equity & Fiscal Responsibility Act of 1982 to suppress the rise in healthcare expenditure to a given rate.

Despite the initial success of the current system in suppressing hospital expenses, the increase in the growth rate of physician remuneration has recently prompted the need for a new payment system. The US Congress has suggested introducing a physician fee schedule (PFS) that determines the remuneration of physicians according to their relative value units (RVUs), which are converted from their professional behaviors according to the quantity and quality of resource inputs.

This approach is referred to as the relative value scale (RVS) payment model. The factors (resource inputs) in the calculation of RVUs include the quantity of labor (working time and labor intensity), necessary medical expenses, and expenses for professional training.

3. Medicare Catastrophic Coverage There were no major reforms to Medicare benefits since its establishment to the 1980s. During this period, there were only short-term reforms to the benefits received by Medicare recipients for home-based care and inpatient services. However, a large-scale, comprehensive Medicare reform for suppressing healthcare expenditure was designed in 1988 and subsequently implemented in 1989.

TABLE 13.1 US Healthcare Expenditures from 1995 to 2009 (Unit: US$billion)

Types of Expenditures and Funding Sources	1995	1996	1997	1998	1999	2000	2001	2002	2003	2004	2005	2006	2007	2008	2009
Total	1,027.3	1,081.6	1,142.4	1,208.6	1,286.8	1,378.0	1,495.3	1,637.0	1,772.2	1,894.7	2,021.0	2,152.1	2,283.5	2,391.4	2,486.3
Funding sources: Residents	146.4	152.9	164.6	180.0	190.7	202.1	209.5	222.8	237.1	248.8	263.8	272.1	289.4	298.2	299.3
Health insurance	682.9	723.5	760.4	794.0	847.1	918.8	1013.5	1119.5	1219.2	1316.2	1410.5	1513.7	1597.5	1681.8	1767.4
Third-party payment and programs	101.1	105.1	110.3	117.1	121.4	124.5	130.9	137.3	148.2	153.9	159.8	168.5	179.5	181.2	186.1
Public health activities	31.0	32.4	34.8	37.5	40.7	43.0	47.5	51.9	53.7	54.0	56.2	62.6	68.8	72.9	77.2
Investment	65.9	67.7	72.2	80.1	86.8	89.6	94.0	105.4	114.0	121.8	130.7	135.2	148.4	157.2	156.2
Types of expenditures															
Health consumption expenditure	961.4	1,013.9	1,070.2	1,128.5	1,200.0	1,288.5	1,401.4	1,531.6	1,658.2	1,772.9	1,890.3	2,016.9	2,135.1	2,234.2	2,330.1
Individual health insurance	872.7	921.7	974.5	1,028.3	1,088.8	1,164.4	1,264.1	1,371.6	1,479.0	1,585.0	1,692.6	1,798.8	1,904.3	1,997.2	2,089.9
Hospital insurance	339.3	350.8	363.4	374.9	393.6	415.5	449.4	486.5	525.8	564.5	606.5	648.3	686.8	722.1	759.1
Physician and clinical services	222.3	231.3	242.9	257.9	271.1	290.0	314.7	340.8	368.4	393.6	419.6	441.6	462.6	486.5	505.9
Other professional services	27.0	29.2	31.7	33.8	35.0	37.0	40.6	43.7	46.8	50.1	53.1	55.4	59.5	63.4	66.8
Dental services	44.5	46.8	50.2	53.5	57.2	62.0	67.5	73.4	76.0	81.8	86.8	91.4	97.3	102.3	102.2
Other health, residential, and personal care	42.1	46.6	50.5	56.2	59.8	64.7	70.7	77.7	84.0	90.7	96.5	102.1	108.3	113.3	122.6
Family health insurance	32.4	35.8	37.0	34.2	32.9	32.4	34.4	36.6	39.8	43.8	48.7	52.6	57.8	62.1	68.3
Continuing community care services	64.5	69.6	74.4	79.4	80.8	85.1	90.8	94.5	100.1	105.4	112.1	117.0	126.5	132.8	137.0
Prescription drugs	59.8	68.1	77.6	88.4	104.7	120.9	138.7	158.2	175.2	190.3	201.7	219.8	230.2	237.2	249.9
Durable medical equipment (DME)	15.9	17.4	19.2	21.3	23.0	25.1	25.1	27.0	27.8	28.9	30.4	31.9	34.4	35.1	34.9
Nondurable medical supplies	25.1	26.0	27.6	28.3	30.6	31.6	32.3	33.3	35.1	35.8	37.2	38.7	41.1	42.3	43.3
Investment	65.9	67.7	72.2	80.1	86.8	89.6	94.0	105.4	114.0	121.8	130.7	135.2	148.4	157.25	156.2
Research	18.7	17.8	19.6	21.5	23.4	25.5	28.5	32.0	34.9	38.5	40.3	41.4	41.9	43.2	45.3
Buildings and facilities	47.2	49.9	52.5	58.6	63.5	64.1	65.5	73.4	79.2	83.3	90.4	93.8	106.4	114.0	110.9

Note: This table does not include the healthcare expenditures of Puerto Rico and other islands; the total healthcare expenditures are classified according to funding sources and types of expenditures.

Source: US Centers for Medicare & Medicaid Services, Office of the Actuary, National Health Statistics Group, 2011.

TABLE 13.2 US Medicare Expenditures from 1967 to 2010 (Unit: US$million)

Types of Services	Year											
	1967	1974	1980	1983	1990	1997	2000	2002	2004	2006	2009	2010
Total payment	$4,239	$11,179	$33613	$53,446	$101,419	$175423	$174,261	$215411	$255,325	$280,672	$318,009	$331,129
Hospital insurance (Part A)	2,967	8,000	23,119	36,314	62,347	114,327	101,663	122,993	139,747	151,917	170,331	176,224
Inpatient services	2,667	7,680	22,297	34,519	56,716	84,563	85,197	99,382	110,550	116,350	125,662	128,728
Professional care facilities and services	274	224	344	428	1,971	11,237	10,621	14,363	17,043	20,387	25,580	27,258
Home-based care services	26	96	478	1,366	3,660	16,487	2,918	4,788	5,479	5,979	6,992	7,252
Hospice services	–	–	–	–	–	2,040	2,927	4,460	6,675	9,201	12,097	12,986
Supplemental medical insurance (Part B)	1,272	3,179	10,494	17,132	39,072	61,069	72,599	92,418	11,5579	12,8755	14,7677	154,906
Physician and other healthcare services	1,217	2,740	8,358	13,660	30,222	43,621	51,474	64,272	79,271	85,305	91,174	95,087
Outpatient services	38	397	1,962	3,443	8,773	17,256	16,787	23,346	30,335	35,411	44,596	47,573
Home-based care services	17	40	175	29	78	219	4,338	4,800	5,973	8,039	11,908	12,245

Note: The expenditures are classified based on types of insurance and healthcare services.
Source: Centers for Medicare & Medicaid Services, Office of Information Services: Data from the Medicare Decision Support Access Facility. Effective 2002 data from the Medicare Data Extract System.

TABLE 13.3   US Population Aged under 65 Years and Their Health Insurance Coverage from 1980 to 2000

Year	Population Aged Under 65 Years (Million)	Uninsured Persons Aged Under 65 Years (Million)	Percentage of Uninsured Persons (%)
1980	199.0	29.6	14.9
1985	209.4	32.7	16.2
1990	214.9	34.5	17.8
1995	216.7	36.0	18.3
2000	219.2	37.8	18.9

Note: The statistics shown in this table are slightly different from those of Table 13.4 due to their different statistical basis.

It is certainly impossible for such a major reform to be accomplished overnight, and for all healthcare issues facing the US to be solved. Currently, we can point to three major issues facing the US healthcare system.

1. In 2002, the US Medical Expenditure Panel Survey (MEPS) reported that 18.9% (or 37.8 million people) of the US population aged under 65 years were uninsured, and this figure was expected to increase in the future (Table 13.3).
2. *Healthcare expenditure for geriatric long-term care.* Medicare does not cover long-term services, which are solely covered by Medicaid despite the rapidly increasing expenses for long-term care due to population aging.
3. *High Medicare out-of-pocket expenses.* Prior to its reform, patients had to bear a share of the Medicare expenses (Table 13.4). Medicare does not cover pharmaceutical expenses, with the exception of drugs required for inpatient care; the expenses for other drugs are almost entirely covered by the patients.

In order to address these healthcare issues, the project team of the US Department of Health and Human Services (DHHS) released a report entitled "Catastrophic Illness Expenses" in November 1986. This report proposed that the first two issues should be solved by private enterprises, private insurance companies, or state governments, while the third issue should be tackled by the federal government. Specifically, the report proposed abolishing or capping out-of-pocket expenses for Medicare and reintroducing drug coverage to Medicare, which would greatly reduce the burden on patients.

The US government drafted a bill based on this report and proposed the Medicare Catastrophic Coverage Act to Congress in February 1987. Both Congress and the government were scheduled to implement the Medicare Amendments of 1987 in January 1988; however, bill review was postponed due to the opposition led by the American Pharmaceutical Manufacturers' Association (AmPharMA), who took issue with the stipulation that Medicare should cover outpatient prescription drugs. The bill was finally passed by the US Senate and rolled out in phases from January 1, 1989.

4. Insured Persons   As noted previously, Medicare is divided into Part A (hospital insurance) and Part B (medical insurance). Almost all Americans over the age of 65 are covered by Medicare Part A. Some individuals who are not automatically covered by Medicare

TABLE 13.4 Medicare Out-of-Pocket Expenses in the US from 1966 to 2000

		Inpatient Expenses (US$)			
Year	Patients' Deductibles	Average Copayment Per Day from Day 61 to Day 90 of Hospitalization (US$)	Average Copayment Per Day from Day 91 of Hospitalization (US$)	Average Copayment Per Day from Day 21 to Day 100 of Hospitalization at Skilled Nursing Facilities (US$)	Part B Deductibles (US$)
1966	40	10	18	5.00	50
1968	40	10	20	5.00	50
1970	52	13	26	6.5	50
1972	68	17	34	8.50	60
1974	84	21	42	10.50	60
1976	104	26	52	13.00	65
1978	144	36	75	18.00	65
1980	180	45	90	22.50	70
1982	268	98	164	32.00	70
1984	385	156	187	51.00	70
1986	458	286	208	62.50	75
1988	640	135	270	68.00	75
1990	809	156	355	78.50	75
1992	948	179	677	88.50	80
1994	1146	216	705	95.00	80
1996	1313	285	846	102.50	80
1998	1467	324	962	105.00	85
2000	1542	369	1078	108.00	85

Note: Part B refers to medical insurance. In addition to the deductibles, patients must cover 20% of the medical expenses.

Part A and do not receive a social pension are eligible to join the program by paying the necessary insurance premiums. The premiums were US$240 per month in 1989 and US$578 per month in 1999. Recipients of Social Security Disability Insurance (SSDI) aged under 65 years are eligible to enroll in Part A after a two-year waiting period. In addition, individuals who require long-term hemodialysis because of kidney transplantation are also eligible to join Part A, irrespective of their age.

Medicare Part B, on the other hand, is a voluntary insurance program. Americans over the age of 65, regardless of whether they have a pension, can enroll in Part B by paying the requisite insurance premiums. The premiums were US$28 per month in 1989 and US$135.5 per month in 2019.

In 1988, there were approximately 28 million elderly adults and 3 million individuals with disabilities who were insured under Part A. Among them, an estimated 6.5 million elderly adults and 800,000 individuals with disabilities benefited from the program.

In 1988, approximately 28.8 million elderly adults and 2.8 million individuals with disabilities were insured under Part B.

(2) Medicare Benefits

1. Part A (Hospital Insurance)

1. *Inpatient charges at hospitals.* Patients who have been admitted to Medicare-designated hospitals, and who receive confirmation from physicians that the necessary healthcare services are unavailable outside of these hospitals, are entitled to the following benefits when hospitalization is deemed necessary by the Utilization Review Committee of the hospital or a PRO. In 2010, the inpatient charges incurred under Medicare Part A were US$128.728 billion.

   Patients who have met their deductibles for a given year are entitled to reimbursement from Medicare Part A for the necessary inpatient expenses (service expenses incurred by Medicare recipients) within that year. In 2000, the deductible for each patient was US$1,542. However, these benefits were the result of reforms since January 1989, in accordance with the Medicare Catastrophic Coverage Act.

   When the initial deductible is met, Medicare pays for all inpatient charges deemed necessary for the first 60 days of hospitalization. From day 61 to day 90, Medicare partially covers the inpatient charges after deducting patient copayments (US$369 per day on average). These out-of-pocket expenses are known as "coinsurance." Medicare does not cover inpatient charges incurred after the first 90 days of hospitalization; however, patients can tap into their lifetime reserve of 60 days, during which they must also pay daily copayments of US$1,078 per day on average, while the remaining balance is covered by Medicare.

   Medicare-covered inpatient services include wards with two to four beds, meals, general care, ICU care, hospital-dispensed drugs, blood transfusions, diagnostic tests, X-rays and radiotherapy, and any other expenses associated with medical appliances, operating rooms, and rehabilitation. Medicare does not cover charges incurred for single rooms.

2. *Nursing home expenses.* Medicare-covered nursing home expenses refer to service expenses incurred for extended inpatient care. As mentioned above, Medicare does not cover expenses for long-term ICFs, but it does cover patients admitted to Medicare-designated SNFs as instructed by physicians and deemed necessary by a PRO. In 2010, the nursing home charges incurred under Medicare Part A were up to US$27.258 billion.

   Inpatient expenses for the first 150 days of nursing home stay per year are covered by Medicare Part A. Patients must share expenses for the first 8 days of hospitalization, but the copayment is established by the US Secretary of Health and Human Services, and is equivalent to about 20% of the average daily expenses in nursing homes in the US. Since 1988, it is no longer necessary for the person requesting to stay at a nursing home to have been discharged from a hospital.

   Prior to the implementation of the Medicare Catastrophic Coverage Act, Medicare covered up to 100 days of nursing home care, during which patients had to pay a certain amount of daily copayments after the first 20 days of hospitalization (US$108 per day on average).

   Inpatient services falling within the scope of Medicare coverage are determined based on Medicare-covered inpatient services.

3. *Home-based care expenses.* Medicare covers home-based care services delivered by nurses, physiotherapists, and other experts for two to three weeks, regardless of the number of visits per week (anywhere from five to seven days per week, with an unlimited number of visits per day). However, Medicare only actually covers expenses for up

to five days per week, according to the Health Care Financing Administration (HCFA) [HCFA has been renamed Centers for Medicare and Medicaid Services (CMS)]. In 2010, home-based care charges incurred under Medicare Part A were up to US$7.252 billion.

Since 1990, in accordance with amendments to the Medicare Catastrophic Coverage Act, Medicare now covers home-based care expenses for seven days per week for up to 38 consecutive days.

4. *Hospice expenses.* Medicare covers people who have a life expectancy of less than six months and have been admitted to a hospice; the benefit periods are 90 days in a year and 180 days in two years. In addition, each Medicare recipient has a lifetime 30-day additional benefit period. Furthermore, in accordance with the Medicare Catastrophic Coverage Act, Medicare also covers hospice care deemed necessary by physicians even after exceeding the total benefit period above (210 days, including the additional 30 days).

Medicare-covered services include nursing, physician services, analgesic drugs, social and healthcare services, consultation services and so on In 2010, hospice care charges incurred under Medicare Part A were up to US$12.986 billion.

2. Part B (Medical Insurance) After patients met an annual deductible of US$85, Medicare Part B covered 80% of the medical expenses calculated retrospectively. Although patients only have to pay 20% of their medical expenses, these expenses were uncapped, and some patients had to pay a high amount of copayment, which led to a number of social issues.

Since 1990, in accordance with the Medicare Catastrophic Coverage Act, Medicare Part B must cover the remaining balance of the copayment once it exceeds US$1,370 (known as the "catastrophic limit"). The US Secretary of Health and Human Services sets the catastrophic limit annually to ensure that the proportion of Part B recipients whose copayment levels exceed this limit is only around 7%.

In addition to the aforementioned deductibles and copayments, the out-of-pocket expenses covered by patients also include deductibles for blood transfusions and a copayment for outpatient psychiatric treatment (US$250). In 2010, the medical expenses incurred under Medicare Part B were up to US$154.906 billion.

Healthcare services covered by Medicare Part B are as follows.

1. *Physician services.* General healthcare services, such as medical care, diagnoses, treatment, surgeries, and consultation, as well as home, office and facility visits.
2. *Home-based care.* Medicare Part B provides patients who are not covered by Part A with the same benefits. Since 1990, in accordance with the Medicare Catastrophic Coverage Act, Part B has covered the service fees for home-based intravenous drips and long-term care for up to 80 hours per year (patients must pay the amount of Part B deductibles and copayments below the catastrophic limit or drug expenses below the out-of-pocket limit).
3. *Other healthcare services.* Outpatient clinics, chiropractic services (such as spinal correction), diagnostic tests (including X-ray), radiotherapy, community healthcare services, drugs (including those that are difficult to obtain in pharmacies), home-based hemodialysis equipment, physiotherapy, speech and language therapies, emergency care services, nursing services, and outpatient transfusions of blood and blood substitute.

TABLE 13.5 Premium surcharge in the US from 1989 to 2003 (Unit: US$)

Year	Premium Surcharge	Year	Premium Surcharge
1989	4.00	1997	10.95
1990	4.90	1998	11.40
1991	5.46	1999	12.50
1992	6.75	2000	13.50
1993	7.18	2001	14.50
1994	8.35	2002	15.70
1995	9.28	2003	16.00
1996	10.16		

3. Outpatient Prescription Drugs Apart from the aforementioned benefits, the prescription drug benefit was reintroduced in accordance with the Medicare Catastrophic Coverage Act. This benefit stipulates that from 1993, for patients who have met the deductible (set such that only 16.8% of recipients would have expenses for outpatient prescription drugs exceeding the deductible), Medicare Part B will cover 80% of the remaining balance for outpatient prescription drugs. Reimbursable drugs primarily include drugs that have been identified as safe and effective by the Federal Food, Drug and Cosmetic Act as well as biologics licensed under the Public Health Act.

As of 2003, the Medicare Part B prescription drug benefit has been implemented on a stage-by-stage basis. The deductible in 2000 was US$850 (which benefits 19.8% of recipients above), and the main targets were immunosuppressants and home-based intravenous drugs. After this deductible was met, Part B covered 50% of the remaining balance of medical expenses (for Medicaid recipients, Part B covered 80% within one year after organ transplantation). In 2001, the deductible was US$880; after this deductible was met, Part B covered 50% of the remaining balance for medical expenses on prescription drugs. In 2002, the deductible was US$962; after this deductible was met, Part B covered 65% of the remaining balance of medical expenses on prescription drugs.

4. Increasing Burden of Medicare Catastrophic Coverage Due to the reforms of the Medicare Catastrophic Coverage Act or the introduction of institutional costs, the reimbursements incurred under Medicare Part B amounted to US$54 billion within five years. As a result, the premiums for Medicare Part B have risen from US$24.80 in 1989 to US$49.00 in 2005, and a premium surcharge of US$18 was added due to the introduction of Medicare Catastrophic Coverage. This premium surcharge has gradually increased annually following the introduction of prescription drug benefits (Table 13.5). The amount of the premium surcharge is calculated to cover 37% of the total expenses incurred by the adoption of these new systems.

To cover the remaining 63% of medical expenses, the US government introduced a supplementary premium that is levied in conjunction with income taxes on high-income insured persons. The supplementary premium is adjusted by the Internal Revenue Service (IRS); as of 1993, this is calculated based on the taxes owed for every US$150 (Table 13.6 and Table 13.7).

TABLE 13.6 Supplementary Premiums in the US from 1989 to 1993 (Unit: US$)

Year	Premiums for Medicare Catastrophic Coverage	Premiums for Prescription Drug Benefits	Total
1989	22.50		22.50
1990	27.14	10.36	37.50
1991	30.17	8.83	39.00
1992	30.55	9.95	40.50
1993	29.55	12.45	42.00

Note: The above supplementary premiums are levied on every US$150 of income taxes owed.

5. Part C and Part D   Service items beyond the scope of the original Medicare coverage and patients' out-of-pocket expenses are known as "gaps in Medicare." In order to increase their received benefits and better meet their individual needs, insured persons can purchase supplementary health insurance from PMI companies or another form of supplementary insurance (Medicare Advantage Plans and Medicare Prescription Drug Plans).

1. *Medicare Advantage Plans.* Originally referred to as "Medicare +Choice" and abbreviated as Medicare Part C, Medicare Advantage Plans offer a range of insurance options, which generally fall into the following four categories:
   1. *Health Maintenance Organization (HMO) Plans.* Patients are only allowed to seek medical attention from HMO-contracted physicians. Patients who wish to consult a specialist require a referral certificate from a primary care physician (PCP).
   2. *Preferred Provider Organization Plans (PPOs).* Similar to HMO Plans, patients who wish to consult a specialist need a referral from a PCP under the PPO. The difference is that patients are allowed to consult physicians outside the PPO network if they are willing to pay additional charges.
   3. *Medicare Private Fee-for-Service (PFFS) Plans.* Patients are allowed to seek medical attention from Medicare-approved physicians and hospitals. The payment terms and covered healthcare services are determined by the PMI companies.

TABLE 13.7 Supplementary Premiums for Different Income Earners under Medicare Catastrophic Coverage in the US from 1989 to 2000 (Unit: US$)

Income	1989	1993	2000
5,000–15,000	0.00	0.00	0.00
15,000–20,000	78.12	116.52	317.72
20,000–25,000	197.88	250.56	589.36
25,000–30,000	306.96	401.28	845.68
30,000–35,000	370.68	702.00	1,089.20
35,000–40,000	678.36	1,021.68	1,625.50
40,000–45,000	800.00	1,050.00	1,950.00

4. *Medicare Special Needs Plans (SNPs)*. Insured persons under Medicare SNPs include Medicare and Medicaid recipients admitted to healthcare institutions (such as nursing homes) due to long-term chronic diseases or physical disabilities. Medicare SNPs must offer Medicare prescription drug coverage. Diabetic patients can purchase this type of insurance in order to access specialized medical care, health education, counseling, nutrition, and exercise programs.

2. *Medicare Prescription Drug Plans (Part D)*. Medicare Part D (includes coverage of generic and brand-name drugs) was implemented on January 1, 2006, to cover not only therapeutic services but also preventive care services, such as medical examinations and prevention of complications from chronic diseases. All individuals can choose whether to purchase Medicare Part D irrespective of their income, health status, and current drug expenses. Policyholders who enrolled before May 15, 2006, were offered lower premium rates, whereas those who enrolled after the time limit were penalized. However, there are three groups who can sign up for Medicare Part D at any time without restriction: (1) Recipients of both Medicare and Medicaid; (2) individuals who have been identified as low-income subsidy recipients; and (3) victims of Hurricane Katrina. Medicare Part D offers two types of insurance plan: a standard plan and a catastrophic coverage plan. The average premium of the standard prescription drug plan is US$37 per month. Once the annual deductible of US$250 is met, Medicare will pay 75% of the drug costs incurred up until an annual cap of US$2,250. The patient has to cover the remaining out-of-pocket drug costs, but if the patient has paid more than US$3,600 in a year, the catastrophic coverage will pay for the remaining 95% of drug costs.

   Actuarial predictions have shown that, in the next decade, Medicare Part D plans will cost a total of US$720 billion. This is likely to attract the participation of several large health insurance companies and pharmaceutical companies.

(3) Medicare Payment Systems

Broadly speaking, there are two types of Medicare payment system: (1) conventional fee-for-service payment systems based on a reasonable charge/cost calculated for each healthcare service; and (2) a prospective payment system (PPS) based on expenses determined by the DRGs of diseases and injuries and the types of treatment (internal or surgical treatment) on a per discharge or per admission basis.

1. Payment Systems for Hospitals The Social Security Amendment Act of 1984 significantly reformed the payment systems for Medicare Part A – namely, the introduction of the momentous DRG/PPS. Under the DRG/PPS, Medicare pays hospitals according to a predetermined price for each DRG (to which each disease is assigned) and the number of discharges.

Hospitals earn profits if they can deliver services at a cost lower than the payment received from Medicare Part A; conversely, they are also required to bear any losses. Under this payment system, hospitals have the opportunity to earn profits while also being required to bear risks, which has led to intense competition among hospitals to improve their service efficiency.

Before the introduction of this payment system, hospitals received reimbursement via the same payment system adopted in Medicare Part B, that is, a fee-for-service payment system based on reasonable costs.

However, the DRG/PPS is not necessarily applicable to inpatient expenses in all hospitals. Even in hospitals where the PPS is applicable, capital costs for facilities and equipment, as well as direct costs for the training of healthcare workers, have remained unchanged; reimbursements are paid based on reasonable costs on a fee-for-service basis.

Hospitals that are not accustomed to the use of the DRG/PPS, including psychiatric hospitals, pediatric hospitals, rehabilitation hospitals, and long-term care hospitals (LTCHs), can still receive reimbursement via the conventional fee-for-service system. However, the US government has taken measures to restrict the increase in medical expenses in these hospitals.

Under the DRG/PPS, Medicare reimburses hospitals for the additional expenses incurred for patients with extremely high medical expenses, the indirect costs involved in training healthcare workers, and hospitals that accept more than the average number of low-income inpatients (i.e., patients who cannot afford the medical expenses). Furthermore, the reimbursement of additional expenses by Medicare under the DRG/PPS is also applicable to special cases in hospitals that serve as regional core hospitals, national or regional referral centers, and cancer treatment centers.

Medicare usually reimburses patients according to the actual cost, while hospitals need to request reimbursement (calculated based on the DRGs) from Fiscal Intermediaries (FI), also known as Medicare Administrative Contractors.

2. Fee Calculation Methods of DRG/PPS　The expenses incurred for patients' use of hospital services are reimbursed via the DRG/PPS based on the type of treatment (internal medicine or surgical); initially, there were 473 DRGs, but this later expanded to 477. The payment amount for each DRG is calculated by multiplying the following factors.

1. Basic payment amount applicable to all DRGs (which varies by region)
2. The relative weighting factor established for each DRG

The basic payment amount is determined as the average expense incurred for Medicare inpatients in the region, while the relative weighting factor is a coefficient indicating the price of each DRG. The relative weighting factors are uniform nationwide, but the basic payment amount varies depending on the location and tier of the hospital.

3. Designated and Nondesignated Physicians　A designated physician is a physician who has agreed to Medicare reimbursement and thus will not impose additional charges other than the statutory out-of-pocket expenses (deductibles and copayments) on patients. Designated physicians must submit their fee requests directly to an FI, and patients need only pay the out-of-pocket expenses to access services that are paid according to the actual costs. In 2000, approximately 74% of Medicare claims were fee requests from designated physicians.

On the other hand, nondesignated physicians might request additional charges beyond Medicare out-of-pocket expenses from patients. Nondesignated physicians have the right to determine the type of patients and treatments that will be subject to additional charges. Medicare reimbursement is directly transferred to the insured persons.

Whether a physician decides to become a designated physician depends on whether they are willing to sign a contract with the US Secretary of Health and Human Services to become a Medicare "participating physician." The contract usually has a fixed-term of 12 months but will renew automatically unless either party gives notice of termination.

Medicare's participating physician and designated physician program was launched in 1984. A physician is free to choose whether to become a designated physician, with the incentive being that designated physicians are given preferential treatment in terms of remuneration calculation or application fees and procedures.

The US government has capped the amount that a nondesignated physician can charge via the Maximum Allowable Actual Charge (MAAC), in order to prevent nondesignated physicians from requesting additional charges that substantially exceed the statutory out-of-pocket expenses for patients and to control healthcare expenditure. Under this limitation, nondesignated physicians whose fees in the previous year exceed the current regional average by more than 15% will have the growth rate of their requested fees controlled to less than 1%. Furthermore, even nondesignated physicians whose requested fees in the previous year were within 15% of the regional average are only allowed to increase by 1% or by a fixed percentage of the difference between the requested fees of the previous year and 115% of the regional average in the current year.

For example, if the requested fees of a physician in 1999 were US$100 and 115% of the regional average fees in 2000 were US$124, the MAAC of the physician in 2000 would be US$106 [US$100+0.25×(US$124 – US$100)].

In summary, despite the introduction of various control measures, such as the MAAC, the US is continuing to experience a significant increase in the healthcare expenditure in recent years. Therefore, the payment system adopted in Medicare Part B requires major amendments.

4. Payment Methods for Home-Based Care Services   In principle, home-based care services are reimbursed according to reasonable costs/charges, but this payment system differs from that for hospitals in some respects. For instance, the average cost for each home visit is determined based on the services delivered, that is, the total service charge is divided by the number of visits for each service to obtain the average cost per visit for calculating the requested fees. All healthcare institutions calculate their requested fees by multiplying the average cost of each service (e.g., special care and family care services) by the number of Medicare-covered home visits.

However, the home-based care services delivered by these healthcare institutions cannot be fully reimbursed via the above calculation method. Hence, the upper quartile of the average cost per visit (obtained via the method described above) is used as the upper limit of the average cost for each service.

5. Payment Methods for Hospice Care Services   Hospice care institutions are reimbursed based on reasonable costs/charges or fees that are calculated based on standards established by the US Secretary of Health and Human Services. However, there is an upper limit to the reimbursement amount (in 2000, this was US$16.50 per patient per day), which increases automatically according to the cost of the market basket.

On the other hand, HCFA reimburses hospice care institutions using the PPS, just as with hospitals. That is, hospice care institutions are reimbursed by Medicare based on a predetermined average daily fee for each patient. However, the reimbursement for hospitals is calculated from the predetermined average daily fee based on DRGs for each discharged patient. In contrast, the reimbursement for hospice care institutions is calculated from the average daily fee based on the content and place of service delivery for each patient. Therefore, the reimbursement amount varies considerably among patients. Furthermore, the HCFA rules classify reimbursement recipients into the following four categories in order to determine the average amount of reimbursement per day.

1. *Routine home care day.* Expenses incurred for home-based hospice care.
2. *Continuous home care day.* Expenses incurred by a specialized institution for continuous home-based hospice care.
3. *Inpatient respite care day.* Expenses incurred for short-term (not more than 5 days) inpatient hospice care.
4. *General inpatient care day.*

6. Payment Methods for the Treatment of Chronic Kidney Disease   As of 1983, the cost of hemodialysis, which requires patients to travel back and forth to a hospital, was deemed necessary and thus fully covered under Medicare. Medicare covers the reasonable costs for hemodialysis at other facilities.

From August 1, 1983, reimbursements were made according to the newly established prospective payment method. Before October 1, 1986, the DHHS stipulated that the average reimbursement amount for a patient who requires hemodialysis was US$131 per treatment, irrespective of whether the hemodialysis is carried out at a hospital, the patient's home, or institutions under the supervision of hospitals. The average reimbursement amount was US$127 per treatment for hemodialysis carried out under the supervision of other independent medical facilities (note that both these amounts are the average base prices for which the exception clause does not apply).

However, the Omnibus Budget Reconciliation Act of 1986 (OBRA, 1986) mandated that the above reimbursement amounts be reduced to US$129 and US$125, respectively, and also be frozen for two years. After the two-year term, the US Secretary of Health and Human Services was given the authority to adjust these amounts according to the regional performance index to reflect the differences in the hemodialysis cost across hospitals and areas. In 2000, these reimbursement amounts increased to US$214 and US$209, respectively.

7. Payment Methods for SNFs   Medicare covers the reasonable costs of SNFs, but there is an upper limit to the reimbursement amount. Specifically, the upper limit is established based on the general inpatient care delivered by hospital-affiliated SNFs and independent SNFs. The SNF cost is calculated as 112% of the sum of the average labor-related and non-labor-related costs.

This payment method has been reformed several times since its introduction. Recently, the Tax Equity and Fiscal Responsibility Act (TEFRA) required the US Secretary of Health and Human Services to enact a uniform reimbursement cap nationwide.

The reimbursement cap for independent SNFs in urban and nonurban areas is calculated as 112% of the average cost. For hospital-affiliated SNFs, the reimbursement cap is calculated as the sum of 50% of the reimbursement cap for independent SNFs and 112% of the average cost of hospital-affiliated SNFs.

The OBRA introduced the PPS into specific SNFs. In the previous year, an SNF with Medicare patients hospitalized for a total of less than 1,500 days was allowed to choose whether to receive Medicare reimbursement, and the amount of this reimbursement was calculated as 105% of the average cost of all SNFs in that region. The prepaid amount was also adjusted depending on whether the SNF was located in urban or nonurban areas.

(4) Medicare Administration and Funding Management

Funding for Medicare Part A and Part B is administered by the Hospital Insurance Trust Fund (HI) and Supplementary Medical Insurance Trust Fund (SMI), respectively.

1. Medicare and the US DHHS The US DHHS is responsible for the management of Medicare, but the business operations of Medicare are administered by the HCFA. The HCFA is a relatively large agency consisting of four offices that assist the Administrator, four principal deputy administrators, and their affiliated departments (Figure 13.3). The HCFA is subjected to major changes every three to four years.

Medicare Administrative Contractors that are charged with ensuring smooth collaboration among DHHS, healthcare institutions and physicians in the daily operation of Medicare services are known as Part A FIs and Part B Carriers.

Part A FIs are HCFA-recognized public or private agencies that play an intermediary role in fiscal administration between the federal government and healthcare institutions, with whom they sign contracts. Each state usually has one FI. The majority of healthcare institutions nominate a single healthcare service company, known as Blue Cross, as their FI.

As for Part B, the US Secretary of Health and Human Services has entered into contracts with insurance companies known as "carriers" (the majority of states nominate a healthcare service company, known as Blue Shield, as their insurance carrier), which agree to reimburse the reasonable costs incurred by physicians under Part B.

Medicare funds spent on FIs and carriers account for about 2.5% of the total Medicare expenditure. The US government is still taking steps to reduce such expenses.

2. Hospital Insurance Trust Fund (HI) The HI is essentially funded by the social security payroll tax paid by employers, employees, and self-employed persons. This tax is levied together with the pension tax. After 2000, the total insurance premium rate was 8.70% of

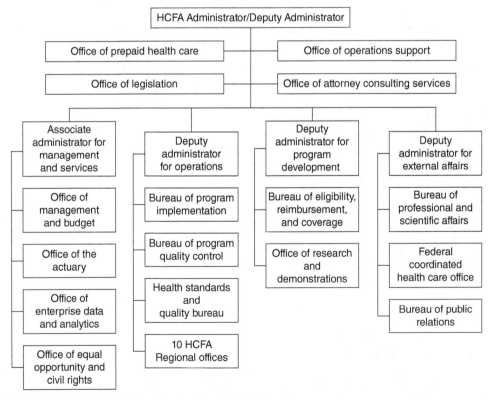

FIGURE 13.3 Organization chart of the US HCFA.

TABLE 13.8 Premium Rates of Medicare Part A in the US from 1978 to 2000

| Year | Insurance Premium Rate (%) | | | Upper Limit of Annual Income Per Capita (US$) | Upper limit of Additional HI Premiums (US$) |
	Annual Income Per Capita	Additional HI Premiums	Total		
1978	5.05	1.10	6.05	17,700	194.70
1980	5.08	1.05	6.13	25,900	271.95
1982	5.40	1.30	6.70	32,400	421.20
1984	5.70	1.30	7.00	37,800	491.40
1986	5.70	1.45	7.15	42,000	609.00
1988	6.06	1.45	7.51	45,000	652.50
1990	6.20	1.45	7.65	47,000	711.60
1992	6.50	1.55	8.05	49,700	755.80
1994	6.50	1.55	8.05	54,200	794.40
1996	6.70	1.65	8.35	61,800	827.10
1998	6.70	1.65	8.35	68,600	882.50
2000	7.00	1.70	8.70	75,000	947.20

the annual income per capita, which includes the premium rate for Part A (7.00%) and an additional 1.70% for HI, as shown in Table 13.8. The upper limit of taxpayers' incomes is set annually and increases with taxpayers' annual income per capita. In 2000, the upper limit of income was US$75,000. Both employers and employees contribute equally to the social security payroll tax, while self-employed persons have to contribute twice as much as employers.

3. Supplementary Medical Insurance Trust Fund (SMI) The SMI is essentially funded by the insurance premiums paid by insured persons aged over 65 years, disabled individuals, and patients with chronic kidney disease, as well as by transfer payments from general funds.

The insurance premiums for Part B are established according to annual estimates at the beginning of the year; however, the following calculation methods, which yielded lower premiums, have been employed in the past.

1. Insurance premiums that are sufficient to cover half the Medicare reimbursement.
2. Multiplying the total insurance premium for Part B collected in the previous year with the annual growth rate of the reimbursement amount to obtain the premium rate for the current year.

These calculation methods successfully suppressed the annual insurance premium, which in turn reduced the total insurance premium collected to less than one-fourth of the total revenue of Part B, as shown in Table 13.9.

Under the most recent US tax reform (i.e., the TEFRA Amendments), the following changes were suggested: (1) removal of the upper limit established using the above-mentioned method (2), which would increase the premium rate (note that a subsequent assessment indicated that this policy was ineffective), and (2) exempting individuals with a personal income tax of less than US$200.

TABLE 13.9　Annual Revenues of Medicare Part B in the US from 1970 to 1989

Funding Source	Annual Revenue (US$)						1989 Revenue Composition (%)
	1970	1975	1980	1985	1988	1989	
Transfers from general funds	928	2,330	6,932	17,898	25,152	32,697	76.40
Interest	12	105	415	1 155	540	556	1.30
Others	936	1,887	2,928	5,524	8,536	9,551	22.30
Total	1,876	4,322	10,275	24,577	34,228	42,804	100.00

(5) Medicare Service Utilization and Quality Management

1. Brief Historical Review　The US government is extremely concerned about the utilization and quality of healthcare services. Medicare was introduced in 1965 and subsequently led to a rapid increase in healthcare expenditure in the 1970s. As a result, the DHHS began to express serious concern about the utilization of hospital services.

To supervise the degree of hospital utilization, the DHHS abandoned the direct approach and adopted an indirect approach by providing grants to organizations to monitor the degree of healthcare service utilization. This indirect approach gave rise to the establishment of PSROs, which were later replaced by PROs.

The Social Security Amendment of 1972 designated PSROs as legal review organizations to be established nationwide for monitoring healthcare services covered under Medicare, Medicaid, and the Maternal and Child Health Program. In order to control the reimbursements under these public healthcare systems, the Social Security Amendment of 1972 stated that the role of PSROs is to determine whether a healthcare service is medically necessary, whether the service quality meets professional standards, and whether a healthcare institution (e.g., a hospital) can provide the service using appropriate facilities and equipment. A total of 188 PSROs have been established by physician groups since 1972, but it was not until 1977 that the system was fully implemented. In 1982, there were a total of 203 PROs (which replaced PSROs) in the US. By 2000, there were 473 DHHS-contracted PROs throughout the US.

As noted earlier, the TEFRA replaced PSROs with PROs in 1982. The fundamental role of PROs is to examine whether a healthcare service is medically necessary. However, the TEFRA – which aimed to introduce the PPS to reimburse Medicare-covered medical expenses – emphasized that the purpose of introducing PROs is also to audit healthcare services, in order to avoid early hospital discharge under the PPS.

Both PSROs and PROs have basically the same objectives and organizational structures. However, unlike the PSROs, PROs are neither necessarily composed of physicians nor non-profit organizations.

2. PROs　Figure 13.4 shows the roles of PROs in the process of Medicare reimbursement.

There are two types of PROs: physician-sponsored PROs and physician-access PROs. The former is primarily composed of at least 20% of the physicians in a given region (mostly at the state level) or 10–20% of physicians in the state with support from other physicians or physician organizations. The latter must sign contracts with at least one specialist from every specialty, who provides peer review services for PROs.

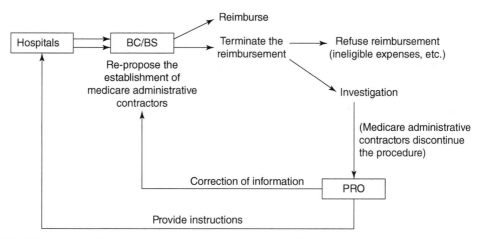

FIGURE 13.4   Medicare reimbursement process in the US.

The TEFRA required the HCFA to prioritize physician-sponsored PROs when signing agreements. Hence, when evaluating the performances of PROs using a point system, the HCFA awarded 100 bonus points to physician-sponsored PROs. Thus, it is clear that physician-sponsored PROs received considerable prioritization because these additional 100 bonus points account for 7% of the point system (out of a total of 1,500 points). As a result, there were 44 physician-sponsored PROs out of a total of 54 PROs, while the remaining were physician-access PROs.

Due to the introduction of the PPS for hospital expenditures, PROs are expected to screen not only for over-provision of healthcare services but also for the insufficient supply of healthcare services, such as an early discharge of patients. However, PROs have been criticized over their biases toward the overprovision of healthcare services.

The basic goals of PROs are as follows:

1. Reduce hospitalization for patients who can receive safe and effective treatment outside the hospital.
2. Reduce inappropriate and unnecessary hospitalization.
3. Reduce inappropriate and unnecessary medical services and examinations for specific physicians and hospitals to prevent the misuse of DRGs.

The PRO contracts mainly focus on reviewing Medicare reimbursements, as part of their implementation of the federal government's policy orientation. The federal government subsidizes 75% of the contract fee for states that have signed contracts with PROs for this purpose.

5. Medicaid for Low-Income Earners

(1) Overview of the Medicaid Scheme for Low-Income Earners

1. Establishment of Medicaid   The US Medicaid scheme emerged in the 1930s during the Great Depression, when health insurance was a prominent issue on the government agenda. During this period, the number of unemployed persons increased dramatically due to the collapse of a large number of industrial and commercial enterprises. Many of these

Americans were unable to afford their daily necessities, much less their medical expenses. To maintain social stability and prevent major social upheavals, the government adopted a number of medical aid measures to resolve some of the more urgent issues. In 1935, the Federal Health Surveillance Agency investigated the healthcare status of the elderly, vulnerable, and impoverished populations in the US and proposed providing medical aid for socially disadvantaged groups. However, the bill was shelved for various reasons.

Since then, the issue of social medical aid was revisited several times in 1952, 1954, and 1959, but was not implemented due to various obstacles. However, the eight-year term spanning the presidencies of John F. Kennedy and Lyndon B. Johnson (both of the Democratic Party) in the 1960s became the peak period for expanding and improving the social welfare and security system since Franklin Roosevelt's New Deal. During John F. Kennedy's presidency, the US government introduced a prepaid health insurance plan that guaranteed absolute freedom of choice. In October 1961, President Kennedy signed into law the Community Health Services and Facilities Act, passed by the US Congress.

In January 1965, President Johnson proposed a universal health insurance bill; following extensive coordination and compromise among the interests and claims of both parties, the original plan was gradually pared down to the Social Security Amendments, which only targeted certain vulnerable groups. In July 1965, the President signed the Social Security Amendments into law, which was implemented a year later in July 1966. These amendments included both Medicare and Medicaid, which provided health coverage for individuals aged over 65 years and impoverished individuals, respectively.

The US government has long considered it necessary to establish a health insurance scheme for low-income earners. In 1942, Rhode Island reported to the federal government that it hoped to use social welfare funds to cover the medical expenses of low-income earners. The US Social Security Administration rejected the request, but in 1949, it proposed the establishment of an extensive social welfare (aid) system that included the Medicaid scheme. However, this proposal was rejected by Congress due to its overly extensive coverage. Other discussions and proposals followed from the 1950s to the early 1960s, but none were passed by Congress or implemented in government agencies.

For example, a Medicare-like Medicaid scheme proposed by the DHHS in 1954 was opposed by the Bureau of the Budget (which later became the Office of Management and Budget) due to its excessive cost. In 1960, the DHHS proposed a Medicaid scheme covering individuals and married couples with household incomes less than US$2,500 and US$2,800, respectively. However, the proposal was also opposed by Congress. Instead, Congress put forward the Kerr-Mills bill, which later became the foundation of the Medical Assistance for the Aged Act.

In 1960, working groups for the health insurance system were set up within government agencies, following which the DHHS brought up the issue of whether Medicaid should be established in conjunction with Medicare. Thus, the framework of the Medical Assistance for the Aged Act was gradually established. The Medical Assistance for the Aged Act was extended from the Kerr-Mills bill and remains in place today.

2. Medicaid Recipients Medicaid is mainly implemented by states and special districts, which have considerable authority over the scope of recipients and benefits. The federal government has also established the following three categories of people who are eligible for Medicaid in each state:

1. *Mandatory categorically needy recipients.* States must include these individuals as Medicaid recipients and cover them via cash benefits, that is, Aid to Families with Dependent Children (AFDC) and Supplemental Security Income (SSI) for low-income individuals who are elderly, blind, or disabled.

The SSI is a standardized federal program, whereas AFDC reimbursement is administered by the states. The AFDC reimbursement criteria vary considerably across different states. For example, in 2000, there was an eightfold difference in AFDC reimbursements for families of four between West Virginia (which had the highest amount at US$2,675 per month) and Alabama (which had the lowest amount at US$334 per month).

Although the SSI is a standardized program implemented by the federal government, states have a degree of freedom in adjusting the requirements for SSI and can make them stricter than those at the national level. The stringency of the criteria for disability and poverty levels is significant but is still not comparable to the Medicaid eligibility criteria of 1972. In terms of the poverty level, Medicaid only covers individuals or families who experience a substantial decrease in income due to medical expenses, in accordance with the "spend down program." Such stringent eligibility criteria have been imposed in 14 states, including Connecticut, Hawaii, and Illinois.

2. *Optional categorically needy recipients.* Each state may decide whether to include these individuals as Medicaid recipients. Optional categorically needy recipients include individuals who meet the requirements for Medicaid in terms of personal incomes and assets (like the mandatory categorically needy recipients) and are eligible for cash benefits, but who are ineligible for these benefits because of family-related factors; and eligible individuals who refuse Medicaid coverage. The states must provide the same benefits as the aforementioned mandatory categorically needy recipients if they wish for these individuals to be covered under Medicaid.

In response to rising infant and child mortality rates in urban areas, state governments began to amend Medicaid laws to include pregnant women, infants, and children who have not received cash assistance, but who meet certain requirements for Medicaid coverage. Specifically, the states included the following groups of people as Medicaid recipients: pregnant women who meet the state's AFDC income and asset eligibility requirements; and children under the age of seven who meet the AFDC household income and asset requirements but are ineligible for AFDC coverage because of their cohabiting parents.

These measures were introduced in accordance with the OBRA of 1986 and 1987. Specifically, the OBRA of 1986 stipulated that pregnant women and infants who meet the state's requirements and fall below the federal poverty level (FDL) could be included as Medicaid recipients from January 1987 onwards. Subsequently, the age limit of children increased by one year annually from 1988, until all children under the age of five were covered. To further expand the coverage of children, this age range was extended to age seven and under by 1991. Furthermore, the OBRA of 1987 loosened the poverty level criteria by including pregnant women and children living in households with incomes below 185% of the federal poverty line (FPL) as Medicaid recipients.

3. *Medically needy recipients.* (1) Apart from considering income and asset criteria, states also cover blind, disabled, and elderly individuals, as well as mother-only families, pregnant women and children, as Medicaid recipients; (2) States also cover individuals who have financial difficulty in seeking medical attention, but are neither mandatory categorically needy recipients nor optional categorically needy recipients because their incomes and assets exceed the states' criteria.

States that provide Medicaid coverage for medically needy recipients are required to cover at least outpatient services for children, home-visit services for pregnant women, and home-based care services. Furthermore, almost all states cover various Medicaid-covered healthcare services for disadvantaged groups who fall beyond the abovementioned scopes.

Nevertheless, to become medically needy recipients, individuals must still meet state-specific income and asset criteria, which are determined by family size and must be standardized for each group. In addition, states cannot establish excessively loose criteria if they wish to receive federal subsidies; that is, the criteria must not be more than 133.3% of the state's AFDC income and asset criteria.

Although the Medicaid scheme has been implemented in all states and special districts for those living in poverty, the personal income criteria vary considerably by state. In 2000, there was a five-fold difference in the reimbursement amount for families of four between Virginia (which had the highest amount at US$2,660 per month) and Tennessee (which had the lowest amount at US$530 per month); the average amount was US$1,168 per month.

Medically needy individuals who become Medicaid recipients generally do not have low incomes from the beginning; instead, the vast majority of them only fall below the FPL after paying for their medical expenses. Hence, personal income after deducting medical expenses (i.e., Medicaid spend-down) is considered when reviewing the income criterion in all states. For example, in a state with an income criterion of US$1,500, a Medicaid applicant who earns US$2,000 per month can become a Medicaid recipient if they spend at least US$500 on medical expenses.

3. Changes in the Composition of Medicaid Recipients Table 13.10 shows the changes in the composition of Medicaid recipients in 1975–2000. There were no major changes in the total number of recipients in the decade after 1977. However, after 1986, the number of recipients increased gradually because of the eligibility expansion by Congress and population aging. The increasing trend became even more significant after 1995.

Among the target groups of Medicaid, the number of elderly and visually impaired recipients decreased slightly, while the number of disabled individuals and single-mother families increased slightly from 1990 to 2000. One factor contributing to the decrease in elderly recipients is the rise in social security retirement benefits, which increased the overall income level of these individuals. Indeed, the poverty rate (i.e., the ratio of the population below the FPL) among Americans aged over 65 years decreased from 15% in 1975 to 11.7% in 2000. The increase in the number of single-mother households over this period was attributed to eligibility expansion. For instance, the system introduced during this period guaranteed that AFDC recipients would receive access to Medicaid benefits for

TABLE 13.10 Number of Medicaid Recipients in Different Target Groups in the US from 1975 to 2000 (Unit: 1,000 people)

Year	Elderly Individuals	Visually Impaired Individuals	Disabled Individuals	Children from Single-Mother Families	Single Mothers	Others	Total
1975	361	109	235	959	452	180	2,296
1980	344	92	281	933	487	149	2,276
1985	306	80	293	975	551	121	2,326
1990	332	91	345	109	654	154	1,685
1995	310	82	356	112	674	164	1,698
2000	308	78	371	134	712	156	1,759

Source: HCFA 2082 data, Bureau of Data Management and Strategy.

TABLE 13.11   Medicaid Recipients from Single-Mother Families in the US from 1975 to 1985 (Unit: million people)

Year	AFDC Recipients		Non-AFDC Recipients		Total	
	Children	Adults	Children	Adults	Children	Adults
1975	8.2	3.9	0.9	0.4	9.1	4.5
1980	8.0	4.0	0.9	0.5	8.9	4.6
1985	8.0	4.2	1.2	0.9	9.2	5.0

Source: HCFA-2082 data, Bureau of Data Management and Strategy.

several months even after they are employed through employment programs despite no longer being eligible for cash assistance.

The changes in recipients and nonrecipients of cash assistance in each target group are shown in Table 13.11 and Table 13.12. Overall, the number of Medicaid recipients receiving cash assistance declined, but not to a significant degree. The number of recipients from single-mother families increased, but only to a limited extent. On the other hand, there was an increase in the number of people for all target groups who did not receive cash assistance but were eligible for Medicaid, which was likely due to the increase in the income level of the elderly population. However, the implementation of cash assistance most likely had some impact in this regard as well.

(2) Medicaid Benefits for Low-Income Earners

1. Benefits   All states must provide at least the following benefits for mandatory and optional categorically needy recipients:

1. Hospital inpatient and outpatient services
2. Biochemical tests and X-ray examinations
3. SNF services for patients aged over 21 years
4. Home-based care services replacing SNF services (e.g., home-visit services and medical supplies delivered by home-based care institutions)
5. Physician services
6. Family planning services
7. Suburban medical services

TABLE 13.12   Number of Elderly and Disabled Medicaid Recipients in the US from 1975 to 1985 (Unit: million people)

Year	SSI Recipients		Non-SSI Recipients		Total	
	Aged Above 65 Years	Aged Under 65 Years	Aged Above 65 Years	Aged Under 65 Years	Aged Above 65 Years	Aged Under 65 Years
1975	2.7	1.8	1.2	0.5	3.9	2.4
1980	2.5	1.8	1.4	0.6	3.9	2.4
1985	2.2	1.8	1.4	0.6	3.6	2.4

Sources: HCFA-2082 data, Bureau of Data Management and Strategy, and the Social Security and Administration, Office of Research and Statistics.

8. Early periodic screening, diagnosis, and treatment (EPSDT) for individuals aged under 21 years
9. Nurse and midwifery services

Although the federal government has established certain standards with respect to the service content above, the administration of Medicaid benefits is essentially the responsibility of the states. Therefore, Medicaid benefits can vary across states.

2. Reimbursement of Inpatient Services   The federal government imposes several regulations and restrictions on healthcare institutions offering Medicaid-covered services for patients.

1. The healthcare institution must be recognized by the state department of health and has to meet state requirements.
2. The healthcare institution must be Medicaid-designated healthcare institution.
3. The treatment and management of inpatients must be performed under the instruction of a physician or dentist.
4. The healthcare institution must have a utilization review plan in effect.

In addition to the above federal regulations and restrictions, almost all states also impose certain restrictions on service content. In 1986, only four states (i.e., Maine, Massachusetts, North Dakota, and South Dakota) had no such restrictions; all other states imposed certain limits on the benefits provided.

1. Eleven states (e.g., Alabama, Florida, Minnesota, West Virginia) limit the length of hospital stay (from a minimum of 12 days to a maximum of 60 days).
2. Nineteen states (e.g., California, Indiana, Maryland) require third-party approval and reviews prior to hospitalization.
3. Seventeen states do not cover all medical procedures, and 10 states do not cover individuals who may be treated via outpatient procedures (e.g., California, Connecticut, Oregon).

Many other restrictions have also been imposed by the respective state governments.

3. Reimbursement of Outpatient Services   The federal government imposes the same regulations for inpatient and outpatient services in hospitals. In addition, 42 states have imposed their own limits on certain benefits, as follows.

1. Eleven states (e.g., Alabama, Arkansas, Hawaii, Tennessee) have limited the number of outpatient visits among Medicaid recipients (from a minimum of 3 visits to a maximum of 48 visits).
2. Fourteen states (e.g., Georgia, Kansas, Kentucky) do not cover conventional health census, experimental treatments, or outpatient psychiatric treatments.
3. Fourteen states (e.g., Michigan, Missouri, Utah) require third-party approval before the implementation of outpatient services.
4. Five states (e.g., Connecticut, Hawaii, North Carolina) impose limitations on psychiatric services.

4. Expanded Medicaid Coverage in Each State Apart from the above mandatory services, the states might choose to provide expanded Medicaid coverage with additional services, including drugs, ICF services, eyeglasses, and inpatient psychiatric services for those aged under 20 years and over 65 years (Table 13.13).

1. *Medicaid drug coverage.* Almost all states, with the exception of Alaska and Wyoming, cover the drug expenses of Medicaid recipients. In 1990, Medicare began covering drug expenses in a phased manner. Before 1990, Medicare only covered the prescription drug expenses of Medicaid recipients.

    Naturally, Medicaid does not cover all drugs administered to patients, but rather imposes strict restrictions for reimbursement. These restrictions can roughly be divided into the following three approaches.
    1. Limiting the number of prescriptions and expenses within a certain period (adopted in 12 states, e.g., Arkansas, Georgia, Maine; most of which allow for 12 prescriptions per month and a few states allow only 3 prescriptions per month).
    2. Limiting the number of supplemental payments (additional drug coverage based on existing prescriptions) within a certain period (adopted in 24 states, e.g., Alabama, Kentucky, Louisiana; these states limit the average number of supplemental payments per existing prescription to five payments in six months).
    3. Limiting the quantity of drugs per prescription per day (adopted in 31 states, e.g., Michigan, Nevada, New Jersey; often limited over a number of days).

    In addition, 37 states either do not cover or only cover a handful of over-the-counter (OTC) drugs, while 16 states have adopted a preauthorization process for certain drugs.

2. *ICF services.* These services are provided to individuals requiring medical care, rehabilitation, or assistive care services upon admission to a healthcare institution other than a hospital or SNF. All 50 states include these services (with 49 states including mentally disabled care facilities and related services) in Medicaid coverage, and 18 states have not established special limits on reimbursements. However, there are some state-imposed restrictions for the following circumstances.
    1. Twenty-two states (e.g., Massachusetts, New York, Wisconsin) have adopted the preauthorization process for inpatient services, among which six states have implemented periodic reviews of preauthorization.
    2. Fourteen states have excluded certain services from Medicaid coverage, such as occupational therapy (OT), physical therapy (PT), and speech therapy, or have imposed restrictions on the use of out-of-state nursing homes.

5. Differences in the Benefits Provided to Different Groups of Recipients Mandatory benefits are provided to categorically needy recipients, but not to medically needy recipients. However, since March 1986, out of 35 states that implement Medicaid for medically needy recipients, 27 began providing mandatory benefits to medically needy recipients as well. Additionally, 23 states provided the same discretionary benefits for both categorically and medically needy recipients. Therefore, these two groups of recipients enjoy almost exactly the same benefits, which also include the mandatory benefits.

TABLE 13.13 Types of Medicaid-Covered Services and the Number of States Covering These Services in the US (Unit: Number of States)

Service Type	Number of States that Cover the Service for Categorically Needy Recipients	Number of States that Cover the Service for Categorically Needy and Medically Needy Recipients	Total
Podiatric services	10	31	41
Ophthalmology services	15	35	50
Chiropractic services	8	20	28
Other professional services	10	25	35
Attendant care services	5	14	19
Clinic services	14	35	49
Dental care services	13	29	42
Physiotherapy services	8	28	36
Occupational therapy services	5	22	27
Speech therapy services	7	26	33
Prescription drugs	14	37	51
Periodontal therapy	9	27	36
Dental filling	12	35	49
Eyeglasses	13	34	49
Diagnostic services	4	19	23
Screening	2	14	16
Preventive care	3	19	22
Rehabilitation	8	26	34
Psychiatric hospital service for patients over the age of 65	14	35	49
Inpatient services	16	25	41
SNFs	9	14	23
ICFs	11	17	28
Geriatric ICF services	18	32	50
Facilities for individuals with mental retardation	9	26	35
Christian nurses	1	5	6
Christian (tuberculosis) sanatoria	5	13	19
SNFs for patient aged under 21 years	15	33	48
Emergency hospital services	15	29	44
Individual care services	7	22	29
Patient transfers	10	28	38
Case management	0	1	1
Hospice care institutions	0	1	1

(3) Funding Sources and Management of Medicaid for Low-Income Earners

1. Federal Subsidies The federal government pays states for a specified percentage of Medicaid expenditures (between 50% and 83%), which is determined using a formula and is inversely related to the state's income per capita – that is, wealthier states receive fewer subsidies, and vice versa. In 2000, the largest federal share of Medicaid expenditures was 79.65%. The federal government also shares 50% of all administrative costs for Medicaid, with the exception of certain administrative functions.

2. Medicaid Expenditure When Medicaid was first established, some studies underestimated its total expenditure, suggesting that it would only increase the total federal expenditure by US$250 million. However, the total spending on Medicaid by federal and state governments was US$1.66 billion in 1966 and US$12.64 billion in 1975. Since then, the expenditure has increased rapidly, reaching US$40.92 billion in 1985, US$99.6 billion in 1995, and US$150.4 billion in 2000. As a result, by 2000, the total Medicaid expenditure accounted for more than 10% of the total US healthcare expenditure.

Medicaid coverage expanded substantially from 1966 to 1975. In 1966, only 26 states had implemented the Medicaid scheme. However, Medicaid expenditure increased with the expansion of Medicaid to the remaining states by 1980, sometimes at an annual rate of 40–50%.

The increasing trend ended between 1976 and 1985, during which the growth rate decreased from more than 10% in the first half of this period to less than 10% in the second half. The reduction in the growth rate was already quite substantial in the first half, as the higher growth rate could be attributed to the 12% inflation rate. After 1981, the implementation of policies to control healthcare expenditure also effectively reduced the growth rate of Medicaid expenditure. Among those policies, the OBRA of 1981 was arguably the most effective, as it reduced the federal share of Medicaid expenditure within three years of its implementation. Furthermore, the introduction of a performance-based reward system into the AFDC effectively suppressed the increase in the number of Medicaid recipients.

The Medicaid expenditures for different target groups in 1996 are shown in Table 13.14. The expenditures were exceedingly high for elderly and disabled recipients, at US$27.87 billion and US$26.55 billion, respectively, accounting for 36.7% and 34.9% of the total expenditure. On the other hand, although the number of children in single-mother families and single mothers accounted for 42.4% and 24.2% of the total number of Medicaid recipients, respectively, their Medicaid expenditures as a share of the total were lower, at 13.7% and 11.8%, respectively. This can be attributed to the lower average amount spent on each recipient.

Healthcare services can be ranked in descending order of Medicaid expenditure as follows: ICF admission fees, hospital inpatient expenses, SNF expenses, and physician charges. Of these, the expenditure for ICFs showed an especially notable increase, whereas the expenditure for physician charges decreased substantially. Furthermore, the expenditure for elderly and disabled recipients increased gradually, whereas the expenditure on single-mother families decreased.

In addition to the ICF admission fees, the overall Medicaid expenditure for elderly recipients increased significantly as well. In fact, Medicaid expenditure for elderly recipients ranked second only to ICF admission fees from 1976 to 1985.

As elderly individuals are often Medicaid recipients, other than reducing ICF admission fees, it is also possible to control the increase in Medicaid expenditure by introducing a deductible mechanism for Medicare Catastrophic Coverage or a reasonable cost-sharing mechanism for prescription drugs.

TABLE 13.14 Medicaid Expenditures for Different Target Groups in the US in 1996

Target Groups	Total Expenditure (US$100 Million)	Share of Total Expenditure (%)	Number of Recipients (1,000)	Share of Total Number of Recipients (%)	Average Expenditure Per Recipient (US$)
Elderly individuals (> 65 years old)	278.7	36.7	3,231.1	13.7	8,617.5
Visually impaired individuals	5.3	0.7	80.6	0.3	6,575.7
Disabled individuals	265.5	34.9	3,101.5	13.1	8,560.4
Single-mother families (children)	104.4	13.7	10,025.6	42.4	1,041.3
Single-mother families (adults)	89.6	11.8	5,723.1	24.2	1,565.6
Others	16.7	2.1	1,472.3	6.2	1,134.3
Total	760.2	100.0	23,634.2	100.0	3,216.5

Source: HCFA, Office of the Actuary, Office of Medicaid Estimates and Statistics. Division of Medicaid Statistics, 1997.

Medicaid expenditure for ICFs for individuals with mental retardation (ICF/MR) also increased significantly. Following the expansion of Medicaid to cover ICF/MR in 1971, Medicaid expenditure for this purpose increased rapidly to US$910 million in 1975 (current price in 1985) and US$3.8 billion in 1995. In fact, it became one of the most expensive services covered by Medicaid, accounting for 14.7% of the total expenditure, even though ICF/MR recipients only accounted for 0.9% of the total number of Medicaid recipients.

3. Medicaid Reimbursement Methods   The US federal government has imposed the following requirements on each state with respect to Medicaid reimbursement: (1) full coverage of reasonable costs of effective and economical hospitals, SNFs, and ICFs; (2) full coverage of high-quality teaching hospitals and facilities with a high proportion of low-income patients; and (3) ample reimbursement of hospitals to ensure patients have access to high-quality healthcare services.

However, the precise reimbursement structure is determined by each state. Therefore, the amount and method of reimbursement vary considerably across states because of differences in their service contents. The reimbursement methods for ICFs and physician services are summarized as follows.

1. *Reimbursement methods for ICFs.* The reimbursement of ICFs is optional but has been implemented in all states. Of the 50 states, 38 have adopted the PPS for the reimbursement of ICFs. This method can be further divided into a prospective facility-specific system and a prospective classification–based system (i.e., the reimbursement amount is determined based on region, facility size, and facility type). The former has been adopted in 31 of these 38 states (e.g., Alabama, Connecticut, New Jersey, and so on), with the remaining 7 states (e.g., California, Louisiana, Texas) adopting the latter.

Only three states (Iowa, Massachusetts, and Tennessee) have adopted the retrospective payment system, while the remaining nine states (e.g., Maryland, Pennsylvania, Wisconsin) have combined the prospective and retrospective payment systems for the reimbursement of ICF expenses.

The standard reimbursement amount varies significantly across states. After excluding Alaska and Hawaii, which have particularly high standard reimbursement amounts, the standard reimbursement per patient in 1999 ranged from US$108.25 per day in Arkansas to US$296.13 per day in New York, with an average actual reimbursement of US$147.23.

2. *Reimbursement methods for hospital services.* Eleven states have adopted the retrospective payment system, while the remaining 39 have adopted the DRG/PPS method or other reimbursement methods.

A total of 10 states have adopted the DRG/PPS method, including Hawaii, Michigan, Ohio, and Pennsylvania.

Many other reimbursement methods are in use, but for most, the reimbursement amount is determined based on the preestablished average daily expenses for each patient or the average expenses for each service item. The states rely on these methods to control their healthcare expenditures.

In accordance with the respective state laws, each state can apply the Medicaid reimbursement method to other health insurance schemes (e.g., Medicare and private insurance). For instance, Maine, Maryland, and New Jersey apply the same reimbursement method as Medicaid to all insurance sold in the state. In contrast, Massachusetts and Rhode Island only apply the same reimbursement method to private insurance. Mississippi, New York, Tennessee, and eight other states apply the same reimbursement method to Medicare.

3. *Reimbursement methods for physician outpatient services.* Broadly speaking, there are two major reimbursement methods for physician services: the reasonable cost method and the fee schedule method. The former has been adopted in 15 states, such as Hawaii, Kentucky, and Texas, while the latter has been adopted in the remaining 35 states, among which 28 (e.g., Connecticut, Florida, Illinois) have adopted a fixed fee schedule, and 7 (e.g., Minnesota, New York) have adopted the RVS method. Six of these 35 states (e.g., California, Michigan, New Jersey) have also introduced a capitation reimbursement method.

4. Medicaid Management Medicaid is a state-implemented program, but all state operations are monitored by the HCFA of the DHHS.

Federal law requires each state to establish an independent executive agency for the management of Medicaid. The executive agency appointed for Medicaid management varies across states, but the business operations of Medicaid are usually administered by the state welfare agency, healthcare agency, or human resources agency. These state agencies might delegate parts of their business operations to other state agencies, or delegate the claims and reimbursement of medical expenses to a management service intermediary or insurance company.

6. Healthcare Cost-containment Policies

(1) Growth Characteristics of Healthcare Expenditure

1. Continuous Growth in Healthcare Expenditure Over the Past 50 Years The US ranks first globally in healthcare expenditure. The total healthcare expenditure increased from US$26.9 billion (US$148 per capita) in 1960 to US$73.2 billion in 1970 and US$247.3 billion in 1980. In 1996, the US healthcare expenditure exceeded US$1 trillion

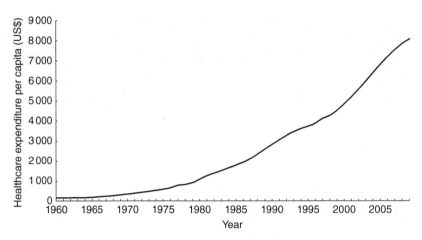

FIGURE 13.5   US Healthcare expenditure per capita from 1960 to 2009. *Source:* US Centers for Medicare and Medicaid Services, 2011.

(US$1.035 trillion) for the first time. In 1998, the US healthcare expenditure reached US$1.1491 trillion (US$4,270 per capita), making it more than twice the average per capita of the other 23 OECD countries (US$2,000) and nearly twice the country ranked second, Switzerland, which is a European welfare state (US$2,740 per capita). Subsequently, US healthcare expenditure increased to US$1.553 trillion in 2002, US$2.3 trillion in 2008 and US$2.5 trillion in 2009 (US$8,086 per capita). Overall, the US healthcare expenditure per capita increased 54-fold from 1960 to 2009, with an average annual growth rate of 9% (Figure 13.5).

2. Growth Rate of Healthcare Expenditure   The US healthcare expenditure recorded a double-digit percentage annual growth before 1990. However, the average annual growth rate dropped to single-digit percentage after 1990 and continued to decline to the lowest point in the past 40 years (4.6%) in 1996, rebounding to only 4.7% and 5.6% in 1997 and 1998, respectively. Although the total healthcare expenditure remained high, its share of the GDP and growth rate has declined due to the effectiveness of cost-containment policies centered on "managed care." In fact, healthcare expenditure increased to a lesser extent than the GDP growth in specific years (e.g., 1996 and 1997). However, the growth rate of the total healthcare expenditure in 2003 (7.7%) was greater than the GDP growth rate (4.9%). By 2008, the growth rate of the total healthcare expenditure still exceeded the GDP growth rate (2.6%) but had dropped to 4.4%.

3. Constantly High Healthcare Expenditure as a Share of the GDP   After undergoing exponential growth for more than three decades, the total healthcare expenditure as a share of the GDP has been relatively stable in recent years. In 1960, the US healthcare expenditure accounted for less than 6% (5.2%) of the GDP; by 1993, this had more than doubled to 13%. After 1993, the total healthcare expenditure as a share of the GDP remained within 13–14% until about 2003, when it increased to 15.3%. It further increased to 16.2% in 2008 (about US$7,681 per capita). In 2009, healthcare expenditure accounted for 17.6% of the GDP, with an expenditure per capita of US$8,160 (Figure 13.6), thus overtaking other traditional industries (e.g., energy, military, and education) to become the largest industry in the US. With regard to the composition of healthcare expenditure, hospital nursing costs accounted for the largest share, followed by physician charges. In 1998, these two items

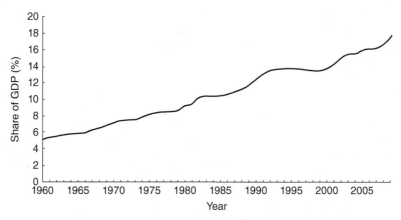

FIGURE 13.6 US healthcare expenditure as a share of the GDP from 1960 to 2009. *Source:* US Centers for Medicare and Medicaid Services, 2011.

accounted for 60.1% of the total healthcare expenditure (hospital nursing costs, 37.6%; physician charges, 22.5%). By 2009, hospital nursing costs and physician services accounted for 31.6% and 31.4% of the total healthcare expenditure, respectively, giving a total of 63.0%. In addition, expenditure for prescription drugs showed the highest growth rate among personal healthcare expenditures, reaching US$90.6 billion in 1998 (or 7.9% of the total healthcare expenditure). After 1995, the total healthcare expenditure and the majority of itemized expenditures grew at a slower rate. However, the expenditure for prescription drugs maintained a double-digit percentage growth: increase of 10.6% from 1994 to 1995, 12.9% from 1995 to 1996, 14% from 1996 to 1997, and 15.4% from 1997 to 1998. Furthermore, the expenditure increased by over 17% for four consecutive years, from 1999 to 2001. More recently, the growth rate for prescription drug expenses has been somewhat attenuated. Statistical analysis by IMS Health showed that in 2010, the sales of prescription drugs in the US was US$307 billion, and its growth rate declined continuously to only 2.3%.

(2) Causes for the Growth in Healthcare Expenditure

1. Increasing Number of Insured Persons The coverage of private and government health insurance plans has continued to expand over the past half century. However, due to the imperfect insurance system and moral hazard, the increase in the number of insured persons as a result of third-party payments has adversely influenced the control of healthcare expenditure. On the one hand, insured persons have an increased tendency to seek medical attention and access healthcare services more frequently; on the other hand, healthcare providers (hospitals and physicians) have become more driven by economic interests to provide as many healthcare services as possible, thereby leading to wastage of healthcare resources and an overly rapid increase in healthcare expenditure.

2. High Reimbursement Levels for Healthcare Providers To encourage the participation of hospitals, physicians, and other healthcare providers in government health insurance plans, the government has legislated that both Medicare and Medicaid reimburse physicians at standard levels and reimburse hospitals on the basis of additional costs. These approaches have also been frequently adopted by private insurance companies, which have led to a rise in the income of healthcare providers.

3. Substantial Expenses for Administration Costs and Civil Litigation The management of the health insurance system comprises four components: transaction costs, profit management, marketing costs, and regulatory and enforcement costs.

Pharmaceutical companies. It is estimated that the marketing cost of drugs accounts for about 25% of their total sales.

Insurance agencies. The diversified and mixed US health insurance system has forced insurance agencies to spend 17–21% of their total expenditure on administration. This is a much higher proportion than in developed countries that have adopted universal health coverage or a single-payer healthcare system. Indeed, insurance agencies in other OECD countries only spend about 5% of their total expenditure or less on administration.

Hospitals. Hospitals in the US spend 25% of their total expenditure on administration. Experts estimate that if administration costs can be reduced to the same level as other countries, the US can save up to US$80 billion per year, equivalent to about one-third of the total healthcare expenditure in all developing countries.

4. Emergence of New Medical Technologies The emergence of new and expensive medical technologies in the late twentieth century has led to a rapid increase in healthcare expenditure. This is a common issue facing Western developed countries. Medical technologies are currently actively promoted and widely utilized in the US. Hence, many economists and insurance agencies believe that the annual growth in healthcare expenditure is primarily attributed to the adoption of new technologies.

5. Population Aging Accelerates the Growth of Healthcare Expenditure As in many other countries, the US is facing accelerated population aging. The most immediate consequence of population aging is the rise in the demand for emergency and long-term care services. Elderly Americans spend 18% of their income on medical expenses, and the growth rate of out-of-pocket expenses is almost twice that of their social security payments.

(3) Theories and Value Orientations for Healthcare Cost Containment

How can the rising healthcare expenditure be controlled? Politicians, scholars, healthcare workers, and the public have long debated this issue and have diverse opinions in this regard. However, there are two main approaches or strategies for healthcare cost containment: containment based on government management and containment based on market competition.

1. Great Emphasis on Governmental Macroprudential Regulation There are three prerequisite assumptions about government intervention in the control of healthcare expenditure. First, as in other industries, the healthcare market harbors numerous flaws, that is, "market failures." These primarily involve the information asymmetry between providers and consumers about healthcare services and the use of a third-party payment system (i.e., insurance), which can induce the demand for healthcare services, thus resulting in overexpenditure, inefficiency, and irrational allocation of healthcare workforce and resources. Second, the healthcare market differs from other markets in various ways, primarily with regard to the unique relationship between providers and consumers of healthcare services and products. Physicians have control of both the supply and demand of healthcare services – that is, they serve as advisors who recommend services that a patient needs, as well as service providers. Without specialized training in cost containment, physicians are rarely aware of the problem of overexpenditure. However, they have an enormous impact on overall healthcare expenditure because they influence not only the purchase decisions of each patient but also the growth in healthcare expenditure for the entire healthcare institution. In addition, the third-party payment system, which heavily relies on private health insurance and government funding, has reduced the awareness of healthcare expenditure among patients and healthcare institutions to a certain extent. Finally, there are three major value orientations in public administration: political responsibility, public participation, and public accessibility to information. Public administration is the process by which the government achieves these three value orientations, which are conducive to the control of the healthcare expenditure.

2. Emphasis on Market Competition Mechanisms   Governmental macroprudential regulation is an inefficient measure as healthcare resources are allocated according to the principle of equality. It is a major factor underlying the growth in healthcare expenditure. Therefore, it is crucial to introduce market competition in order to ensure the effective allocation of healthcare resources. In response to the "moral hazard" of the third-party payment system and its consequent exacerbation of the growth in actual expenses, some market reformers have begun demanding the remodeling of the market incentive mechanism. They suggest providing consumers with multiple options that have a genuine impact on healthcare expenditure, thereby creating a fair and competitive market and promoting market competition in order to control healthcare expenditure. Based on social values that focus on individual creativity and freedom of choice, as well as the risks of large companies and a large government, those who advocate for perfect competition believe that efficiency and innovation can be enhanced through competition. They also encourage decentralization and diversification and believe that a competitive market is more stable than a noncompetitive market because the former is capable of responding to constantly changing market conditions.

Although macroprudential regulation and market competition theoretically occupy diametrically opposite positions, they are not necessarily completely incompatible with one another. In fact, the combination of both approaches could be an ideal cost-containment approach. The former emphasizes stimulation, while the latter emphasizes government guidance and recognition. It is extremely difficult for macroprudential regulation to achieve established goals against the market trend by depending solely on legislation. Therefore, it is crucial to enhance market stimulation, competition, and choice while implementing regulatory strategies, as well as to prevent the rigidity that arises from regulating the highly complicated healthcare system. The weakening of market strength is unavoidable, and it is impossible to create a healthcare market free from government intervention; thus, it is perhaps inevitable that macroprudential regulation will be selected as an alternative, which had led to the establishment of "managed competition."

The US has arguably the most abundant resources for theoretical research globally. Based on rigorous research and analysis, the world's top universities and research institutions have proposed an ideology that places equal emphasis on macroprudential regulation and market competition. This ideology has exerted a significant impact on the international community.

(4) Specific Measures for Healthcare Cost Containment

1. Cost-Containment Plan   The US federal government has adopted a middle way of cost containment comprising both management and competitive cost-containment measures. However, in general, the federal government is more biased towards regulatory measures.

Currently, three main approaches have been adopted in the management and supervision of healthcare expenditure: institutional and service management, utility management, and premium and benefits management. Based on these three management approaches, the federal government has introduced three types of cost-management plans at different points in time: the certificate of need (CON), PSRO, and PPS.

The CON is a supply-side cost-management plan requiring hospitals to prove the presence of social needs and obtain expense approval prior to the expansion of their facilities, medical equipment, and healthcare services, with the aim of reducing unnecessary healthcare investment. The CON also established strict market entry regulations, whereby new medical practitioners could only enter the healthcare market if there is new demand.

PSROs were developed to ensure more rational healthcare resource utilization. They refer to local PROs responsible for assessing and supervising healthcare services delivered to Medicare and Medicaid patients. These organizations also determine the necessity, professional quality, and delivery mode of these services. They aim to reduce the national healthcare expenditure by preventing unnecessary treatment and services.

The PPS is a cost-control measure that first classifies patients based on their diagnostic results, or DRGs (of which there are currently 468 in the US) to predetermine the standard fees for each group of patients and their diseases, based on which the hospitals are reimbursed.

2. Managed Care Plan   As a competitive PPS-based health insurance model, HMOs control healthcare expenditure using the following three approaches: (1) establishing an incentive mechanism to stimulate the restructuring of healthcare institutions and the integration of more expensive inpatient services with cheaper outpatient services; (2) introducing competition into the traditional healthcare delivery system to encourage competition among healthcare institutions; and (3) choosing the best prices offered among HMOs through market mechanisms.

In general, HMOs collect a certain amount of fees in advance (capitation payments), after which they provide their registrants with various necessary healthcare services. There is a similarity between HMOs and PPS in terms of the incentive mechanism for cost containment. That is, healthcare institutions are encouraged to improve their efficiency by reducing unnecessary treatment and wastage, which allow them to gain more profits. Additionally, the insurance premiums are reduced alongside the reducing cost of healthcare institutions, thereby enhancing the market competitiveness of HMOs.

PPOs, on the other hand, are a health insurance plan that aims to limit treatment options offered to health insurance beneficiaries. They grant health insurance beneficiaries access to healthcare services at designated healthcare institutions via hard regulations or economic strategies. These healthcare institutions are generally selected based on their prices, thus physicians or hospitals with less expensive services or fewer expected services are more likely to be chosen. Furthermore, healthcare institutions must strive to reduce unnecessary treatments through obtaining utility assessments and modifying treatment regimens. In addition, some PPOs designate certain physicians that provide basic healthcare services as "gatekeepers" whose approval is required for beneficiaries to receive specialist treatments.

Aside from relying on market competition and economic stimulation for cost reduction, the healthcare services provided by prepaid group practices, such as HMOs and PPOs, must be assessed and monitored to prevent unnecessary treatment. This concept of cost containment is known as "managed care."

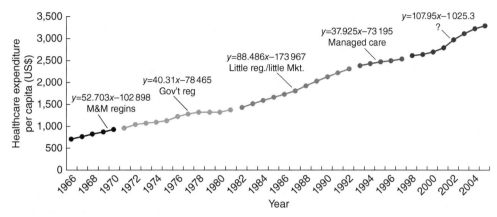

FIGURE 13.7 Strategies for healthcare cost containment in the US (US healthcare expenditure per capita from 1906 to 2005). *Source:* Stuart Altman, "Growing Healthcare Spending: Can or Should It Be Controlled to Prevent a Health System 'Meltdown'?," Brandeis University. Note: The data have been corrected for inflation.

The fundamental difference between conventional medical practice and managed care is the presence of managers, who are responsible for supervising and controlling the transactions between physicians and patients. In general, there are five managed care approaches for cost containment. (1) Reimbursement restrictions, such as when the federal government reimburses Medicare expenses for healthcare institutions based on DRGs. (2) Preauthorization for healthcare services; for instance, the manager must be consulted prior to a surgical operation. (3) Assigning GPs who provide basic healthcare services as gatekeepers in order to control patients' accessibility to specialist treatments. (4) "Skill reduction," which involves assigning undertrained healthcare workers to provide certain services, such as having nurses examine patients before they see the physicians. (5) Encouraging physicians to reduce utilization of healthcare services via economic measures.

Figure 13.7 uses healthcare expenditure per capita as the parameter to show the strategies for healthcare cost containment in the US from 1906 to 2005. The piecewise function graph shows that the fourth curve (i.e., managed care) has the lowest slope. This indicates that managed care, which was implemented in the 1990s, gave rise to the most desirable outcome in controlling US healthcare expenditure.

(5) Outcomes of Healthcare Cost-Containment Policies

1. Cost-Control Plan The actual implementation outcomes have shown that neither the CON nor PSRO has significantly reduced hospital expenses or total healthcare expenditure. This is mainly because they did not break the monopoly of physicians or improve the information asymmetry in the healthcare sector. As a result, these cost-management organizations were instead controlled by their subjects and failed to exert an effect on cost containment.

On the other hand, the most significant characteristic of the PPS, which sets it apart from the CON and PSRO, is the incentive mechanism for controlling for healthcare expenditure. The fixed reimbursement rates allow hospitals to obtain more profits by changing their therapeutic methods or reducing the length of hospital stay, thereby improving therapeutic efficiency and reducing costs. Conversely, hospitals must bear the losses if their costs exceed the predetermined reimbursement rate. Therefore, this system encourages and forces hospitals to be more concerned with healthcare expenditure so as to improve their efficiency and control their expenses.

Following the introduction of the PPS, the number of inpatients and the length of hospital stay have both decreased, leading to significantly attenuated growth in hospital expenses compared to before its introduction. Nevertheless, the national healthcare expenditure continued to rise, mainly because of the shift in emphasis of the supply side to other healthcare fields, such as raising the charges for outpatient and home-based care services.

2. Managed Care Plan Managed care plans, represented by HMOs and PPOs, developed rapidly with the support of the government and employers. Statistics showed that in 1995, there were 571 HMOs with 58 million registrants and 1,036 PPOs with nearly 50 million registrants in the US. Taken together, more than 100 million Americans had registered under managed care plans. However, there are some obstacles to the successful development of these plans, especially in recent years, which are largely the result of the vigorous debate between theorists and consumers. Specifically, a large number of reports indicate that consumers are consistently less satisfied with managed care plans compared to FFS plans, mainly because the former limits consumers' freedom of choice and affects the quality of healthcare services to a certain extent. Healthcare providers are also dissatisfied with these plans because they hinder physicians' freedom to diagnose and treat individuals based on patients' conditions. Therefore, providers must constantly argue with the management team of the insurance agencies over treatment regimens. As a result, expenses are a prerequisite for therapeutic processes. Even though these plans can partially limit healthcare expenditure, the resources are almost completely drained by management and network expansion costs. Thus, increasing doubts have been cast on the outcomes of managed care plans.

The implementation outcomes of managed care plans can also be affected by population aging and the development of new technologies. This is because managed care plans aim to reduce unnecessary treatments, while population aging and new medical technologies both lead to an increase in the number of essential treatments, thereby limiting the potential effect of these plans. Managed care plans have been serving as a cost-containment measure for about 20 years. However, they have had a much weaker impact on the total healthcare expenditure compared to initial expectations.

(6) Social Impact of Healthcare Cost-containment Policies

Cost-containment measures might be able to reduce healthcare expenditure within a short period of time, but their long-term effects on social goals should not be overlooked. In particular, it is not advisable to achieve economic goals at the expense of social goals.

First, the immediate social impact of cost-containment measures is the reduced accessibility of impoverished and uninsured individuals to healthcare services. Medicare and Medicaid are government-funded public health insurance schemes accounting for the largest share of healthcare expenditure in the US. Therefore, both of these schemes have taken the brunt of the government's cost-containment measures. The reduction in Medicare and Medicaid budgets and the strict hospital reimbursement policy have excluded or delayed some impoverished and elderly groups from receiving healthcare services. There is abundant evidence to suggest that cost-containment measures, especially those concerning Medicaid, have reduced accessibility of impoverished individuals to healthcare services.

Moreover, the number of uninsured persons has increased because of the reduction in Medicaid and employer group insurance. Statistics show that there were 43 million uninsured Americans in 2001. These individuals will be faced with a difficult situation once they fall ill. Unlike other industrialized countries, however, the US does not have universal health coverage; thus, it cannot guarantee minimum health coverage for all citizens. As a result, impoverished and uninsured individuals only have access to free medical aid or charity healthcare. Some teaching hospitals provide a large volume of free healthcare services, but intense market competition and strict cost-containment measures have greatly reduced the delivery of such charity healthcare. Increasingly, such institutions are shifting away from charitable motives to a more commercial orientation. Consequently, uninsured and impoverished patients are constantly transferred from one hospital to another like hot potatoes. Overall, the US lacks a safety net consisting of a well-established health insurance system, a network of public hospitals and clinics, and charity healthcare to ensure that all Americans have access to basic healthcare services.

Second, the cost-containment measures will also have a negative impact on biological and medical research, as well as medical education. The growth of HMOs and PPOs might keep patients away from more expensive teaching hospitals, which might influence their incomes. Furthermore, Medicare PPS revenue has increased at a lower rate than inflation, which has been generally unfavorable to medical education and research unless alternative funding sources can be identified. The reduction in Medicare funding allocation and the increase in NIH investment in accordance with the health reform plan formulated by the Bush administration both suggest that the US government has recognized the seriousness of this issue.

Third, cost-containment measures have influenced the quality of healthcare services. Most cost-containment measures are designed to target inefficiency and waste in the healthcare system. Once these factors have been identified and eliminated, it may be too optimistic to claim that the reduction in healthcare expenditure is not due to the compromise of healthcare quality. Recent studies have suggested that it has become extremely difficult to significantly influence healthcare expenditure by merely reducing wastage and improving service efficiency. It is, therefore, crucial to establish a surveillance mechanism to ensure the quality of healthcare services and prevent the adverse effects of cost-containment measures.

Finally, federal and state budgetary pressures are expected to further broaden the gap in reimbursement rate between patients with public health insurance and patients with private health insurance, thereby affecting the accessibility and quality of healthcare services for vulnerable groups. This issue is expected to become increasingly difficult to solve over time.

7. Plan and Progress of Obamacare

(1) Background and History of the Patient Protection and Affordable Care Act (i.e., Obamacare)

In 2007, the US healthcare expenditure as a share of the GDP was 16.2% and fiscal expenditure was 49.54%. This was a heavy fiscal burden on the US and the most expensive healthcare system in the world. Despite the alarming growth of healthcare expenditures, the health status of Americans is lagging behind that of many other developed countries. The US is also the only developed country in the world that does not have universal health coverage, and medical debt is the main reason for bankruptcy among American families. Statistics have shown that there are 50 million uninsured Americans, accounting for approximately one-sixth of the total US population. In other words, the US still has relatively low health insurance coverage. Furthermore, a widely observed phenomenon in the US healthcare system is the tremendous time and energy spent by physicians on affairs related to health insurance, medical authorization, and medical litigation, with less attention given to the quality of healthcare services. Thus, the overall operational efficiency of the system is lower, and it has become more difficult to ensure the quality of healthcare services.

Currently, the US spends about US$2,500 billion annually on healthcare. Healthcare costs are poorly controlled, with experts estimating that at least one-third of delivered healthcare services are unnecessary. With the support of various medical and healthcare groups, such as insurance agencies, hospitals, physicians, pharmaceutical companies and labor unions, President Barack Obama proposed a reform plan to cut taxes by US$836 billion (US$736 billion for middle-class families and US$100 billion for small enterprises) over the next decade. This reform plan also aimed to reduce healthcare costs and expand the coverage of health insurance by including around 50 million previously uninsured Americans. The current situation in the US is as follows: About 15.3% of Americans are uninsured, and the remaining 84.7% are insured (59.3% covered by employer group insurance, 13.2% by Medicaid, 8.9% by private insurance, and 3.7% by TRICARE).

In March 2009, President Barack Obama held the White House Health Care Summit to call for a congressional proposal on the 2009 health reform plan. President Obama then put forward a US$787 billion economic stimulus package (known as the American Recovery and Reinvestment Act, ARRA), which contained additional cuts to expenditures and taxes. This act also increased investment in health, including some healthcare plans, to help overcome the global economic crisis at the time. The ARRA was estimated to take two to three years to have any beneficial effect on the quality and cost-effectiveness of healthcare services. The US government passed the ARRA later in 2009.

The first step of the ARRA was to inject US$634 billion within 10 years into health reform, including the expansion of health coverage to uninsured Americans and the control of US healthcare expenditure. The government also appointed new leaders in several health-related departments, such as the DHHS, HRSA, and CDC.

Before 2010, the US government allocated about US$1.1 billion to the funding of comparative studies, including US$400 million for the NIH, US$300 million for the US Agency for Healthcare Research and Quality (AHRQ), and US$400 million for the DHHS. Furthermore, the number of children covered by the State Children's Health Insurance Program (SCHIP) increased from 7 million to 11 million through increasing cigarette taxes.

(2) Main Points of Obamacare

1. Basic Goals of Obamacare Obamacare was drafted with the aim of "reducing healthcare costs and ensuring universal access to available and affordable healthcare services." In the Obama-Biden Plan, President Obama proposed a blueprint of Obamacare containing the following three goals.

1. *Cost reduction.* This can be achieved through three measures: (1) Adopting an advanced health information technology (HIT) system. (2) Ensuring the best healthcare services for patients, including preventive care and chronic care services. (3) Reforming the market structure, promoting competition, and providing employers with federal reinsurance against emergency and major illnesses, thereby preventing them from being unable to afford medical expenses arising from catastrophic illnesses or being refused coverage by commercial insurance companies.

2. *Universal, affordable, and attainable healthcare.* This can be achieved via the following measures: (1) Ensure broad eligibility for all health insurance plans. Insurance companies should provide comprehensive health coverage for insured persons at a fair and consistent premium rate, regardless of their current and previous health status. (2) Establish a National Health Insurance Exchange to help Americans and businesses purchase commercial health insurance. In addition to the existing private insurance companies, this system would allow for the establishment of a public health insurance plan, thereby ensuring the accessibility of all Americans to health coverage (either under the newly established public health insurance or licensed private insurance companies). (3) Provide a new pretax payroll deduction for families who are unable to afford insurance premiums and encourage small enterprises to cover up to 50% of health insurance premiums for their employees via tax credits. (4) Require large enterprises to either offer health insurance coverage for a certain proportion of their employees or pay a minimum fee to the health insurance system. Some models employ a "pay or play" penalty, such that enterprises either provide minimum basic coverage for their employees or contribute a certain amount of the fees to the government fund to help more Americans obtain health coverage. (5) Provide health insurance coverage to all children. (6) Expand the scope of Medicaid and SCHIP recipients. (7) Allow some flexibility for states in health reforms.

3. Promote and enhance preventive public healthcare by emphasizing the accountability and close cooperation of individuals, families, schools, and employers with the healthcare sector and federal and state governments, thereby creating conditions to allow and encourage a healthier lifestyle among Americans.

2. Goals and Provisions of Obamacare   The primary goals of Obamacare were to expand the coverage of health insurance, reduce healthcare costs, and improve service efficiency. The specific provisions of Obamacare are as follows:

1. *Expanding the coverage of public health insurance and raising subsidies for low- and middle-income families.* Obamacare aimed to loosen the eligibility criteria for Medicaid to include all nonelderly Americans with incomes below 33% of the FPL; the original plan only included elderly individuals eligible for social welfare. The federal and state governments would jointly administer and share the cost of Medicaid and SCHIP in order to establish a health insurance safety net for low-income and vulnerable groups. In addition, the US government also provided tax credits and cost sharing reduction (CSR) subsidies for low- and middle-income earners and families, which gave the biggest tax cuts in American healthcare history for individuals and families.

2. *Providing employers with options and subsidies to cover the health insurance premiums of their employees.* All enterprises must purchase group health insurance for their employees or participate in public health insurance. Employers will be penalized if any employee must rely on federally funded insurance schemes. Enterprises with fewer than 50 employees are exempt, and enterprises with fewer than 25 employees can receive government subsidies. Large enterprises with more than 50 employees are exempt from paying any health insurance premiums for the top 30 highest paid full-time employees. In addition, the government will support employers who provide health insurance for their retirees aged 55–64 years with a reinsurance plan.

3. *Establishing a new national insurance market and strengthening the supervision of insurance companies.* Obamacare has prohibited the discrimination of insurance companies

618 ■ Commercial Health Insurance and Medical Savings Accounts Systems

against applicants based on existing conditions, health status, gender, and so on. Furthermore, it has sought to create a competitive insurance exchange market such that individuals and small enterprises will be able to afford health insurance like large enterprises. The US government has authorized the DHHS and the National Association of Insurance Commissioners (NAIC) to conduct an annual review in order to identify unreasonable increases in premium rates.

4. *Increasing the capital injection for basic healthcare facilities and transforming the reimbursement mechanism for healthcare providers.* Obamacare aimed to increase the capital injection for community healthcare centers to improve the quality of primary healthcare and expand regional coverage of health insurance. Community healthcare centers play a vital role in providing high-quality healthcare services. Currently, there are approximately 1,250 community healthcare centers providing preventive and primary care services for around 20 million Americans in the US.

    The government has increased funding for the training of physicians, nurses, and other healthcare providers. Presently, about 65 million Americans live in communities without basic healthcare facilities, and it is expected that an additional 165,000 healthcare workers are needed to meet the healthcare demands of this population. Obamacare proposed solving the shortage of basic healthcare services by injecting further capital, as necessary, into the recruitment of healthcare workers.

5. *Other aspects.* Obamacare also aims to prevent chronic diseases and improve the health status of the general public; improve the transparency and integrity of medical procedures; impose a crackdown on wastage, fraud, and abuse of healthcare resources; provide access to innovative therapeutic methods for patients; and provide community residential assistance and support services.

The Medicare Payment Advisory Commission (MedPAC) has made the following recommendations to Congress: reduce the Medicare reimbursement rate for home-based care by 5.5%, but ensure that the reimbursement levels for existing nursing and rehabilitation hospitals remain unchanged; increase the prospective payment for outpatient services and the reimbursement rate for inpatient services according to the increase in the hospital market price index; introduce a hospital quality incentive program and allocate 1% of the expenditure to indirect medical education (IME) programs; increase the reimbursement amount for PCPs while reducing the reimbursement amount of Medicare Advantage; standardize the reimbursement standards between supplementary health insurance and conventional FFS payments, such that it is only possible to raise the reimbursement standards by providing services with better outcomes; increase the reimbursement rate for physicians by 1.1%; and establish the "budget-neutral payment system" to increase the remuneration for PCPs while reducing the remuneration standards for specialists.

(3) Responses and Evaluations from Various Parties

The US Congressional Budget Office (CBO) estimated that this health reform bill will reduce the US deficit by a total of US$143 billion from 2010 to 2019 and is expected to further decline by a total of US$1.2 trillion over the following 10 years. Hence, the health reform is expected to have a major impact on the government financing of the US. At present, there are about 50 million US permanent residents under the age of 65 who are not covered by any health insurance scheme. This population is expected to increase by 4 million in the next decade based on the current healthcare system. Obamacare is seeking to cover 16 million more eligible Americans under Medicaid and SCHIP. Together with individuals who will be included in other health insurance plans, it is expected that there will be 32 million more insured individuals in the US health insurance system. In other words, the nationwide coverage of the US health insurance system will increase from 81% to 92% (or 94%, if illegal immigrants are excluded from the estimation) within 10 years, which is akin to universal health insurance.

President Obama learned from the failures of President Bill Clinton in promoting health reform during his presidency from 1992 to 2000. He invited the six major health insurance groups to make a joint commitment to the health reform strategy, thereby reducing the obstacles to its achievement. Although it is difficult to predict how the healthcare system will fare over the next 10 years, experts are expecting an annual increase in healthcare expenditure of about 7%, which would far exceed the economic growth rate. Nevertheless, Obamacare has taken a major step toward achieving universal health coverage.

Paul Krugman, who was awarded the 2008 Nobel Prize in Economics, said that the US insurance and healthcare markets are dominated by private insurance agencies and private hospitals. As a result, the US healthcare system is inefficient, as the increase in healthcare costs does not translate into increased healthcare value. Based on a comparison between the US, Canada, and France, he suggested that public health insurance is more effective than private health insurance, as it is more feasible to control healthcare expenditures in a single-payer system. He also analyzed the US TRICARE system and suggested that healthcare expenditure could be more effectively controlled via the direct provision of healthcare services by the government.

Inevitably, these healthcare reform measures have faced opposition from some Republican grassroots organizations, who claim that such reforms will lead to bankruptcies in the insurance industry, leaving Americans with no other option but to select government-sponsored health insurance. These organizations have stated that it is impossible for a monopolistic organization to deliver good-quality healthcare services and that a monopolistic system will limit personal choice. Alain Enthoven, a renowned professor from Stanford University, has stated, however, that health insurance agencies had guaranteed that they would support the health reforms 15 years ago but had gone back on their word.

A total of 31 commercial organizations, including the US Chamber of Commerce and the Business Roundtable, jointly sent a letter of opposition to Congress. In this letter, they called the 1000-page draft legislation of Obamacare a "job killer" and claimed that "mandatory insurance" will increase the cost of recruiting new employees. Instead, enterprises should be given the freedom to decide via "market forces" the types of benefits provided to their employees. They also stated that the government-run insurance companies will undermine the US healthcare system, as it is inevitable that such companies will have a "profit-seeking tendency."

A poll conducted jointly by the *Washington Post* and ABC Television Network in July 2009 revealed that 49% of respondents agreed with President Obama on the need for health reform, which was lower than the support received in April 2009 (57%). Another poll showed that only 22% of the respondents believed that the implementation of Obamacare would actually improve their healthcare situation. Many opposition groups criticized that this Democratic health reform would give rise to "death panels" of bureaucrats that control the lives and deaths of Americans.

A commentary in the *New York Times* claimed that Democrats were trying to make the vast majority of insured Americans believe that the existing healthcare system serves the interests of enterprises rather than patients, which roused anger among insurance companies. Although these companies did support some of the major reforms proposed by the Democrats, including prohibiting refusals or premium surcharges based on previous health status, they strongly opposed the establishment of public insurance plans that would compete with private insurance agencies. The vast majority of Americans are unaware of the total cost of employer-sponsored health insurance schemes. Therefore, it was much simpler for the Democrats to focus on the greed of insurance companies than to explain that the current healthcare expenditure has exceeded sustainable levels.

The Economist, a UK publication, reported that Rahm Emanuel, President Obama's chief of staff, was able to soften the president's insistence on this plan. Ultimately, several concessions were made in response to the strong opposition of insurance lobbying groups. Rahm Emanuel also suggested that the public insurance plan should be introduced after the reform failure of the commercial insurance market.

SECTION II. THE MEDICAL SAVINGS ACCOUNT SYSTEM IN SINGAPORE

Singapore is a tropical city-state and island country in Southeast Asia at the southernmost tip of the Malay Peninsula. In 2013, Singapore had a total land area of approximately 712.4 km^2 and a total population of 5.3992 million, of which 3.7717 million were citizens. Of its citizens, 74.1% were Han Chinese. The demographic structure of Singapore from 1957 to 2010 is shown in Table 13.15. In 2012, the life expectancy at birth in Singapore was 82.1 years (79.9 years for males and 84.5 years for females).

Singapore is a young city-state that became independent from colonial rule in 1963. Prior to its independence, a national health service (NHS) system similar to that of the UK had been implemented. After gaining independence, Singapore gradually developed a unique universal healthcare system that combines the public and private systems and is committed to the dual goals of equality and efficiency. The WHO Annual Report 2000 indicated that Singapore's healthcare system was ranked sixth out of 191 countries for its overall performance and efficiency. Specifically, Singapore was ranked 30th in health status, 26th in health system responsiveness, and 101st in equity in health financing. In addition, its healthcare expenditure per capita was US$876, of which US$286 was funded by the government. In 2012, Singapore's healthcare expenditure per capita was US$2,426, and its total healthcare expenditure accounted for 4.7% of the GDP.

Following World War II, Singapore achieved tremendous economic and social development and emerged as a newly industrialized country. Throughout its development, Singapore has continually learned from Western developed countries, while also paying careful attention to avoid the issues facing these countries. In the healthcare sector, Singapore noticed the dilemma of rising healthcare expenditure in Western welfare states. In order to prevent these mistakes, Singapore began to reform its healthcare and insurance systems in the 1980s by increasing the level of personal responsibility in healthcare. Singapore's outstanding achievements in reforming its healthcare system are internationally recognized and have inspired a number of countries in their own reforms.

1. Healthcare System

(1) Organizational Structure of Public Health

Healthcare in Singapore is the shared responsibility of the Ministry of Health (MOH), the Ministry of the Environment and Water Resources (MEWR), and the Ministry of Manpower (MOM), as well as the private sector. The Singapore MOH has five professional boards: the

TABLE 13.15 Demographics of Singapore from 1957 to 2012

Year Item	1957	1970	1980	1990	1999	2000	2001	2010	2012
Permanent residents (1,000 people)	1,445.9	2,074.5	2,282.1	2,705.1	3,217.5	3,263.2	3,319.0	3,771.7	5,312.4
Sex ratio	111.7	104.9	103.2	102.6	100.6	99.8	99.0	97.4	–
Population distribution by race (%)									
Chinese	75.4	76.2	78.3	77.3	76.9	76.8	76.7	74.1	–
Malay	13.6	15.0	14.4	14.1	14.0	13.9	13.9	13.4	–
Indian	9.0	7.0	6.3	7.1	7.7	7.9	7.9	9.2	–
Others	2.0	1.8	1.0	1.1	1.4	1.4	1.5	3.3	–
Median age (Years)	18.8	19.7	24.4	29.8	33.7	34.2	35.0	–	–
Age structure (%)									
0–14 years	42.8	38.8	27.6	23.2	22.3	21.5	21.4	17.3	16.5
15–64 years	55.0	57.9	67.5	70.8	70.4	71.2	71.2	73.7	73.8
>65 years	2.1	3.3	4.9	6.0	7.3	7.3	7.4	9.0	9.7
Total fertility rate (%)	6.41	3.07	1.82	1.87	1.47	1.59	1.42	1.15	1.30
Crude death rate (%)	7.4	5.2	4.9	4.8	4.5	4.5	4.4	4.4	4.5

Singapore Medical Council (SMC), Singapore Dental Council (SDC), Singapore Pharmacy Council (SPC), Singapore Nursing Board (SNB), and Traditional Chinese Medicine Practitioners Board (TCMPB).

1. Three Ministries
1. *Ministry of Health (MOH).* The MOH is mainly responsible for formulating healthcare policies; participating in the planning and development of government and private healthcare institutions; providing preventive, therapeutic, and nursing services; and undertaking the legal supervision of the pharmaceutical industry. The main tasks of the MOH are health promotion and disease prevention, which are accomplished by ensuring Singaporeans' accessibility to healthcare services that meet their needs at an affordable rate. The MEWR is responsible for public health and environmental health, while the MOM is responsible for occupational health and prevention of occupational diseases. The Ministry of Education is responsible for the healthcare of children and students.

    The MOH is responsible for managing the preventive, therapeutic, and rehabilitation services in Singapore, formulating national health policies, coordinating the planning and development of the public and private healthcare sectors, and establishing health standards. The MOH Holdings, established in 1987, is a government-owned, MOH-controlled holding company for public hospitals.

    The primary aims of the health policies of Singapore are as follows: (1) promote a healthy lifestyle to enhance the physical health of Singaporeans; (2) emphasize personal responsibility towards healthcare and reduce patients' expectations of limited healthcare resources and capacity, in order to prevent overdependence on national welfare or health insurance; (3) provide high-quality and economical basic healthcare services; (4) encourage competition to improve the efficiency of healthcare services; (5) intervene in the pharmaceutical market to suppress the overly rapid increase in drug consumption and costs. In short, the ultimate goal of these policies has been to provide Singaporeans with a wide range of modern and efficient healthcare services and ensuring that they can access good-quality and affordable healthcare, thereby improving their overall health status and building a healthy nation.
2. *Ministry of the Environment and Water Resources (MEWR).* The MEWR is responsible for environmental health services (e.g., urban drainage, sewerage, and waste treatment systems); the control of air and water pollution, toxic chemical emissions, infectious disease sources, infected persons and parasitic outbreaks; and the safety of the food supply.
3. *Ministry of Manpower (MOM).* The MOM is responsible for addressing health issues facing workers of various industries and professions.

2. Healthcare Concept
1. The main operational goal of Singapore's healthcare system is to maintain the health status of its population through healthcare planning and improving healthy standards of living. The system encourages citizens' personal responsibility towards their own health by using public health education programs to help them choose healthy lifestyles. Specifically, members of the public are made aware of the adverse effects of unhealthy habits, such as smoking, alcoholism, irregular eating patterns, and lack of physical exercise. Child immunization programs are also performed by polyclinics against various infectious diseases, such as tuberculosis, polio, diphtheria, pertussis, tetanus, measles, mumps, rubella, and hepatitis B. In addition, health surveillance programs are implemented to enable early diagnoses of some common diseases such as cancer, heart disease, hypertension, and diabetes.

2. The government of Singapore provides high-level subsidies for public hospitals and clinics to ensure universal access to high-quality and affordable basic healthcare services. Although basic healthcare services include many high-quality and emerging medical technologies, they do not cover nonessential healthcare services, cosmetic surgery, or experimental healthcare services that are not widely used. All private hospitals, clinics, clinical laboratories, and nursing homes in Singapore must be licensed by the MOH to practice and must provide healthcare services in compliance with MOH requirements.

3. Singapore's healthcare delivery system operates on the basis of personal responsibility and government subsidy. Patients must share their medical expenses, with higher grades of services incurring higher out-of-pocket costs. Furthermore, copayments are required even for highly-subsidized wards to prevent overuse and wastage of healthcare resources. For instance, the government subsidizes up to 80% of medical expenses for patients admitted to lower-class wards in public hospitals.

4. Singaporeans are also encouraged to take responsibility for their own health through medical savings. Medisave is a national medical savings account system allowing employed individuals to set aside 6–8% of their salaries into a Medisave account, which can be used to meet future hospitalization expenses for themselves or their family members. The government has also established MediShield to cover medical expenses in the event of major illnesses or chronic diseases. Another government program, Medifund, was developed to provide a safety net for impoverished individuals who cannot afford their medical expenses. As a result, no Singaporeans can be denied admission to public hospitals due to their inability to afford medical expenses. In Singapore, the average waiting time for elective surgery is two to four weeks, whereas patients who require acute and emergency care services are typically served immediately without having to join a waiting list.

(2) Healthcare Provision System

Singapore has a dual healthcare provision system that combines the public and private sectors. The public system is administered by the government, whereas the private system is operated by private hospitals and GPs. The overall healthcare provision system includes primary healthcare services provided by private clinics and public polyclinics and secondary and tertiary specialist care services provided in both private and public institutions. Primary healthcare services are mainly provided by private hospitals, private practitioners, public hospitals and polyclinics, whereas inpatient services are mainly provided by public hospitals. More specifically, private practitioners provide 80% of primary health services, while the remaining 20% is provided by polyclinics. Conversely, public hospitals are responsible for providing 80% of relatively expensive hospital services, while the remaining 20% is provided by private healthcare institutions.

1. Primary Health Services   Since attaining self-governance in 1959, the government of Singapore began implementing large-scale immunization programs for the prevention of tuberculosis, smallpox, diphtheria, and polio; these have continued in each subsequent election year. The government also launched Child Nutrition Singapore, which is a program to prevent poor development caused by malnutrition among children. In order to fulfill its promise of making primary health services more accessible to the public, the government delegated the provision of such services from large-sized polyclinics – which received about 2,400 outpatient visits per day – to 26 healthcare outlets and 46 maternity and child care hospitals in 1964. Two years after Singapore achieved independence, the MOH declared that healthcare deserved significant attention and ranked it fifth on the national agenda, after national security, employment, housing, and education.

Currently, 82% of primary health services are provided by about 800 healthcare institutions distributed across Singapore. These are all private institutions that utilize a fee-for-service payment system and include 1,128 GPs. The government has integrated the outpatient departments of all public hospitals to form 16 modern polyclinics that provide one-stop services for people of all ages. These services include immunization, health promotion, health screening, women's health, family planning, nutrition counseling, home-based care, and rehabilitation, psychological counseling, dental services, pharmaceutical services, X-rays, laboratory testing and so on. Each service is charged at a relatively reasonable price of S$7 per adult and S$3.5 for minors under the age of 18 and seniors over the age of 65, which is much cheaper than that of private hospitals (which charge an average of S$19 per visit). Patients can freely choose between public polyclinics and private hospitals, but most Singaporeans prefer the latter. This implies that most citizens can afford the expenses for primary health services and wish to receive personalized healthcare services.

In addition, a considerable number of Singaporeans choose alternative medicine, especially traditional Chinese medicine (TCM), for their treatment. Given that about 12% of patients sought medical attention at TCM clinics, in 1994, the government appointed the MOH Committee of TCM to review the practice of TCM. The committee is also responsible for formulating provisions to regulate TCM practitioners and ensuring the safe use of medications by the public. These provisions specifically stipulate the training program and registration methods of TCM practitioners and established the MOH Chinese Pharmacopeia.

School health services represent an important area of primary health services, which involve the provision of health checkups, immunization, and health promotion services to students. Students who require further examination after receiving health checkups in school can be referred to the Student Health Center of the Institute of Health. Immunization has always been a centerpiece of school health services and is intended to improve the overall health status of students by preventing common childhood diseases, such as tetanus, rubella, measles, tuberculosis, and polio. In 2000, school health services covered 93% of the service volume for its target population. A survey conducted in Singapore showed that 60% of teenagers and young adults aged 15–24 years are susceptible to hepatitis B. In 1987, the National Childhood Immunization Program initially considered providing a nationwide hepatitis B vaccination, although this was ultimately not implemented. Hence, nearly all children over the age of 13 years in Singapore did not receive this vaccination. To prevent these individuals from contracting the hepatitis B virus, chronic hepatitis, and liver cancer, the MOH administered hepatitis B vaccinations to specific groups of adolescents and young adults over a period of four years (2001 to 2004), which included students in the third year of secondary school, second year of junior college, third year of centralized institutes, all polytechnic and university students, and full-time military personnel.

2. Hospital Services

1. *Overview.* In 2000, there were 21 acute hospitals and 5 specialty centers, providing a total of 11,798 beds in Singapore. Of these beds, 81% (9,556 beds) were provided by 13 public hospitals and specialty centers, while the remaining 19% (2,242 beds) were provided by 13 private hospitals (Table 13.16 and Table 13.17). As of 2010, there were 22 hospitals and 6 specialty centers in Singapore, with a total of 10,283 beds, of which 8,881 beds were provided by 15 public hospitals and specialty centers. These specialty centers provide specialized healthcare services and consist of the National Cancer

TABLE 13.16 Distribution of Hospital Beds in Public Healthcare Institutions in Singapore

Singapore Health Services (SingHealth)		National Healthcare Group (NHG)	
Hospitals or Specialty Centers	Number of Beds	Hospitals or Specialty Centers	Number of Beds
Singapore General Hospital	1,434	National University Hospital	957
Changi General Hospital	801	Tan Tock Seng Hospital	1,314
KK Women's and Children's Hospital	898	Alexandra Hospital	404
National Cancer Center	85	Institute of Mental Health / Woodbridge Hospital	3,114
National Heart Center	186	National Skin Center	–
Singapore National Eye Center	–	National Neuroscience Institute	–
National Dental Center	–		

Center, Singapore National Eye Center, National Heart Center, National Neuroscience Institute, National Skin Center, and National Dental Center of Singapore. However, among these, the National Eye Center, National Skin Center, and National Dental Center of Singapore provide outpatient services only. Patients requiring inpatient care may choose to be admitted to the affiliated hospitals of these centers. The remaining 1,402 beds are distributed among the 13 private hospitals.

2. Coverage of hospital services:
   1. *Inpatient services.* In 2000, 8 hospitals and 3 specialty centers (National Cancer Center, National Heart Center, and Institute of Mental Health) admitted a total of 390,370 patients, accounting for 78% of the total admissions in Singapore; the remaining 22% of patients were admitted to the 13 private hospitals. In 2000, the

TABLE 13.17 Distribution of Hospital Beds in Private Healthcare Institutions in Singapore

Singapore Health Services (SingHealth)		National Healthcare Group (NHG)	
Hospitals or Specialty Centers	Number of Beds	Hospitals or Specialty Centers	Number of Beds
Mount Elizabeth Hospital	505	Ren Ci Hospital	294
Gleneagles Hospital	328	St. Andrew's Community Hospital	1,314
Eastshore Hospital	157	St. Luke's Hospital for the Elderly	224
Mount Alvernia Hospital	303	Kwong Wai Shiu Hospital	30
HMI Balestier Hospital	62	Adam Road Hospital – Psychiatry	49
Johns Hopkins Singapore Clinical services	14	Raffles Surgi Center	25
Thomson Medical Center	191		

Source: MOH of Singapore, 2001.

8 hospitals and 3 specialty centers showed a 4% increase in total admissions compared to the previous year (373,502 patients). Most patients admitted to public hospitals were children aged 0–4 years or elderly adults over 65 years. The only women's and children's hospital in Singapore – KK Women's and Children's Hospital – had the greatest number of admissions (68,430 patients), followed by the largest emergency care hospital (i.e., Singapore General Hospital) with 62,296 patients.

2. *Emergency services.* All public hospitals, with the exception of Ang Mo Kio Community Hospital and Woodbridge Hospital, provide accident and emergency services. In 2000, the hospital departments providing these services received a total of 556,583 admissions, of which 85% (474,922 admissions) were due to accidents. There are four private emergency hospitals, namely, Mount Elizabeth, Gleneagles, Mount Alvernia, and Eastshore, which provide 24-hour emergency care services. However, they tend to avoid admitting patients with major trauma.

3. *Outpatient services.* In 2000, the specialist outpatient clinics of public hospitals and five specialty centers (i.e., Singapore National Eye Center, National Cancer Center, National Neuroscience Institute, National Heart Center, and National Skin Center) admitted a total of 2.74 million patients. Among them, the Singapore National Eye Center had the highest number of admissions (342,953 patients), followed by the National Skin Center (286,097 patients).

4. *Rehabilitation services.* Five community hospitals (Ang Mo Kio Community Hospital, Ren Ci Hospital, St. Andrew's Community Hospital, St. Luke's Hospital, and Kwong Wai Shiu Hospital) provided rehabilitation services. Ang Mo Kio Community Hospital has long been the only public community hospital to provide late-stage rehabilitation services for postoperative and acute patients (e.g., stroke patients) discharged from public emergency hospitals. The objective of rehabilitation services is to maximize patients' self-care abilities and enable more rapid community reintegration. The other four community hospitals are government-funded healthcare institutions operated by Voluntary Welfare Organizations (VWOs), which provide healthcare services for elderly and chronically ill patients living in the community.

3. *Restructuring of public healthcare institutions.* Hospital restructuring is mainly intended to reduce inefficiencies in public healthcare institutions. The establishment of the National University Hospital in 1985 marked the beginning of the restructuring of public healthcare institutions in Singapore. Other hospitals were restructured between 1990 and 1992. In 2000, polyclinics, which are the main public providers of outpatient services, underwent restructuring. In other words, the public healthcare institutions that provide 80% of inpatient services and 20% of outpatient services have been completely restructured over time. The restructured public hospitals are currently administered by a state-owned company, MOH Holdings, which initially did not participate in hospital management. Later, however, it began to employ integrated management of certain aspects of hospitals, such as computer systems, human resources, and hospital logistics, to achieve economies of scale. Unfortunately, this approach has given rise to a lack of incentive mechanisms among hospitals to improve the centrally managed services by MOH Holdings, and these hospitals did not meet MOH Holdings requirements. More seriously, this approach also caused MOH Holdings to become a monopolistic provider of health services. To address this monopoly, the Singapore Medical Group (SMG) was established.

Health reforms and hospital restructuring have enabled hospitals in Singapore to achieve a very high quality of healthcare, advanced medical equipment, and more stringent management. Improvements to hospital management and service quality are primarily attributed to the introduction of incentive mechanisms and an emphasis on employee training quality, which has achieved good outcomes in hospitals. In other words, the key to the success of the Singaporean healthcare system lies in hospital management.

4. Administrative management of hospitals

   1. *Tangible facilities in hospitals.* Hospitals in Singapore have their own characteristic architecture and tend to be closely integrated with their surroundings. Their buildings have been jointly designed by architects and health experts to meet basic human needs, with good lighting, ventilation, and greenery. Furthermore, they keep in step with global medical advancements, offering modernized, smart, and networked medical facilities. Hospitals are equipped with automated sliding doors and windows, automated corridor monitoring systems, and automated conveyor systems. Laboratory specimens, urgently-needed drugs, medical records, and X-ray films can be transported to designated locations using transport boxes. In addition, hospitals have implemented medical gas pipelines, diversified communications, transmission automation, and high-speed collection, processing, and delivery of information. These hardware facilities have helped greatly improve the quality of healthcare services in hospitals.

   2. *Intangible facilities in hospitals.* Hospitals in Singapore attach great importance to "people-centered and detail-oriented" services, based on the notion that respect for patients is essential. Such patient-centered values are mainly focused on commitment, compassion, respect, integrity, cooperation, openness, and technical excellence. Hospitals in Singapore group their services into five tiers based on need: essential services, expected services, desired services, unexpected services, and implausible services. The service outcomes are rated in terms of four levels: "I feel I can trust you," "I feel cared for," "I feel at home," and "I feel very special." Singaporean hospitals have a strong awareness of maintaining healthcare quality and as such implement comprehensive quality management that covers "all employees, all processes, and all tasks." They use the ISO 9002 and ISO 14001 systems as the main standards of quality management and employ a "quality promotion" model that requires primary-level employees to have a sufficient comprehension of the diversity and variability of hospital management, in order to encourage their active participation in such management.

      Healthcare workers at all levels must comply with the standards enforced by these hospitals. A quality assurance committee of senior physicians, nurses, and administrative staff is formed in each hospital and is chaired by the hospital director. This committee, in turn, comprises subcommittees for emergency care, pharmacy, nosocomial infections, nursing, wards, ethics, and so on, each with their own standards of healthcare services. For instance, the waiting time for outpatient appointments, treatment, and emergency care must not exceed 5 days, 30 minutes, and 15 minutes, respectively. Other standards include the following: the incidence of nosocomial infections must be zero; reoperation within 3 days of primary surgery is considered a medical problem; patients must be readmitted in case of aseptic incision infection; hospitals must maintain complete medical records; hospitals must provide holistic nursing care for patients; patient falls in the hospital are automatically considered the result of medical malpractice; all drugs used in the hospitals must be WHO-approved; and nurses must follow up with each discharged patient via telephone about their rehabilitative status within one week of discharge. The committee also holds two quality assessment meetings and six quality control demonstration meetings annually.

3. *People-centered management.* Hospital leaders are experts in hospital management and are responsible for providing high-quality and value-for-money healthcare services to patients; encouraging continuous improvement in their employees and ensuring employees' welfare; and serving their country in the pursuit of universal healthcare. Hospitals in Singapore tend to have a strict organizational structure with a clear hierarchy, in which each personnel has clearly defined roles and responsibilities. They have adopted a people-centered management style, attaching great importance to employees' opinions and cultivating team spirit. Multiple channels are used to obtain feedback from patients and members of the public, as feedback, especially in the form of criticism and complaints, is considered essential for improving hospital services. Patients who are dissatisfied with certain healthcare workers may lodge a complaint with the MOH and relevant hospital, and the hospital then immediately requests a written explanation from the personnel concerned. General issues are typically handled by having discussions or issuing warnings to the personnel concerned. Serious issues, on the other hand, are investigated and handled by the Disciplinary Committee of the MOH, which then forwards the investigation results to the patient in a timely manner. Healthcare workers, particularly physicians, generally have a strong sense of self-discipline as they tend to be respected by the public and possess a high social status and income. Additionally, most healthcare workers do not dare to violate medical regulations or compromise their professional ethics due to the severe penalties that they may face. All hospital work is centered on this principle, and workers at all levels strive to serve their patients. In fact, hospital staff are advised to "serve patients like they would their own mothers" to maintain the quality of hospital services. Moreover, hospitals tend to be equipped with facilities that are convenient for patients. For instance, Singaporean hospitals rarely have long queues, and many possess open-door pharmacies, which are found on every floor of outpatient clinics and in certain wards. Many hospitals also have supermarkets, while maternity and children's hospitals often have photography studios. Nurses conduct all the admission and discharge procedures in hospital wards. All equipment for examination and treatment, with the exception of large-sized equipment, are delivered to the bedside of patients for their convenience.

   Hospitals in Singapore also send between 400 and 600 letters each month to discharged patients, seeking their opinions on how to improve hospital performance. Patients who make particularly critical comments in a given month may be invited to provide more detailed opinions at a dinner attended by executive directors, department heads, and the physicians and nurses concerned. Hospitals are constantly striving to understand patients' demands so as to improve their services and better meet these demands.

4. *Building good patient-physician relationships*: Healthcare workers generally strive to maintain a good professional image by adhering to strict norms regarding their dress code, generosity, words and deeds, and interactions with others. Singapore has a relatively sound legal system, and citizens generally have very strong legal awareness. During the process of medical treatment, patients have the legal rights to access healthcare and relevant health information, make decisions about their medical treatment, maintain their privacy, and to appeal.

   In patient infringement disputes, hospitals generally apply a reverse burden of proof. In order to protect the legal rights and interests of hospitals, employees, and patients, hospitals have developed a comprehensive set of rules and regulations and employ numerous information-recording forms that must be filed to provide reliable legal evidence. Healthcare workers must always pay attention to the relevant laws and regulations when engaging in medical or nursing activities; in particular, they must strive to protect patients' rights and interests while also protecting themselves by producing clear and detailed medical records. When medical disputes do occur, they are channeled to a specialized hospital department so that healthcare workers can better devote themselves to fulfilling their required tasks.

5. *Overall quality training of employees.* Besides requiring prospective employees to have graduated from relevant professional institutions and to pass a national qualifying examination, hospitals in Singapore also demand that these individuals possess sufficient dedication, team spirit, altruism, and diligence. Each new employee is required to undergo a three-day training course before starting their position. Furthermore, employees must receive no less than 50 hours of quality training each year – this includes senior-level experts who are trained by the Singapore Service Quality Center (SQC, an agency founded by Singapore Airlines and SPRING Singapore to provide training for individuals working in the service industry).

Hospitals spend about 5% of their personnel expenses to send employees to quality training at SMRT Corporation Ltd., McDonald's, and various hotels. Furthermore, they attach great importance to the professional knowledge training of their healthcare workers. Hospitals often organize symposiums and seminars, invite scholars to give presentations on academic reports, and encourage employees to participate in training courses organized by the MOH and in various local and foreign academic activities. Hospitals also send some of their employees to 9- to 12-month training courses at foreign hospitals or universities every year. Employees who wish to be sponsored for such training courses must pay around S$2,000 as a deposit and sign a contract to work in the hospital for at least five years after returning from their training. In addition, hospitals carry out continuing education for nurses. There are two types of nurses, registered nurses and assistant nurses, each with different focuses on continuing education. Continuing nursing education consists of short-term courses held by nursing schools and in-service professional education. Each year, hospitals recommend that some nurses take part in a full-time course to help improve their professional knowledge and skills, thus enabling them to provide more meticulous and high-quality services.

3. Dental Health Services   Dental health services include school dental services and community dental services. They aim to prevent the onset and spread of dental diseases and maintain the dental health of schoolchildren and community residents.

Initially, the community dental services in Singapore were provided by 10 dental clinics. Following the restructuring of the public healthcare provision system on October 1, 2000, community dental services were also restructured, such that the Bedok, Geylang, Tampines, and Queenstown dental clinics were integrated into SingHealth, whereas the Bukit Batok, Choa Chu Kang, Jurong, Hougang, Toa Payoh, and Woodlands dental clinics were integrated into the National Healthcare Group (NHG). Furthermore, school dental services were administered by the Health Promotion Board (HPB) of the MOH.

School dental services are provided to all schoolchildren by 184 primary school dental clinics, 6 mobile dental clinics, and the School Dental Center of the Institute of Health. These services are also provided to preschool children, with the aim of reminding parents and teachers about the prevention and treatment of dental diseases.

In 2000, the government launched a three-year update plan for primary school dental clinics to upgrade their medical equipment. This plan was implemented in parallel with the primary school building renovation plan launched by the Ministry of Education. By 2000, the government had completely renovated seven clinics, while four clinics were either still in the process of renovation or relocated to newer facilities. In 2001, school dental services were extended to cover secondary school students. A 6-year plan was implemented, which aimed to establish 20 mobile dental clinics and 53 permanent dental clinics in secondary schools.

4. Healthcare Services for the Elderly

1. *Administrative agencies.* The government of Singapore attaches great importance to elderly care. In June 2000, the MOH established the Elderly and Continuing Care Division by merging the Elderly Care Division and the Elderly Policy and Development Division, in order to centralize the administration of all elderly care institutions in Singapore. The government also provides financial support for VWOs and is responsible for providing palliative care and mental health services. In addition, the government has established the Inter-ministerial Committee on Health Care for the Elderly (IMCHCE) to provide advice on the drafting of relevant policies. Specifically, the IMCHCE is mainly responsible for assessing the healthcare needs of elderly adults, determining whether their needs can be met and whether they are able to afford the expenses for required services, and making reasonable and feasible recommendations about issues related to elderly care.

2. *Types of services.* Singapore has a wide range of elderly care institutions that provide varying types of services, including community hospitals, long-term care hospitals, nursing homes, and community healthcare institutions (Table 13.18). In general, the scope of elderly care does not cover acute care, which is mainly provided by primary care physicians and specialists in acute hospitals. Elderly care services are typically provided by community hospitals and nursing homes. Community hospitals primarily serve individuals who require long-term inpatient care or who were transferred from acute hospitals for continuing rehabilitation services (especially elderly patients). On the other hand, nursing homes tend to serve a relatively wider range of elderly individuals.

   Long-term care hospitals serve patients who cannot walk because of chronic diseases, such as coronary heart disease, diabetes, and cancer, as well as patients who

TABLE 13.18 Types and Providers of Elderly Care Services in Singapore

Types of Elderly Care Services	Service Providers
Primary care	Private general practice
	Public polyclinics
Secondary and tertiary care	Hospitals and specialty centers
Transitional care	Community hospitals
Life assistance services	Nursing homes
Community-based day care	Day rehabilitation centers
	Day care centers for patients with dementia
Home-based care	Home-based medical care
	Home-based nursing care
Others	Advisory agencies
	Personal wellness centers

TABLE 13.19 Services Provided by Different Types of Elderly Care Institutions in Singapore

Types of Services	Quantity
Community hospitals	4 hospitals with a total of 430 beds
Nursing homes	24 VWOs and 26 private nursing homes with a total of about 5,700 beds (VWOs and private nursing homes accounted for 67% and 33% of beds, respectively)
Day rehabilitation center (including senior care centers and comprehensive service centers)	23 VWO-run institutions providing 1,100 beds
Day care centers for patients with dementia	5 VWO-run institutions
Home-based medical care	6 VWO-run institutions
Home-based nursing care	7 VWO-run institutions
Home-based assistance care services	6 VWO-run institutions

require long-term medical and nursing care services. In addition, as certain risk factors for chronic diseases can be eliminated through a healthy lifestyle, some health promotion institutions can also be categorized as elderly care institutions.

The services provided by different types of elderly care institutions are shown in Table 13.19.

3. *Financial assistance.* Among the elderly care institutions, some are government funded, some are privately operated, and others are VWO operated. As the population ages, the number of adults who can contribute to labor productivity decreases, which also leads to a corresponding decrease in Singapore's tax revenues. However, without the necessary government subsidies, the availability and sustainable development of elderly care will be compromised. Therefore, the government of Singapore provides financial and material resources to a certain extent in order to support these elderly care institutions.

In 2000, the government of Singapore established the ElderCare Fund, which is dedicated to funding the construction of elderly care facilities and subsidizing VWO-operated institutions. The government has injected S$500 million into this fund, and this is expected to reach S$2.5 billion by 2010. The establishment of the ElderCare Fund has enabled the government to provide operating subsidies to elderly care institutions solely using the interest earned on this fund, thus precluding the need to increase taxes. This has ensured the smooth provision of elderly care services.

Since July 1, 2000, nursing homes in Singapore have begun implementing a three-tier subsidy scheme based on means testing, with the aim of reducing health-care subsidies for high-income families. The specifics of this three-tier subsidy scheme are as follows: a 70% healthcare subsidy is provided to families with a per capita weekly household income of S$0–300; a 50% subsidy is provided to families with a per capita weekly household income of S$301–500; and a 25% subsidy is provided to families with a per capita weekly household income of S$500–700. This subsidy scheme has significantly increased the number of subsidized families compared to the previous two-tier subsidy scheme (which covered 75% of publicly funded patients) or the subsidy program that covered 50% of low-income families.

In addition to financial support, the MOH, the Urban Development Committee and the Housing and Development Board have jointly reserved 17 plots of land for the construction of elderly care institutions and for lease to VWO- or privately-operated institutions for the next decade. The government of Singapore has sought to increase the number of beds in private nursing homes in order to meet the needs of Singaporeans.

4. *Service management.* The government of Singapore also introduced a series of policies intended to provide full financial support, while also improving the regulation and management of elderly care institutions. Although elderly care institutions were previously distributed across Singapore, most of them operated independently of each other. In July 2000, the MOH proposed an elderly care blueprint encouraging the collaboration of elderly care institutions to establish a comprehensive and high-quality healthcare provision system, which could ensure the access of elderly individuals to comfortable and cost-effective elderly care services. Specifically, the government linked acute hospitals with the elderly care divisions of community hospitals and nursing homes, enabling them to lead the development and improvement of other service agencies in the region. Approved community hospitals and nursing homes were also permitted to provide other services, such as day rehabilitation, home-based medical care, and home-based nursing care services. In addition, the government began offering additional development funds for some of these service agencies.

To ensure the service quality of elderly care services, the MOH requires community hospitals and nursing homes to meet certain industry entry standards. Relevant personnel and elderly care providers must jointly formulate guidelines for new or existing service agencies (e.g., nursing homes, day rehabilitation centers, day care centers for patients with dementia, home-based medical and nursing care services), such that these agencies can establish or improve their elderly care services.

The MOH has also established several review committees for the assessment and monitoring of service delivery in elderly care institutions, as well as for the formulation of guidelines and standards for the development of elderly care services. For instance, the review committee for primary care providers of psychiatric and geriatric psychiatric services and the community hospital review committee are responsible for evaluating the daily operations in relevant service agencies as well as providing constructive suggestions on their development and improvement. Additionally, health-related poverty-alleviation organizations are responsible for establishing standards for public shelters and health-related poverty alleviation.

In recent years, the MOH has adopted the proposal of the IMCHCE and launched a training program for home-based care workers. During its trial period, 43 volunteer nurses from restructured hospitals and general hospitals participated in this home-based care worker training program, which was organized by the Nanyang Institute of Technology (NIT) and the Tsao Foundation, and the program demonstrated excellent outcomes. In January 2000, this program was officially implemented at the Kim Seng Community Center. Two courses were held in one year, and 47 home-based care workers received training. This program has gradually expanded to other community centers. Furthermore, the MOH has taken several other measures to improve the professional skills of healthcare providers and the service quality of the relevant institutions. Examples include incorporating two home-based elderly care courses into the training program for home-based care providers, educating volunteers on the risk factors of disability in the elderly so that they can refer patients to the relevant healthcare departments in a timely manner, and listing geriatrics as a compulsory course for medical graduates.

(3) Status of Healthcare Workers

1. Overview   A report entitled "Affordable Health Care: A White Paper" published by the Singaporean government noted that a surplus of specialists might increase healthcare demand, as has been observed in some countries. Currently, the government of Singapore invests more than S$200,000 to train one physician, which is far higher than that for other students in higher education. Furthermore, the number of medical students has been increasing each year, which has made it necessary to limit the number of enrollees to fewer than 150 per year. The number of specialists in the physician population must be controlled, and medical schools should emphasize primary care rather than focus solely on technical improvement. Table 13.20 shows the distributions of physicians, dentists, nurses/midwives, and pharmacists between public and private institutions in Singapore in 2010, and the ratio of these professionals to the total population.

2. Specialist Qualifications

1. *Overview.* The Medical Registration Act of 1997, which was implemented on April 3, 1998, stipulated that all medical practitioners in Singapore must complete a registration process before they are entitled to the title of "specialist" and are qualified to practice specialist services. This registration process is administered by the SMC, and the results are published in the government gazette.

    Medical practitioners who wish to register as specialists must obtain a Certificate of Specialist Accreditation issued by the Specialists Accreditation Board (SAB), which was established in accordance with the Medical Registration Act of 1997. The SAB is responsible for defining the medical scope of each specialty; administering the first part of the specialist registration process; and reviewing the qualifications, experience, and other registration criteria of applicants.

2. *Application process for specialist accreditation.* Each applicant can apply for only 1 of the 35 recognized specialties when submitting an application form. Upon receiving the application, the SAB determines whether the applicant meets the requirements for

TABLE 13.20   Distribution of Healthcare Workers in Singapore in 2010

Healthcare Workers	Institution	Number of Workers	Healthcare Workers	Institution	Number of Workers
Physicians	Public healthcare institutions	4,987	Nurses/midwives	Public healthcare institutions	17,613
	Private healthcare institutions	3,292		Private healthcare institutions	6,965
	Number of physicians: Total population	1:580		Number of nurses: Total population	1:170
Dentists	Public healthcare institutions	339	Pharmacists	Public healthcare institutions	712
	Private healthcare institutions	1,021		Private healthcare institutions	931
	Number of dentists: Total population	1:3370		Number of pharmacists: Total population	1:2800

Source: MOH of Singapore, 2012.

becoming a specialist. After obtaining a specialist accreditation certificate, the medical practitioner must submit an application to the SMC for specialist registration. Medical practitioners who are refused registration by the SMC may submit a written appeal to the MOH within one month; the decision of the Minister of Health is final.

3. *General requirements for specialist applications.* Applicants must be SMC-registered medical practitioners who have obtained the relevant basic specialist qualifications, and must have undergone accredited specialist training programs in Singapore or abroad. Applicants wishing to participate in specialist training programs abroad are advised to submit their program arrangements to the SAB in order to determine whether it has been approved for the specialist registration procedure in Singapore. Otherwise, they must undergo a training program in Singapore. The applicant's history of training abroad is given due consideration when applying for training in Singapore.

    An accredited training program must guarantee the ability of trainees to handle specialized medical tasks independently upon completion of the program. The length of training varies across specialties from five to seven years and can generally be divided into two stages: basic specialist training and advanced specialist training. The former takes at least three years, during which trainees must obtain a basic specialist qualification. The latter takes two to four years, depending on the specialty, and a formal assessment is performed upon completion of the training program. Furthermore, the training coordinator must give written confirmation of training completion so that the trainee can apply for specialist accreditation and registration. In general, all specialist training programs in Singapore are designed in accordance with this framework. Trainees are only allowed to receive advanced specialist training after they have successfully completed the basic specialist training.

    On the other hand, foreign training programs often do not fully comply with this framework, and individuals who are trained abroad may have to be reassessed when applying for accreditation. The SAB will directly approve an application if the assessment indicates that the applicant does, in fact, meet the requirements. Otherwise, the SAB will reject the application and request that the applicant be retrained. For both basic and advanced specialist training, the length of the training of part-time trainees is converted to its full-time equivalent, and the remaining training hours must be completed on a full-time basis. Trainees are encouraged to actively participate in research activities and seminars during their training and must spend about 20% of their time during advanced specialist training conducting accredited research projects. However, the time spent on research activities during basic specialist training is not counted as training hours. In addition to the specified course contents, certain general pharmaceutical and therapeutic topics should also be incorporated into all training programs, such as medical ethics, medical laws, communication skills, organization and implementation of healthcare services, and understanding the development of medical specialties and their relationship with other disciplines. In addition, trainees should keep training logs, and the program coordinator must submit a training progress report to the program director in a timely manner.

4. *After completing the specialist registration process.* Registered specialists should continue to receive medical education in order to regularly update their knowledge and professional skills. Furthermore, they are not excluded from practicing in other medical fields, as there is extensive overlap among these fields.

3. Typical Content of Annual Planning by the MOH

1. *Enhancing primary care services.* The Singapore MOH Annual Report 2001 stated that the MOH will focus on providing primary care services to the elderly. Elderly adults who require healthcare services but live far away from polyclinics may seek help from private practitioners to facilitate their access to primary care services.

2. *Enhancing training for physicians.* This covers training for medical officers as well as basic and advanced specialist training. Untrained officers must temporarily engage in general tasks until passing the examination. The MOH will also continue to provide continuing medical education (CME) in order to regularly update the skills and service quality of medical practitioners.

3. *Ensuring service quality.* The MOH further enhanced the issuance of medical licenses and the accreditation of medical qualifications via strict law enforcement and account auditing. The MOH also ensures that the feedback channels for complaints about healthcare services are kept open by initiating clinical audits and accreditation systems based on the quality indicator (QI) project.

4. *Salary adjustment.* In light of the shortage of nursing staff and the increasing demand for nursing services, the government of Singapore raised the salaries of nursing staff in June 2000, with the aim of attracting secondary school graduates to join the nursing profession and retaining existing nursing staff. The government spent a total of S$33 million on salary adjustments, which led to a 13% increase in nurses' wages. Furthermore, nurses' allowances have been increased accordingly to encourage their engagement in urgently needed round-the-clock services. In addition to salary adjustments, the nursing profession has been restructured to increase the number of clinical nurse specialists, case management nurses, and nurse trainers, thereby making nursing work more professional and challenging. These measures have helped trigger greater professional enthusiasm among nursing staff. In addition, physicians' salaries were adjusted in July 2000, resulting in a 25% wage increase among medical officers, registrars, and associate consultants. A new assessment structure was also introduced into the remuneration assessment system, whereby senior physicians were given greater salary increases to retain them in public healthcare institutions for a longer period of time. The overall increase in physician salaries was 22%.

5. *Return-to-Nursing (RTN) Training Scheme.* Nursing work requires continual improvement in skills and expertise in order for nursing staff to keep pace with the advancement of medical technologies. Therefore, it is necessary to improve the skills of nonpracticing nursing staff before they return to nursing tasks. In August 2008, the RTN Training Scheme was implemented in three healthcare institutions, namely, Changi General Hospital, KK Women's and Children's Hospital, and the National Heart Center. The training course covered both the theoretical and clinical aspects of nursing and lasted for two to three months. Its aim was to provide nursing staff with basic and professional nursing qualifications. Upon completion of the training course, the nurses were then evaluated and licensed by the respective healthcare institutions. In 2000, the first batch of 15 nursing staff received retraining under the RTN scheme, following which, another 36 nursing staff completed the training course during the first half of 2001 in various healthcare institutions. The training scheme has attracted an increasing number of applicants, primarily because it is a government-funded program, and the healthcare institutions that provide it have flexible working hours.

2. Reforms of the Public Hospital System

(1) Reform Background

The ideologies that guide the healthcare policies in Singapore include promoting a healthy lifestyle and improving the physical health of Singaporeans; promoting personal responsibility towards health and avoiding overreliance on state welfare or health insurance; providing good and affordable basic healthcare services to Singaporeans; introducing competition and market mechanisms to improve the quality and efficiency of healthcare services; and introducing government intervention whenever market mechanisms fail to reduce healthcare expenditure.

The reform of the public hospital system in Singapore can be traced back to the early 1980s. The total healthcare expenditure in Singapore accounted for about 3% of the GDP at that time, which was much lower than the share in Western developed countries. However, Singapore was still experiencing a very rapid increase in healthcare expenditure at that time – the average annual growth rate was 7.9% from 1973 to 1979, and showed no sign of deceleration. The government acknowledged that the rise in healthcare demand was inevitable following the increase in life expectancy and income per capita, and that healthcare expenditure would become a heavy burden. Hence, the government began considering preventive measures before healthcare expenditure became a serious problem. In 1983, the government released the National Health Plan (NHP), which primarily aimed to establish a medical savings plan (Medisave) for the coverage of personal medical expenses. At the same time, the government also began reforming the public hospital system.

Several issues facing public hospitals in Singapore further prompted the government to reform the public hospital system. Prior to the reform, public hospitals generally lacked effective incentive mechanisms, exhibited low efficiency, experienced severe talent loss, and constantly faced workforce shortages. Furthermore, the healthcare expenditures in public hospitals continued to rise despite government control over the service prices in these institutions. In addition, it was difficult for public hospitals to adapt to a competitive healthcare market, as they were unable to rapidly and flexibly respond to changes in market demand for healthcare services and facilities. As a result, the public became increasingly dissatisfied with public hospitals.

Singapore was also affected by the global trend of privatization in the late 1970s and early 1980s. Economic stagflation, rising unemployment, and increased social welfare expenses facing Western countries in the 1970s challenged the Keynesian prescription of government intervention. Hence, governments began changing their roles in the economy and shifting toward privatization. In their pursuit of improving economic benefits, even healthcare services in the social and public sectors underwent privatization.

In 1984, the MOH of Singapore announced a plan to reform government-run public hospitals, giving them greater autonomy, in order to improve their efficiency and service quality through market competition. Public hospitals with greater administrative autonomy would have greater flexibility to foster innovation and motivation among their employees. The government also aimed to improve the working conditions and the environment in public hospitals in order to increase employee service efficiency and provide more humane services for patients.

(2) Reform Process

The health reform process can be divided into two stages.

1. The first stage of the reform was the pilot stage. In 1985, the hospital restructuring plan was piloted at the newly established National University Hospital (NUH), which

was privatized as NUH Co., Ltd. As a subsidiary of the government-controlled Temasek Holdings Pvt. Ltd., the main objective of NUH Co., Ltd. was to "provide the best service quality to patients at the lowest possible cost." It was given considerable autonomy, allowing it to introduce innovative and cost-effective management methods and systems in order to motivate and attract outstanding employees. The restructured hospital also received government subsidies to provide healthcare services to those living in poverty at below-cost prices, thereby helping it fulfill its responsibilities to the community.

2. The second stage of reform began in 1987 and revolved around expanding the hospital restructuring plan to other public hospitals. The government established the wholly-owned MOH Holdings to take over all the restructured hospitals. In general, public hospitals were restructured into hospital companies that subsequently joined MOH Holdings as subsidiaries over a short period (six months to one year). All reformed hospitals were still considered public hospitals that provide healthcare services in compliance with government healthcare policies; however, they changed their administrative approaches and became autonomous legal entities under the Singapore Companies Act. In the early stages of hospital reform, the government took certain measures that were more in keeping with privatization; in fact, the term "privatization" was initially used to refer to this plan, whereas "restructuring" was only adopted later. The early stage of reform gave rise to many issues, however, such as rising healthcare expenditure and the reluctance of public hospitals to provide basic healthcare services; this invited much criticism from the public. Given the enormous political sensitivity of privatization and the problems arising from the reform, the government changed some of its measures and enhanced its own ability to intervene in the healthcare market. As a result, the reform did not ultimately lead to privatization.

(3) Reform Contents

The reform of the public hospital system was centered on restructuring public hospitals, which were formerly administered directly by the MOH, into autonomous healthcare companies. The MOH piloted the indirect management of these restructured hospitals via the newly established MOH Holdings. Consequently, Singapore's healthcare system, which originally comprised the MOH and public hospitals, now consists of the MOH, MOH Holdings, and restructured hospitals. This reform not only altered the structure of the healthcare system but also changed the roles and responsibilities of each party (Figure 13.8).

1. Functions of MOH Holdings The MOH Holdings was established in 1987 by the MOH, which retains 100% of its ownership. The fundamental mission of MOH Holdings is to provide high-quality, cost-effective healthcare services via its subsidiary hospitals. The MOH Holdings has two major roles: (1) holdings, that is, it acts as the holding company of the restructured hospitals; and (2) business operations, that is, it serves as a purchasing group to benefit from the economies of scale in the procurement of medical supplies, drugs, and logistical services.

1. Holdings
    1. Ensure that MOH Holdings and its subsidiary hospitals operate in compliance with national laws and financial regulations.
    2. Ensure that MOH Holdings and its subsidiary hospitals have good financial operations through internal audits and enhanced financial monitoring.
    3. Monitor and assess the operational status of MOH Holdings and its subsidiary hospitals via performance audits based on key performance indicators and industry standards.

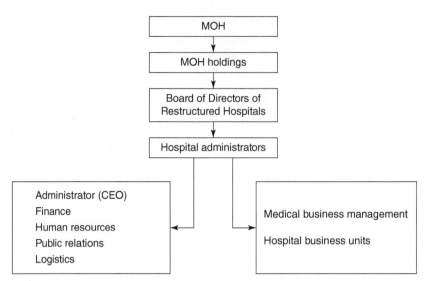

FIGURE 13.8 Organizational structure of the restructured public healthcare system in Singapore.

---

    4. Formulate a revenue utilization plan to fund the newly launched businesses of MOH Holdings. As a holding company, MOH Holdings is entitled to a reasonable return on investment, which can be used for its further development.

    5. Establish the major policies of MOH Holdings and determine the policy orientation for the development of subsidiary hospitals, thereby ensuring the full and rational utilization of healthcare resources.

    6. In consultation with the MOH, MOH Holdings appoints a board of directors and a chief executive officer (CEO) for each subsidiary hospital, determines the salary and bonus plan of the CEO, and reviews their reward and punitive measures.

  2. Business operations

    1. Benefit from economies of scale through the centralized procurement of medical supplies, drugs, and equipment, and the centralized management of hospital logistical services.

    2. Recruit and administer special professionals required by hospitals but who are in low demand; the cost of hiring these professionals is shared among subsidiary hospitals.

    3. Benefit from the economies of scale and reduce costs in other aspects.

2. Functions of Restructured Hospitals The restructured hospitals have their own boards of directors, which are led by chairmen who in turn make up the board of directors of MOH Holdings. Restructured hospitals have dual hierarchies of administration: an administrative hierarchy comprising executives and a professional hierarchy comprising medical professionals.

1. MOH policies allow restructured hospitals to have administrative authority over their operations, including the hiring of personnel and the determination of salaries.

2. The hospitals are nonprofit organizations that provide the best health service output via the most efficient allocation and utilization of healthcare resources.

3. The hospitals have the right to change their own operations, service content, and service processes.
4. Internal audits of hospital financial operations are conducted using commercial accounting.
5. Hospitals must consult with the MOH as to which decisions require MOH approval and which decisions do not require MOH participation.
6. Hospitals must maintain a reasonable balance between competition and mutual cooperation in terms of quality and efficiency of services.
7. Hospitals must seek to develop at a reasonable speed rather than focus on undermining the interests of their competitors.

3. Functions of the MOH   The MOH requires restructured hospitals to focus on basic healthcare services in order to ensure the affordability of such services for both the government and citizens. Furthermore, the restructured hospitals must remain efficient to curb the rising costs of healthcare services. Owing to the unique features of the healthcare market, the greater autonomy of restructured hospitals has led to the government to impose a more defined and transparent regulatory scope. Restructured hospitals should be given the autonomy they deserve while complying with the established rules. The government serves two functions: regulation and procurement, which specifically involves the following.

1. The government is responsible for establishing revenue caps on restructured hospitals, determining which services are funded by patient self-payments and government subsidies, and preventing fee transfers across different registered wards.
2. The government stipulates that the board of directors of restructured hospitals should conduct cost assessments with the aim of cost recovery, and report its results to the MOH.
3. The government defines the service and environmental standards that must be achieved by all classes of wards.
4. The government establishes the upper limit of charges incurred by different classes of hospital wards.
5. The government stipulates that the annual revenue growth rate of hospitals must be determined based on "consumer price index + X," where X is adjusted according to various factors, such as the advancement of medical technologies and the growth in productivity.
6. The government also specifies the total number of beds and the proportion of beds in different ward classes in each restructured hospital.
7. The government is responsible for controlling and coordinating the development of various specialties and the introduction of new medical technologies into hospitals.
8. The hospitals are reimbursed at varying rates according to the type of outpatient visit and the class of wards used.
9. The government must clearly define the expected therapeutic outcomes for certain types of diseases or healthcare services and negotiate the prices of these services with restructured hospitals.
10. The government also establishes standards for services and waiting times, and penalizes hospitals that do not meet these service standards via subsidy reduction.

In addition, the MOH also supervises and manages MOH Holdings, which primarily involves the handling of its diversified business activities, revision of its corporate charter, the issuance of new stocks and loans, advice on mergers, the sale or transfer of assets, establishment of new subsidiaries, termination and dissolution of companies, adjustment of medical expenses, appointment of directors, and so on.

(4) Evaluation of the Reform

The reform of the hospital management system led to the separation between ownership (state ownership) and management (private limited company) in public hospitals. Before 1984, public hospitals in Singapore were administered directly by the government, as with the British model. However, the patients, hospitals, and government were dissatisfied with this system due to its inefficiency, lack of enthusiasm among personnel, and poor service quality in hospitals. Therefore, the government has adopted a series of measures since 1985 to effectively reform its hospital and healthcare systems. The government of Singapore restructured all its affiliated hospitals (including eight acute hospitals and six specialist hospitals) to form wholly government-owned hospitals that operate as private limited companies.

After restructuring, the government shifted administrative authority over the restructured hospitals to these private limited companies, which are led by a board of directors comprising representatives from all parties involved. The board of directors is responsible for formulating development plans, guidelines, and policies for the restructured hospitals, while the government is responsible for reviewing and approving the hospital fee standards and use of funds for the procurement of large-scale equipment and infrastructure projects. Each hospital is also appointed an administrative director, who is fully responsible for hospital administration and is accountable to the board of directors. Hospitals have authority over regular promotion, salary increases, and dismissal of personnel; income and expenditure; hospital operations; and administrative management. The reform also introduced a commercial accounting system that provides a more accurate picture of operating expenses and gradually adopts more financial principles and responsibilities.

The restructured hospitals receive yearly subsidies from the government for providing healthcare services, the amount of which is based on the number of patients served (similar to nonprofit hospitals). The government provides policy guidance to hospitals through the MOH. The government delegates authority to hospitals for micromanagement issues, such as reimbursement and remuneration, but hospitals still require government approval for certain sensitive issues, such as price adjustment. As a result, hospitals are given greater administrative autonomy without losing their basis in social welfare. A two-way referral system within the medical cluster also enables government polyclinics to better fulfill their functions, thus improving the quality of healthcare services while reducing medical expenses via cooperation among healthcare providers at various levels. The complementary nature of hospitals within the cluster also helps reduce redundant construction, thereby ensuring the optimal development of hospital service volume, and prevent the excessive expansion of healthcare capacity.

The restructuring of public hospitals in Singapore has enabled the complete separation of ownership and management. This clarifies the ownership structure of hospitals and the roles of the government, which in turn has further improved the quality and efficiency of healthcare services. The reform has resulted in a significantly higher number of outpatient visits in government hospitals, bed utilization rates of more than 85%, and an average length of stay of less than six days. The reform has also achieved a 90% public satisfaction in the quality of hospital healthcare services and improved the overall healthcare standard in Singapore. Furthermore, public hospitals in Singapore are equipped with hardware facilities comparable to those in Europe and the US. They are clean, quiet, spacious, almost as comfortable as hotels, and have green garden-like environments. All hospital departments are also managed through computer network systems.

1. The Robustness of Public Hospitals as Improved Via the Introduction of Competition Mechanisms The restructured public hospitals entered the healthcare market as independent companies, competing with other healthcare institutions under government guidance. This competitive environment forced them to focus on improving their service quality, expanding their scope of services, and reducing their healthcare costs, all of which improved their overall robustness and the quality of the healthcare services delivered to patients. The government has given patients the freedom to choose their preferred hospitals and class of wards and subsidizes the hospitals based on the service volume provided, thereby triggering greater enthusiasm among hospitals and physicians to deliver quality services.

2. Hospitals are Capable of Competing with Greater Administrative Autonomy Restructured public hospitals are no longer directly administered by the government, which has greatly expanded their autonomy, giving them the authority to hire employees and determine the salaries of said employees, thereby inducing employee enthusiasm and preventing the loss of talent to a certain extent. Additionally, hospitals now are able to respond rapidly to changes in the healthcare market and consumer demand, thus avoiding the bureaucratic inefficiency previously encountered under the direct administration of the government. These changes have enabled hospitals to compete with each other.

3. The Changes in Patient Flow Have Reduced the Burden on the Government An increasing number of patients have turned to private hospitals in the years following the restructuring of public hospitals. A possible reason is more comfortable and personalized services offered by private hospitals. The increase in the patient flow towards private hospitals suggests that the multilevel needs of patients are being met. It also implies that the financial pressure on the government has been eased because of the decrease in government subsidies for patients. Moreover, the establishment of MOH Holdings and the delegation of authority to the restructured hospitals have reduced government responsibility for public hospitals.

4. Positive Role of MOH Holdings MOH Holdings is a buffering agency between the government and public hospitals. It not only guarantees the administrative autonomy of restructured hospitals but also enables rational allocation and effective use of healthcare resources through gradual adjustment. Group purchasing by MOH Holdings benefits from the economies of scale in the procurement of medical supplies and drugs, which reduces the cost of healthcare services in restructured hospitals. Furthermore, MOH Holdings appoints special professionals (e.g., senior management personnel and computer engineers) to serve in subsidiary hospitals, thus sharing the cost of hiring these professionals while also improving the management capabilities of these hospitals. The socialization of hospital logistical services provided by MOH Holdings (acquired through group purchasing or provided by a centralized organization) has also greatly alleviated the burden and administrative complexity of hospitals.

5. Rising Administrative Costs of the Government Hospital restructuring has increased hospital autonomy and enhanced the competition in the healthcare market, which in turn has made the hospitals more robust. However, the healthcare market still requires considerable government intervention as it is an imperfectly competitive market. In the early stages of hospital system reform, there was an increase in profitable, high-level health-care services and a reduction in nonprofitable, basic healthcare services. The government faced increasing political pressure as the public became dissatisfied with the rising price of healthcare services in hospitals. This situation improved when the government enhanced its control over restructured hospitals and the healthcare market by implementing measures such as price-cap regulation and controlling and coordinating the development of specialties and hospital beds. However, these actions have undoubtedly imposed greater regulatory costs on the government.

6. Issues Arising from Competition with Private Hospitals Competition with private hospitals in the healthcare market has prompted public hospitals to improve their efficiency. However, private hospitals occupy a relatively favorable position due to their lower government regulation and inclusion under Medisave coverage. For instance, they are allowed to offer only highly profitable healthcare services, whereas public hospitals must offer nonprofitable basic services as well. Furthermore, private hospitals can attract medical experts from public hospitals by offering higher salaries, which has led to a loss of talent in public hospitals. On the one hand, it has adversely affected the medical education and research activities of public hospitals. On the other hand, it has also prompted public hospitals to increase their wages to retain talented personnel, thus increasing both the workforce costs and overall healthcare costs in public hospitals.

7. Quality Issues in Healthcare Services In market competition, hospitals may sometimes reduce their costs at the expense of service quality, which may not be readily noticed or monitored due to information asymmetry in the healthcare market. Despite enhanced government control over the cost and prices of healthcare services, the oversight and quality assurance of healthcare services remain relatively inadequate.

(5) Further Reforms

In 2000, public healthcare institutions in Singapore were divided into two medical clusters based on their geographical locations and size – Singapore Health Services (SingHealth) located in the east and the National Healthcare Group (NHG) located in the west. These two medical clusters are equal in size and receive an equal amount of government subsidy. Each cluster consists of a tertiary hospital, a regional hospital, a specialist hospital, several national centers, and a number of primary care clinics. The annual turnover of each cluster is close to S$1 billion. These two clusters were established to promote internal competition among public healthcare institutions.

Table 13.21 shows that SingHealth consists of four public hospitals, seven polyclinics, and four national centers, while the NHG consists of four public hospitals, nine polyclinics, and two national centers.

The director of each medical cluster is appointed by the MOH, while the board of directors consists of the heads of the member institutions. Both medical clusters have different management and incentive mechanisms. For example, the NHG pays half-month to one-month bonuses each year to subsidiary hospitals that show excellent performance. In addition, both clusters employ the balanced scorecard approach in managing their subsidiaries.

In 2001, the MOH signed an agreement with these two medical clusters stipulating the amount of MOH subsidies they will receive, as well as the quantity and quality of services

TABLE 13.21 Public Medical Clusters in Singapore

Medical Clusters	Healthcare Institutions in Clusters
Singapore Health Services Pte. Ltd.	4 hospitals
	7 polyclinics
	4 national centers
National Healthcare Group Pte. Ltd.	4 hospitals
	9 polyclinics
	2 national centers

that each cluster must deliver. For instance, the agreement established acceptable ranges for appointment and clinic waiting times: The average appointment waiting time for subsidized patients is 14 days, and waiting times exceeding 42 days are considered a failure; similarly, the average clinic waiting time is 30 minutes, and waiting times exceeding 75 minutes are considered a failure. The agreement also strictly defines the fines levied on hospitals that fail to meet the established standards. In addition, the agreement stipulates that both clusters must limit the rate of increase in expenses for subsidized patients. The MOH has also imposed total revenue control on each medical cluster; in other words, government subsidies are reduced in proportion to the total expenditure of the cluster that exceeds an upper limit.

3. Health Security and Health Insurance

The healthcare system in Singapore is based on the medical savings component (known as Medisave) of the Central Provident Fund (CPF), which provides the most basic health coverage to all CPF members. In addition, the government of Singapore has closely integrated Medisave with commercial health insurance to cover the medical expenses for major illnesses. The government has also assumed the responsibility of providing subsidies and a safety net for healthcare security. Specifically, it subsidizes the medical expenses of low-income patients admitted to general wards and has established healthcare funds that provide medical assistance to those living in poverty. Singapore has effectively achieved universal health coverage through the establishment of this multilevel healthcare system.

Currently, the social security systems in most countries operate based on the joint responsibility of governments, enterprises, and individuals. Among them, some schemes are jointly funded by individuals and enterprises, with the government only acting as a supervising entity that performs macroprudential regulation, for example, in Southeast Asian countries, such as Singapore, Malaysia, and Indonesia. Despite the rapid economic development of these countries in recent years, they have implemented a self-help model of social security based primarily on the use of personal or family savings, due to the traditional mindset that families should play a dominant role in ensuring social security. Therefore, it is crucial to briefly introduce the CPF before discussing the health security system in Singapore.

(1) Overview of CPF

1. Contents of CPF   The CPF obligates all employers and employees to allocate a certain percentage of their salaries to a CPF account. The CPF Board then credits the contribution plus the interest payable to the personal account of each member on a monthly basis.

The interest is computed according to the balance in each citizen's CPF account. The CPF exempts only foreign workers from paying this contribution. Self-employed individuals, with the exception of taxi drivers and barbers, are allowed to participate in the CPF voluntarily; all other Singaporeans are obligated to become CPF members. As a result, there are more than two million CPF members, equivalent to a coverage rate of 85% of the total population. The CPF was initially established as a retirement savings system, which gradually evolved over several decades into a social security system meant to meet the various needs of Singaporeans, including retirement, housing, healthcare, and social welfare.

1. *Retirement, disability, and later-life plans.* From the establishment of CPF in 1955 until about 1968, a CPF member could apply to use CPF savings at the age of retirement (age 55) or on other grounds, such as migrating to a foreign country, incapacitation, or death (CPF savings will be distributed to the nominated beneficiaries). Members are still eligible to withdraw their funds even if they continue to work after the age of 55 years.

   In 1987, the CPF established the Retirement Sum Scheme, which required retired employees (aged 55 years) to set aside a minimum sum of S\$31,600 (S\$47,000 for a married couple) when withdrawing funds from their CPF, in order to support a basic standard of living during retirement. This is to prevent CPF members from exhausting all their savings.

   The same year, the CPF also established the Retirement Sum Topping-Up Scheme (RSTU), which allowed members who retire with less than S\$30,000 in their CPF account to receive top-ups via transfers from their children's CPF savings or via cash top-ups. Members are given three options regarding the remaining S\$30,000 in their CPF accounts: (1) They may continue to keep it in their CPF accounts and receive about S\$200 per month (S\$237 in 1987) by the age of 60 years until these savings are exhausted (generally for 15–20 years). Upon the death of the CPF member, any remaining CPF savings will be distributed to their nominated beneficiaries. (2) They may deposit the savings in an authorized bank (with higher interest rates), which will distribute the deposits as described above. (3) They may use the savings to purchase an annuity plan from a designated insurance company, which will issue about S\$300 per month to them from the age of 60 years for the rest of their life. However, any remaining balance will not be returned to their family upon their death.

   In 1989, the CPF established the Dependents' Protection Scheme (DPS), a nonmandatory low-cost insurance scheme that requires members to pay an annual premium that varies with age. The DPS benefit (S\$30,000) is paid out to insured members or to their dependents in the event of total permanent disability or death.

2. *Housing plan.* The Public Housing Scheme (PHS) was introduced in 1968 to allow low-income CPF members to use their CPF savings to purchase Housing and Development Board (HDB) flats. Members with insufficient savings could apply for a loan and pay the installments using contributions to their CPF accounts. Subsequently, the CPF established the middle-income housing program and Private Properties Scheme in 1975 and 1981, respectively. Additionally, the CPF introduced the Home Protection Scheme (HPS), which is compulsory for members who purchase HDB flats using loans. It enables members to pay off their loans in the event of their death or total permanent disability, thus protecting them from losing their HDB flats (the flats are transferred to their children in the event of their death). At present, 90% of CPF members have their own houses.

3. *Healthcare plan.* In 1984, the Medisave scheme was established to allow CPF members to pay a certain amount of inpatient expenses for themselves and their dependents using their CPF savings. However, Medisave can only cover general inpatient expenses and is far from sufficient to cover large inpatient expenses for patients with major illnesses. Therefore, MediShield (currently known as MediShield Life) was established in 1990. MediShield is an optional, low-cost health insurance plan whereby the CPF Board withdraws a small fee from the accounts of MediShield members for social pooling and adjustment. Medisave covers a portion of inpatient expenses for patients with major illness, while the remaining balance is covered by MediShield Life.

   In addition, the CPF established Integrated Shield Plans (IPs) to cover 80% of inpatient expenses. IPs are currently limited to members under the age of 65 years; expansion of this scheme to members over the age of 65 years is still being investigated, as doing so is expected to lead to a substantial increase in healthcare expenditure. In addition, the following schemes have also been established.

4. In 1978, the Singapore Bus Services (SBS) Ltd. Share Scheme was established, which enabled members to use their CPF savings to purchase SBS shares, allowing them to enjoy transport privileges and dividends, as well as higher interest rates than that of the CPF.

5. The Company Welfarism through Employers' Contributions (COWEC) Scheme was established in 1984. Singapore was undergoing rapid economic development during this period, which led to higher turnover rates. The COWEC sought to improve enterprise cohesiveness by allowing employers to withhold parts of their employees' salaries and redistribute them to their employees as bonuses. The COWEC is not a mandatory scheme and has only been implemented in several large companies thus far.

6. In 1986, the Approved Investment Scheme (AIS) was established to enable members to retain a certain basic amount of CPF savings for investment in unit trusts, stocks, gold, and so on. The member is responsible for any risk arising from the investment, but the return on investment, including the initial capital, must be deposited back into their CPF account.

7. In 1989, the CPF Education Scheme was introduced to enable CPF members to use their CPF savings to cover the cost of their own or their children's higher education. This scheme does not cover members seeking to study abroad. After graduation and joining the workforce, members must immediately begin repaying their loans, with interest, to their CPF accounts.

8. The Self-Employed Scheme was established in 1992.

9. The Enhanced Investment Scheme (EIS) was introduced in 1993.

2. Fund Raising and Operations

1. *CPF.* The CPF is jointly funded by both employers and employees. The government exempts the CPF from taxation and guarantees payouts. The contribution rate of the CPF is proposed by the National Wages Council (NWC, which is affiliated with the MOM), after giving due consideration to economic growth and wage increases, and is only implemented after approval by the government. In general, the CPF contribution rate is increased when there are significant economic growth and wage increases. Conversely, the contribution rate is reduced during an economic recession or challenging times for enterprises.

When the CPF was first established in 1955, it had a relatively low contribution rate (equivalent to 10% of the employee's total salary, which is shared equally between employers and employees). Later, in 1968, the contribution rate was increased to about 13% of the employee's salary (with the employers and employees contributing 6.5% each). Subsequently, the contribution rate increased rapidly, peaking at 50% (with employers and employees contributing 25% each) in 1984. The rapid increase during this period was attributed to the increased affordability among members because of increasing wages and rapid economic development. The introduction of the PHS prompted the government to accumulate more funds for the construction of public houses and CPF members to increase their savings in order to purchase public housing. Additionally, converting part of members' salaries into CPF savings enabled the effective control of inflation. However, the overly rapid increase in the contribution rate led to an economic recession and severe inflation in Singapore because of increased labor, production, and service costs. Therefore, the contribution rate was reduced from 50% to 35% in 1986; specifically, the employers' share was reduced from 25% to 10%, while the employees' share remained unchanged. As a result, there was a rebound in economic growth because of cost reduction. The contribution rate gradually increased again after 1988, and the share between employers and employees has been adjusted accordingly.

Both employers and employees contribute an equal rate most of the time, with only a few exceptions. The adjustment in the contribution rate depends not only on the needs of the CPF itself but also on economic affordability and the competitiveness of enterprises in the international market. Since July 1988, the CPF has reduced the contribution rate for employees aged over 55 years (a reduction that increases with age) in order to encourage the hiring of elderly employees.

An actuarial analysis carried out by the CPF has suggested that the contribution rate must be increased to at least 40% (with employers and employees contributing 20% each) in order to guarantee that members have an income equivalent to 20–40% of their final salary after retirement, own a house, and can cover S$15,000 of medical expenses.

At present, the CPF contribution rate is about 40% of the employee's salary (with the employers and employees contributing 18.5% and 21.5%, respectively). In 1993, the CPF received a total of S$10.1 billion from members, and the total CPF savings was about S$52.3 billion. The provident funds collected by the CPF are calculated and credited to the personal account of each member on a monthly basis. Currently, the personal account of each CPF member is divided into three parts: (1) the Ordinary Account, which is equivalent to 30% of the salary and is used for housing, investment, education and so on; (2) the Medisave Account, which is equivalent to 6% of the salary and is used for inpatient expenses and critical illness insurance; and (3) the Special Account, which is equivalent to 4% of the salary and is used for retirement-related and emergency purposes. Generally, the SA cannot be used before retirement.

2. *CPF interest rates.* The CPF is mainly invested in government securities. From 1955 to 1962, the interest rate paid to members was about 2.5%, which increased to 5% in 1963 and later to 6.5% between 1974 and 1985. During this period, the CPF interest rates were sometimes higher or lower than the bank interest rates. However, when the CPF interest rate was lower than the bank interest rates, the CPF received considerable criticism from its members. Therefore, since March 1986, the CPF began to

match its interest rate with those of banks. The interest earned for the CPF account is not subject to taxation, unlike the interest earned for bank accounts. Since 1955, the CPF interest rate has been slightly higher than the inflation rate (the annual average inflation rate from 1966 to 1987 was 3.7%), which has ensured that the CPF has not been devalued but has increased in value instead. In terms of long-term development, Singapore is expected to experience a 4% economic growth and a 4% increase in salaries and interest rates. Similar to bank interest rates, the CPF interest rate is adjusted twice annually (in April and October). The interest is calculated on a monthly basis and deposited into the personal account of members annually.

3. *CPF operation.* The CPF Board invests and operates in accordance with the Central Provident Fund Act and the Trust Investment Act. The CPF is mainly invested in government securities, while the remaining balance is invested in the financial markets. For example, in 1987, CPF savings reached about S$31.4 billion, S$29.8 billion of which was invested in government securities; in 1990, CPF savings reached S$39 billion, S$32 billion of which was invested in government securities. More specifically, CPF savings can be invested in the following areas: government securities, Monetary Authority of Singapore deposits, transferable certificate of deposit, bonds, unit trusts, and bank fixed deposits. The CPF Board has commissioned five investment experts to fulfill this task, who submit monthly investment reports to the Board and hold an investment meeting quarterly in order to report on their investment performance and formulate investment plans for the next quarter.

4. *Administration of the CPF.* The CPF is administered centrally by the CPF Board. It is an affiliate of the MOM, which formulates and oversees the implementation of relevant policies. The CPF Board operates independently and does not receive intervention from other departments. The CEO is responsible for the CPF under the leadership of the CPF Board. The chairman and CEO are appointed by the MOM and hold three-year terms. The CPF Board comprises 11 members, including a chairman and 10 board members (2 government representatives, 2 employer representatives, 2 employee representatives, and 4 experts). It meets once every two months in order to make decisions on major issues. There are two committees under the CPF Board that handle specific policy issues: the Staff and Finance Committee and Planning and Decision Committee.

The CPF Board is an independent quasi-government organization comprising a CEO (who is responsible for daily tasks), a deputy CEO, and 6 groups containing a total of 700 staff: (1) the Services Group, which is responsible for the formulation and implementation of member service plans; (2) the Employer and Finance Group, which is responsible for ensuring that payments from employers are on schedule and for the dissemination of information to employers; (3) the Human Capital Management Group, which is responsible for staff allocation and adjustment; (4) the Administrative Group, which is responsible for daily tasks and public relations; (5) the Information Group, which is responsible for information and investment issues; and (6) the Internal Audit Group.

(2) Basic Health Security System

The health security system of Singapore primarily consists of Medisave and MediShield. In addition, the government has implemented several other universal health coverage schemes, such as MediShield Plus and ElderShield.

1. Medisave   The Medisave scheme is a national medical savings scheme, which was launched on July 1, 1993. It is compulsory by law for all employed and self-employed persons. Medisave is linked with the CPF, which, as noted earlier, consists of three accounts for each member: the Ordinary Account, Medisave Account (MA), and Special Account. Medisave helps residents to set aside part of their income into their MAs to cover their future inpatient expenses, especially their healthcare needs in old age. Specifically, these savings are used to cover future inpatient expenses for themselves or their immediate family members, as well as some of the more expensive outpatient tests and drugs. The Medisave contribution rate is set not only to meet the basic healthcare needs of Singaporeans, but also to prevent inappropriate increases in healthcare needs, excessive utilization of healthcare services, and wastage of healthcare resources due to "overfunded" MAs. To this end, the government has imposed an upper limit on the monthly contribution to Medisave. Access to Medisave is also restricted by capping the payment for medical expenses, such as inpatient expenses per day per bed (annual caps have also been applied to some service items). To ensure that families with insufficient Medisave savings have access to basic healthcare services, the government allows for a "deficit" in MAs that must be repaid afterwards at the same interest rate as the CPF. Upon the death of a Medisave member, any remaining Medisave savings are distributed to nominated beneficiaries without being subject to inheritance tax.

2. MediShield   This is a basic health insurance scheme for major illnesses, which was launched in 1990. It aims to address issues related to the high medical expenses incurred by CPF members with major or chronic illnesses. This scheme has imposed age restrictions – only members up to a maximum age of 70 years are covered, but this age limit has since been reviewed and was eventually raised to 75 years. MediShield comprises three plans: Integrated Shield Plans (IPs), Plan B, and Plan A. The annual premiums for these three plans increase with age. Additionally, the plans have their own daily claim limits for inpatient and surgical expenses. MediShield premiums can be paid via cash transfers from member's MA. Note that while MediShield covers both inpatient and expensive outpatient expenses (e.g., hemodialysis, radiotherapy, and chemotherapy for cancer patients), it does not cover members with preexisting conditions 20 months prior to MediShield enrollment. MediShield only covers medical expenses that exceed a certain amount (i.e., the claim limit or deductible). For instance, the MediShield claim limits for Class C wards in public hospitals is S$500, while those for other classes of wards in public hospitals or authorized private hospitals may reach upwards of S$1,000. In total, MediShield covers 80% of the medical expenses, while the remaining 20% are covered by members.

3.MediShield Plus   MediShield Plus is a health insurance scheme based on MediShield but has a higher level of protection. CPF members can freely choose to purchase this scheme for themselves and their dependents, and may allocate a maximum of S$660 of their Medisave savings to pay for MediShield Plus premiums; the remaining balance of the premiums must be paid in cash. MediShield Plus has a higher premium rate than MediShield, and as a result, provides greater benefits. For instance, inpatients can choose to be admitted to a higher ward class (Class A or B1). MediShield Plus can be further divided into Plan A and Plan B. The annual premiums of Plan A range from S$60 to S$1,200 depending on the age of the insured person. The claim limits of Plan A are S$500 per day for inpatient expenses and S$5,500 for surgical charges. On the other hand, the annual premiums of Plan B range from S$36 to S$720, depending on the age of the insured person. The claim limits of Plan

B are S$300 per day for inpatient expenses and S$4,500 for surgical charges. This health insurance scheme was designed to meet the needs of CPF members with better economic statuses and a greater demand for the standard of inpatient services.

4. ElderShield   This is a special health insurance scheme formulated and introduced by the Singapore MOH in 2002; as the name suggests, this scheme was intended to benefit the elderly population. ElderShield is a severe disability insurance scheme that provides financial insurance for elderly CPF members requiring long-term care. CPF members can pay for the premiums of this scheme using their MAs. There are three types of ElderShield plans available: the Regular Premium Plan, 10-Year Premium Plan, and Single Premium Plan. There are significant differences among these plans in terms of the premiums and benefits, which are closely associated with the age of the insured person. For example, in 2002, an insured person who purchased ElderShield at age 40 had to pay S$175 per year until age 65. All insured persons are entitled to a compensation of S$300 per month for a maximum of five years in the event of severe disability.

To ensure that ElderShield can adapt to the changing needs of Singaporeans, the MOH reformed this scheme in 2007, as follows: (1) The amount of compensation was increased from S$300 per month to S$400 per month, while the maximum period of compensation was extended from five years to six years, with a corresponding increase in the premium rate. (2) Insured persons can now set aside a maximum of S$600 from their MAs for the purchase of "ElderShield Supplements," which complement their basic ElderShield plan. These supplementary plans provide insured persons with additional benefits, which are determined by the premiums paid. Provision of the above-mentioned insurance plans has been delegated by the MOH to three commercial insurance companies: Aviva Ltd., Great Eastern Life Insurance, and NTUC Income Insurance Co-Op., Ltd.

(3) Medical Aid and Subsidies from the Government

The government of Singapore has emphasized personal responsibility in healthcare expenditure via the establishment of the Medisave scheme. It has also introduced a commercial health insurance mechanism, which provides individual or group insurance schemes, in order to protect individuals against major illnesses. On the other hand, the government has also attached great importance to the establishment of healthcare facilities and is continually increasing the capital injection for health coverage, with the aim of achieving universal health coverage. The government has also established various medical aid programs and subsidies to assist low-income earners.

1. Medifund   The Medifund scheme was established in April 1993. The government invested an initial capital of S$200 million and has continued to inject S$100 million into the fund annually depending on the sustainable growth of the economy. Only the interests generated from this endowment fund are distributed to all public hospitals, each of which has a government-appointed Medifund Committee. Individuals living in poverty who are unable to afford their medical expenses can apply for assistance via the Medifund Committee, which reviews, approves, and distributes the funds. About 3% of patients admitted to Class B2 and C3 wards apply for this fund, and the approval rate is 99.6%. Patients who choose to be admitted to higher-class wards are not eligible for Medifund coverage. Furthermore, Medifund prioritizes Singaporeans born before 1940.

Medifund is a government-funded, welfare-based medical aid fund that provides a safety net for impoverished patients who are unable to afford their medical expenses. The main eligibility criteria for receiving Medifund coverage are as follows: The patient must be admitted to a Class B2 or C ward in a Medifund-approved healthcare institution, or the patient must be receiving government-subsidized outpatient surgeries or treatments; and both the patient and their family must have difficulty affording medical expenses and have exhausted both their own and their family's Medisave savings.

The assistance provided by the Medifund scheme depends on patients' economic status and medical expenses. Medifund is administered by the MOH, but Medifund-approved hospitals and other healthcare institutions are responsible for handling patient applications. Each Medifund-approved hospital or healthcare institution has a Medifund Committee, which reviews the eligibility of applicants and determines the amount of funds they will receive. Medifund is an endowment fund that has thus far accumulated about S$1.5 billion and is expected to gradually increase to about S$2 billion in the future.

2. Government Subsidies for Basic Healthcare Services

1. *Community Health Assist Scheme (CHAS).* The CHAS is a MOH-sponsored medical allowance scheme piloted in October 2000 that subsidizes the treatment of certain diseases among the elderly and impoverished. The CHAS stipulates that individuals aged over 65 years with a household monthly income per capita of S$700 or below, or who are Public Assistance (PA) scheme cardholders, are eligible to apply for a Community Medical Benefit (CMB) card. For private clinics, this scheme only covers treatments for minor illnesses, such as colds, coughs, headaches, red eyes, and otitis. Patients seeking medical attention from CHAS clinics only need to pay S$4 for the consultation fee and S$0.7 for each packet of medicine. This scheme was further extended in January 2009 to cover outpatient, drug, and laboratory testing fees for Pioneer Generation cardholders who have diabetes, hypertension, and hypercholesterolemia, and are receiving chronic care services at CHAS private clinics. Currently, a total of 450 private clinics and 190 dental clinics in Singapore participate in this scheme. About 25% of households have a monthly income per capita of less than S$700, and about 300,000 Singaporeans are aged over 65 years, of whom, 19,000 benefit from this medical allowance scheme. The government is considering whether to further relax the CHAS eligibility criteria in the future to cover more individuals.

2. *Government subsidies for inpatient expenses in general wards.* The government of Singapore also covers varying proportions of inpatient expenses in general wards based on the class of wards and patients' income levels. About 80% of public hospital beds (including 10-bedded Class C wards and 6-bedded Class B2 wards) are entitled to higher government subsidies. On the other hand, the remaining 20% of public hospital beds receive either lower subsidies (4-bedded Class B1 wards) or no subsidies at all (single-bedded Class A wards). The Inpatient Affordability Survey conducted by the MOH in March 2008 revealed that the daily medical costs for Class A, B1, B2, and C wards were S$244, S$200, S$128, and S$115, respectively. The government provides the highest subsidy (80% of inpatient expenses) for Class C wards, followed by Class B2 (65%) and B1 wards (20%). The majority of retirees and homemakers, who lack typically an income, are entitled to the above-mentioned government subsidies upon hospitalization. Middle- to high-income earners admitted to Class B2 and C wards are entitled to subsidies that cover at least 50% of their inpatient expenses. Patients with higher incomes are not eligible for such government subsidies, regardless of the class of wards. Therefore, the Inpatient Affordability Survey, which reflects the financial ability of an individual, will only affect individuals whose residential home prices rank in the top 20% in Singapore when they were hospitalized.

TABLE 13.22   Ward Classes in Singapore (Unit: %)

Ward Class	Patients' Share of Medical Expenses	Government's Share of Medical Expenses
Class C (8–12 beds, no air conditioning)	20	80
Class B2 (6 beds, no air conditioning)	35	65
Class B1 (4 beds, air conditioning)	80	20
Class A (1–2 beds, air conditioning)	100	0

Source: MOH of Singapore, 2003.

The MOH stipulated that from January 2009, government subsidies will only be provided after an assessment of the inpatients' economic status. A Singaporean with an average monthly income of S$3,200 or below can continue to receive 65% and 80% inpatient subsidies in Class B2 and C wards, respectively.

Government subsidization of the healthcare sector is limited to public hospitals, which account for 58% of the total hospital expenditure. The fee standards for public hospitals are established by the government. Public hospital wards are categorized into four classes: A, B1, B2, and C (Table 13.22). Although they have different accommodation conditions, they are treated equally in terms of medical services and share the same group of physicians, thereby ensuring a similar quality of healthcare services across different ward classes. In addition, the government has stipulated that the number of beds in general wards (Class B2 and C wards) must account for more than 70% of the total number of hospital beds. The fees for hospitalization, examinations, surgery, drugs, outpatient care, and emergency care are all controlled by the government, with a particular emphasis on controlling the fees for Class B2 and C wards and subsidizing outpatient and emergency care. The government not only takes into account the multilevel healthcare demands of different groups but also shifts the country's subsidy orientation to meet the healthcare demands of the majority of patients. In addition to the Medisave scheme, patients must pay a proportion of their medical expenses in general wards, thereby embodying the principle of mutual aid among individuals, the government, and society.

4. Healthcare Funding Policies

(1) Healthcare Funding Sources

1. Public Sources of Healthcare Funding

1. *Taxation.* Taxation is the key source of healthcare funding. A personal income tax is levied on Singapore residents at a progressive rate ranging from 2% to 28%. Corporate tax is levied at 26% on the profits made after deducting government subsidies. The total tax revenue of Singapore in 1995 was S$19.6 billion.
2. *Medifund.* The origin and function of Medifund have been outlined previously. Medifund is applicable to all Singapore residents who need medical subsidies, and the amount of subsidies received by each applicant varies according to their individual

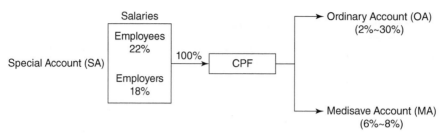

FIGURE 13.9 Capital flow of CPF accounts in Singapore.

circumstances. The applicants must have been or will be admitted to Class B2 and C wards or have received treatment at government-subsidized outpatient clinics, and are unable to afford their medical expenses. With annual capital injections, the Medifund balance increased from the initial capital of S$200 million in 1993 to S$600 million in 1998. Every public hospital with a Medifund Committee is authorized to review and approve Medifund applications.

2. Private Healthcare Funding There are various sources of individual and organizational healthcare funds, including government-administered Medisave, MediShield, personal savings, and private insurance.

1. *Medisave.* This is essentially an extension of the CPF that covers 85% of the total population of Singapore. Currently, Singaporeans must contribute 40% of their income to the CPF, of which 22% is contributed by employees and the remaining 18% by employers. Of this 40% contribution, 6–8% is deposited into MAs (Figure 13.9 and Table 13.23). However, there is an upper limit to the amount transferred to their MAs (S$7,200) in order to prevent surplus capital accumulation and misuse of healthcare resources.

   Medisave covers a maximum of S$300 per day for routine medical expenses in public and private hospitals. Medisave also covers surgical charges with limits ranging from S$150 to S$5,000, depending on the individual circumstances of each patient. However, these surgeries must fall within the scope of coverage designated by the MOH. In 1996, the average inpatient charges for Class C and A wards in public hospitals were S$530 and S$2,700 per day, respectively; whereas Class A wards in private

TABLE 13.23 Three Types of CPF Accounts in Singapore in 1998 (Unit: %)

Age of Employees	Share of Salary Deposited into the Account			
	OA	SA	MA	Total
35 years and below	30	4	6	40
36–44 years	29	4	7	40
45–54 years	28	4	8	40
55–59 years	12	–	8	20
60–64 years	7	–	8	15
65 years and above	2	–	8	10

hospitals charged S$4,100 per day. The cost-sharing mechanism of this scheme has prevented the misuse of MAs. Furthermore, Medisave covers certain more expensive outpatient services, such as outpatient surgeries, radiotherapy, chemotherapy, hemodialysis, *in vitro* fertilization, and hepatitis B vaccination.

MA holders may use their Medisave funds for themselves and their families. Family members may use their Medisave funds to jointly pay for a single medical bill. Medisave also provides lifelong protection. MA holders can start withdrawing funds from their accounts after the age of 55 but must keep at least S$16,000 in the account. In 1997, there were 2.6 million MA holders, who collectively had saved about S$17 billion.

2. *MediShield.* MA holders aged over 75 years are automatically covered under MediShield unless they withdraw voluntarily from the scheme. MediShield is an insurance scheme that targets patients with major or chronic illnesses. MA holders may use their Medisave funds to pay MediShield premiums for themselves and their spouse or dependents. The premiums range from S$12 to S$240 per year.

The principle of copayment (using a predetermined deductible) has been adopted for MediShield to prevent moral hazard and overutilization of MediShield funds. The MediShield deductibles for Class C and B2 wards are S$500 and S$1,000, respectively. MediShield Plus is divided into Plan A and Plan B, which covers medical expenses in private hospitals or inpatient charges for Class A and B wards in public hospitals. The deductibles of Plan A and Plan B are S$4,000 and S$2,500, respectively, and cover inpatient, drug, and diagnostic fees. By the end of 1995, MediShield covered 1.5 million people, accounting for 87% of CPF members and their families; there were 43,919 claims in total, most of which were claims for cancer and chronic kidney disease. Together, these claims cost S$23.6 million.

3. *Private health insurance.* In addition to these two government-administered schemes, individual or group private health insurance can also serve as the source of healthcare funding. Private health insurance includes group insurance (which covers about 750,000 employees and their families) and individual insurance (where the premium is paid by the policyholder's employer). Employers' payment of employees' insurance premiums used to be regarded as office expenses that were exempt from taxation. However, the government became concerned that the tax exemption would lead to an increase in healthcare expenditure. Therefore, in 1994, the tax exemption was adjusted to about 2% of employees' salaries, and the government began encouraging employers to utilize this tax exemption to increase their share of the MA copayment.

Private insurance companies are given the freedom to provide insurance services to insured persons, but MOH approval is required if these insurers want insured persons to use their Medisave funds to pay for their private insurance premiums. Furthermore, they must provide insurance schemes that align with the government's policy goals and objectives (e.g., applying the principle of copayment).

4. *Direct payment.* Even after participating in Medisave, MediShield, and employer-sponsored private health insurance, Singapore residents must still cover deductibles and copayments for their medical expenses. People often pay cash for these expenses and for the purchase of prescription drugs.

(2) Analysis of Income and Expenditure of the Healthcare System

1. Healthcare Funding Models

1. *Total healthcare funding*: According to the healthcare funding sources in Singapore described in Table 13.24, 70% of all funds were contributed by individuals or groups

TABLE 13.24 Healthcare Funding Sources in Singapore from 1986 to 1995

Year Item	1986	1987	1988	1989	1990	1991	1992	1993	1994	1995
Total funding (a) (S$million)	1,312	1,412	1,645	1,747	2,050	2,314	2,687	2,816	3,132	3,545
Public funding sources (b) (S$million)	414	449	506	502	524	631	770	767	873	1,142
Private funding sources (c) (S$million)	898	963	1,139	1,245	1,526	1,683	1,917	2,049	2,259	2,403
MAs (d) (S$million)	105	141	170	179	208	231	238	250	276	296
Other private funding sources (e) (S$million)	793	822	969	1,066	1,318	1,452	1,679	1,799	1,983	2,107
Ratio (%)										
b/a	31.55	31.80	30.76	28.73	25.56	27.27	28.66	27.24	28.27	32.21
c/a	68.45	68.20	69.24	71.27	74.44	72.73	71.34	72.76	72.13	67.79
d/a	8.00	9.99	10.33	10.25	10.15	9.98	8.86	8.88	8.81	8.35
e/a	60.44	58.22	58.91	61.02	64.29	62.75	62.49	63.88	63.31	59.44
Growth rate (%)										
a	–	7.62	16.50	6.20	17.34	12.88	16.12	4.80	11.22	13.19
b	–	8.45	12.69	–0.79	4.38	20.42	22.03	–0.39	13.82	30.81
c	–	7.24	18.28	9.31	22.57	10.29	13.90	6.89	10.25	6.37
d	–	34.29	20.57	5.29	16.20	11.06	3.3	5.04	10.40	7.25
e	–	3.66	17.74	10.01	23.64	10.17	15.63	7.15	10.23	6.25

Source: MOH of Singapore, 1997.

from 1986 to 1995. Since the 1980s, the burden of raising healthcare funds began shifting towards the private sector. By 1990, private funds accounted for 74.4% of the total healthcare funding in Singapore. By contrast, from 1986 to 1995, Medisave funds accounted for 8–10% of the total healthcare funding, while government funds accounted for one-third. During this period, the share of government funding fell below 30% for six years.

2. *Public healthcare funding.* The government's healthcare funding is mainly derived from the fiscal revenue, nearly 80% of which is contributed by taxation. In 1995, the government's total fiscal revenue was S$24.8 billion, of which S$19.6 billion came from various forms of taxes; the remaining balance came from fees or other incomes. In addition to fiscal revenue, public healthcare funds also came from the interest income generated from the Medifund capital sum. In 1995, the interest income of Medifund was S$9.8 million, which accounted for less than 1% of the public health funding.

3. *Private healthcare funding.* Table 13.25 shows that private healthcare funding is derived from Medisave, MediShield, employer-sponsored insurance, and privately purchased insurance. Specifically, in 1986 and 1995, Medisave accounted for more than 10% of total private healthcare funding; this share exceeded 14% in the late 1980s but dropped to approximately 12% in the 1990s. Since 1990, MA holders have been able to use funds from their MA to purchase MediShield health insurance. However, in 1994 and 1995, the MediShield premiums only accounted for less than 1% of the total private healthcare funding.

Other sources of private healthcare funding include employer- or employee-paid private health insurance and direct payments. In general, direct payments are cash payments made by patients for routine healthcare services as well as for copayments of MA and other insurance schemes. Together, these sources account for more than 85% of the total private healthcare funding.

2. Patterns of Healthcare Expenditure

1. *Total healthcare expenditure.* In 1995, Singapore spent nearly S$3.545 million on healthcare, which was 42 times that in 1960 and 2.7 times that in 1986 (Table 13.26). The total healthcare expenditure consisted of direct and indirect payments made by the government, individuals, and organizations for healthcare services; management of health insurance schemes; health education; construction of medical facilities, and so on.

As shown in Table 13.26, since 1960, the total healthcare expenditure as a share of the GDP ranged from 3% to 4%, which is lower than that of other developed countries. For instance, the total healthcare expenditure as a share of the GDP among the Economic Cooperation Organization (ECO) countries was 8.8% in 1985 and 10.4% and 1995. The share in Singapore has been declining since 1986, reaching 2.96% in 1989. This trend of decrease was a result of the health reforms of the 1980s, such as the introduction of Medisave, hospital restructuring, and various cost-containment measures.

2. *Public healthcare expenditure.* This refers to government funding allocation for healthcare services, management of health insurance schemes, health education, and construction of medical facilities. The total public healthcare expenditure in 1995 was S$114.2 million (Table 13.27), which was 2.7 times the amount in 1986. However, the growth rate in expenditure has not been consistent. In fact, there was negative growth in 1989 and 1993, whereas in other years, the growth rate was in the double digits, possibly due to the establishment of new medical facilities. The public healthcare expenditure as a share of the GDP declined from 1.05% in 1986 to 0.99% in 1988,

TABLE 13.25 Private Sources of Healthcare Funding in Singapore from 1986 to 1995

Year Item	1986	1987	1988	1989	1990	1991	1992	1993	1994	1995
Total private healthcare funding (a) (S$million)	1,312	1,412	1,645	1,747	2,050	2,314	2,687	2,816	3,132	3,545
MAs (b) (S$million)	414	449	506	502	524	631	770	767	873	1,142
MediShield (c) (S$million)	898	963	1 139	1,245	1,526	1,683	1,917	2,049	2,259	2,403
MediShield Plus (d) (S$million)	105	141	170	179	208	231	238	250	276	296
Other private funding sources (e) (S$million)	793	822	969	1,066	1,318	1,452	1,679	1,799	1,983	2,107
Growth rate (%)										
a	–	7.62	16.50	6.20	17.34	12.88	16.12	4.80	11.22	13.19
–	–	8.45	12.69	-0.79	4.38	20.42	22.03	-0.39	13.82	30.81
c	–	7.24	18.28	9.31	22.57	10.29	13.90	6.89	10.25	6.37
d	–	34.29	20.57	5.29	16.20	11.06	3.3	5.04	10.40	7.25
e	–	3.66	17.74	10.01	23.64	10.17	15.63	7.15	10.23	6.25
Ratio (%)										
b/a	31.55	31.80	30.76	28.73	25.56	27.27	28.66	27.24	28.27	32.21
c/a	68.45	68.20	–	–	–	–	–	–	0.69	0.98
d/a	8.00	9.99	–	–	–	–	–	–	0.03	0.13
e/a	88.31	58.22	58.91	61.02	64.29	62.75	62.49	63.88	63.31	59.44

Source: MOH of Singapore, 1997.

TABLE 13.26 Total Healthcare Expenditure in Singapore from 1960 to 1995

Year Item	1960	1970	1980	1986	1987	1988	1989
Total expenditure (a) (S$million)	85	203	635	1,312	1,412	1,645	1,747
GDP (b) (S$million)	2,150	5,805	25,091	39,264	43,145	51,082	58,943
Population (c) (million)	1.6	2.1	2.4	2.5	2.6	2.6	2.6
Growth Rate (%)							
(a)	–	138.82	212.81	106.61	7.62	16.50	6.20
(b)	–	170.00	332.23	56.49	9.88	18.4	15.39
(c)	–	31.25	14.29	4.17	4.00	0.00	64,7035
Ratio (%)							
a/b	3.95	3.50	2.53	3.34	3.27	3.22	2.96
Expenditure per capita (S$)	53.13	96.67	264.58	524.80	543.08	632.69	671.92

Year Item	1990	1991	1992	1993	1994	1995	
Total expenditure (a) (S$million)	2,050	2,314	2,687	2,816	3,132	3,545	
GDP (b) (S$million)	67,879	75,266	80,940	94,223	108,505	121,081	
Population (c) (million)	2.7	2.8	2.8	2.9	2.9	3.0	
Growth rate (%)							
(a)	17.34	12.88	16.12	4.80	11.22	13.19	
(b)	15.16	10.88	7.54	16.41	15.16	11.59	
(c)	3.85	3.70	0200	3.57	0.00	3.45	
Ratio (%)							
(a)/(b)	3.02	3.07	3.32	2.99	2.89	2.93	
Expenditure per capita (S$)	759.26	826.43	959.64	971.03	1,080.00	1,181.67	

Source: MOH of Singapore, 1997.

TABLE 13.27 Public Healthcare Expenditure in Singapore from 1960 in 1995

Year Item	1960	1970	1980	1986	1987	1988	1989
Expenditure (a) (S$million)	33	81	223	414	449	506	502
GDP (b) (S$million)	2,150	5,805	25,091	39,264	43,145	51,082	58,943
Growth rate (%)							
(a)	–	175.31	85.65	8.45	12.69	–0.79	4.38
(b)	–	332.23	56.49	9.88	18.4	15.39	15.16
(a)/(b) (%)	3.95	3.50	2.53	3.34	3.27	3.22	2.96

Year Item	1990	1991	1992	1993	1994	1995	
Expenditure (a) (S$million)	524	631	770	767	873	1 142	
GDP (b) (S$million)	67,879	75,266	80,940	94,223	108,505	121,081	
Growth rate (%)							
a	20.42	22.03	–0.39	13.82	30.81	30.81	
b	10.88	7.54	16.41	15.16	11.59	11.59	
a/b (%)	0.772	0.838 4	0.951 3	0.814 0	0.804 6	0.94	

Source: MOH of Singapore, 1997.

TABLE 13.28 Public Healthcare Expenditure and Total Government Expenditure in Singapore from 1960 to 1995

Year Item	1960	1970	1980	1992	1993	1994	1995
Public healthcare expenditure (a)	33	81	223	770	767	873	1,142
Total government expenditure (b)	223	982	3,651	12,280	12,550	14,100	15,600
(a)/(b) (%)	14.80	8.25	6.11	6.27	6.11	6.19	7.32

Note: The unit for public healthcare expenditure and total government expenditure is S$million.
Source: MOH of Singapore, 1997.

whereas in 1991, 1992, and 1995, the growth rate of public healthcare expenditure exceeded the economic growth rate of Singapore.

Table 13.28 shows that healthcare expenditure has accounted for less than 10% of the total government expenditure since 1970, which indicates that the Singapore government did not allocate excessive resources to the healthcare industry.

3. *Private healthcare expenditure.* This refers to individual and organizational expenditure for healthcare services. Table 13.29 shows that the total private healthcare expenditure in 1995 was S$2.403 million, which was more than twice that in 1986. From 1986 to 1995, this expenditure accounted for approximately 2% of GDP. The share of private healthcare expenditure out of the total consumption expenditure of Singapore has been increasing since 1986, reaching 5.26% in 1992. This increase might be due to the introduction of Medisave, which led to the greater utilization of previously unaffordable medical facilities.

(3) A Commentary on the Health Insurance Model

Singapore has implemented a series of policies to control the expenditure of the overall healthcare system, and one of its key policies is the copayment of medical expenses. The government of Singapore has intervened in the healthcare delivery system without hesitation, from its pricing to the determination of service standards. A white paper issued by the government in 1993 clearly states that "direct government intervention is required as the market force is insufficient to control medical expenses" and "medical expenses will eventually be passed on to citizens regardless of the fundraising approach used. Premiums are still paid by citizens, regardless of whether payroll deduction or taxation is adopted." Therefore, the issue currently facing the healthcare system of Singapore is not who should ultimately bear these expenses but rather how to balance a number of expected goals, specifically, service equality, freedom of choice, and affordability.

1. Government's Financial Burden of Healthcare In the 1980s, the government of Singapore shifted much of the financial burden of healthcare to the private sector. For many years, the government contributed only about 30% of the healthcare expenditure, which accounted for less than 1% of its total expenditure. The resulting financial surplus was used for healthcare subsidies or the provision of free healthcare services to people living in poverty.

TABLE 13.29 Private Healthcare Expenditure in Singapore from 1960 to 1995

Year Item	1960	1970	1980	1986	1987	1988	1989
Private healthcare expenditure (a)	52	122	412	898	963	1,139	1,245
GDP (b) (S$million)	2,150	5,805	25,091	39,264	43,145	51,082	58,943
Total consumption (c)	1,922	3,920	12,911	18,405	20.541	23,911	26,710
Growth rate (%)							
(a)	–	237.70	117.96	7.24	18.28	9.31	22.57
Ratio (%)							
(a)/(b)	2.42	2.10	1.64	2.29	2.23	2.23	2.11
(a)/(c)	2.71	3.11	3.19	4.88	4.69	4.76	4.66
Year Item	1990	1991	1992	1993	1994	1995	
Private healthcare expenditure (a)	1,526	1,683	1,917	2,049	2,259	2,403	
GDP (b) (S$million)	67,879	75,2636	80,940	94,223	108,505	121,081	
Total consumption expenditure (c)	30,762	33,398	36,436	42,056	46,571	49,577	
Growth rate (%)							
(a)	10.29	13.90	6.89	10.25	6.37	6.37	
Ratio (%)							
(a)/(b)	2.25	2.24	2.37	2.17	2.08	1.98	
(a)/(c)	4.96	5.04	5.26	4.87	4.85	4.85	

Note: The unit for private healthcare expenditure, GDP, and total consumption expenditure is S$million.
Source: MOH of Singapore, 1997.

2. Advantages and Disadvantages of the Medisave Scheme

1. *Advantages of Medisave.* Medisave does not need to be administered by an independent agency as it is part of the CPF. This scheme encourages individuals and their families to utilize their Medisave funds in a responsible and careful way. The use of deductibles and copayments has also prevented the excessive utilization of healthcare resources. Employers and employees collectively account for about 60% of the total healthcare expenditure, with Medisave only accounting for about 10%. Medisave gives patients the freedom to choose their preferred hospitals and wards and facilitates their ability to pay for hospital charges, including charges for higher-class wards in public hospitals and wards in private hospitals.

2. *Disadvantages of Medisave.* Medisave gives patients the freedom to decide how to pay for their medical expenses. However, patients may not have access to complete information about medical charges or be able to correctly analyze the information they receive, which could potentially lead to the misuse of these funds. In addition, this scheme might grant patients access to healthcare services they cannot actually afford. Relevant surveys have found that if patients had to fully cover their medical expenses, approximately 24% of patients admitted to Class A wards could only afford 40% of their medical expenses based on their monthly incomes.

3. Control of Healthcare Expenditure   There have been several years (e.g., 1990, 1992, and 1995) where the growth rate of healthcare expenditure in Singapore exceeded its economic growth rate. However, Singapore's healthcare expenditure as a share of the GDP still ranged from 3% to 4% for those years, which was lower than that of other ECO countries. In fact, in 1995, the average healthcare expenditure as a share of the GDP for ECO countries was 10.4%. Therefore, the future sustainability of healthcare funding in Singapore remains optimistic. Moreover, the government of Singapore has been extremely cautious in regulating the prices of healthcare services in order to control their supply.

5. Healthcare Cost-Containment Mechanisms

The government of Singapore has attempted to control healthcare expenditure through the following two approaches: (1) Enhanced construction and management of public hospitals by the government in order to form a healthcare system dominated by public healthcare institutions. The government has striven to reduce healthcare expenditure through various approaches, such as infrastructure construction, inpatient subsidies, and drug procurement through tendering. (2) Stipulating appropriate caps for the use of CPF funds depending on different circumstances in order to reduce healthcare expenditure on both the supply side and the demand side.

(1) Enhanced Construction and Management of Public Hospitals

1. Restructuring Public Healthcare Institutions and Enhancing Competitive Mechanisms
Statistics compiled by the MOH of Singapore showed that, by the end of 2006, Singapore had 29 hospitals and specialty centers with a total of 11,545 beds. Of these beds, 72% were in 13 public healthcare institutions, including 7 public hospitals (5 general hospitals, 1 women's and children's hospital, and 1 psychiatric hospital) and 6 national centers (specializing in oncology, cardiology, ophthalmology, dermatology, neurology, and dentistry). By the end of 2010, there were 15 public healthcare institutions (including public hospitals and specialty centers) and 13 private hospitals in Singapore. Patients admitted to public hospitals may choose different types of ward within the permissible range. In 2006, the average length of hospital stay in Singapore was 4.7 days, while the average bed occupancy rate was about 75%.

As mentioned earlier, the government of Singapore has restructured all public hospitals and specialty centers. The ownership of these institutions still belongs to the government, but they have adopted a management system similar to that of private enterprises. The restructured hospitals receive government subsidies for the healthcare services delivered to patients and are administered like nonprofit organizations with ample policy guidance from the government via the MOH. The government has also established community hospitals to serve convalescent patients or elderly adults who do not require treatment at general hospitals.

To introduce moderate competitive mechanisms into public healthcare institutions and reduce the adverse effects of excessive competition among healthcare institutions, in October 2000 the government grouped all public healthcare institutions into two major medical clusters – the NHG (also known as the Western Group) and SingHealth (also known as the Eastern Group). The former consists of four hospitals, one national center, nine polyclinics, and three specialist research institutes, including the NUH and Tan Tock Seng Hospital. The latter consists of three hospitals, five national centers, and nine polyclinics, including Changi

General Hospital, Women's and Children's Hospital, and Singapore General Hospital. Each medical cluster provides a comprehensive range of services, from primary care at polyclinics to secondary care or higher in various types of hospitals.

These two medical clusters are solely responsible for administering their subordinate institutions, using a management system similar to that of private enterprises. Each medical cluster has its own board of directors, which nominates and appoints the CEO. The CEO is supported by a chief operating officer, chief financial officer, and so on, who are responsible for the general operations and other affairs in their respective healthcare institutions. This system enables the government to have direct control over these public healthcare institutions under the national healthcare system, thereby ensuring that the relevant government policies can be fully implemented in these institutions. All hospitals purchase drugs in bulk through open tendering to effectively reduce the purchase prices of drugs. Additionally, healthcare institutions within each medical cluster collaborate with each other to achieve economies of scale. The healthy competition between these two clusters helps facilitate innovation and improvement in the quality of healthcare services and strives to ensure the affordability of medical expenses.

2. Disclosure of Healthcare Service Information   The MOH of Singapore advocates for the management and control of medical expenses using market forces. Thus, the MOH strives to ensure transparency of information regarding the efficiency and standards of each healthcare institution by publishing indicators concerning medical charges and service quality whenever appropriate. This enables well-informed patients to choose a healthcare institution that offers better service quality at a lower charge. As a result, the MOH has effectively controlled healthcare expenditure by using competition to reduce the medical costs and charges imposed by healthcare institutions.

3. Sharing of medical Equipment Among Healthcare Institutions   Some hospitals in Singapore, especially private hospitals and ordinary clinics, cannot afford expensive medical equipment, such as X-rays or nuclear magnetic resonance (NMR) imaging systems (e.g., computed tomography scanners). Therefore, they share medical equipment with other hospitals or rent this equipment from related healthcare institutions, thereby reducing their own medical costs and charges. This approach has been effective in containing the medical expenditures in many healthcare institutions throughout Singapore.

(2) Supply Side and Demand Side Restrictions of Healthcare Services

1. Medisave Claim Limits for Outpatient Expenses   The CPF stipulates that MAs can be used to pay for the following 12 outpatient expenses: Hepatitis B vaccination, artificial insemination, hemodialysis, radiotherapy or chemotherapy for cancer patients, antiretroviral therapy for AIDS, hyperbaric oxygen therapy, outpatient intravenous antibiotic therapy, immunosuppressants for organ transplant patients, and treatment for four chronic diseases (diabetes, hypertension, lipid disorder, and stroke). Among them, patients with the four chronic diseases must pay S$30 as a deductible and 15% of the balance of their outpatient expenses, while the remaining balance can be paid using their MAs. The MA of each CPF member can be used to cover the outpatient expenses for the above 12 diseases or treatments, but there is a claim limit of S$300 per year. Furthermore, they can also use their family's MAs to pay for their outpatient expenses, with a claim limit of S$300 per year for each account.

2. Medisave Claim Limits for Inpatient Expenses   The government has imposed strict limits on Medisave claims for inpatient expenses in order to ensure that CPF members retain adequate savings in their MAs for their future healthcare needs, especially after retirement and in old age. The specific claim limits are as follows:

Internal medicine and surgical charges. S$450 per day for inpatient and treatment charges, including a maximum of S$50 for physician's daily ward round fees and a separate fixed limit for surgical charges.

Approved outpatient surgeries. S$300 per day for inpatient and treatment charges, including a maximum of S$30 for the physician's daily ward round fees and a separate fixed limit for surgical charges.

Surgical operations. The fixed claim limit for each surgical operation is determined according to the complexity of the operation.

Psychiatric treatment. S$150 per day for inpatient and treatment charges, including a maximum of S$50 for the physician's daily ward round fees and an annual limit of S$5,000.

Admittance to approved community hospitals. S$150 per day for inpatient and treatment charges, including a maximum of S$30 for the physician's daily ward round fees and an annual limit of S$3,500.

Admittance to approved convalescent hospitals. S$50 per day for inpatient and treatment charges, including a maximum of S$30 for the physician's daily ward round fees and an annual limit of S$3,000.

Admittance to approved hospices. S$160 per day for inpatient and treatment charges, including a maximum of S$30 for the physician's daily ward round fees.

Singapore Gamma Knife Center. S$7,500 for each treatment session and S$150 per day for inpatient and treatment charges.

Daycare for elderly adults in approved day care centers. S$20 per day for daycare charges and an annual limit of S$1,500.

Hospital birth. Medisave covers prenatal care, childbirth, and inpatient charges with a claim limit of S$450 per day for inpatient charges, plus an additional limit depending on the type of delivery (e.g., S$900 for vaginal birth and S$1,850 for Caesarean section).

3. Rules of Expense Settlement   The Medisave claims made by CPF members in compliance with the relevant laws and policies must be settled directly between the CPF and hospitals. For patients enrolled in MediShield, MediShield Plus, or private health insurance, the remaining balance of their medical expenses after the settlement is covered by the claim limits of these three schemes (in the aforementioned order). If there remains an unpaid balance after applying these claims, patients must pay the rest in cash. Patients who are not enrolled in the above three schemes must make cash payments to cover the remaining balance of their medical expenses after the Medisave claim. However, patients who cannot afford their medical expenses can apply for medical aid, which is mainly provided by the government-established Medifund to eligible patients in accordance with the relevant provisions. In general, hospitalized patients must sign a Medical Claims Authorization Form (MCAF) to use their MAs. Furthermore, they must pay a deposit, which will be used to cover any remaining balance if their medical expenses exceed the claim limit. However, this deposit can be waived for patients admitted to Class B2 or C wards if their Medisave savings are sufficient to serve as the deposit. Upon discharge, hospitals then submit the medical bill to the CPF to claim the amount to be paid by the patient. The CPF deducts the payable amount from the MA in compliance with relevant regulations and issues an account statement to the patient. Patients admitted to Class B2 or C wards in restructured hospitals can overdraft their MAs in order to pay for medical expenses.

Currently, the CPF-established MediShield has been entrusted to five private insurance companies: NTUC Income Insurance Co-Op., Ltd. (hereinafter referred to as Income Insurance), Great Eastern Life Insurance, Aviva Ltd., AIA, and Prudential Plc. Income Insurance integrates MediShield into its IncomeShield scheme. The inpatient expenses of CPF members who have purchased the IncomeShield scheme must be covered by Income Insurance as the first payer. For patients who have obtained insurance from other private insurance companies (e.g., employer-paid insurance), these insurance companies must transfer the insurance claims to Income Insurance, who serves as the final payer. This payment rule was established by the government to protect the interests of CPF members.

Despite the various measures adopted by the government of Singapore, the containment of healthcare expenditure is challenging. Currently, medical expenses have risen to the point where they far exceed the ability of most citizens to pay. Statistics show that the average medical expenses at public hospitals for Class A, B1, B2, and C wards in 2006 were S$3,830, S$3,193, S$1,284, and S$1,112, respectively, which increased by 10.3%, 16.7%, 17.4%, and 29.6% compared to the previous year. Specifically, the medical expenses for Class C and B2 wards, which have higher subsidies, have relatively high growth rates, whereas the medical expenses for the nonsubsidized Class A wards have much lower growth rates. In other words, the growth rate of medical expenses in these different ward classes is directly proportional to the level of government subsidy. This, to a certain extent, reflects how hospitals are taking advantage of government subsidies to obtain greater profits by substantially raising the medical charges of lower-class wards (which are selected by most patients).

In terms of healthcare cost containment, the government has established daily claim limits for Medisave only for inpatient expenses and some outpatient expenses. The remaining balance of medical expenses is entirely borne by the patients or their private insurance companies. However, there are no restrictions on expenses for prescription drugs, medical examinations, or treatments. Overall, there is a lack of effective control over medical expenses, which are reimbursed using patients' CPF accounts or insurance claims based solely on the medical bills provided by hospitals.

The MOH of Singapore once attempted to reduce medical charges by promoting competition among hospitals via the mandatory disclosure of pricing in hospitals. However, the actual outcomes of this approach were counterproductive, as most services delivered in the healthcare system remained expensive for a number of complex reasons, including the different interests of various parties with the healthcare system. The counterproductive outcomes might also have been due to a lack of awareness among patients, who knew that their medical expenses would be borne or subsidized by insurance companies or their employers. Furthermore, patients might also lack medical knowledge and have no choice but to follow the medical instructions of their physicians.

CHAPTER FOURTEEN

Improved Health Systems in Hong Kong and Taiwan

 ## SECTION I. THE HEALTH SYSTEM IN HONG KONG

Hong Kong is located on the southeastern coast of China, covering an area of 1,104 km², which includes Hong Kong Island, Kowloon, the New Territories and four outlying islands. The GDP of Hong Kong in 2013 was approximately US$274 billion, which was a 2.9% increase from the previous year, and its income per capita was US$38,123.50. The proportion of elderly adults in Hong Kong has been increasing over the past 50 years. In 2013, the population of Hong Kong was 7,187,500, of which about 14% were elderly adults aged over 65 years. The health outcomes of Hong Kong are comparable to those of Western developed countries. In 2013, the life expectancies of men and women in Hong Kong were 81.1 and 86.7 years, respectively; the infant mortality rate was 1.7 per 1,000 live births, and the maternal mortality rate was 0.

After World War II, Hong Kong experienced rapid socioeconomic development. In 1964, the British authorities in Hong Kong issued a white paper entitled "The Development of Medical Services in Hong Kong" to encourage the construction of public hospitals and clinics, and to provide affordable healthcare services to individuals living in poverty. Ten years later, in 1974, the British Authorities in Hong Kong published a second white paper, entitled "The Further Development of Medical Services in Hong Kong." This paper proposed various policies, such as the regionalization of government and subvented hospitals; promotion of healthcare development in new towns; establishment of new medical, dental, and nursing schools; and improvement of the ratios of the number of hospital beds and healthcare workers to the population size. Since then, the public healthcare service system has expanded.

In the 1980s, Hong Kong adopted a dual-track healthcare model comprising both public and private healthcare institutions. Patients were given the freedom to choose between public and private healthcare institutions, but a two-way referral system was strictly enforced in the public healthcare system to control the total service volume based on disease urgency and queuing. For historical reasons, the public healthcare system of Hong Kong has been significantly influenced by the UK National Health Service (NHS), such that healthcare services are nearly free of charge. The medical expenses of public healthcare institutions are covered by the government via taxation, enabling all residents to receive public healthcare services (mainly inpatient services) at very little expense to themselves. On the other hand, private clinics and hospitals strive to attract patients by providing higher-quality services. A fixed salary system, without personal bonuses, was adopted by public hospitals in Hong Kong, in which the preferment relies on the availability of vacancies and job performance, and healthcare workers cooperate as a team when treating patients. Patients who wish to seek outpatient services from specialists in hospitals must be referred by their primary care physicians. However, in the event of an emergency, they may visit the emergency department of a hospital, which is completely free of charge. The distribution of public hospitals (including government and subvented hospitals) is shown in Table 14.1. Physicians are usually trained in public hospitals, but may serve in private hospitals after passing relevant qualifying examinations. Private practitioners have their own clinics that lack a fixed referral system. Most private hospitals have been established in urban areas, and have no fixed department. They rely on patient referrals from private practitioners.

Similar to the challenges facing the UK NHS, a number of issues have begun to emerge in Hong Kong's healthcare system, such as the lack of management knowledge and skills in the Department of Health (DH), lack of social supervision in public hospitals, inadequate control over subvented hospitals, and low system-utilization efficiency. Since the 1990s, Hong Kong began reforming its healthcare system and established the Hospital Authority (HA), which is an independent, statutory body responsible for managing all public hospitals in Hong Kong. These health reforms were the concepts of New Managerialism that were promoted with reference to the trends of other countries. The reforms achieved the true separation of ownership and management, and its outcomes have gradually been recognized by the international community in recent years.

TABLE 14.1 Distribution of Public Hospitals in Hong Kong in the 1980s

Territory	Leading Hospital	Other Hospitals
Hong Kong Island	**Queen Mary Hospital**	**Tsan Yuk Hospital**, Ruttonjee Hospital, Grantham Hospital, Alice Ho Miu Ling Nethersole Hospital, Tung Wah Hospital, Tung Wah Eastern Hospital, and so on
Kowloon	**Queen Elizabeth Hospital and Kwong Wah Hospital**	**Kowloon Hospital**, Hong Kong Buddhist Hospital, and Wong Tai Sin Hospital
Kowloon East	United Christian Hospital	Haven of Hope Hospital and Lady Trench General Outpatient Clinic
Kowloon West	**Princess Margaret Hospital and Kwai Chung Hospital**	Caritas Medical Center, Yan Chai Hospital, and **Lai Chi Kok Hospital**
New Territories East	**Prince of Wales Hospital**	**Shatin Hospital, Fanling Hospital**, and Cheshire Home Shatin
New Territories West	**Tuen Mun Hospital and Castle Peak Hospital**	Pok Oi Hospital

Note: Boldface text indicates public hospitals, and normal text indicates subvented hospitals.

In the twenty-first century, the Hong Kong government has striven, through the maintenance and continuous development of its healthcare system, to implement a healthcare policy such that "no one should be prevented through lack of means from obtaining adequate healthcare." The World Bank stated that among the health reform experiences of various regions, Hong Kong is a good example of health reforms that have achieved effective outcomes while also maintaining appropriate control over its healthcare system.

1. Health System

(1) Healthcare Management System

1. Department of Health (DH)   The Health, Welfare and Food Bureau (HWFB) is the health administrative department in Hong Kong, which is affiliated with the Chief Secretary for Administration. It has jurisdiction over five departments – the Social Welfare Department, DH, Government Laboratory, Food and Environmental Hygiene Department, and the Agriculture, Fisheries and Conservation Department (Figure 14.1). Among them, the DH serves as a consultant for health affairs to the Government of the Hong Kong Special Administrative Region (SAR) and is also responsible for implementing healthcare policies and other statutory duties. Its main functions include advising the government on health affairs, regulating the provision of healthcare services, prevention, and control of diseases, managing port health controls, and promoting public health. It is responsible for protecting the health of the public through the provision of health promotion, disease prevention, medical and nursing care, and rehabilitation services (Figure 14.2).

2. Hospital Authority (HA)   The HA is not affiliated with any government administrative agency; rather, it is an independent statutory body established in 1990 under the Hospital Authority Ordinance (see Figure 14.2). It is responsible for establishing public healthcare institutions in order to ensure the provision of effective public healthcare services.

The HA is the sole legal entity of public healthcare institutions in Hong Kong. Its chief executive is nominated by the Hospital Authority Board (HAB) and appointed by the Secretary for Health, Welfare and Food.

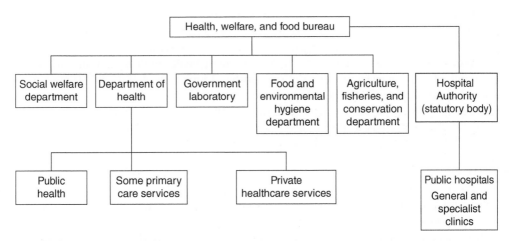

FIGURE 14.1   Organizational structure of healthcare administration in Hong Kong.

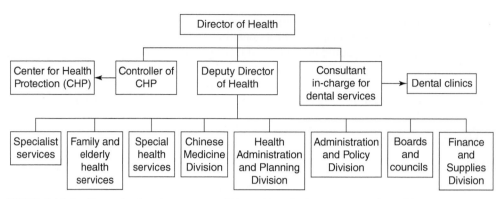

FIGURE 14.2 Organizational structure of Hong Kong's Department of Health.

Although the HA is not directly affiliated with the HWFB, the latter still has full administrative authority over the HA and employs strong management approaches to effectively oversee it. First, the chairman and members of the HA's highest governing body – that is, the HAB – are appointed by the chief executive of Hong Kong. Furthermore, both the Secretary for Health, Welfare and Food and the Director of Health are members of the HAB. Second, about 92% of funding for the HA is by the government through the HWFB. Finally, the HA is accountable to the HWFB and must submit quarterly and annual reports.

(2) Health Service System

1. Healthcare Service System The public healthcare institutions affiliated with the HA include 41 public hospitals (27,784 beds), 74 general clinics, and 48 specialist clinics, with a total of 27,784 beds. The most well-known public hospitals in Hong Kong are Tung Wah Hospital, the Sai Ying Pun Jockey Club Polyclinic, and Alice Ho Miu Ling Nethersole Hospital. Public healthcare institutions provide approximately 29% of all outpatient services and 91% of all inpatient services in Hong Kong. On the other hand, the private healthcare institutions of Hong Kong consist of 12 private hospitals (3,438 beds; see Table 14.2) and numerous private clinics, which altogether account for 71% of all outpatient services and 9% of all inpatient services. In addition, there are 31 nursing homes in Hong Kong, which have a total of 2,945 beds. Similar to Germany, hospitals in Hong Kong only provide emergency care and inpatient services; none of them have an outpatient department. Inpatients primarily consist of emergency cases and clinic referrals.

As of the end of 2007, there were 75,800 registered health professionals in Hong Kong, including 119,000 physicians and 37,700 registered nurses (including 4,700 midwives), which is equivalent to 10.94 health professionals (1.73 physicians and 5.34 nurses) per 1,000 people. The physician-to-nurse ratio was 1:3.09. Although the number of physicians per 1,000 people in Hong Kong was less than half that in Shanghai, Hong Kong had a significantly higher number of healthcare workers per 1,000 people and a more reasonable physician-to-nurse ratio.

The HA organizes its 41 hospitals into seven hospital clusters (Table 14.3): Hong Kong East Cluster (7 hospitals), Hong Kong West Cluster (7 hospitals), Kowloon East Cluster (3 hospitals), Kowloon Central Cluster (6 hospitals), Kowloon West Cluster (7 hospitals), New Territories East Cluster (7 hospitals), and New Territories West Cluster (4 hospitals). Each hospital cluster is headed by a Cluster Chief Executive, and includes a large-sized, leading general hospital, several specialist hospitals, and several public clinics. HA funds are

TABLE 14.2 Distribution of the 12 Private Hospitals in Hong Kong

Territory	Number of Hospitals	Names of Hospitals
Hong Kong Island	6	Canossa Hospital (affiliated with Caritas Hong Kong), Matilda International Hospital, Hong Kong Central Hospital, Hong Kong Adventist Hospital, St. Paul's Hospital (colloquially known as the [Hong Kong] French Hospital), and the Hong Kong Sanatorium and Hospital
Kowloon	4	Precious Blood Hospital (affiliated with Caritas Hong Kong), Evangel Hospital, St. Teresa's Hospital (colloquially known as the [Kowloon] French Hospital), and Hong Kong Baptist Hospital
New Territories	2	Hong Kong Adventist Hospital – Tsuen Wan and Shatin International Medical Center Union Hospital

TABLE 14.3 Seven Regional Hospital Clusters under the Hong Kong Hospital Authority

Cluster	Number of Hospitals	Cluster Hospitals
Hong Kong East Cluster	7	Pamela Youde Nethersole Eastern Hospital, Tung Wah Eastern Hospital, Tang Shiu Kin Hospital, Ruttonjee Hospital, St. John Hospital, Cheshire Home (Chung Hom Kok), and Wong Chuk Hang Hospital
Hong Kong West Cluster	7	Tsan Yuk Hospital (Obstetrics), Tung Wah Hospital, Tung Wah Group of Hospitals Fung Yiu King Hospital, The Duchess of Kent Children's Hospital at Sandy Bay, MacLehose Medical Rehabilitation Center, Grantham Hospital, and Queen Mary Hospital
Kowloon East Cluster	3	United Christian Hospital (Kwun Tong), Haven of Hope Hospital (located in Tseung Kwan O), and Tseung Kwan O Hospital
Kowloon Central Cluster	6	Queen Elizabeth Hospital, Kowloon Hospital, Hong Kong Buddhist Hospital, Hong Kong Red Cross Blood Transfusion Service, Hong Kong Eye Hospital, and Rehab-aid Center
Kowloon West Cluster	7	Kwong Wah Hospital, Tung Wah Group of Hospitals Wong Tai Sin Hospital, Our Lady of Maryknoll Hospital, Caritas Medical Center (Cheung Sha Wan), Princess Margaret Hospital, Kwai Chung Hospital (Psychiatrics), and Yan Chai Hospital (Tsuen Wan)
New Territories East Cluster	7	Cheshire Home Shatin, Bradbury Hospice, Shatin Hospital, Alice Ho Miu Ling Nethersole Hospital (Tai Po), Tai Po Hospital, North District Hospital, and Prince of Wales Hospital
New Territories West Cluster	4	Tuen Mun Hospital, Pok Oi Hospital (Yuen Long), Castle Peak Hospital (Psychiatrics), and Siu Lam Hospital (Psychiatrics)

Note: Queen Mary Hospital (Li Ka Shing Faculty of Medicine, University of Hong Kong) is located in Pok Fu Lam, Hong Kong West; Prince of Wales Hospital is a teaching hospital (affiliated with the Faculty of Medicine of the Chinese University of Hong Kong) located in Ma Liu Shui, the Sha Tin District, New Territories East.

allocated to individual healthcare institutions through these hospital clusters. Each cluster manages its own resource allocation, and there is a clear division of functions among its healthcare institutions, with no overlap in departments. Additionally, each cluster has one hospital dedicated to the provision of rehabilitation services.

2. Disease Prevention and Control   The DH is responsible for disease prevention and control in Hong Kong. Since the outbreak of severe acute respiratory syndrome (SARS), the HA has attached great importance to the prevention and treatment of infectious diseases. Recently, the HA has begun focusing on the development of community-oriented healthcare services and disease prevention because of the financial burden caused by greater healthcare expenditure. To further enhance the prevention and control of diseases in Hong Kong, the Center for Health Protection (CHP) was established under the DH in June 2004. It comprises six branches: Surveillance & Epidemiology Branch, Infection Control Branch, Public Health Laboratory Services Branch, Public Health Services Branch, Emergency Response and Information Branch, and Program Management and Professional Development Branch. The functions of the CHP can be summarized as the "3Rs" – real-time surveillance, rapid intervention, and responsive risk communication. Specifically, this involves the surveillance of infectious diseases; formulating strategies for controlling communicable diseases; formulating risk communication strategies; establishing partnerships with healthcare professionals, community organizations, scholars, other government agencies, and local and international agencies to jointly control infectious diseases; formulating and reviewing contingency plans to effectively cope with the outbreak of communicable diseases; formulating, supporting, implementing, and assessing initiatives for the prevention and control of such diseases (including nosocomial infections); and outlining applied research to support the prevention and control of infectious diseases. In the long term, the CHP is also striving to attain control over the management of environmental risks and noncommunicable diseases.

(3) Incentive Mechanisms for Healthcare Workers

1. Types of Healthcare Workers   Physicians in Hong Kong can be categorized into medical officers (MO), senior medical officers (SMO), and consultants (CONS). Medical graduates who have obtained a medical license by passing the qualifying examination are granted the title of "Doctor of Medicine" and can serve in hospitals as MOs. After three years of clinical practice, they are eligible for a three-year specialist training program (pending their passing a qualifying examination), six months to two years of which will be spent studying abroad. Upon completing this program, they are considered qualified specialists but still have the title of MO. Specialists can be promoted to become SMOs, and subsequently CONS, depending on the availability of job vacancies.

   Nurses in Hong Kong can be categorized into student nurses (SNs), enrolled nurses (ENs), and registered nurses (RNs). Students who have enrolled in nursing schools are known as SNs. They become ENs after graduating from nursing school and RNs after passing the qualifying examination. Practicing nurses can be promoted to specialist nurses, but will still have the title of RN. On the other hand, nurses who perform management duties can be promoted to the position of chief nurse, ward nurse manager, department nurse manager, or general manager (nursing).

2. Economic Incentive Measures   Prior to the establishment of the HA, there was no standardized salary system for healthcare workers. Healthcare workers in government-run public hospitals were paid on a monthly basis in accordance with the salary structure of civil servants and were entitled to civil service benefits, such as paid vacations, travel, education for their children, housing subsidies, medical subsidies, and pensions. On the other hand, there was no standardized salary structure for healthcare workers in hospitals operated by religious or charitable organizations. Furthermore, they generally had lower salaries than did those in government-run hospitals.

After the HA took over control of public hospitals, a standardized salary system was established for healthcare workers in 1993. Although hospital staff members in government-run public hospitals were given the freedom to choose between the new salary system and the salary structure of civil servants, about 60% chose the former. Furthermore, this new salary system was adopted by hospitals operated by religious and charitable organizations. This new system was formulated based on actuarial methods. The original civil service benefits were abolished, and all salary payments are now made in cash. The salary can be divided into three parts: (1) *Basic salary*, which is similar to the standards used for civil servants, whereby hospital staff members are provided with a salary based on a fixed framework according to their pay grade, which changes annually. Hospital staff members are grouped into 49 pay grades based on their position. (2) *Additional allowance (cash allowance)*, which is based on the original civil service benefits; it is calculated as a percentage of the basic salary of healthcare workers. (3) *Special allowances*, which are used to compensate staff for performing special tasks, such as the Extraneous Duties Allowances, Hardship Allowance, Shift Duty Allowance, and Typhoon Allowance.

3. Characteristics of Economic Incentive Mechanisms

1. *Clearly defined standards.* Public hospitals in Hong Kong have clearly defined salary standards for healthcare workers, with a standardized salary range for different positions and standardized criteria for salary increases. Furthermore, the salary system is highly transparent, such that hospital staff members are well aware of not only their own salary standards but also those of other staff members.
2. *Salaries unaffected by hospital revenues.* The salaries of healthcare workers in Hong Kong's public hospitals are funded by the government, and thus are unaffected by the operation, cost, and price of the healthcare services provided in hospitals. There are no bonuses or gray income for healthcare workers in public hospitals.
3. *Wide income gap between physicians and nurses.* For instance, in 1998, a newly graduated nurse earned approximately HK$23,000 per month, whereas a newly graduated physician earned approximately HK$55,000 per month. The incomes of the highest-paid nurses and physicians were approximately HK$42,000 and HK$118,000 per month, respectively. Although the incomes of both nurses and physicians have since increased, there is still a clear gap between them.

(4) Centralized Drug Procurement

1. Methods and Procedures for Drug Procurement   The HA spent a total of HK$2.38 billion on pharmaceutical expenditures in 2008–2009, which accounted for 8% of its total expenditure. This is considered low when compared to other countries in the world. The ability of the HA to meet the healthcare demands of residents to the maximum extent under a limited budget is inseparable from its drug procurement policy. According to the procurement system of the Hong Kong government, all government departments can directly purchase items costing less than HK $50,000 per year, whereas items costing more than this amount are subject to centralized procurement by the government. Commonly used items are purchased by the Government Supplies Department, whereas special items are purchased by the respective government departments (or their affiliated public agencies). For example, vehicles are purchased by the Government Fleet Division, ships are purchased by the Hong Kong Marine Department, and drugs used in hospitals are purchased by the HA using the following drug procurement methods.

1. *Direct purchase.* Drugs that cost less than HK$50,000 per year can be directly purchased by the respective hospitals in compliance with the Material Supply and Management Manual issued by the government of the Hong Kong SAR. From 2007 to 2008, the hospitals in Hong Kong directly procured a total of 1,702 types of drugs, accounting for 54% of all types of drugs used in hospitals. However, the cost of drugs purchased directly accounted for only about 7% of the total pharmaceutical expenditure.
2. *Standing quotation, that is, competitive negotiation.* For drugs that cost less than HK$1 million per year, the HA collects information on their overall utilization and invites suppliers to provide quotations. Then, the HA determines the pricing and suppliers for drug procurement via negotiations, thereby reducing the costs that could have arisen from separate negotiations by individual hospitals. From 2007 to 2008, the hospitals in Hong Kong purchased a total of 603 types of drugs via centralized bidding, which accounted for 19.3% of all types of drugs used in hospitals and 21% of the total pharmaceutical expenditure.
3. *Bulk supplies contract, that is, centralized tendering and procurement.* Drugs that cost more than HK$1 million per year are purchased via tendering. Brand-name drugs are purchased through sole-source procurement, whereas generic drugs are purchased via open tendering, mostly using a two-year contract. The HA considers tendering the most suitable procurement approach for achieving the economies of scale and maximizing cost-effectiveness. The HA attaches particular importance to the openness and fairness of the procurement process and encourages competition among suppliers. It also requires suppliers to offer the highest possible discounts via centralized procurement. Furthermore, the HA imposes penalties on suppliers for breach of contract to ensure the quality of the drugs provided. From 2007 to 2008, hospitals in Hong Kong purchased a total of 634 types of drugs via bulk supply contracts, which accounted for 20.3% of all types of drugs used in hospitals and about 72% of the total pharmaceutical expenditure. The HA is relatively flexible with regard to procurement approaches, which are essentially selected based on the volume of drugs used. The procurement approach is changed when the amount of drugs used in the previous year exceeds the acceptable range of the original procurement approach. Regardless of the procurement approach used, the HA has strict requirements for ensuring the quality of drugs.

There are four departments or agencies under the HA that are responsible for the tendering and procurement of drugs. They adhere to the following basic procedures (Figure 14.3): (1) The Chief Pharmacist's Office assesses the types and quality of drugs, and proposes the items for tendering; (2) The Central Drug Procurement Section is responsible for formulating and implementing the procurement procedures; (3) The Tender Evaluation Team is responsible for verifying, appraising, and recommending the tenders; and (4) The Central Tender Board approves the recommended tender.

2. Quality Management and Strategies in Procurement
1. *Risk management of drug quality.* During the tendering process, the HA determines (1) the drug safety signals for overseeing drug use in clinical practice; and (2) the drug recall mechanism, whereby suppliers must recall drugs with quality issues and must clearly state the recall location, recall timing, and compensation method

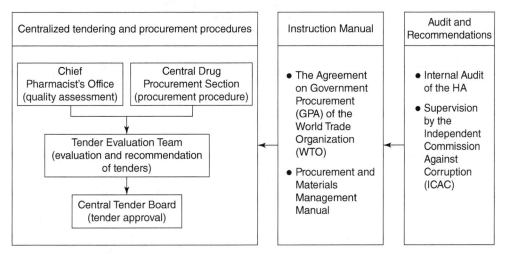

FIGURE 14.3 Division of functions and procedures for the centralized tendering and procurement of the Hong Kong HA.

during the tendering process. The HA can request detailed quality information of drugs they intend to purchase, including manufacturer information, drug registration information, past sales data, and other detailed quality-related data. According to the "WHO Certification Scheme on the Quality of Pharmaceutical Products Moving in International Commerce," the HA can request suppliers to submit supplementary reports on whether a given generic drug has the same efficacy as its brand name counterpart. In addition, the HA has also established the Drug Selection Committee (DSC), which works independently to evaluate the quality of drugs. The quality management of purchased drugs is mainly carried out via the periodic sampling of contract drugs for quality testing. Moreover, the HA has established a drug complaint system, whereby in-depth and detailed testing is conducted in a timely manner on drug samples that have received complaints, in order to prevent possible quality issues. In addition, the HA carries out long-term monitoring of international drug information and promptly takes the relevant steps in Hong Kong once quality-related issues are reported for a certain drug elsewhere in the world.

2. *Drug procurement strategies.* The HA strives to remain up to date with the current market and adjusts its procurement strategies accordingly. Suppliers of generic drugs are selected via open tendering, whereas brand-name drugs are purchased via centralized, sole-source procurement based on the total amount of drugs used. The HA also pays close attention to the price trends of brand-name drugs that have the same therapeutic effect. Brand-name drugs with low or rapidly declining prices are prioritized and purchased in bulk.

For brand-name drugs with expired patents, but for which the preparation processes and other technologies remain under patent protection, the HA carries out an investigation of the feasibility of shifting to their generic counterparts. This survey involves the following:

1. Proactively check the structure and the term of the patents for the brand name and generic drugs
2. Assess the risks associated with shifting to the use of the generic drug

3. Seek foreign patent attorneys to evaluate the risks
4. Request disclaimer protection from the contracted suppliers

The HA adopts the use of the generic drug as soon as possible if this survey reveals that no issue will arise from doing so. This process is known as a "gray zone survey" and is one of the key cost containment measures. For example, the molecular patent of simvastatin expired in 2003, and its generic counterpart appeared the same year. The HA immediately launched a gray zone survey, which revealed that it would be feasible to begin widespread use of the generic counterpart. As a result, around HK$23 million was saved in the year following the shift, representing an 80% decrease in expenses compared to the previous year. In addition, the shift from atorvastatin to generic simvastatin saved a total of HK$15 million.

The HA also attaches great importance to the use of information technology to improve its procurement procedures. It has created online drug formulary guidelines and established a computerized outpatient prescriptions entry system to obtain comprehensive data for drug procurement. These data are especially useful for analyzing current drug use trends in order to select the appropriate procurement approach. The prescription entry system also helps to enhance supervision and ensure that hospitals comply with the appropriate regulations and standards for the utilization and purchase of drugs. Furthermore, it also can facilitate auditing and oversight by improving the drug risk management mechanism.

2. Reforms in Public Hospital Management

(1) Reform Background

Prior to the establishment of the HA, the British authorities in Hong Kong played the dual roles of manager and owner for all public hospitals. Hospitals were directly funded and administered by the Hospital Services Department, and all employees of public hospitals were considered to be civil servants. However, the Hospital Services Department faced various issues, such as poor hospital management, low patient satisfaction, and the wastage and inadequacy of healthcare resources. These issues attracted the attention of the British authorities, who then began actively reforming Hong Kong's healthcare system.

In 1985, the British authorities in Hong Kong commissioned the Australian consultancy firm, WD Scott & Co to review Hong Kong's hospital administrative system. That same year, WD Scott & Co published a report entitled "The Delivery of Medical Services in Hospitals," which suggested that the British authorities in Hong Kong lacked flexibility and were also restricted by the Civil Service Regulations. Furthermore, subvented hospitals perceived that they were being treated unfairly. The report made several recommendations to the British authorities, including establishing an independently-administered hospital system, recovering the costs of hospital services, and increasing the number of higher class wards (Class B), followed by establishing a hospital authority separate from the government framework and civil service system that oversees the public healthcare system, abolishing regional offices, and delegating greater authority to hospitals. The government was also advised to introduce the CEO system to hospitals, enhance social supervision, and introduce a modern management system and relevant talents, in order to improve the service quality and operational efficiency of hospitals. After three years of public consultation, the British authorities in Hong Kong promulgated the Hospital Authority Ordinance.

In 1989, the provisional HA released a report proposing to recover 15–20% of the cost of hospital services. In the following year, the Hong Kong government published a report entitled "Health for All, the Way Ahead: Report of the Working Party on Primary Health

Care," which reiterated the government's healthcare policy – "no one should be prevented through lack of means from obtaining adequate healthcare services." The HA was officially established on December 1, 1990, to take over public hospitals and related healthcare institutions, which were previously administered by the DH. It is now the second-largest public agency after the government.

(2) Functions and Missions of the HA

1. Functions of the HA   The main functions of the HA are as follows: (1) Provide recommendations to the government regarding the public demand for hospital services and the necessary resources for meeting those demands. (2) Provide recommendations to the Secretary for Health, Welfare, and Food on appropriate fees for the public's use of hospital services. (3) Establish public hospitals. (4) Administer and develop the public hospital system. (5) Promote, assist, and participate in the education and training of HA staff, as well as research on hospital services. The HA has delegated the authority for decision making and resource allocation to hospitals, such that the hospital directors are responsible for resource allocation, administration, service development, routine operations, and financial management.

2. Missions of the HA   The main missions of the HA are as follows: (1) To provide appropriate public hospital services to meet the different healthcare needs of patients, and to improve the hospital environment with patients' best interests in mind. (2) To create the image that hospitals are dedicated to caring and serving their patients, highly efficient, committed to making the best use of resources, and highly cooperative, thereby encouraging public's participation in hospital affairs and making hospitals more directly accountable to the public. (3) To provide reasonable remuneration, fair treatment, and a challenging work environment for all employees, in order to attract, motivate, and retain high-quality and efficient talent. (4) To advise the government on the provision of adequate, internationally recognized, high-quality, and highly efficient public hospital services based on the demand for public hospital services and the necessary resources for meeting this demand. (5) To collaborate with both foreign and local healthcare agencies and other related organizations in order to benefit the people of Hong Kong.

(3) Governance Framework of the HA

1. Hospital Authority Board (HAB)   The HAB is the highest governing body of the HA, whose chairman and members are directly appointed by the government of the Hong Kong SAR. HAB members come from all walks of life, including entrepreneurs, deans of medical schools, public officials, legal professionals, community representatives, and so on. According to the Hospital Authority Ordinance, the HA must have a chairman, who is not a civil servant; no more than 3 civil servants and 4 chief administrative staff; and no more than 23 other members, none of whom are civil servants. In addition to the chairman, the HA currently comprises 25 members (including the Chief Executive); among whom, the representatives of public officials are the Director of Health, the Secretary for Health, Welfare and Food, and the Secretary for Financial Services and the Treasury. There are 11 committees under the HAB: the Audit and Risk Committee, Finance Committee, Human Resources Committee, Information Technology Services Governing Committee, Medical Services Development Committee, Supporting Services Development Committee, Public Complaints Committee, Staff Appeals Committee, Executive Committee, Central Tender Board, and Emergency Executive Committee.

2. Regional Advisory Committees (RACs) There are three RACs in Hong Kong, including the Hong Kong Regional Advisory Committee, the Kowloon Regional Advisory Committee, and the New Territories Regional Advisory Committee. Each RAC comprises HAB members, representatives of the Director of Health, community members, and hospital representatives. RACs are primarily responsible for advising the HA on healthcare demands in their respective regions. The Chief Executive of the HA and hospital administrators in each region must report regularly to these RACs.

3. Hospital Governing Committees (HGCs) There are currently 38 HA-affiliated hospitals with HGCs. These committees serve as the boards of directors of these hospitals and are responsible for reviewing the periodic management reports submitted by the chief administrative officer (CAO) of the hospitals, monitoring the hospitals' operational and financial performance, participating in the decision-making and governance functions of hospitals, and organizing hospital and community partnership activities. Hospital CAOs must regularly report to the HGCs.

4. Head Office The Head Office is the main body of the HA responsible for determining its policy orientation and coordinating overall strategic planning, management, and support. The Head Office is headed by the Chief Executive and comprises eight divisions: the Cluster Services Division, the Quality and Safety Division, the Strategy and Planning Division, the Finance Division, the Corporate Services Division, the Human Resources Division, the Information Technology and Health Informatics Division, and the Group Internal Audit. The overall functions of the Head Office include governance support, institutional development, and implementation of shared services and professional development training. There are eight senior leadership positions under the Chief Executive: Director of Cluster Services, Director of Strategy and Planning, Director of Quality and Safety, Director of Finance, Head of Corporate Services, Head of Human Resources, Chief Internal Auditor, and Head of Information Technology and Health Informatics.

5. Clusters and Hospitals The HA has organized all public hospitals into seven clusters based on their geographical locations; each cluster comprises three to seven hospitals and is headed by a Cluster Chief Executive, who is usually also the director of the leading hospital within that cluster. The Cluster Chief Executive is assisted by a service executive and a cluster manager in performing various tasks related to medical affairs, financial affairs, human resources, nursing, and support services. Each hospital is headed by a CAO (equivalent to the hospital president), who is assisted by a general manager and managers of various hospital affairs.

The management framework of Hong Kong's HA is shown in Figure 14.4.

(4) Operational Strategies of the HA

The overall objective of the HA is to establish a coherent healthcare system via joint efforts with other community healthcare agencies, in order to achieve the best healthcare outcomes and meet the healthcare demands and expectations of the community. To this end, the HA has formulated five operational strategies.

1. Establishing an Outcome-Based Healthcare System This strategy involves formulating guidelines for the allocation of healthcare resources based on the health status

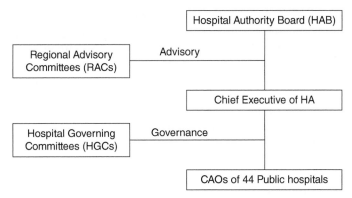

FIGURE 14.4 Regulatory framework of Hong Kong's HA.

and healthcare needs of the public, in order to provide healthcare services in a systematic, step-by-step manner and thereby achieve optimal outcomes with limited healthcare resources. The first step in this strategy is to identify the health status and healthcare needs of the public. To do this, the HA obtains information about "killer diseases" affecting the residents of Hong Kong via the public hospital information system, which provides a clear focus for understanding healthcare issues. This is followed by analyzing the main factors affecting health and years of potential life lost (YPLLs) to identify the problems that must be prioritized.

2. Establishing a Coherent Healthcare System   Healthcare services in Hong Kong are divided into primary, secondary, and tertiary services, which also include emergency care services and continuing care services (i.e., rehabilitation and long-term hospitalization). Among them, secondary and tertiary healthcare services are mostly provided by the HA, whereas primary healthcare services are mainly provided by private healthcare institutions (which also perform a small proportion of secondary and tertiary services). On the other hand, continuing care services are almost entirely performed by the HA. Given these circumstances, the HA formulated this strategy to form a cooperative network with other healthcare providers (including patients' families, community groups, welfare groups, private organizations, and so on) to provide patients with more comprehensive, coherent healthcare services.

3. Collaborating with the Community in Decision Making and Provision of Healthcare Services   The Hospital Authority Ordinance clearly stipulates that community representatives must be included in each HA committee in order to ensure that healthcare administrators regularly interact with the public and strive to enhance their mutual understanding. The HA committees include hundreds of independent members of the public with varying expertise, backgrounds, experience, and perspectives. These members influence and participate in the decision-making processes of the HA, and have helped reduce the gap between hospitals and communities. The HA also regularly reviews the public's viewpoints and patients' satisfaction with healthcare services. There are special teams consisting of managers and healthcare workers at both the Head Office and within individual hospitals to investigate, follow-up, and reply to each complaint received in order to maintain the public's satisfaction with healthcare services. Additionally, these complaints also serve as a basis for service improvement and the formulation of administrative policies by the HA.

4. Providing Comprehensive Healthcare Services and Continuous Quality Improvement (CQI) Via Multidisciplinary Collaboration   This strategy aims to focus on the development of first-line healthcare service teams and equip them with the necessary expertise and skills to provide patients with comprehensive healthcare services by introducing concepts and training related to modern healthcare management and adopting multidisciplinary collaboration. HA managers have recognized that the success of the HA is dependent on an organizational culture that promotes teamwork and CQI. Hence, the HA encourages staff to engage in CQI in all aspects of their work. As mentioned above, the majority of hospitals under the HA have their own HGCs, whose decision-making and discussion mechanisms are highly conducive to the implementation of this strategy.

5. Promoting the Development and Innovation of Infrastructure to Support Service Improvement   Besides being committed to the development of medical technologies, the HA pays close attention to the development and innovation of infrastructure. For example, it strives to systematically improve hospital facilities and management to ensure patients' comfort and convenience; ensures the strict compliance of all basic projects to various quality assurance procedures and introduces health and safety management standards; develops and improves the medical information system to provide clinical decision support to healthcare workers; reforms logistical support services to improve the service quality and cost-effectiveness of public hospitals; and formulates a standardized financial management information system to increase the consistency of internal data standards, thus facilitating interhospital comparison as well as more effective planning and management of healthcare resources.

3. New Development Ideas of the Hospital Authority

(1) Introduction of Corporatized Management

Learning from the reform experiments of the public sector in other countries, the government of the Hong Kong SAR has attempted to combine the advantages of public and private sectors. Under the guidance of the World Bank's theoretical framework of the four organization types (government budget units, independent operating units, enterprise units, and corporate units), the government hoped to achieve the following outcomes through the corporatization of the HA: more flexible responses to social changes; increased efficiency and competitive enthusiasm; introduction of advanced management methods; establishment of market and consumer cultures; introduction of cost concept, saving incentives, and social supervision; and effective sharing of government responsibilities.

1. Reform Process   The corporatization of the HA was achieved through the following processes: implementation of various legislative procedures; introduction of the three levels of governance in social supervision (central, territorial, and hospital levels); transfer of management rights by the government and charitable organizations but retention of governance rights; continued government control of overall funding, fee standards, and healthcare policies; and delegating specific operations, such as remuneration, job titles, staffing, financial usage, service development, and accident compensation, to the discretion of the HA.

2. Separation of Governance and Management   The separation of governance and management in the healthcare service management system of Hong Kong is reflected on two levels: At the macro level, the HWFB is responsible for policy and fund governance, while the HA is responsible for hospital management, policy implementation, and service delivery. At the micro level, this separation is manifested within the HA itself. The HAB is responsible for governing the orientation and strategy of the HA, whereas the administrative staff members are responsible for the management of services and policies. Through the accountability system, the administrative staff report to the HAB, while the HA reports to the HWFB.

3. Ample Delegation of Authority　Hospital clusters are collectively administered by the HA, but are given ample authority. The Cluster Chief Executive can determine the allocation of healthcare resources in their region to more clearly define the roles of each hospital in the cluster, thereby ensuring that they support and complement each other through mutual cooperation. Thus, hospitals within each cluster can be further categorized, based on the nature of their services, into emergency and rehabilitation hospitals, and one or two rehabilitation hospitals are located within the vicinity of each emergency hospital. According to this collective management model, the Cluster Chief Executive acts as a chief executive officer, while the directors of each hospital are like chief business officers. Each cluster also delegates extensive authority to the CAO in each hospital to ensure that administrators have the power to address problems themselves during the delivery of frontline services.

4. New Culture of Corporatized Management　This involves: clearly defined authority and responsibilities; flexible allocation of government funding by the Cluster Chief Executive; giving hospitals a certain level of authority over human resources and financial management within a specific budget range; open recruitment for all administrative positions, with contractual terms and annual performance assessment; the accountability of the administrative team to the governance framework (i.e., social supervision); and the responsibility of the Head Office for planning, supervision, business support, and ensuring fairness in human resource management.

(2) Advocating for a Patient-Centered Culture

1. Introducing the Customer Concept　Hospitals have allowed customers to participate in the establishment of quality standards and strive to respect their dignity, privacy, environment, attitudes, interpretations, choices, and accessibility.

2. Establishing a Complete Patient Complaint System　Hospitals have created a full-time position for a patient relations manager, established the Patient's Charter and implemented a two-tier complaints-handling mechanism.

3. Staff Training　Hospitals try to put themselves in patients' shoes to understand patients' needs, and to conduct staff training for etiquette and communication skills.

4. Hardware Support　Hospitals have added sufficient signage and screens for patients, and have improved the hospital environment by adding air-conditioning, convenience stores, higher-quality building materials, and emergency exits.

5. Measures that Benefit the Public　Hospitals have improved the appointment system, shortened waiting times, improved hospital bed utilization, and reduced overcrowding in hospital wards.

6. Holistic Therapy Hospitals pay greater attention to continuity of treatment, community followups, and the psychological and social needs of their patients.

(3) Improving Productivity and Efficiency

1. Full Utilization of Hospital Beds and Facilities Hospitals complement each other in order to reduce duplication. Furthermore, there is a clear division of functions between emergency and rehabilitation hospitals to establish clinical referral relationships.

2. Cost Reduction via Collective Procurement The HA has adopted centralized procurement using a standard drug formulary, employed collective procurement for consumables, and has exercised strict control over the purchase of large equipment, selecting standard equipment models to tender multiyear contracts.

3. Closing, Merging, and Relocating Urban Hospitals The HA has to continually cope with opposition from residents, employees, and HGCs. Furthermore, it organizes the closing and merging of hospitals to increase their cost-effectiveness.

4. Hospital Cluster System The HA has organized all public hospitals in Hong Kong into seven clusters to promote synergy; the administrative and support departments have been streamlined; and hospitals have taken over and utilized regional public clinics to reduce their own burden and enhance community care.

5. Strategic Planning The HA reviews its objectives and social functions; inspects data trends and makes predictions; discusses its own strengths, weaknesses, opportunities, and threats (SWOT analysis); and formulates its main strategies.

6. Annual Planning The HA utilizes multifunctional management tools, including work planning, financial planning, improvement tools, and accountability tools; responds to key strategies and ideas; examines its achievements and failures over the previous year; and lists the plans and measurable goals for the coming year. The HA is a large-scale agency that relies on highly standardized operations. The operating expenses of each hospital cluster are funded by the Head Office, thus unifying the procurement of medical supplies (e.g., medical equipment and drugs) and support services (e.g., food production and material chain management). Furthermore, the HA utilizes the same set of regulations (financial, personnel-related, and so on) and information platform to reduce duplicate resource allocation and improve its overall efficiency.

7. Enhanced Productivity Program (EPP) Based on the assumption that there is always room for improvement in productivity, the budget allocation for hospitals can be reduced by 1–3% each year to enhance competition among hospitals for marginal resources via new programs. Furthermore, the HA has established an internal audit system to prevent fraud and provides a platform for mutual learning of advanced practices.

(4) CQI Implementation

1. Public Welfare Nature of Public Hospitals The role of public hospitals is to provide high-quality healthcare services to the public, rather than to profit hospitals or physicians. Furthermore, the role of public healthcare services is not only to achieve effective therapy during hospitalization but also to improve the health status of the overall population. Integrated and coherent treatments, community care, quality of life, and patient choice are becoming increasingly important due to the rise in population aging and the prevalence of chronic diseases.

2. Quality Concepts of the HA   The HA has adopted the following quality concepts: the customer concept, which includes internal customers; collaboration with other caregivers to establish a coherent healthcare system; cultivation of CQI to reduce medical errors, improve medical procedures, measure healthcare outcomes, and establish a continuous improvement cycle; and combining CQI with planning and performance assessment systems.

3. Macro-level Measures for Quality Improvement   The macro-level measures include the aforementioned patient-centered measures; establishment (or relocation) of hospitals and clinics to new towns to reduce regional disparities; extended availability of limited, high-end healthcare services (e.g., brain surgery) in all hospitals throughout Hong Kong via clinical relationships; use of EPP for resource allocation to improve rehabilitation and emergency services, as well as conserving healthcare resources and applying for new funds to develop community care services for the elderly and psychiatric patients.

4. Regulated Leadership   Regulated leadership involves overcoming inadequate coordination among hospitals; unifying the information system to make patients' medical records available to all hospitals; centrally controlling hospitals' operational/financial information; utilizing collective procurement of drugs and instruments; implementing a hospital cluster system based on geographical location to enable complementarity of services and avoid vicious competition among hospitals; and releasing an overall work plan each year that details the status of healthcare resources and establishing measurable quality objectives for the coming year, and requiring explanations if these objectives are not achieved.

4. Health Security System

(1) Healthcare Funding System

The healthcare expenditure of Hong Kong increased from HK$67.565 billion in 2003 to HK$73 billion in 2008. In 2008, the public healthcare expenditure was HK$37.4 billion, accounting for 14.3% of total government expenditure and 2.3% of GDP. The private healthcare expenditure in Hong Kong was about HK$35.6 billion, which is comparable to that of public healthcare. Private expenditure was mainly attributed to the medical expenses incurred by private hospitals and clinics.

In 2008, the HA earned a total of HK$30.4 billion, of which 92% came from the government's allocated budget, 6% from healthcare service charges, and 2% from other income sources (including nonhealthcare income and social donations). This tax-funded, welfare-oriented healthcare system ensures the equal access of taxpayers to healthcare services that are nearly free of charge, and thus reflects a higher level of fairness and accessibility. The HA spent about 80% of its income on salaries and the remaining 20% on other items, such as drugs and medical equipment.

The HA experienced a fiscal deficit for the first time in 2001. In 2004, its fiscal deficit reached approximately HK$374 million. The chief executive of the HA, William Ho Shiu-wei, stated that the cumulative fiscal deficit of the HA would reach HK$7.3 billion by 2008–2009 if the public healthcare expenditure remained unchanged over the next few years.

In 2009, the actual expenditure of the HA reached HK$36.6 billion, while the government budget allocation to the HA was only HK$32.7272 billion.

The Health Protection System of Hong Kong is based on the UK NHS. Public healthcare institutions in Hong Kong charge very low medical fees (Table 14.4). For instance, emergency departments charge only HL$100 per admission (since 2002, previously free of charge), while specialist clinics charge HK$100 for the first visit and HK$60 for each subsequent visit. From May 1, 2003, patients who seek medical attention at specialist clinics, children's assessment centers, genetic counseling clinics, or AIDS clinics are charged HK$10 each for the visit. Inpatient rehabilitation and psychiatric care services cost HK$68 per day, but inpatients with financial difficulties can apply for fee waivers. Additionally, private GPs charge about HK$150 per visit. Therefore, it is evident that Hong Kong residents enjoy a very high degree of health security; however, this has also placed a heavy financial burden on the government.

(2) Medical Aid (Relief) Policies

1. Fee Relief Mechanisms for Public Hospitals and Clinics   After revising the fee structure in public hospitals and clinics, the HA began to implement its fundamental principle regarding the role of government in healthcare: "no one should be prevented through lack of means from obtaining adequate healthcare services."

Accordingly, patients receiving Comprehensive Social Security Assistance (CSSA) are exempted from medical charges in public medical institutions, provided that they show a valid medical relief certificate issued specifically to CSSA recipients. In addition, to cover three groups of non-CSSA recipients, namely, low-income earners, chronically ill patients, and impoverished elderly patients, the government has formulated measures to enhance the current medical relief mechanism to prevent these groups from experiencing a heavy economic burden. The enhancement of the existing relief mechanism was based on the following principles: (1) Announcement of vulnerable groups that should be the focus

TABLE 14.4   Medical Charges for Eligible Patients in Public Healthcare Institutions

Service	Item	Fee (HK$)	Cost (HK$)	Subsidy Rate (%)
Emergency department		100 per admission	700	86
Inpatient services	Inpatient charges for emergency beds	100 per day*	3790	97
	inpatient charges for other Types of Beds	68 per day	1,460	95
Specialist outpatient services	First visit	100 per admission	530	81
	Subsequent visit	60 per visit	120	89
	Drugs	10 per drug type		92
General outpatient services	First visit/subsequent visits	45 per visit	250	82

Note: *This daily inpatient charge (HK$100) covers the following services: medical consultation, medical tests, nursing care, drugs, accommodation, and three meals a day. The charges for noneligible patients only aim to recover the cost.

of funding and healthcare services that impose a heavy economic burden on patients; (2) Establishment of objective and transparent eligibility criteria for receiving medical relief in public healthcare institutions and consideration of both economic and noneconomic factors when determining these criteria; (3) Ensuring that the enhanced mechanism is accessible to the public while keeping administrative and operating costs low.

Non-CSSA recipients who cannot afford their medical expenses because of financial difficulties may apply for medical relief from the Medical Social Services Units of public hospitals and clinics, as well as the Integrated Family Service Centers or Family and Child Protective Services Units of the Social Welfare Department (SWD). Medical social workers and social workers in the Integrated Family Service Centres (IFSCs) or the Family and Child Protective Services Units (FCPSUs) process these applications and assess the eligibility of applicants on a household basis. Factors considered include the economic, social, and medical conditions of the applicants that can be attributed to their illness.

1. *Economic factors.* Patients meeting both of the following economic criteria can apply for medical relief based on an enhanced mechanism (patients who do not meet these criteria can also provide other factors for consideration to the medical social workers/ SWD social workers): (1) Patient's monthly household income does not exceed 75% of the median monthly household income applicable to their household size (Table 14.5), and (2) patient's household net worth (excluding the self-occupied property of the household) is lower than the specified upper limit applicable to their household size (Table 14.6). In addition, since most elderly members do not have any income and rely on their personal savings, the upper limit of the net worth of households with elderly members is higher than that of households without an elderly member.
2. *Noneconomic factors.* In addition to assessing the patient's economic status in terms of monthly household income and total net worth, the medical social workers/SWD social workers must also take noneconomic factors into consideration. These include (1) the clinical condition of the patient (determined according to the frequency of using public healthcare services and the severity of the illness); (2) whether the patient is a disabled individual, a single parent with dependent children, or a member of another vulnerable group; (3) whether the medical relief can help solve the patient's family issues; (4) whether the patient is facing difficulties in affording public healthcare expenses due to any other special expenses; and (5) other social factors.

TABLE 14.5 Monthly Household Income Based on Household Size (Unit: HK$)

Household Size	Median Monthly Household Income	75% of Median Monthly Household Income	50% of Median Monthly Household Income
1	7,200	5,400	3,600
2	15,000	11,250	7,500
3	20,500	15,375	10,250
4	26,500	19,875	13,250
5	34,100	25,575	17,050
≥6	39,000	29,250	19,500

Source: General Household Survey (GHS) conducted by the Census and Statistics Department (C&SD) as of the third quarter of 2011.

TABLE 14.6 Upper Limit of Household Net Worth for Medical Relief (Unit: HK$)

Household Size	Upper Limit of Net Worth (without Elderly Member)	Upper Limit of Net Worth (with One Elderly Member)	Upper Limit of Net Worth (with Two Elderly Members)
1	30,000	150,000	–
2	60,000	180,000	300,000
3	90,000	210,000	330,000
4	120,000	240,000	360,000
5	150,000	270,000	390,000

Note: The upper limit for the net worth of households with elderly members (aged over 65 years) is increased by about HK$120,000 for each elderly member. In general, patients will be considered for full medical relief if their monthly household incomes do not exceed 50% of the median monthly household income applicable to their household size.

When taking into account the aforementioned noneconomic factors, the medical social workers/SWD social workers aim to ensure that elderly adults and chronically ill patients who regularly use public healthcare services will receive medical relief whenever necessary. Additionally, each application is handled on a case-by-case basis, as it is impossible to list all the relevant social factors. The standards and guidelines for medical relief are reviewed periodically to ensure that all patients in need have access to appropriate healthcare services.

3. *Validity period of medical relief.* Medical relief assessed and approved by medical social workers/SWD social workers may be valid for a single instance or over a certain period. In the latter case, the medical social workers/social workers determine the length of the validity period (maximum of 12 months) based on the actual needs and circumstances of the patient. The medical social workers/SWD social workers also preapprove medical relief for specialist outpatient charges on a case-by-case basis for the convenience of chronically ill patients who must frequently visit specialist outpatient clinics. Additionally, for the convenience of all medical relief recipients, the medical relief certificate issued by medical social workers is applicable not only to the public hospitals/clinics where the patient typically receives inpatient or outpatient services, or where the certificate is issued but also to other hospitals/clinics providing the same services as the HA and DH, including for inpatient services, outpatient services, and community healthcare services.

2. Pharmaceutical Assistance Program of the Samaritan Fund (SF)   The SF was founded to provide financial assistance to patients who must pay for self-financed medical items or new technologies that they require for their treatment, but that are not covered by the medical charges of public hospitals/clinics. Based on the principle of "no one should be prevented through lack of means from obtaining adequate healthcare services," the SF strives to provide as much financial assistance as possible to patients in need.

1. *Eligibility criteria.* To be funded by the SF, the patient must be an HA patient who meets the following criteria. (1) *Clinical criteria.* According to prevailing SF clinical guidelines, the clinical indications and commencement of treatment must be approved by a designated physician. (2) *Residency status.* The patient must be an eligible person based on the definition outlined in the government gazette. (3) *Financial criteria.* The

patient must pass the household-based financial assessment conducted by medical social workers.

2. *Financial assessment.* The financial assessment involves tallying the incomes, expenses, and assets of the patient and family members living in the same household. The annual disposable financial resources are calculated as the sum of the annual household disposable income plus the household's disposable assets. The annual household disposable income is calculated as the annual household gross income minus all allowable deductions. The annual household gross income includes salary, pensions, financial contributions from relatives, income generated from the patient's household assets and properties, and compensations. The Normal Disability Allowance, Higher Disability Allowance, Old Age Allowance, Higher Old Age Living Allowance, and any subsidies and loans from the Financial Assistance Scheme for Post-Secondary Students (FASP) are not considered as part of the household income.

   The allowable deductions include rental or mortgage payments for the previous 12 months, management fees for land taxes, government rent and self-occupied properties (the sum of the above items is capped at 50% of the annual household gross income), payroll taxes, personal allowances for patients and family members in the same household (Table 14.7), child custody expenses, provident fund contributions, school fees for children under the age of 21 years at secondary level or below (other school-related expenses, such as for school activities and accommodation, are not considered allowable deductions), and medical expenses for public hospitals/clinics (except for pharmaceutical expenses subsidized by or for which applications for subsidies have been submitted to the SF and/or Community Care Fund Medical Assistance Program).

3. *Disposable assets.* These include total cash owned by patients and their cohabiting family members during the application as well as their savings accumulated through different methods, investments in stocks and shares, insurance (including investment-linked insurance policies and dividends from life insurance policies, but excluding the cash value under a life insurance policy), valuable possessions, real estate (e.g., land, car parks, and housing units within and outside Hong Kong), lump-sum compensation, and other realizable assets. Self-occupied properties and tools of their trade are excluded from the calculation.

TABLE 14.7 Personal Allowances for Family Members Cohabiting with Patients (Unit: HK$)

Household Size (Number of Family Members)	Total Personal Allowance
Patient (lives alone)	5,540
Patient + 1 cohabiting family member	9,500
Patient + 2 cohabiting family members	12,410
Patient + 3 cohabiting family members	15,620
Patient + 4 cohabiting family members	19,030
Patient + 5 cohabiting family members	21,180
Patient + ≥ 6 cohabiting family members	22,780

Note: Personal allowances are adjusted once every year according to the Consumer Price Index A and every five years according to the latest Household Expenditure Survey conducted by the Census and Statistics Department.

4. *Patients' share of drug expenses.* The patient's share of the drug expenses is determined based on their disposable financial resources and the estimated drug expenses of the year. The latter is determined by multiplying the drug price per unit by the total consumption units. After determining the patient's annual disposable financial resources, the patient's share of drug expenses is capped according to a progressive calculation table. The patient must cover all drug expenses if their estimated drug expenses of the year fall below the maximum payable share, whereas the SF covers any outstanding balance if their estimated drug expenses of the year exceed the maximum payable share.

(3) Characteristics of the Health Security System

1. The Government Mainly Provides Healthcare Services Directly   Public hospitals in Hong Kong are fully funded by the government, and physicians working in these hospitals are entitled to civil service benefits. In other words, public hospitals are government-affiliated, nonprofit institutions with fundamentally different characteristics from institutions that offer social health insurance under a third-party payment system. The direct provision of healthcare services by the government of Hong Kong has prevented the utilization of medical expertise to gain profits, facilitated the implementation of the government's policy guidelines in hospitals, and reduced hospital administrative costs. However, hospitals are also affiliated with the government through the HA, which negotiates with public hospitals on behalf of the public about the funding allocation for the type and scope of services they offer. On the other hand, the HA is also responsible for managing hospitals to ensure their stable operation, while also providing job and welfare protection for hospital employees. Therefore, the HA is the spokesperson for both public healthcare demand and the interests of hospitals and doctors. Unfortunately, when there are conflicts between the interests of hospitals and the public, the HA may favor the interests of the hospitals at the expense of the public due to the superior social, political, and economic status of the medical community.

2. Emphasizing Accessibility and Equality in Healthcare   Accessibility and equality in healthcare are often considered macro-level indicators of a healthcare system. In Hong Kong, the healthcare system places particular emphasis on accessibility and equality. In terms of accessibility, this system has: (1) *policy accessibility*, whereby there is universal coverage of all Hong Kong residents by the healthcare system; and (2) *geographical accessibility*, which ensures that all Hong Kong residents can reach a service site within 30 minutes regardless of where they live and are provided with ambulances to meet their emergency needs in a timely manner. As for equality, in terms of funding, Hong Kong's healthcare system is funded via taxation, which is relatively fair from a social point of view as high-income taxpayers make greater contributions to taxation. In terms of treatment level, all Hong Kong residents pay the same fees and receive the same healthcare services in public hospitals regardless of their economic status. However, from a micro-level perspective, there is inequality in the level of treatment provided by the Hong Kong's healthcare system as charging the same for medical services across all income levels implies that differing degrees of burden will be placed on households with different income levels.

3. Funding Allocation Based on Hospital Services   The DH and HA are fully aware of the importance of health education and primary healthcare services and have made significant improvements to health education and health promotion in Hong Kong. However, the development of primary healthcare services is currently unsatisfactory because of the small number of primary healthcare workers, especially family medicine specialists – presently, there are only about 120 qualified family medicine specialists in Hong Kong. In addition, the general public still prefers seeking medical attention in hospitals because of their overall lack of understanding of the advantages of family medicine. Many community healthcare services in Hong Kong, such as health promotion and health education, still rely on hospitals. Additionally, the needs of hospitals are often prioritized when establishing development plans and allocating resources for healthcare services. This hospital-centered service provision has naturally facilitated the development of hospitals. In recent years, the numbers of inpatients and emergency outpatients have experienced double-digit increases in growth rates. This has increased the work pressure of healthcare workers, which has hampered the overall quality improvement in healthcare services. In addition, healthcare funding has not yet achieved the maximum benefits for Hong Kong residents.

5. Hong Kong's Health System Reforms in the Twenty-First Century

(1) Emerging Trends and Issues

1. Challenges Caused by Population Aging   The challenges brought by population aging cannot be ignored: In 2005, Hong Kong had 834,700 residents aged over 65 years, which increased to 890,350 in 2009 and 912,100 in 2010. It is estimated that in the next two decades, there will be one elderly adult (aged over 65 years) out of every four Hong Kong residents. The trends in population growth and aging in Hong Kong are shown in Figure 14.5. The most significant consequences of population aging are increasing healthcare expenditure, fiscal deficits, and increasing pressure arising from a greater demand for healthcare services, resource exhaustion, and a greater burden of disease.

2. Fiscal Deficit Crisis Facing the HA   There are three main reasons for the fiscal deficit facing the HA: (1) Population aging and medical advancement have led to an increase in healthcare demands. In 1999–2003, the growth rate of the elderly population was four times that of the total population of Hong Kong. Moreover, the HA's average medical expenditure for the elderly population was six times that of patients under the age of 65 years. (2) As a result of the 1997 Asian financial crisis, public expenditure of Hong Kong has been reduced due to government budget cuts. The HA has estimated that healthcare demand will increase by around 2.5% each year on average (excluding the impact of technological advancement), whereas the healthcare budget has only increased by 1% over the past three years. In fact, in 2004–2005, the budget was even reduced by HK$960 million compared to that in 2003–2004. In 2009–2010, the government of Hong Kong budgeted HK$32.7272 billion for healthcare. (3) Hong Kong has a high level of health protection – 80% for outpatient services, 98% for inpatient services, and 100% for emergency care services, as well as certain psychiatric services and services for individuals with intellectual disability. This has led to the overutilization of healthcare resources.

3. Greater Pressure Facing Public Healthcare Institutions in Service Delivery   In recent years, the gradually strengthening management practices of the HA have greatly improved the service quality of public healthcare institutions, thereby leading to an increase in their market share from 85% to 94%; accordingly, the share of the healthcare market for private hospitals has shrunk. As a result of the affordable and high-quality services they offer, public hospitals and clinics saw an overwhelming surge in patients, including those with high incomes who are capable of affording their own medical expenses. The resultant heavy workload and the salary reduction policy implemented in the past few years have significantly affected employee morale in public hospitals. Furthermore, new medical graduates have experienced greatly reduced benefits, employment instability, and strike actions.

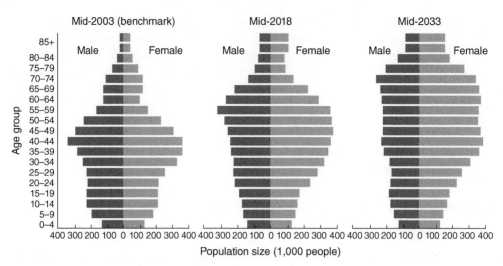

FIGURE 14.5 Trends in population growth and aging in Hong Kong. *Source*: Census and Statistical Department of the Hong Kong Special Administrative Region (2005).

4. SARS and H1N1 Outbreaks Prompted New Requirements for Disease Prevention and Control in Hong Kong The outbreak of atypical pneumonia (known as severe acute respiratory syndrome, SARS) in 2003 had a significant social and economic impact on Hong Kong, during which there was a total of 1,755 cases. Public demand prompted investigations by the SARS Expert Committee and the Hospital Authority Review Panel on the SARS Outbreak, in order to identify issues with the disease prevention and control system, hospital construction, infection control measures, emergency responses, and information systems in Hong Kong. Furthermore, sporadic cases of the H1N1 virus have also presented challenges for the disease prevention and control system of Hong Kong.

(2) Main Policy Adjustments

1. Repositioning Public Healthcare Services to Promote the Rational Distribution of Patients To reduce the burden of service provision on public healthcare institutions, the Hong Kong HWFB has undertaken the repositioning of public healthcare services and determined the following four priority areas: (1) acute and emergency care services; (2) services for low-income earners and vulnerable groups; (3) care for diseases requiring high-cost, high-tech, and cross-disciplinary specialist treatments; and (4) training for healthcare professionals.

In order to promote an efficient use of medical resources, the Hong Kong government has introduced corresponding policies to promote patient diversion. In terms of outpatient services, patients with stable conditions are referred to private healthcare institutions for treatment. Furthermore, the collaboration between public and private medical institutions has been strengthened to facilitate greater exchange of medical records and the referral of patients who are capable of paying private practitioners. A pilot program was implemented, which allowed patients to receive two to three specialist visits and then to return to GPs for followups after their health condition improved. For inpatient services, a patient distribution mechanism has been established to prioritize cancer and emergency patients over nonemergency patients on the waiting list.

2. Strengthening the Management of Healthcare Institutions to Reduce their Operating Costs   The HA implemented the EPP to reduce the operating costs and improve the operational efficiency of healthcare institutions. This was mainly achieved via the following four measures: (1) Collective procurement, whereby the purchase of large-scale medical devices is controlled through regional planning, and the operating costs are reduced by implementing the collective procurement of drugs, consumables, medical equipment, information technology equipment, and building maintenance contracts. (2) The nursing care model was altered to reduce patients' dependence on expensive inpatient services and shifted to focus on preventive care, day care, and community care, thereby saving healthcare resources and ensuring their optimal use. (3) The role of clinical coordination has been strengthened, thus fully utilizing the roles of various medical staff coordinators and enhancing collaboration, while also systematically introducing safe and effective medical technologies. (4) The human resource management system has been reformed through the collective salary reduction for civil servants, outsourcing of noncore business activities, and introduction of a voluntary early retirement program. (5) Administrative expenses have been reduced to 5% of the total expenditure.

3. Reforming Healthcare Funding Policies to Promote the Sustainable Operation of the Public Healthcare System   By the end of 2000, the HWFB promulgated the Consultation Document on Health Care Reform, entitled "Lifelong Investment in Health." This document proposed the following six recommendations for reforming healthcare funding policies: (1) Reforming the hospital fee system to improve the cost-sharing mechanism and making limited adjustments of the fee standards in public medical institutions; (2) Implementing a population-based funding model by the HA to promote community-based treatment and disease prevention; (3) Introducing a mandatory personal savings scheme, which requires Hong Kong residents aged 40–65 years to set aside 1–2% of their income to cover their medical expenses after the age of 65 years; (4) Conducting studies on the feasibility of the long-term care insurance scheme; (5) Undertaking the fourth consultation on the healthcare funding program, which encourages Hong Kong residents to purchase approved health insurance products via government funding; (6) Increasing the budget allocation for the HA to HK\$34.1231 billion in 2010–2011, equivalent to a 4.3% increase compared to the previous year.

4. Developing Community-Oriented Service Models to Strengthen Overall Healthcare Services   In recent years, the HA has emphasized the development of community-oriented service models, promoted cross-departmental and cross-institutional collaboration, prioritized public health, and improved overall service efficiency. First, the HA promoted the development of family medicine by providing GPs with community health service training in Community Geriatric Assessment Teams, emergency departments, rehabilitation and mental health clinics, and Elderly Health Centers and Maternal and Child Health Centers established by the DH. Second, the DH, HA, and various volunteer organizations have jointly organized health programs for Hong Kong residents, such as smoking cessation and cervical cancer screening programs. Third, the HA has strengthened the development of day care and community care services. It has standardized patient education on healthcare for diabetes, respiratory diseases, hypertension, heart disease, stroke and kidney diseases, in order to improve patients' self-care ability and the capability of community caregivers. Furthermore, the HA has launched many other programs to develop community-oriented services, such as the Extended Care Patients Intensive Treatment, Early Diversion and Rehabilitation Stepping Stone (EXITERS) program (to facilitate the re-integration of psychiatric patients into the community), the Elderly Suicide Prevention Program, a pilot program for providing nursing care services in nonhospital settings, and the Elderly Health Care Voucher Scheme.

5. Improving the Disease Control and Prevention System to Enhance Control of and Resilience Against Infectious Diseases Hong Kong has undertaken a series of measures since the SARS outbreak to improve its disease prevention and control system, which mainly involves the following nine aspects: (1) reforming the organizational structure of the HA and establishing the CHP; (2) conducting renovation projects for 14 major acute care hospitals, including outfitting them with ventilation and air filtration devices, personal protective equipment, and necessary drugs, in order to strengthen the control of infectious diseases; (3) revising the contingency plans for outbreaks of infectious diseases and other major accidents; (4) strengthening the cooperation between the HA and DH in terms of information sharing and human resource management; (5) undertaking the collaboration among the HA, DH, and Hong Kong Police Force to jointly establish a new Communicable Disease Information System; (6) enhancing training for infection control using government-established staff training and welfare funds; (7) objectively reviewing the treatment of SARS patients via enhanced clinical research and exchanges to formulate evidence-based medical practices; (8) formulating a comprehensive rehabilitation follow-up plan for SARS patients to monitor the development of possible complications, dysfunctions, and psychological conditions; (9) strengthening collaboration and information exchange between public and private healthcare institutions, and requiring public healthcare institutions to provide training courses for private practitioners. The exchange of medical records between public and private healthcare institutions should be encouraged through government investment in the establishment of an electronic medical record platform.

SECTION II. THE HEALTH SYSTEM IN TAIWAN

Taiwan is the largest island in China, surrounded by a subtropical ocean and located on the continental shelf on the southeastern coast of mainland China. It is divided into 7 cities and 16 counties. In 2013, the island of Taiwan had an area of 36,000 km^2 and a total population of about 23.37 million.

In 2012, the average life expectancy of Taiwanese residents was 79.9 years (male: 76.7 years; female: 83.3 years). In 2011, its GDP per capita was US$37,403, and its healthcare expenditure per capita was US$2,479, which accounted for 6.6% of the GDP.

Taiwan implemented its universal health insurance scheme (National Health Insurance, NHI) on March 1, 1995. It was one of the first regions to achieve universal health coverage. Taiwan's universal, high-quality, and cheap public healthcare system is regarded as a model of universal health coverage. Since its establishment, this health insurance scheme has achieved extensive coverage, high quality, high accessibility, low premium rates, and high public satisfaction. Currently, the health insurance scheme has reached 99% coverage, while the remaining 1% of uncovered individuals is mainly those living abroad and inmates.

1. Overview and Features of the Health System

(1) Healthcare Management System

The major government agencies in Taiwan comprise the National Assembly, Office of the President, Executive Yuan, Legislative Yuan, Judicial Yuan, Examination Yuan, and

Control Yuan, among which, the Executive Yuan is considered the highest administrative body. It consists of 8 ministries and 26 councils and commissions, departments, bureaus, and institutions, including the Department of Health (DOH). At present, Taiwan's health administration can be divided into two levels: central and local (county and city). At the central level, the DOH is the highest health administrative agency, which is responsible for health administrative affairs and the guidance, supervision, and coordination of local health authorities. In terms of local health authorities, Taipei and Kaohsiung special municipalities, along with the 23 other counties and cities, have their own health bureaus responsible for the provision of various healthcare services within their respective jurisdictions. Each health bureau oversees a number of health clinics (which are located in townships) and health centers (which are located in remote areas). There are currently 5 health bureaus and 369 health clinics in Taiwan.

The DOH comprises the Medical Administration Office, Drug Administration Office, Food Hygiene Office, Planning Office, Central Office, and Healthcare Team. It also has a number of subsidiary agencies, including the National Health Insurance Administration, Centers for Disease Control, Health Promotion Administration, Food and Drug Administration, Bureau of Controlled Drugs, Department of Chinese Medicine and Pharmacy, NHI Supervisory Committee, NHI Dispute Mediation Committee, NHI Medical Expenditure Negotiation Committee (NHI-MENC), National Health Research Institutes, Center for Drug Evaluation (CDE), Joint Commission of Taiwan (JCT), and Taiwan Drug Relief Foundation, as well as 28 DOH-established hospitals, 5 psychiatric nursing homes, 4 institutes for the control and prevention of chronic diseases, and 1 nursing home for patients with rickets.

It is worth noting that the Joint Commission of Taiwan (JCT), which was jointly established in 1999, is an important agency for hospital administration in Taiwan. It is a corporation that is jointly funded by the DOH, the Taiwan Medical Association, the Taiwan Hospital Association, and the Taiwan Non-Governmental Hospitals and Clinics Association. It has the following main functions: (1) it is authorized by the DOH for hospital accreditation in Taiwan (i.e., grade assessment); (2) it enhances medical quality management and advises on hospital management; (3) it conducts training programs for healthcare workers.

(2) Healthcare Service Providers

Healthcare institutions in Taiwan include hospitals and clinics. The past 15 years have seen a developing trend towards more intensive, large-scale hospitals, whereas the number of clinics has been gradually increasing. The number of hospitals decreased from 787 in 1999 to 514 in 2009, whereas the number of clinics increased from 15,322 to 19,792 over the same period. The specific classification of healthcare institutions in Taiwan is shown in Table 14.8.

TABLE 14.8 Overview of Healthcare Institutions in Taiwan in 2009 (Categorized by Institution Type)

Item	Public	Private	Total
Hospitals	80 (15.6%)	434 (84.4%)	514 (100%)
Clinics	461 (2.3%)	19,661 (97.7%)	20,122 (100%)
Subtotal	541 (2.7%)	20,095 (97.3%)	20,636 (100%)
Number of beds	46,580 (29.7%)	110,160 (100%)	156,740 (100%)

Hospitals in Taiwan can be classified according to their grade or ownership type. Hospitals are classified by the JCT into three grades: medical centers, regional hospitals, and district hospitals, which account for 4.5%, 16.5%, and 79.0% of all hospitals in Taiwan, respectively. Medical centers are all considered Class A teaching hospitals. Regional hospitals can be classified into Class A teaching hospitals, Class B teaching hospitals, and non-teaching hospitals. District hospitals can only be classified into Class B teaching hospitals and nonteaching hospitals. When classified by ownership type, hospitals are divided into public or private hospitals. Public hospitals are funded and operated by the government, and include DH-affiliated hospitals, municipal hospitals, hospitals affiliated with public medical colleges, military hospitals, and veterans hospitals. Private hospitals mainly include investor-owned hospitals, hospitals founded by religious organizations, and private hospitals founded by physicians. Since the 1990s, the heavy demand by private hospitals for fair competition and the lack of public support for the operating mechanism of public hospitals have caused the government to gradually reduce its subsidization of public hospitals, which has substantially increased their financial burden. To this end, the DOH has adopted various measures, such as merging, operation commissioning, and administrative corporatization, in order to undertake the diversified operations planning of public hospitals.

(3) Characteristics of the Healthcare System

1. The Health Administrative Department is Responsible for the Delivery and Funding of Healthcare Services   The DOH of Taiwan has several affiliated agencies, such as the Health Promotion Administration, the Centers for Disease Control, the Food and Drug Administration, the Medical Administration Office, and the Nursing and Health Care Office. They are responsible for monitoring the provision of healthcare services, food, and drugs, as well as the direct management of 28 DOH-affiliated hospitals. The National Health Insurance Administration (NHIA) is another affiliated agency of the DOH, which specializes in the collection, payment, and management of health insurance funds, as well as the approval and allocation of public funds for healthcare services via a top-down system. In addition, the DOH has established a preparatory team to study the feasibility of establishing a long-term care insurance scheme. In summary, Taiwan has a highly unified health administration system with clearly defined legislative bodies. In 2012, the DOH was upgraded to the Ministry of Health and Welfare.

2. The Healthcare System has Diversified Healthcare Service Providers and Relies Mainly on Social Capital   Currently, Taiwan has established diverse delivery patterns for healthcare services, and social capital is showing good developmental momentum. In 2009, public healthcare institutions accounted for 2.7% of the total number of healthcare institutions (with public hospitals accounting for 15.6% of the total number of hospitals and public clinics accounting for 2.3% of the total number of clinics), and contributed about 29.7% of the total number of beds in Taiwan. On the other hand, private healthcare institutions accounted for 97.3% of the total number of healthcare institutions (with private hospitals accounting for 84.4% of the total number of hospitals and private clinics accounting for 97.7% of the total number of clinics), and contributed about 70.3% of the total number of beds in Taiwan. Detailed data in this regard are shown in Table 14.8.

3. Healthcare Funding is Integrally Managed Solely by the NHI   In 1995, Taiwan integrated more than 10 health insurance schemes into its compulsory NHI system, which currently covers 99% of the population. This system is fully managed by the NHI, which acts as the sole insurer. Insurance premiums are jointly paid by employers and employees, while the government provides subsidies, with a particular focus on individuals who are unable to afford the premiums. In addition, tobacco surtaxes offer a supplementary source of healthcare funding. Health insurance expenditure as a share of the total healthcare expenditure has gradually increased over the years, from 39.8% in 1994 to 53.6% in 2008. The share of private expenditure (including the expenditure on supplemental insurance for individuals and enterprises) was reduced from 44.9% to 40.8%. Furthermore, the share of the government budget directly spent on public healthcare institutions fell from 15.2% to 5.6%. In addition to health insurance funding, the NHI administers the auditing and payment of public health programs, such as the prevention and control of infectious diseases.

4. The Healthcare Payment Method is a "Baton" that Guides Patients' Health-Seeking Behaviors and Regulates the Flow of Healthcare Resources   The universal health insurance of Taiwan covers all types of healthcare services, including outpatient, emergency, inpatient, rehabilitation, nursing, and home-based care services, irrespective of whether these are Western medicine, Chinese medicine, or dentistry services. Patients need only pay a portion of the medical expenses. Designated healthcare institutions account for 92% of all healthcare institutions in Taiwan. Payment of medical expenses is mainly made via a fee-for-service system under a global budget in combination with other payment systems, such as the diagnosis-related group (DRG) payment system. In terms of payment standards, these are more favorable to primary healthcare institutions, referred patients, outpatients, and short-term inpatients, which guide patients to seek medical attention at the nearest clinics or other primary healthcare facilities. This has led to the gradual establishment of a primary referral system that allows both physicians and patients to jointly control the length of hospital stay and the rational allocation of healthcare resources.

5. Government Subsidy Focuses on the Demand Side While Gradually Reducing the Direct Subsidy to the Supply Side   Prior to the implementation of the universal health insurance system, only about 60% of Taiwanese participated in health insurance, with the remaining 40% seeking medical attention at their own expense. In order to ensure that these individuals did not incur excessive medical charges, both the central and local governments established public hospitals by subsidizing their basic construction, purchase of equipment, and basic salaries of existing employees. However, after the implementation of a universal health insurance system, which has more than 99% coverage, it was possible to reimburse medical expenses according to prescribed payment scopes and standards. In addition, the application of equal reimbursement standards for public and private hospitals has brought about considerable competitive pressure on public hospitals. Accordingly, the number of public hospitals in Taiwan declined from 95 in 1995 to 80 in 2009 through restructuring, mergers, operation commissioning, and build-operate-transfer (BOT) financing. During this period, the healthcare expenditures of both the central and local governments were mainly used to subsidize the insurance premiums of low-income earners and veterans, while direct subsidies to public hospitals were gradually reduced. These governments now mainly subsidize the one-time investments in the construction of public hospitals.

6. Improving Hospital Service Quality and Overall Management Level Via Healthcare Quality Evaluation   The DOH of Taiwan began evaluating hospital quality in 1978. In recent years, the DOH has placed even greater emphasis on patient-centered care, and mainly evaluates the implementation of care measures in hospitals, including the hospital's consideration of patients' physical, psychological, and socioeconomic conditions, follow-up measures for patients who cannot be treated in hospitals, staff's respect for patients and their families, and the various cultural and personal differences. These systematic and regulatory measures have effectively motivated public and private hospitals to improve their quality management and cultural development and to promote the optimization of patient-centered service procedures, in order to provide patients with optimal services and convenience.

In addition, an interconnected medical information system has been established in Taiwan that serves as an information platform for the internal management of healthcare institutions and supervision by the government.

2. National Health Insurance (NHI)

(1) Overview of the NHI

1. Development of the NHI

1. *Former health insurance systems.* The former health insurance systems in Taiwan can be classified into three major categories: Labor Insurance, Civil Service Insurance, and Farmer's Health Insurance. The Ministry of Labor and respective municipal authorities in Taiwan served as the "central authority" and "local authorities," respectively, of the Labor Insurance. The business operation of this system was delegated to the Bureau of Labor Insurance, which was affiliated with the local authorities, and supervised by the Labor Insurance Management Committee. Labor Insurance was provided to workers (insured persons) by their affiliated institutions or groups (group insurance applicant). The Civil Service Insurance was administered by the Examination Yuan. Its business operation was entrusted to the Insurance Department of the Central Trust of China (subordinate to the Ministry of Finance), under the supervision of the Public Service Insurance Supervisory Committee, which was jointly established by the Examination Yuan and other agencies. Civil Service Insurance was provided to civil servants and teachers in private schools (including their dependents and retirees) by their affiliated agencies or schools. Finally, the Farmer's Health Insurance scheme was jointly administered by the Ministry of the Interior (which acted as the central authority), as well as the respective provincial and county (municipal) authorities (which acted as the local authorities). Its business operation was entrusted to the Commission Management Bureau, under the supervision of the Farmer's Health Insurance Supervisory Commission of the Ministry of the Interior. The Farmer's Health Insurance was provided by the Grassroots Farmers Association to the farmers.

   Although all three systems were considered examples of social insurance, they differed considerably from each other and were implemented at different times. By the time that the NHI scheme was implemented in Taiwan, the Labor Insurance scheme had been in operation for nearly 45 years, since the promulgation of the Labor Insurance Act in March 1950. Prior to this Act, the authorities had also launched 13 social insurance schemes targeting different groups of people. In 1994, however, the retirement insurance, sickness insurance for retired civil servants, retirement insurance for private school employees, and sickness insurance for spouses of retired private school employees were merged into a single sickness insurance system for retired public servants, school employees, and their dependents. The number of insured persons for each of these insurance schemes increased alongside the continuous expansion of their coverage and the increase in the total population. By the end of 1994, there were around 12,172,080 insured persons under those schemes, accounting for

57.08% of the total population (as shown in Table 14.9). Since the implementation of the NHI (first-generation NHI) on March 1, 1995, the aforementioned comprehensive insurance schemes (i.e., the Civil Service Insurance, Labor Insurance, Farmer's Health Insurance, retiree insurance for private school employees, and retirement insurance), along with the remaining five insurance schemes, were ultimately incorporated into the NHI

2. NHI in Taiwan

   1. *First-generation NHI.* With sustained and rapid economic development in Taiwan, the region's income per capita has been increasing continuously, and its overall standard of living has improved, which has enabled the public to attach increasing importance to physical and mental health. At the same time, the emergence of various issues related to social stability, such as social welfare and social insurance, prompted the Taiwanese authorities to review the various social insurance systems and resulted in the emerging demand for universal health coverage in Taiwan. In addition, the continuous increase in average life expectancy and population aging in Taiwan also led to the increasing concern regarding elderly care. Before the

TABLE 14.9 Number of Insured Persons under Various Health Insurance Schemes and Their Share of the Total Population Before the Implementation of the NHI

Types of Insurance	Number of Insured Persons	Share of the Total Population (%)
Civil service insurance	1,796,739	8.48
Civil servants insurance	581,311	2.74
Sickness insurance for the dependents of civil servants	985,002	4.65
Insurance for private school employees	44,102	0.21
Sickness insurance for the dependents of private school employees	45,153	0.21
Retirement insurance	2,173	0.66
Sickness insurance for retired public servants, private school employees and their dependents	139,050	0.01
Labor and farmer insurance system	10,302,279	48.6
Labor insurance	8,415,244	39.7
Farmer's health insurance	1,740,653	8.21
Health insurance for representatives, legislators, village chiefs, and community chiefs	27,174	0.13
Health insurance for low-income households	119,208	0.56
Total number of insured persons	12,099 072	57.08
Total number of uninsured persons	9,097,133	42.92
Total number of insured persons (including military insurance)	12,579,072	59.35
Total number of uninsured persons (including military insurance)	9,097,133	42.95
Total population	21,196,205	100

Note: The total number of insured persons under the Military Insurance was approximately 480,000.
Source: Yang Zhi-Liang, *Health Insurance* (4th ed.) (Taiwan, China: Chuliu Book Company, 170).

implementation of the NHI in 1995, more than 9 million Taiwanese were uninsured, most of whom were children under the age of 14 years and elderly adults over the age of 65. This placed a heavy burden on their families and themselves. Hence, it is evident that health coverage had become the centerpiece of social welfare needs. It was this social context, coupled with the aforementioned economic growth and the government's clear willingness to fiscally support a universal health insurance initiative, that led to the establishment of the first-generation NHI. Since then, the NHI has served as the best catalyst of universal health insurance.

The NHI, which covers both urban and rural areas, was implemented in Taiwan in accordance with the principles of "phased development," "prioritization," "mandatory," and "group-based." "Phased development" refers to the batch enrollment of uninsured persons into the health insurance system to avoid placing a substantial burden on the healthcare system, employers, and the government. "Prioritization" refers to the prioritized inclusion of vulnerable groups, such as low-income earners and disabled individuals, into the NHI, thus replacing social assistance with social insurance, in order to supervise healthcare quality and prevent wastage of healthcare resources. This was followed by prioritizing formal employees for NHI participation to prevent them from participating as residents. "Mandatory" refers to the mandatory participation in health insurance of all individuals living in Taiwan for more than six months, in order to prevent "adverse selection" (i.e., the imbalance in income and expenditure of an insurance scheme resulting from the majority of insured persons having a poor health condition). Finally, "group-based" refers to the implementation of employer-based group health insurance for employees and their unemployed family members, as well as community-based group health insurance for other residents. It aims to ensure comprehensive insurance coverage and reduce administrative costs. Premiums are set based on the insured person's income, household size, and number of dependents, and are shared among the insured person, their employer, and the government. To facilitate the implementation of the NHI, Taiwan promulgated the National Health Insurance Act, two subregulations, and 58 NHI-related operations specifications. The competent authority of the NHI is the DOH, which established the NHIA to manage the specific operations of the NHI. The NHI covers outpatient services in Western medicine, Chinese medicine, and dentistry, inpatient services, preventive care, childbirth, and so on.

The NHI has achieved tremendous success in providing universal health insurance in Taiwan since its implementation in 1995. It includes the entire Taiwanese population in a health insurance system that has high coverage of healthcare services, low variability in reimbursements, and high contracting rates. The NHI has resolved some of the major difficulties facing vulnerable groups in Taiwan, and it is also a social policy with the highest degree of public satisfaction in Taiwan.

2. *Second-generation NHI.* The healthcare quality and average life expectancy in Taiwan have improved continuously since the implementation of the NHI. Furthermore, public satisfaction with the NHI has shown an increasing trend: from 1995 to 2005, the degree of satisfaction increased from 65.4% to 72.3%, finally reaching 78.5%. However, despite its overall success, the NHI began facing a few worrying issues and challenges. For example, issues with the equity of the premium structure and the lack of an effective mechanism for consumer management became increasingly prominent, along with the emergence of financial crises and financial gaps. These problems gave rise to a number of critical situations for the first-generation

NHI, prompting Taiwan's authorities to further reform and adjust the healthcare resource allocation and the decision-making processes of the NHI.

The planning for NHI reform began in 2001, but owing to multiple setbacks, the reform was only approved by the Executive Yuan and Legislative Yuan in January 2006. The amendments to the National Health Insurance Act (i.e., the second-generation NHI) were formally passed by the Executive Yuan on April 8, 2010 and the Legislative Yuan on January 4, 2011. The main differences between the first-generation and second-generation NHI are shown in Table 14.10.

2. Current Operating Model of the NHI   The current NHI in Taiwan is the result of integrating the Labor Insurance and Civil Service Insurance. In essence, it is a mandatory social insurance scheme provided and operated by Taiwan's authorities. The organization, beneficiaries, reimbursement, and service provision of the NHI are briefly analyzed as follows.

1. *Organization of the NHI.* The NHI comprises insurers, insured persons, group insurance applicants, and healthcare providers. In Taiwan, the competent authority of the NHI is the DOH. In addition to establishing the NHIA as the sole insurer, the DOH also supervises insurance activities and conducts studies and provides advice on issues related to insurance policies and regulations. The DOH has also established the NHI Dispute Mediation Committee for investigating disputes related to claims between group insurance applicants and healthcare providers. In addition, the NHI-MENC and NHI Actuarial Committee have been established for the negotiation and distribution of healthcare expenditure and the actuarial ratemaking of insurance premiums.

   There are currently four parallel units under the DOH responsible for maintaining NHI operations: the NHI Supervisory Committee, which is responsible for overseeing all the insurance-related activities of the NHI; the NHI Dispute Mediation Committee, which is responsible for investigating disputes related to the NHI; the NHI-MENC, which is responsible for the negotiation of NHI expenditures; and the NHIA, which is responsible for NHI implementation.

   The NHIA is the unit responsible for implementing the NHI and is considered the center of overall NHI operations. In order to achieve the effective administration of the NHI and improve its operational efficiency for the convenience of the public, the headquarters of the NHIA have been charged with overseeing all NHI-related activities, including planning, supervision, research and development, staff training, and information management. There are six divisions under the Headquarters of the NHIA that directly handle insurance underwriting, premium collection, review of reimbursement for medical expenses, and the management of contracted healthcare institutions.

2. *NHI beneficiaries.* At present, the NHI covers all individuals who meet the requirement for household registration in accordance with the National Health Insurance Act (with the exception of inmates and individuals who have been missing for six months). This principle of insurance enrollment aims to prevent adverse selection and ensure universal health coverage. In the past 20 years since the implementation of the NHI, all Taiwanese are compulsorily insured under this healthcare system. According to Article 8 of the National Health Insurance Act and the Enforcement Rules of the National Health Insurance Act, NHI beneficiaries include insured persons and their dependents. Insured persons can be further classified into the six categories shown in Table 14.11.

TABLE 14.10   Differences between Second-Generation and First-Generation NHI

System Aspects	First-Generation NHI	Second-Generation NHI
Healthcare quality	There is no explicit stipulation regarding information about healthcare quality. Payments are based on service volume.	Information about healthcare quality is provided for the convenience of the public when seeking medical attention. Reimbursement incentives are provided for high-quality, acclaimed services. There a special unit responsible for healthcare quality
Information disclosure	Not stipulated.	Both the NHIA and healthcare institutions must periodically publish information about healthcare quality. Hospitals above a certain size must publish their financial reports; in the event of major violations, the names of the healthcare institutions, healthcare workers concerned, and perpetrators, as well as the details of the violation are announced to the public.
Relationship between income and expenditure	The separation of the NHI Supervisory Committee and the NHI-MENC hindered the simultaneous consideration of income and expenditure.	The merging of the NHI Supervisory Committee and NHI-MENC enabled simultaneous consideration of income and expenditure, and the implementation of a financial accountability system.
Premium calculation	Insured persons are classified according to their occupations into 6 categories and 14 subcategories with varying premium contribution rates. Premiums are determined based on recurring salary (excluding nonsalary incomes) and household size (i.e., families with larger households have greater burdens).	Insured persons are no longer classified based on their occupations; premiums are determined based solely on the gross household income, which has reduced the burden on larger households.
Administrative efficiency	Premium amounts must be changed or adjusted in the event of a change in occupation or salary adjustment.	No adjustment procedure is required in the event of a change of occupation or salary adjustment.
Healthcare coverage after returning to Taiwan	Residents living abroad who have joined the NHI in the past may rejoin the NHI and enjoy the benefits immediately upon returning to Taiwan.	Residents living abroad who have joined NHI in the past may rejoin the NHI four months after their household registration in Taiwan, with the exception of those who had joined the NHI at some point in the past two years.
Coverage of medical treatment abroad	Medical expenses incurred abroad for unexpected and emergency injuries and illnesses are reimbursable.	Medical expenses incurred abroad for special injuries or illnesses listed by insurers are reimbursable.
Whistleblower rewards	Not stipulated.	Whistleblowers are entitled to receive financial rewards within an amount equivalent to 10% of the penalties imposed for confirmed violations.

TABLE 14.11   Classification of Insured Persons under the NHI

Category	Insurance Beneficiaries
Category 1	1. Employees of public and private enterprises and agencies 2. Full-time supply staff or public officials in public agencies and public or private schools 3. Employed persons other than the above two types of insured persons 4. Employers or self-employed persons 5. Professional and technical freelancers
Category 2	1. Individuals who are members of occupational unions with no specific employer or who are self-employed 2. Expatriate personnel other than those who have joined the National Chinese Seaman's Union or Master Mariners Association
Category 3	1. Members of the Farmers' Association and Taiwan Joint Irrigation Association, or workers aged over 15 years engaged in agricultural activities 2. Class A members of the National Fisherman's Association with no specific employer or who are self-employed, or workers aged over 15 years engaged in fishery activities
Category 4	Dependents of volunteer officers, noncommissioned officers and soldiers, household representatives with a military assistance certificate or military dependents, and military school students
Category 5	Members of low-income households as defined by the Social Assistance Act
Category 6	1. Veterans and household representatives of survivors of veterans 2. Heads or representatives of households other than the insured persons and dependents prescribed in subparagraphs 1–5 and the preceding clause of this subparagraph

3. *NHI premium rate.* The premium rate of NHI increased from 4.25% in 1995 (when the NHI was first implemented) to 4.55% in 2002. The premium rate was further increased to 5.17% in 2010 due to population aging, the application of new technologies, and rising medical expenses for major illnesses, all of which led to a significant income loss for the NHI.

   Military servicemen, low-income households, and veterans are fully exempted from paying premiums by the government. For the remaining insured persons, monthly premiums are calculated based on their insurance category and monthly salary, as follows: Monthly NHI premiums = Monthly income × NHI premium rate × contribution rate × (1 + number of dependents). The contribution rate of the NHI premiums varies depending on the category of insured person and is shared among the insured person's affiliated organization, administrative authorities, and insured persons, as shown in Table 14.12.

4. *NHI benefits.* The NHI retains the same scope of reimbursement that previously existed, which includes outpatient care (for Western medicine, Chinese medicine, and dentistry), inpatient care, emergency care, drugs, various medical tests, and certain preventive care services. Compared to the previous health insurance system, the most distinctive feature of the NHI is its addition of a copayment system. This copayment varies according to the tier of the healthcare institution and is higher for treatments without a referral.

   Currently, the copayment system has also been implemented for drug and inpatient expenses. For instance, outpatients must contribute NT$50 when seeking treatment at primary care clinics. If they are referred to district hospitals, regional hospitals, or medical centers, they must contribute NT$50, NT$140, and NT$210, respectively. However, if they seek medical treatment without referrals, these copayments are increased to NT$80, NT$240, and NT$360, respectively (Table 14.13).

TABLE 14.12 Contribution Rates of NHI Premiums (Unit: %)

	Types of NHI Beneficiaries		Insured Persons	Group Insurance Applicant	Government
Category 1	Civil servants, public officials, and employees of public schools	Insured persons and their dependents	30	70	0
	Employees of private schools		30	35	35
	Employees of public enterprises and agencies		30	60	10
	Other employees with specific employers				
	Employers, and self-employed persons		100	0	0
	Professional and technical freelancers				
Category 2	Professional workers and expatriate sailors	Insured persons and their dependents	60	0	40
Category 3	Fishermen, farmers, and members of Taiwan Joint Irrigation Association	Insured persons and their dependents	30	0	70
Category 4	Military servicemen, military school students, survivors of military veterans, and men enlisted for military substitute service	Insured persons	0	0	100
Category 5	Members of low-income households	Members	0	0	100
Category 6	Veterans and their dependents	Insured persons	0	0	100
		Dependents	30	0	70
	Regional population	Insured persons and their dependents	60	0	40

TABLE 14.13 Copayments for Outpatient Services Covered by the NHI (Unit: NT$)

Level of Medical Institution	Copayments for Outpatient Services		Copayments for Emergency Care Services
	Without referral	With referral	
Medical centers	360	210	450
Regional hospitals	240	140	300
District hospitals	80	50	150
Primary care clinics	50	50	150

NHI beneficiaries must cover 20% of medical expenses incurred for outpatient or emergency care services. However, they must cover 30%, 40%, and 50% when seeking treatment without a referral in district hospitals, regional hospitals, and medical centers, respectively. Deductibles are applied for beneficiaries who make more than 12 outpatient visits per year over two consecutive years.

As for inpatients, those admitted to acute care wards must cover 10%, 20%, and 30% of their inpatient expenses for hospital stays of ≤30 days, 31–60 days, and more than 60 days, respectively. Patients admitted to chronic care wards must cover 5%, 10%, 20%, and 30% of inpatient expenses for hospital stays of ≤30 days, 31–90 days, 91–180 days, and more than 180 days, respectively (Table 14.14).

The copayment ceiling for beneficiaries who are hospitalized for less than 30 days in acute care wards or less than 180 days in chronic care wards for the same illness is determined by the authorities.

In addition, the NHI has established copayment ceilings and exemptions in order to reduce the burden of the copayment system on low-income earners. Beneficiaries with major injuries or who have experienced childbirth, as well as those living in aboriginal areas and outlying islands, are exempt from copayments for preventive care services. The authorities also cover the out-of-pocket expenses incurred by members of low-income households (as defined by the Social Assistance Act and who are eligible for referral). However, the NHI does not cover healthcare services already covered by the government according to the law and specific healthcare services. To ease the financial burden on the public, the NHI has established the following copayment ceilings for inpatient expenses: NT$29,000 for each hospital stay in the same year due to the same illness and NT$48,000 per year for hospital stays of less than 30 days in acute care wards.

TABLE 14.14 Copayments for Inpatient Services Covered by the NHI

Category	Length of Hospital Stay	Copayment Ratio (%)
Acute care wards	≤30 days	10
	31–60 days	20
	More than 60 days	30
Chronic care wards	≤30 days	5
	31–90 days	10
	91–180 days	20
	More than 181 days	30

5. Healthcare expenses and payment methods
   1. *Healthcare expenses.* In 2005, the NHI spent a total of NT$408 billion on health-care expenses, of which hospital services (including outpatient hemodialysis) accounted for 64.97%, Western medicine primary care services (including outpatient hemodialysis) accounted for 21.24%, outpatient dental services accounted for 7.66%, and outpatient Chinese medicine services accounted for 4.25%. From 2005 to 2010, the proportion of hospital expenses increased, whereas the proportion of outpatient services (Chinese and Western medicine) decreased. In 2010, the healthcare expenditure of Taiwan was NT$493.932 billion, of which hospital services (including outpatient hemodialysis), Western medicine primary care services (including outpatient hemodialysis), outpatient dental services, and outpatient Chinese medicine services accounted for 66.71%, 20.88%, 7.24%, and 3.98%, respectively (Table 14.15).
   2. *Payment methods.* In 2002, the NHI fully implemented a global budget payment system (GBPS), whereby the global budget for healthcare expenditures for outpatient dental services, outpatient Chinese medicine services, Western medicine primary care services and hospital services was determined via the calculation of point values. The GBPS has achieved excellent control over the growth in healthcare expenditure. The NHI gradually changed its payment method from the previously adopted "fee-for-service payments" (i.e., payments are made according to service volume) and "per diem payments" (i.e., payments are made according to length of hospital stay) to "pay-for-performance" (i.e., payments are made according to service quality) and "case-based payment" (i.e., DRGs), and is now gradually promoting the GBPS. Its aim is to improve the quality and effectiveness of medical and nursing care services in the most cost-effective manner. The currently adopted GBPS, whereby the global budget is calculated using point values, is described in more detail in the third part of this section.
6. *Provision of healthcare services.* The NHI employs an old-fashioned contract system, whereby the NHIA serves as the insurance provider, while healthcare services are provided by contracted public/private hospitals and clinics. NHI statistics have shown

TABLE 14.15 Composition of Healthcare Expenditure in Taiwan From 2005 to 2010

Item	Year					
	2005	2006	2007	2008	2009	2010
Healthcare expenditure (NT$million)	408,000	423,691	441,615	460,102	478,074	493,932
Hospital services (including outpatient hemodialysis) (%)	64.97	65.20	65.52	66.11	66.75	66.71
Western medicine primary care services (including outpatient hemodialysis) (%)	21.24	21.24	20.99	21.01	20.99	20.88
Outpatient dental services (%)	7.66	7.59	7.45	7.36	7.30	7.24
Outpatient Chinese medicine services (%)	4.25	4.20	4.163	4.07	4.03	3.98
Others (%)	1.87	1.87	1.90	1.45	0.93	1.19
NHI expenditure as a share of the GDP (%)	3.51	3.46	3.40	3.52	3.73	3.63

that by the end of 2008, there were 18,829 NHI-contracted healthcare institutions, accounting for 91.87% of the total number of healthcare institutions in Taiwan. Additionally, there were 4,080 NHI-contracted pharmacies and 863 NHI-contracted home-based care and specialist hospitals. The separation of prescribing and dispensing policy implemented in the NHI is detailed in the fourth part of this section (entitled "Drug Administration System").

(2) Achievements of the NHI

1. Improved Healthcare Equality and Accessibility Since its implementation in 1995, the NHI has achieved a 99% coverage rate, fulfilling its primary goal of universal health coverage.

Furthermore, it has maintained both the equality and accessibility of healthcare services by ensuring lower medical expenses. In 2000, the Economist Intelligence Unit (EIU) published the Global Access to Healthcare Index, which ranked Taiwan second only to Sweden in terms of health indicators, healthcare expenditure, healthcare resources, and healthcare quality. In 2002, the fairness of financial contribution (FFC) index of Taiwan was 0.989, which was the highest among all WHO members. In 2011, a comparison of Taiwan with OECD countries in terms of the GDP and national healthcare expenditure (NHE) showed that Taiwan spent an average of US$2,479 per capita each year, which was much lower than that of the US (US$8,508). Furthermore, the NHE accounted for 6.6% of the GDP in Taiwan (Table 14.16).

2. Main Health Indicators of Taiwanese Residents Have Reached the Levels of Other Developed Countries and Areas According to the World Competitiveness Rankings developed by the International Institute for Management Development (IMD, Lausanne, Switzerland), in 2006 Taiwan ranked 21st among 61 countries and areas in meeting the social demand for infrastructure. In the same year, the average life expectancy and infant mortality rate in Taiwan also reached the levels of developed countries or areas. A comparison of average life expectancy and infant mortality rates between Taiwan and selected developed countries or areas in 2012 is shown in Table 14.17.

TABLE 14.16 Comparison of the GDP and NHE between Taiwan and OECD Countries in 2005 and 2011

Country or Area	2005		2011	
	Average Annual Healthcare Expenditure Per Capita (US$)	NHE as a Share of the GDP (%)	Average Annual Healthcare Expenditure Per Capita (US$)	NHE as a Share of GDP (%)
United States	6,347	15.2	8,508	17.7
France	3,306	11.1	4,118	11.6
Germany	3,251	10.7	4,495	11.3
Canada	3,460	9.9	4,522	11.2
Japan	2,474	8.2	3,415	10.0
South Korea	1,263	5.9	2,198	7.4
Taiwan	949	6.14	2,479	6.6

TABLE 14.17 Comparison of Average Life Expectancy and Infant Mortality Rate between Taiwan and Selected Developed Countries in 2006 and 2012

	2006			2012		
Country or Area	Average Life Expectancy of Females (Years)	Average Life Expectancy of Males (Years)	Infant Mortality Rate (per 1,000 live births)	Average Life Expectancy of Females (Years)	Average Life Expectancy of Males (Years)	Infant Mortality Rate (per 1,000 live births)
Taiwan	80.8	74.5	5	83	76	3.7
US	80.4	75.2	6.8	81	76	6.1
Germany	81.8	76.2	3.9	83	78	3.3
Japan	85.5	78.5	2.8	87	80	2.2
France	83.9	78.7	4.2	85	79	3.5
UK	81.1	76.9	5.1	83	79	4.0

3. Comprehensive Care for Vulnerable Groups and Reduction of the Financial Burden on Taiwanese Residents Since the NHI is a compulsory insurance scheme, the NHIA has proposed numerous concessionary measures for premium payments, with the aim of protecting the right to access healthcare among those who are unable to afford the premiums and other economically disadvantaged groups. As of June 30, 2008, the NHIA has spent NT$6.64 billion to subsidize around 1.39 million recipients, including low-income earners, elderly people aged over 70 years, children under the age of 3, and unemployed individuals. It also spent a further NT$8.29 billion in subsidizing around 600,000 low-income households. Furthermore, for patients with major injury and diseases (e.g., cancer, chronic mental illnesses, kidney diseases that require hemodialysis, congenital diseases) that require expensive treatments, the NHIA exempts them from paying for the treatments for these conditions as long as they can provide evidence of their disease or injury. Full reimbursement is provided by the NHI for DOH-listed essential medicines for the treatment of rare diseases. Furthermore, an application for full reimbursement can also be made for drugs not listed by the DOH. In Taiwan, healthcare resources are fairly limited in many mountainous areas, as their geographical locations have hindered the willingness of healthcare workers to serve in these areas. Furthermore, primary care physicians are unable to meet the demand for expensive equipment and specialist care in these areas. Therefore, the NHIA introduced the Integrated Delivery System (IDS) in 1999 to facilitate the delivery of healthcare services to these remote areas. The IDS program has achieved an average satisfaction rate of 91% (99% in some counties) among those living in remote areas.

4. Controlling the Growth of Healthcare Expenditure via the DRG-Based Payment System and GBPS Due to the rapid increase in healthcare expenditure under the fee-for-service payment system, the NHI has gradually shifted its payment method to a DRG-based system and the GBPS. For the GBPS, before the start of each year, the future total healthcare expenditure is negotiated between healthcare providers and consumers to establish a set range for the volume and content of particular services. In this way, both healthcare providers and consumers can jointly reduce the demand for healthcare services and enhance preventive care measures. Since the full implementation of the GBPS, the NHIA has successfully kept the growth rate of healthcare expenditure below 5%.

5. Steady Increase of the NHE The advancement of medical technology has led to the increasing prices of healthcare services, while population aging in Taiwan has resulted in a growing elderly population, which has increased the demand for healthcare in society as a whole. Therefore, the healthcare expenditure of the NHI has also increased gradually every year. However, the NHI has effectively suppressed the growth in healthcare expenditure by reviewing the services provided by healthcare institutions and implementing the medical expenses reporting system. Specifically, the annual growth rate in healthcare expenditure per capita in Taiwan decreased from 15% before the implementation of the NHI in 1995 to about 7% in 2012.

6. Improved Management Efficiency Through Digitization NHI-contracted healthcare institutions account for 91.17% of all healthcare institutions in Taiwan. The implementation of the NHI IC card system has made it very convenient to access healthcare services, as patients only need to bring their NHI IC cards when seeking medical attention throughout Taiwan. The NHI IC card plays an important role in NHI management, as it contains the cardholder's personal information, including identification codes for major injury and disease, validity period, medication records, allergy records, and so on. Thus, it allows physicians to access the patients' most up-to-date medical and physician examination records, so as to avoid unnecessary repeated examinations and medication duplication.

(3) Problems Encountered in the Implementation of the NHI

1. Financial Imbalances in the NHI Despite receiving considerable acclaim in the international community, the NHI has encountered a number of financial problems that have gone unresolved due to repeated financial crises. These financial problems are the result of population growth and population aging, along with the advancement of medical technologies, the emergence of new drugs, and the expansion of NHI coverage. In 2006, the *Southern Weekly* reported that the NHI faced a risk of bankruptcy because it has remained in a state of deficit since 1995; specifically, the annual growth rate of its income was 4.58% and that of its expenditure was 5.71%.

2. Inflexible premium rate The National Health Insurance Act stipulates that the premium rate of the NHI can be adjusted in a timely manner to maintain a good financial balance. However, due to the unique political system of Taiwan, only two slight adjustments have been made to the NHI premium rates. Although the adjustment of premium rates temporarily curtailed the financial gap of the NHI, it also led to a decline in public satisfaction.

3. Spending NHI Income on Inflated Drug Prices The NHI spends an unreasonable amount of its revenue on the price gap of drugs, that is, the difference between procurement prices paid by hospitals and NHIA reimbursement prices for drugs prescribed to NHI beneficiaries; this is known as the "black hole of drug pricing." Several price cuts have been made by the NHIA to specific drugs but these have yielded insignificant outcomes. This is because when new drug prices were established, hospitals began considering substitute drugs to boost their own profitability and maximize their benefits. Therefore, price cuts are not only incapable of eliminating this black hole of drug pricing, but also have failed to protect public health.

4. Severe Wastage of Healthcare Resources Despite the implementation of the GBPS, Taiwan still faces severe wastage of healthcare resources. Since the implementation of NHI,

Taiwanese residents increasingly began to seek medical attention in hospitals, purchase medicines, and undergo physical examinations. Furthermore, it was common to observe wastage resulting from unnecessary hospitalization, surgeries, and endoscopic examinations. Therefore, the wastage of healthcare resources is an important issue that needs to be resolved by the NHI.

3. Point-for-Service Global Budget Payment System

Under the GBPS, the payer (demand-side) and the healthcare provider (supply-side) negotiate and determine the total NHI expenditure (global budget) for a specific range of healthcare services within a certain period in the future (usually one year), in order to control the healthcare expenditure within the budget. Taiwan's GBPS is a capped global budget system, such that the cost of each healthcare service is reflected in point values. The amount payable for each point value is calculated via retrospective pricing; that is, the global budget is divided according to the total number of service points collected. The implementation process of the GBPS can be divided into three major parts: the determination of global budget amount, allocation of the global budget, and settlement using point values.

(1) Determination of the Global Budget

Article 47 of the National Health Insurance Act stipulates that the global budget of the NHI must be predetermined each year by the relevant administrative agencies six months before the start of the next year. This global budget is submitted to the Executive Yuan for approval after receiving advice from the NHI Committee.

1. Global Budget Negotiation Platform   The National Health Insurance Act stipulates that the NHI-MENC shall serve as the platform for the negotiation of the global budget. It consists of nine representatives each from the healthcare providers (supply-side), insured persons and experts (demand-side), and relevant administrative agencies (government). NHI-MENC representatives must be reelected every two years. In the NHI-MENC meeting, supply- and demand-side representatives engage in peer negotiation on the amount (rate) that payers are willing to spend on the healthcare services (reimbursement scope) delivered by healthcare providers.

2. Global Budget Negotiation Process

1. *The DOH determines the global budget for healthcare expenditure.* Nine months before the start of each year, the DOH determines the recommended lower limit of the global budget growth rate. The recommended upper limit is then determined in consultation with the public, while taking into account factors such as policy promotion measures, overall economic status, the public's ability to pay, and overall healthcare expenditure. The global budget is then submitted to the Executive Yuan for deliberation seven months before the start of the new year.
2. *The Executive Yuan approves the global budget.* At six months before the start of each year, the Council for Economic Planning and Development (CEPD) of the Executive Yuan completes its deliberations on the recommended global budget submitted by the DOH, then determines the upper and lower limits of the global budget growth rate, and establishes the policy instructions for the next year. The detailed procedure for determining the global budget is shown in Figure 14.6.

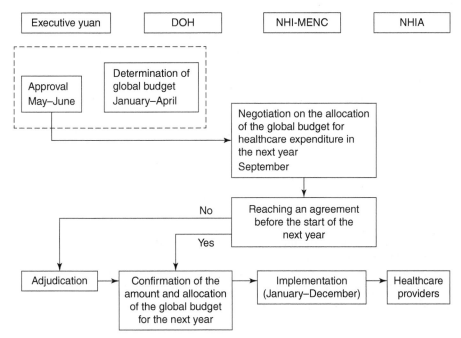

FIGURE 14.6 Procedures for determining the global budget of healthcare expenditures in Taiwan.

3. *Determining the lower limit of the global budget growth rate.* The lower limit of the growth rate for the global budget is nonnegotiable and is calculated by taking into account the following three factors: projected population growth rate, demographic transition rate, and rate of change in health service cost index (HSCI).

(2) Allocation of the Global Budget

Global budget allocation comprises two steps: sector allocation and regional allocation.

1. Sector Allocation of the Global Budget The approved global budget is allocated to four sectors of healthcare services: outpatient dental services, outpatient Chinese Medicine services, Western medicine primary care services, and hospital services. Additionally, the proportion of the global budget allocated to hemodialysis is separate from that for Western medicine primary care services and hospital services; hemodialysis is now categorized as "other services" and is specifically funded by the NHIA. The formula for determining the sector allocation of the global budget is as follows: Global budget of healthcare expenditure for the next year = Total expenditure for general healthcare services in the current year × (1 + growth rate of nonnegotiable factors + growth rate of negotiable factors) + expenses for specially funded items in the sector. The nonnegotiable factors, negotiable factors, and specially funded items are described as follows.

1. *Non-negotiable factors.* Nonnegotiable factors, also known as healthcare cost and demographic factors, include the rate of change in the HSCI, the annual growth rate of the insured population, and the demographic transition rate. When negotiating the global

budget for the next year, the growth rates of these factors are calculated using a formula comprising the same three factors used to determine the lower limit of the global budget growth rate. However, these growth rates vary across sectors. The growth rate of the non-negotiable factors for each sector in 2011 is shown in Table 14.18.

2. *Negotiable factors.* Negotiable factors are the factors that must be negotiated in the process of determining the global budget. During the negotiation, healthcare providers propose a specific growth range for each factor and give their reasons for selecting this range; the range undergoes amendment and confirmation with payer representatives before an agreement is reached. Negotiable factors include changes in the scope of insurance coverage (reimbursable services), improvements in the quality of healthcare services and health status of NHI beneficiaries, changes in the frequency of service utilization, the impact of policy changes and policy incentives, and improvements in healthcare service efficiency.

3. *Specially funded items.* The specific implementation of specially funded items is proposed by healthcare providers during their negotiation with payer representatives on the global budget for the next year. Subsequently, special funds are allocated according to the actual implementation of these items. These special funds cannot be spent on other healthcare services and are not considered in the expenditures of the base year when determining the global budget for the next year.

2. Regional Allocation of the Global Budget   The NHIA comprises six divisions based on the administrative regions of Taiwan (i.e., the Taipei Division, Northern Division, Central Division, Southern Division, Kaoping Division, and Eastern Division). In order to ensure a good balance in healthcare resources, the approved global budget for each sector is allocated to the six divisions under the NHIA after adjusting for their demographic structures and standardized mortality rates. After determining the global budget allocation for each division, the quarterly global budget is determined according to the distribution and ratio of healthcare expenditure in each administrative region in the previous year.

3. Settlement of the Global Budget Using Point Values   At the start of each year, healthcare institutions report their medical point values to the respective NHIA divisions before February 20, which are calculated based on various payment methods (e.g., fee-for-service,

TABLE 14.18 Growth Rates of Nonnegotiable Factors for All Sectors in 2011 (Unit: %)

Item	Outpatient Dental Services	Outpatient Chinese Medicine Services	Western Medicine Primary Care Services	Western Medicine Hospitals	Overall Global Budget
Annual growth rate of insured population	0.336	0.336	0.336	0.336	0.336
Demographic transition rate	−0.197	0.579	0.886	2.064	1.602
Rate of change in the HSCI	0.865	0.973	−0.767	−0.353	−0.298
Growth rates of nonnegotiable factors	1.006	1.893	0.455	2.053	1.644

Note: Growth rate of nonnegotiable factors = (1 + Demographic transition rate + Rate of change in HSCI) × (1 + Annual growth rate of insured population).

value-based pricing, per diem payment, capitation, and DRGs). The NHIA of each division then provides all healthcare institutions with a temporary payment of health insurance costs within 15 days after reporting the point values. This payment is determined according to the point values reported by each healthcare institution, the estimated amount payable for each point value, and reduction rates based on reviews of the first three months after reporting the point values.

In the fourth month of each quarter, the NHIA divisions deduct the total amount payable for the purchase of drugs and healthcare services reported by healthcare institutions from their quarterly global budgets for healthcare. The remainder of the quarterly budget is then divided by the total point value reported in each division to obtain the amount payable for each point value, also known as the "floating" point value (Table 14.19). Subsequently, the NHIA divisions release their updated floating point values, which are used to recalculate the quarterly amount payable to healthcare institutions. The overpaid amount will be refunded while the underpaid amount will be replenished accordingly.

4. Drug Administration System

(1) Overview of the Drug Administration System

The National Health Insurance Act was promulgated in Taiwan on August 9, 1994. Under the framework of the GBPS, this act allows for the separation of prescribing and dispensing; determining the share of the global budget allocated for drugs; determining the shares of pharmacy services and drug charges for outpatient services; and establishing the pricing standards and reimbursement scopes for drugs. The NHI's total expenditure for drugs accounted for a relatively consistent share of the total healthcare expenditure. From 1999 to 2009, the share of drug expenditure remained between 24.4% and 25.4%.

The DOH is responsible for all healthcare services provided in Taiwan. Specifically, the Drug Administration Office and the NHIA are primarily responsible for drug administration, whereby the former is responsible for all drug-related laws, regulations, and administrative affairs, and the latter is responsible for the NHI drug formulary and pricing. The DOH is also responsible for the approval, oversight, funding, pricing, and reimbursement of drugs.

In Taiwan, the Food and Drug Administration of the DOH is responsible for approving the marketing of new drugs. Since 1998, new drugs must undergo technical assessments by the

TABLE 14.19 Floating Point Values of the Regional Global Budget for All Sectors in the First Quarter of 2011

Item	Taipei Division	Northern Division	Central Division	Southern Division	Kaoping Division	Eastern Division
Global Budget for Outpatient Dental Services	0.9559	1.0695	0.9595	1.0275	0.9638	1.1522
Global Budget for Outpatient Chinese Medicine Services	0.9958	0.9790	0.9249	1.0044	1.0333	1.3727
Global Budget for Western Medicine Primary Care Services	0.7918	0.7892	0.8154	0.8819	0.8275	0.9922
Global Budget for Hospital Services	0.8164	0.8791	0.8841	0.8671	0.8692	0.8521

CDE in terms of quality, safety, and efficacy. On the other hand, the NHIA of the DOH is responsible for deciding whether a new drug is eligible for reimbursement. The decision is made based on comparative efficacy studies; budget impact analysis; pharmacoeconomic cost-effectiveness or cost-efficiency analysis; and ethical, legal, and social implications (ELSI) analysis.

(2) Overview of Drug Expenditure

The NHI in Taiwan reimburses up to 15,879 types of drugs. Funding for drug reimbursement comes from insurance premiums contributed by the government, employers, and insured persons, but the exact share of contribution depends on the circumstances of each case. The government fully covers drug expenses for vulnerable groups, such as low-income households. Expenses for insured drugs account for 30% of the total drug expenditure in Taiwan. The expenses for insured drugs in Taiwan in the past years are shown in Table 14.20.

Drug expenditure accounted for about 25% of total healthcare expenditure and 1.3% of GDP. The top 50 brand-name drugs accounted for about 30% of total drug expenditure, while the top 200 brand-name drugs accounted for 50%. Brand-name drugs and generic drugs accounted for about 30% and 70% of the total drug expenditure, respectively. Imported drugs and locally manufactured drugs accounted for 65% and 35% of the total drug expenditure, respectively. On August 1, 1999, a copayment system was introduced for insured drugs to encourage more careful utilization of healthcare resources among NHI beneficiaries. According to this system, drug charges below NT$100 were exempted from copayment, but NHI beneficiaries had to contribute NT$20 for every additional NT$100 increase in drug expenses, with a copayment cap of NT$100; this cap was further increased to NT$200 from September 1, 2002, onward.

(3) Drug Pricing

The National Health Insurance New Drug Listing and Pricing Guidelines and National Health Insurance Drug Pricing Benchmarks came into effect in March 2010. According to these guidelines, new drugs are defined as new applications of drugs with new ingredients,

TABLE 14.20   Increase in Expenses for Insured Drugs in Taiwan From 1995 to 2007

Year	Drug Expenditure (NT$100 Million)	Annual Growth Rate (%)
1995	439	15.53
1996	489	11.33
1997	496	1.51
1998	555	11.87
1999	668	20.35
2000	790	18.14
2001	880	11.47
2002	922	4.72
2003	944	2.38
2004	1,033	9.47
2005	1,113	7.73
2006	1,141	2.52
2007	1,170	2.54

dosage forms, routes of administration, or therapeutic compounds. Head-to-head comparisons with the best commonly used drugs or indirect comparisons among clinical studies must be conducted for newly licensed drugs. Drugs that have been shown to have significantly better therapeutic efficacies and validated by medical experts are entitled to international price referencing (IPR), whereby the drug price is set with reference to the median of 10 countries worldwide (the UK, Germany, Japan, Switzerland, the US, Belgium, Australia, France, Sweden, and Canada). The detailed classification and pricing of drugs are shown in Table 14.21.

There are various pricing methods for the second category of new drugs. For example, the drug price can be set with reference to the lowest price among the 10 countries or the price set in the country of origin. The drug price can also be determined via IPR and price-per-dose methods. On the other hand, the price of compounded drugs can be determined by multiplying the sum of the NHI price for each component by 70% or calculated from the price of the primary active pharmaceutical ingredient.

Examples of IPR calculation methods for drug pricing are shown in Table 14.22. For instance, the price ratio of a new drug (Drug A) to its reference drug (Drug B) is calculated as A/B. If we assume that only 6 out of 10 countries are available for the price comparison between the reference and new drugs, as the new drug has not been marketed in 3 countries (i.e., the price is unavailable), while the price of the reference drug is unavailable in the remaining country.

Thus, the equation for calculating the price of new drugs payable by the NHI is as follows: The price of new drugs payable by NHI = the price of the reference drug (B) paid by the NHI × the median price of the new drug in other countries.

Another drug pricing method is the price-per-dose method, whereby the unit price of the new drug is calculated based on the therapeutic dose of the new drug as well as the therapeutic dose and unit price of the reference drug.

The price-per-dose method takes into account the advantages of the new drugs when pricing, which further improves the pricing standard. The first case is where there

TABLE 14.21 Principles of Classification and Pricing for New Drugs in Taiwan

Categories of New Drugs	Characteristics	Principles of Pricing
Category 1	Innovative drugs	The price is set with reference to the median of 10 countries, or 1.1 times the median cost of these 10 countries for drugs that have been shown to have good efficacy and safety according to local clinical trials of a certain scale. If there are ≤5 countries available for IPR, the IPR shall be conducted once a year (in the fourth quarter), thereafter until there are ≥5 countries available for referencing.
Category 2A	Drugs shown to exhibit moderate improvement in clinical value compared to the best available drugs	The median of 10 drug prices is taken as the upper limit. A 10% price hike is permitted for drugs that have exhibited significant efficacy and safety by local clinical trials of a certain scale. A 10% increase in the maximum price is permitted for drugs that have been subjected to pharmacoeconomic assessment.
Category 2B	New drug with similar clinical value to existing reference drugs	–

TABLE 14.22 IPR Calculations

Country or Area	Price of the New Drug (A)	Price of the Reference Drug (B)	Ratio ((A)/(B))
US	639.50	480.33	1.33
Japan	–	252.20	–
UK	390.91	230.42	1.69
Canada	–	198.50	–
Germany	455.00	256.32	1.77
France	458.72	240.92	1.90
Belgium	403.05	–	–
Sweden	–	200.78	–
Switzerland	420.60	262.95	1.59
Australia	365.21	188.89	1.93
Taiwan	320.00	185.00	1.73

is objective evidence showing that the new drug has greater therapeutic efficacy than the reference drug, then a maximum price hike of 15% is allowable. The second case is where there is objective evidence showing that the new drug is safer than the reference drug; then a maximum price hike of 15% is allowable. The third case is where the new drug is more convenient than the reference drug (e.g., a longer dosing interval, more convenient route of administration, more stable therapeutic efficacy, easier safety monitoring, safer packaging, and so on); then a maximum price hike of 15% is allowable. In addition, a maximum price hike of 15% is also allowable for a new drug manufactured with dosages for children.

5. Challenges Facing the Health System in Taiwan

The healthcare system in Taiwan has evolved over the years. The NHI, which has been in operation for almost two decades, enables more convenient, better-quality, and more afford-able healthcare services with greater coverage and satisfaction for all residents of Taiwan.

(1) Financial Imbalance in NHI Funding

On the one hand, it is difficult to continually raise the NHI premium rate in conjunction with increasing economic development and the higher incomes of insured persons. Furthermore, there is also limited revenue from other sources. On the other hand, a financial imbalance in NHI funding is inevitable because of population aging, emerging novel medical technologies, and the continuous expansion of NHI coverage. A financial imbalance in the NHI arose in the third year of its implementation, but it was somewhat alleviated after several measures were adopted. However, a second crisis occurred in 2001–2003, while a third one emerged in 2004. This can be seen from the trends in healthcare expenditure and GDP in Figure 14.7. From 2001 to 2002, healthcare expenditure showed a growth rate of over 7%, which was significantly higher than that of the GDP. In 2009, each resident of Taiwan paid for an average of 32.4 physician visits per year, which was much higher than that of Germany (10.5 physician visits), another country that has implemented universal healthcare coverage.

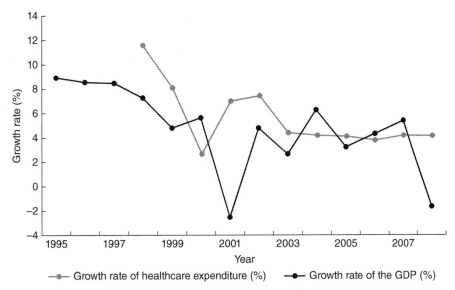

FIGURE 14.7 Growth rates of healthcare expenditures and GDP in Taiwan in 1995–2008.
Source: NHI-MENC, NHIA.

Statistics indicate that in 1997–2009, the NHI had a much greater average annual growth rate in expenditure (5.27%) than income (4.02%). Currently, countermeasures against the financial imbalance in NHI funding are actively being studied. In general, the main objectives of these studies include expanding the premium base of the NHI under the principle of ensuring fairer contributions from insurance premiums; enhancing the diversified pay-for-performance payment system to protect and improve the quality of healthcare services; enhancing the public disclosure of service quality and financial reports for healthcare institutions; merging the NHI Supervisory Committee and NHI-MENC to improve administrative efficiency; and establishing a link between income and expenditure to promote a balance between them in the NHI funding.

(2) Increasing Operational Pressure on Hospitals

Due to the frequent financial crises in the NHI, the administrative authorities of Taiwan, especially the NHIA, have been constantly improving the NHI payment system through various measures. These include promoting the implementation of the DRG-based and pay-for-performance payment systems, and enhancing the oversight of healthcare institutions (e.g., increasing the penalty imposed on hospitals for the violation of rules and regulations). Furthermore, these circumstances are driving hospitals to improve their internal management by emphasizing internal quality management and supervision, while also controlling service costs to achieve financial balance (even a slight surplus). However, it is often difficult for hospitals to balance service quality and healthcare expenditure in order to meet patients' demand for high-quality services while also meeting their own profit goals. This is due to the considerable difficulty in controlling costs and the barrage of complaints against paying higher healthcare expenses.

(3) Rigid Management System in Public Hospitals

Public nonprofit organizations in Taiwan, including public hospitals, have all adopted a unified management and dispatching system. According to this system, personnel affairs are administered by the Department of Personnel Administration, while financial affairs are administered by the Department of Finance. Hence, hospitals have complicated staff mobility procedures and budgeting of income and expenditure. As a result, it is difficult for public hospitals to compete with private hospitals because the hospital directors lack authority in personnel and financial affairs. In recent years, an appointment system has been adopted to recruit new employees while retaining existing public officials; however, this is still in the preliminary stages.

PART FOUR

IV

Characteristics of Health Systems in Developing Countries

CHAPTER FIFTEEN

Definition of Developing Countries and Challenges in Health Systems

 ## SECTION I. DEFINITION AND STRUCTURAL FORMATION OF DEVELOPING COUNTRIES

1. Concept and Definition of Developing Countries

Developing countries are generally considered to be the conceptual opposite of developed countries, and they are also known as less developed countries or underdeveloped countries. This term usually refers to countries with lower levels of socioeconomic development and living standards that are still in the process of transitioning from traditional agricultural societies to modern industrial societies. There is currently a lack of a unified definition of developing countries, and even organizations such as the World Bank, the World Trade Organization (WTO), and the United Nations Conference on Trade and Development (UNCTAD) have failed to provide a clear conceptual definition. The international community previously regarded a country's participation in the Organisation for Economic Co-operation and Development (OECD) as an indication of being economically developed. However, with the subsequent participation in the OECD of Mexico, Chile, and other developing countries, it became difficult to uphold this consensus.

From a historical perspective, the term "developing countries" generally refers to emerging democracies that were previously colonies, semi-colonies, or dependent territories and that have gained political independence and now possess national sovereignty after a struggle for independence.

From a political perspective, another concept that is closely related to that of developing countries is that of Third World countries. However, the political concept of the "Third World" ceased to exist after the end of the Cold War and the disappearance of bipolar international relations. Nevertheless, the term Third World is still widely used as a conceptual aggregate of developing countries. More than 130 UN member states in Asia, Africa, Latin America, and other regions are classified as Third World countries.

From the perspective of economic development, the evaluation criteria for developing countries are usually per capita gross national product (GNP), per capita gross national income (GNI), and national gross domestic product (GDP). Countries with lower GDPs per capita, where economic development has not yet reached the level of developed countries, are regarded as developing countries. According to the *World Development Report 2002* by the World Bank, in 2000, the average GNI per capita was US$420 in low-income countries, US$1,140 in lower-middle-income countries, and US$4,620 in upper-middle-income countries; the average value in developed countries was US$1,230. All countries with GNIs per capita of US$755 or less were classified as low-income countries, with GNIs per capita of US$756 to US$2,995, US$2,996 to US$9,265, and US$9,266 and above corresponding to lower-middle income, upper-middle income, and high-income countries, respectively.

From a comprehensive perspective, economic development is not a necessary and sufficient condition for developed countries. For example, although Saudi Arabia, Kuwait, the United Arab Emirates, Brunei, and other oil-producing countries have high GNIs per capita, they are also considered undeveloped. Although Japan and Israel were not wealthy in the 1950s, they were considered developed countries. Moreover, the concepts of poverty and wealth are constantly changing and can only truly be understood within a context of mutual comparison and dynamic development. To ensure a comprehensive determination, the United Nations Development Program (UNDP) adopted the Human Development Index (HDI) to classify developed and developing countries. The HDI is calculated based on three indicators: (1) the level of population health, mainly measured by average life expectancy; (2) the level of education and knowledge, mainly measured by indicators such as the literacy rate and the enrollment ratio in tertiary, secondary, and primary education; and (3) the quality of life, measured using GDP per capita.

Regardless of the definition criteria used, developing countries account for more than 70% of the world's land area and total population. Not only do they have a vast territory, immense populations, extensive markets, and rich natural resources, they also occupy many strategic areas. Therefore, developing countries occupy a crucial strategic position in terms of economic, trade, and military affairs. A US company, Goldman Sachs, first proposed the concept of BRIC countries in a report entitled "Building Better Global Economic BRICs" (Global Economics Paper No. 66) published in 2001. The BRIC countries are the four major emerging markets, namely, Brazil, Russia, India, and China. The report predicted that these four developing countries would occupy key positions in the future global economic landscape. In 2010, South Africa was officially included as a member in the BRIC cooperation mechanism, and the term "BRIC" was changed to "BRICS." As major emerging markets, the BRICS countries cover 25% of the world's territorial land area, 40% of the global population, 20% of global GDP, and 15% of global trade, and they contribute about 50% of global economic growth. Since China's economic reform, its average economic growth rate has exceeded 9% each year. Since the 1990s, India has experienced an average economic growth rate of about 6% each year. Since the twenty-first century, the average economic growth rates of Russia and Brazil have been around 6% and 3–4.9% each year, respectively, both of which are higher than the average levels of Western countries and the world. The rapid economic growth of these four countries has been accompanied by their ever-increasing international influence.

In summary, the developing world is composed of countries and areas with the following characteristics. These countries and areas are either former colonies and dependent territories, countries that have long implemented highly centralized planning systems, or countries with particular natural resource endowments (e.g., crude oil) that can bring about high income levels, but they have uniform economic structures, low degrees of modernization, and low levels of sociocultural evolution. Precisely for the reasons above, these countries have dualistic socioeconomic structures and underdeveloped market economies. They are still in or have not yet entered the process of industrialization and, thus, form a group of countries with clear differences from developed countries.

2. Social Formation and Structure of Developing Countries

Marxism provides scientific insights and general theories related to social formation and structure that are indispensable to the analysis of social development. These theories possess significance for both philosophy and general sociology. They formulate the concept of social formation based on the general trend of development in human history. Social formation refers to the qualitative, determinate type of society that a social system adopts at a given stage of historical development. Marxist sociology stems from the social relations formed among humans in their production activities. The first of these relations is the material relations of production, which can further be viewed as the basic and primitive relations that determine all other relations. Once we isolate the relations of production from all social relations and view them as the most basic relations that form the structure and skeleton of society, then we can obtain a completely objective standard, which in turn enables us to compare the histories of different regions and peoples within the same framework.

(1) Social Formation of Developing Countries

A social formation is the concrete form in which a society exists. It is a society that divides human history into specific stages of development for investigation and examination. The types of social formations found among the numerous developing countries can mainly be summed up by the characteristics below.

First, after breaking free from colonialism and imperialism, developing countries have largely embarked on the path of national independence during the same historical period. However, these countries have adopted different formations on the ladder of social progress. For example, in the African region, some sub-Saharan countries have remained in the slavery formation, in which tribal land ownership exists and tribal or commune chiefs have control over the land. In contrast, the majority of Latin American countries still implement the feudal system. In addition to the social formations of slavery and feudalism, a considerable proportion of developing countries have taken the direction of capitalism, whereas in Asia, Europe, and Latin America, some developing countries have taken the path toward socialism. Moreover, some countries have also defined socialism as their future development goal.

Second, among the types of social formations of developing countries, many countries also exhibit distortions of certain formations or transitional states from one formation to another. For example, the tribal ownership system in sub-Saharan countries is significantly different from the slavery system that had existed previously. Developed product economies have emerged in Asian and Latin American countries where feudal land ownership still prevails. Among countries with socialist formations, which primarily have public ownership of the means of production, there are in fact numerous ownership relations and means of distribution. In countries that have adopted capitalism or socialism as their directions of development, the transitional natures of their social formations are even more prominent.

Third, in the evolution of social formations, many developing countries may even bypass certain formations and directly adopt new formations. Certain ethnic groups or countries with tribal ownership systems do not necessarily have to undergo the feudal ownership system but instead may skip forward to the capitalist formation; certain ethnic groups or countries with feudal or semi-feudal formations may bypass the capitalist stage of development and directly take the path toward socialism.

The diverse, transient, and transitional nature of social formations in developing countries is mainly influenced by factors such as the effects of the global historical era, the control of the imperialist neo-colonial system, and interactions among developing countries. In their shared political and economic struggles, the vast number of developing countries have influenced each other in terms of material technologies, production relations, political systems, and ideologies, which has resulted in the emergence of different social formations among developing countries.

It is precisely due to the many particularities of the social formations of developing countries that their social development should be based on their national realities. They should not be too eager to achieve success and should certainly avoid blindly imitating the models of developed countries but should instead adopt gradual approaches and select the most appropriate social, political, economic, and cultural development strategies.

(2) Social Structures of Developing Countries

The social structures of developing countries generally share the following characteristics.

In terms of economic structure, the first characteristic is a relatively low level of GDP per capita. Currently, the GDP per capita of developing countries is about US$4,000. Although China is the world's second largest economic body, its GDP per capita is only one-tenth that of Japan's, and, hence, China is undoubtedly still a developing country. The second characteristic is a large population living in poverty. According to the latest "World Development Indicators" published by the World Bank on April 17, 2013, the top three countries and areas with the most people living in extreme poverty were Sub-Saharan Africa, India, and China, which are all developing countries or areas. The population living in poverty in developing countries has increased from 1 billion in 1990 to 1.3 billion today. These individuals live in the poorest countries in the world and have incomes of less than US$1 per person per day. Up to 80 million people in developing countries do not have any access to healthcare services, 840 million are malnourished, and 260 million are unable to attend school. In the poorest areas of Africa, the poverty incidence (the proportion of the total population living below the poverty line) has been increasing continuously. Currently, about half of the 630 million people in Africa are struggling at the starvation line. The third characteristic of developing countries is a large share of agriculture. As a whole, the vast majority of the population in developing countries lives in rural areas, generally accounting for 80% of the total population, whereas the rural population only accounts for 35% of the population or less in developed countries. The agriculture labor force in developing countries accounts for 66% of the labor force, whereas that of developed countries only accounts for 21% of the labor force. In terms of agricultural output as a share of GNP, that of developed countries is 8%, whereas that of developing countries is 32%. The fourth characteristic is a low level of exports. The export volume of developing countries is less than 30% of the global total, and primary products, which have relatively low technological content, account for 80% of export products. Moreover, the domestic sites of export production are largely controlled by foreign capital.

In terms of the political structure, the first feature is poor administrative stability. The political management of most developing countries is concentrated in industrial areas, major cities, and certain key regions. For example, during the 1980s in Africa, apart from Egypt, Tunisia, Morocco, Lesotho, and Somalia, virtually no other single nation-states were formed. The continuous conflicts among ethnic groups, tribes, and religions in many countries have made it impossible for central governments to implement effective administrative jurisdiction. The second feature is a turbulent political situation. As economic growth leads to new economic benefits for certain social groups and economic losses for other social groups, the daily lives and values of these members of society undergo rapid changes given their newly acquired or lost wealth. These changes easily induce people to form organizations to change the existing political system. The third feature is a low degree of democracy. Feudal oligarchies and military dictatorships are still common among developing countries. For example, countries such as Thailand, Indonesia, Pakistan, Afghanistan, Turkey, Egypt, Nigeria, Mexico, Nicaragua, Brazil, Chile, and Argentina have all implemented military dictatorships. This type of political power not only easily leads to political coups but is also inclined toward the overconcentration of power. The fourth feature is serious political corruption. For example, Rafael Trujillo profited US$400 million during the 20 years he was in power in the Dominican Republic, the wealth of the Somoza family in Nicaragua was such that they could buy half of all the land and factories in the country, and Ferdinand Marcos of the Philippines secretly pocketed large sums of public funds from the state treasury.

In terms of group structure, most developing countries have a dualistic structure that consists of a lower-level group and emerging upper-level groups. With the development of industrialization and urbanization, this group structure also underwent social differentiation. The original insular nature of rural areas was destroyed, causing lower-level groups to flood into the cities, thereby producing new relations, concepts, and values. The differentiation of the classes intensified with industrialization and economic development, and the degree of social inequality continued to worsen.

The education and health development of developing countries are generally lagging behind. In some countries, the rate of illiteracy is still relatively high in the population. Despite the increasing availability of tertiary education in recent years, the migration of talent is a serious issue due to the lack of planning. Most countries have poor healthcare professions, rampant diseases, a lack of medication and treatments, and slow development in science and technology.

3. Proposal of Representative Countries and Its Implications

Due to the current lack of a unified definition for developing countries, this book follows the principles of representativeness and a balanced distribution to select typical developing countries in Asia, Africa, Europe, and America; the leading countries of each region are represented by their respective BRICS countries. Specifically, seven countries were selected from Asia: China, India, Thailand, Vietnam, Philippines, Armenia, and Kyrgyzstan. Three countries were selected from Africa: South Africa, Egypt, and Morocco. Four countries were selected from Europe: Russia, Hungary, Czech Republic, and Bulgaria. Four countries were selected from America: Brazil, Cuba, Chile, and Mexico.

The selection of the developing countries that this book has chosen to investigate was based on the full consideration given to the economic, social, population, and health development of each country on the four continents. The social security systems in each of the four continents have their own unique characteristics, and it is of great value to study them separately. For example, Latin American countries are faced with growing poverty and defects in their social insurance systems. Eastern European countries have experienced regressions in the privatization of the reforms to their social insurance systems. The distorted welfare systems of southern European countries have affected their levels of income equality and have held back their economies. Low-income countries in Africa and Asia have been striving to achieve universal health insurance. Studying these healthcare systems with different characteristics will provide an excellent reference for China to develop its own unique healthcare security system.

SECTION II.HEALTH SYSTEMS AND HEALTH STATUSES OF DEVELOPING COUNTRIES

1. Exploration of Universal Health Security Systems

(1) Universal Health Coverage

Achieving universal coverage in health security is currently a major global trend. By comprehensively surveying the features of the historical development of health security worldwide, we know that the goal has always been to improve health security coverage until universal coverage is achieved. This understanding is of significant referential value to developing countries, where healthcare is generally still in its infancy. As a crucial step in the process of achieving universal health coverage (UHC) in developing countries, the universal coverage of healthcare security can be based on the path to attaining UHC.

UHC was a theory proposed by the WHO in recent years and was the theme of the World Health Report 2013, "Research for Universal Health Coverage." WHO Director-General Margaret Chan stated in her speech at the 65th World Health Assembly that UHC is the only powerful concept that must be mentioned in public health.

UHC was established based on the declaration in the 1948 Constitution of the WHO that health is a basic human right and the universal health agenda defined in the 1978 Declaration of Alma-Ata. Its goal is to ensure that everyone has access to the health services they need without suffering financial hardships. The theory of UHC believes that equality is the most crucial aspect, and it is hoped that all countries, especially developing countries, will not only track the progress of the overall national population but will also promote equality within different groups (e.g., by income level, gender, age, place of residence, immigration status, and ethnicity).

UHC has a direct impact on the health of the population. Access to health services ensures greater productivity in the population, which in turn enables people to actively contribute to their families and communities. It also ensures that children are able to attend school. In addition, protective measures against financial risks can prevent people from being impoverished due to out-of-pocket payments for health services expenses. Therefore, UHC is a key component of sustainable development and poverty reduction. It is also a key element in reducing social inequality and a sign of the government's commitment to improving the welfare of its citizens.

In order to achieve UHC, we must also recognize that all departments play crucial roles in guaranteeing human health, including the transport, education, and urban planning departments.

The theme of the World Health Report 2010 was "Health Systems Financing: The Path to Universal Coverage." The report listed several recommendations for the appropriate strategies that should be adopted by countries at different stages of development to maximize service coverage and reduce financial risks.

The realization of UHC is also a topic of significant concern worldwide. The WHO pointed out that achieving UHC in a community or a country requires the following essential factors:

1. A robust, efficient, well-functioning health system that can meet key health needs through integrated, people-centered healthcare services (including services for HIV, tuberculosis, malaria, noncommunicable diseases, and maternal and child health). This system includes the provision of information encouraging the public to stay healthy and prevent diseases, early health status detection, the capacity for disease treatment, and the rehabilitation of patients.
2. The establishment of a system of financing health services to ensure that individuals do not experience financial hardships when using health services.
3. Access to basic drugs and technology for the diagnosis and treatment of medical problems.
4. Well-trained and enthusiastic healthcare workers with the full capacity to deliver services and meet the needs of the patients based on the best available evidence.

The promotion and protection of health contributes to the enhancement of human well-being and is a facilitator of sustainable socioeconomic development. Thirty years ago, the Declaration of Alma-Ata stated that "primary health care for all people" contributes not only to a better quality of life but also to world peace and security. However, numerous factors can influence health. The WHO defines the Social Determinants of Health (SDH) as the factors affecting health that result from the basic structure and social conditions of social stratification within the living and working environments of the people that are beyond the direct causes of diseases. These factors are the "causes of causes" of diseases and include all the social conditions in which people live and work, such as poverty, social exclusion, and living conditions. Based on this definition, we can see that the methods to promote and maintain health have exceeded the purview of the health sector. The conditions in which people grow, live, work, and age have an immense impact on life and death. Education, housing, food, and employment issues all have impacts on health. This notion eventually resulted in the theory of Health in All Policies (HiAP).

(2) Health in All Policies (HiAP)

In China, the majority of functions in healthcare security do not come under the jurisdiction of the health sector. Hence, to achieve the universal coverage of healthcare security, it is necessary to fully implement the contents of HiAP. HiAP was first proposed by the Finnish EU Presidency in 2006 and aims to achieve common goals through intersectoral cooperation. It reiterated the importance of public health in policies and structural factors that affect health. In 2013, the Eighth Global Conference on Health Promotion was held in Helsinki, Finland, with HiAP as the theme of the conference. In her speech at the conference, WHO Director-General Margaret Chan stated that the social determinants of health are exceptionally broad and that policies in other sectors can have profound effects on health. When addressing the problems of health, we should make full use of the HiAP strategy and lend the strength of multisectoral collaboration to protect health policies from the effects of commercial interests. The conference reviewed and adopted the Helsinki Statement and Health in All Policies: Framework for Country Action, which called on all countries to place an emphasis on the social determinants of health and to provide organizational and technical measures to support the implementation of the HiAP strategy.

2. Transition of Health Statuses in Developing Countries

Developing countries have had extremely poor health statuses in the past. Rural children were severely undernourished and were afflicted by infectious diseases and diarrhea.

According to the World Health Statistics 2014, the life expectancy in Angola in 2012 was 51 years, the infant mortality rate was 100 deaths per 1,000 births, and the under-five mortality rate was 164 deaths per 1,000 births. In stark contrast, during the same year, the life expectancy in Japan was 84 years, the infant mortality rate was 2 deaths per 1,000 births, and the under-five mortality rate was 3 deaths per 1,000 births. If only cross-sectional comparisons are made, then these data clearly indicate the major differences between the two extremes of developing and developed countries. However, we should not ignore the fact that the health statuses of many developing countries have improved significantly. In 1960, 34 countries had life expectancies lower than 40 years of age, and only a few had life expectancies that exceeded 70 years of age. However, by 2012, more than 120 countries had life expectancies over 70 years of age. In 1960, nearly 50 countries had infant mortality rates above 150 deaths per 1,000 births. By 2012, apart from Angola and the Republic of Congo, all countries were within 100 deaths per 1,000 births. In 1960, only three countries had infant mortality rates below 20 deaths per 1,000 live births. By 2012, more than half of the countries had fewer than 20 deaths per 1,000 live births. Figures 15.1 and 15.2 show that the under-five mortality rates of low-income and lower-middle-income countries decreased by around half and that their life expectancies have also increased. See also Table 15.1. On October 26, 1979, the WHO declared that smallpox had been eradicated throughout the world. Polio has disappeared in the Western hemisphere and has significantly decreased in other parts of the world. An effective vaccine against hepatitis B has been developed, and an effective treatment for filariasis was discovered. The first health revolution in public health has smoothly transitioned to the second revolution in public health and medicine. With the rapid pace of urbanization and industrialization, the risks faced by the population include tuberculosis, psychiatric disorders, and sexually transmitted diseases, with increasing risks of injuries and illnesses related to crime, motor vehicles, and the workplace. Since 1985, the proportion of the urban population in developing countries has increased from 30% to 50%. In countries that are undergoing health status transitions, cancer mortality has increased from 7% to 14%, and cardiovascular disease mortality has increased from 19% to 35%. Chronic diseases are characterized by long durations and high costs. In order to improve the

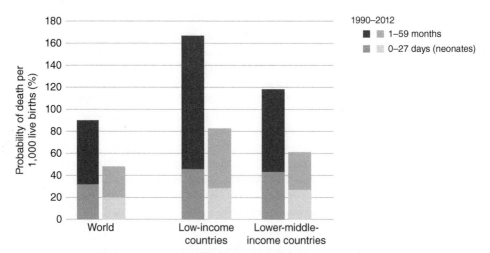

FIGURE 15.1 Under-five mortality rates of the world, low-income countries, and lower-middle-income countries in 1990 and 2012. *Source:* World Health Statistics, 2014.

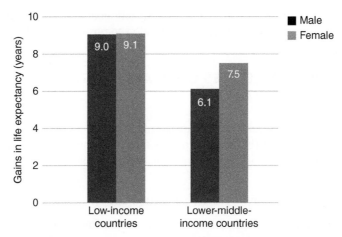

FIGURE 15.2 Years gained in life expectancy by gender in low-income countries and lower-middle-income countries in 1990–2012. *Source:* World Health Statistics, 2014.

TABLE 15.1 Health Indicators of Some Developing Countries in 1990–2012 (Partial Years)

Indicators	Country	Year 1990	1995	2000	2005	2010	2012
Life expectancy (years)	Afghanistan	49	52	55	57	60	61
	Angola	41	42	45	49	51	51
	Chile	73	75	77	78	79	80
	China	69	70	71	74	75	75
Under-five mortality rate (%)	Afghanistan	17.9	14.9	13.6	11.9	10.6	10.0
	Angola	22.6	22.5	21.7	20.5	18.2	17.3
	Bangladesh	14.4	11.4	8.8	6.7	4.9	4.3
	Bolivia	12.3	10.0	7.7	5.8	4.4	4.1
	China	5.4	4.8	3.7	2.4	1.6	1.4
	India	12.6	10.9	9.1	7.5	1.6	1.4
Crude death rate (%)	Afghanistan	1.6	1.4	1.2	1.1	0.9	0.8
	India	1.1	1.0	0.9	0.8	0.8	0.8
	Angola	2.4	2.2	1.9	1.7	1.5	1.4
DTP3 immunization rate (%)	Afghanistan	25	20	24	58	66	71
	Angola	24	24	31	47	91	91
	Ethiopia	49	57	27	44	63	61
	Ghana	51	70	80	84	94	92

Source: World Bank, 2013.

quality of life and promote human health and longevity, the third health revolution, health promotion, was included in the agenda. As a result, the goal of medicine began shifting from being disease-centered to being health-centered, and its objectives have gradually shifted from fighting diseases and death to fighting premature death, maintaining and promoting health, and improving the quality of life. Thus, the specific goals of the third health revolution are to promote self-care and family care and to develop community-based health services.

SECTION III. CHALLENGES OF HEALTH SYSTEMS IN DEVELOPING COUNTRIES

Although we recognize the series of achievements attained by developing countries, we must also acknowledge that the health statuses of developing countries are still far from perfect. The following are the main challenges facing the transition in health status.

1. Inadequacies in Overall Health Resources

Many developing countries lack healthcare workers and infrastructure and, hence, cannot provide their people with high-quality services. Most countries implement a mixed system of health services provided by public and private institutions. However, the public system still has a monopoly over health service provision and, therefore, prevents social capital from increasing the health resources of society. The World Health Report 2006 pointed out that there is a lack of healthcare workers worldwide, and although this shortage is global, it is most prominent in poor developing countries. For example, one-third of full-time healthcare workers work in North American regions, such as the US and Canada, where the number of healthcare workers per 1,000 people is 24.8, whereas that of Africa is only 2.3. The shortage of healthcare workers is most severe in Sub-Saharan Africa, where the population accounts for 11% of the global population and the disease burden accounts for 24% of the global total but the number of healthcare workers only accounts for 3% of the total. In terms of infrastructure, the healthcare institutions, equipment, human resources, and drug supplies of nearly all developing countries are biased toward the top of the pyramid in the healthcare system, whereas rural areas are poorly equipped, have backward infrastructure, and lack human resources. Furthermore, public investment is overly concentrated in tertiary hospitals located in major cities, which has exacerbated the inequality and low effectiveness of healthcare services.

2. Poor Implementation of Health System Reforms

From a global perspective, the reform of the medical and health system is a major issue that is difficult to resolve in both developed and developing countries. Healthcare system reform is a global problem, and its progress is challenging even in the US. Before US President Barack Obama took office, he promised to implement thorough reforms to the health system. However, it was a major challenge for him to prevent the increase in the fiscal burden and also guarantee public welfare and healthcare efficiency, and this issue has plagued previous US administrations for several decades. This challenge exists in both developed and developing countries because healthcare services are a type of professional technical service with a high degree of information asymmetry and an ultimate goal of being safe and effective. Regardless of whether greater dependence is placed on the government or the market, these are only the means to achieve the ultimate goal of healthcare. According to current global trends, guaranteeing public welfare is the most basic aim of healthcare. On this basis, gradual improvements in efficiency and quality can be achieved through increased investment and refined mechanisms. Reforming the medical and health system is a project of social system engineering. Based on the experiences of all countries and of history, we can see that healthcare reform is a global problem. Thus, the governments and people of all countries must fully acknowledge the long-term, arduous, and complicated nature of healthcare reforms.

3. Uneven Distribution of Health Statuses and Human Resources

Countries that are in a state of health status transition include most countries in South America, several countries along the Pacific coast (e.g., Thailand, Malaysia, and Indonesia), and some countries in central and eastern Europe. Most countries in Africa are still in a pretransition state; that is, they have high birth rates, high infant mortality rates, relatively low life expectancies, poor environmental health, and high rates of fatal infections. Furthermore, there are vast differences in the healthcare workforce among different countries. In Thailand, there are 3.9 physicians and 20.8 nurses and midwives per 10,000 people. In Hungary, there are 29.6 physicians and 63.9 nurses and midwives per 10,000 people. Many developing countries require medical students to serve in primary care for one to five years after graduation. However, such attempts often fail due to insufficient incentives, thus leading to losses of talent in prevention, rehabilitation, nursing, and emergency care, which are areas where demand has been increasing. The strongest disciplines of medical schools in developing countries are usually basic science and clinical medicine, whereas disciplines such as primary healthcare, preventive medicine, public health education, and clinical epidemiology are relatively weak. At present, a number of medical schools in developing countries have modified their courses substantially. However, sustained development is still needed to rectify the long-term disadvantaged positions of these disciplines.

4. Low Willingness to Invest in Adult Healthcare

Due to political, economic, and equality issues, the funding and technologies provided by government planning and nongovernmental organizations are generally more inclined toward supporting maternal and child healthcare. In contrast, governments lack the same willingness to invest in adult healthcare. First, the achievements in health status transition have benefited from economic growth and increased investment in healthcare. However, the frequent occurrence of financial and economic crises (e.g., the global recession from the late 1970s to the early 1980s and the global financial crises of 1997 and 2007) has hindered this trend, as the increase in debt and inflation has led to cutbacks in healthcare investments. Second, the economic benefits of improving adult health are low. Using the US dollar to represent the gains in healthy life expectancy per person per year, the average spending on medical and social programs for maternal and child health was US\$5–\$50, whereas that on adult interventions (prevention or treatment) was consistently higher. Third, there has been limited "transfer" of investments in adult healthcare. If low-cost investments in maternal and child health can lead to gains in healthy life expectancy of several decades, then it is difficult to motivate people to invest their limited resources in adult healthcare, which may only lead to gains of several years. Finally, the majority of developing countries are still struggling with improving the three major health indicators. Both domestic and international pressures point to the need to incorporate the three major unaccomplished indicators in the agenda.

5. Low Input into Health Research

Most of the world's diseases (including chronic diseases) occur in developing countries. However, the majority of research on health issues is carried out in developed countries, where the focus is on the health issues of these countries. Stephen Matlin, the former Executive Director of the Global Forum for Health Research, stated during the 11th Global Forum for Health Research that low- and middle-income countries face multiple challenges in health research. In 2003, global investment in health research was nearly US$126 billion, but only a small proportion was used to address the health issues of developing countries. Only 5% of research funding in developing countries was spent on researching various health issues. However, these countries account for 90% of the total global burden of disease. Such research may emphasize prevention, with a focus on developing new or improved vaccines, parasite control, and occupation health; this research may also emphasize clinical medicine, with a focus on the efficacy of new diagnosis and treatment techniques. As health research does not bring about immediate changes in health status, it is of crucial significance to change the old attitudes held by governments and private donors. As the health issues of developing countries are becoming more similar to those of developed countries, the opportunities for collaboration in research will increase.

6. Overdependence on Aid May Weaken the Government's Sense of Responsibility Toward National Health

"Charitable" organizations play a role in the international health community through the provision of funding, knowledge, and technology by a variety of organizations. These organizations include international organizations (e.g., the WHO and the United Nations Children's Fund [UNICEF]), governmental organizations (e.g., the US Agency for International Development), various religious voluntary organizations, various foundations, and private voluntary organizations (e.g., The Hope Foundation). Most of these organizations have specific aid areas or program focuses, and they provide direct services or support to the implementation of related programs. The majority of developing countries, especially low-income countries, have insufficient financial reserves, weak public health systems, outdated infrastructure, and long-term dependence on external donations. In some areas, receiving aid has become the only means for maintaining health.

CHAPTER SIXTEEN

Comparison of Healthcare and Social Security Systems in BRICS Countries

 SECTION I. COMPARISON OF SOCIOECONOMICS AND HEALTH RESOURCES IN BRICS COUNTRIES

1. Origin of BRICS Countries

In 2001, the former chief economist of Goldman Sachs, Jim O'Neill, first proposed the concept of BRIC countries, which included the four largest emerging markets in the world, namely, Brazil, Russia, India, and China. The acronym formed from the names of the four countries (BRIC) was associated with the word "brick." In December 2010, the BRIC countries unanimously agreed to incorporate South Africa as an official member of the BRIC cooperation mechanism. Thus, the BRIC countries became the BRICS countries.

Developed countries have completed the process of industrialization and urbanization. The continuous improvement in their levels of socioeconomic development is accompanied by relatively comprehensive healthcare systems with high service levels. In contrast, BRICS countries are emerging market economies that are undergoing social transformations and rapid economic development. Thus, a gap remains between these countries' healthcare services and the health needs of their inhabitants. As developing countries, the BRICS countries have numerous similarities in terms of their historical, political, and economic systems; economic development processes; and population sizes. Therefore, an in-depth analysis and exploration of the healthcare systems in BRICS countries can provide ideas and policy suggestions for China's current healthcare reform process, which aims to establish a healthcare system that better suits China's national conditions. Thus, the healthcare systems of BRICS countries can serve as more direct references for China as it deepens its healthcare system reforms.

2. Health Resources of BRICS Countries

As shown in Table 16.1, China's total GDP has always ranked first among the BRICS countries. However, from 2000 to 2010, Russia had the fastest GDP growth rate. Brazil had the highest GDP per capita, followed by Russia, whereas China ranked fourth, with a relatively low level of GDP per capita. However, China ranked second in terms of growth rate. China consistently ranked first in terms of total healthcare expenditure and its growth rate. In 2013, Russia had the highest healthcare expenditure per capita, whereas China ranked fourth among the BRICS countries, with relatively low expenditure per capita. However, China had the fastest growing healthcare expenditure per capita, followed by Russia, and then Brazil. Total healthcare expenditure as a share of GDP and its growth rate were relatively low in China, as it ranked fourth for both. As for government healthcare spending as a share of total healthcare expenditure, China ranked fourth in 2000 but leapt to second in 2013 with a cumulative increase of 16 percentage points, far higher than the increases in other BRICS countries. China consistently ranked second in terms of government healthcare spending as a share of total government spending and its corresponding growth rate was ranked third; Brazil's corresponding growth rate was the highest among the BRICS countries (6.6 percentage points), followed by that of South Africa in second (1.5 percentage points).

As shown in Table 16.2, among the BRICS countries in 2012, Russia had the most physicians per capita (43.1/10,000 people), followed by Brazil (17.6/10,000 people), with China ranking third (14.6/10,000 people) and India ranking last (6.5/10,000 people). Considering just the BRICS countries, Russia also had the most nurses and midwives per capita (85.2/10,000 people), followed by Brazil (64.2/10,000 people), with China ranking third (15.1/10,000 people) and India ranking last (10.0/10,000 people). Among the BRICS countries, Russia had the most hospital beds per capita (97.0/10,000 people), followed by China (39.0/10,000 people), with Brazil ranking third (23.0/10,000 people) and India ranking last (9.0/10,000 people). Finally, among these countries, Russia had the most psychiatric beds per capita (11.1/10,000 people), followed by South Africa, with Brazil ranking third, China ranking fourth, and India ranking last.

These comparisons indicate that Russia's healthcare resources are far ahead of those of the other BRICS countries. However, studies have shown that Russia's healthcare level, service

TABLE 16.1 Healthcare Expenditures of BRICS Countries in 2013

Items Related to Healthcare Expenditure	China	Russia	India	Brazil	South Africa
GDP (US$100 million)	92,400	20,970	18,770	22,460	3,506
GDP per capita (US$)	4,433	10,710	1,419	10,978	7,266
Total healthcare expenditure (US$100 million)	4,991	1,742	1,520	1,968	458
Healthcare expenditure per capita (US$)	373	1,227	126	1,009	915
Total healthcare expenditure as a share of GDP	5.0	6.5	3.7	9.0	8.7
Government healthcare spending as a share of total healthcare expenditure (%)	54.3	58.7	28.2	47.0	46.6
Personal out-of-pocket expenses as a share of total healthcare expenditure (%)	45.7	41.3	71.8	53.0	53.4
Government healthcare spending as a share of total government expenditure (%)	12.1	9.7	6.8	10.7	12.4

TABLE 16.2 Healthcare Resources of BRICS Countries in 2012

Item	China	Russia	India	Brazil	South Africa
Total population (100 million people)	13.51	1.44	12.37	1.98	0.51
Percentage of population over 65 years of age (%)	9.00	13.00	5.00	7.00	
Number of physicians per 10,000 people	14.60	43.10	6.50	17.60	7.60
Number of nurses and midwives per 10,000 people	15.10	85.20	10.00	64.20	—
Number of hospital beds per 10,000 people	39.00	97.00		23.00	20.00
Number of psychiatric beds per 10,000 people	1.40	11.10	0.20	1.90	2.20

quality, and health conditions are relatively poor given the wealth of its healthcare resources. Many of its hospitals and clinics have poor management and equipment, and some even lack a quality management system. India has significant urban–rural and interregional differences in the health levels of its residents. The services provided by the public healthcare sector are insufficient to meet its residents' needs. India was once rated by the WHO as the country with the lowest degree of healthcare coverage. Brazil is the largest country in Latin America and the country with the largest wealth gap in the world. However, over a long period of time, Brazil has gradually established a relatively comprehensive Unified Health System, a strict and meticulous two-way referral process, and a strong network of community health services, all of which have enabled the health status of Brazilians to approach that of citizens of developed countries. This experience undoubtedly provides China with useful ideas to resolve the issue of equality in healthcare. However, due to the lack of emphasis on hospital quality and efficiency, Brazil's hospitals consume up to two-thirds of the total healthcare budget of the Brazilian government. South Africa is facing issues such as inadequate healthcare resources and service provision and low service efficiency in public healthcare institutions. The South African government has opted to implement the restructuring of private institutions to improve the services provided by public institutions.

Studies have shown that China has a moderate level of health resources among the BRICS countries, but its number of hospital beds per capita is relatively high. China has the highest total healthcare expenditure and the fastest growth rates of total healthcare expenditure and healthcare expenditure per capita among the five countries. Its total healthcare expenditure as a share of GDP is relatively low and also has a low growth rate. Its total healthcare expenditure as a share of total government healthcare spending, however, is increasing at a relatively fast pace. Since the Chinese economic reform, the Chinese government has fully relaxed its interventions and control in the field of healthcare. Healthcare institutions have taken responsibility for their own profits and losses, and government investments have gradually decreased. All healthcare institutions, including public healthcare institutions and even public health institutions, implemented independent financial accounting and management methods. Various healthcare institutions gradually moved toward full competition, and the price formation mechanisms of healthcare services were also mainly determined by market supply and demand. Healthcare institutions often adopted enterprise management models. Economic indicators were evaluated and even contracted at every level to fully link personal income with business income. The unreasonable distribution and structure of health resources led to simultaneous issues of waste and shortages.

About 80% of health resources in China are concentrated in cities, two-thirds of which are concentrated in major cities. The share of certain high-end medical equipment in these major cities has reached or surpassed the levels of developed countries, which clearly indicates a surplus. To recover the costs of these investments and pursue higher returns, healthcare institutions began arbitrarily using large-scale medical equipment for patients and frequently conducting indiscriminate or duplicate examinations, all of which increased patients' burdens. At the same time, the public health institutions below the county level, especially those in rural villages, lacked basic medical equipment and adequate conditions. The marketization of public healthcare institutions was not consistent with the characteristics of healthcare development and became a major feature of China's healthcare reform. This reform process ultimately led to the problem of expensive and inaccessible healthcare, which was widely criticized by the public. At present, private healthcare institutions account for a very small market share in China and mainly provide primary healthcare services and general services for treatment and diagnosis. Development in the private healthcare market faces many restrictions, as sound and orderly market mechanisms have not been formed and the functions of the government and the market in the healthcare system have not been clearly defined.

SECTION II. COMPARISON OF HEALTH INSURANCE SYSTEMS IN BRICS COUNTRIES

The healthcare security system and citizens' health levels are important indicators of a country's levels of political, economic, and social development. The development of the healthcare system is a gradual and progressive process in all countries and always involves starting from scratch and developing from a low to a high level. This process is intimately linked to economic development. Due to their low levels of economic development, developing countries have mostly established multi-modal, composite health security systems that are based on their actual conditions but that also draw on the successful experiences of other countries.

By systematically investigating the BRICS countries, which have similar socioeconomic development levels and population structures to those of China, we can identify the common characteristics of the healthcare systems of these countries.

1. Establishment of Universal Healthcare Security Systems

This characteristic refers to the establishment of a basic healthcare security system through state legislation and institutional arrangements to guarantee that all citizens have access to a certain level of free healthcare services.

In 1949, India adopted its first constitution, which stipulates that all citizens shall enjoy free basic healthcare. Since 2005, the Indian government has implemented the National Rural Health Mission to fully guarantee that children, women, and poor individuals in impoverished areas have access to high-quality and efficient healthcare services. The government has established a three-tier healthcare network in rural areas that includes subcenters, primary health centers, and community health centers. The most basic healthcare coverage is provided to the majority of farmers through the Universal Immunization Program and the free treatment programs in public hospitals. Furthermore, there are three forms of rural health insurance in India: organizations for agricultural product processing companies that help collectively insure farmers with insurance companies; nongovernmental organizations that help members design collective insurance schemes with insurance companies; and health and welfare programs for trade unions of the informal economy. Public financing in India is mainly raised through taxation at various levels of government, nontax revenues, and social insurance premiums. There are two main types of social insurance: the Employees' State Insurance Scheme and the Central Government Insurance Schemes. As the government's share of healthcare expenditure is relatively low, personal out-of-pocket expenses are the main source of health funds.

In 1986, the Brazilian government drafted a new constitution and established the national Unified Health System (Sistema Único de Saúde, SUS), which views protecting the basic health rights of all citizens as a key responsibility of all levels of government. The new constitution stipulates that it is the responsibility of the state and the government to provide every citizen with free healthcare services and that protecting the health of all citizens is a key obligation of the state and the government. Everyone is equal under the SUS, and the services provided range from preventive care and disease treatment to rehabilitation care, with the goal of simultaneously meeting the different healthcare needs of different groups. A three-tier management system is implemented among the federal, state, and municipal governments, all of which have clearly defined responsibilities. Each region has an SUS management committee, and residents of a committee's region participate in its management. The implementation of the national SUS enabled Brazil to achieve major progress in its health system reforms. The public service system is centered on primary healthcare, and the financing system is mainly based on general taxation. This system differs from the financing system recommended by the World Bank, which is based on social health insurance. The financing system is also the most prominent feature that distinguishes Brazil's healthcare system from those of the majority of Latin American countries. Brazil's funding method is public financing, which means that health funds are jointly raised by the federal, state, and municipal governments, which also jointly provide basic healthcare services to Brazilian citizens. The system places a special emphasis on the functions of the municipal government in healthcare management. Private health insurance is a supplement to the SUS through which private health insurance companies provide insured persons with various health insurance schemes to meet the needs of different social classes. In addition, all levels of government are required to establish healthcare committees consisting of citizen representatives who participate in the formulation of healthcare policies and monitor their implementation. Brazil stipulated through legislation that the government must assume full responsibility for national fiscal expenditure on healthcare, and explicit provisions were made regarding the share of healthcare expenditure that shall be borne by the state and municipal governments as a percentage of total fiscal expenditure. Specifically, that of state governments shall not be lower than 12%, and that of municipal governments shall not be lower than 15%. Market-based operations drive Brazil's private health insurance. Its premiums are collected based on disease risk, and its focus is on items that are not covered by the SUS. Hence, it is a useful supplement to the free healthcare programs.

China implements a "three vertical and three horizontal" healthcare security system that can be divided into the main tier, the supplementary tier, and the basic tier. The main tier forms the bulk of China's healthcare security and has the largest number of insured persons and the most extensive coverage. This tier includes the Urban Employee Basic Medical Insurance, the Urban Resident Basic Medical Insurance, and the New Rural Cooperative Medical Insurance. Currently, at an institutional level, China has preliminarily established the basic framework for a multitier healthcare security system. This framework is based mainly on basic medical insurance and is complemented by various forms of supplemental health insurance and backed by social medical assistance as a bottom line. The population covered by basic medical insurance includes urban employees and urban residents (e.g., students, children, elderly persons without income, and incapacitated persons), whereas rural residents have access to health insurance coverage through the New Rural Cooperative

Medical Care Scheme. Basic health insurance follows the principle of "low levels and broad coverage" because "broad coverage" implies that the health security provided can only be at a "low level." Since 2009, the Chinese government has gradually promoted new reforms of the healthcare system that have been further strengthened by advocating government leadership and public welfare. Thus, China's healthcare system has ushered in a new era.

The implementation of the Russian health insurance law, entitled "On Compulsory Health Insurance in the Russian Federation," led to the establishment of the Federal Compulsory Medical Insurance Fund and promoted the adoption of compulsory health insurance. Its main sources of funding are compulsory and voluntary health insurance contributions. As in the case of China's Urban Employee Basic Medical Insurance, in Russia, companies and employees must each contribute part of the insurance premiums. Specifically, companies or employers must contribute 3.6% of an employee's total wages, and the employee must contribute 1.80% of his total wages.

2. Encouraging the Development of Private Healthcare Institutions and Commercial Health Insurance

This characteristic implies not imitating the models of developed countries but instead focusing on national conditions and designing a health security system that targets different income groups and encourages the development of private healthcare institutions and commercial health insurance.

Brazil implements a universal, unified, and free basic healthcare system. The government runs public hospitals and community health centers, which provide free basic healthcare services to all citizens. The system covers about 700,000 people, which includes all low-income groups and rural residents in the country. As the conditions and security levels provided by free healthcare are fairly low, commercial health insurance and private healthcare institutions co-exist with the universal free healthcare system. Based on their personal income levels, citizens can voluntarily purchase and use the healthcare services of private hospitals. The majority of high-income individuals, who account for about 30% of the total population, are enrolled in private health insurance.

India's free universal healthcare refers to the most basic healthcare services provided by government-run public hospitals. Due to insufficient government investment, the conditions and standards of public hospitals are relatively poor. Thus, patients of greater financial means often choose to seek medical treatment from private hospitals. As commercial health insurance is underdeveloped in India, residents must bear relatively high out-of-pocket medical expenses. India also has 45,000 private healthcare institutions, and, in 2000, these institutions accounted for 93% of all healthcare institutions in India, 64% of all hospital beds, and 80–85% of all physicians. Furthermore, private healthcare institutions have continued to increase in number and have essentially monopolized the vast majority of outpatient services in urban and rural areas. Thus, we can conclude that India's private healthcare services occupy a dominant position in terms of both the number of institutions and the size of the population served.

In Russia, each state has established funds at the corresponding level as new sources of nonbudgetary funding to increase the budget and establish a consolidated financing mechanism. This funding provides comprehensive coverage for accessible healthcare services but also gives patients the freedom to choose their service providers and insurance. The main sources of funding for the compulsory health insurance fund are the compulsory insurance premiums provided by companies and funding from the federal government. Of these sources, premium contributions account for more than 90% of the total funding for compulsory health insurance. The wages of healthcare workers are paid by the country, whereas patients' medical and meal expenses during hospitalization are covered by health insurance. With the economic recovery of the Russian Federation in recent years, the Russian government has gradually expanded its investment in the healthcare sector. However, individuals must still bear relatively high levels of medical expenses. Due to its insufficient investment in the health sector, the Russian government has been encouraging the public to purchase commercial health insurance and use the services of private healthcare institutions.

South Africa has a vast and growing private health sector. In the early 1990s, the private financing of healthcare costs accounted for about 60% of all financing, but less than one quarter of the population had access to health services in the private sector. The largest funding medium in the private sector was the health insurance schemes, which were supported by nonprofit associations funded by employers and employees. The government provided subsidies through the tax deductions of premiums contributed by employers. Since the late 1980s, health insurance premiums and spending on benefit payments have been growing at an annual rate that is two to three times higher than inflation, and the co-payment rates borne by members of the health insurance schemes have also been increasing substantially. Thus, the number of members enrolled in health insurance schemes grew at a slower rate from the late 1980s to the early 1990s, eventually leading to decreases in the number of members and in the coverage rate (the coverage rate fell from 17% in 1996 to 16% in 1998). Since the 1980s, the health insurance schemes began implementing risk stratification, which led to more detailed risk sharing within the health insurance schemes and a gradual increase in the burdens of high-risk individuals. In contrast, actual health expenditure in the public sector was mostly stagnant in the 1980s and 1990s. However, the dependence of low- and middle-income groups on public services has begun to increase for reasons such as population growth, rising costs, risk stratification in the private sector, and the "elimination" of insured patients in the public sector once their benefits have been consumed.

3. Emphasis on the Construction of Primary Healthcare Services

According to the economic principles concerning the nature of public goods, quasi-public goods, and private goods, among healthcare services, the primary healthcare system is a type of public good or quasi-public good. It is not difficult to see that governments should provide primary healthcare services and that improving the primary healthcare system can also help to reduce a country's disease treatment costs. All BRICS countries have attached great importance to the construction of the primary healthcare system and have established strict referral and basic drug systems to control healthcare costs and improve service efficiency.

In 1988, due to powerful democratic movements and the promotion of the National Health Assembly, Brazil proposed the reform concept of "universal coverage, equality, continuity, and integration" and created the SUS. This program altered the past focus on disease and began to emphasize family health services. Not only does it provide traditional health services, but it also pays greater attention to the growing problems of food safety, undernutrition, and the health of the living environment. Free family health services are a prominent feature of Brazil's current primary public healthcare system. However, Brazil's universal SUS also faces certain problems that are difficult to solve. (1) The demand for public healthcare services has surpassed its supply. The government's limited financial investment is unable to guarantee that the demand for public health services, such as primary healthcare, disease prevention, and basic treatments, can be met. (2) Healthcare service networks are lacking in rural areas. Although the Family Health Program, Regionalization Program, and other programs are currently underway, nearly 10% of Brazil's population still has difficulty accessing health services. (3) Public healthcare services are of poor quality, and the supply of drugs is inadequate. However, Brazil has established a health service network and a two-way referral system. The free healthcare system is based on community healthcare institutions, which provide local residents, especially the elderly, women, and children, with free access to primary healthcare services within their communities. A community-based first-visit system was established such that patients must first seek medical treatment within their communities. When a patient with a complex condition needs to be transferred to a hospital for treatment, the community healthcare institution contacts the referral office directly to arrange for a visit to a general or specialist hospital. The referral system has effectively enhanced the utilization rate of community healthcare institutions, improved the efficiency of general hospitals, and controlled the rise in healthcare costs. China can draw on this valuable experience.

In January 2005, the Indian government launched the National Rural Health Mission (2005–2012) to address the poor conditions of the rural health industry. Its focus was on resolving a series of issues influencing national health, such as toilets and environmental sanitation, safe drinking water, the control of infectious diseases, and nutritional intake. The Indian government established a three-tier health service system that covered both rural and urban areas, and 60% of the national health service network consisted of public healthcare institutions. Of these institutions, 150,000 were primary healthcare institutions, providing basic preventive and general outpatient healthcare services; 7,500 were secondary healthcare institutions, providing simple inpatient healthcare services; and only 120 were tertiary healthcare institutions, mainly providing specialist inpatient services to wealthy individuals. However, due to insufficient fiscal investment, India's primary healthcare system is still fraught with many serious problems. (1) In rural areas, not many health centers have been established in remote and impoverished regions; regions with primary health centers lack necessary facilities, healthcare workers, and basic drugs; and rural health officials and healthcare workers often fail to fulfill their responsibilities. (2) In urban areas, the health status of the floating population is poorer than that of rural residents; the coverage rate of primary health centers is far lower than that in rural areas; and public hospitals generally face issues such as severe shortages of medical equipment and drugs and dissatisfactory referral channels.

In the late 1950s, China established and developed a primary healthcare system during a time of extreme poverty. Prior to the economic reform, cooperative medical care covered approximately 90% of the rural population, which essentially guaranteed the health levels of most citizens and was praised by UNESCO. However, with the weakening of the collective economy, the coverage rate of rural medical care dropped from 90% in 1978 to 5% in 1990, and the rural public healthcare system was on the verge of collapse. Under these circumstances, the focus of healthcare work gradually shifted from rural to urban areas, with a greater emphasis on treatment and less emphasis on prevention. Since the SARS outbreak in 2003 and especially from 2005 to the present, the Chinese government has begun to pay close attention to the reconstruction of the public health system, with a new focus on a comprehensive primary healthcare service system to promote the gradual equalization of basic public health services. In 2009–2011, five requirements were proposed as new healthcare reforms, one of which was to promote the gradual equalization of basic public health services.

Despite the differences in the specific contents of the healthcare systems of the BRICS countries and the continuous improvements made according to socioeconomic development, changes in the disease spectrum, and changes in citizens' healthcare needs, the basic functions of these healthcare systems remain largely consistent. All of these systems embody the principles of strengthening government investment and supervision, rationally allocating healthcare resources, promoting equal access to healthcare services, strengthening health education, reducing disease costs, controlling healthcare costs, standardizing healthcare procedures, improving healthcare service quality, and continuously improving health levels. All of them focus on guaranteeing the basic health rights of citizens and continuously improving the health levels of citizens as the overall goals of establishing a healthcare system. In addition, these countries have also established financing mechanisms based on government taxation, social insurance, and individual expenses, with public healthcare institutions making up the main body of the healthcare delivery system to ensure the public nature of basic healthcare services. Private healthcare institutions are important supplements to the system, introducing the competitive effects of market mechanisms, and commercial health insurance has also been introduced to satisfy the multi-level and diversified healthcare needs of the populations.

SECTION III. COMPARISON OF HEALTH SYSTEMS IN BRICS COUNTRIES

The experiences of developed countries have shown that marketization not only improves the efficiency of healthcare services but could also contribute to social equality, that is, "managed marketization." Managed marketization has been the major trend of global healthcare system reforms. The healthcare systems of developing countries, as represented by the BRICS countries, are also managed but involve different forms of management.

1. From Models of Centralized Government Management to Commercial Fund Management

Prior to its healthcare reforms, Russia inherited the centralized management model of the Soviet Union, in which the government played a substantial role in various social insurance schemes, including health insurance. After the healthcare reform, Russia's healthcare management system underwent a major transformation. (1) Health insurance companies: according to the relevant provisions in the Health Insurance Act of 1991, health insurance companies are independent operational entities that are not governed by the government's health administration agencies and healthcare institutions. Health insurance companies serve as insurers and are responsible for paying the medical expenses of insured persons. They reserve the right to choose the healthcare services provided to insured persons by healthcare institutions. In addition, they are able to inspect and monitor the quality of the healthcare services provided by healthcare institutions and, if necessary, claim compensation and impose fines on healthcare units. (2) Compulsory health insurance funds: administratively, the compulsory health insurance funds are not affiliated with the health administration agencies. They are independent, quasi-governmental commercial credit agencies implementing a commercial operating fund management model. These funds signify the emergence of a new entity in healthcare system reforms. Not only do compulsory health insurance funds serve the function of distributing funds to health insurance companies, but they also directly allocate funds to healthcare institutions. In addition, they are responsible for the centralization, allocation, and utilization of health insurance funds. Although the Russian healthcare management system, which consists of health administration agencies, compulsory health insurance funds, and health insurance companies, has adopted a decentralized management model, it has surpassed the official vertical and horizontal decentralization and is distinctively characterized by its commercial fund management model. In addition, Russia also implemented the separation of prescribing and dispensing, which prevented drug wastage and "covering medical expenses with drug sales."

In 2004, the Russian government initiated comprehensive reforms to promote the super-ministry system and strived to reduce the number of government departments. The Ministry of Social Development and the Ministry of Health were merged to form the Ministry of Health and Social Development, which was responsible for both social development and healthcare. This merge allowed a wider range of departments to participate in addressing healthcare issues and greatly improved coordination. In May 2000, Putin signed a decree to further strengthen the authority of the central government in the health sector, and seven new federal districts replaced the nine territories that were formed after the reforms of 1993. The central government appointed representatives to manage healthcare affairs and formulate health policies, revoked the authority of the territories, and implemented vertical management in practical operations. In addition, the functions of the Ministry of Health were modified, the existing epidemic prevention network was expanded, and the prevention and control of infectious diseases (e.g., HIV/AIDS) were strengthened to protect the physical health of the people.

2. "Super-Ministry System" Bureaucratic Management

India has established a relatively comprehensive health administration system based on its national conditions. The Ministry of Health and Family Welfare has two relatively independent subordinate departments: the Department of Health and Family Welfare and the Department of Indian Traditional Medicine. The former is fully responsible for disease prevention, maternal and child healthcare, family planning, basic healthcare services, medical education and scientific research, and pharmaceutical production, circulation, and use. The latter is responsible for the management of Indian traditional medicine. The design of this management system avoids the obstacle of policy coordination between departments due to the division of duties, differing goals, and varying emphases, thereby enhancing the system's management efficiency.

Brazil's healthcare management is further characterized by its rational bureaucratic division of labor. (1) Administrative management: Brazil has established a "super-ministry" health administration system that "integrates healthcare, health insurance, and drugs." The Unified Health System comes under the unified leadership of the Ministry of Health, state health departments, and municipal health departments. Although the Director of the Drug Regulatory Agency is appointed by the President, he reports to the Minister of Health and is responsible for supervising the production and circulation of drugs. The health administration agencies, medical councils at all levels, and private health insurance agencies are responsible for the oversight of healthcare behaviors. In addition, Brazil has a large primary health inspection team. (2) Physician management: physicians in most states are managed by the Brazilian Medical Association and are private practitioners. (3) Service management: the two-way referral and the zoning and grading systems of public hospitals have ensured that health resources are fully and rationally utilized. (4) Drug administration: the National Drug Plan of 1998 involved the implementation of an administration system for basic drugs, which were provided free of charge through the public health system.

The health service system in South Africa has adopted a three-tier management model spanning the central, provincial, and municipal levels. The central level is responsible for unified policy formulation and overall planning as well as supervising, managing, and assessing whether the distribution of social welfare funds meets the requirements of the central government. The provincial (across a total of nine provinces) and municipal levels are responsible for implementation. The central government established the Department of Social Development mainly to provide social security services to the general population and to provide services for vulnerable, disabled, low-income, and impoverished individuals. The Department of Social Development has offices in all nine provinces to coordinate with the local development of social security work. In addition to the Department of Social Development, other governmental departments in South Africa are involved in providing social security for South Africa's citizens. The first is the Department of Health, which is responsible for health and maternity insurance and improving the residential environments of black citizens. The second is the Department of Labor, which is responsible for unemployment benefits; the unemployed are able to receive four to six months of unemployment benefits. The third is the Department of Transport, which is responsible for determining the compensation for injuries from traffic accidents. Black individuals live in black areas with high rates of traffic accidents, and the Department of Transport is responsible for setting up traffic accident insurance policies.

3. Multipronged Management

In China, the government is the most important healthcare service provider, and the public healthcare institutions in China are all vectors of the government for the delivery of healthcare services to the population. Since the reforms of the 1980s, which involved delineating the fiscal responsibilities of the central and local governments and enabling hospitals to absorb their own profits and losses, the Chinese healthcare system has mainly featured the following characteristics. (1) Self-governance of administrative departments: the Ministry of Human Resources manages the medical affairs of government agencies and public institutions. The Ministry of Labor and Social Security administers the Urban Employee Basic Medical Insurance. The Ministry of Health is in charge of public health, and the New Rural Cooperative Medical Scheme introduced at the turn of the twenty-first century has also been incorporated within the Ministry of Health's administrative system. The General Administration of Quality Supervision, Inspection, and Quarantine, which was established in 2001, has assumed certain public health administration functions. The Food and Drug Administration, which was formed in 2003, is responsible for the public safety of food and drugs. (2) The presence of numerous superior administrative agencies that has control over hospitals: the hospitals include those directly under the Ministry of Health and Health Departments, those operating in various industry systems, those run by large-scale industrial and mining enterprises, and those affiliated with the military system, as well as township health centers and health clinics under the jurisdiction of local governments. (3) Overmanagement by the government: many public hospitals are closely related to the government's health administrative departments and are subject to micromanagement by the government. Although hospitals are nominally public, they are unable to provide every citizen with equal access to services, nor can they effectively participate in market competition. (4) Undermanagement by the government: the lack of separation between prescribing and dispensing and the coverage of medical expenses with drug sales are, in fact, the result of government inaction. Due to their relative alienation from social healthcare institutions, especially individual healthcare institutions, health administrative departments do not provide the necessary management of individual healthcare institutions, which has led to market confusion and other issues.

Based on the experiences of other BRICS countries, the level of economic development is not the only factor involved in achieving universal healthcare coverage, as universal coverage can also be accomplished through effective institutional arrangements that aim to resolve or alleviate various social issues, such as inaccessible or expensive healthcare. Both India and Brazil have established basic health security systems that guarantee that all citizens have access to a certain level of healthcare services for free. These systems have undoubtedly been of great benefit to the poor. In addition, governments can implement medical assistance systems specifically for the poor who have fallen ill and do not have the financial ability to pay for treatment. By providing special assistance and support and organically integrating medical assistance with the overall social security system, a government can provide the poor with real and effective assistance.

SECTION IV. PERFORMANCE EVALUATION OF HEALTH SYSTEMS IN BRICS COUNTRIES

1. Differences in Health System Reforms

Within the health security systems of the BRICS countries, the health-related indicators, including the extent of coverage, the level of security, beneficiary groups, the national income level, the income level per capita, the labor force ratio, and the protection of health laws, are closely related. A comparison of these health systems is shown in Table 16.3.

The data indicate that, in general, the BRICS countries have basically implemented free (or partially free) healthcare systems. However, these publicly funded healthcare systems are, in fact, vast hierarchical systems that do not have transaction costs but do generate a large amount of expenses. The healthcare systems of the BRICS countries generally have the following shortcomings: a lack of supervisory mechanisms, leading to the serious waste of public healthcare resources; fully state-funded systems, causing a lack of competition and low labor efficiency; and, in particular, a lack of cost-constraining mechanisms, resulting in increasing financial burdens.

In terms of healthcare system reforms, those of China and Brazil are mainly based on high degrees of national macroeconomic control together with appropriate coordination with market mechanisms. Russia's reforms involve using market incentives and national regulations to jointly promote the improvement of health performance. India, somewhat in reference to certain US models, mainly relies on spontaneous market self-regulation, which enables consumers to choose the improvements made to health system performance. Judging from the indicators and the effectiveness of healthcare service quality, all countries have attached great importance to service quality and have combined the overall goal of healthcare service with the evaluation framework of performance assessment to continuously improve the quality and performance of healthcare services. From the perspective of management goals, India has mainly emphasized flexible, timely, and reasonable decision-making at all levels; Brazil has focused on gradually improving the construction of the medical information system; Russia has emphasized improvements to the level of health performance management; and China has attached great importance to the effective integration of multiple health resources (policies, funds, equipment, manpower, and so on) to improve performance levels, thereby establishing and gradually improving the health system and its mechanisms.

Based on this comparison, we can see that the basic functions of the healthcare systems in the BRICS countries are largely consistent. Countries with different political systems differ

TABLE 16.3 Comparison of Health Systems in the BRICS Countries

Country	Who Ranking	Government Spending	Healthcare Expenditure	Funding Situation	Health Service System
India	43rd in the assessment of health financing and distribution equality; 153rd in health level; 112th in comprehensive health system performance	Public health spending only accounts for 0.9% of GDP, far lower than the average level of low-income countries (2.8%) and the average global level (5.5%)	5.3% of GDP	Public financing mainly takes the form of taxation at all government levels, direct fiscal spending, and social health insurance; personal out-of-pocket medical expenses account for 93.8% of private financing, and medical expenses paid under various insurance schemes account for 0.8% of private financing	Central-level healthcare institutions, state-level healthcare institutions, local healthcare institutions, community-based healthcare institutions, primary health centers, and subcenters; there are currently 3,500 urban health centers
Brazil	188th in the assessment of health financing and distribution equality	According to the law, the federal government must allocate 1–2% of GDP for healthcare expenditure, and the growth rate of the health budget cannot be lower than that of GDP; the healthcare expenditures of the state and municipal governments should not be less than 12% and 15% of total fiscal expenditures	7.6% of GDP	Health financing is based on general taxation; sources of funding include corporate income tax, consumption tax, business tax, and social insurance tax paid by certain groups; commercial insurance covers 25–30% of the population	The government-run Unified Health System, which includes community hospitals and large hospitals, public health laboratories, pharmaceutical factories, medical research institutions; private hospitals and other supplementary healthcare systems account for 80% of all healthcare institutions
Russia	130th in the assessment of health financing and distribution equality	Total government health spending accounts for 64.2% of total healthcare expenditure and 10.2% of total government spending	5.4% of GDP	A health insurance fund that covers more than 1,000 commonly used drugs free of charge was established; individuals bear part of operation costs in different proportions based on different circumstances	Divided into the federal, federal district (state), and municipal (district) levels

(continued)

TABLE 16.3 (Continued)

Country	Who Ranking	Government Spending	Healthcare Expenditure	Funding Situation	Health Service System
China	139th in healthcare expenditure per capita, 144th in overall health system performance; 188th in equality of health service financing	Government health spending accounts for 27.23% of total healthcare expenditure, social health spending accounts for 34.57%, and personal health spending accounts for 38.19%	5.1% of GDP	Mainly financed through budgets at all government levels and various health insurance premiums	Government-run public healthcare institutions account for 93% and private healthcare institutions account for about 6%
South Africa	44th in total healthcare spending as a share of GDP	Government health spending accounts for 46.6% of total healthcare expenditure	8.7% of GDP	About 40% borne by the government	Free universal coverage but with long waiting times and few physicians

in terms of their healthcare systems and the related legislation but also continue to improve given rapid socioeconomic development and the changing healthcare services needs of residents. Nevertheless, the basic functions of the healthcare systems in all BRICS countries have embodied the principles of strengthening government intervention, promoting equal accessibility, rationally allocating resources, responding to population aging, reducing disease risk, controlling healthcare costs, enhancing service quality, and improving health performance. The starting point of these policies is protecting the basic health rights of citizens, and their goal is to continuously promote the health of their citizens.

The 2009 winner of the Nobel Prize for Economics, Elinor Ostrom, proposed a conceptual analytical evaluation framework to help public policymakers formulate more accurate assessments. This framework clearly defines the main factors influencing the formulation and operation of policies and reflects the interrelations among these factors. Ostrom proposed that a precondition for the development of public policies is to clearly define this analytical evaluation framework. Therefore, based on the balance between equality and efficiency that she proposed, we have formulated a framework for evaluating the operational performance of healthcare systems, as shown in Table 16.4.

Table 16.4 demonstrates the correlation between equality and efficiency in healthcare system reforms. Under normal circumstances, public and private healthcare institutions often coexist in a health system. If the private service system is replaced by the public service system, then equality will increase, but since public hospitals lack competition, efficiency will be reduced. In contrast, if the public service system is replaced by the private service system, then the profit motivations of private hospitals will result in a decrease in equality. In terms of the management model, adopting the commercial operational model of marketization can improve efficiency but makes it more difficult to guarantee equality. In contrast, the super-ministry management model that is biased toward centralization can concentrate resources and address the issues of efficiency to a large extent but makes it more difficult to guarantee equality. However, if there is a fierce power game between local departments and the central government, then the super-ministry management model can also lead to efficiency loss.

As shown in Table 16.5, the evaluation of equality and efficiency in the BRICS countries indicates significant differences. These differences are most prominent in the gains and losses of primary healthcare, the financing of healthcare services (social insurance and general taxation), the supplementary and alternative private services systems, and management models (commercial operation, super-ministry system, and multipronged control). These factors are closely related to the development levels of the BRICS countries with regard to social, economic, and political (governing concepts of the ruling party) factors, health resources and their conditions, residents' health needs and the degree of distribution, population quality, cultural levels, and so on.

By analyzing the characteristics of the healthcare systems in other BRICS countries, we can see that these countries, which are currently undergoing accelerated urbanization and industrialization, each have their own unique healthcare systems. The development of a healthcare system is a gradual and progressive process that requires a country to learn and draw on the experiences of other countries, especially countries at similar development levels, in order to continuously improve. Not only should the reforms of the healthcare system guarantee the health of the people, but the level of healthcare services is also an important yardstick for measuring a country's socioeconomic development. Hence, the focus of China's healthcare system reforms includes providing better health security for the vast majority of the population and promoting the equal and rational distribution of healthcare resources.

TABLE 16.4 Analytical Framework of Healthcare System Reforms

Item	Primary Healthcare		Healthcare Service Funding		Private Service System		Commercial Operation	Management Model	
	Gain	Loss	Social Insurance	General Taxation	Supplementary	Alternative		Super-ministry System	Multipronged Control
Equality	+	−	+	+	+	−	+/−	−	−
Efficiency	+	−	+	−	+	+/−	+	+/−	−

Note: "+" indicates "present," "−" indicates "absent."

TABLE 16.5 Comparison of the Outcomes of Health System Reforms in the BRICS Countries

Indicator		China		Russia		India		Brazil		South Africa	
		Equality	Efficiency	Equality	Efficiency	Equality	Efficiency	Equality	Efficiency	Equality	Efficiency
Primary healthcare	Gain/Loss	–	–	–	–	+	–	+	–	–	–
Healthcare service funding	Social insurance	+	–	+	–	+	–	+	–	+	–
	General taxation										
Private service system	Supplementary	–	–	+	–	+	+	+	+	–	–
	Alternative										
Management model	Commercial operation	–	–	+	–	+	+	+	+	+	+
	Super-ministry system										
	Multipronged control										

2. Comparison of Health System Performances

The WHO published an article entitled "Relative Health Performance in BRICS over the Past 20 Years: The Winners and Losers" in its 2014 briefing. The study found that the health performances of the BRICS countries differed markedly in 1990–2011.

Years of life lost (YLL) was used as a direct indicator to evaluate the population's disease burden, and data from the BRICS countries were compared with those of the top-performing countries and countries with similar income levels. The findings were as follows.

1. Brazil showed a significant improvement in health performance; India's improvement was more modest; the health performances of South Africa and Russia showed substantial declines; and China's health performance improvement remained low relative to its rapid economic growth.

2. There were significant differences among different age and sex subgroups in the five countries. The health statuses of women were generally poorer compared to those of men. Children in India had the worst health performance. Most of South Africa's population has seen worsening health performance in the past 20 years. The health status of elderly people is worse than that of young people.

3. With regard to different income levels, Russia had the highest income level per capita but the poorest health performance, with no substantial improvements in 20 years. Although China's income level per capita is half that of Russia's, it has substantially outperformed Russia in terms of health performance. India's income level is lower than that of South Africa, and that of Brazil is comparable to South Africa, but both exhibited better health performance than that of South Africa.

CHAPTER SEVENTEEN

Insights from Health System Reforms in Developing Countries

 SECTION I. COMMON CHALLENGES IN THE DEVELOPMENT OF HEALTH SYSTEMS

1. Limited Funding Sources and Insufficient Investment

Theoretically speaking, the funding sources for public hospitals should include the government budget, reimbursements from health insurance funds, direct payments by patients, and charitable donations. As developing countries are constrained by their economic development and financial resources, they tend to have very limited financial investment and charitable donations, as well as relatively low levels of health insurance funding and benefits. Furthermore, low-income groups in these countries are usually unable to afford their medical expenses. Besides directly reducing the ability of the government, society, and individuals to cover medical costs, the lack of capital investment often becomes the root cause for the shortage of healthcare resources (e.g., medical facilities, equipment, technologies, human resources, and drugs) and poor healthcare quality, which in turn give rise to numerous interrelated, nested problems.

2. Imbalances in Regional and Vertical Resource Allocation

In addition to the shortage of healthcare resources and poor healthcare quality resulting from insufficient capital investment, finding ways to improve the scientific and rational allocation of resources has become a common difficulty facing developing countries, for the following reasons. (1) Imbalances in vertical resource allocation: High-quality resources are concentrated in large-sized specialist hospitals, whereas primary healthcare institutions often face a shortage of healthcare resources. (2) Imbalances in regional allocation: There is a large gap in resource allocation between urban and rural areas and even between urban and suburban areas. (3) Imbalances in resource allocation across specialties: The contradiction between the supply and demand of healthcare resources is more prominent for rehabilitation, elderly care, mental healthcare, and maternal and child healthcare.

The insufficient emphasis on primary care services and excessive concentration of healthcare resources in a handful of large-size and specialist hospitals have restricted the development of primary care institutions, preventive care, and general medicine, which has caused the public to become overly or even blindly dependent on large-size hospitals and the professional titles of medical experts. As a result, there is confusion among the roles held by different levels of healthcare institutions, leading to the simultaneous existence of disorderly expansion and functional reduction, thereby reducing the operational efficiency of the entire healthcare system.

Rural healthcare is another noteworthy issue in developing countries. The majority of such countries have relatively low industrialization and urbanization. As with other public services, such as transportation and education, these conditions have led to an excessive concentration of limited healthcare resources in densely populated urban areas. There is a substantial gap between rural and urban areas in terms of the quantity and quality of the medical facilities. Furthermore, rural residents have much lower economic and geographical accessibility to public and basic healthcare services than do urban residents, which has an adverse impact on the country's degree of social equality and the credibility of its leaders.

3. Lack of Incentive and Restraint Mechanisms in Public Healthcare Institutions

Healthcare systems have unique industrial characteristics when compared to other service industries. Therefore, there are higher requirements for the conceptual skills and knowledge structure of administrators in the macro-level planning and organization of healthcare systems, as well as the micro-level operation and management of healthcare institutions.

From a management perspective, improving managerial quality must progress through several stages and is constrained by the nature of the industry or organization and its institutional environment. Healthcare systems in developing countries often focus on planning and tend to implement regulatory measures through administrative orders. In addition, there is a blurred boundary between the government and the market in these systems. It can be difficult for conventional management approaches to create effective incentive and restraint mechanisms for public healthcare institutions because of issues of information asymmetry and monopolies, which are especially prominent in the healthcare market. Other issues with public healthcare institutions, such as inefficiency, poor service quality, staff indifference, and "gray income," have been extensively criticized in developing countries.

4. Lagging in the Funding and Payment of Health Insurance

Healthcare funding has three core functions: income generation, financial risk management, and service procurement. In developing countries, the implementation of health insurance schemes often faces the following challenges with regard to levying premiums on households to generate adequate economic resources.

(1) Insurance Registration

Incomplete registration information of the population can make it more difficult to identify target groups that fall within the coverage scope of insurance schemes.

(2) Individual Choice

Governments are often only able to collect premiums from the salaries of formal employees, which makes it difficult to implement a compulsory social health insurance scheme for all residents. International experience suggests that the relative scale of formal and informal employment channels is a key determinant of a country's ability to achieve universal health coverage. Many developing countries lack effective measures for mandating or encouraging a large number of informal freelancers to participate in compulsory health insurance.

(3) Premium Collection

The amount of premiums collected in developing countries is limited because of the relatively low proportion of formal economic organizations that participate in social insurance. Inadequate understanding of social insurance and behaviors of adverse selection have both hampered the willingness of target groups to pay their premiums. Furthermore, a large number of impoverished individuals are unable to afford their insurance premiums in developing countries. Research has shown that the primary cause of the reluctance of many people in developing countries to purchase health insurance is their lack of understanding of the concept of insurance. The secondary reason is the government's lack of requirements and effective supervision of the solvency of insurance companies, which have led to relatively low public trust in insurance companies. The third reason is related to the individual's willingness to pay. Individuals are more willing to participate in an insurance scheme when they experience identifiable health issues that give rise to catastrophic medical expenses but are less willing to pay for premiums to protect them against possible health risks.

(4) Progressive Premium Rates

The lack of accurate income data impedes the implementation of progressive premium rates in developing countries.

Health insurance schemes in developing countries encounter several challenges when attempting to achieve efficient and equal redistribution of resources in their financial risk management:

1. *Size and quantity of risk pools.* The spontaneous emergence of numerous small-scale funds and the social diversity associated with employment and household registration have led to an increase in the number of voluntary funds that are limited in size. The low public credibility and insufficient management and institutional capacities of government or national insurance schemes have had an adverse impact on the quantity and size of mandatory funds.
2. *Risk equalization.* The healthcare sector accounts for a low share of the fiscal budget, and thus there is a lack of adequate public resources to subsidize unemployed groups. Furthermore, the inadequacy of social solidarity in developing countries has led to a lack of horizontal subsidies from rich individuals to poor individuals, healthy individuals to patients, and employed individuals to unemployed individuals.
3. *Coverage.* The direct provision of healthcare services through a national health plan reduces the need for universal health insurance or comprehensive protection via insurance.

Health insurance schemes in developing countries also encounter several challenges when purchasing healthcare services to achieve effective use of scarce resources:

1. *Target groups for the purchase of healthcare services.* It is often difficult to identify vulnerable groups.
2. *Types of services to purchase.* The lack of cost-effectiveness data impedes improvement in capital utilization efficiency.
3. *Selection of healthcare providers.* Healthcare markets tend to have varying levels of monopoly, which limits the range of suppliers for selection.
4. *Payment methods.* The lack of management and institutional capacities limits the role of the pay-for-performance system.
5. *Prices.* The lack of cost-effectiveness data restricts the price transparency of both public and private healthcare providers.

5. Ineffective Use of Health Insurance Funds

The institutional environment of developing countries often restricts the role of health insurance funds in the health security system. These institutional environmental factors include insufficient institutional capacity, incomplete legal systems, ineffective or insufficient enforcement of regulatory instruments, rigid administrative procedures, and difficulty in changing informal rules.

For example, most developing countries allocate their healthcare budgets to public hospitals in urban areas, while these public hospitals, especially tertiary hospitals, primarily provide healthcare services to urban residents, who tend to be more affluent. This, in turn, leads to inequalities in the utilization of healthcare services between urban and rural residents. Another example is that many developing countries do not fully utilize insurance mechanisms for risk pooling or their implementation of insurance mechanisms is limited to civil servants or formal employees. This implies that the health insurance funds mainly benefit middle-class groups, who are more affluent, rather than impoverished or other vulnerable groups, who are in urgent need of healthcare coverage.

6. Inadequate Efficiency and Capacity of Health Insurance Management

In some developing countries, health insurance funds are characterized by their miniaturization, community orientation, and decentralization, which pose various issues related to their scale, coverage, and benefits. Many government-run health insurance schemes are, in theory, administered by semi-autonomous agencies. However, as in the case of state-owned and state-operated healthcare institutions, the rigid and hierarchical incentive mechanisms of such agencies can have adverse effects on these insurance schemes. This issue is more pronounced in countries where insurers are able to gradually establish their own extensive network of healthcare providers, which can reduce any benefits from the separation of purchasing and provision of healthcare services. In other countries, employment-based health insurance funds tend to be adversely affected by the fragmentation of risk pools and procurement groups, rather than benefiting from the greater competitive pressure.

The management characteristics of health insurance funds constitute the fourth factor affecting the implementation of health insurance schemes in developing countries. Such countries often have inadequate management capacities in terms of responsibility allocation, governance mechanisms, line management, customer service, and so forth.

Mandatory health insurance schemes, in particular, lack the necessary management skills. For instance, the insurers may serve multiple roles at the same time, acting as the representatives of the government, service users, and service providers, which lead to conflicting incentive and remuneration structures. Moreover, health insurance schemes often lack appropriate management tools such as effective information technology, communications, and the necessary systems required for effective financial management, human resource management, health information tracking, and service utilization review.

In summary, the fundamental issues facing the healthcare funding mechanisms in developing countries are: (1) insufficient tax revenues and incomplete channels to provide ample resources for the healthcare industry via government subsidies, user contributions, and donations; (2) the direct provision of healthcare services by government-run public institutions, commercial health insurance, and other forms of funding arrangements are unable to effectively protect patients against economic risks associated with illnesses; (3) new management approaches supported by integrated healthcare funding and procurement systems in the public sector have failed to overcome the shortcomings of bureaucracy; (4) institutional, organizational, and management rigidity. These fundamental issues have also driven governments in some developing countries to implement mandatory health insurance schemes.

Due to the lack of capacity in the public sector, many countries have largely failed in their efforts to improve the health security system through the public sector, which has ultimately resulted in healthcare systems that only serve the interests of those who control and manipulate the national discourse. As a rule, the public sector in these countries is incapable of effectively providing public goods and implementing income and risk redistribution. Furthermore, the absence of effective legal and economic systems can lead to considerable uncertainty and risk in healthcare, which can have a profound impact on the behaviors of patients, healthcare institutions, and communities, thus leading to a vicious cycle of insufficient investment, inadequate governance, and lack of functional coordination in the healthcare industry.

 ## SECTION II. KEY ISSUES FACING THE HEALTH SYSTEM IN CHINA

1. Equality – The Coexistence of Wastage and Shortage of Healthcare Resources

Since the marketization of the healthcare industry in China, all levels of government have shifted the majority of the pressure for capital investment to healthcare institutions. Profit-seeking is an instinctive reaction by market players, including healthcare institutions, whose flow of resource investment is closely associated with the rate of return. Within this context, public hospitals have gradually shifted away from social welfare to become monopolistic, for-profit agencies. However, basic healthcare services are quasi-public goods with social welfare features, thus making it impossible for healthcare providers to completely avoid this social responsibility. Therefore, this disorderly and excessive marketization of the healthcare system in China has inevitably led to issues of inequality in the allocation of healthcare resources.

This inequality is further compounded by limited government investment, which precludes the government's ability to compensate for market shortfalls or correct market failures. Instead, the government is blindly bound to market forces, which has led to a further distortion of resource allocation. Therefore, the healthcare industry in China is currently facing the co-occurrence of market and government failure, which has resulted in the concentration of both market-oriented and government-oriented healthcare resources in cities and developed areas. In contrast, people living in rural areas, underdeveloped areas, and rural–urban fringes tend to have inadequate access to advanced healthcare services, equipment, and even healthcare institutions.

2. Accessibility – Deviations in Service Focus and Technology Orientation

The accessibility of healthcare services includes geographical and population accessibility, as well as the accessibility associated with the demand side's ability to pay. These, in turn, have given rise to the prominent issues of inaccessible and expensive healthcare services, respectively. Here, we discuss the issue of expensive healthcare services, as the issue of inaccessibility has been gradually alleviated alongside economic development, financial enrichment, and increased willingness to reform the healthcare system.

Although there are many reasons behind the rise in healthcare expenditure in recent years (e.g., commodity price), the most prominent are institutional factors, such as price system, reimbursement mechanism, and payment system. The most direct manifestation of this issue is the gradual deviation of service focus and technology orientation from basic social needs. Based on China's healthcare characteristics and national circumstances, a rational choice for its healthcare system is to focus its healthcare services for disease prevention and control and its technology orientation for the development of appropriate technologies and essential drugs. During the era of planned economy, China managed to successfully and persistently uphold these principles. However, in recent years, there have been major deviations in service focus and technology orientation because of the active pursuit of healthcare institutions in their economic interests. In particular, they tend to focus on therapeutic services and new and advanced technologies rather than on preventive services and appropriate technologies.

3. Coordination – The Decentralization and Fragmentation of Different Healthcare Resources

An ideal healthcare system is a hierarchical, networked system whereby the different levels, types, and ownerships of healthcare institutions follow the rational division of labor and patients comply with the principles of receiving first treatment in the community, hierarchical referral, and two-way referral. Such a healthcare system optimizes its potential to effectively utilize limited healthcare resources, thus providing continuous and coordinated healthcare services, such as preventive, diagnostic, therapeutic, nursing, and rehabilitation services, in a more cost-effective manner.

However, the opposite is observed in China. Thus, there is decentralization in the power to conduct, supervise, and operate the investments of different levels and types of hospitals, and the system has a complicated network of interest relationships. This has led to numerous isolated and fragmented units based on local interests rather than a continuous, coordinated, and patient-centered healthcare system. These conditions have adversely affected the efficiency and quality of the entire healthcare system, which can easily lead to a vicious cycle.

4. Marginalized Groups and Blind Spots in Social Insurance Coverage

Currently, China has essentially established the framework for a universal basic health security system, whereby urban employees, urban unemployed persons, rural residents, and urban and rural disadvantaged groups are covered by the Urban Employee Basic Medical Insurance (UEBMI), Urban Resident Basic Medical Insurance (URBMI), New Rural Cooperative Medical Scheme (NRCMS), and Urban and Rural Medical Assistance (URMA), respectively. As of the end of June 2010, these basic health security schemes have covered more than 90% of the total population, of whom 390 million are covered by the UEBMI and URBMI, while 833 million are covered by the NRCMS. Thus, theoretically speaking, universal health coverage has essentially been achieved in China. In addition, the promulgation of the Social Insurance Law has placed these health insurance schemes under legal protection. However, the reality of the situation in China is not as optimistic.

A large number of flexible and independent forms of informal employment exist in China. Hence, although the legal coverage includes a significant proportion of the population, they generally have very low effective access to healthcare services. The UEBMI and publicly funded healthcare systems in some areas mainly cover individuals employed by national agencies and institutions, as well as enterprises with more standardized labor relations. Although the URBMI was established for unemployed residents living in urban areas, it is a voluntary, government-sponsored community-based health insurance with a very high potential risk of adverse selection among insured persons. Moreover, it lacks the ability for risk pooling among insured persons of different health statuses and income levels since insurance premiums are levied at a single price, which is contrary to the primary objective of universal health coverage.

Similar to other developing countries, China has a vast, nonstandardized job market characterized by high labor intensity, long working hours, and poor living and sanitary conditions among workers. Furthermore, workers are unable to access legal welfare benefits and have no bargaining power with employers. Many of them also lack the resources needed to change their fates, which implies that they are susceptible to a vicious cycle of poverty and illness. In addition, because of its unique dual economic system, unfavorable conditions for small- and medium-sized private enterprises, low levels of social insurance coordination, and difficulties in interregional transfer of insurance, China has a large population of freelancers who do not have a permanent employment contract with employers and are forced to or voluntarily decline insurance coverage. Therefore, rural residents engaged in short-term seasonal work at construction sites, housekeeping staff, and part-time employees of micro- and small-sized enterprises or individual industrial and commercial households are all marginalized groups that fall beyond the coverage of social security. This is a common phenomenon that has resulted in a far lower level of effective healthcare accessibility than the theoretical coverage of the UEBMI. Furthermore, it is difficult to effectively oversee and regulate this scheme through labor inspection.

5. Increased Healthcare Demand and Inadequate Health Security

Based on official statistical data and academic literature, the framework for a basic health security system has been established in China, and its coverage is rapidly increasing. This has effectively improved the economic accessibility to basic healthcare services and significantly increased the utilization rate of outpatient and inpatient services among insured persons. However, when considered in relation to the basic healthcare demands of insured persons, the current health security system remains inadequate in its capacity to protect patients against the economic risks associated with illness. The excessively high out-of-pocket expenses borne by insured patients have severely limited the ability of the social health insurance scheme to reduce the financial burden on patients and families.

Due to the effects of multiple factors, such as population aging and advancements in medical technology, every country in the world is facing the problem of increased healthcare expenditures, including China. It is inevitable that the public will demand the improvement of health benefits after (or upon) the expansion of health security coverage. This demand is likely to conflict with socioeconomic development and limited government subsidies, thereby influencing the balance and sustainability of health insurance funds. This is particularly the case for China, whose citizens are "getting old before getting rich." Therefore, government agencies that are responsible for UEBMI, URBMI, NRCMS, social relief, healthcare, civil affairs, etc., often find it necessary to make compromises between different goals. This results in a social health insurance system that provides basic, low-level and broad coverage, which is often unable to protect patients against the economic risks associated with illnesses, thus attracting public criticism of the health security system.

According to data published by the Ministry of Health (MOH) (currently known as the National Health and Family Planning Commission, NHFPC), out-of-pocket medical expenses borne by patients accounted for 40.4% of the total healthcare expenditure in China. Some studies on the three major health insurance programs in China found that some patients declined treatment due to their household's inability to afford the copayment, which has led to the problematic phenomenon where "the poor subsidize the rich." For households that have incurred catastrophic medical expenses, their economic losses were still devastating even after receiving financial compensation from the NCMS. A survey on the URBMI pilot areas (including pilot cities in Fujian Province and Wuhan City of Hubei Province) revealed that about 75% of insured persons believed that the URBMI has not significantly alleviated the financial burden on patients' families because of the excessively high copayments. The NCMS has established a personal medical account for each insured person to help pay for their outpatient expenses. However, the savings in these personal accounts are extremely limited and are merely a drop in the ocean compared to the outpatient medical expenses for patients with chronic diseases, who do not require hospitalization but do require long-term medical examination and medication.

6. Flaws in Management Capacity and Institutional Design

Immense management capacity is required to achieve a highly efficient and sustainable social health insurance system that is capable of covering China's enormous population of approximately 1.3 billion. Over the years, China has been reforming its healthcare system through trial-and-error (i.e., pilot testing and institutionalization) and constantly discovering and resolving new issues in the process of exploration and application. Just as new problems always replace the old, the solutions must also be constantly updated. However, since policies must exhibit a certain level of stability, there is always a slight lag in the implementation of solutions in relation to the issues concerned. This has caused certain institutional contradictions to become increasingly severe over time, and their negative effects have gradually shifted from being implicit to explicit in nature. Policymakers, researchers, and the general public are acutely aware of the need for greater convergence and integration of the currently decentralized urban and rural health security schemes, in order to improve social equality, management efficiency, and public experience. Both the Party and the current government have issued key documents proposing clear reform goals, but progress has been slow. The flaws in institutional design have severely hampered the management capacity of the administrative departments and business agencies of the social health insurance system, specifically in the two major aspects of funding and supervision.

(1) Low Hierarchies and Decentralized Funding

Low hierarchies and decentralized funding can have numerous adverse consequences for the sustainability, equality, and operability of social health insurance.

Risk pooling is an essential aspect of social health insurance, whereby medical expenses are shared among insured persons of varying levels of health and economic risk. Ideally, this risk is transferred from unhealthy individuals to healthy individuals and from low-income earners to high-income earners. The sustainability and benefits of health insurance schemes are closely related to their risk pooling capability. According to the statistical law of large numbers, the risk pooling capability of an insurance scheme depends on the scope of its funding.

Presently, the health insurance schemes in China have relatively low hierarchies of coordination. Specifically, the UEBMI and URBMI are generally coordinated at the prefectural level, while the NRCMS is generally coordinated at the provincial level, with around 7,000 coordination units. Furthermore, it is difficult for voluntary insurance schemes such as the URBMI and NRCMS to prevent adverse selection, which impedes the transfer of risks from unhealthy to healthy individuals. Additionally, individuals insured by the UEBMI generally have higher incomes than those insured by the URBMI and NRCMS. These three basic health insurance schemes are isolated from each other in terms of funding and utilization, which impedes the transfer of risks from low-income to high-income earners. The use of personal medical accounts also reduces the risk-pooling capability and equality of these health insurance schemes to a certain extent.

In addition to influencing the sustainability of these insurance schemes, the low hierarchies and decentralized funding also weaken the bargaining power of payers in the purchase of services from designated healthcare institutions. Since funding and procurement activities are decided and carried out by different levels and departments of administrative bodies and agencies (payers), it is difficult for a single payer to impose effective incentives and constraints regarding the quality and cost control of healthcare services via negotiations with designated healthcare institutions, especially third-tier hospitals, which have technological and regional advantages.

Furthermore, China is currently experiencing rapid urbanization and economic transformation, with unprecedented scopes and densities of population, capital, technology, and information flow. Hence, the interregional transfer and continuation of social health insurance have become an urgent need for the majority of insured persons. Because of the low hierarchy of coordination and decentralization, the portability of social health insurance shows very poor operability. This not only undermines the enthusiasm of marginalized groups to participate in social health insurance, and increases the information, time, and economic costs for insured persons during reimbursement procedures but also greatly increases the management and coordination costs of social (health) insurance agencies and other relevant agencies. On a higher level, it also adversely affects the free flow and optimal allocation of the labor force, thereby solidifying or even aggravating regional and socioeconomic gaps, while also reducing macroeconomic efficiency.

(2) Multiple Supervisory Authorities with Weak Supervision

The unclear division of jurisdictions and responsibilities between the funding, payment, and supervisory systems of health insurance with the organizational, delivery, and supervisory systems of healthcare services is a key issue affecting the further development and improvement of the health protection system in China. In fact, it has led to a number of adverse consequences, such as increasing costs and difficulties in implementing horizontal coordination and reducing vertical implementation, oversight, assessment, and account-ability of policies. Furthermore, one of the biggest problems currently facing China's reform of the healthcare system is that even though the reform vision proposed by the central government seems to be meeting the actual needs and expectations of the public, there is considerable opposition to the promotion of deeper reforms. In fact, reform appears to pres-ently exist mainly in the form of documentation and meetings, which is partially because of the overly extensive interest adjustments that are involved. In particular, the management system and operating mechanism of health security cannot yet fundamentally suppress nonstandardized healthcare services and unreasonable growth of medical expenses.

The management agencies for health insurance funds have become passive payers rather than strategic purchasers due to their lack of motivation and ability to negotiate prices, as well as the lack of effective oversight over the quality of healthcare services and the practices of healthcare institutions. Under the fee-for-service method, designated health-care institutions are able to take advantage of their monopolistic position in location, tech-nology, and information to encourage insured patients to choose nonessential healthcare services, leading to the common occurrence of overmedication, overtreatment, overtesting, and overdiagnosis. However, in some areas where a global budget payment system (GBPS) based on the fee-for-service system is implemented, overtreatment appears to coexist with undertreatment in China's system, along with deeper-level hospital–patient and hospital–insurance conflicts. In order to fundamentally resolve these issues, management agencies must not solely rely on technological innovation in payment methods; they must also clearly define the relationship between the healthcare system and health security system, so as to improve their institutional designs and management capacities. In addition, management agencies also should rationally design the management roles, organizational structure, affil-iation, separation of power, and management mechanisms of the health security system in order to establish a scientific and rational management system.

Owing to the long-term impact of the urban–rural dual economy, this duality has also emerged in health security, with different types of health protection systems being imple-mented in urban and rural areas. Specifically, the UEBMI and URBMI are administered by the Ministry of Human Resources and Social Security, the NRCMS is administered by the MOH, and the URMA is administered by the Ministry of Civil Affairs (MCA). Even though this duality facilitates the enthusiasm and professional advantages of these ministries, it can easily lead to a lack of cross-sectoral coordination.

These ministries often formulate health protection policies based on their own expertise, schemes, and target recipients, which has resulted in varying standards and benefit levels among different insurance schemes. This has led to conflicting policies as well as varying eli-gibility criteria and benefits among the different schemes. As a result, these schemes cannot fully meet the needs of insured persons for identity conversion and interregional healthcare, as well as the unification of the future health security system. For example, the separation of management agencies and information systems, as well as the competition for insurance resources, have led to the widespread phenomenon of overlapping coverage and duplicate reimbursement among urban and rural residents. According to relevant statistics, the over-lapping coverage accounted for about 10% of the total insured population in urban and rural areas. Assuming that the financial subsidy for each insured urban and rural resident is RMB120, this is equivalent to a total duplicate reimbursement of RMB12 billion.

In addition, owing to the fact that health security management agencies are affiliated with the administrative department of health insurance, the multidepartmental supervision of health security is inevitable, which causes considerable inconvenience to both urban and rural residents, along with substantial wastage of resources. Each health security scheme is administered by its own management agency or team and has established its own information network system. This has resulted in not only overlapping agencies but also represents a massive obstacle to the unification of basic health insurance schemes in the future because of inconsistent data standards among different schemes.

SECTION III. EXPERIENCES AND INSIGHTS FROM HEALTH SYSTEM REFORMS IN DEVELOPING COUNTRIES

1. System Planning – Optimized Integration of Health Resource Allocation

Over the past few decades, many developing countries, such as Indonesia, Brazil, Colombia, Costa Rica, Tunisia, Czech Republic, Hungary, Poland, and several Soviet republics, have reformed the management structure of their public hospitals and achieved good progress. These countries have gradually realized that the scientific planning of their system structure must emphasize not only regional health plans, which are frequently prioritized in conventional system planning but also the structural optimization of various types and levels of healthcare resources within the same region. This structural optimization may serve as a potential handhold for the further mobilization and exploitation of limited resources and is a challenging phase that nevertheless must be overcome in health system reforms.

1. *Optimizing the regional allocation of healthcare resources.* Governments should attach great importance to regional health plans, and may shift the focus of public financing to areas with inadequate markets and social funds by either maintaining the current level of funding or even discontinuing funding in areas where the market and social funds are sufficient. When allocating new public funds to healthcare institutions, the government should focus on rural areas, remote areas, rural–urban fringes, and the central and western regions.

2. *Optimizing the vertical allocation of healthcare resources.* Hospital groups and medical clusters are useful attempts at establishing a continuous and well-coordinated healthcare system. The health administrative department should establish a cross-administrative and cross-ownership medical cluster within each unified planning area, comprising tertiary and secondary general hospitals and community healthcare centers. The overall outcomes of regional healthcare systems can be improved by strengthening the patient-centered service concept; clarifying the functional roles of tertiary hospitals, secondary hospitals, and community healthcare centers; improving the coordination, continuity, and integrity of healthcare services; and emphasizing the entire process of treatment and continuous health management.

2. Primary Care – Fully Utilizing the Role of Family Physicians

In order to cope with the issues of population aging and shifts in the disease spectrum, while also improving the efficiency of resource allocation and utilization, developing countries often turn to the development of general medicine, recruitment of family physicians, and improvement of primary care services. The governments of these countries must play an active role in increasing the availability of primary care services, as these are typically lacking in the healthcare market. Governments not only need to increase their capital investment in order to increase the capacities and construction of existing primary care institutions but also have to guide and facilitate the coordination with large-sized and specialist hospitals to improve their market competitiveness. Furthermore, despite the difficulties in reintroducing the concept of "first treatment in the community," this is an essential measure in the long run.

In this respect, Thailand and Vietnam (both of which are located on the Southeast Asian Indochinese Peninsula) can be considered two opposing examples. In Thailand, the social health insurance system utilizes a fixed-point healthcare policy, whereby insured persons are not allowed to seek medical attention directly from upper-tier hospitals without being referred by primary care centers. On the other hand, the majority of patients in Vietnam flock to hospitals in the main cities, causing long hospital queues from morning to midnight, which has led to an overburdened and inefficient system.

Recently, India launched the National Rural Health Plan (NRHM) to establish a primary care subcenter for every 5,000 people, a primary health center for every 30,000 people, and a community health center for every 100,000 people. The main goal of the NRHM is to improve the rural health infrastructure, optimize the allocation of healthcare resources by improving the tertiary care network, and enhance the operational efficiency of the entire healthcare system. The NRHM is worthy of reference in other developing countries, especially China, which also has vast rural areas and populations.

3. Nongovernmental Healthcare Institutions – Guiding the Development of Private Healthcare Institutions

By fully relaxing its control over the flow of social capital into the healthcare service industry, governments can create an institutional environment with fair competition among all healthcare institutions (including private, public, nonprofit, and for-profit medical institutions). Governments have also invested more public resources against market shortfalls and market failures, thereby ensuring the balanced development of the entire healthcare system.

Governments have begun promoting the privatization of healthcare services via the separation of ownership and management under the premise that it will gradually improve a health insurance scheme to the point that it can serve as a third-party payer for healthcare services. Encouraging the establishment of healthcare institutions via social capital and vigorously developing private healthcare institutions are considered effective approaches for expanding the funding sources in healthcare. This is especially effective in sectors without technological monopolies, such as primary care (i.e., community healthcare services). Retired physicians, GPs, and voluntary medical teams are allowed to open clinics in densely populated urban areas and even in some economically developed rural areas. Furthermore, social capital also facilitates the vitalization of healthcare resources that are dispersed across various primary care institutions. Market entry barriers should not be imposed on large-sized hospitals that are established using domestic and foreign social capital.

Currently, in both theory and practice, many developing countries are exhibiting a worrying tendency to perceive the restoration of a planned economy as an effective approach for enhancing social welfare, and to equate government-guided healthcare institutions with government-run and even government-controlled healthcare institutions. In many countries, relevant administrative departments tend to equate social welfare in the healthcare system with state-run and state-administered public healthcare institutions, thereby seeking to further strengthen their long-held monopolistic position. At the same time, the development of private hospitals and other private healthcare institutions has been widely ignored, discriminated against, or even suppressed. Health administrative departments in some countries even secretly expect private healthcare institutions to fend for themselves. All the aforementioned circumstances not only fail to promote the restoration of public welfare in the healthcare industry but also will eventually produce the next reform dilemma.

All highly standardized and competitive healthcare services with good performance measurability should be provided in a market-oriented manner as far as possible. The procurement of healthcare services by the government should be conducted via competitive tendering, whereby all types of healthcare providers – whether they are public, private, nonprofit, or for-profit healthcare institutions – should be treated equally in competing for government procurement contracts.

It should be noted that many of the aforementioned issues are not independent or fragmented but are interrelated and interdependent. Hence, the government should adhere to the principles of systems theory in their practice and devise an overall plan that does not neglect any type of healthcare institution.

4. Policy Orientation – Emphasis on Equality and Supporting Vulnerable Groups

The WHO and many developing countries have proposed that the goal of achieving universal coverage is to alleviate the financial burden of medical treatments on the public and thereby break the vicious cycle between illness and poverty. The explicit policy preference for vulnerable groups in some representative countries is undoubtedly useful for social progress, as it reflects the fairness and inclusiveness of the government's social management and public services. Health security is a quasi-public good that retains certain features of social welfare and requires an appropriate amount of investment and support from the government. In some developing countries, government involvement and support are essential for achieving universal health coverage and improving the accessibility of vulnerable and marginalized groups to healthcare services.

Unlike developed countries, which often rely on social health insurance for healthcare funding, the health security systems of developing countries are mainly funded through fiscal revenue and patients' out-of-pocket payments. As a result, these systems are imperfect, with many rural, vulnerable, and marginalized groups showing poor economic accessibility to healthcare services. Thus, insurance becomes an important fundraising strategy for overcoming financial difficulties and achieving key health policy goals, such as the important indicators of the Millennium Development Goals. From a global perspective, most developing countries have so far failed to resolve health security issues in rural areas. Only a handful of countries, such as Mexico, Brazil, Thailand, India, and Senegal have resolved these issues to varying degrees using different approaches. A common feature across the health security systems of these countries is the clearly defined responsibilities of the government in capital investment and social management in the healthcare industry, with an emphasis on social equality. Using India as an example, which is another major player in Asia like China, the most important feature of its health security system is the effort to maintain the equality and rationality of healthcare resource allocation, thereby ensuring a social health insurance system with maximum coverage. This feature is commendable and highly valued in developing countries. In the World Health Report 2000, which ranked the WHO's member states according to a health status assessment, India ranked 43rd in terms of equality in healthcare fundraising and allocation, which was far higher than China (ranked 188th).

In Thailand, government investment has become the main funding source for rural health insurance. In Brazil, the Family Health Strategy, which is jointly implemented and monitored by the federal and state governments, was specifically established for rural populations in conjunction with implementing a unified universal health insurance system. Since India gained independence, its government has been committed to establishing a free rural health insurance system based on the principle of providing free healthcare services to impoverished groups. Furthermore, the government launched various public health programs, such as the Universal Immunization Program (UIP), and provided free treatment in public hospitals, in order to ensure the access of vulnerable groups (especially the vast majority of farmers) to basic health security. The National Health Insurance plan in India targets impoverished groups and informal workers, such as mobile street vendors and construction workers, in order to provide them with free healthcare services. In addition, the government of India has established unique health insurance systems for informal sectors and workers to prevent large insurance companies from excluding rural residents because of their dispersed residences, inconsistent incomes, and limited insured amounts. To achieve this goal, the government established rural health micro-insurance organizations, which serve as a unit to purchase health insurance policies from formal insurance companies. This approach has not only reduced the transaction cost of insurance companies but also ensured the access of farmers to formal healthcare services. In other words, it benefits the health and safety of these vulnerable groups, while also enhancing social cohesion in India.

It is evident from the international experience that there is no single model or approach to achieving universal health coverage. Health protection systems in developing countries have been constantly evolving due to various factors, such as historical and economic development, social and cultural values, and the political system. To ensure that marginalized groups are included in the scope of health security coverage, China must rationally adopt diversified funding mechanisms and coordinate various types of existing social health insurance. Doing so will, in turn, ensure universal access to essential and affordable healthcare services.

The government should play a key role in defining each health security subsystem to encourage and stimulate its development. Furthermore, the government should establish a top-level legal framework that has absorptive capacity to guarantee adequate funding and comprehensive healthcare rights. This framework should include effective supervision and also consider the patients' need and ability to pay.

5. System Design – Payment System Reforms and Fund Supervision

Health security systems, especially social health insurance, can improve the economic accessibility of insured persons, particularly the impoverished and vulnerable, to healthcare services through fundraising and risk pooling. It is a common trend for the social health insurance in developing countries to shift the target recipients of public subsidies from the supply side to the demand side, in order to improve the efficiency and quality of healthcare services. Such a shift allows a clear division of responsibility for the fundraising and management of social insurance funds, and the delivery of healthcare services. Fund managers purchase, in the form of contracts, healthcare services required by insured persons from independent healthcare providers, who in turn are accountable for the quality of their services.

Some Asian and African countries, such as India, Indonesia, the Philippines, Vietnam, Rwanda, and Ghana, have established an independent agency for the procurement of healthcare services in their health security systems. This agency gives healthcare service payers full negotiating power, thus establishing the appropriate incentive and restraint mechanisms for healthcare providers.

Countries such as Brazil and Egypt have adopted a single universal health insurance system. China, on the other hand, has implemented three health insurance schemes – the UEBMI, URBMI, and NCMS. Despite the inevitability, necessity, and rationality of these three schemes, they have considerable limitations when it comes to ensuring the equal right to basic health security and the effective allocation of social healthcare resources. Such limitations must be overcome, which can be achieved by integrating these three schemes into a single health insurance system. Presently, the social health insurance in China is administered by the Ministry of Human Resources and Social Security (MOHRSS), NHFPC, and their affiliated agencies. The involvement of multiple agencies has increased the administrative and social costs and influenced the system's operational effectiveness. It is necessary to merge these agencies to better integrate the health insurance system, thereby saving costs and improving effectiveness.

The health insurance system in the Philippines utilizes a strict referral mechanism, encouraging insured patients to first seek medical attention in primary care hospitals, which entitles them to 100% reimbursement; seeking treatment in secondary hospitals and tertiary hospitals only entitles patients to 50% and 10%–20% reimbursement, respectively, while the remaining out-of-pocket expenses must be paid by the patients themselves. The health insurance system in the Philippines could serve as a useful reference for a systematic referral hierarchy in China, which ensures "first treatment in the community," "two-way referrals," and "hierarchical referrals," concepts that have long been advocated but have not yet been established.

Imposing effective constraints against the overutilization of unnecessary medical technologies induced by healthcare providers plays a key role in ensuring effective resource utilization in the health security system. In recent years, health reforms in developing countries have been focusing on adjusting the cost-sharing mechanism, reforming the payment method, and introducing competitive mechanisms, in order to control rising healthcare expenditures. China must further improve its governance in terms of regulatory mechanisms and fund management.

6. Sustainable Funding – Advocating a Multichannel Model of Increasing Revenue and Reducing Expenditure

The progressive development in the scope and level of health security coverage is a process that cannot be rushed. The maturation of the health security system in all countries is an upward spiral, from its establishment and development to its continuous reform. In general, the level of health protection improves gradually, expanding its scope of coverage from industrial workers to the entire workforce and finally to all citizens.

Most countries simultaneously employ all forms of existing funding models: taxation and budgeting, national health insurance, social health insurance, community health insurance, and commercial health insurance. However, there is often a lack of coordination among these funding models, leading to issues of healthcare equality and quality. The majority of countries that have successfully achieved universal health coverage have adopted two methods: (1) direct establishment of public healthcare institutions using public funds as the main funding source and absorbing social capital for supplementation and integration (e.g., Sri Lanka and China); and (2) subsidizing social health insurance via tax revenue (e.g., China and Mongolia). Although there is a correlation between national income and health coverage rate, this correlation is not inevitable. There could be considerable variations in the achievement of health security across countries with the same level of economic development. According to data published by the International Labor Organization (ILO) in 2008, countries with very similar GDP per capita can have surprisingly different health coverage rates. For instance, the health coverage rate of Bolivia (US$890) was 66%, whereas that of Guinea-Bissau (US$920) was 1.6%; similarly, the health coverage rate of Ghana (US$320) was 18.7%, whereas that of Togo (US$330) was 0.4%.

The government of China has to learn from the lessons of other developing countries to ensure that the health benefits of its social health insurance can meet actual healthcare demands. Healthcare expenditure must be strictly controlled based on the ability of insurance funds to pay, in order to ensure the sustainability of the health security system. On the one hand, it is necessary to establish a vertical multilevel and horizontal multichannel health security system with high risk-pooling capacity. More specifically, the three levels of health security (basic health insurance, supplemental health insurance, and medical assistance for the poor) should be consolidated vertically, while the three funding channels (public funding, charitable donations, and commercial health insurance) must be expanded horizontally. On the other hand, the government should also fully utilize payment methods in leveraging its negotiation advantage with third-party payers in "group procurement" and enhancing its supervisory role, thereby improving the utilization efficiency of health insurance funds.

Brazil's experience suggests that a comprehensive health insurance system must include commercial health insurance. The government of Brazil has consistently encouraged its citizens to purchase commercial health insurance plans, which are contracted insurance plans requiring policyholders to sign contracts on the terms of the insurance company. Insurance companies provide three levels (high, medium, and low) of protection, and the number of covered healthcare services increases with the premiums. Insurance companies reimburse medical expenses according to the age, health status, and coverage scope of the insured person. Insurance companies also sign contracts with private and public hospitals. Those insured by commercial health insurance do not need to pay any fees in designated private hospitals within the coverage scope stipulated in their contract. All medical expenses incurred are settled between the insurance company and the hospital. Insurance companies also reimburse the major surgeries of insured patients in public hospitals, such as liver and kidney transplantations.

Countries such as Brazil and Egypt provide medical aid to impoverished patients and those who have difficulties for other reasons. Despite their different approaches, the medical aid systems of these countries share the characteristics of wide coverage and substantial reimbursement. In the light of their experiences, China should expand the scope of its medical aid to include not only major illnesses but also common diseases. Furthermore, the government of China should increase the reimbursement amount of medical aid. In addition to reimbursing most of the drug expenses, the medical aid scheme also should cover most of the diagnostic charges. Both the coverage scope and reimbursement amount should be increased to allow impoverished individuals and those living in difficulty for other reasons to receive medical aid in a timely manner.

It is worth mentioning that the establishment and improvement of the health security system is not a panacea for resolving all issues related to the funding and delivery of healthcare services in developing countries. It is almost inevitable that the process of reforming the health security system will have drawbacks and risks of varying degrees and scopes, thereby rendering it impossible to achieve the expected outcomes overnight. Thus, this process requires policymakers to possess the wisdom to select the appropriate reform approaches, a global outlook to achieve good coordination among various stakeholders, and the boldness for the strong enforcement of reform measures.

V

Health Systems in Developing Countries

CHAPTER EIGHTEEN

Health Systems in Seven Asian Countries

SECTION I. THE HEALTH SYSTEM IN CHINA

1. Overview of Socioeconomics and National Health

(1) Political and Economic Situations

China, officially the People's Republic of China (PRC), is located in Eastern Eurasia along the western coast of the Pacific Ocean. It is a socialist country under the people's democratic dictatorship, which is led by the working class and based on an alliance between workers and farmers. China is the third largest country in the world, covering a land area of approximately 9.6 million km². The coastline of the mainland is about 180,000 km and that of its islands is about 140,000 km. The total area of the inland sea and territorial waters is about 4.7 million km² and contains more than 7,600 islands (of which Taiwan is the largest, covering an area of 35,798 km²). China shares land borders with 14 countries and maritime boundaries with 8 countries. In terms of administrative division at the provincial level, China is divided into 4 municipalities, 23 provinces, 5 autonomous regions, and 2 Special Administrative Regions (SARs). China is a multiethnic country with 56 officially recognized ethnic groups, of which Han Chinese accounts for the majority (91.51%) of the total population. Standard Mandarin is the official national language of China.

China is the second largest economy, as well as the largest trading nation, steel producer, agricultural country, and grain-producing country in the world. Furthermore, it has the fastest economic growth and largest foreign exchange reserve worldwide. China is the second most attractive country for foreign investment and is an important member of many international organizations. China is considered a potential new superpower. The National Bureau of Statistics (NBS) reported that the gross domestic product (GDP) of China in 2013 was RMB 56.88 trillion, which was an increase of nearly RMB5 trillion (7.7%) compared to the previous year when calculated at constant prices; this increase is equivalent to the total economic output in 1994. China's GDP exceeded that of Japan for the first time in 2010, ranking second only to the US; within the subsequent three years, China's GDP was twice that of Japan. On August 15, 2012, the NBS reported that in 2003–2011, China's economy showed an average annual growth rate of 10.7%, indicating significant increases in social productivity and comprehensive national power (CNP). The per capita of the GDP China has also increased rapidly alongside the steady growth in total economic output. In 2011, the per capita GDP of China was RMB35,083; after deducting price factors, this is equivalent to 1.4 times that of 2002 and an average annual growth rate of 10.1%. Based on the average exchange rate, the per capita GDP of China rose from US$1,135 in 2002 to US$5,432 in 2011 and US$6,750 in 2013.

(2) Population and Health Status Development

China is the most populous country in the world. As noted in the "National Population Census Regulation" and the "Notice of the State Council on Carrying out the Sixth National Population Census," China began its sixth national population census at the standard time of 0:00 on November 1, 2010. Upon its completion, the census revealed that the total population of China (including the 31 provinces, autonomous regions, municipalities, and active servicemen) was approximately 1.371 billion. Compared to the fifth national population census (1.266 billion), which began at 0:00 on November 1, 2000, this figure represents an increase of 5.84% (73.9 million) over 10 years, which is equivalent to an average annual growth rate of 0.57%. The male and female populations accounted for 51.27% (687 million) and 48.73% (653 million) of the total population in China, respectively. As for age distribution, individuals aged 0–14 years, 15–59 years, and ≥60 years accounted for 16.60% (222 million), 70.14% (940 million), and 13.26% (178 million) of the total population, respectively, among which, the population of individuals aged ≥65 years was 119 million, accounting for 8.87% of the total population in China. Compared to the fifth national population census in 2000, the proportion of the population aged 0–14 years decreased by 6.29%, whereas the proportion of the population aged 15–59 years, ≥60 years, and ≥65 years increased by 3.36%, 2.93%, and 1.91%, respectively. It is evident from this data that China's family planning policy had achieved significant outcomes over the past decade in controlling the birth rate, but China has also entered a stage of population aging. In accordance with the 2014 "Decision of the Central Committee of the Communist Party of China (CCCPC) on Some Major Issues Concerning Comprehensively Deepening the Reform," the decision was made to adhere to the basic national policy on family planning but to allow married couples to have a second child if one of the parents was an only child. The aim of which was to gradually improve the birth planning policy and promote the long-term balanced development of the population.

Based on the key indicators of national health status, China's residents show a high level of health among developing countries. In 2012, the average life expectancy of China was 75.2 years (Figure 18.1). The maternal mortality rate decreased from 51.3 deaths per 100,000 live births in 2002 to 24.5 deaths per 100,000 live births in 2012 (Figure 18.2).

In addition, the infant and under-five mortality rates have shown continual decline. The former decreased from 29.2% in 2002 to 10.3% in 2012, while the latter decreased from 34.9% in 2002 to 13.2% in 2012 (see Figures 18.3 and 18.4). These statistics indicate that China has achieved United Nations Millennium Development Goal 4 in advance of its deadline.

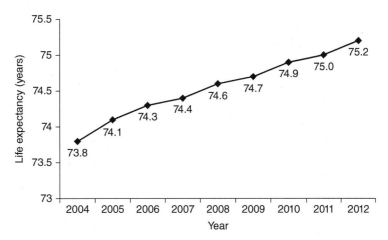

FIGURE 18.1 Average life expectancy in China in 2004–2012. *Source*: China Health Statistics Yearbook, 2013.

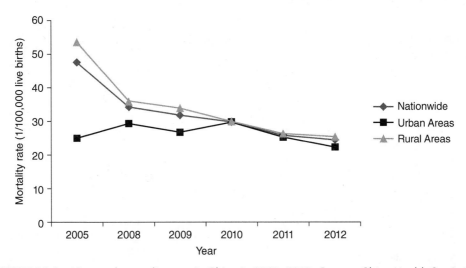

FIGURE 18.2 Maternal mortality rate in China in 2005–2012. *Source*: China Health Statistics Yearbook, 2013.

2. Healthcare System

The healthcare system in China comprises several subsystems, including: (1) service organizations responsible for the delivery of preventive care, healthcare, medical care, and rehabilitation services, as well as healthcare supervision and law enforcement, medical education, and scientific research; and (2) government health administrative agencies that are charged with the oversight of these service organizations. The healthcare system includes healthcare organizations in the narrow sense, such as institutions that provide medical, preventive, and healthcare services and conduct medical research. It also includes other healthcare institutions in the broader sense, such as manufacturers of blood and blood products, biologics, drugs, and medical supplies and devices; drug inspection agencies; nongovernmental health academic organizations (e.g., societies, associations, research societies,

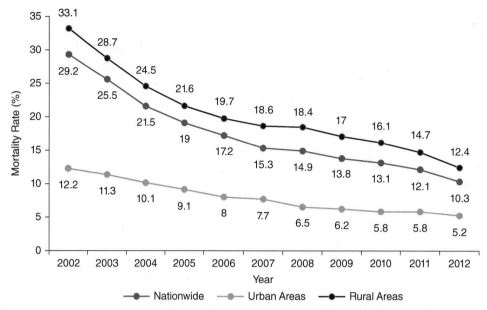

FIGURE 18.3 Infant mortality rate in China in 2005–2012. *Source*: China Health Statistics Yearbook, 2013.

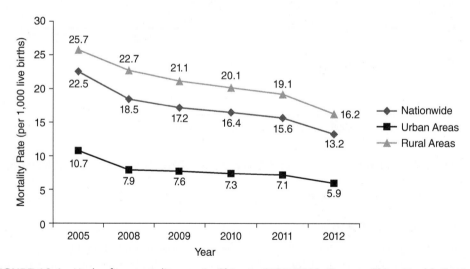

FIGURE 18.4 Under-five mortality rate in China in 2005–2012. *Source*: China Health Statistics Yearbook, 2013.

foundations); and intermediary organizations (e.g., the Medical Technology Assessment and Accident Appraisal Committee). The composition of the healthcare system in China is shown in Figure 18.5.

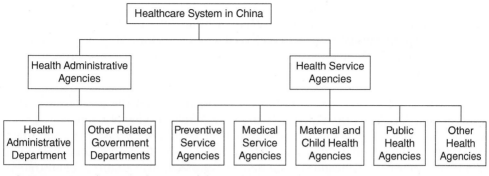

FIGURE 18.5 Schematic diagram of the healthcare system in China.

(1) Management Levels in Organizations

1. National Health Administration   The National Health and Family Planning Commission (NHFPC) of the PRC is a department established by the State Council for the administration of healthcare-related affairs. Drawing on the principles of health services formulated for a new era – specifically, focusing on rural healthcare, prioritizing preventive care, equal emphasis on Chinese and Western medicine, relying on science and education, mobilizing public participation, promoting public health, and serving socialist modernization – the Ministry of Health (MOH) has made a number of successive adjustments to its internal organization since 1998. Presently, the MOH comprises 21 divisions (departments, bureaus, and offices), including the General Office; the Department of Human Resources; the Department of Planning and Information; the Department of Finance; the Department of Legal Affairs; the Department of System Reform; the Office of Health Emergency; the Chinese Center for Disease Control and Prevention; the Department of Medical Administration; the Department of Community Health; the Department of Maternal and Child Health Care; the Department of Food Safety Standards, Risk Surveillance and Assessment; the Bureau of Supervision; the Department of Drug Policy and Essential Drugs; the Department of Community Guidance for Family Planning; the Department of Family Planning and Family Development; the Department of Family Planning Service and Management for Migrant Population; the Department of Publicity; the Department of Science, Technology and Education; the Department of International Cooperation; and the Bureau of Healthcare; as well as the Committee of the Communist Party of China at the MOH. There is also the State Administration of Traditional Chinese Medicine, which is the health administrative department responsible for regulating Traditional Chinese Medicine (TCM).

2. Local Health Administrative Departments   In accordance with the layout of the national health administrative departments, all levels of local government, including provincial, prefectural, autonomous regional, and municipal governments, as well as their prefectural-level cities, counties, and townships, have their own local health administrative agencies (offices or divisions). A department (division) of TCM has also been established in each local health administrative agency in order to administer local TCM affairs.

3. Related National And Local Government Departments As healthcare is part of a large number of sectors, in addition to health administrative departments, many other government departments participate in the oversight and administration of the healthcare industry as well, and this involvement extends vertically to the relevant department of the local governments.

In addition to the MOH, the main regulatory authorities also include more than 10 ministries or departments, such as the Ministry of Finance (MOF), the Ministry of Human Resources and Social Security (MOHRSS), the State Administration of Commodity Prices, the State Administration of Industry and Commerce (SAIC), the Ministry of Civil Affairs (MCA), the General Administration of Quality Supervision, Inspection and Quarantine (AQSIQ), the Ministry of Education (MOE), and the State Medical Insurance Administration, as well as the Food and Drug Administration. These ministries or departments, including the military, have their own hospitals. A number of other agencies affiliated with all levels of government (including provincial, prefectural, and autonomous regional, as well as their prefecture-level cities, counties, and townships) also participate or intervene in local healthcare affairs.

(2) Healthcare Service System

China has established a health system that covers both urban and rural areas. This system comprises four parts: (1) Public health system: This includes the professional public health networks responsible for disease prevention and control, health education, maternal and child health, mental health, health emergency response, blood collection and supply, health supervision and family planning. It also includes the healthcare system that is based on primary care service networks and is responsible for the provision of public health services. (2) Healthcare system: This consists of three-tier rural healthcare networks that are led by county-level hospitals in rural areas and is based on township health centers and village clinics. It also includes new urban healthcare systems that coordinate various levels and types of hospitals with community health service (CHS) agencies in urban areas. (3) Health security system: Its main body consists of basic health security, which is complemented by various types of supplemental and commercial health insurance. Basic health security includes the Urban Employee Basic Medical Insurance (UEBMI), Urban Resident Basic Medical Insurance (URBMI), New Rural Cooperative Medical Scheme (NRCMS), and Urban and Rural Medical Assistance (URMA) schemes, which cover the urban employed population, urban unemployed population, rural residents, and disadvantaged groups in urban and rural areas, respectively. (4) Drug supply security system: This system governs the production, circulation, price management, procurement, distribution, and use of drugs. The number of healthcare institutions in China is shown in Table 18.1.

Based on China's socioeconomic development and its healthcare services' specific attributes, the government adheres to the basic principles of ensuring access to basic healthcare services, improving community healthcare services, and establishing a sound supporting mechanism. In other words, the government is duty-bound to ensure the universal access to essential healthcare services, especially for low-income earners. On the other hand, market and social capitals play a crucial role in ensuring access to nonessential healthcare services, which primarily aim to meet the multilevel, diversified demands of the public. The scope of essential healthcare services is expected to expand gradually alongside the country's economic development and increasing financial security.

TABLE 18.1 Number of Healthcare Institutions in China in 1999–2012

Healthcare institutions	1999	2000	2001	2002	2003	2004	2005	2006	2007	2008	2009	2010	2011	2012
Total	1,017,673	1,034,229	1,029,314	1,005,004	806,243	809,140	882,206	918,097	912,263	891,480	916,571	936,927	954,389	950,297
Hospitals	16,678	16,318	16,197	17,844	17,764	18,393	18,703	19,246	19,852	19,712	20,291	20,918	21,979	23,170
General hospitals	11,868	11,872	11,834	12,716	12,599	12,900	12,982	13,120	13,372	13,119	13,364	13,681	14,328	15,021
TCM hospitals	2,441	2,453	2,478	2,492	2,518	2,611	2,620	2,665	2,720	2,688	2,728	2,778	2,831	2,889
Specialist hospitals	1,533	1,543	1,576	2,237	2,271	2,492	2,682	3,022	3,282	3,427	3,716	3,956	4,283	4,665
Primary care institutions		1,000,169	995,670	973,098	774,693	817,018	849,488	884,818	878,686	858,015	882,153	901,709	918,003	912,620
Community Healthcare Centers (CHCs)				8,211	10,101	14,153	17,128	22,656	27,069	24,260	27,308	32,739	32,860	33,562
Township health centers	49,694	49,229	48,090	44,992	44,279	41,626	40,907	39,975	39,876	39,080	38,475	37,836	37,295	37,097
Village clinics	716,677	709,458	698,966	698,966	514,920	551,600	583,209	609,128	613,855	613,143	632,770	648,424	662,894	653,419
Outpatient departments (clinics)	226,588	240,934	248,061	219,907	204,468	208,794	207,457	212,243	197,083	180,752	182,448	181,781	184,287	187,932
Professional public health institutions		11,386	11,471	10,787	10,792	10,878	11,177	11,269	11,528	11,485	11,665	11,835	11,926	12,083
Centers for Disease Control and Prevention	2,763	3,741	3,813	3,580	3,584	3,588	3,585	3,548	3,585	3,534	3,536	3,513	3,484	3,490
Specialist hospitals (clinics) for disease prevention and treatment	1,877	1,839	1,783	1,839	1,749	1,583	1,502	1,402	1,365	1,310	1,291	1,274	1,294	1,289
Maternal and child health hospitals (clinics/stations)	3,180	3,163	3,132	3,067	3,033	2,998	3,021	3,003	3,051	3,011	3,020	3,025	3,036	3,044
Health surveillance clinics (centers)				571	838	1,284	1,702	2,097	2,553	2,675	2,809	2,992	3,022	3,088

Notes:

1. The decrease in the number of CHCs in 2008 was attributed to the reclassification of approximately 5,000 rural CHCs in Jiangsu Province as village clinics.

2. Since 2002, the headquarters of medical colleges and universities, drug inspection agencies, frontier health and quarantine stations, and non-MOH family planning service stations have not been included in calculating the number of healthcare institutions.

3. Before 1996, "health centers" referred to "township health centers" and outpatient clinics did not include private clinics.

Source: China Health Statistics Yearbook, 2013.

(3) Healthcare Workers

At the end of 2012, there were 9.116 million healthcare workers in China, which was an increase of 500,000 (5.8%) compared to the previous year. Among them, there were 6.667 million healthcare technicians, 1.094 million rural physicians and healthcare workers, 319,000 other technicians, 373,000 management personnel, and 654,000 skilled workers. Among the healthcare technicians, there were 2.616 million medical (assistant) practitioners and 2.497 million registered nurses, who collectively showed an increase of 473,000 (7.7%) compared to 2011. The number of medical (assistant) practitioners per 1,000 people was 1.94, and the number of registered nurses per 1,000 people was 1.85; the number of public health professionals per 10,000 people was 4.96 (Table 18.2 and Table 18.3).

(4) Healthcare Funding Structure

China has multiple sources of healthcare funding, including general taxation, social health insurance, commercial health insurance, residents' out-of-pocket expenses, and so forth. In 2012, China's total healthcare expenditure was RMB2784.68 billion, and its healthcare expenditure per capita was RMB2056.60, accounting for 5.36% of the GDP. The average annual growth rate of the total healthcare expenditure from 2005 to 2012 was 18.16% (calculated based on constant prices). Personal out-of-pocket expenses declined from 52.2% in 2005 to 34.4% in 2012, during which the levels of risk protection and redistribution of the healthcare funding system continued to increase. In 2011, both hospitals and outpatient clinics spent a total of RMB1,808.94 billion, while public health institutions spent RMB204.067 billion, accounting for 71.74% and 8.09% of the total health expenditure,

TABLE 18.2 Number of Healthcare Workers in China in 2005–2012 (Unit: 10,000 people)

Indicator	2005	2008	2009	2010	2011	2012
Total	664.7	725.2	778.1	820.8	861.6	911.6
Healthcare technicians	456.4	517.4	553.5	587.6	620.3	667.6
Medical (assistant) practitioners	204.2	220.2	232.9	241.4	246.6	261.6
Medical practitioners	162.3	179.2	190.5	197.3	202.0	213.96
Registered nurses	135.0	167.8	185.5	204.8	224.4	249.7
Pharmacists	31.1	33.1	34.2	35.4	36.4	37.7
Technicians	26.9	30.5	32.36	33.9	48.8	36.4
Others	59.3	65.9	68.9	72.2	78.1	81.2
Rural physicians and healthcare workers	91.7	93.8	105.1	109.2	112.6	109.4
Rural physicians	86.4	89.4	99.5	103.2	106.1	102.3
Other technicians	22.6	25.5	27.5	29.0	30.6	31.9
Management personnel	31.3	35.7	36.3	37.1	37.5	37.3
Skilled workers	42.8	52.7	55.8	57.9	60.6	65.4

Notes:
1. Since 2008, healthcare workers include those who have been reemployed by the same unit for more than six months.
2. Healthcare technicians also include civil servants with a health inspector certification.
Source: China Health Statistics Yearbook, 2013.

TABLE 18.3   Number of Healthcare Technicians per 1,000 People in China in 2005–2012 (Unit: Person)

Indicator	2005	2008	2009	2010	2011	2012
Healthcare technicians	3.50	3.90	4.15	4.39	4.61	4.94
Urban areas	5.82	6.68	7.71	7.62	7.77	8.55
Rural areas	2.69	2.80	2.94	3.04	3.20	3.41
Medical (assistant) practitioners	1.56	1.66	1.75	1.80	1.83	1.964
Urban areas	2.49	2.68	2.83	2.97	2.95	3.19
Rural areas	1.26	1.26	1.31	1.32	1.33	1.40
Medical practitioners	1.19	1.35	1.43	1.47	1.50	1.58
Urban areas	2.23	2.45	1.60	2.74	2.73	2.96
Rural areas	0.82	0.92	0.96	0.95	0.96	1.00
Registered nurses	1.03	1.27	1.39	1.53	1.67	1.85
Urban areas	2.10	2.54	2.82	3.09	3.23	3.65
Rural areas	0.65	0.76	0.81	0.89	0.98	1.09

Note: For the total number of healthcare technicians, the number of permanent residents is used as the denominator; for the number of healthcare technicians in urban and rural areas, the number of households is used as the denominator.
Source: China Health Statistics Yearbook, 2013.

respectively. The expenses for urban hospitals, county hospitals, CHCs, and township hospitals accounted for 64.13%, 21.28%, 5.17%, and 9.3% of the total hospital expenditure, respectively (Table 18.4).

From the perspective of international trends, total healthcare expenditure as a share of the GDP tends to increase with the country's level of economic development. In 2010, total healthcare expenditure as a share of the GDP was an average of 6.2% in low-income countries and 8.1% in high-income countries. Among the five BRICS countries, the shares for Brazil and India were 9% and 8.9%, respectively. In contrast, China's share was only 5.36%, indicating that its healthcare expenditure still has considerable room for growth.

3. Health Security System

The government of China has attached great importance to the establishment of a health security system. The Publicly-Funded Medical Insurance and Labor Medical Insurance schemes were established in the early stages of the founding of New China. Later, in the 1960s, the Rural Cooperative Medical Scheme (RCMS) was established. The establishment and subsequent improvement of these schemes played a crucial role in protecting the health of employees and farmers in China. In the 1990s, China began initiating health reforms, which actively and steadily promoted the establishment of various health security systems and have made significant progress to date. For example, the UEBMI has progressed steadily over the years, covering more than 318 million people by the end of 2008. In October 2002, the government of China introduced several policies to establish the NRCMS. Since 2003, this scheme has been piloted and gradually promoted nationwide. It now covers up to 833 million insured persons across all agricultural counties (districts) in China. The NRCMS is

TABLE 18.4 China's Total Healthcare Expenditure and its Composition in 2005–2012

Indicator	2005	2008	2009	2010	2011	2012
Total healthcare expenditure (RMB10,000)	8,659.9	14,535.4	17,541.9	19,980.4	24,345.9	27,846.8
Government expenditure on healthcare (RMB10,000)	1,552.5	3,593.9	4,816.3	5,732.5	7,464.2	8,366.0
Social expenditure on healthcare (RMB10,000)	2,586.4	5,065.6	6,154.5	7,196.6	8,416.5	9,916.3
Out-of-pocket payments (RMB10,000)	4,521.0	5,875.9	6,571.2	7,051.2	8,465.3	9,564.6
Composition of total healthcare expenditure (%)	100	100	100	100	100	100
Government expenditure on healthcare (%)	17.9	24.7	27.5	28.7	30.1	30.0
Social expenditure on healthcare (%)	29.9	34.9	35.1	36.0	34.6	35.9
Out-of-pocket payments (%)	52.2	40.4	37.5	35.3	34.8	34.4
Total healthcare expenditure as a share of the GDP (%)	4.68	4.63	5.15	4.98	5.15	5.36
Healthcare expenditure per capita (RMB)	662.3	1,094.5	1,314.3	1,490.1	1,807.0	2,056.6
Urban areas (RMB)	1,126.4	1,861.8	2,176.6	2,315.5	2,697.5	2969.0
Rural areas (RMB)	315.8	455.2	562.0	666.3	879.4	1,055.9
Elasticity coefficient of healthcare consumption	0.87	1.72	2.32	0.65	1.41	

Notes:
1. This table shows the accounting data of the total healthcare expenditure. Only the preliminary accounting data are shown for the total healthcare expenditure in 2012.
2. Calculated at the price of the year.
Source: China Health Statistics Yearbook, 2013.

benefiting a growing number of farmers, which is playing an increasingly important role in reducing or alleviating the economic burden caused by illness.

The overall framework of the health security system in China is composed of three horizontal and three vertical tiers. As shown in Figure 18.6, the three vertical tiers form a main portion of the three horizontal tiers. In other words, the UEBMI, URBMI, and NRCMS together constitute the most fundamental part of the health security system and provide basic health insurance to their beneficiaries. The "bottom horizontal tier" mainly refers to medical assistance provided to low-income or disadvantaged groups, whose healthcare needs are mainly met via the URMA.

The "top horizontal tier" mainly targets patients with a greater demand for healthcare services, which can be met through various supplemental health insurance schemes, including commercial health insurance, enterprise supplemental health insurance, critical illness supplemental health insurance, and civil service medical assistance (Table 18.5).

Currently, China has preliminarily established a basic framework for a multitier health security system at the institutional level. The main component of this framework is basic health insurance, which is complemented by various supplemental health insurance schemes and social medical assistance. Basic health insurance covers urban employees and residents (including students, children, elderly adults without income, and individuals

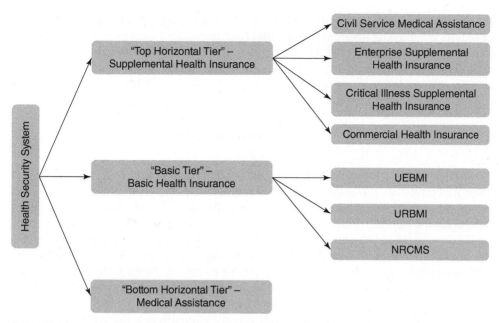

FIGURE 18.6 Schematic diagram of the health security system in China.

who have lost the ability to work), whereas the NRCMS covers rural residents. Basic health insurance adheres to the principle of "low-level, broad coverage." Specifically, in order to achieve "broad coverage," basic health insurance can only offer a "low level" of protection.

Therefore, given the limited level of protection offered by basic health insurance, the demand for greater, more flexible health security can only be met through the use of supplemental health insurance schemes. Aside from offering financial subsidies to address the issue of medical expenses among civil servants, the government of China has also encouraged employers to establish supplemental health insurance schemes, where economically feasible, in order to partially cover medical expenses that have exceeded the reimbursement limit of basic health insurance, thereby alleviating the burden on employees. Thus, various forms of supplemental health insurance schemes have been established, such as

TABLE 18.5 Composition of Social Health Insurance for Urban Employees and Residents in China in 2008 and 2011 (Unit: %)

Item	Total		Urban Areas		Rural Areas	
	2008	2011	2008	2011	2008	2011
UEBMI	12.7	14.8	44.2	47.4	1.5	2.9
Publicly-Funded Medical Insurance	1.0	0.7	3.0	2.2	0.3	0.2
URBMI	3.8	9.5	12.5	25.1	0.7	3.8
NRCMS	68.7	69.5	9.5	13.4	89.7	89.9
Other social health insurance schemes	1.0	0.3	2.8	0.9	0.4	0.1
Uninsured persons	12.9	5.2	28.1	10.9	7.5	3.1

Sources: 2008 National Health Services Survey (NHSS) and 2011 Phased Evaluation of China's Health Care System Reform.

enterprise supplemental health insurance or critical illness supplemental health insurance. In addition, commercial insurance companies have introduced a number of supplemental health insurance products to fill the gap between commercial health insurance and basic health insurance, in order to better alleviate the high medical charges incurred by individuals with different levels of needs. As a result, commercial health insurance has become the main provider of supplemental health insurance.

(1) Urban Employee Basic Medical Insurance (UEBMI)

1. Development Background and Process   One of more notable outcomes of UEBMI reform in China was the establishment of a complete policy system for health insurance in the late 1990s, which was centered on the "Decision of the State Council on Establishing the UEBMI" (hereinafter referred to as the Decision). This policy system consists of four aspects: policies for basic health insurance, management system, basic framework of multi-tier health insurance, and ideas for reforming the healthcare system. The Decision was formulated by summarizing the "Opinions on Piloting the Reform of the Employee Medical Insurance" and the "Opinions on Piloting the Expansion and Reform of the Employee Medical Insurance" issued by the four ministries of the State Council in 1994 and 1996, respectively. The Decision was subsequently promulgated by the State Council in December 1998. The introduction of this document marked the establishment of a health insurance policy system with a new institutional framework, which provided the policy basis and operational specifications for the implementation of the new system. Following the promulgation of the Decision, the UEBMI scheme was gradually promoted in urban areas nationwide.

2. Basic Characteristics   The UEBMI is a social insurance system established to compensate employees for economic losses due to the risk of illness. The UEBMI's health insurance fund relies on premium contributions by employers and individuals. Under this scheme, medical expenses incurred by insured persons can be reimbursed to a certain extent by health insurance agencies, in order to avoid or reduce economic risks faced by employees due to illness, treatment, and so forth.

By the end of August 2004, pilot projects and reforms of the UEBMI had been conducted successively across 4 municipalities, 340 prefecture-level cities, and over 2,000 counties (cities); up to 118 million individuals were insured under this scheme. By the end of 2005, 137.83 million individuals were insured under the UEBMI, including 100.22 million employees and 37.61 million retirees, which were equivalent to increases of 9.77 million and 4.02 million compared to the previous year, respectively. By the end of September 200, 149.66 million individuals were insured under the UEBMI, accounting for 52.95% of the total number of eligible urban employees (282.63 million) nationwide. By the end of 2012, 264.67 million individuals were insured under UEBMI.

3. Coverage Scope and Premium Payment Methods   Participation in the UEBMI is compulsory for all employers in urban areas, including enterprises (e.g., state-owned enterprises, collective enterprises, foreign-invested enterprises, private enterprises), agencies, institutions, social organizations, and private non-enterprise units, as well as their employees. The participation of township and village enterprises (TVEs) and urban sole proprietors, as well as their employees, in this scheme must be decided by the respective provincial, autonomous regional or municipal governments.

In principle, the social pooling units of the UEBMI are the administrative divisions at the prefectural level or above (including prefectures, municipality, and leagues) but can sometimes be a county (or county-level city), and social pooling is generally implemented throughout the entire municipalities of Beijing, Tianjin, and Shanghai (these social pooling units are hereinafter referred to as "pooling regions"). All employers and their employees must participate in the UEBMI in their respective pooling regions according to the principle of territorial administration, in order to ensure the implementation of uniform policies and the uniform collection, use, and management of UEBMI funds. Transregional enterprises in railways, electricity, freight transport, and other industries with high production mobility, as well as their employees, can participate in the basic health insurance at different pooling regions in a relatively centralized manner.

The UEBMI premiums are jointly paid by employers and employees. Employers' contributions are controlled at about 6% of their employees' salaries, while employees' contributions are generally equivalent to 2% of their salaries. The contribution rates of both employers and employees can be adjusted in accordance with China's economic development.

4. Outcomes The prototype of a multitier health security system, based mainly on the basic health insurance system, was preliminarily established, which formed the basic characteristics of the new system. At the beginning of the twenty-first century, both the civil service and critical illness medical assistance schemes were gradually introduced in more than 90% of urban areas in China. In addition, numerous enterprises that had the ability to participate in the insurance schemes began developing various types of supplemental health insurance. Thus, the prototype of a multi-tier health security system was preliminarily established, which was mainly based on the basic health insurance system and supplemented by the civil service medical assistance, critical illness medical assistance, and enterprise supplemental health insurance schemes. This gradually evolved into a new system with characteristics that differed from those of the original Publicly-Funded Medical Insurance and Labor Medical Insurance schemes.

With regard to the type of insurance, the UEBMI involves shifting from the previous "employment-based insurance" to "social insurance" and establishing a model for social pooling and personal accounts. In terms of its financing mechanism, the UEBMI has shifted from the previous approach, whereby medical expenses were fully covered by the government and enterprises, to one that utilizes joint premium contributions from employers and employees, which increases employees' awareness of cost savings to a certain extent. In terms of the health protection level, the UEBMI aims to meet basic healthcare demands and has established various cost-containment mechanisms, such as copayments, deductibles, and reimbursement caps, thereby fundamentally altering the previous lack of personal accountability and constraints in the payment of medical expenses. With regard to the coverage of the UEBMI, this has been expanded from employees of agencies, institutions, and collective enterprises to employees of all urban employers, including all enterprises, agencies, institutions, social organizations and private nonenterprise units, as well as employees of TVEs and sole proprietors. With regard to its management system, the UEBMI employs a localized, socialized management system that transcends the previous boundaries of Publicly-Funded Medical Insurance and Labor Medical Insurance schemes, as well as those of employers with different ownerships (Table 18.6).

TABLE 18.6   Differences Between the UEBMI and the Publicly Funded Healthcare and Labor Insurance Medical Schemes in China

Item	UEBMI	Publicly Funded Medical Insurance and Labor Medical Insurance
Type of insurance	Use of social pooling and personal accounts (social insurance), thus embodying the principle of social equality	Employment-based insurance
Funding mechanism	Joint premium contributions between employers and employees, which has increased employees' cost awareness to a certain extent	Employees' medical expenses are fully covered by the government and enterprises without a constraint mechanism for both physicians and patients
Protection level	Aims to meet basic healthcare demands with a lower protection level and stipulation of deductibles and reimbursement caps	Patients do not have to pay or only have to pay a small proportion of their medical expenses (such as registration fees)
Coverage	All employers in urban areas, including enterprises (state-owned enterprises, collective enterprises, foreign-invested enterprises, private enterprises), agencies, institutions, social organizations, private nonenterprise units and their employees, as well as employees of TVEs and sole proprietors.	Only limited to employees of agencies, institutions and collective enterprises
Management system	Employs a localized, socialized management system that transcends the previous boundaries of the Publicly-Funded Medical Insurance and Labor Medical Insurance schemes, as well as those of employers with different ownerships	The Publicly-Funded Medical Insurance is administered by the MOH and Labor Medical Insurance is administered by the Ministry of Labor.

(2) Urban Resident Basic Medical Insurance (URBMI)

1. Development Background and Process   China began establishing the UEBMI in 1998, which was followed by the initiation of NRCMS pilot projects and the establishment of the URMA. At this point, the majority of individuals not included within the institutional arrangements for health security are unemployed urban residents. Thus, the government devised URBMI pilot projects with the primary aim of exploring possible policies and approaches that would encourage informal employees (i.e., flexible employees, employees of nonpublic economic organizations, agricultural workers, and other migrant workers) and unemployed persons (elderly adults and minors living in urban areas) to enroll in health insurance within a unified institutional framework, thereby expanding the coverage scope of urban basic health insurance. The URBMI is based on social pooling and government funding, rather than the previous employment-based insurance, whereby funding was operated in a closed manner within the employment units. The URBMI also expands the scope of urban basic health insurance from employees of public economic sectors to employees of all sectors and nonemployed persons in urban areas.

Unlike the UEBMI (gradually established since 1998) and NRCMS (gradually implemented since 2002), the URBMI is still at the initial stages of piloting and expansion of pilot sites. Alongside the preliminary development of the UEBMI and on the basis of the transition from the UEBMI to the URBMI in certain regions, the State Council decided to launch the URBMI pilot projects from 2007 onward, with the goal of achieving universal health coverage for both urban and rural residents in China. Thus, in July 2007, the State Council issued the "Guiding Opinions of the State Council on the Pilot Program for the Urban Resident Basic Medical Insurance." This document proposed the expansion of URBMI pilot projects in 2008, aiming to cover more than 80% of cities by 2009 and to fully implement the URBMI by 2010, thereby gradually covering all urban nonemployed residents nationwide. The aim of the URBMI pilot projects is to explore and improve the policy system for urban basic health insurance; to form a rational financing mechanism, sound management system, and standardized operating mechanism; and to gradually establish a health insurance system for urban residents dominated by the comprehensive coverage for critical illnesses.

With regard to the future arrangements for the URBMI pilot projects, on August 23, 2007, Hu Xiaoyi, the State Council's Director of the Department of Urban Resident Basic Medical Insurance and the Vice-Minister of Labor and Social Security, noted in his interview on the PRC's official website (www.gov.cn) that: the URBMI is a scheme that will benefit 240 million people. Hence, the plan is to launch URBMI pilot projects in 79 cities in 2007; further expand the pilot projects in 2008; cover more than 80% of cities in 2009; and achieve full coverage in 2010.

2. Basic Characteristics   The URBMI is a mandatory, government-led scheme that forms part of China's social health insurance. It is mainly funded by residents (families) via premium contributions and supplemented by appropriate subsidies from the government. It aims to meet the healthcare demands of urban residents based on the principle of consistency between premium contribution standards and benefit levels (Table 18.7).

3. Insurance Benefits   The URBMI fund is mainly used to cover medical expenses incurred by insured residents for inpatient and outpatient services for critical illnesses and outpatient emergency services. The scope and standards of reimbursement are based on the URBMI drug formulary, treatment regimens, and the scope and standards of the healthcare services and facilities (which might be adjusted depending on the economic conditions across different provinces, autonomous regions, and municipalities).

TABLE 18.7   Status of the UEBMI and URBMI in China in 2005–2012

Indicator	2005	2008	2009	2010	2011	2012
UEBMI						
Number of insured persons (10,000)	13,783	19,996	21,937	23,735	25,227	26,467
Number of employed persons (10,000)	10,022	14,988	16,411	17,791	18,949	–
Retirees (10,000)	3,761	5,008	5,527	5,944	6,279	–
Fund income (RMB100 million)	1,405.3	3,040.0	3,672.0	3,955.4	4,945.0	–
Fund expenditure (RMB100 million)	1,078.7	2,084.0	2,797.0	3,271.6	4,018.3	–
Cumulative balance (RMB100 million)	1,278.1	3,432.0	4,276.0	4,741.2	5,683.2	–
URBMI						
Number of insured persons (10,000)	-	11,826	18,210	19,528	22,116	27,122

Source: China Health Statistics Yearbook, 2013.

1. *Deductibles.* The deductibles (i.e., threshold fees) of the URBMI are similar to those of the UEBMI – RMB 980 in tertiary hospitals, RMB 720 in secondary hospitals, and RMB 540 in primary hospitals.
2. *Medical management.* The URBMI follows the principle of "first treatment appointed institutions" and utilizes a two-way referral system. CHCs, specialist hospitals, hospital–pharmacy cooperatives, secondary healthcare institutions, and primary healthcare institutions are designated as the appointed healthcare institutions for initial treatment. On the other hand, tertiary general hospitals and specialist hospitals are designated as referral healthcare institutions. URBMI-insured residents must first seek medical attention at an appointed healthcare institution, which in turn refers patients to a referral hospital for inpatient treatment whenever necessary. Patients return to the formerly appointed healthcare institution after their condition stabilizes. In other words, when insured residents fall ill, they will initially seek medical attention at appointed CHCs or small-sized hospitals. If their condition does not improve, these CHCs or small-sized hospitals refer them to large-sized hospitals. Once their conditions have improved, patients will be referred immediately back to the former institutions.
3. *Reimbursement rate.* The proportion of medical expenses that can be reimbursed is determined by the tier of the healthcare institution, whereby primary (including CHCs), secondary, and tertiary institutions have reimbursement rates of 75%, 60%, and 50%, respectively. However, after two years of continuous premium contributions, these reimbursement rates can be increased to 80%, 65%, and 55%, respectively. In other words, the reimbursement rates are higher when seeking treatment at a lower-tier hospital.
4. *Basic insured amount.* The reimbursement cap of the URBMI is RMB16,000 per person per calendar year. However, this may be increased to RMB20,000 per person per year for patients with certain "outpatient critical illnesses," including chronic renal failure (outpatient hemodialysis treatment), malignant tumors (outpatient radiotherapy and chemotherapy), antirejection therapy after organ transplantation, systemic lupus erythematosus, and aplastic anemia.

(3) New Rural Cooperative Medical Scheme (NRCMS)

1. Development Background and Process   In 2002, during the process of establishing and improving the UEBMI, the Central Committee and the State Council held the National Rural Health Conference. Subsequently, on October 19, 2002, the Central Committee and State Council issued the "Decision on Further Strengthening Rural Health Work" (hereinafter referred to as the "Decision on Rural Health Work"), which outlined the following objective: "To establish a rural healthcare service system and rural cooperative medical scheme that meet the requirements of a socialist economic system and rural socioeconomic development by 2010." The Decision on Rural Health Work represents a major decision by the Central Committee and State Council in establishing a new rural cooperative medical scheme in China. It explicitly states that it is necessary to "establish a new rural cooperative medical scheme and medical assistance scheme primarily to pool funds for critical illnesses" in order to ensure that all rural residents have access to primary care services.

The NRCMS is an important aspect of China's health reform, as it has had a direct impact on the health and interests of hundreds of millions of farmers in China. Its establishment was a major decision made by the central government in its efforts to resolve the Three Rural

Issues. Furthermore, it has also played a significant role in implementing a more scientific outlook on development, ensuring coordinated urban–rural development, and creating a more moderately prosperous society.

As the main rural health insurance scheme in China, the NRCMS has been, in general, shown to benefit insured rural residents, healthcare providers, and the government through pilot projects from 2003 to the termination of pilot projects announced by the State Council in January 2007, and is currently in the process of full implementation. Medical expenses incurred by rural residents can be reimbursed to a certain extent under the NRCMS. This has improved the accessibility and utilization of healthcare services in rural areas and alleviated the direct economic burden of medical treatment, which has increased the trust of rural residents in the NRCMS. The operations of the NRCMS fund are considered safe, which ensures that its system operations are relatively stable. The NRCMS has increased the income, annual number of visits, utilization rate of hospital beds, service capability, and service efficiency of rural healthcare institutions, especially township hospitals. Furthermore, it has also promoted the development of rural healthcare services and has played an active role in alleviating illness-related poverty among rural residents, as well as promoting their accessibility to basic healthcare services. Naturally, the specific operating mechanisms and management measures of the NRCMS still require gradual adjustments and improvements to best fit current developments, the wishes of rural residents, and the actual operating conditions. However, the results from the first comprehensive assessment of the NRCMS in the first three years of its implementation showed that it is successful, feasible, and consistent with the actual conditions of rural areas and the wishes of most rural residents in China (MOH, 2006).

2. Basic Characteristics   The NRCMS is a voluntary, rural mutual aid medical scheme established, guided, and supported by the government and has multiple sources of funding, including premium contributions from individuals, support from collectives, and subsidies from governments.

Statistics have shown that, by December 31, 2005, there were 678 NRCMS pilot counties in 31 provinces (autonomous regions and municipalities), which accounted for 23.7% of the total number of counties (county-level cities and districts) and covered 236 million rural residents. By June 30, 2006, there were more than 1,400 pilot counties (county-level cities and districts), which accounted for 50.7% of the total number of counties (county-level cities and districts), covering 396 million rural residents. In 2007, the NRCMS covered around 86% of all counties and more than 700 million rural residents were enrolled. At this point, the central government decided to transition from pilot projects to full implementation, with the goal of achieving NRCMS coverage for all rural counties (county-level cities and districts) by 2008, according to the current deployment of the State Council. By the end of 2012, a total of 2,566 counties (county-level cities and districts) had launched the NRCMS, covering 805 million insured persons, resulting in an enrollment rate of 98.3%. In 2012, the total amount of NRCMS funds raised was RMB248.47 billion, which is equivalent to RMB308.50 per capita. The NRCMS spent a total of RMB240.8 billion on 1.745 billion reimbursements, of which 85 million were made for inpatient services and 1.541 billion were made for general outpatient services.

The NRCMS is a basic health security system for rural residents that maintains a high level of coverage while also significantly increasing the amount of funding. As noted earlier, in 2012, the enrollment rate in the NRCMS was 98.3%, while its funding level per capita increased from RMB246.20 in 2011 to RMB308.50 in 2012 (equivalent to an increase of RMB62.30). The number of reimbursements also grew alongside the expansion of

NRCMS coverage, which increased from 1.315 billion in 2011 to 1.745 billion in 2012. The management of the income and expenditures of the NRCMS fund was enhanced, such that in 2012, the balance rate was 3.1%, which suggested that the NRCMS had a balanced fund with a slight surplus.

3. Insurance benefits

1. *Target beneficiaries.* The target beneficiaries of critical illness insurance are participants of the URBMI and NRCMS.
2. *Coverage scope.* There is continuity in the coverage scope for critical illness insurance with that of the URBMI and NRCMS. Specifically, the URBMI and NRCMS provide basic health insurance as specified in each policy; on top of which the critical illness insurance reimburses all qualified out-of-pocket expenses remaining after insured persons who have incurred catastrophic medical expenses have been reimbursed under the URBMI or NRCMS. "Catastrophic medical expenses" are defined as the annual cumulative qualified medical expenses that have exceeded the annual disposable income per capita of urban residents or net income per capita of rural residents in the previous year, as reported by the local statistical department; the specific amount is determined by the local governments. "Qualified medical expenses" refers to actual and reasonable medical expenses (stipulated as nonreimbursable items) incurred by the patients; the specific amount is determined by the local governments. Local governments can also begin providing the critical illness insurance by starting with diseases that impose a heavier burden on patients (Table 18.8).
3. *Protection level.* In order to protect urban and rural residents from catastrophic medical expenses, the reimbursement policy for critical illness insurance was established to maintain a reimbursement rate of at least 50%. Different bands of reimbursement rates were formulated based on the level of medical expenses incurred, such that, in principle, a higher rate of reimbursement will be provided for higher levels of medical expenses. Furthermore, the reimbursement rate for critical illness insurance can be gradually increased alongside improvements in funding, management, and protection levels, in order to minimize the financial burden of medical expenses.

TABLE 18.8 Status of the NRCMS in China in 2005–2012

Indicator	2005	2008	2009	2010	2011	2012
Number of NRCMS-participating counties (districts and cities)	678	2,729	2,716	2,678	2,637	2,566
Number of insured persons (100 million)	1.79	8.15	8.33	8.36	8.32	8.05
Enrollment rate (%)	75.7	91.5	94.0	96.0	97.5	98.3
Total funds raised for the current year (RMB100 million)	75.4	785.0	944.4	1,308.3	2,047.6	2,484.7
Funding per capita (RMB)	42.1	96.3	113.4	156.6	246.2	308.5
Fund expenditure for the current year (RMB100 million)	61.8	662.0	922.9	1,187.8	1,710.2	2,408.0
Number of reimbursements (100 million)	1.22	5.85	7.59	10.87	13.15	17.45

Source: China Health Statistics Yearbook, 2013.

Ensuring the smooth transition among basic health insurance, critical illness insurance and medical assistance for catastrophic diseases, establishing a notification system for critical illnesses, enabling the timely retrieval of information on the reimbursement status of patients with critical illnesses, and enhancing policy continuity will help prevent illness-related poverty. The appointed healthcare institutions, medications, and treatment scope for RMAS are established in accordance with the relevant policies and regulations regarding basic health insurance and critical illness insurance.

4. Outcomes

1. The responsibilities of governments at all levels were increasingly clear in the process of establishing the NRCMS. First, the government's fundraising responsibilities were clarified, and the funding standards for each level of government were stipulated. Second, the government's administrative responsibilities were clarified, which specifically involved the establishment of administrative agencies and funding management; moreover, NRCMS administration was included as part of the public affair responsibilities of local governments. Currently, the NRCMS has essentially been fully established, and is equipped with various administrative systems focusing on implementation methods, fund management, accounting, auditing, and periodic publicity. Additionally, the NRCMS has been continuously improved via pilot projects, which have laid an excellent foundation for the institutionalization, standardization, and legalization of the NRCMS. In terms of fund management, the NRCMS fund is a close-ended fund that utilizes various supervisory mechanisms, including administrative, financial, auditing, and democratic supervision, which together ensure the operational safety of the NRCMS fund.

2. Since the implementation of the NRCMS, the utilization rate of healthcare services (particularly inpatient services) among insured rural residents has increased significantly. NRCMS-insured rural residents tend to have higher utilization rates of outpatient and inpatient services than uninsured rural residents. Specifically, the two-week consultation rates among insured and uninsured rural residents were 21.9% and 18%, respectively. Compared to areas that did not participate in NRCMS, the two-week outpatient consultation rate of participating areas showed an increase of 33.2%, and their hospitalization rate increased by 52.7%. In addition, the two-week nonconsultation rate decreased by 10.7%, and the percentage of nonhospitalized patients who should have been hospitalized decreased by 15%. In short, the NRCMS has improved the accessibility and utilization rates of healthcare services among rural residents.

3. The result of a nationwide survey revealed that: the NRCMS has benefited 57.6% of households; 83% of insured inpatients were reimbursed, at an average reimbursement amount of RMB784 per visit and a reimbursement rate of 23.2%; the average out-of-pocket inpatient expenses after reimbursement was RMB3,013, which was 12–13% less than uninsured rural residents (MOH, 2007). Furthermore, in 2004, the average inpatient expenses as a share of the net income of rural residents decreased from 89% before reimbursement to 65% after reimbursement. These data indicate that NRCMS reimbursements have reduced the financial burden of rural residents due to medical expenses to a certain extent.

4. Since the implementation of the NRCMS, there has been increasing awareness of its benefits among rural residents, which has led a steady growth of its enrollment rate. The majority of rural residents believed that the NRCMS is an excellent scheme that is capable of reducing the financial burden imposed by medical expenses to a certain

extent. In addition, most rural residents showed favorable responses to the measures adopted to facilitate their access to healthcare services and the reimbursement of their medical expenses. An assessment of NRCMS pilot projects in 2005 revealed that about 90% of insured rural residents expressed a willingness to continue their participation in the NRCMS the following year, while 51% of uninsured rural residents expressed a willingness to join the NRCMS the following year (MOH, 2006).

5. The institutional framework and basic principles of the NRCMS in terms of its organizational system, funding mechanism, fund management, and supervisory management were gradually established on the basis of historical lessons and pilot experiences in order to meet the actual needs of most rural residents. During the piloting process, the implementation plan of the NRCMS was formulated according to the socioeconomic characteristics of each region and adjusted in a timely manner according to the actual operational conditions and responses of the rural residents. For example, the scope and rate of reimbursement were adjusted to enable more effective fund utilization, such that the utilization rate of the NRCMS fund among the first batch of pilot counties increased from 71% in 2004 to 91% in 2005. Furthermore, all participating counties have also actively improved their reimbursement methods to facilitate more effective reimbursement of medical expenses incurred by rural residents and reduce reimbursement costs, which have received favorable responses from rural residents.

6. In 2003–2005, township health centers in NRCMS-participating counties showed a significant increase in annual income, annual number of visits, hospital bed utilization rate, and average annual number of visits per healthcare technician, while the rate of increase was higher than that of nonparticipating counties. Furthermore, in NRCMS pilot counties, the average annual growth rates for the number of outpatient visits and hospital discharges in county hospitals were 6.56% and 11.87%, respectively, while those of township health centers were 8.85% and 8.58%, respectively. There were also significant increases in the utilization rate of hospital beds, with county hospitals and township health centers in pilot counties showing average annual growth rates of 5% and 10%, respectively, which were significantly higher than those of similar healthcare institutions nationwide the same period (MOH, 2007). Based on the needs of establishing the NRCMS, many provincial governments also began increasing their capital investment, enhancing their rural healthcare institutions and healthcare teams, and actively promoting the reforms of the internal operating mechanism and human resource allocation system in township health centers, with the aim of improving the conditions and quality of healthcare services provided in their healthcare institutions. However, county hospitals remained the largest beneficiaries of the NRCMS, receiving about 40% of the allocated funds.

7. Following implementation of the NRCMS, the government established a reimbursement drug list and a strict referral system. The government also began employing stricter regulatory measures during the implementation of the NRCMS, such as a diagnosis-related group (DRG)-based payment system. These measures have restricted medical malpractice among healthcare providers and controlled the growth of medical expenses to some extent. In addition, the implementation of the NRCMS was conducive to the standardized management of healthcare institutions, which has significantly improved the quality of statistical data collection and medical records of primary care institutions and helped promote computerized management in these institutions.

(4) Urban and Rural Medical Assistance (URMA)

URMA is a medical assistance scheme with multiple funding sources (e.g., government subsidies, charitable donations) that subsidizes medical expenses incurred by rural households enjoying the "Five Guarantees" (food, clothing, housing, medical care, and burial expenses or compulsory education for minors), impoverished rural households, urban residents covered by the Minimum Livelihood Guarantee (MLG) system but who have not joined the UEBMI, UEBMI-insured persons who are still overwhelmed by financial burden, and other disadvantaged groups (the Rural Medical Assistance Scheme can also subsidize its recipients to participate in their local NRCMS).

With the acceleration of health reforms and the separation of corporate social responsibility, urban residents began shifting from the use of employer-based insurance to social insurance. Thus, certain responsibilities for the provision of welfare and assistance were transferred from employers to the government and society. Moreover, the collective welfare and assistance capabilities of rural areas were hampered to a degree by the implementation of the household responsibility system, especially after the implementation of rural tax reform. Thus, the Rural Cooperative Medical Scheme gradually lost its effectiveness in rural areas, whereas the healthcare issues facing the urban poor became increasingly prominent during the transition from the Publicly-Funded Medical Insurance and Labor Medical Insurance schemes to a social health insurance system. Therefore, against this backdrop, the improvement of medical assistance schemes for disadvantaged groups in rural and urban areas quickly became an urgent issue that needed to be addressed.

The medical assistance system in China was first introduced in rural areas. In 2002, the Central Committee and the State Council jointly formulated and promulgated the "Decision on Further Strengthening Rural Health Work," which proposed for the first time the establishment of a Rural Medical Assistance Scheme that helps impoverished rural households to cover their medical expenses due to critical illnesses and subsidize their participation in the NRCMS. In 2003, the MCA, MOH, and MOF jointly promulgated the "Opinions on the Implementation of Rural Medical Assistance Scheme" (MCA [2003] No. 158), which clarified that the RMAS is a medical assistance scheme with multiple funding sources (e.g., government subsidies, charitable donations) for "rural households enjoying the Five Guarantees" and impoverished rural households. The goal was to establish a standardized and comprehensive medical assistance scheme for rural areas nationwide by 2005, thereby effectively improving the health status of rural populations in China. In 2005, the General Office of the State Council forwarded the "Notice of Opinions on the Establishment of a Pilot Program for the Urban Medical Assistance Scheme" (GOSC [2005] No. 10) to the MCA and several other ministries. The same year, a series of policy documents were issued in succession, including the "Opinions on Strengthening the Administration of Urban Medical Assistance Funds" (MOF & MCA [2005] No. 39) and the "Notice on Accelerating the Implementation of a Rural Medical Assistance Scheme" (MCA [2005] No. 121). As a result, an urban and rural medical assistance system characterized by institutionalized management, standardized operations, universal coverage, broad income sources, appropriate standards, and continuity with related assistance schemes, was gradually established. The introduction of URMA and its related schemes further expanded the scope and level of medical assistance coverage, thus effectively alleviating the difficulties faced by impoverished residents in seeking medical attention.

In 2006, the Rural Medical Assistance Scheme was fully implemented in all agricultural counties (county-level cities and districts) in China. By 2008, the Urban Medical Assistance Scheme had essentially been established in all counties (county-level cities and districts) nationwide. In the process of establishing URMA, a "government-led, MCA-headed" administrative system with "cross-departmental cooperation and social participation," as well as a fund management system were established in each region to ensure the earmarking of its funds (Table 18.9).

Medical assistance schemes for impoverished populations have been successively established and implemented in both urban and rural areas in China. Funds have also been actively raised to preliminarily explore a feasible medical assistance model. In addition, a medical assistance model that meets the specific national circumstances of China was preliminarily explored nationwide during the establishment of the various medical assistance schemes. Medical assistance schemes in some areas focus on critical illnesses as well as common diseases and outpatient services. Furthermore, the timing of medical assistance provision has gradually shifted from posttreatment to during and pretreatment. In terms of fund settlement, the application and processing procedures have been simplified via the direct transfer of payments from the MCA to the healthcare agencies. Additionally, the threshold for aid has been relaxed by reducing the deductibles and the proportion of copayment. In terms of service provision, the feasibility of using CHCs as platforms for service provision has been explored. In terms of system continuity, various approaches, such as advance payments and disbursements, have been adopted to ensure that disadvantaged groups receive appropriate compensation for NRCMS deductibles and copayments that they are unable to afford.

(5) Critical Illness Insurance for Urban and Rural Residents

1. Basic Characteristics Critical illness insurance reimburses catastrophic medical expenses incurred by urban and rural residents due to critical illnesses. Its aim is to ensure that the vast majority of the population does not fall into poverty due to illness, which is an issue of great concern to the public. On August 30, 2012, the National Development and Reform Commission (NDRC), MOH, MOF, MOHRSS, MCA, and China Insurance Regulatory Commission (CIRC) jointly issued the "Guiding Opinions on the Provision of Critical Illness Insurance for Urban and Rural Residents," which specifically targets URBMI- and NRCMS-insured persons facing a heavy financial burden due to critical illnesses. This proposal aimed

TABLE 18.9 Status of the URMA in China in 2005–2012

Indicator	Year					
	2005	**2008**	**2009**	**2010**	**2011**	**2012**
Number of URMA recipients (10,000)	970	5,278	6,295	7,556	8,519	8,051
Urban residents (10,000)	115	1,086	1,506	1,291	2,222	2,077
Rural residents (10,000)	855	4,192	4,789	5,635	6,297	5,974
URMA expenditure (RMB100 million)	11.0	68.0	97.2	133.0	187.6	203.8
Urban residents (RMB100 million)	3.2	29.7	37.3	49.5	67.6	70.9
Rural residents (RMB100 million)	7.8	38.3	59.9	83.5	120	132.9

Note: This table only includes the number of government-funded medical assistance recipients (excluding those under social medical assistance schemes).
Source: China Health Statistics Yearbook, 2013.

to introduce market mechanisms to establish critical illness insurance schemes with reimbursement rates of at least 50%, which will alleviate the financial burden of urban and rural residents due to critical illnesses.

The annual medical expenses incurred by patients are considered catastrophic if they exceed the annual disposable income per capita of urban residents or the net income per capita of rural residents in the previous year; the exact amount is determined by the local governments.

2. Funding Sources and Management　The funding criteria for critical illness insurance were scientifically and rationally determined based on a number of factors, including local socioeconomic development, fundraising capability, affordability of catastrophic medical expenses incurred for critical illnesses, the reimbursement level of basic health insurance, and the protection level of critical illness insurance. Specific proportions or amounts of the URBMI and NRCMS funds are set aside as funds for critical illness insurance. In areas with surpluses in the URBMI and NRCMS funds, these surpluses are pooled to form the critical illness insurance funds; whereas in areas with insufficient or no surpluses, pooling will be undertaken during the annual increase in the fundraising of the URBMI and NRCMS, thereby gradually improving the multisource funding mechanism of the URBMI and NRCMS. It is also possible to undertake the social pooling of critical illness insurance at the municipal (prefectural) or to explore uniform policies at the provincial (district and county-level city) level to achieve unified organization and implementation, thereby enhancing its resistance to risk. Areas with favorable conditions are also able to explore and establish a unified critical illness insurance system that covers employees, urban residents, and rural residents.

According to the provisions of the aforementioned document, the funds for the critical illness insurance is derived from the surpluses of existing health insurance funds and its management is entrusted to commercial insurance companies, that is, critical illness insurance is purchased from commercial insurance companies. For a commercial insurance company to offer critical illness insurance, it must have operated as a provider of health insurance in China for more than five years; be equipped with a comprehensive service network and sufficient expertise in health insurance; have full-time service personnel with medical backgrounds; and be able to perform separate accounting for its critical illness insurance. In addition, commercial insurance companies that offer critical illness insurance must also control their profitability to within a reasonable range and provide "one-stop" real-time settlement services, so as to ensure that the public has convenient and timely access to the benefits of critical illness insurance.

3. Pilot Progress　On October 25, 2013 (10 a.m.), the MOHRSS held a press conference on its progress in the third quarter of 2013. During this conference, the MOHRSS spokesman Yin Chengji said that the MOHRSS has actively promoted pilot projects of critical illness insurance for urban and rural residents. In total, 23 provinces have proposed implementation plans for critical illness insurance and 120 pilot cities were identified. Subsequently, the Chair of the NHFPC, Li Bin, mentioned during the 2014 "National Lianghui" that 28 provinces in China had begun conducing pilot projects of critical illness insurance for urban and rural residents, 8 provinces of which have fully implemented the insurance scheme.

In 2013, rural health security in China has shifted its focus toward critical illnesses. Critical illness insurance now covers around 20 types of diseases, with reimbursement rates ranging from 70% to 90% for inpatient expenses. These diseases include childhood leukemia, congenital heart disease, end-stage renal disease, breast cancer, cervical cancer, severe mental illnesses, drug-resistant tuberculosis, AIDS-related opportunistic infection, hemophilia, chronic myeloid leukemia, orofacial cleft, lung cancer, esophageal cancer, gastric cancer, Type 1 diabetes, hyperthyroidism, acute myocardial infarction, cerebral infarction, colon cancer, and rectal cancer.

4. Progress of Health System Reforms

(1) Development Background

The progress of health reforms in China has always followed on economic reforms. Therefore, despite being an important component of social policy, health reforms in China have clearly lagged behind its economic reforms. Song Xiaowu mentioned in his speech at the China Symposium on the Macroeconomic and Reform Trends in March 2006 that most economic reforms in China have centered on reforming state-owned enterprises, which have resulted in an unequal access to social security or public goods among different social groups (e.g., between employees or state-owned and non-state-owned enterprises). This, in turn, led to the uneven provision of healthcare public goods in society. In addition, there is uneven socioeconomic development across different regions in China, and the reform of its health-care system is relatively complicated, as it involves different health security systems for urban and rural employees from different economic categories, as well as healthcare institutions and drug distribution channels that were established under different circumstances. Thus, the introduction of a market economy led to the diversification of stakeholders and the withdrawal of the government's complete intervention in the healthcare market in its management methods. Furthermore, due to the government's unfamiliarity with the special rules of the healthcare market, there was a lack of government responsibility and the inadequate provision of public goods and services, which naturally resulted in the distorted development of the healthcare system.

In the early stages of the founding of New China, the functions of the healthcare system were clearly defined under the planned economic system. As a result, the system attained noteworthy achievements in a number of different aspects, such as healthcare services and preventive care. However, due to the impact of socioeconomic development and comprehensive national power, as well as the "unification of government affairs," the healthcare system had numerous problems of varying severity that were related to medical technologies, service quality, and infrastructure. Therefore, in order to meet the needs of economic development, social progress, and improvements in the health status of the Chinese population, China continuously explored new avenues of development in its healthcare system and successively implemented a series of health reforms, the most noteworthy of which began in 1985. China has made great strides after more than two decades of reforming its healthcare system.

(2) Reform Process

The different medical disciplines in China have long lacked clearly defined scopes, such that even the classification between public health and healthcare services is unclear, while the functions of relevant health departments and boundaries of related policies are also constantly blurred. Therefore, healthcare and public health are often not strictly distinguished and tend to be considered together during the reform process of China's health system.

(3) Outcomes and Issues

Since the Chinese economic reform, the healthcare industry in China has shown a number of great achievements, including: the expansion of healthcare teams; establishment of a healthcare service system; improvement of medical technologies; significant improvement in the capacity of drug production and supply; significant increases in health status; and the establishment of a legal system for healthcare. These achievements have played an important role in socioeconomic development, social progress, and improving the health status of the Chinese population. These outcomes are mainly reflected in the important indicators of national health status, which indicate that Chinese residents have a relatively high level of health among developing countries. In 2012, the average life expectancy in China was 75.2 years. The maternal mortality rate decreased from 51.3 deaths per 100,000 live births in 2002 to 24.5 deaths per 100,000 live births in 2012. The infant and under-five mortality rates have also continuously declined: The former decreased from 29.2% in 2002 to 10.3% in 2012, while the latter decreased from 34.9% in 2002 to 13.2% in 2012, thus fulfilling the United Nations Millennium Development Goals in advance of their due dates (Table 18.10).

In terms of the health security system, the universal coverage of healthcare services has essentially been achieved through the implementation of the various health insurance and public health plans, which have greatly improved equality in healthcare.

In particular, following the major success of controlling the SARS outbreak, all levels of government have increased their capital investment to accelerate the development of public health, rural healthcare, and community healthcare in urban areas. Furthermore, breakthroughs in the NRCMS and URBMI have laid an excellent foundation for deepening the health reform in China. It is, however, important to note that there remains a prominent gap between the current healthcare development in China with public healthcare demands and coordinated socioeconomic development. The following problems are of particular importance: uneven healthcare development in urban and rural areas; unreasonable resource allocation; relatively poor performance of public healthcare, rural healthcare, and community healthcare services; an imperfect health security system; nonstandardized production and circulation of drugs; an imperfect hospital management system and operating mechanism; insufficient government investment in healthcare; overly rapid increases in medical expenses; and heavy financial burden imposed on patients due to medical expenses. These issues have led to strong public dissatisfaction.

The current outcomes of health reforms in China also demonstrate that there remain various challenges in implementing health reforms due to the prominent contradiction between the current healthcare system and the increasing public demand for healthcare services.

On July 17, 2014, the NHFPC held a meeting of the steering group for the formulation of the Thirteenth Five-Year Plan, which focused on the development of healthcare and family planning policies and their full implementation. Counselor Li Bin pointed out in this meeting that China currently faces multiple health-related issues and challenges, such as urbanization, population aging, industrialization, rapid globalization, and increasing burden of chronic noncommunicable diseases (NCDs). He anticipated that some of the more deep-seated issues will become even more prominent following the expansion of health reforms.

Due to China's rapid population aging and increasing prevalence of NCDs, the need for further health reforms is becoming increasingly urgent. NCDs account for 80% of the disease burden in China, and this is expected to increase alongside the progress of urbaniza-

TABLE 18.10 Timeline of Health Reforms in China

Time	Reform Content
1985	The State Council approved the MOH's "Report on Several Policy Issues Related to Health Reforms," which proposed the undertaking of reforms, relaxation of policies, simplification of bureaucratic procedures, decentralization of decision-making, creation of multiple funding sources, and broadening the scope of healthcare development, in order to achieve good outcomes in health work.
1988	The State Council promulgated the MOH's "Three Determinations" plan, which defined the basic functions of the MOH, thus shifting from direct management to indirect management over directly owned enterprises and institutions.
1989	The State Council approved the MOH's "Opinions on Issues Related to Expanding Medical and Health Services," which proposed: the active implementation of various forms of contract responsibility systems; performing paid part-time services; further adjustments in the fee standards for healthcare services; performing paid services in preventive care institutions; implementing the principles of "supporting the construction of township health centers with the economic strength of township enterprises" and "supporting healthcare-related tertiary industries through the establishment of township health centers"; and the active development of the healthcare industry via a three-year tax exemption for healthcare enterprises. The MOH also officially issued notices and methods for implementing hospital hierarchical management.
1990	MOH established a group for drafting the "Outline of Health Development and Reforms in China (1991–2000)." This outline was redrafted 12 times based on continuous solicitation of opinions, discussions, and revisions. This process played a significant role in increasing the in-depth understanding of health reforms among various sectors.
1991	The seventh National People's Congress put forward guidelines for health work in the new era: focus on preventive care, reliance on technological advancement, mobilization of social participation, equal emphasis on Chinese and Western medicine, serving public health, and focus on rural healthcare.
1992	The State Council issued the "Several Opinions on the Deepening of Health Reform," which was implemented by the MOH based on the principle that the government is responsible for establishing hospitals, which in turn have to rely on themselves to generate income. Hospitals were required by the MOH during the National Health Conference to achieve positive results with regards to "supporting the construction of township health centers with the economic strength of township enterprises" and "supporting healthcare-related tertiary industries through the establishment of township health centers." This policy stimulated hospitals to generate revenues in order to make up for their insufficient income. It also influenced the role of healthcare institutions in public welfare. This led to the greater prominence of the "difficulties in seeking medical attention" among the public.
1997	The Central Committee and the State Council jointly issued the "Decision on Health Reform and Development," which explicitly stated the mission and ideology for health work in China. The Decision also put forward the general objectives for health reforms, including reforming the UEBMI, healthcare management system, and operational mechanism of healthcare institutions, as well as actively promoting the development of community healthcare services (CHS).
2000–2004	Several reform measures, such as the "Opinions on the Implementation of Classification Management in Urban Healthcare Institutions," "Opinions on the Subsidy Policy for Healthcare Enterprises," and "Interim Measures on the Management of Drug Revenue and Expenditure in Hospitals" were promulgated. The debate between a market-led and government-led healthcare sector also deepened gradually, especially after the SARS outbreak. Reform of hospital ownership was the clearest context at this stage.
2005	The Development Research Center of the State Council published the latest health reform report in *China Youth Daily*, which concluded through a review of the health reform in previous years that the health reform in China had been essentially unsuccessful.

TABLE 18.10 *(Continued)*

Time	Reform Content
2007	The 17th National Congress of the Communist Party of China proposed for the first time that the institutional framework of the healthcare system with Chinese characteristics comprised the following four main components: public health service system, healthcare service system, health security system, and pharmaceutical supply system.
2009–2011	The "Opinions of the Central Committee and the State Council on Deepening the Health Reform" and the "Notice of the State Council on Issuing the Plan on Recent Priorities in Carrying out the Health Reform (2009–2011)" were issued. Health reforms continued to adhere to the basic principles of "ensuring access to basic healthcare services, improving CHS, and establishing a sound supporting mechanism." The health reform focused on five key reforms of the healthcare system, ensuring universal coverage of basic health insurance for both urban and rural residents and thus significantly improving the health security level. The health reform also ensured the universal coverage of the National Essential Medicine System at the primary care level. Comprehensive reform of primary care institutions was implemented, including the introduction of a new operating mechanism. Additionally, the health reform ensured that the primary care service system was completely established and demonstrated significantly improved service capabilities. The health reform also ensured the effective delivery of essential and major public health services, with a higher degree of equalization. The pilot projects of public hospital reforms were expanded continuously, with substantial progress being made in the comprehensive reform of institutional mechanisms to improve their convenience and promote greater benefits to the public.
2013	"Several Opinions on Facilitating the Development of Non-Governmental Healthcare Institutions" was promulgated. This policy proposed prioritizing the establishment of nongovernmental, nonprofit healthcare institutions using social capital in order to accelerate the formation of a nongovernmental healthcare system that is mainly composed of nonprofit healthcare institutions and supplemented by for-profit medical institutions. The health reform continued to improve the management and quality of nongovernmental healthcare institutions and drove the large-scale, multilevel development of nonpublic healthcare institutions, thus enabling the greater division of labor, cooperation, and mutual development between public and nonpublic healthcare institutions.

tion. However, China's current healthcare service system remains centered on therapeutic services. Furthermore, its current reimbursement and incentive mechanisms have largely failed to promote cost-effective and health-promoting medical practices. At present, one of the key challenges is to free the healthcare system from its reliance on hospital services and revitalize the primary care system, thereby improving the coordination of primary care institutions with secondary and tertiary healthcare institutions.

In addition, the healthcare system in China is also facing a number of issues related to the efficiency and equality of healthcare services. Previous surveys have suggested that supplier-induced demand is a considerably widespread and serious issue in China. Supplier-induced demand refers to unnecessary consumption by patients due to the influence (or even coercion) of healthcare providers, who use their expertise for their own benefit. In China, supplier-induced overconsumption of healthcare services includes overprescription, antibiotic overuse, overdiagnosis, and unnecessary surgery, which not only leads to the wastage of limited healthcare resources but also results in a number of adverse effects on the health of consumers. On the other hand, the decline in healthcare equality is mainly reflected by the unbalanced healthcare expenditure between urban and rural areas and among different regions. About 80% of healthcare resources in China are concentrated in cities, of which two-thirds are allocated to hospitals in major cities. Moreover, healthcare resources in China are mainly concentrated in secondary and tertiary hospitals, whereas healthcare resources allocated for primary and rural healthcare services are severely inadequate, which has led to an increasingly unbalanced allocation of healthcare resources. In terms of health security, more than three-quarters of the total healthcare expenditure is allocated to urban residents. Nearly 80% of the rural population and 50% of the urban population (i.e., nearly three-quarters of the total population) have not yet enrolled in any health insurance scheme, making them ineligible for government assistance in the event of illness.

Current healthcare services can no longer meet the varying demands of patients with different income levels. In recent years, China has established a series of health security systems and expanded the overall coverage of health security. However, due to the limited level of health security, there remains a large gap in the degree of health security among different populations and regions, especially in terms of healthcare equality. Most general hospitals in China are developing toward a "large-scale and comprehensive" model, but this largely fails to meet the varying patient demands as these hospitals tend to offer similar levels and types of services. Therefore, hospitals make no clear distinction between public health services (e.g., planned immunization, infectious disease control, maternal and children healthcare, environmental health, and health education), essential healthcare services (i.e., healthcare services for the vast majority of common and recurring diseases), and nonessential healthcare services that are mainly provided through marketization. This, in turn, implies that hospitals are unable to adequately meet the healthcare demands of different population groups.

(4) Future Reform Directions

On May 28, 2014, the Medical Reform Office of the State Council stated in a press conference on deepening health reforms that future health reforms will focus on public hospitals, in order to further promote the continuity among the healthcare, health insurance and pharmaceutical industries; improve the essential medicine system; provide a new operating mechanism for primary care institutions; and promote reforms in other related fields. Specifically, the main focus of future health reforms will include:

1. *Accelerate the reform of public hospitals.* This mainly involves addressing issues such as the unreasonable planning of public hospitals, poor public welfare, incomplete management system, nonstandardized medical procedures, and lack of comprehensive reforms.

   Furthermore, the implementation of a family physician system and medical cluster system will also be accelerated. Family physicians mainly provide basic healthcare services in the form of proactive services and home visits, which will help to clearly define the responsibilities and service scopes of healthcare workers in CHS agencies, while also enabling the CHS model to become more scientific and beneficial to the public. This will ultimately help to achieve a new "universal, full-course, and comprehensive" healthcare management model that ensures the "universal access to medical records, family physicians, and health literacy," thereby enabling family physicians to truly fulfill their functions as "gatekeepers" of residents' health. On the other hand, the feasibility of a new urban healthcare system based on regional medical clusters will be explored through comprehensive reforms of the management model, health insurance payment model, and urban residents' treatment-seeking model in healthcare institutions, which aim to improve the overall allocation and utilization efficiency of healthcare resources and effectively control healthcare expenditure, thereby providing the public with safer, effective, convenient, inexpensive, and continuous basic healthcare services.

2. *Actively promote the establishment of nongovernmental healthcare institutions.* The health reforms will focus on addressing the challenges in certain aspects of nongovernmental healthcare, including market entry, talents, land, capital investment, and service capabilities, where there are inadequate policy implementation and insufficient support. Priority will be given to supporting nonprofit healthcare institutions sponsored by social capital, in order to establish a nongovernmental healthcare system that mainly comprises nonprofit healthcare institutions and supplemented by for-profit healthcare institutions. The main tasks include lowering the market entry requirements, optimizing a policy environment for the establishment of nongovernmental healthcare institutions, and encouraging physicians to serve in multiple healthcare institutions. The health reform will also involve facilitating the implementation of points of contact for nongovernmental healthcare institutions and pilot projects for the reform of public hospitals.

3. *Promote the establishment of a universal health insurance system.* The health reform will focus on resolving issues related to the imperfections in the funding mechanism, health security mechanisms for critical illnesses, supervisory mechanism for healthcare services, and deeper reforms of payment methods, thus further consolidating the universal health insurance system in China. Furthermore, the health reform will serve to promote the integration of basic health insurance for urban and rural residents, improve the funding mechanism, reform the health insurance payment system, improve the critical illness insurance scheme, promote the management of fee settlement for interregional healthcare services, and develop commercial health insurance.

Reforms will be implemented on the health insurance payment system. This will involve summarizing the local experiences in reforming the health insurance payment system, improving control over the total reimbursement amount paid by health insurance, accelerating the reform of payment methods, and establishing and improving the incentive and restraint mechanisms of health insurance schemes on medical behaviors. The health reform will also focus on improving the payment system for public hospitals in pilot counties and cities. The reform may further promote the establishment of negotiation mechanisms between health insurance agencies, healthcare institutions, and pharmaceutical suppliers, as well as payment mechanisms for the procurement of healthcare services.

In addition, the health reforms will promote the management of fee settlement for interregional healthcare services. This will involve accelerating the improvement of pooling levels in basic health insurance, enhancing the pooling quality, and encouraging the implementation of province-level pooling. Pilot projects for establishing a national settlement platform will be launched based on standardized provincial-level platforms for interregional medical fee settlement. For the benefit of retirees who relocate to other regions, the reform will focus on promoting real-time, cross-provincial (district and county-level city) medical fee settlement services. Furthermore, health insurance agencies in each pooling region may also explore different approaches (e.g., autonomous negotiations and commissioning to commercial insurance companies) to resolve issues related to cross-provincial (district- and county-level city) medical fee settlements.

4. *Improve the essential medicine system and the new operating mechanisms of primary care institutions.* The health reform will attach great importance to issues such as the unbalanced implementation of primary healthcare reform policies, poor timeliness and shortage of drug dispensation, and inadequate service capabilities.

5. *Regulate the circulation of drugs.* The health reform will focus on solving issues related to uncontrolled circulation of drugs, uncontrolled competition, and low service efficiency. A new order for the circulation of drugs will be established by fully utilizing the role of market mechanisms.

6. *Promote the implementation of related reforms.* In light of issues such as the low efficiency of certain public healthcare services, lagging informatization, poor supervisory capability of the healthcare industry, and imperfect assessment mechanisms, the health reforms can be further enhanced by promoting reforms in related fields and increasing their comprehensiveness, systematicity, and interoperability, thereby promoting greater synergy among these reforms.

Medical informatization, in particular, should be vigorously promoted. With the aim of promoting the informatization of public health, medical care, health insurance, drugs, and financial supervision, a unified, highly efficient, and interconnected healthcare information system will be gradually established by integrating healthcare resources, enhancing information standardization, and constructing a public service information platform. Furthermore, the standardization of health information technology will be promoted, and the use of electronic health or medical records for residents will be implemented. Telemedicine services for remote rural areas will also be enhanced by making full use of available resources.

In addition, the healthcare industry will be developed through extensive social mobilization and numerous measures. This will involve mobilizing the enthusiasm and creativity of social forces, promoting the injection of social capital, expanding the supply of healthcare services, innovating the healthcare service models, and increasing consumers' spending power. These, in turn, will help to satisfy the multilevel, diversified healthcare needs of the public; create a new impetus for socioeconomic transformation and development; and create the necessary conditions for facilitating holistic human development.

SECTION II. THE HEALTH SYSTEM IN INDIA

1. Overview of Socioeconomics and National Health

(1) National Circumstances of India

The Republic of India is a federal state that has adopted a parliamentary system modeled after the Westminster system. The country has a total land area of approximately 2.98 million km^2. The Constitution of India grants all states in the country a high degree of autonomy and stipulates that both the central and state governments are formed via elections.

India has shown relatively slow economic development since its independence. However, the initiation of economic liberalization in 1991 accelerated its economic growth, which reached 10.55% in 2010. India's GDP has increased substantially, from US$477.6 billion in 1990 to US$1.877 trillion in 2013 (World Bank). By increasing its industrial exports and innovative technologies, such as information technology, biopharmaceuticals, nuclear technology, space satellites, and lunar exploration, India has transformed from being one of the poorest countries in the twentieth century to becoming a major global economy in the twenty-first century.

India implements 12 years of free and compulsory primary and secondary education, and only charges nominal tuition fees for higher education. India has achieved a school enrolment rate of 84.9% among minors aged 6–14 years. However, the illiteracy rate among adults in India is around 38.0%.

(2) Population and Health Status

The Indian population comprises 10 major ethnic groups and numerous ethnic minorities. Almost all Indians are religious, with 82.0% being Hindu and 12.0% being Muslim. There are numerous other religions in India as well, including Christianity, Sikhism, Buddhism, and Jainism.

The World Bank reported that as of 2013, the total population of India was 1.252 billion. The Indian population is expected to surpass that of China by 2020, at which point it will become the most populated country in the world.

Since its independence, the burden of infectious diseases in India has been alleviated to a certain extent due to socioeconomic development and greater use of vaccines and antimicrobial agents. However, infectious diseases still account for about 30% of the total disease burden in India. Only a handful of infectious diseases are prioritized in the vertical disease control program run by the central government. The program has successfully controlled the spread of human immunodeficiency virus (HIV) and leprosy but has failed to achieve desirable outcomes for the control of tuberculosis, malaria, and visceral leishmaniasis. The majority of other infectious diseases not included in the vertical program has been neglected and lack formal monitoring or control at the population level. Thus, the public healthcare network has been overwhelmed because of the prevalence of preventable infectious diseases or other diseases, which has led to the emergence of a largely unregulated commercial healthcare industry, thereby increasing the household financial burden due to healthcare expenditures.

India has a vast population living under the poverty line. As a result, approximately 51.8% of pregnant women and 74.3% of children under the age of three years suffer from iron deficiency anemia. Furthermore, nearly 47% of children suffer from moderate to severe growth retardation. The living environments of impoverished groups lack basic sanitation facilities and sewerage systems, while only 20% of rural households have toilets. Owing to the lack of proper drainage systems and public toilets, open defecation and urination are common phenomena in India, even in the capital city of New Delhi. Therefore, many Indian residents are highly susceptible to malaria, tuberculosis, diarrhea, and pneumonia. India currently has the greatest number of patients with tuberculosis in the world and has 5.1 million HIV/AIDS patients (second only to South Africa), 3.1 million of whom live in rural areas.

As India is currently undergoing rapid economic development, the overall life expectancy of India's population has been increasing continually, and the lifestyle of its citizens has changed gradually. Hence, India is also facing numerous challenges due to chronic NCDs, such as cardiovascular diseases, cancer, blindness, and mental illness, which have become increasingly severe health issues. It is expected that by 2020, the burden of NCDs will account for 57% of the total disease burden in India, while that of infectious diseases will account for 24% and injuries 19%.

Over the past 50 years, the health status of Indian residents has improved at a faster rate than that of residents in most other low-income developing countries. The average life expectancy of males and females increased from 57 years and 58 years in 1990 to 64 years and 68 years in 2012, respectively. In 2012, the healthy life expectancy at birth in India was 57 years. In addition, the under-five mortality rate declined from 126 deaths out of 1,000 in 1990 to 56 deaths out of 1,000 in 2012, while the maternal mortality rate declined from 560 deaths per 100,000 live births in 1990 to 190 deaths per 100,000 live births in 2013.

The World Health Report 2000 ranked India 112th in terms of the overall performance of its healthcare system, 118th for its overall health status, and 43rd for its funding equality, thus placing India among one of the developing countries with the highest rankings.

In 2009, India was ranked 134th among 182 countries in the Human Development Index due to its inadequate investment in healthcare and education. The Ministry of Health and Family Welfare does not have a department dedicated to public health. Furthermore, there is no department charged with public health affairs at the state level, with the exception of Tamil Nadu.

2. Healthcare Organizations and Regulatory Systems

In 1949, India adopted its first constitution, which stipulates that all citizens shall have access to free healthcare. Therefore, the government of India has established a free universal health system and a public healthcare system.

(1) Regulatory System of the Health Administration

The Ministry of Health and Family Welfare (MOHFW) is responsible for the formulation and implementation of national healthcare policies and family planning programs in India. The MOHFW comprises two independent departments: the Department of Health and Family Welfare and the Department of Ayurveda, Yoga and Naturopathy, Unani, Siddha and Homoeopathy (AYUSH). The Department of Health and Family Welfare is not only responsible for national public health programs (e.g., disease prevention), but also for the management of healthcare services, drug regulatory policies, and essential drug policies, as well as the management of primary care institutions and teaching hospitals.

The MOHFW has established the following three affiliated agencies to effectively implement its policies and programs: the Family Welfare Training & Research Centre (located in Mumbai), Homoeopathic Pharmacopoeia Laboratory (Ghaziabad), and Pharmacopoeia Laboratory for Indian Medicine (Ghaziabad). In addition, there are 34 autonomous statutory bodies and 3 public sector undertakings (PSUs), such as the Indian Council of Medical Research (ICMR) and the All India Institutes of Medical Sciences (AIIMS), which are responsible for medical research and medical postgraduate education in India, respectively.

The first category of employees under the MOHFW is politicians, which only includes the Minister of Health and Family Welfare. The Minister is appointed by the political party that won the national election and is accountable to parliament. The second category is civil servants, including the directors of the Department of Health and Family Welfare and the Department of AYUSH, who are considered deputy ministers accountable to the Minister of Health and Family Welfare and are responsible for the administration of their respective departments. The second category also includes various civil servants under the directors, such as the additional secretary and joint secretary. The third category is technical officers, including director generals, director professors, associate professors, specialist grades, chief medical doctors, senior medical officers, and medical officers.

According to the Constitution of India, state governments are mainly responsible for providing healthcare services to residents, while the central government is mainly responsible for the organization and coordination of policy development, funding for healthcare programs, healthcare service supervision, and training of the healthcare workforce. To maximize the advantages of the central government in policy development and program planning and to minimize the interregional disparities in government health investment resulting from the differences in economic development among the states, the central government is also tasked with designing and developing national programs for the control of key diseases, maternal and child healthcare programs, family planning programs and rural healthcare programs, as well as fundraising to implement these programs, in order to ensure the equal distribution of national public goods, such as public health services and basic healthcare services. On the other hand, local governments are required to utilize their familiarity with local circumstances, residents, and consumers, in order to modify and implement the programs launched by the central government based on their local conditions.

In response to various issues concerning the funding and delivery of healthcare services in India, the central government established the National Commission on Macroeconomics and Health (NCMH), which made the following recommendations: (1) fully integrate secondary and tertiary health insurance; (2) substantially increase public expenditure on healthcare; and (3) create a competitive environment for healthcare providers.

(2) Healthcare System

1. Public Healthcare System   The public healthcare system in India is divided into five levels of hospitals: national, state (provincial), regional, district, and village. Although there are far fewer public hospitals at each level than there are private hospitals, the former provides free healthcare services for all residents, including meal expenses for inpatients. Free healthcare services are mainly provided by community health centers, primary health centers, subcenters, as well as public hospitals in major cities.

Public hospitals are facing a number of problems, such as financial shortage, poor management, and poor conditions. Due to the lack of accountability toward patients, communities, and public goals, these public hospitals often have issues related to poor healthcare quality, insufficient supply, indifferent attitudes, and corruption, which have given these hospitals poor creditability and a bad reputation. The shortcomings of public hospitals in India are mainly manifested as: the shortage of pharmaceutical supplies and diagnostic tests, long waiting time, poor attitude among physicians, and poor hospital environment. However, public hospitals in India are mostly visited by low-income earners who have relatively low requirements for healthcare conditions and prefer inexpensive therapeutic services. Therefore, public hospitals serve as "stabilizers" for social equality and poverty relief. Owing to the National Rural Health Mission (NRHM), there have been improvements in the infrastructure and facilities of public hospitals, and an increase in the number of healthcare workers. Nevertheless, the lack of accountability among public hospitals remains a challenge that needs to be resolved.

2. Private Healthcare System   The proportion of private healthcare institutions in India is rapidly increasing. They serve as the main venues for outpatient and inpatient treatment and are predominantly outpatient clinics. In recent years, the number of private healthcare institutions accounted for 93% of all healthcare institutions in India. Furthermore, the number of hospital beds in private healthcare institutions accounted for 64% of the total number of hospital beds, and it is estimated that 80–85% of physicians in India work in private healthcare institutions.

Most private healthcare institutions are for-profit organizations, while the majority of nonprofit organizations are charitable private healthcare institutions and specific departments in some large-sized private hospitals. Private hospitals tend to employ high-quality healthcare workers, and many physicians have postgraduate degrees from famous medical colleges, such as the Royal College of Physicians in the UK. In addition, private hospitals typically have more advanced medical equipment and management approaches. Hence, the quality of healthcare services and medical expenses of private hospitals are often much higher than those of public hospitals. Therefore, patients with better economic conditions are usually admitted to private hospitals.

Private hospitals in India possess the following characteristics:

1. The vast majority are for-profit private sole proprietorships.
2. Most private hospitals are relatively small, with an average of 23 beds.
3. There is no difference in the distribution of private hospitals between developed and underdeveloped regions, indicating that they target patients of varying income levels.
4. Most private hospitals do not have full-time physicians. They mostly rely on part-time specialists and general practitioners (GPs). Most part-time physicians also work in public hospitals, and mostly consist of obstetricians and gynecologists, GPs, general surgeons, and pediatricians. However, laws in India differ among states. For example, the Rajasthan health authorities prohibit physicians who work in public hospitals from serving part-time in private hospitals, but allow them to establish their own private practices. As a result, specialists from public hospitals might be on par with those who serve in private hospitals.
5. Most private hospitals do not purchase large-scale medical equipment, such as MRI and X-ray machines, and generally refer patients to diagnostic centers for medical examinations.
6. Private healthcare institutions impose substantially higher charges than do public institutions. The outpatient and inpatient charges in private hospitals are four to five times those of public hospitals. Furthermore, private hospitals usually charge a registration fee of about ₹500, which is equivalent to the one-month living expenses of an impoverished individual. Private hospitals normally rely on cash payments made by patients because insurance companies rarely cover private hospital services, and the health insurance coverage in India is very low. The medical charges imposed by private hospitals include physician charges and hospital charges. Owing to the lack of government-set fee standards, the former is determined by physicians themselves by taking into account the economic status of patients and whether they are covered by health insurance. Physicians, in turn, must pay rent to their hospitals based on the size of the wards they rent, at a rate determined by their negotiations with the hospital; the exact rate depends on various factors, such as the reputation and negotiation skills of the physicians. Hospital charges, on the other hand, refer to additional fees imposed by hospitals based on the economic status of patients.
7. Private hospitals offer numerous outpatient and tertiary specialist services, rather than general specialist or surgical services.
8. The service quality of most private hospitals is not guaranteed. This is because more than 50% of Indian private practitioners are traditional Indian healers who are not educated in Western medicine but often prescribe Western medication. Furthermore,

numerous private clinics lack the necessary equipment and personnel; offer health-care services, such as surgery, without obtaining certification; and provide services not based on their own capabilities but rather on the profitability of the services. There is also a lack of legal standards for private healthcare institutions, as well as their staff and services. In addition, the private hospitals in some major cities provide high-quality and advanced healthcare services at lower prices, thereby attracting foreign patients seeking inpatient and surgical services in India. As a result, "medical tourism" has become a unique and important service export that brings in US$330 million per year in India. Private healthcare institutions account for about 82% of outpatient services, 56% of inpatients, 46% of hospital childbirth deliveries, 40% of prenatal check-ups, and 10% of planned immunization.

Private practitioners are extremely common in India, but the scope and quality of their services vary considerably. Compared to public healthcare institutions, private healthcare institutions attach greater importance to therapeutic services rather than vaccination and prenatal care services. In rural India, there are numerous unqualified allopathic physicians who may charge as little as one-third the amount charged by qualified allopathic physicians. Most qualified physicians serve in urban areas. However, in recent years, medical franchises have begun to expand their target markets to small cities. Due to the lack of regulatory management of private practitioners, almost anyone in India can start a medical practice. Almost all physicians in public healthcare institutions also work in private practices or as consultants in private healthcare institutions.

(3) Rural Healthcare System

Since its independence in 1947, the government of India has strived to establish a rural healthcare system that provides free healthcare services to impoverished individuals.

The government enhanced its rural healthcare infrastructure during the Sixth Five-Year Plan (1982–1987) and the Seventh Five-Year Plan (1987–1992). Furthermore, the government also attempted to establish a three-tiered healthcare network, which consists of a subcenter for every 5,000 people, a primary health center (PHC) for every 30,000 people, and a community health center (CHC) for every 100,000 people. By the end of 2004, there were 145,000 subcenters (60% of which were funded by the federal government), 23,000 PHCs, and 3,222 CHCs in India.

Subcenters are the peripheral institutions of PHCs and CHCs, where healthcare services are delivered by primary healthcare workers. In general, a subcenter is equipped with only one nurse or midwife, who is responsible for child immunization, prenatal and postnatal visits, family planning services, and health education, and generally do not provide medical services. Each subcenter is responsible for providing healthcare services to 3,000–5,000 villagers in surrounding villages. They are the connection points between communities and healthcare services. Their operating costs are fully supported by the MOHFW.

A PHC generally comprises more than 10 healthcare workers, including a medical officer (MO), three to four medical graduates, laboratory technicians, radiologists, maternal and child care workers, and nurses. Each PHC also has four to six observation beds. In addition to outpatient services, PHCs are responsible for providing preventive services, such as planned immunization programs and Directly Observed Treatment, Short-course (DOTS) for tuberculosis. Although PHCs are equipped with the basic facilities for inpatient services, they rarely provide inpatient and specialist services. In short, PHCs play a very similar role to that of township health centers in China. Both the federal and state government are jointly responsible for the establishment and maintenance of PHCs. They serve as the first point of connection between rural areas and the healthcare officials of local governments. Each PHC serves as a referral unit for six adjacent subcenters, but patients with severe conditions or who require hospitalization can only be admitted to CHCs or district hospitals. PHCs are primarily responsible for providing therapeutic, preventive, health promotion, and family welfare services, as well as supervising their respective six subcenters.

CHCs are primary hospitals equipped with hospital beds, and are mainly responsible for providing specialist and inpatient services. Both the federal and state governments are jointly responsible for the establishment and maintenance of CHCs. CHCs are equipped with complete medical facilities and adequate healthcare workers. They act as referral hospitals for every four PHCs and patients who cannot be treated by CHCs are referred to district hospitals.

The three-tiered rural healthcare network provides free healthcare services for the general public, specifically covering registration fees, physical examination fees, hospitalization fees, treatment fees, emergency care expenses, and even meals for inpatients. However, prescription charges are not covered (Table 18.11).

In summary, subcenters are public healthcare agencies managed and operated by healthcare assistants rather than physicians. PHCs are the lowest tier healthcare institu-

TABLE 18.11 Tiers and Positioning of Healthcare Institutions in India

Service Tier and Name of Institutions	Number of Beds	Covered Population (10,000)	Service Providers
Village health volunteers	0	0.1	Social health activists who have undergone short-term training and certification. They are volunteers who receive limited subsidies.
Subcenters	0	0.5	Healthcare technicians who are responsible for various tasks, such as midwives and nurses.
PHCs	4–6	3.0	MOs (physicians), healthcare supervisors, and healthcare technicians.
CHCs (primary hospitals)	20–50	10.0	Provide the most basic specialist services, such as internal medicine, surgery, gynecology, and pediatrics.
Subdistrict hospitals (secondary Class B hospitals)	50–100	50.0	Provide other basic specialist services (excluding internal medicine, surgery, gynecology, and pediatrics), such as otorhinolaryngological and dermatological services.
District hospitals (secondary Class A hospitals)	150–300	100.0	Provide secondary services for specialties such as internal medicine, surgery, gynecology, and pediatrics.
State (Federal) hospitals (tertiary hospitals)	300–1 500	>100.0	Various types of advanced healthcare services.

tions, wherein healthcare services are provided by physicians. Patients who require further observation may remain in PHCs but can also be referred to CHCs, whereas more complicated cases are transferred to higher-tier hospitals.

(4) Traditional Indian Medicine

Traditional Indian medicine has a history of more than 5,000 years, and has numerous separate branches, such as Ayurveda, yoga, naturopathy, Unani, siddha, and homeopathy. Traditional Indian medicine plays an important role in disease prevention, health promotion, and treatment in India. Currently, there are 718,000 registered traditional health practitioners in India, that is, about seven traditional health practitioners per 10,000 people. There are around 450 traditional Indian medical schools (99 of which can enroll postgraduate students) and 8 national research institutes, which together receive an annual enrollment of 25,000 students and train a total of 2,128 postgraduates. In addition, there are 3,100 traditional Indian medical hospitals with a total of 53,296 hospital beds, 22,635 traditional Indian pharmacies, and 9,493 traditional Indian pharmaceutical manufacturers in India. A survey by the National Institute of Medical Statistics (NIMS) revealed that 37.8% of the Indian population prefers to utilize traditional Indian medicine when they fall ill. As it is effective, inexpensive, convenient, and generally free of side effects, Indian residents often seek out traditional Indian medicine for common diseases, particularly chronic diseases, such as gastrointestinal diseases, arthritis, skin diseases, respiratory diseases, and gynecological diseases.

3. Healthcare Funding and Payment Systems

(1) Healthcare Funding

The healthcare system in India is funded by the central, state, and local governments, among which, state governments are the main contributors, providing about 90% of healthcare funds. On the other hand, the central government is responsible for funding national family planning programs; efforts to control infectious diseases such as leprosy, malaria, and tuberculosis; immunization; nutritional improvement; and some academic and research institutions.

Conventionally, India has had a relatively low level of healthcare expenditure. In 2008–2009, it accounted for only about 4.1% of the GDP, equivalent to a per capita healthcare expenditure of about US$40. The Indian population accounts for more than 16% of the world's total population, but accounts for less than 1% of the world's total healthcare expenditure. In the first decade of the twenty-first century, public expenditure on healthcare accounted for only about 1% of the GDP. Regarding the composition of the total healthcare expenditure, the central, state, and local governments accounted for about 20%, while personal medical expenses accounted for around 70%.

From 2004 to 2005 to 2008 to 2009, the total healthcare expenditure of India increased by 64%, during which the government's share increased by more than twice. The central government significantly increased its investment during that period. In 2008–2009, the government spent about 5% of its total expenditure on health insurance (Table 18.12).

Healthcare funding in India comprises five major components:

1. The first component is out-of-pocket household expenses, which are almost entirely spent on purchasing healthcare services from private healthcare institutions; however,

TABLE 18.12 Composition of Healthcare Funding Sources in India for Selected Years

Item	2004–2005		2008–2009	
	Source (₹ Million)	Percentage (%)	Source (₹ Million)	Percentage (%)
Central government	90,667	7	223,857	10
Central expenditure (excluding health insurance)	44,997		90,137	
Transfer payments to states	37,670		113,720	
Health insurance expenditure	8,000		20,000	
State and local government healthcare expenditure	172,465	13	362,957	17
Noninsurance expenditure	171,465		352,957	
Health insurance expenditure	1,000		10,000	
Total public healthcare expenditure	283,085		586,814	
External aid	30,495	2	37,016	2
Private healthcare expenditure	1,004,135	78	1,573,935	72
Out-of-pocket expenditure	928,388		–	
Health insurance expenditure	21,717		68,740	
Others	94,030		–	
Total healthcare expenditure	1,337,763	100	21,197,765	100

Note: The total healthcare expenditure accounted for 4.25% and 4.13% of the GDP in 2004–2005 and 2008–2009, respectively.
Source: World Bank report, "Government-sponsored Health Insurance in India: Are You Covered?," 2012.

a small proportion is used to pay for the registration fees in public healthcare institutions. The heavy burden of household medical expenses is considered one of the greatest causes of poverty in India. About 80% of outpatient and 60% of inpatient services are provided by private healthcare institutions. As a result, about 77% of the total healthcare expenditure is channeled to private healthcare institutions (including charitable healthcare institutions and other nonprofit healthcare institutions).

2. The second component is tax-funded public healthcare institutions (which account for 20% of the total healthcare expenditure). Such institutions should, in principle, be available to the entire Indian population. Most of the funds for these institutions are derived from the MOHFW and the health secretariat of each state. However, public medical schools and their affiliated hospitals are jointly funded by the central and state governments. Additionally, there are a few independent public healthcare institutions and nonprofit hospitals that also receive funding from the central and state governments. The public healthcare system, which consists of primary, secondary, and tertiary healthcare institutions, is mainly operated by state governments. It provides 20% and 40% of the total outpatient and inpatient services in India, respectively. The utilization of inpatient services varies considerably across different states in India.

In general, tax revenue is the main funding source for healthcare spending by both the central and state governments. Most of this revenue is allocated to public healthcare institutions to provide citizens with free or highly subsidized healthcare services. The bulk of the central government's healthcare budget is allocated by the MOHFW to all states through various national health programs. Although the healthcare budget of the central government has increased significantly, the share of transfer payments allocated to the states out of the MOHFW's budget began declining drastically since the 1990s. It was only until 2005, when the central government launched the NRHM, that the share of healthcare expenditure out of the total public expenditure rose to 40%.

The healthcare funds raised by each state as a share of the GDP vary among the different states, ranging from 0.6% to 1.5% in 2008–2009. The healthcare expenditure of state governments accounts for 58% of the total public healthcare expenditure. However, there are still disparities among the different states. Conventionally, most states do not place sufficient importance on healthcare expenditure.

3. The third component is the social health insurance schemes for employees in the private sector, civil servants, military personnel, and railway workers, which account for 4.1% of all healthcare funding. These are mandatory insurance schemes, which are funded by employers and individuals via payroll taxes and supplemented by government subsidies. However, some schemes are fully subsidized by the government or state-owned enterprises. For example, health insurance schemes for military and railway workers are fully subsidized by the government, whereas semi-state-owned enterprises in the coal and petroleum industries fully subsidize health insurance premiums for their employees. Insured persons can receive healthcare services in healthcare institutions owned or operated by their health insurance schemes or contracted private healthcare institutions.

4. The fourth component is private voluntary health insurance (PVHI), emerged in India during the 1980s and underwent rapid development in the early twenty-first century. In 2008–2009, PVHI accounted for 3% of the total healthcare expenditure. The products provided by insurance companies are primarily intended for inpatient services provided by private healthcare institutions. The commercial health insurance market can be roughly divided into two broad categories: the employer-sponsored group market and the retail market for individual and family plans. In 2010, there were approximately 60 million insured persons covered by PVHI schemes, accounting for 5% of the total population of India.

5. The fifth component is the government-sponsored health insurance schemes (GSHISs), which emerged after 2005. These schemes are fully subsidized by the government and have a broad coverage, mainly targeting individuals living in poverty.

The remaining healthcare expenditure comes from private companies, external agencies, and other organizations. Even though companies make up a considerable proportion of healthcare funding, these funds are not channeled directly to commercial or social health insurance schemes but are used to pay for medical departments established within the enterprises or to reimburse medical expenses incurred by employees.

Data from the World Bank indicate that medical expenses account for an average of 5.8% of the total household expenses and 10.5% of nonfood expenses in India. Furthermore, about 14% of rural households and 12% of urban households spend more than 10% of their total annual expenses on healthcare. In a comparison between India and its neighboring developing countries, the financial burden of healthcare in Indian households was higher than that in Sri Lankan households but lower than were those in Chinese, Bangladeshi, and Vietnamese households. The composition of household medical expenses showed that drug expenses accounted for 45–55% and 70–80% of inpatient and outpatient expenses, respectively.

(2) Health Insurance Schemes

The GSHISs in India originated from the Employees' State Insurance Scheme (ESIS), which was implemented by the central government in the late 1940s to cover blue-collar workers in the private sector, and the Central Government Health Scheme (CGHS), which was launched in the 1950s to cover civil servants and their families. These two health insurance schemes covered a relatively comprehensive range of healthcare services and utilized a risk-sharing mechanism adopted by traditional social insurance schemes. The schemes were funded by premium contributions from both employers and employees via payroll taxes, and supplemented by government subsidies. Other health insurance schemes for railway workers, military personnel, and civil servants also emerged soon after India gained independence (Table 18.13).

In 2003, the central government of India launched the Universal Health Insurance Scheme (UHIS) as a method of reimbursing inpatient expenses. It can be purchased voluntarily from any state-owned insurance company at a highly subsidized price. However, as of 2008–2009, the UHIS only covered 3.7 million insured persons. Yeshasvini is another health insurance scheme launched that same year by the Department of Cooperation in Karnataka for members of the rural cooperative societies in that state.

Both these health insurance schemes provided valuable lessons for establishing the new generation of GSHISs. Specifically, a number of the following approaches were adopted and promoted in the new GSHISs: (1) the government subsidizes partially or most of the insurance premiums incurred by the demand side; (2) cashless hospitalization coverage is provided; (3) services are provided by contracted public and private hospitals; (4) providers are paid through prospective, case-based "package" rates; (5) the coverage is designed to target informal employees and those living in poverty; and (6) health insurance companies or third-party administrators (TPAs) serve as intermediaries for administrative functions.

At the turn of the century, India's commercial health insurance industry was relatively small, accounting for only 2% of inpatient expenditure in India. However, by 2008–2009, commercial health insurance companies bore nearly 10% of the inpatient expenditure in India. This proportion was even higher for hospitals in major cities, where insurance companies and TPAs contributed about 30% of the total hospital revenues. In the 2000s, the number of network hospitals increased rapidly to approximately 10,000 hospitals. GSHISs also began tapping into the network hospitals of commercial health insurance in the late 2000s, which facilitated the expansion of the GSHISs. With the rapid development of commercial insurance and the introduction of TPAs, the "cashless" settlement method emerged and was subsequently adopted by all GSHISs. The reimbursement of medical expenses is settled between TPAs or insurance companies and hospitals, while patients need only cover their copayments or out-of-pocket expenses. GSHISs also benefited from the fierce competition within the commercial health insurance market. For example, insurance companies might offer an exceedingly low price in the tendering process to secure a GSHIS contract.

In addition, Andhra Pradesh and Himachal Pradesh transformed the previous Chief Minister's Relief Fund into a more standardized and institutionalized health insurance scheme, which has since been considered for implementation in other states.

As of 2012, the main GSHISs included the ESIS, Rashtriya Swasthya Bima Yojana (RSBY) Scheme, CGHS, Rajiv Aarogyasri (Andhra Pradesh, AP), Yeshasvini (Karnataka,

TABLE 18.13 Comparison of Major Characteristics Among Gshiss in India

Name of Scheme	ESIS	CGHS	Yeshasvini Co-operative Farmers' Health Care Scheme	Rajiv Aarogyasri Community Health Insurance Scheme	RSBY Scheme	Chief Minister Kalaignar's Insurance Scheme	Vajpayee Arogyashri Scheme	RSBY Plus Scheme	Apka Swasthya Bima Yojana (ASBY) Scheme (In Planning)
Year of Initiation	1952	1954	2003	2007	2008	2009	2009	2010	2011 – 2012
Geographical Area	Certain regions in India	25 cities in India	Karnataka	Andhra Pradesh	Certain states in India	Tamil Nadu	Certain regions in Karnataka	Himachal Pradesh	Delhi
Target population	Employees of formal private sector enterprises	Employees and retirees of the central government, and other specific groups	Members of rural cooperative societies	Impoverished households or households with annual income below ₹75,000	Impoverished households or other target groups	Impoverished households or households with annual income below ₹72,000 and other specific groups	Impoverished population residing in covered areas	Insured persons of RSBY Plus Scheme	Insured persons of RSBY Plus Scheme
Number of insured persons (10,000)	5,540	300	300	70	70	36	7.5	0.8	0.65 families
Unit of enrollment	Household	Household	Individual	Household	Household	Household	Household	Household	Household
Covered service items	Comprehensive	Comprehensive	Inpatient services, surgical secondary healthcare services, and more than 1,200 surgical procedures	Inpatient services, tertiary healthcare services, and 938 inpatient treatment regimens, including postdischarge follow-ups	Inpatient services and secondary healthcare (including maternity care services)	Inpatient services, tertiary healthcare services, and 400 inpatient treatment regimens	Inpatient services, tertiary healthcare services, 402 service packages, and 50 postdischarge follow-up service packages	Inpatient services, tertiary healthcare services and 326 inpatient treatment regimens	Inpatient services, tertiary healthcare services and designated inpatient treatment regimens
Cap	No Limit	No Limit	₹200,000 per individual per year	₹150,000 per household per year + ₹50,000 buffer per year	₹30,000 per household per year	₹100,000 per household every four years	₹150,000 per household per year + ₹50,000 buffer per year	Subsidizes ₹175,000 beyond the RSBY cap	₹150,000 per household per year

(continued)

TABLE 18.13 (*Continued*)

Name of Scheme	ESIS	CGHS	Yeshasvini Co-operative Farmers' Health Care Scheme	Rajiv Aarogyasri Community Health Insurance Scheme	RSBY Scheme	Chief Minister Kalaignar's Insurance Scheme	Vajpayee Arogyashri Scheme	RSBY Plus Scheme	Apka Swasthya Bima Yojana (ASBY) Scheme (In Planning)
Minimum number of beds in network hospitals	100 beds in major cities and 50 beds in other regions	100 beds in major cities and 51 beds in other regions	50 hospital beds and 3 intensive care unit (ICU) beds	50	10	30	50	50	50 hospital beds
Total number of network hospitals (public and private)	148 independently owned and operated hospitals and 400 contracted private hospitals	562 private hospitals and all public hospitals	543 hospitals (including 30 public hospitals)	241 private hospitals and 97 public hospitals	8111 hospitals (including 2,507 public hospitals)	692 hospitals (including 56 public hospitals)	94 hospitals (including 8 public hospitals)	16 hospitals	–
Funding source	Premium contribution based on employees' salaries (employees: 1.75%; employers: 4.75%)	Central government budget and premium contributions based on employee's salaries	Premium contribution (insured persons: 58%; state government: 42%)	Fully funded by the state governments via the healthcare budget and a tax levied on alcohol sales	75% and 25% from the central and state governments, respectively. In some states, the central government contributes 90% while insured persons contribute ₹30	Fully funded by the state government	Fully funded by the state government	Fully funded by the state government	Fully funded by the state government
Total expenditure in 2009–2010 (₹100 million)	199	160	5.5	120	35	51.7	–	–	–
Number of hospitalizations in 2009–2010	417,498	–	66,749	319,446	400,000	–	–	–	–

Note: This table includes statistical data up to 2010.
Source: World Bank report, "Government-sponsored Health Insurance in India: Are You Covered?," 2012.

KA), Vajpayee Arogyashri (Karnataka, KA), Kalaignar (Tamil Nadu, TN), RSBY Plus Scheme (Himachal Pradesh, HP), and ASBY (Delhi). The first three of these schemes are implemented by the central government, while the latter six are implemented by state governments. Prior to the implementation of these schemes, public funds were almost entirely allocated to government-owned and government-run healthcare institutions.

In 2010, these GSHISs covered about 240 million individuals, which is equivalent to around 19% of the total population. If we consider commercial insurance and other types of health insurance schemes, then there were more than 300 million insured persons, which is equivalent to more than 25% of the total population. GSHISs that were recently implemented mainly target populations living below the poverty line and working in the informal sector; however, these newer GSHISs have adopted varying standards for the poverty line. The RSBY Scheme, as well as some state-level schemes, have adopted the standards of the Central Government Planning Commission, while other state-level schemes have adopted looser standards and have a theoretical coverage of 80% of the vulnerable population and 50% of the total population. The ESIS targets formal private sector employees who earn no less than ₹150,000 and their dependents. The CGHS covers civil servants employed by the central government.

The main aim of newly implemented GSHISs is to provide financial protection to those living in poverty against the economic risks of catastrophic health issues. The definition of catastrophic health issues is related to inpatient healthcare services. The RSBY Scheme primarily covers secondary healthcare services, while most state-level schemes target tertiary healthcare services. Most of the newly implemented schemes place a strong emphasis on surgery, whereas outpatient services typically fall outside of the scope of coverage. However, there are considerable differences in the covered services and benefits among the different GSHISs, and most have established an annual reimbursement cap. The ESIS and CGHS are the only exceptions, as both cover preventive and primary care services, and have not established an annual reimbursement cap.

In 2009–2010, the expenditure of the aforementioned nine GSHISs was about ₹58 billion, which was about 8% of the total government healthcare expenditure. The total health insurance expenditure (including commercial, community-based, and other insurance schemes) of that same year amounted to ₹160 billion, which is 6.4% of the total healthcare expenditure (estimated at ₹2.5 trillion). At that time, government-led healthcare institutions still accounted for 90% of the total public healthcare investment.

There is a significant variation in the utilization rate of healthcare services among the different GSHISs due to a number of reasons, such as their differing service items and payment methods. Some of the state-level schemes cover only tertiary inpatient services with low utilization rates and high costs, and their hospitalization rate is only 5% among all insured persons. The RSBY Scheme covers most secondary inpatient services, resulting in a hospitalization rate of up to 25% among insured persons. On the other hand, commercial health insurance schemes have much higher hospitalization rates (up to 64%) among insured persons than GSHISs owing to potential adverse selection and moral hazards, as well as the lack of effective cost containment mechanisms.

GSHISs use package rates to purchase inpatient services from network healthcare institutions. The ESIS and CGHS also use itemized budgets and salaries to pay their own healthcare institutions and employees. A package rate is defined as a simplified case-based payment system, whereby reimbursements are made according to a single fee or price ceiling for all the material and labor costs required for a predefined treatment or procedure.

The majority of GSHISs are still in the preliminary stages of development, and almost all of them have yet to develop a sound institutional architecture to ensure robust governance and management. All recently implemented GSHISs have introduced intermediaries, such as commercial insurance companies and TPAs, to fulfill most of the managerial functions on behalf of the government departments. In recent years, the rapid development of commercial health insurance in India has improved the handling capacities of insurance companies (e.g., their technological level, management experience, and professional talent) needed to operate the GSHISs, whereas the government systems still the lack incentive and capacity to perform these same functions. Hence, the newly implemented GSHISs have effectively utilized the capacity of commercial insurance companies to create collaborative models between private healthcare institutions and the GSHISs, which is unique to India.

GSHISs are also faced with various issues, such as induced demand, unreasonable charges, and fraud, as well as a lack of systematic and active antifraud measures. However, there is a growing trend for GSHISs to adopt antifraud measures; for instance, as a result of these measures, the RSBY Scheme dissolved their service agreements with 54 hospitals in September 2010.

Most GSHIS-contracted hospitals are private healthcare institutions. GSHISs primarily focus on the reimbursement of tertiary inpatient services, for which public healthcare institutions have a limited capacity to provide. Furthermore, most insured persons prefer private hospitals when seeking medical attention, which suggests that private hospitals might have a higher share of service utilization out of all network hospitals. Most public hospitals, especially district and subdistrict hospitals, provide extremely limited healthcare services for insured persons, with the exception of a few large-sized tertiary public healthcare institutions. Under the current management system in India, most public hospitals are incapable of competing with private hospitals. Almost all public hospitals lack the necessary autonomy and flexibility to manage their own affairs and are essentially completely dependent on the hierarchical control of state health authorities for budgeting and investment decisions.

According to the World Bank, the GSHISs in India have introduced a demand-side purchasing plan to public healthcare funding, which has the following innovative features: (1) clearly defined rights; (2) separation of purchasing from funding; (3) focus on low-income groups; (4) effective use of information and communication technologies, including the electronic registration of insured persons and tracking of service utilization; (5) patients' right to choose their preferred healthcare institutions; (6) package rates for payments; and (7) the extensive involvement of the private sector in insurance, management, and service delivery.

In recent years, the health insurance system in India has placed considerable attention to vulnerable groups. The government has actively explored innovation in the health insurance system to ensure that the vast majority of the population is covered by social health insurance. In fact, three types of health insurance have been introduced in the informal sector: group insurance for the contract farmers of agro-processing companies; group insurance for members of nongovernmental organizations (NGOs); and healthcare and welfare programs by the trade unions of the informal sector. These three insurance schemes mainly cover critical illnesses with low incidence rates but high medical expenses.

1. Group Insurance for Contract Farmers of Agro-Processing Companies   This scheme was established in 1975 by the Tribhuvandas Foundation to facilitate hospital insurance coverage among dairy farmers in the Kheda district of Gujarat. The scheme currently covers 634 out of 960 villages within this district. The Tribhuvandas Foundation collects ₹10 as an annual premium from each participating household or ₹1 as a monthly premium. There are also relief mechanisms for these premiums: The poorest households are exempt from paying premiums, and those who cannot afford the full premium are subject to a reduced rate. Premiums are paid on a voluntary basis and collected through milk producer cooperatives. Premiums, medical revenues, interest incomes, and capital injection from milk producer cooperatives account for 28%, 27%, 22%, and 4% of the funding for this foundation, respectively. The out-of-pocket expenses borne by patients accounted for an average of 23% of the total medical expenses. Members of the foundation are provided with free primary care and outpatient services in network healthcare stations and hospitals. The payout ratios for healthcare services delivered by non-network healthcare institutions that meet the referral criteria range from 20% to 100%.

2. Healthcare and Welfare Programs by Trade Unions of the Informal Sector These trade unions mainly serve impoverished groups living in Mumbai. They place great emphasis on collaborating with the National Federation of Indian Women and National Slum Dwellers Federation (NSDF) in establishing various programs, such as savings plans, consumer cooperatives, ration shops, and housing cooperatives. In 1997, the unions negotiated and collaborated with the Oriental Insurance Company (OIC) to establish a special insurance scheme for impoverished groups, whereby a married couple is eligible to receive health security with an annual premium of ₹30. This is a comprehensive insurance scheme that covers not only inpatient expenses but also the loss of property and tools, as well as accident casualties and other major events. The scheme imposes a relatively low loan threshold, and premiums are collected from the interest paid by borrowers, who account for about 60% of insurance beneficiaries.

3. Group Insurance for Members of NGOs The Self-Employed Women's Association (SEWA) is a trade union that was established in Ahmedabad in 1972. It is a nonindustrial organization that aims to increase the economic, social, and political status of self-employed women and general female workers in India. Since 1992, the SEWA has been working with the Life Insurance Corporation (LIC) and United India Insurance Company (UIIC) to develop an insurance scheme that provides health protection against major health risks to all its members at a favorable price. At present, the SEWA is the only traditional cooperative insurance organization in India, and has a total of 215,000 members living across six states (Table 18.14).

In 2003–2004 to 2009–2010, the population coverage of all the GSHISs increased by more than fivefold, which was mainly attributed to the inclusion of low-income earners. The population coverage of commercial health insurance showed a fourfold increase during that same period. Given that the main GSHISs cover about 243 million people, it is estimated that more than 300 million people in India – or about one-fourth of the total population – are covered by some form of health insurance. Furthermore, based on current trends as well as the growing political and economic support from government agencies, we can make a conservative estimation that there will be more than 630 million insured persons by 2015, or about half of the total population of India. This expected expansion in coverage is mainly derived from three sources: the RSBY Scheme, commercial health insurance, and state-sponsored health insurance schemes. Of these, the RSBY Scheme is expected to cover nearly 60 million households (and approximately 300 million insured persons) by 2015 and will account for the largest share of the observed growth in insurance coverage. GSHISs and commercial health insurance companies are continuing to focus on expanding their coverage. However, the benefits vary considerably among the different types of insurance, with the majority of insured persons receiving very limited benefits and a small minority

TABLE 18.14   Population Size of Health Insurance Coverage in India in 2003–2010 and Growth Projections (Unit: Million)

Insurance Scheme	2003–2004	2009–2010	2015
Central government schemes			
ESIS	31	56	72
CGHS	4.3	3	3
RSBY Scheme	Not yet launched		
State government schemes			
Andhra Pradesh	Not yet launched	70	75
Tamil Nadu	Not yet launched	40	42
Vajpayee Arogyashri (Karnataka, KA)	Not yet launched	1.4	33
Yeshasvini Co-operative Farmers Health Care Scheme (Karnataka, KA)	1.6	3	3.4
Total (GSHISs)	37.2	243	528.4
Commercial health insurance	15	55	90
Total	55	300	630
(including other health insurance schemes)			

enjoying extensive benefits. It is perhaps inevitable that the next stage of expansion in insurance coverage will occur in a more decentralized and fragmented manner. This may eventually lead to the use of different risk pools for various groups, based on factors such as employment status (e.g., formal employment vs. flexible employment) and socioeconomic status, which will have an impact on the equality of financial protection and the efficiency of service procurement and delivery.

The newly implemented GSHISs aim to protect impoverished groups against catastrophic health events. Hence, they generally only cover inpatient services but not outpatient services. Therefore, comprehensive benefits, including preventive and primary care services, are only provided by earlier schemes, such as the ESIS and CGHS, which mainly provide outpatient services through their own healthcare institutions (Table 18.15).

The new-generation GSHISs, with the exception of the RSBY Scheme, tend to place especially greater emphasis on the reimbursement of surgical procedures. Furthermore, the reimbursement scope of these schemes is defined based on service packages. An annual household reimbursement cap has been established for all GSHISs, with the exception of the ESIS and CGHS. Therapeutic services in cardiology, neurology, nephrology, cosmetic surgery, oncology, and general surgery account for 60% of the total number of service packages, whereas those for pediatrics, obstetrics, and gynecology account for only 9%. Among all specialties, surgery accounted for most inpatient service packages (96%). In addition to providing clearly defined service packages, the RSBY Scheme, ESIS, and CGHS also cover other inpatient services and provide reimbursements on a fee-for-service basis according to their respective rules and payment methods.

TABLE 18.15 Healthcare Service Package and Reimbursement Cap of GSHISS in India in 2009–2010

Insurance Scheme	Benefit Type	Number of Inpatient Packages	Coverage Extension to Other Healthcare Services	Annual Reimbursement Cap (₹)
ESIS	Comprehensive	1,900	Yes	No annual or lifetime cap
CGHS	Comprehensive	1,900	Yes	No annual or lifetime cap
RSBY Scheme	Inpatient, secondary	727	Yes	30,000/Household
Rajiv Aarogyasri Community Health Insurance Scheme	Inpatient, tertiary	938	No	150,000/Household + 50,000 Buffer
Vajpayee Arogyashri Health Insurance	Inpatient, tertiary	402	No	150,000/Household + 60,000 Buffer
Chief Minister Kalaignar's Insurance Scheme	Inpatient, tertiary	412	No	100,000/Household, cumulative over 4 years
Yeshasvini Co-operative Farmers Health Care Scheme	Inpatient, secondary	1,229	No	200,000/Person
RSBY Plus Scheme	Inpatient, tertiary	326	No	Additional 175,000 after exceeding RSBY cap
ASBY Scheme	Inpatient, tertiary	–	No	Additional 150,000 after exceeding RSBY cap

The geographical accessibility of healthcare services is an important factor affecting insured persons who seek medical attention. Hence, healthcare accessibility for insured persons who live in remote areas or far away from networked hospitals is an issue that remains to be resolved.

The hospitalization rate among persons with commercial health insurance is two- to three times that of the national average. This indicates the presence of significant adverse selection, moral hazard, and overutilization, which the insurance companies are unable to resolve. In addition, the GSHISs rely heavily on commercial insurance companies in terms of management operations. The insurance companies can then pass on additional costs incurred by the above issues to the government agencies of the respective schemes through price renegotiations. Data from monitoring systems of these schemes have indicated that the delivery and utilization of unnecessary healthcare services has become an increasingly serious issue. For example, data from the RSBY Scheme showed that some hospitals provided far more than the expected number of hysterectomy procedures or simultaneous hysterectomy and ovarian salpingectomy in order to obtain additional reimbursement claims. Monitoring data from the Rajiv Aarogyasri Scheme showed that supplier-induced demand is evident in some treatment procedures, such as appendectomy, hysterectomy, laminectomy/discectomy, and extracorporeal shockwave lithotripsy. Additionally, some schemes might have led to excessive investment in tertiary inpatient services and expensive medical technologies in hospitals, while neglecting the importance of outpatients and preventive care services.

Health insurance is playing an increasingly important role in India's healthcare funding system. The World Bank has estimated that the total health insurance expenditure in India amounted to ₹160 billion in 2009–2010, which was 6.4% of the country's total healthcare expenditure. In 2003–2004, the CGHS and ESIS were the predominant schemes among all GSHISs; the other schemes were still in the early stage of implementation or had not been implemented at that point. During this period, the expenditures of the GSHISs were also slightly higher than those of their commercial counterparts. By 2009–2010, however, the expenditures of the GSHISs and commercial health insurance schemes had increased by nearly four and six times, respectively. The World Bank estimated that by 2015, the total health insurance expenditure in India will account for 8.4% (₹380 billion) of the total healthcare expenditure, with commercial health insurance accounting for 45% of the total health insurance expenditure. Furthermore, if there are more state-sponsored health insurance schemes or the growth rate of the expenditure in the public healthcare system decreases, the government expenditure on health insurance as a share of the total healthcare expenditure will exceed 10% before 2015 (Table 18.16).

(3) Payment Methods

Payment methods are powerful tools that allow buyers to influence the behaviors and performance of service providers. A payment method with scientific incentive mechanisms can guide providers toward cost containment, increased efficiency, and improvements in quality; conversely, it could also lead to supply-side distortions, such as cost shifting, care denial, and overtreatment. Rate setting (i.e., the pricing of a service or service package) is a core element of all payments methods.

TABLE 18.16 Trends and Predictions for the Expenditures of Various Health Insurance Schemes in India (Unit: ₹ 10 Million)

	Year		
Insurance Scheme	2003–2004	2009–2010	2015
Central government schemes			
ESIS	767	1,990	4,500
CGHS	700	1,600	3,500
RSBY Scheme	–	480	4,000
State government schemes			
Andhra Pradesh	–	1,200	1,500
Tamil Nadu	–	517	720
Vajpayee Arogyashri (Karnataka, KA)	–	–	660
Yeshasvini Co-operative Farmers Healthcare Scheme (Karnataka, KA)	11	55	80
Total (GSHISs)	1,478	5,842	14,960
Commercial health insurance	1,800	7,000	17,500
Total	4,500	16,000	38,000
(including other health insurance schemes)			

1. Advantages And Disadvantages Of Package-Based Rates Package-based rates have been adopted to a greater or lesser extent by GSHISs for reimbursing inpatient expenses incurred by providers. Package-based rates are a simplified case-based pricing method comprising a single fee or close-ended payment tied to a set of inputs and services required for a predetermined treatment or surgical procedure. The inputs and services generally include bed charges (including ICU or operating room charges), service charges for healthcare workers (consultation, surgery, anesthesia, etc.), diagnostic facilities, drugs, and consumables. The package-based rates for some schemes also include public transport costs for patients, outpatient screening before admission, and postdischarge drugs for a certain number of days. The operation of package-based rates is relatively simple. Reasonable prices can help to control costs, improve service efficiency, and reduce the risk of fund liabilities. In order to gain the potential service volume offered by GSHISs, many healthcare institutions are willing to accept package-based rates that are much lower than the fee-for-service charges incurred by uninsured patients (Table 18.17).

However, there are also some shortcomings for package-based rates: (1) almost all schemes employ a single price structure across their coverage areas. The reimbursement rates are not adjusted for labor and input prices among different regions (e.g., Tier 1, 2, or 3 cities), thereby resulting in overpayment in some regions and underpayment in others. For example, the fee-for-service charges in Tier 2 cities can be less than one-fifth the charges in Tier 1 cities, while an appendectomy in Tier 3 cities can cost less than one-half of the charges in Tier 1 cities. Furthermore, shared or general wards in Tier 1 cities might charge 15–20 times the rate in smaller cities. (2) A single fee that fails to make up for the costs might cause hospitals to favor more lucrative service packages. In the absence of adequate control, package-based rates might also fail to completely prevent fraud. (3) Hospitals prefer low-risk cases and are reluctant to take in patients with severe illnesses because the rates are not adjusted according to the severity of illnesses, unexpected complications, or treatment complexity. (4) Most schemes lack a standardized definition and description of the service packages. For example, a service package for cataract surgery or benign prostatic hyperplasia might not specify the surgical methods, consumables, length of hospital stay, diagnostic methods, or drugs to be provided by hospitals. Service packages that are not clearly defined allow for considerable flexibility in hospitals, which might lead to cheaper, more short-lived, or inferior quality implants and drugs, or cause premature hospital discharge. This could have an adverse impact on healthcare quality and health outcomes.

2. Package-Based Rates and Market Prices The mechanism for formulating package-based rates lacks empirical evidence and is not linked with market prices or costs. The reimbursements issued by different schemes for the same service package may vary significantly. A single hospital can sign service agreements with several GSHISs and commercial insurance companies, which may provide widely different income levels for the same services. This may cause hospitals to provide better services to wealthy patients who participate in schemes with higher reimbursement rates. Some healthcare institutions, particularly large-sized hospitals in major cities, refuse to serve patients insured by certain GSHISs, as they claim that these schemes offer reimbursement rates that are much lower than their costs.

In cases where the reimbursement rate is indeed lower than the cost, healthcare institutions may attempt to make up for the lost income through illegal charges or inducing a demand for out-of-pocket services. For example, some healthcare institutions require patients themselves to pay for drugs and service items covered by insurance schemes.

TABLE 18.17 Healthcare Service Packages Covered by Health Insurance in India in 2010 Based on Diagnosis-Related Groups and Internal Medicine/Surgery Classification

Disease Group	Internal Medicine/Surgery	RSBY Scheme	Chief Minister Kalaignar's Insurance Scheme	Yeshasvini Co-Operative Farmers Health Care Scheme	Vajpayee Arogyashri Scheme	ESIS And CGHS	Rajiv Aarogyasri Community Health Insurance Scheme	RSBY Plus Scheme
Heart diseases	Surgery	Not covered	24	135	134	85	109	109
	Internal medicine	–	1	–	–	–	11	–
Kidney diseases	Surgery	109	9	212	21	129	54	54
	Internal medicine	–	–	–	–	–	5	–
Neurology	Surgery	50	70	67	55	38	67	67
	Internal medicine	–	–	–	–	–	12	–
Cosmetic surgeries	Surgery	131	29	295	8	109	68	20
	Internal medicine	–	–	–	–	–	0	–
Gastrointestinal diseases	Surgery	73	37	167	Not covered	123	55	55
	Internal medicine	–	–	–	–	–	19	–
Tumors	Surgery	23	121	Not covered	106	11	132	–
	Internal medicine	–	57	–	60	3	62	12
Eye diseases	Surgery	41	14	152	–	36	26	–
	Internal medicine	–	–	Not covered	Not covered	–	–	Not covered

Category	Type							
ENT diseases	Surgery	71	3	124	–	50	23	–
	Internal medicine	–	–	–	Not covered	–	–	Not covered
Obstetric and gynecological diseases	Surgery	46	5	60	–	75	17	–
	Internal medicine	–	–	–	Not covered	–	–	Not covered
General surgeries	Surgery	148	10	117	11	26	79	0
	Internal medicine	–	–	–	–	–	–	–
Pediatric diseases	Surgery	31	56	10	7	22	57	Not covered
	Internal medicine	–	–	–	–	–	67	–
Others	Surgery	4	Not covered	18	Not covered	–	29	Not covered
	Internal medicine	–	–	7	–	24	46	–
Total	–	727	412	1,229	402	731	938	326
Percentage (%)	Surgery	100	86	100	86	96	77	96
	Internal medicine	0	14	<1	14	4	23	4

4. Health System Reforms

The government of India is directly responsible for establishing public healthcare institutions and for determining the public health and basic healthcare services that each level of public healthcare institution should provide. The government also ensures that the most basic level of equipment and appropriate technologies are available for laboratory tests, examinations, and treatment. It also formulates a list of essential medicines that can be provided to patients free of charge. The operating costs of secondary and tertiary hospitals are mainly borne by state governments. Conversely, the central government is responsible for the construction and operation of subcenters, PHCs, and CHCs, thereby ensuring that public hospitals are able to provide basic healthcare services.

Public hospitals in India need not generate their own income as they are not responsible for constructing or developing their own infrastructure. As a result, they have no intrinsic motivation to increase their medical charges and patient burden. In addition, they have no incentive to encourage physicians to provide excessive services, as physicians themselves are civil servants who receive fixed salaries based on their performance. Therefore, despite the extremely poor inpatient conditions in Indian public hospitals, where more than 10 or even 20 patients might share a public hospital ward that is not likely to be equipped with air-conditioning or toilets, these hospitals still play a crucial role in health security. They serve as a social buffer, ensuring equal access to basic healthcare services by preventing impoverished individuals from falling into debt or financial crisis by offering free services. However, the conditions and quality of healthcare services of public healthcare institutions often fail to meet patient demands, which have hindered its service utilization. Even impoverished individuals now frequently utilize services in private healthcare institutions, which account for 10% of planned immunization services, 27% of prenatal checkups, 37% for hospital childbirth deliveries, 40% of inpatient services, and 69% of outpatient services.

After 1991, public hospitals underwent autonomous reforms due to the influence of the economic reform. For example, public hospitals in Rajasthan underwent user fee reforms, which included increasing the registration fee and imposing partial charges for certain laboratory tests and drugs. However, the reform of public hospitals in India remains in its infancy. Furthermore, it has an imperfect management system. For instance, charges are imposed on patients without cost-based pricing, without reasonable budgeting or periodic auditing; there are no clearly defined criteria or validity period for relief policies of the poor; and certain ineligible patients, such as civil servants and medical students, are included in fee exemptions. In addition, many users find public hospital charges unacceptable because they are used to the free services provided by such hospitals; more importantly, most users are unable to afford the out-of-pocket expenses. In fact, the most important reason for mismanagement is that public hospitals lack the motivation to impose fees because of the government's stringent controls on their use of extra revenues. For example, the government prohibits public hospitals from using their fee income for equipment repairs or staff bonuses, and stipulates that imposing fees that exceed a certain amount requires government approval. Furthermore, the government employs separated income and expenditure management systems for hospital income. As a result, the implementation of public hospital fee policies has faced many obstacles, with most hospitals collecting less than 10% of the expected medical charges. Therefore, the implementation of user fees in the autonomous hospital reforms is clearly a double-edged sword. On the one hand, if these fees are used to improve hospitals conditions or benefit healthcare workers, it may prompt hospitals to ignore their own fundamental roles and deviate from the initial reform goals in pursuit of profits. On the other hand, hospitals and physicians who face too many restrictions are not motivated because of their lack of decision-making power.

The key areas of health reforms in India are: (1) Increasing the organic integration of the central, state, and local governments to improve health outcomes, with a particular emphasis on women and vulnerable groups living in underdeveloped states and regions, so as to achieve the United Nations Millennium Development Goals. (2) Strengthen the collaboration among partners in the healthcare industry to form a healthcare system comprising the public sector, private sector, NGOs, and community organizations. (3) Establish healthcare funding policies and funding mechanisms (e.g., social health insurance) that favor impoverished groups.

With reference to its experiences in rural healthcare, the MOHFW developed a seven-year program, the NRHM (2005–2012), which covers 650,000 villages and 780 million rural residents. The aim of the NRHM was to improve the rural healthcare system in India, especially in underdeveloped areas, by providing accessible, affordable, responsible, effective, and reliable healthcare services for impoverished and disadvantaged groups living in rural areas. The NRHM targets all rural areas in India, with a particular focus on 18 states. Its main strategies and measures are as follows:

1. *Promote social participation via decentralization.* The implementation of the NRHM was delegated to district and village committees to help improve their management capacities. Furthermore, communities were responsible for the control and management of public healthcare programs, which has promoted social participation among local residents in NRHM activities.
2. *Capacity building.* The service quality and adequacy of essential medicines in subcenters, PHCs, and CHCs were improved in order to enhance the management and service capacities of these healthcare institutions. The NRHM aims to increase the number of CHCs from 3,215 to 6,500; PHCs from 22,974 to 25,000; and subcenters from 143,000 to 175,000.
3. *Adoption of flexible, patient-directed funding policies.* The sources of capital investment have been expanded to fully utilize the role of NGOs. The MOHFW has implemented the horizontal integration of programs for disease prevention and maternal and child healthcare, in order to reduce overlaps and improve service efficiency. The healthcare funding capacity of the NRHM has also been improved through expansion of the health insurance funding plan to secure the financial support needed for reform.
4. *Human resource management.* After being trained in villages for one year, accredited social health activists (ASHAs) are eligible to provide basic preventive healthcare services to rural residents using small medicine boxes containing dozens of essential medicines. The NRHM also provided an adequate number of professional technicians to ensure the 24/7 availability of emergency services in PHCs. A number of multiskilled personnel have also been trained to perform various tasks in each PHC.
5. *Enhanced supervision and management of healthcare institutions.* The regulations and standards of primary care services have been established to enable the inspection and supervision of healthcare institutions. In addition, independent, district- and community-level supervisory committees have also been established to oversee the quality of healthcare services.

The government of India is also seeking to increase its policy and financial support for traditional Indian medicine, enhance basic research and industrial development, and establish pharmaceutical quality standards and certification systems in India. This will help facilitate the integration of traditional Indian medicine into the national healthcare service system, as well as the entry of Indian herbal medicine into the pharmaceutical markets of developed countries, such as the European Union and the US.

5. Outcomes, Characteristics, and Challenges

India has always had a clear vision of the development and reform of its healthcare industry. In brief, limited government funds are to be equally allocated to those most in need of healthcare services. Impoverished and vulnerable groups are the main beneficiaries of government healthcare subsidies and social security. In fact, the government of India has always shown a policy preference toward impoverished groups, who have always been served by public hospitals. The healthcare system of India strives to ensure the stable operation of public hospitals as well as to encourage the healthy development of private hospitals. The coexistence of public and private hospitals also ensures the healthcare accessibility of both rich and poor patients.

The rural healthcare system in India still harbors numerous shortcomings in its actual operations, such as the inadequate coverage of subcenters and health centers, poor-quality infrastructure, and the lack of healthcare workers and medical supplies, all of which have hindered the delivery of public healthcare services that rely on these basic criteria. However, it is undeniable that the rural healthcare system has reduced the financial burden on rural families and enhanced social equality.

The three types of health insurance schemes introduced for the informal sector in India have overcome the difficulties of covering low-income earners and individuals with uncertain income, who fall beyond the scope of conventional insurance schemes. Community- and collective-based group insurance schemes have not only reduced the transaction costs of insurance companies in providing formal insurance services to informal employees but also improved the risk pooling capacity of each community or collective by linking them with insurance companies. Therefore, these insurance schemes are not only beneficial to the health and income security of insured persons but also have helped to enhance community and societal cohesion.

In terms of health system performance, over the past decade, India has achieved tangible results in reducing the infant mortality rate. Unfortunately, its achievements in reducing malnutrition, maternal mortality rate, adult mortality rate, and the prevalence of infectious diseases are dwarfed by those of neighboring countries, such as Bangladesh and Nepal. In addition, there are significant variations in the health outcomes in India among different regions and groups (in terms of social class and ethnicity), indicating an overall lack of healthcare equality.

The current challenges facing the public healthcare system of India are: (1) there are shortages in healthcare institutions, facilities, capital, and talents. In fact, the predicted shortages in CHCs, PHCs, and subcenters are 68%, 31%, and 29%, respectively, while the shortages in physicians, assistant nurses and midwives, multiskilled healthcare workers, pharmacists, and healthcare technicians are 39%, 17%, 47%, 22%, and 18%, respectively. (2) There are shortages in drugs and medical supplies. (3) There is lax management, lack of enthusiasm among employees, poor service attitude, inconsistent healthcare quality, and low service efficiency.

Due to the imbalances in socioeconomic development between urban and rural areas, there are substantial disparities in the health statuses of residents of India. The healthcare system attaches great importance to the use of advanced healthcare technologies for urban elites, but lacks adequate and effective public health infrastructures that are essential for disease control in all communities. The infant mortality rate in rural areas (75%) was found to be 70% higher than the rate in urban areas (44%), while the under-five mortality rate in rural areas (103.7%) was 64.3% higher than the rate in urban areas (63.1%). A comparison between Kerala (which has good healthcare performance) and Rajasthan (which has poor healthcare performance) indicates that the infant mortality rate in Rajasthan (81.0%) was 4.8 times that in Kerala (14.0%), while the maternal mortality rate in Rajasthan (607 deaths per 100,000 live births) was almost 6.9 times that in Kerala (87 deaths per 100,000 live births).

Hospitalization is the main cause of poverty among Indian residents. Although Indian residents have the right to free healthcare services provided by the government, a vast number of patients remain exposed to illness-related financial risks. This is due to the limited resources of the public healthcare system, which can only provide the most basic healthcare services, causing a large number of patients to seek medical attention in private hospitals at their own expense. Moreover, patients who receive free healthcare services in public hospitals still face heavy indirect financial burdens due to the loss of income during hospitalization and treatment. Currently, roughly a quarter of all inpatients fall into poverty due to illness in India.

SECTION III. THE HEALTH SYSTEM IN THAILAND

1. Overview of Socioeconomics and National Health

Thailand, officially the Kingdom of Thailand, is a Southeast Asian country bordered to the east by Laos and Cambodia, to the south by the Gulf of Siam and Malaysia, and to the west by Myanmar and the Andaman Sea. Originally known as Siam, the country was renamed "Thailand" on May 11, 1949. The new name is based on the word "Tai," which means "freedom," as Thailand is the only Southeast Asian country to never have been colonized. The country's official language is Thai, which is written in the Thai alphabet and is considered the native language of about 50 million citizens of Thailand. The vast majority of Thais – more than 90% of the total population – practice Theravada Buddhism. Thailand has 76 first-level administrative divisions, including 75 provinces and the capital city (Bangkok). Thailand is considered a lower middle-income country with an extremely wide wealth gap. It has a free-market, export-oriented economy that greatly relies on foreign markets, particularly those of the US, Japan, and European countries. In the 1980s, Thailand experienced rapid economic growth due to its rapidly developing manufacturing industry, especially electronics. The country was listed as a middle-income economy in 1996. However, following the financial crisis of 1997, Thailand fell into economic recession and only began its recovery in 1999. Since 1961, Thailand has formulated five-year National Economic and Social Development Plans, with the ninth plan beginning in 2002. In recent years, Thailand has achieved significant economic growth. In July 2003, Thailand achieved full settlement of its debts with the International Monetary Fund (IMF), which had amounted to US$17.2 billion during the financial crisis, two years in advance of its deadline. At the end of 2010, the foreign debts and foreign-exchange reserves of Thailand amounted to US$96.5 billion and US$172.1 billion, respectively. In 2010, the GDP of Thailand was ฿4.5958 trillion, with a GDP growth rate, inflation rate, and unemployment rate of 7.8%, 3.3%, and 1.04%, respectively. In 2013, the GDP of Thailand was US$38.73 billion.

Thailand is a democratic nation with a constitutional monarchy, whereby the king serves as the head of state. Thailand is divided into 6 regions, 76 provinces (including two specially governed districts: Bangkok and Pattaya), 146 cities, 984 districts, 7,159 subdistricts, and 65,170 villages. The capital city of Thailand is Bangkok. The total population of Thailand was approximately 67.01 million in 2013, nearly one-third of which consisted of people who were Thai with Chinese ancestry or Thai Chinese. Individuals aged over 60 years account for 9.3% of the total population. In 2003, the average life expectancies for males and females in Thailand were 69.97 and 74.99 years, respectively, which were slightly higher than those in China. The infant mortality rate was 22 per 1,000 live births, and the maternal mortality rate was 12.9 deaths per 100,000 live births. In 2009, the average life expectancies for males and females in Thailand were 66 years and 74 years, respectively. The mortality rate of adults aged 15–59 was 205 deaths per 1,000 people, while the under-five mortality rate was 14 deaths per 1,000 people. In 2010, the purchasing power parity (PPP) per capita of the total healthcare expenditure was US$331. The total healthcare expenditure as a share of the GDP was 3.9%, of which 55.8% and 31.4% came from public and private resources, respectively. In Thailand, the number of physicians per 10,000 people was 2.98 (2004), and the number of hospital beds per 100,000 people was 22 (2002). In 2000–2010, Thailand had an average of 3 physicians, 15 nurses and midwives, 1 dentist, 1 pharmacist, and 22 hospital beds per 10,000 people. In 2012, the average life expectancies for males and females in Thailand were 70.9 years and 77.6 years, respectively.

2. Healthcare System

(1) Healthcare System and Service Provision

The healthcare system of Thailand is comprised of two components: public healthcare institutions and private healthcare institutions. The former dominates the system, accounting for approximately 70% of all healthcare institutions. The main types of healthcare institution in Thailand are as follows.

1. Regional Hospitals   The Ministry of Public Health (MOPH) divides Thailand into 12 health districts, each comprising 7–10 provinces and containing at least one regional hospital with 500–1,000 beds for inpatient services. There are 25 regional hospitals nationwide.

2. Provincial General Hospitals   There are currently 67 provincial general hospitals, each with more than 120 hospital beds (typically ranging from 300 to 500 beds). They provide inpatient services to residents in their respective provinces.

3. Community Hospitals   There are 725 community hospitals (i.e., district hospitals) in Thailand, each of which has 10–120 beds and serves 50,000–100,000 people. In general, there are only a handful of physicians in these hospitals, who provide comprehensive healthcare services (including inpatient services) and technical support to subdistrict health centers and rural PHCs.

4. Subdistrict Health Centers   These are the most basic unit of service delivery at the district level. Each subdistrict health center provides primary healthcare services, such as therapeutic and preventive services to 3,000–5,000 people, and is operated by three to five college-educated healthcare workers. Currently, there are 9,738 subdistrict health centers in Thailand,

5. Rural PHCs   There are currently 72,192 rural PHCs organized by community volunteers to provide primary care services and promote health awareness among rural residents. The government provides a nominal operating subsidy of ฿180 per month to each volunteer.

6. Private Hospitals and Clinics   There are 436 private hospitals and 14,403 private clinics in Thailand, most of which are commercial institutions.

Healthcare services in Thailand can be further divided into three levels: primary, secondary, and tertiary care services. Primary care services are usually provided by community hospitals, subdistrict health centers, and rural PHCs, among which the subdistrict health centers serve as the main service providers. Secondary care services are primarily provided by provincial general hospitals, community hospitals, and private hospitals. Tertiary care services are mainly provided by regional hospitals and large-sized hospitals in Bangkok (including several large-sized private hospitals).

(2) Healthcare Management System

Thailand's healthcare management system consists of two levels: the central level (i.e., the MOPH) and the provincial level (i.e., provincial health offices, PHOs). To improve its healthcare management, Thailand has also clustered its 76 provinces into five health districts: Bangkok and the Northern, Northeastern, Central, and Southern districts. Each district is administered by a regional health office in order to regulate provincial healthcare affairs.

As the main national agency for healthcare affairs, the MOPH is responsible for formulating laws and regulations related to public health, healthcare, food, drugs etc.; financial allocation of subsidies; national planning of health development strategies; and macro-level regulation, supervision, and technical guidance for local healthcare services. MOPH comprises 10 departments: the Office of the Minister, Office of the Permanent Secretary, Department of Medical Services, Department of Health, Department of Disease Control, Department of Medical Sciences, Food and Drug Administration, Department of Mental Health, Department of Thai Traditional and Alternative Medicine, and Department of Health Service Support. It also contains two subordinate units: the Government Pharmaceutical Organization and Health Systems Research Institute. After 2002, the departments of the MOPH were reorganized; apart from the Office of the Minister, they were grouped into three clusters of three departments each, each of which is administered by a Deputy Secretary. For instance, the Department of Medical Services, Department of Thai Tradition and Alternative Medicine, and Department of Mental Health were organized into the Bureau of Health Service System Development. Nevertheless, the departments remain relatively independent from each other in terms of planning, human resource allocation, asset management, and foreign relations, with a clear division of responsibilities.

The provincial level is primarily administered by PHOs, whose Medical Chiefs are appointed by the Office of the Permanent Secretary of the MOPH. PHOs are responsible for implementing MOPH policies and administering public healthcare institutions within individual provinces. Furthermore, they also provide supervisory and technical support for district health offices, which are mainly responsible for coordinating between community hospitals and subdistrict health centers in delivering healthcare services to local residents.

In accordance with the National Health Security Act, the following three major agencies were established to oversee the enforcement of the law: the National Health Security Board (NHSB), Health Service Standard and Quality Control Board (HSSQCB), and National Health Security Office (NHSO). The NHSB is responsible for determining the content and standards of healthcare services, healthcare funding, and management standards for compensations made for no-fault liability. The NHSB is also responsible for encouraging local governments and NGOs to engage in the management of the Universal Coverage Scheme (UCS, also known as the "30-Baht Scheme"). The HSSQCB is primarily responsible for controlling, supervising, and supporting the quality and standards of healthcare institutions, as well as proposing treatment fee standards, management procedures, and compensation for no-fault liability. Finally, the NHSO serves as an administrator, with a focus on ensuring the achievement of UCS goals. In addition to playing this secretarial role, the NHSO is responsible for collecting and analyzing implementation data, beneficiary registration, healthcare provider registration, fund management, reimbursement procedures, oversight of service quality, accelerating management procedures, and so forth. The NHSO establishes local health committees at the provincial level to serve as purchasers of healthcare services and to sign procurement contracts with healthcare providers on behalf of the public. In areas without local health committees, these responsibilities are delegated to PHOs. Beneficiaries must register with designated CHCs to join the 30-Baht Scheme and obtain a card. Any beneficiary is allowed to register with a nearby subdistrict health center and can select one community hospital as the secondary care provider. In the event of illness, beneficiaries must initially seek medical attention at their registered subdistrict health center, and are not allowed to directly visit secondary or tertiary hospitals without a referral issued by PHCs (except in cases of emergency or accident). See Figure 18.7.

3. Health Insurance System

The total healthcare expenditure of Thailand has increased significantly over the past 30 years, from ฿25.3 billion in 1980 to ฿298 billion in 2000. In 2002, the per capita healthcare expenditure was ฿2,738 (approximately US$68.40). The central government has also gradually increased its investment in healthcare, as reflected by the increase in the MOPH's budget from 4.2% of the national budget in 1989 to 6.2% in 2002. After the implementation of the 30-Baht Scheme, the healthcare expenditure of the central government increased

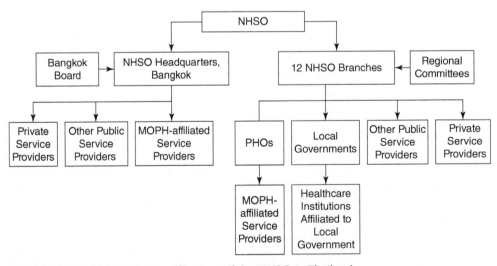

FIGURE 18.7 Administrative affiliations of the NHSO in Thailand.

by about 10%. Healthcare funds are allocated by the MOPH to PHOs or equivalent service providers based on local demand. Furthermore, employees of public healthcare institutions, including subdistrict health centers, are considered civil servants; thus, their salaries are paid using MOPH-allocated funds.

A vertical management system has been adopted in the healthcare system of Thailand, whereby the MOPH implements a central budget for all healthcare-related funds that are allocated to public healthcare institutions or for healthcare-related affairs nationwide. Because of its vast capital injections, which provide security to the salary and welfare of civil servants, the government has considerable control over healthcare planning.

(1) Overview of the Development of the Health Insurance System

In the 1960s, Thailand established the Civil Servant Medical Benefit Scheme (CSMBS) for civil servants and their dependents. Subsequently, in the 1970s and 1980s, the Medical Welfare Scheme (MWS) and Voluntary Health Card Scheme (VHCS) were successively established in order to cover impoverished individuals, senior citizens, children, and disabled individuals. Thailand expanded its health coverage between the 1990s and 2000s. In 1991, the social health insurance (SHI) was established for formal sector employees. In 1997, the Constitution of Thailand was amended to emphasize health as a basic human right. In the meantime, the coverage scope of the Workmen's Compensation Fund (WCF), which is funded by employers, employees, and the government, was expanded to include all private sector employees, while a capitation payment system was adopted for reimbursing hospitals. In addition, free healthcare services provided to the poor were reformed into a public aid system, while the global budget payment system (GBPS) was converted to a capitation payment system for reimbursing hospitals. At this point, the total coverage rate of all health security schemes in Thailand was about 60%.

In 2001, Thailand's government proposed the UCS, that is, the 30-Baht Scheme, which covers all residents apart from civil servants, formal sector employees, and their dependents, with the aim of replacing the MWS and VHCS. Residents are entitled to free preventive services, but are charged ฿30 (equivalent to about RMB6) for outpatient and inpatient services (excluding cosmetic surgeries, organ transplantation, and hemodialysis). This fee is waived for impoverished groups, elderly adults aged over 60, children aged under 12, disabled individuals, veterans, and monks. Currently, the CSMBS, SHI, and UCS cover 10%, 12%, and 74% of Thailand's population, respectively. In November 2002, the government of Thailand passed the National Health Security Act, which established the NHSO under the MOPH. The NHSO is responsible for the central administration of the UCS as well as the gradual takeover of the management of the CSMBS and SHI. The NHSO board is chaired by the Minister of Public Health.

In 2001, Thailand became the first lower-middle income country to achieve universal health coverage. The 30-Baht Scheme is a universal health insurance scheme that covers all Thai residents apart from civil servants and formal sector employees. Funds for the 30-Baht Scheme are allocated based on certain standards by the central government to the PHOs, which in turn allocate the funds to the corresponding healthcare institutions. Beneficiaries only need to pay ฿30 to receive basic healthcare services, including outpatient and inpatient services, in network healthcare institutions. During the preliminary stages of the 30-Baht Scheme, it covered previously uninsured and low-income groups, who accounted for more than 30% of the total population, and by 2002, its coverage increased to 80% of the total population.

(2) Basic Health Security System

The health security system of Thailand is divided into three categories: the first is mandatory, employer-sponsored health insurance. The second is the VHCS for rural residents, which can be joined by all rural residents except for those who are entitled to free healthcare services or are voluntarily participating in private health insurance schemes. Each household is entitled to one health card, and are required to pay ฿500 (equivalent to US$20), with the remaining ฿500 being subsidized by the government. Cardholders are eligible to receive healthcare services in health centers or community hospitals when they fall ill. Patients may be referred to provincial hospitals for treatment whenever deemed necessary by their primary care institutions. Each household is entitled to a maximum of eight visits per year (multiple treatment sessions for the same illness are considered as a single visit, with a maximum allowable reimbursement of ฿2,000 per visit; patients have to cover the remaining balance after exceeding this reimbursement limit). The VHCS has enabled the integration of preventive and therapeutic services as its service contents include both basic health insurance and preventive care. The final category is the free healthcare services provided to civil servants, state-owned enterprise employees, monks, elderly adults aged over 60, children aged under 12, disabled individuals, and impoverished individuals. Furthermore, the government issues certificates of free healthcare to rural residents below the poverty line (single individuals with a monthly income of less than ฿200 or households with a monthly income of less than ฿2,800). These beneficiaries account for 14% of the rural population in Thailand.

4. Health System Reforms and Evaluation

(1) VHCS and CHS System

The population census in 2000 revealed that some 41 million Thais lived in rural areas, accounting for around 69% of the total population. The past few years have seen significant improvement in the rural economy and society of Thailand, but there is still a substantial gap between rural and urban areas.

In terms of health status, rural areas in Thailand generally have a higher prevalence of disease than do urban areas. Nonetheless, the prevalence of several major life-threatening diseases, such as respiratory, digestive, cardiovascular, cerebrovascular, and infectious diseases, has decreased significantly in rural areas. There are also differences between urban and rural areas in several health-related behaviors, such as smoking and alcoholism. Specifically, urban areas have a lower prevalence of smoking and alcoholism than rural areas, and this gap is widening. On the other hand, the child mortality rates in urban and rural areas have both declined significantly, but the rate of decline was lower in rural areas than in urban areas. In 1966, the child mortality rate in rural areas was higher than urban areas by 26%; by 1996, the rate in rural areas was 85% higher than that in urban areas.

1. VHCS   The VHCS was implemented in rural areas by the government of Thailand to achieve the ultimate goal of "Health for All by the Year 2000" and to encourage greater community participation in healthcare. The VHCS is a voluntary health insurance scheme that fully utilizes local resources in the delivery of healthcare services and community development. It operates an improved referral system that promotes the full utilization of healthcare resources and enhances self-help and self-management abilities at the community level.

The VHCS has progressed through the following four stages in Thailand:

Stage 1: From June 1983 to June 1984, the MOPH conducted pilot studies on a health insurance scheme based on a prospective payment system (PPS) in 18 villages across 7 provinces, with an emphasis on the provision of maternal and child healthcare.

Stage 2: From 1984 to 1985, this scheme was officially named the VHCS, and its pilot projects were further expanded to include at least two villages in each province, with a voluntary coverage rate of at least 70% in each village.

Stage 3: From 1985 to 1987, the price and utilization rate of the VHCS was studied to facilitate the establishment of a VHCS fund, to which each household and single individual contributed ฿300 and ฿200 per year, respectively (children were given a ฿100 discount). The remaining half of the premium was covered by the MOPH.

Stage 4: From 1988 to the present, VHCS subsidies in the government budget were investigated and reformed. Health cards were purchased voluntarily by each household. Households with fewer than five members were charged ฿500 per year (accounting for 3–5% of their annual household income) and the MOPH covering the remaining half. Households with more than five members were charged separately for their purchase of the VHCS (the premium contributions of both the government and rural households rose to ฿1,000 after the financial crisis in 1997). VHCS premiums were publicized and collected from each household by CHCs via village health volunteers (VHVs).

The VHCS is valid for one year and has to be repurchased after the expiration date. Village officials and VHVs are entitled to VHCS benefits without having to pay the premiums. In addition, rural households with a monthly income of less than ฿2,800 are considered impoverished households and, therefore, might be exempted from paying the premiums. Households with VHCS health cards are entitled to free healthcare services in CHCs and regional hospitals by showing their health cards and ID cards. Patients who cannot be treated by CHCs may be referred to secondary or tertiary hospitals. Critically ill patients admitted to special wards are entitled to a 10% discount on all ward charges. Each household is entitled to a maximum of eight visits per year using the health cards, with a reimbursement cap of ฿2,000 per visit and ฿16,000 per year. Patients must cover the remaining balance after exceeding the reimbursement cap. The VHCS is administered by provincial VHCS committees; for the VHCS to be implemented in a given village, the village must have a minimum household participation rate of 35%. The committees standardize the health cards and determine the service coverage and referral system for cardholders in public hospitals. In addition, a large number of VHVs (usually one VHV per 10 households) have been trained, who are affiliated with CHCs and are mainly responsible for providing health education and preventive services, as well as promoting the VHCS. During the preliminary stage of VHCS implementation, the VHCS fund was administered by a committee comprising the village leader and four individuals elected by the villagers. After the 1990s, the VHCS fund was administered at the regional level, which increased their scope of social pooling and capacity for risk resistance. The regional committees deposited a portion of VHCS funds into the Bank for Agriculture and Agricultural Cooperatives (BAAC) at an interest rate of 5% (the inflation rate in Thailand from 1980 to 1990 was 3.4%). The VHCS fund is used to reimburse healthcare institutions on a fee-for-service basis. In general, the VHCS allocates 60% of its funds to hospitals above the regional level, 30% to regional hospitals and CHCs, and 10% to management costs.

The VHCS has the following four basic characteristics:

1. The VHCS covers both basic healthcare and preventive care, thus enabling better integration of preventive and therapeutic services.
2. The VHCS takes into account both equality and efficiency. Due to its gradual implementation via pilot projects and the participation of local and foreign experts, it has become a comprehensive and cost-effective scheme in terms of its funding approaches and standards, fund management, referral system, scope of coverage, etc.
3. Strong government support is the key to the success of the VHCS implementation. The government of Thailand provides a ฿1,000 subsidy to each household for the payment of VHCS premiums and encourages VHVs to promote the VHCS. Furthermore, the government has stipulated that the training and support of VHVs, as well as the implementation of primary healthcare services are the core tasks of regional hospitals and CHCs. Hence, it can be seen that the government has played an indispensable role in providing financial support and organizational leadership.
4. The integration of the VHCS and CHS has stabilized the community-based healthcare funding channels. The VHCS is an important community-based funding approach that ensures the access of rural residents to basic healthcare services and the development of the CHS. The systematic management of the VHCS has improved the continuity and accessibility of CHS in rural areas.

2. Rural CHS   The development of rural CHS is closely associated with the VHCS. The primary healthcare program initiated in the 1970s enabled the implementation of the basic contents of CHS in rural areas; however, this program lacked continuity. Then, the VHCS was launched in 1985 and had covered more than 30 million cardholders by the end of the 1990s, which was more than 70% of the total rural population of Thailand. The integration of community healthcare funding into the healthcare system has greatly improved the continuity of CHS.

1. *Rural healthcare system and CHS network.* The rural CHS system in Thailand has a clear hierarchical structure, in which healthcare institutions at each level have clearly defined roles and responsibilities. Despite having varying roles, all healthcare institutions, from the provincial to the village level, are responsible for providing primary healthcare services. Provincial healthcare institutions are mainly responsible for providing technical support to primary care institutions, such as accepting referred patients and training primary healthcare workers. Since the population of each district in Thailand is only about 50,000 to 100,000, community hospitals (district hospitals) are equivalent in size to township health centers in the rural areas of China. Hence, they are actually comprehensive healthcare institutions geared toward the prevention and treatment of diseases. The modern operating model and management approach of CHS in Thailand are mainly embodied in these community hospitals. On the other hand, rural CHCs are a type of subdistrict health center equipped with healthcare workers who have only been trained for two to three years; thus, they are only capable of providing therapeutic services for minor illnesses, and are mainly responsible for preventive services. The operating costs of rural CHCs, including employees' salaries, building construction, and equipment costs, are primarily funded by the government.
2. *Rural CHS institutions and their functions.* In general, rural CHS institutions in Thailand include community hospitals, CHCs, and village health stations. In general, there are approximately 30 beds in community hospitals, which have relatively well-equipped clinical departments as well as various departments for maternal and child healthcare,

preventive care, information management, and so forth. They tend to have a high degree of digitization in their information management. Apart from focusing on inpatient services, community hospitals are responsible for the management of VHCS-related information – they have information systems for storing information related to healthcare services and the medical expenses of cardholders in subdistrict and village healthcare institutions. In addition, the medical conditions of patients are recorded into this information system during each visit to community hospitals, thereby ensuring the continuity of community hospital services.

In general, community hospitals have 30–50 employees, mainly consisting of nurses and healthcare technicians, with only three to five licensed physicians, whose salaries are usually several times higher than those of other healthcare workers. Rural CHCs are subdistrict healthcare institutions that are similar to urban CHCs in terms of infrastructure and size, and serve approximately 5,000 residents. Rural CHCs are generally staffed with one physician who has been trained for two to three years, one midwife, and one nurse. Their main tasks include health promotion, disease prevention, treatment of common diseases, and providing guidance to village health stations. Furthermore, rural CHCs must operate in compliance with the standards established by the MOPH under the support and guidance of community hospitals. In addition, rural CHCs and subdistrict governments jointly recruit about 20 community healthcare volunteers per subdistrict. Their main responsibility is to assist healthcare workers in community hospitals and CHCs in providing out-of-hospital services, such as health promotion, home-based care, planned immunization, and the verification and management of the VHCS. Village health stations are only established in remote rural areas with 500–1,000 residents. Each village health station is staffed with only one community healthcare worker, who is paid by the government to perform various tasks, such as health promotion, disease prevention, and simple therapeutic procedures.

3. *Support and operation of rural CHS.* Rural CHS in Thailand are mainly characterized by the VHCS, government funding, emphasis by local governments, and full utilization of community healthcare resources. Community hospitals, which serve as important institutions for rural CHS, are directly administered by district governments rather than district health offices. This suggests that the government attaches great importance to healthcare services. The VHCS plays a vital role in rural CHS, not only ensuring the access of rural residents to basic healthcare services but also embodying the fundamental characteristics of rural CHS. Most healthcare institutions in Thailand are located in rural areas. The incomes of rural healthcare workers and healthcare facilities are mainly funded by the central and local governments, which guarantee the stability and development of rural healthcare institutions. To ensure an adequate supply of physicians in rural healthcare institutions, the government of Thailand has proposed the provision of 300 physicians per year specifically for rural areas by requiring medical students to sign contracts to work in public hospitals for two to four years after graduation. To support this program, the government has also established a network of local clinics and hospitals to help train medical students. Medical schools have been established across the country and medical students receive considerable subsidies from the government throughout their studies. Additionally, medical students tend to undertake internships at their future workplaces, which help to familiarize them with their future work environment. This program has greatly increased the proportion of medical students in rural areas. The government of Thailand has also encouraged

physicians to serve in remote and rural hospitals by adding an additional ฿10,000 to their salaries. In addition, it is crucial for CHCs to have a large number of VHVs, who not only facilitate the daily tasks of healthcare workers but also serve as a bridge between CHS agencies (i.e., medical professionals) and communities (i.e., residents).

(2) The 30-Baht Scheme

After more than three decades of development, various health security schemes in Thailand had covered more than 60% of the population by 2000. However, this meant that roughly 30% of Thailand's population was still uninsured, and the utilization efficiency of healthcare resources was still unsatisfactory. In light of this situation, the government of Thailand implemented the UCS (the 30-Baht Scheme), which was based on previously implemented health security schemes.

The 30-Baht Scheme is a universal health insurance scheme that covers all Thais apart from civil servants and formal sector employees. The 30-Baht Scheme fund is allocated by the central government based on specific standards to the provinces. The PHOs, in turn, allocate the funds to the corresponding healthcare institutions according to their human resources (wages), preventive services, therapeutic services, etc. Beneficiaries are entitled to basic healthcare services, including outpatient and inpatient services, for a nominal fee of ฿30 in networked healthcare institutions.

1. Basic Healthcare Services of the 30-Baht Scheme Beneficiaries of the 30-Baht Scheme are entitled to the following services for a fee of only ฿30: (1) preventive services and health promotion services, including physical examination, planned immunization, family planning, maternal and child care, AIDS prevention, oral disease prevention, and so on; (2) outpatient and inpatient services, including medical examination, treatment, and rehabilitation, as well as drugs listed in the National List of Essential Drugs (NLED) and medical supplies; (3) childbirth deliveries (not more than twice); (4) hospital meals and accommodation; (5) treatment for common oral diseases, such as dental extraction. However, the following patients and treatments fall beyond the scope of the 30-Baht Scheme: (1) patients with mental illnesses who are hospitalized for more than 15 days; (2) treatment and rehabilitation of drug addicts; (3) assisted reproductive treatments and artificial insemination for infertility; (4) cosmetic surgeries; (5) organ transplantation; (6) experimental treatments and hemodialysis.

2. Administration of the 30-Baht Scheme The National Health Commission, which is chaired by the Minister of Public Health, was established to formulate policies related to the 30-Baht Scheme. The NHSO was also established to serve under the MOPH as the fund manager of the 30-Baht Scheme. Specifically, it is responsible for allocating funds to provinces according to their healthcare needs, as well as overseeing their fund utilization. The NHSO establishes local health committees at the provincial level to serve as purchasers of healthcare services and sign procurement contracts with both public and private healthcare providers on behalf of the public. In areas without local health committees, these responsibilities are delegated to PHOs. Beneficiaries of the 30-Baht Scheme are allowed to register with a single nearby subdistrict health center, and to select a community hospital as the secondary care provider. In the event of illness, they can seek medical attention at the registered subdistrict health center, and cannot directly visit secondary or tertiary hospitals without obtaining a referral from their PHCs (i.e., the subdistrict health center), except in the case of an emergency or accident. Otherwise, the beneficiary must cover the resulting medical charges at their own expenses.

3. Funding and Payment Method of the 30-Baht Scheme Funds for the 30-Baht Scheme are mainly from the structural adjustments made to the national healthcare expenditure. After allocating funds for building infrastructure, procuring large-scale medical equipment, medical research, and the prevention and treatment of diseases (e.g., AIDS), the central government allocates all remaining healthcare funds (including newly added funds equivalent to nearly 10% of the total healthcare fund) to the 30-Baht Scheme.

In general, the National Health Commission reimburses healthcare institutions via two payment systems: a capitation payment system for outpatient and inpatient services, or a capitation payment system for outpatient services and a DRG-based GBPS for inpatient services. However, the payment methods might vary across different provinces during actual implementation.

4. Implementation Outcomes of the 30-Baht Scheme The implementation of the UCS in Thailand has changed not only the central government's method of budget allocation to provinces but also the funding approaches of public hospitals. The healthcare budget was previously allocated to provinces or public hospitals based on their expenditure in previous years. However, this method was replaced with a method of allocating the budget based on the size of the served population. This latter method of budget allocation has improved the equality of budget allocation across different provinces. In addition, the attempt to adjust the budget allocation according to age and disease burden has ensured that the budget is better allocated according to the local healthcare needs in each province. Allocating funds according to health or healthcare needs can further enhance the equality of budget allocation and can serve as an indicator of allocation equality. The method of allocating the healthcare budget based on the size of the population served is also able to force public hospitals to redistribute their human resources. Therefore, this method of government budget allocation is worth recommending. The improvements in budget allocation and provider payment systems have helped to accelerate the health reforms in Thailand.

The use of a capitation payment system has prompted public hospitals to improve their service efficiency. The capitation payment system helps reduce the irrational allocation of healthcare workers among different regions, promote equality in budget allocation, and improve hospital efficiency. Specifically, the capitation payment system has influenced the redistribution of the healthcare workforce. Since the implementation of the UCS, MOPH policymakers have recognized the irrational distribution of public healthcare services, facilities and healthcare workers, and have therefore attempted to redistribute the healthcare workforce among public healthcare institutions by adopting the capitation payment system. However, this resulted in numerous uncontrollable outcomes due to inadequate preparation. In areas with a surplus of healthcare workers, the healthcare workers began complaining that they were being treated unfairly under the new payment system. The inclusion of their salaries in the capitation budget caused them to resent the policy due to a sense of job insecurity. On the other hand, in areas with a shortage of healthcare workers, the considerable increase in budget allocation was still incapable of attracting the necessary healthcare workers.

In light of such circumstances, the MOPH delegated the management of human resource expenditure to PHOs and used contingency funds to supplement hospitals with inadequate budgets. These measures helped to temporarily alleviate the financial pressure. However, this approach also shifted the focus to fresh graduates, which may delay the redistribution of the healthcare workforce. Furthermore, this approach has also given rise to several new issues. There is evidence that the number of physicians who resigned from public hospitals increased significantly in 2002. In 2000, the number of physicians who resigned from public hospitals was only 2%, which increased to 2.5% in 2001 and 4.6% in 2002. Most of the physicians who resigned were young physicians with civil servant status.

The budget allocation is affected by the capitation payment system. Prior to the implementation of the capitation payment system, the healthcare budget was allocated to provinces based on historical allocations. The number of public healthcare institutions, including the number of hospital beds and healthcare workers in public hospitals, was the main factor influencing budget allocation. The irrational distribution of healthcare institutions and healthcare workers was a major issue facing Thailand's healthcare system, as most physicians served in high-income areas. This earlier budget allocation approach exacerbated the inequality among provinces, as high-income areas would receive above-average healthcare budgets due to their higher number of physicians. The implementation of the UCS, which employs capitated budget allocation, has improved the equality of the budget allocation throughout the country. Evidently, budget allocation based on the average per capita should not be the ultimate goal of budget allocation, because healthcare needs vary among different communities in different areas. The bias in budget allocation toward wealthy areas is unreasonable because impoverished populations often have greater healthcare needs because of their poor health status. Implementing budget allocation based on the size of the population served can alleviate this inequality to a certain extent. However, due to the current irrational allocation of the healthcare workforce, this approach will eventually lead to inadequate budgets in some healthcare institutions, thus requiring an additional budget to maintain their operations.

The MOPH utilized the contingency fund to help solve this issue. In 2003, the adjusted capitated budget was adopted, leading to a gradual reduction in budget gaps among the provinces due to the differences in the number of healthcare institutions and facilities. The MOPH proposed that the contingency fund could be used as a tool to improve the efficiency of public hospitals. To achieve a better allocation and utilization of the contingency fund, the MOPH established the "Guidelines for Healthcare Workforce Management in Universal Health Insurance," which must be complied with by public hospitals applying for the contingency fund. Before granting the contingency funds, a national expert group must conduct an in-depth analysis of the financial and management information of each hospital. This national expert group engages in a discussion with the hospital management team, and upon reaching an agreement, both parties submit proposals to the MOPH for improving hospital efficiency. The total income of each hospital (including the contingency fund) must not exceed 90% of its annual expenditure in 2002. This implies that the service efficiency should be improved by at least 10% from its existing level.

The CHS system in Thailand has made major contributions to the expansion of health coverage, guidance of healthcare funding, improvement in healthcare service efficiency, and the prevention and treatment of AIDS. Thailand's healthcare is jointly funded through government budget injection and community fundraising. The former accounts for about 36% of the total amount of healthcare funds. The government's substantial capital injection to the CHS falls not only on the supply side, such as the salary of employees or the construction and deployment of facilities but also on the demand side, mainly through the Low-Income Card Scheme. The WHO refers to the CHS system in Thailand as "a new health reform idea for achieving universal health coverage based on a market economy." This system has also provided useful insights for the delivery of CHS in China, specifically with regard to the development of a health security system and the prevention of AIDS.

SECTION IV. THE HEALTH SYSTEM IN VIETNAM

1. Overview of Socioeconomics and National Health

Vietnam, officially, the Socialist Republic of Vietnam, is a country located in the eastern part of the Indochinese Peninsula, covering an area of about 329,500 km². Vietnam is bordered by China to the north, Laos and Cambodia to the west, and the South China Sea to the east and south, with a coastline of more than 3,260 km. Its capital city is Hanoi. Vietnam has a population of approximately 87.84 million, with around 54 different ethnic groups, among which the Kinh account for about 86% of the total population. The main language of Vietnam is Vietnamese, and its main religions are Buddhism, Catholicism, Hoahaoism, and Caodaism.

Vietnam is a developing country that established diplomatic relations with China on January 18, 1950. The economic reform and liberalization of Vietnam began in 1986. A comprehensive strategic partnership was signed between China and Vietnam in 2008. After nearly three decades of reform, Vietnam has maintained rapid economic growth, as evidenced by the continuous expansion of its total economic volume. The country's tendency toward a more coordinated economic structure in its tertiary industry and its continuously increasing economic liberalization have led to the domination of state-owned enterprises and the joint development of various economic sectors. During the 1996–2000 five-year plan, the average annual GDP growth rate of Vietnam was 6.7%, while the average annual growth rates of the primary, secondary, and tertiary industries were 5%, 12.2%, and 6.4%, respectively. Food production increased at an annual average of 1.3 million tons, among which rice and coffee exports ranked the second and third highest in the world, respectively. In 2001, the main indicators of economic development in Vietnam included the following: its GDP, which was approximately US$32.5 billion, total private investment, which increased by 16% (about US$10 billion, equivalent to 30.8% of GDP), and foreign investment capital, which was approximately US$2.2 billion, with more than 400 new foreign investment projects. China is Vietnam's largest trading partner – they had a bilateral trade volume of US$50.4 billion in 2012, which was a 25% increase compared to the previous year. In 2012, the GDP of Vietnam had increased by 5.03% compared to the previous year, specifically, 4.64% in the first quarter, 4.8% in the second quarter, 5.05% in the third quarter, and 5.44% in the fourth quarter. This increase in GDP was attributed to growth in the agricultural, forestry, and fishery industry, which grew by 2.72% and contributed 0.44% to the GDP growth; the industrial and construction industry, which grew by 4.52% and contributed 1.8% to the GDP growth; and the service industry, which grew by 6.42% and contributed 2.7% to the GDP growth. Vietnam's GDP reached US$171.4 billion in 2013.

Vietnam has established an education system consisting of early childhood education, primary education, secondary education, higher education, teacher education, vocational education, and adult education. In 2000, the government of Vietnam announced that it had essentially achieved universal compulsory primary education, and in 2001 it began working on the universalization of nine-year compulsory education. In 2009–2010, there were approximately 17.49 million university, secondary, and primary school students, as well as 810,300 teachers in Vietnam. There were 376 higher education institutions throughout the country.

Vietnam is ranked 13th globally in terms of population, which reached 86.5 million people in 2008 and 89.7 million people in 2013. However, Vietnam's per capita income and various health-related indicators are far lower than are those in many other countries. Its enormous population has also led to an exceedingly high population density of about 227 people per km², which is five times the world average. In 2013, the annual population growth rate was 0.99%, birth rate 16.47%, mortality rate 6.18%, net migration rate −0.39%, sex ratio at birth (male births: female births) 1.07:1, and infant mortality rate 23.61%. The average life expectancy was 71.33 years (males: 68.52 years; females: 74.33 years), while the total fertility rate was 1.86 infants per woman. In 2003, it was estimated that the HIV/AIDS infection ratio was 0.4%, the total number of HIV/AIDS patients was 220,000, and the number of HIV/AIDS deaths among adults was 9,000. In 2012, the average life expectancy at birth in Vietnam was 75.6 years (males: 71.1 years; females: 80.4 years).

2. Healthcare System

(1) Healthcare System of Vietnam

Healthcare services in Vietnam are based on the service model of the Soviet Union and China, whereby free universal healthcare is provided across the country in established primary healthcare units. In 1992, Vietnam formulated a five-year plan (1990–1995) corresponding to the global health sector strategy established by the WHO in order to achieve universal health coverage by 2000. The five-year plan included: a provincial hospital with 300–500 beds for referred patients in each province with 1–2 million residents; at least one general hospital with 100–200 beds in each region or large town with about 150,000 residents; and 5–10 hospital beds for each community with an average population of 2,000–5,000 people (Vietnam has around 10,000 communities in total).

Healthcare workforce allocation is based on existing and planned hospital beds. In 1990, there were 26,954 physicians, equivalent to 40.7 physicians per 10,000 people; 46,961 healthcare assistants (all of whom had completed short-term training in vocational medical schools), equivalent to 70.9 healthcare assistants per 10,000 people; and 13,391 trained midwives, equivalent to 2.02 midwives per 10,000 people.

According to the conference proceedings of the 2007 Summary of Healthcare Services and 2008 Development Plan conference held by the Ministry of Health (MOH) of Vietnam in mid-January of 2008, there were 13,400 public hospitals in Vietnam, which in total offered around 151,671 beds (with a utilization rate of 110%), and 30,000 private health-care institutions (66 private hospitals, 300 private medium-sized polyclinics, and 45,000 private practices). The private healthcare institutions founded the Association of Private Medical Practice (*Hoi Hanh Nghe Y Tu Nhan*) in mid-December of 2007. The MOH statistics in 2013 indicated that there were 157 private hospitals in total, including 151 locally invested hospitals and 6 foreign-invested hospitals. There were also more than 30,000 small-sized private clinics, including 30 polyclinics, 87 birth centers, 30 foreign-invested clinics, and 29 clinics with foreign physicians; the rest were specialist clinics and healthcare institutions.

(2) Healthcare Management System in Vietnam

The healthcare management system in Vietnam comprises the MOH, which consists of 16 departments and bureaus, and a number of subordinate units, including state-owned pharmaceutical companies, eight medical research institutes, and eight medical schools. The healthcare funds in Vietnam are allocated directly by the Ministry of Finance (MOF). In the event of insufficient funds, the country can apply for medical aid directly from international aid agencies, such as the United Nations (UN) and the Swedish International Development Agency (SIDA). These foreign aid funds are administered by a separate committee. With the exception of some provincial and municipal public hospitals, the majority of healthcare institutions within the Vietnamese public healthcare system are outdated, obsolete, and severely understaffed. Hence, the vast majority of residents living in district-level cities and townships prefer provincial public hospitals as their first stop for medical care because of the overall lack of trust in local healthcare institutions. As a result, hospitals in Ho Chi Minh City and Hanoi are regularly overwhelmed with patients, many of whom start queuing at midnight or in the early morning to seek medical attention. Vietnam's Prime Minister, Nguyễn Tấn Dũng, while attending the 13th Medical Association of Southeast Asian Nations (MASEAN) Conference held by the MOH of Vietnam in Hanoi in November 2007, said that the MOH had inspected and rectified the country's medical networks in order to promote the adoption of open-door policies in the healthcare industry. The government promised to continue injecting capital into the industry in order to establish further tangible and intangible assets; promote the training of healthcare workers; and improve the development of specialized healthcare programs in provincial, district, and township healthcare institutions. Furthermore, the government also began encouraging the establishment of joint ventures between private and public healthcare institutions to provide healthcare services.

In early 2008, the government of Ho Chi Minh City passed a plan to establish hospitals (each with 500–1,000 beds) in four suburbs of the city: the Thủ Đúc, Bình Chánh, Hóc Môn, and Củ Chi districts. The hospital establishment plan was formulated in response to the central government's decision to prohibit the establishment of new schools and hospitals in downtown Hanoi and Ho Chi Minh City, as well as to relocate existing schools and hospitals to suburbs in order to reduce urban traffic congestion.

Dr. Nguyen Van Chau, the head of the Department of Health of Ho Chi Minh City, informed the media in early August 2008 that the department had completed land consolidation as reserves for the construction of suburban hospitals, and had begun to invite the participation of local and foreign investors. It is estimated that Ho Chi Minh City will need at least 8,377 hospital beds before 2015 in order to serve approximately 3 million suburban residents. The government has received about 20 investment proposals for hospital construction from companies in Singapore, the US, and various Asian countries. Singapore Health Services Pte. Ltd. (SingHealth), AsiaMedic Limited, and Parkway Group Healthcare Pte. Ltd. have all visited Ho Chi Minh City and expressed their willingness to invest. Most of these investors were interested in the investment environment in the western suburbs (Bình Tân and Tân Phú districts). Shangri-la Healthcare Investment Pte. Ltd. (Singapore) was licensed in early July 2008 to establish the Hi-Tech Healthcare Park in the Bình Tân district.

The Hi-Tech Healthcare Park covers an area of 37 hectares and is a US$400 million joint venture between Shangri-la Healthcare Investment Pte. Ltd. (contributing 70% of the total capital) and the Vietnam-based Hoa Lam Services Co. Ltd. (contributing 30%). It consists of a hospital with 1,750 hospital beds (equipped with various departments, such as the diagnostic department, oncology department, cardiology department, and obstetrics and gynecology department, as well as rooftop helipads) along with a number of nursing schools and restaurants. Construction began at the end of 2008, and the Hi-Tech Healthcare Park is expected to be opened by the end of 2010; however, construction is expected to be completed in 2015.

The healthcare system of Vietnam has achieved great success over the past few years. The United Nations Development Program (UNDP) reported that the human development index (HDI) of Vietnam has increased rapidly over the past few decades, from 0.582 in 1985 to 0.603 in 1990, 0.646 in 2000, and 0.704 in 2003. Furthermore, in terms of the HDI rankings, from 1985 to 2003 Vietnam moved from seventh to sixth (overtaking Indonesia) among the ASEAN countries; from 32nd to 28th among all Asian countries; and from 122nd to 108th among all 177 countries worldwide. Its improvement was most prominent in 2003, as its HDI ranking overtook four Asian countries and showed the fastest increase in Asia.

The average life expectancy of Vietnam has improved greatly as well over the past few years, from 65.2 years in 1995 to 67.8 years in 2000 and 70.5 years in 2003. The average life expectancy index of Vietnam is 0.76, which is 1.4 times that of its per capita GDP index. This increase in average life expectancy has been attributed to increases in the per capita GDP, improvements in healthcare services, and decreases in neonatal mortality rate, perinatal mortality rate, under-five mortality rate, and neonatal mortality rate among vaccinated low-body-weight (birth weight less than 2,500 g) infants. In addition, the availability of physicians in each commune has exceeded the goal of the 2005 and even the 2010 healthcare plan. Tetanus and polio have also been eliminated among newborn infants.

3. Health Insurance System

Prior to 1986, healthcare services in Vietnam were fully funded by the government, which utilized the national budget to fund the construction of hospitals, purchase equipment, reimburse medical expenses incurred by patients, and pay the salaries of healthcare workers serving in the central and local healthcare systems. However, after entering the reform phase, the healthcare sector faced numerous challenges because of the termination of government subsidies, which led to a severe shortage of financial resources needed to maintain the activities of the public healthcare sector. Additionally, the rapid development of the private healthcare sector has triggered a new round of reforms of the public healthcare sector. Specifically, the healthcare sector has shifted from relying completely on government subsidies and control to more dependence on the private sector. The government has also enacted numerous policies, laws, and regulations related to healthcare development during this period, particularly in relation to medical expenses, health insurance, and healthcare services for the poor.

Presently, the health insurance system of Vietnam comprises three components: compulsory health insurance (CHI), voluntary health insurance (VHI), and healthcare funds for the poor (HCFP). Insured persons are given access to healthcare services in public hospitals as well as private hospitals that cooperate with health insurance agencies. In 2007, there were 1,087 public hospitals and medical centers, and 106 private hospitals throughout Vietnam participating in these health insurance schemes. By 2010, there were 2,767 participating healthcare institutions, which ensured the timely access of around 106 million insured persons to diagnostic and therapeutic services.

(1) Compulsory Health Insurance (CHI)

The premiums of the CHI are contributed by both employers and employees at 2% and 1% of employees' monthly salary, respectively. The scheme covers inpatient services for insured persons, including medical care, laboratory testing, X-ray examinations, and other imaging diagnostic tests, as well as some expensive, high-end healthcare services, such as open-heart surgery. The list of reimbursable drugs under this scheme is very extensive and comparable to that of developed countries. Insured persons who fall ill are entitled to a sickness allowance equivalent to 75% of their salaries. Furthermore, insured persons who have joined the scheme for more than 15 and 30 years are able to take 30 and 40 days of sick leave per year, respectively. Insured persons with hazardous occupations who have participated in the scheme for at least 15 years, 15–30 years, and more than 30 years are eligible to take 40, 50, and 70 days of sick leave per year, respectively.

(2) Voluntary Health Insurance (VHI)

VHI covers students and other individuals outside the scope of CHI coverage. In 2007, the VHI premium rates for urban residents, rural residents, urban students, and rural students were đ160,000–đ320,000, đ120,000–đ240,000, đ60,000–đ120,000, and đ50,000–đ10,000, respectively. VHI-insured persons can freely choose their premium rates. This scheme provides both inpatient and outpatient services for insured persons. Outpatient fees below đ100,000 are entitled to full reimbursement, while fees above 100,000 are entitled to 80% reimbursement. Inpatient fees below đ20 million are entitled to 80% reimbursement. Furthermore, VHI-insured students who seek medical treatment for the first time are entitled to additional reimbursement equivalent to 17.4% of their total medical charges.

(3) Health Care Funds for the Poor (HCFP)

Since 1989, the Vietnamese government has provided financial assistance to the HCFP scheme. In 2002, the Vietnamese government provided the entire impoverished population with health insurance subsidies to cover premiums for the Free Health Insurance card (HI card) and critical illness assistance. In 2003, the government invested đ512 billion into this scheme, which increased to đ1,450 billion in 2006. The HCFP scheme was incorporated into the CHI in 2005. Impoverished individuals who can afford and have paid at least đ60,000 in insurance premiums are entitled to CHI coverage, as well as more than 11% and 17% reimbursement for their outpatient and inpatient expenses, respectively. The annual premium rose to đ130,000 in 2008. In 2010, up to 65 million people nationwide have received the HI card (a form of social insurance). Currently, this scheme is operating smoothly across 64 provinces and cities nationwide. It has significantly reduced the financial burden of disease treatment on impoverished groups and narrowed the gap in access to healthcare services.

(4) Health Insurance Fund Management in Vietnam

1. Fundraising The Vietnam Social Insurance (VSI) fund is mainly made up of employer contributions, government allocation, investment income, and charitable donations. With the expanding insurance coverage and increasing minimum wage, the premium contribution and accumulated amount of the VSI fund have been increasing continuously in Vietnam. The average growth rate of the VSI fund from 2003 to 2006 was 26.33%. See Figure 18.8.

2. Reimbursement The reimbursement of health insurance funds in Vietnam utilizes the pay-as-you-go (PAYGO) system, which ties the premium contribution to the reimbursement level, and allows the premium contribution to be adjusted based on the minimum

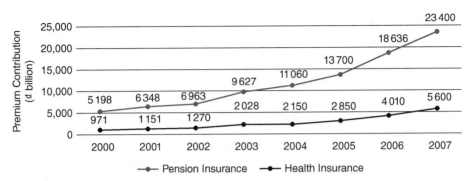

FIGURE 18.8   Pension insurance and health insurance contributions in Vietnam from 2000 to 2007. *Source*: Compiled from VSS (Vietnam Social Security) announcements.

wage and consumer price index (CPI). The increasing number of VSI beneficiaries and the level of minimum wage have led to the continuous increase in fund expenditures.

3. Capital Operation   The VSI fund has mainly been invested in banks and government bonds; for example, according to data published by the VSS in 2007, 41.37% of the fund has been invested in commercial banks, 18.24% in state finance, 23.05% in government bonds, 15.85% in development banks, and 1.48% in others.

The revenue of the VSI fund increased from ₫824.16 billion in 2000 to ₫4081 billion in 2006, with an average annual growth rate of only 7.58%. However, the VSI fund has spent a considerable amount on management costs, which accounted for 3.59% of its revenue in 2006, and 4% in subsequent years. It is difficult for the VSI fund to maintain its long-term, stable development after the deduction of management costs and financial losses due to CPI increases (which grew by 6.9% and 12% in 2006 and 2007, respectively) from its investment income. It is estimated that the fund's expenditures will exceed its income by 2020 (Table 18.18).

4. Health System Reforms and Evaluation

(1) Evaluating the Implementation and Effects of the Policy on Partial Hospital Fees

In 1994, the government issued a decree on hospital fees, which was subsequently implemented in 1995. Under this decree, hospital fees are priced according to the actual situation of each province and healthcare institution. This policy on partial hospital fees has reaffirmed the socialized guidelines that enable the diversification of healthcare activities and the mobilization of people's contributions to healthcare. Similar to health insurance, hospital fees play an important role in determining healthcare expenditure. Hence, this policy has also reduced the financial burden placed on the government. Hospital fees (including the reimbursement made by health insurance) account for 40% of the total hospital expenditure and about 14% of the total healthcare expenditure. In addition, charging hospital fees allows healthcare institutions to set aside government subsidies for the provision of free healthcare services to VSI target groups, such as impoverished groups, ethnic minorities, and critically ill patients who require long-term treatment, in order to reduce their financial burden (Table 18.19).

TABLE 18.18 Expenditure of the Vsi Fund from 2000 to 2008

Year	2000	2001	2002	2003	2004	2005	2006	2007	2008
Total expenditure (đ million)	1,335	1,936	2,572	3,972	4,865	6,759	10,780	14,465	21,360
Total income (đ million)	5,196	6,347	6,962	11,480	13,238	17,195	23,573	27,594	30,939
Growth rate of expenditure (%)	42.00	44.99	36.94	47.42	28.32	38.92	59.48	34.18	47.66
Expenditure/total income (%)	25.69	30.50	36.94	33.03	36.75	39.39	45.73	52.42	69.03
Income/expenditure (annual)	3.89	3.28	2.71	3.03	2.72	2.54	2.19	2.08	1.98

Source: Compiled data from VSS Announcements.

TABLE 18.19 Composition of Hospital Income Sources in Vietnam from 1998 to 2003

Year	Total Income (đ Billion)	Government Budget (đ Billion)	Hospital Fees and Health Insurance		
			Hospital Fees (đ Billion)	Health Insurance (đ Billion)	Share of Total Income (%)
1998	2,720	1,450	703	567	46.7
1999	2,940	1,560	828	552	46.9
2000	3,560	1,990	727	843	44.1
2001	3,910	2,220	877	813	43.3
2002	4,420	2,540	941	939	42.5
2003	5,100	2,900	1,050	1,150	43.1

Source: The MOH of Vietnam (2004).

(2) Evaluation of Decree No. 58/1998 on CHI and VHI

1. Implementation of CHI and VHI In 1998, the government issued Decree No. 58, which introduced the CHI and VHI. Health insurance provides an extremely important source of direct funding for medical examinations and treatments, which in turn is conducive to protecting population health and improving healthcare institutions, particularly community hospitals. However, health insurance in Vietnam is still unable to meet its healthcare demands or achieve sufficient coverage for compulsory insurance. There have been numerous difficulties in encouraging participation in compulsory insurance. Much like hospital fees, health insurance plays an important role in the socialization and diversification of healthcare services, as both help increase the income of the healthcare sector and reduce the financial burden on the government. Moreover, health insurance is the embodiment of the moral and spiritual value of mutual aid in Vietnam, enhancing the people's sense of mutual responsibility by enabling them to support each other through difficult times via mutual care.

At the end of 2007, Vietnam introduced the VHI, which increased the public's opportunity to participate in health insurance by revoking the following previous provisions: that an insurance scheme must be purchased for all members of a family; at least 10% of households in each block or township must participate in the scheme; at least 10% of students in each school must participate in a scheme; and the scheme must be introduced by the local government and accepted by the national health insurance fund agent. The decree requires urban residents, rural residents, urban students, and rural students to pay đ320,000, đ240,000, đ120,000, and đ100,000 as their annual premium contributions, respectively. The Vietnamese government also allocates đ800 billion per one million people each year (initially đ900,000 per person each year) to subsidize their health insurance premiums.

The Health Insurance Law was implemented on July 1, 2009, and its applicability was expanded to 25 different population groups in Vietnam, including disabled individuals and AIDS patients. According to this law, the government must allocate a budget to fully subsidize the insurance premiums of economically disadvantaged groups, children under six years of age, and beneficiaries of the national care policy, as well as to partially subsidize the insurance premiums of low-income households and students (university and secondary school students). Furthermore, all participants of health insurance schemes are given access to the highest quality services that can be provided by the healthcare community, including advanced diagnostic equipment, disease prevention, and functional rehabilitation.

However, this law could only be implemented progressively because of the lack of implementation rules. For example, the law was only implemented for secondary school and university students on January 1, 2010; residents engaged in agriculture, forestry, fisheries, and salt production since January 1, 2012; dependent children of insured persons (employees), members of industrial cooperative societies, and self-employed households since January 2014; and other groups since July 1, 2009. Furthermore, the law also expanded the use of HI cards for children under six years of age (who previously used free health cards), which allow the full reimbursement of medical expenses. According to the implementation process of the Health Insurance Law, health insurance schemes had covered 87.5% of Vietnamese by the end of 2018.

2. Basic Items of the CHI and VHI The Health Insurance Law stipulates that health insurance schemes must either fully reimburse or share the medical expenses incurred by patients seeking medical attention at registered healthcare institutions or specialist departments. Medical expenses incurred by retirees, disability allowance recipients, ethnic minorities, and economically disadvantaged groups are entitled to 95% reimbursement from the health insurance fund, while all other groups are entitled to 80% reimbursement. In addition, HI cardholders can only register in public healthcare institutions, private hospitals, and private polyclinics at the district or township (ward) level for their first visits. The registration of cardholders in provincial (municipal) and central hospitals for their first visit must be approved by the MOH. In 2010, health insurance premiums were raised to 4.5% (from 3%) of the personal income of Vietnamese residents. It is expected that, after July 1, 2010, the primary healthcare institutions will be overwhelmed by millions of township residents who are required to return from provincial and municipal public hospitals (especially in Ho Chi Minh City and Hanoi), where they initially registered for their first visit, to healthcare institutions in their hometowns or the areas in which they are employed (except as otherwise specified by MOH).

As of the first quarter of 2009, more than 3 million residents in Ho Chi Minh City were enrolled in health insurance (including employees of state-owned enterprises, employees of foreign-invested enterprises, military personnel, civil servants, teachers, and the general public who purchased VHI schemes) and had registered for their first visit in one of 100 local healthcare institutions. Among them, approximately 1.4 million residents had registered in local public hospitals across 24 districts; approximately 1.3 million residents had registered in 16 municipal public hospitals; and about 370,000 residents had registered in private polyclinics, private hospitals, and government-affiliated health stations. However, none of these residents had registered in ward health stations (*tram y tế phường*) or commune health stations (*tram y tế xã*). It remains unclear how many residents need to return to their hometowns for registration, as the government has not yet issued implementation rules for the Health Insurance Law and the MOH has not yet established the criteria for registering in provincial and municipal healthcare institutions.

The Social Insurance Agency of Ho Chi Minh City reported that only a handful of residents were willing to register for their first visits in ward and commune health stations, and there was a rush to register in urban public hospitals across 24 districts after the Health Insurance Law came into effect. In early 2009, the Social Insurance Agency conducted a survey and found that the maximum number of HI cardholders that can be admitted to those healthcare institutions was 2.1 million (equivalent to an increase of 705,100 patients).

Health insurance coverage has increased continuously over the past few years: in 1993, health insurance schemes covered only 5.3% of the total population, which increased to 16.5% in 2002 and 18.5% (equivalent to 14.8 million people) in 2003. Data from the Vietnam Health Insurance Agency showed that as of the end of 2004, there were 17.5 million insured persons (includes CHI and VHI), accounting for 22% of the total population; by 2006, this had increased to 35 million insured persons (25 million CHI-insured persons and 10 million VHI-insured persons), accounting for 40% of the total population. During that same period, the income from health insurance increased rapidly.

Both CHI and VHI schemes have not only expanded their coverage but also begun to target impoverished and socially disadvantaged groups. This has afforded many benefits to both providers and users of healthcare services. Specifically, these health insurance schemes protect patients from being overwhelmed by medical expenses when they are unable to work or have a normal life owing to illness. The schemes have also prevented individuals who are close to the poverty line from falling below that line due to a terminal or critical illness. The health insurance premiums of these schemes are much lower than are the medical fees charged by hospitals. As a result, patients and their families no longer need to single out affordable healthcare services and can have greater access to better specialist treatment. As for service providers (hospitals), the greatest benefit to them is that physicians, who provide healthcare services, can focus on examining patients and selecting the most effective treatments for them rather than whether they can afford their medical expenses. In other words, the physician–patient relationship is not adversely affected by financial or economic factors. Hence, physicians can employ the most suitable treatments for their patients. The health insurance premiums collected by the MOH can be reinvested in the purchase of medical supplies, equipment, and high-end technologies in order to deliver better healthcare services to the public.

The existence of third-party payers (health insurance companies) has prevented the MOH from serving as both the main provider and user of health services, thereby creating a fairer competitive environment that is financially beneficial to healthcare institutions. The government has also reduced the amount of subsidies given to healthcare institutions and has gradually shifted towards providing direct subsidies to healthcare users in the form of "subsidized outputs."

3. Problems Facing the CHI and VHI

1. Under the current regulations, health insurance schemes cannot attract the participation of the private sector. This can be attributed to not only the characteristics of these schemes but also the personal health examinations and treatments they cover. It may also be attributed to the fact that health insurance is still a heavy financial burden. Hence, private sector enterprises that contract with health insurance agencies must pay higher medical expenses than public sector institutions. Private sector enterprises also believe that the insurance reimbursement rate is too low to fully cover medical expenses incurred by patients or other charges incurred during medical examinations and treatments. Therefore, it is easy to understand why the private sector is reluctant to participate in health insurance schemes.

2. The CHI and VHI schemes have also failed to attract a sufficient number of insured persons because of their premium and reimbursement systems. Impoverished individuals are unable to afford the health insurance premiums, as premiums are the same across all regions, regardless of whether the regions are wealthy or poor. There is also a lack of trust in health insurance among people who can afford the premiums, as making direct payments is more effective than using health insurance when they seek medical attention. Thus, they do not believe that they need health insurance, as most do not require public

healthcare services when they are healthy and many do not benefit from healthcare insurance even after falling ill. People who live in poverty, on the other hand, may not be aware of their own interest in health insurance because of the lack of information and are generally unable to afford the insurance premiums. As a result, these individuals are also not interested in health insurance, leading them to have a much lower enrollment rate in health insurance than wealthier individuals: only 6% of the poorest 20% of Vietnamese have health insurance, whereas 29% of the richest 20% of Vietnamese do. Furthermore, the poorest population group accounts for only 8% of the total number of insured persons, while the richest group accounts for 37% (Figure 18.9).

3. Health insurance premiums are lower than the expenses for medical examinations and treatments. This is partly due to the regulations on hospital fees, including the health insurance premiums paid by various sectors.

4. There are too few reimbursable drugs and tests available under the CHI and VHI. The schemes reimburse only basic medical tests and not advanced medical tests. As for drug expenses, the schemes only reimburse listed essential medicines. However, the treatment of some diseases, particularly special diseases, often requires special drugs, but which are nonreimbursable under these health insurance schemes.

5. Due to their current approaches, the CHI and VHI have largely failed to serve their redistributive functions between wealthy and poor provinces. There tend to be very few insured residents in poor provinces and many insured residents in wealthy provinces, thereby allowing healthcare institutions to increase their incomes. Therefore, the goal of achieving mutual support between poor and wealthy groups has been hindered by geographical barriers. The amount of health insurance funds estimated by the National Health Support Project has also shown similar results: insured persons were found to be mainly concentrated in major cities (29%), while those living in the Mekong Delta and mountainous provinces accounted for only 10% and 11%, respectively. Health insurance schemes that can only cover a certain group of people are likely to widen the inequalities between poor and wealthy groups, as well as between poor and wealthy provinces. Therefore, the health insurance schemes must adjust the subsidies allocated to each region, in order to ensure equality.

6. The lack of knowledge and understanding of health insurance is also one of the main factors hindering growth in the number of insured persons. There are many people who do not know what health insurance is, how it is purchased, and what its benefits are (Table 18.20).

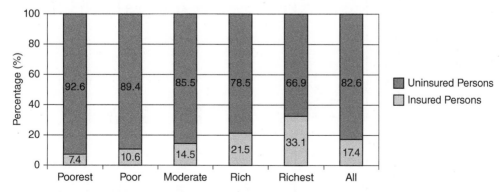

FIGURE 18.9 Distribution of health insurance coverage among different income groups in Vietnam in 2002. *Source*: VSI National Health Survey 2002.

TABLE 18.20 VSI Survey on the Reasons for not Participating in Health Insurance Among Vietnamese Residents (Unit: %)

Item	Reasons for not Participating in Health Insurance						
	Lack of Knowledge About Health Insurance	Economic Factors	Residents Do Not Know Where to Buy Health Insurance	Residents Are Healthy and Do Not Feel the Need to Buy Health Insurance	Poor Public Healthcare Services	Others	Total
Overall	57.3	10.4	25.2	3.1	1.0	3.2	100
Income							
Poorest	71.8	10.7	14.6	0.8	0.2	1.9	100
Poor	58.0	13.4	23.0	2.3	0.7	2.7	100
Moderate	53.5	11.7	27.3	3.4	0.9	3.2	100
Rich	52.3	8.9	29.8	4.0	1.1	4.0	100
Richest	45.7	5.3	35.6	5.9	2.5	5.0	100
Areas							
Urban	45.4	9.1	33.0	5.3	2.1	5.1	100
Rural	59.7	10.6	23.6	0.7	0.7	2.8	100

Source: 2002 VSI Social Survey.

7. Maintaining a financial balance is the main challenge facing health insurance in Vietnam. In 2006, the health insurance deficit had reached đ1.5 trillion, which prompted the government to supply temporary funds; by 2007, these funds were insufficient. Without an appropriate solution, this may eventually lead to a serious financial crisis (Table 18.21).

(3) Decision No. 139/QD-TTg for Impoverished Individuals and Its Evaluation

Decision No. 139/QD-TTg (hereinafter referred to as "Decision 139"), issued by the Vietnamese Prime Minister in 2002, is a milestone in policymaking on medical examinations and treatments for impoverished individuals. In fact, Decision 139 was drafted as part of the government's new vision of healthcare for impoverished individuals. Under this decision, the MOH no longer provides subsidies but is permitted to spend the funds on healthcare for beneficiaries, especially impoverished individuals. Specifically, Decision 139 benefits impoverished individuals in the following two ways: (1) greater access to public healthcare services, and (2) reduced financial burden on hospitals. In addition, this Decision allowed provincial governments to establish healthcare funds to provide financial assistance for the examination and treatment expenses incurred by impoverished individuals in public healthcare institutions. Decision 139 also increased the efficiency and responsibility of provincial governments in funding and providing public healthcare services, thereby reducing the financial pressure of provincial governments while increasing the demand for higher quality public healthcare services. For these reasons, Decision 139 was supported by both the local governments and citizens of Vietnam. Healthcare funds have been established in all centrally controlled provinces and cities to cover the examination and treatment expenses incurred by impoverished individuals in public healthcare institutions. These subsidies take the form of issuing HI cards that cover đ70,000 per person per year and reimbursing the actual examination and treatment expenses incurred by impoverished patients. CHI beneficiaries must pay 20% of their medical expenses (this copayment mechanism was revised in 2005), while impoverished patients with HI cards are exempt from paying their medical charges. About 75% of the budget for medical examinations and treatments comes from the government, whereas the remaining 25% comes from international organizations, donors, charitable organizations, and local and foreign NGOs.

1. *Positive outcomes.* As numerous impoverished individuals receive examinations and treatments in provincial hospitals, Decision 139 has made effective contributions to the healthcare of impoverished individuals, thereby ensuring greater healthcare and social equality, as well as greater political stability. In 2003, the MOH reported that 11 million Vietnamese benefited from Decision 139, which accounts for 77% of the

TABLE 18.21 Financial Comparison of Vietnamese Health Insurance Funds in 2006

Type of Health Insurance	Number of Insured Persons	Insurance Expenditure (đ per person per year)	Deficit in 2006 (đ billion)
VHI	10,000,000	120,000–160,000	900
CHI	24,500,000	300,000–500,000	600

Source: VSI (2006).

total number of beneficiaries. Among them, 25% of beneficiaries had HI cards, and 52% received insurance reimbursements for actual medical expenses. In 2004, the Vietnamese government invested an additional đ64.6 billion in healthcare, in order to improve the healthcare status of more than 13 million impoverished individuals. The MOH of Vietnam reported that the government spent đ11.5 billion in the first half of 2004 to purchase health insurance for more than 3 million impoverished individuals (this amount accounted for 18% of the total funds allocated by the Vietnamese government to improve the healthcare status of impoverished individuals). In addition, the Vietnamese government has spent đ14.5 billion on reimbursing the actual medical expenses of more than 7.6 million Vietnamese, which accounted for 23% of the funds allocated by the Vietnamese government to improve the healthcare status of impoverished individuals. Overall, the implementation of Decision 139 has improved the share of investment in healthcare at the communal and provincial levels, thereby promoting the establishment of healthcare networks and improving the quality of basic healthcare services.

2. *There are still many shortcomings that must be overcome.* The approach adopted by Decision 139 for improving the healthcare status of impoverished individuals is not a one-size-fits-all approach. That is, in some provinces, Decision 139 is implemented by reimbursing impoverished individuals for their actual medical expenses, and in other provinces, it is implemented by purchasing HI cards for these individuals, while both approaches are employed in some provinces. However, the reimbursement amount for actual medical expenses is quite low, and basic health insurance does not cover all medical expenses incurred by impoverished individuals during the examination and treatment process. It can also be difficult to reimburse actual medical expenses in central hospitals because of the complicated reimbursement process, with its numerous terms and conditions. It can also be difficult to ensure that government funding is allocated to those most in need of it. For instance, the current definition of "impoverished population" was proposed by the Ministry of Labor, but the definition of impoverished population under Decision 139 was created by the Ministry of Social Affairs. As a result, there might be lengthy delays in truly identifying "disadvantaged households" when providing reimbursements. The financial allocation for reimbursing examination and treatment expenses incurred by impoverished individuals remains inadequate. This is because many provinces had only established their own healthcare funds at the end of 2003 (one year before Decision 139 was passed). In addition, healthcare funds continue to have a very limited number of funding sources. Information asymmetry has also hindered numerous impoverished individuals from understanding the status of healthcare funds in Vietnam, which is another reason for their low utilization rates. Moreover, the cross-sectorial collaboration presented another major difficulty during the process of implementing Decision 139. This is because the decision was implemented by a single healthcare institution in many provinces, which meant that the collaboration among individual sectors was especially crucial. Finally, Decision 139 only describes the healthcare for individuals who are close to but not yet below the poverty line, although this group of people is also in great need of healthcare funds.

3. *Currently, two approaches have been employed to help solve the healthcare issues in Vietnam.* Two years after the implementation of Decision 139 (which provides medical assistance to impoverished individuals), the MOH reported that numerous provincial governments preferred the direct reimbursement of medical expenses over the purchase of health insurance. However, both approaches have their advantages and disadvantages.

(1) The direct reimbursement of medical expenses has been selected by many provincial governments due to the following advantages: (i) there are numerous provincial health insurance schemes that do not provide health coverage at the communal level (particularly in some remote mountainous areas), which makes direct reimbursement of medical expenses significantly more advantageous; (ii) the direct reimbursement of medical expenses is more feasible because the government is unable to purchase health insurance on behalf of all residents; (iii) each province has a wide variety of health insurance beneficiaries, which presents numerous obstacles to the full implementation of health insurance. However, the direct reimbursement of medical expenses also has several shortcomings: (i) it is difficult to set the eligibility criteria for beneficiaries under this approach in many provinces. As a result, there are a large number of residents who are in great need of direct reimbursement but who fall beyond the coverage scope of Decision 139; (ii) there are numerous obstacles to the direct reimbursement of medical expenses in central hospitals; (iii) it is difficult to determine the reimbursement amount of medical expenses and the utilization of healthcare funds, as a large-scale institution is needed to administer the use of healthcare funds; (iv) impoverished individuals often find the reimbursement procedure too complicated; (v) impoverished individuals are unsure of their right to access health insurance benefits, as many provinces only issue proofs of medical examination instead of HI cards. (2) Some provincial governments purchase HI cards for impoverished individuals for the following reasons: (i) HI cards can increase the confidence of impoverished individuals in the health insurance scheme and make them feel more privileged, as they are distinguished from other "ordinary" patients. Therefore, they have more opportunities and conditions to access healthcare services; (ii) impoverished individuals are generally more concerned about their status as beneficiaries of health insurance; hence, having health insurance will enable them to receive all tiers of healthcare services more smoothly; (iii) when seeking medical treatment in central hospitals, health insurance is more convenient than the direct reimbursement of medical expenses; (iv) currently, each of Vietnam's provinces has a comprehensive health insurance system that gives beneficiaries equal access to healthcare services, which helps to reduce the financial burden on healthcare funds; (v) local governments first determine the eligibility of each beneficiary before issuing HI cards to ensure fair and error-free financial allocation; (vi) the remaining balance in HI cards is brought forward for the following year instead of being used for other purposes. However, there are also many problems with the use of HI cards: (i) it is impossible for such health insurance to cover all urban and rural areas, especially in mountainous areas, remote areas, and some special areas, which is why many local governments select the direct reimbursement of medical expenses; (ii) it is extremely difficult to identify eligible health insurance beneficiaries and issue HI cards to all residents; (iii) the amount insured is very low (đ60,000–đ80,000 per person per year); (iv) it is still difficult for those residing in mountainous areas, remote areas, and some special areas to keep and carry their HI cards.

An overall comparison of the advantages and disadvantages of the two approaches adopted by the Vietnamese government to improve the health status of impoverished individuals indicates that health insurance better meets the requirement of socioeconomic development and generally outperforms the direct reimbursement of medical expenses. Furthermore, it enables more effective management of healthcare institutions and healthcare finances. Therefore, it may be necessary for the government to replace the direct reimbursement system with the health insurance system gradually over a long period of time. In addition, one of the strategic goals of the Vietnamese government is to achieve universal health coverage by 2010.

 ## SECTION V. HEALTH SYSTEM IN THE PHILIPPINES

1. Overview of Socioeconomics and National Health

The Philippines, officially the Republic of the Philippines, is an archipelagic country in Southeast Asia. It is situated in the western Pacific Ocean, facing Taiwan to the north, across the Bashi Channel; Indonesia to the south, across the Celebes Sea; Vietnam to the west, across the South China Sea; and is bounded by the Philippine Sea to the east. It consists of 7,107 islands, covering a total area of 299,700 km². The northern region of the Philippines has a tropical maritime climate, while the southern region has a tropical rainforest climate. Hence, it is usually hot, humid, and high in precipitation. The Philippines has rainy summer and autumn seasons, and the northern region of Visayas is prone to typhoons. The annual average temperature of the Philippines is 27°C, with an annual precipitation of 2,000–3,000 mm. The Philippines has a high forest cover, accounting for more than 40% of the country's total land area. The Philippines is divided into three main geographical areas: Luzon, Visayas, and Mindanao. As of April 2018, the Philippines comprise 18 regions. The Philippines is a major member of the Association of Southeast Asian Nations (ASEAN) and one of the 21 member-states of the Asian-Pacific Economic Cooperation (APEC). As of the end of 2018, the Philippines had a population of around 106.65 million. The Philippines has one of the fastest-growing populations worldwide, having an annual population growth rate of 1.6% from 2010 to 2019. In terms of the age distribution, children aged under 15 years and elderly adults aged over 60 years account for 31% and 5% of the total population, respectively. The urban population accounts for 49% of the total population. The ethnic majority of the Philippines is Malays, including Tagalogs, Ilocano, Kapampangan, Visayas, and Bikol, who account for more than 85% of the total population. It also contains several ethnic minorities and foreign descendants, such as the Chinese, Arabs, Indians, Spanish, and Americans, as well as a large number of indigenous peoples. More than 70 languages are spoken in the Philippines, among which Tagalog-based Filipino is considered the national language, while English is also an official language. The Philippines has a long history of colonization. It was ruled by Spain for more than 350 years (1542–1899), followed by the US, which ruled for nearly 50 years (1899–1946). It was taken over by Japan during World War II and gained independence from Japanese rule after the war. Under the influence of colonialism, the Philippines became the main Christian hub in Asia, with 90% of Filipinos practicing Christianity (80% of Filipinos practice Catholicism), thus accounting for nearly 60% of the Christian population in Asia.

The Philippines is a low-middle income country. World Bank statistics show that that the GDP of the Philippines in 2012 was US$250.2 billion, with an annual GDP growth rate of 6.3%. The gross national income (GNI) of the Philippines was US$2,470. In 2009, 26.5% of the population of the Philippines lived below the poverty line. Using 2009 as an example, the country's GDP was ₱7669.144 billion and the total healthcare expenditure accounted for 3.6% of its GDP.

The 2013 HDI Report revealed that the HDI of the Philippines was 0.654, ranking it 114th among the 187 countries in the world, which indicates a moderate HDI.

The WHO World Health Statistics 2012 showed that in 2009, the average life expectancy of the Philippines was 70.0 years (male: 67 years; female: 73 years), while the infant and under-five mortality rates in 2010 were 23 and 27 deaths per 1,000 live births. In 2008, the mortality rates of communicable diseases, chronic noncommunicable diseases, and injuries in the Philippines were 231 deaths per 100,000 people, 599 deaths per 100,000 people, and 55 deaths per 100,000 people, respectively.

In general, the overall health status of Filipinos has greatly improved over the past 20 years. From 1990 to 2010, the under-five and maternal mortality rates in the Philippines declined at annual rates of 29% and 99%, respectively. Moreover, the annual reduction rates in the percentage of the population without potable water and healthcare services were 8% and 26%, respectively. From 2000 to 2009, the annual reduction rates of HIV and TB were 9.5% and 275%, respectively.

However, the Philippines has relatively poor healthcare equality. Data in 2008 showed that there were significant differences between the highest and lowest wealth quintiles in the under-five mortality rate (17 per 1,000 live births vs. 59 per 1,000 live births), antenatal care coverage (93% vs. 61%), and professional birth delivery rate (94% vs. 26%).

2. Healthcare System

(1) Organization and Supervision of Healthcare Services

The Department of Health (DOH) of the Philippines is a national healthcare policymaker and regulatory agency, which gives it comprehensive technical authority over healthcare. The DOH is mainly responsible for: (1) health guidance; (2) health promotion and capacity building; (3) and providing specific services as an administrator. In other words, the DOH is responsible for formulating national plans, healthcare technical standards, and guidelines. In addition to overseeing healthcare services and products provided by healthcare institutions, the DOH also serves as a special tertiary healthcare provider, technical assistance provider, and stakeholder.

(2) Provision of Healthcare Services

The healthcare system of the Philippines comprises two major entities: public and private healthcare institutions. The healthcare system is dominated by the latter, particularly in urban areas, whereas healthcare institutions in rural areas are mainly run by the government. The government pays public hospitals via budgets while also allowing them to earn additional income by providing healthcare services. However, the service fees charged by physicians are not tied to their workloads, as the total service income is managed and evenly distributed by the hospital. Physicians are remunerated for their services based on salaries. Public hospitals usually charge lower medical fees than private for-profit hospitals. The Philippine General Hospital is the most representative public hospital in the Philippines. In addition to for-profit hospitals, private healthcare institutions include a large number of charitable healthcare institutions that usually provide healthcare services to impoverished individuals for free or for a very small voluntary payment. The Chinese community in the Philippines has organized numerous charitable healthcare institutions to provide medical assistance for those living in poverty.

(3) Accreditation of Healthcare Institutions and Distribution of Hospital Beds

Healthcare providers are accredited and regulated by the DOH, but the Philippine Health Insurance Corporation (PhilHealth) has also established an independent accreditation procedure for healthcare institutions. The total number of accredited beds in public hospitals is larger than that in private hospitals, but private hospitals have the majority of PhilHealth-accredited beds.

1. DOH-Accredited Healthcare Institutions and Hospital Beds Table 18.22 shows the number of DOH-licensed hospitals in the Philippines, among which private hospitals account for two-thirds and primary hospitals (i.e., relatively small-sized primary hospitals) account for half of the total number of DOH-licensed hospitals.

Public hospitals account for more than half of the total number of DOH-accredited hospital beds (Table 18.23). Among these hospitals, 54% of DOH-accredited beds are provided by tertiary referral hospitals. More than one-third of DOH-accredited beds are located in public hospitals in the capital area, whereas only 27% of DOH-accredited beds are in private hospitals in the capital area.

Primary public healthcare services are provided by Rural Health Units (RHUs), which are also accredited by the DOH and given the Sentrong Sigla stamp as a sign of valid certification.

Following the enactment of the Local Government Code (LGC) in 1991, the ownership of RHUs was delegated to local chief executives as part of the decentralization process.

2. PhilHealth-Accredited Healthcare Institutions and Hospital Beds In addition to DOH accreditation, PhilHealth has established its own independent accreditation procedure. Under this procedure, hospitals are also classified into primary, secondary, and tertiary hospitals. Table 18.24 shows the number of PhilHealth-accredited hospitals in 2005, categorized according to ownership and tier.

The data clearly indicate that secondary hospitals seem to be overloaded. Currently, PhilHealth does not control the quantity or structure of hospital accreditation. As a result, all hospitals that meet certain basic standards are eligible for accreditation.

PhilHealth-accredited beds are predominantly found in private hospitals (55.1%), whereas DOH-accredited beds are mainly found in public hospitals (53.2%). PhilHealth has also accredited 18 teaching hospitals and a number of mobile surgical clinics that can perform outpatient surgeries (Table 18.25).

In 2000, PhilHealth began accrediting RHUs after the implementation of the outpatient consultation and diagnostic package (OCDP), which applies only to impoverished individuals and subsidized items. PhilHealth pays local government units (LGUs) to provide the OCDP at ₱300 per participant. However, currently, there are still no PhilHealth-accredited private hospitals at the primary healthcare level. By the end of 2004, PhilHealth had accredited a total of 749 RHUs to provide the OCDP.

In addition to the OCDP, PhilHealth has launched several other services in recent years, such as the maternal service packages (e.g., normal spontaneous deliveries) and TB-DOTS packages. PhilHealth has also established a new accreditation procedure, whereby hospitals must provide these new service packages. This represents a strategic

TABLE 18.22 Number of DOH-Accredited Hospitals in the Philippines in 2003 (Unit: Hospitals)

DOH-Accredited Hospitals	Primary Hospitals	Secondary Hospitals	Tertiary Hospitals	Total
Public hospitals	327	250	82	659
Private hospitals	465	377	164	1006
Total	792	627	246	1665

Note: Hospitals are categorized according to ownership and tier.
Source: Data retrieved from the official website of the Philippine DOH.

TABLE 18.23 Number of DOH-Accredited Hospital Beds in the Philippines in 2003 (Unit: Beds)

DOH-Accredited Hospital Beds	Primary Hospitals	Secondary Hospitals	Tertiary Hospitals	Total
Public hospitals	6,775	14,261	24,242	45,258
Private hospitals	6,428	11,328	21,293	39,049
Total	13,183	25,589	45,535	84,307

Note: Hospitals are categorized according to ownership and tier.
Source: Data retrieved from the official website of the Philippine DOH.

shift by PhilHealth – from focusing only on the reimbursement of inpatient expenses to improving the health status of insured persons and the quality of preventive services, in order to avoid the need for expensive inpatient services. This shift has changed the behavior of healthcare providers, who now attach greater importance to preventive services. However, these services overlap with the public health and primary healthcare services provided by the DOH, and the healthcare investments made by the DOH has increased; for instance, the capital injection in 2002 was more than three times that of PhilHealth subsidies (Table 18.26).

In 2005, PhilHealth performed its first review of the accreditation of all three tiers of hospitals. This re-accreditation process was relatively lax compared to the initial accreditation, which was pass/fail. For previously accredited healthcare institutions that failed to meet certain requirements for contract renewal (e.g., the lack of facilities for specific functions), PhilHealth issued temporary accreditations and permitted them to reapply for contract renewal. As for institutions that did not meet its criteria for healthcare workers, PhilHealth reduced the number of approved hospital beds, service volume, and protection level for insured persons.

3. Distribution of Healthcare Workers The DOH is responsible for the registration of healthcare professionals. Physicians, nurses, nursing personnel, midwives, and healthcare administrators can be trained in the Philippines. However, due to the general lack of formal learning and practical training, most of them are unable to practice outside the Philippines, in countries they choose to migrate. Despite the large-scale overseas migration of healthcare technicians from the Philippines, this country still has a higher number of healthcare technicians per capita than do many other countries and areas (Table 18.27).

TABLE 18.24 Number of PhilHealth-Accredited Hospitals in 2005 (Unit: Hospitals)

PhilHealth-Accredited Hospitals	Primary Hospitals	Secondary Hospitals	Tertiary Hospitals	Total
Public hospitals	291	231	80	602
Private hospitals	389	389	178	956
Total	680	620	254	1,558

Note: Hospitals are categorized according to ownership and tier.
Source: Data retrieved from the official website of the Philippine DOH (https://www.doh.gov.ph).

TABLE 18.25 Number of PhilHealth-Accredited Hospital Beds in 2005 (Unit: Beds)

PhilHealth-Accredited Hospitals Beds	Primary Hospitals	Secondary Hospitals	Tertiary Hospitals	Total
Public hospitals	4,213	10,160	17,782	32,155
Private hospitals	4,055	10,753	21,801	36,609
Total	8,268	20,913	39,585	68,764

Note: Hospitals are categorized according to ownership and tier.
Source: Data retrieved from the official website of the Philippine DOH (https://www.doh.gov.ph).

3. Health Security System

(1) Development of Health Security System

The Philippines promulgated the Philippine Medical Care Act (Republic Act No. 6111) on August 4, 1969. At the time, there was no unified form of organization, and the funding sources were diverse, which included government taxes, compulsory insurance, the prospective payment system (PPS), private insurance, and fee-for-service payments. This act mainly targeted formal employees and did not cover impoverished individuals and workers in the informal sector. Furthermore, the insurance schemes established by this act faced a number of issues, including the slow expansion of their coverage over the past two decades, limitation of reimbursements only to inpatient expenses, duplicate management, unreasonable insurance premiums, and service contents that fail meet social needs. Therefore, it became clear that the health insurance system in the Philippines was in dire need of reforms (Table 18.28).

In 1969, the Philippine Medical Care Act was adopted as the basis of the social security system (SSS), which was subsequently amended in 1987 and 1991. In 1995, PhilHealth was established to implement the Philippine National Health Insurance Act (Republic Act No. 7875), with the aim of achieving universal health coverage within 15 years through the principles of mutual aid, equality, rationality, quality assurance, and clear division of responsibilities. PhilHealth, which is affiliated to the DOH, was endowed with certain rights and obligations to implement the content of the Philippine National Health Insurance Act. All previously implemented health insurance schemes were gradually incorporated into the National Health Insurance Act and administered by the state-owned PhilHealth. The National Health Insurance Act stipulates that all Filipinos who can afford the premiums may become insurance beneficiaries, and abolished the eligibility restrictions imposed by the Government Service Insurance System (GSIS) for government employees and the SSS for private sector employees. Moreover, the National Health Insurance Act has also expanded

TABLE 18.26 PhilHealth Accreditation of Providers of New Service Packages in 2004

Healthcare institutions	Providers	Accredited	Pending	Rejected
Maternity health centers	76	74	1	1
TB-DOTS centers	31	29	2	0
Independent dialysis clinics	19	8	1	0

Source: Data retrieved from the official website of the Philippine DOH.

TABLE 18.27 Number of Healthcare Workers in the Philippines in 2010

Healthcare Workers	Total	Number Per 1,000 People
Physicians	93,862	1.15
Nurses and midwives	488,434	6
Pharmacists	49,667	0.61
Dentists	45,903	0.56

Source: Data retrieved from the official website of the Philippine DOH.

the coverage scope of benefits beyond inpatient services. Nevertheless, on top of its role as a purchaser of clinical services, PhilHealth still needs to continue exploring different avenues to promote healthcare development in the Philippines.

In the Philippines, the SSS is a compulsory insurance scheme that requires the participation of all employees. Under this scheme, both insured persons and their dependents are entitled to the most basic health security. In addition, most unemployed persons can participate voluntarily in this scheme. The Philippine National Health Insurance Program (NHIP) is a nonmandatory scheme that employers and employees can join voluntarily.

TABLE 18.28 Development of the National Health Insurance Program in the Philippines

Date	Event
Stage 1	Coverage of formal employees
August 4, 1969	The Philippine Medical Care Act (Republic Act No. 6111)
1972	The Philippine Medical Care Commission was established and a compulsory health insurance program was introduced for formal employees.
1991	Local Government Code (LGC): Service delivery for impoverished groups
Stage 2	Shift to universal health coverage
1995	PhilHealth established to implement the Philippine National Health Insurance Act (Republic Act No. 7875)
1999	The DOH introduced the Health Sector Reform Agenda (HSRA)
October 1999	Implementation of pro-poor programs
July 2000	Implementation of OCDP
December 2001	Implementation of Plan 500 program (for impoverished households)
February 2002	Implementation of relative value scale (RVS) 2001
April 2003	Implementation of TB-DOTS service package
May 2003	Implementation of maternal and SARS service packages
July 2003	Collaboration with other organizations to cover workers of the informal sector
	Accreditation of mobile surgical clinics
February 2004	Plan 5/25 program: Massive increase in coverage of impoverished households

Source: Retrieved from the official website of PhilHealth (http://www.philhealth.gov.ph), 2004.

Insurance coverage has increased steadily since 1972. However, its progress is fairly slow for impoverished individuals and workers of the informal sector. As in other countries, the inclusion of these two groups is extremely crucial for PhilHealth to achieve universal health coverage.

(2) Healthcare Funding

In the Health Sector Reform Agenda (HSRA) issued by the DOH in 1999, healthcare funding is a reform priority and driving force of the PhilHealth.

The total healthcare expenditure of the Philippines accounted for 3.6% of its GDP (₱7669.144 billion) in 2009. Furthermore, the government expenditure on healthcare accounted for 35.1% of the total healthcare expenditure and 7.1% of the fiscal expenditure. From 1998 to 2009, there was a decrease in government expenditure as a share of the total healthcare expenditure compared to private expenditure (Figure 18.10).

In 2009, government expenditure accounted for only 35.1% of the total healthcare expenditure, of which 27.5% was funded via social health insurance. The vast majority of the total healthcare expenditure was borne by the private sector (accounting for 64.9%), of which about 83.6% was from out-of-pocket payments, and 10.6% was from prepaid plans. One of the objectives of the HSRA was to increase the share of PhilHealth reimbursement to 25% of the total healthcare expenditure by 2004; however, this share was only 9% in 2002. PhilHealth reimbursement is also an increasingly important source of government funding, as its share of government expenditure rose from 8.9% in 1998 to 27.5% in 2009 (Table 18.29).

(3) National Health Insurance Program (NHIP)

The NHIP was first implemented in 1972, and the Philippine Medical Care Commission served as its main policymaker, healthcare accreditation department, and arbitrator. The GSIS for employees of state-owned enterprises and SSS for private sector employees were

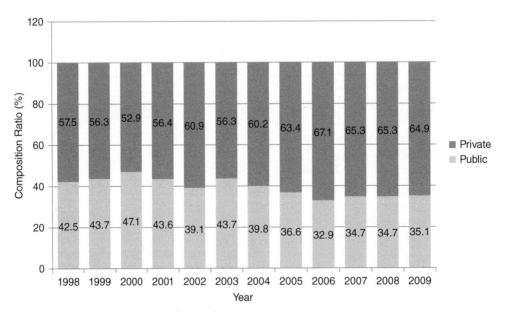

FIGURE 18.10 Funding composition of total healthcare expenditure in the Philippines from 1998 to 2009. *Source*: Data retrieved from the official website of the Philippine DOH.

TABLE 18.29 Composition of Government and Personal Healthcare Expenditures in the Philippines from 2003 to 2009 (Unit: %)

Year	Social Health Insurance as a Share of Government Healthcare Expenditure	Out-of-Pocket Payments as a Share of Personal Healthcare Expenditure	Prepaid Plans as a Share of Personal Healthcare Expenditure
2003	21.8	78.2	10.5
2004	23.8	77.9	12.1
2005	31.6	80.3	10.5
2006	25.8	83.5	9.7
2007	22.3	83.7	9.8
2008	21.7	82.5	12.2
2009	27.5	83.6	10.6

Source: Data retrieved from the official website of the Philippine DOH (https://www.doh.gov.ph).

responsible for the registration, premium collection, and reimbursement of the NHIP. However, these roles and responsibilities were transferred to PhilHealth after the agency was established.

The chairperson for the board of directors of PhilHealth is the Philippine Secretary of Health, and the executive members of PhilHealth are given full autonomy in their operations. PhilHealth must comply with the administrative instructions of the Office of the President, but not with the DOH. PhilHealth can also determine its own salary structure within a certain range and can set aside 12% of all premium income each year for management costs (including salaries). The salaries of the chairperson and CEO of PhilHealth must be approved by the Office of the President. Furthermore, the chairperson and CEO of PhilHealth are responsible for establishing salary caps for the entire organization. PhilHealth has served 80 million Filipinos since its establishment. It aims to provide sustainable, affordable, and progressive social health insurance services to ensure universal access to high-quality healthcare services. PhilHealth is the funding medium to ensure the sustainability of the NHIP, which includes: (1) universal health insurance; (2) ensuring that insured persons can benefit from their affordable premiums; (3) enhancing contact with customers via close partnerships; and (4) providing effective internal information and management systems to improve the quality of healthcare services. The core principle of the NHIP is to achieve social harmony via a mechanism of mutual aid, whereby the poor are supported by the rich, patients are supported by healthy individuals, and the unemployed are supported by the employed. The NHIP aims to comprehensively promote healthcare development so as to ensure that all Filipinos can afford and access basic necessities, healthcare services, and other social services.

1.NHIP Coverage   NHIP coverage has increased steadily since its implementation in 1972. As shown in Figure 18.11, the straight line represents the total Philippine population, and the white area below that line roughly coincides with the proportion of the population who are uninsured. It can be seen from Figure 18.11 that NHIP coverage was initially limited to private sector employees. From 1986 to 1987, the number of NHIP-insured persons declined drastically, while the number of privately insured persons decreased from 2.36 million to 1.62 million. These decreases may have both been due to the regime changes during that period. There are four PhilHealth programs: the regular program for employees, the

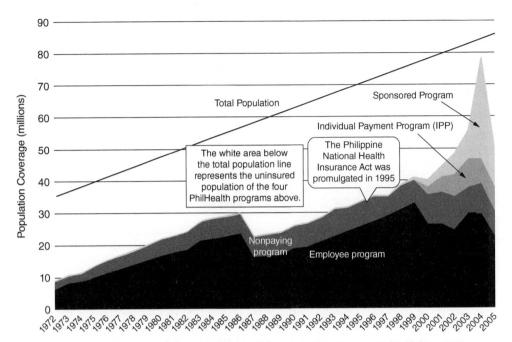

FIGURE 18.11   Number of NHIP-insured persons in the Philippines from 1972 to 2005.
Source: Retrieved from the official website of PhilHealth (http://www.philhealth.gov.ph).

sponsored program for impoverished individuals, the individual payment program (IPP), and the nonpaying program.

1. *Employee Program.* The Implementing Rules and Regulations (IRR) for RA7875 stipulate that: participation in the NHIP is compulsory for all government and private sector employees, including domestic workers and overseas Filipino workers (OFWs). The National Health Insurance Act stipulates that all salaried workers must set aside 2.5% of their monthly salary as insurance contributions, which is shared equally between employers and employees. The monthly salary cap is set at ₱25,000, but this cap has increased significantly in recent years to improve the fairness and equality of healthcare funding.

   Although premiums are automatically deducted from employees' monthly salaries, compliance is still a major issue, particularly in the informal sector. The Office of the Actuary has estimated that about 70% of its target population does not pay their monthly premiums.

   The PhilHealth premiums were raised in 2013. Specifically, the monthly insurance premium increased from ₱100 to ₱150 for self-employed persons, while it increased from ₱50 to ₱87.50 for employees who earn ₱8,000 or less per month. The monthly insurance premium for employees who earned ₱8,001–₱34,999 per month was equivalent to 1.25% of their salaries. Furthermore, the monthly insurance premium for employees who earned ₱35,000 or above per month increased from ₱375 to ₱437.50. The premium contributions of employers increased by an equal amount for all these income levels.

2. *Impoverished/Sponsored Program.* This program was initiated by LGUs to enroll impoverished individuals into PhilHealth as well as to review their eligibility. LGUs pay an annual premium of ₱1,200 on behalf of these individuals, but this amount is subject to change over time and with the level of the LGU. For example, LGUs of Class 4–6 cities need only pay 10% of the annual premium for the first two years, and the remaining balance is borne by the central Department of Budget Management.

During the Philippine national elections of 2004, health coverage for impoverished individuals was a hotly debated issue. After being reelected to office, President Gloria Macapagal Arroyo launched Plan 5/25, which aimed to enroll 5 million households (equivalent to 25 million individuals) into PhilHealth. The resulting expenditure was funded by the Philippine Charity Sweepstakes Office (PCSO) instead of the LGUs. Although largely considered a political show for winning votes, this program was nevertheless successful in increasing the number of insured persons, thereby expanding the coverage to impoverished populations, and became a top priority in the political agenda

However, Plan 5/25 had certain shortcomings. In particular, the variability in the definition of impoverished groups gave rise to certain technical challenges. Since the premiums for the OCDP are shared by LGUs, LGUs receive ₱300 as an OCDP capitation payment for impoverished individuals eligible for the OCDP. However, individuals covered by Plan 5/25 are not entitled to this OCDP capitation payment as there is no cost sharing with LGUs under Plan 5/25. In addition, some LGUs no longer share in the premium contributions because they expect the central government or PCSO to fully cover these expenses.

Although the number of insured impoverished individuals has increased steadily over the years, whether this growth is sustainable in the future remains unclear. Some achievements have been made in the continuous funding of the sponsored program through tobacco taxes, but certain future variables cannot be accounted for, particularly because this program is closely associated with specific politicians and elections.

Another approach being considered by PhilHealth is by deducting the premiums from the share of domestic taxes allocated to LGUs, which is similar to the deduction of annual premiums from the monthly salaries; however, this approach is not politically feasible. A new legislation has been enacted, which stipulates that 4% of the incremental revenue from the value-added tax (VAT) will be earmarked as funds for the sponsored program, and these funds will be used to cover part of the expenditures paid by local governments. However, this special fund only lasted until 2008. From 2005 to 2010, funds from tobacco taxes were earmarked to provide PhilHealth with 2.5% of the incremental revenue from VAT each year (equivalent to about ₱100 million per year), which were used to cover the premiums paid by the corresponding central department for impoverished individuals.

These efforts have had positive effects on the health coverage of impoverished groups. However, the centralization of funds for the sponsored program was relatively slow after the introduction of PCSO funds in 2004, suggesting that local governments were not prioritizing the improvement of PhilHealth coverage for impoverished individuals.

3. *IPP.* Individuals who are not covered by the employee program and sponsored program can join the NHIP voluntarily via the PhilHealth IPP. Broadly speaking, the IPP targets nonimpoverished workers in the informal sector, and charges the same annual

insurance premium as the sponsored program (₱1,200). The International Labor Organization (ILO) estimates that workers in the informal sector account for 50% of the working population in the Philippines.

A major issue facing workers in the informal sector is the payment of insurance premiums on schedule. Although most IPP members pay their premiums on a quarterly basis (i.e., ₱300 every three months), about two-thirds do not pay their premiums on schedule. For example, some might pay their premiums in the first and third quarters of the year, but fail to pay in the second quarter. The variable income of this employment sector has led to unstable funding, intermittent financial protection, and management difficulties among insurers.

PhilHealth is currently considering dividing IPP members into several groups with different premiums, with the aim of getting more able members to pay a higher amount of premiums (it is assumed that there is heterogeneity among IPP members, who would be divided into relatively rich and relatively poor groups).

4. *Nonpaying program.* This program aims to cover retirees who have paid their insurance premiums to PhilHealth for at least 10 years (120 months) according to law. PhilHealth has become increasingly concerned about the financial burden facing this high-risk group, as they do not have any sources for healthcare funding – that is, they do not have to pay any insurance premium and the government does not contribute premiums on their behalf.

In 2004, the proportion of members in the sponsored program rose drastically from 16% to 48%. At the end of 2004, PhilHealth estimated that the NHIP has reached a national coverage of 81%. However, the official figure on NHIP coverage released in September 2005 was only 63%. This could be attributed almost entirely to the reduced enrollment rate among impoverished individuals (Figure 18.12).

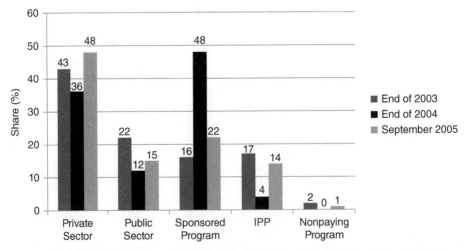

FIGURE 18.12 Changes in the membership of the nonpaying program in the Philippines from 2003 to 2005. *Source*: Data retrieved from the official website of the Philippine DOH (https://www.doh.gov.ph).

2. Insurance Benefits   Most NHIP benefits are mainly associated with inpatient services. The implementing rules and regulations of PhilHealth are:

1. *Inpatient services.* (1) Meals and accommodation; (2) healthcare professionals' fees; (3) fees for prescriptions, diagnostic testing, and other medical examinations; (4) fees for the use of surgical and medical facilities; and (5) prescription drugs.
2. *Outpatient services.* (1) Fees of healthcare professionals; (2) fees for prescriptions, diagnostic testing, and other medical examinations; (3) personal preventive services; and (4) prescription drugs.
3. Health education packages.
4. Emergency care and transportation services.
5. Other appropriate and economical healthcare services provided by insurance companies.

PhilHealth excludes the following services from its benefits packages:

1. The fifth and subsequent childbirths for conventional delivery methods).
2. Nonprescription drugs and equipment.
3. Treatment for alcohol abuse and dependency.
4. Optometry services.
5. Noneconomical services defined by insurance companies.

These benefits are available in all PhilHealth-accredited hospitals nationwide. Furthermore, these benefits have different reimbursement caps depending on the hospital tiers, which in turn have different ward and professional fees, as shown in Table 18.30. Generally speaking, PhilHealth Regional Offices can adjust their benefit packages according to their local areas given that they do not change the total expenditure.

In recent years, PhilHealth has launched several new service packages (Table 18.31), such as the Maternity Care Package (MCP) for normal deliveries introduced in 2003. PhilHealth-accredited providers are entitled to receive ₱4,500 per case, regardless of the length of hospital stay, of which ₱2,000 is allocated to the healthcare workers while the remaining ₱2,500 is allocated to the medical facility, which is expected to cover meals and accommodation, drugs, diagnostic tests, operating theatre expenses, and other basic healthcare services.

In 2003, the PhilHealth also launched the outpatient TB-DOTS benefit package, which provides ₱4,000 per case for accredited DOTS facilities to cover outpatient diagnostic procedures, consultation services, and antituberculosis drugs. After patients have completed the intensive phase of treatment, accredited DOTS facilities are entitled to receive ₱2,500, while the remaining ₱1,500 is paid after the completion of the maintenance phase. In 2003, PhilHealth extended the reimbursement of hemodialysis services to freestanding dialysis centers and launched the SARS package in response to the SARS outbreak, which has a reimbursement cap of ₱50,000 per case.

3. Financial Situation   PhilHealth is currently in good financial shape. It has been legally authorized to retain up to two years of benefit reimbursements as a reserve. In practice, however, PhilHealth has retained far more – in 2004, it had reserved four years of benefit reimbursements. Figure 18.13 shows that, to a certain extent, PhilHealth faces limited risks with regard to benefit reimbursements. The figure also shows that both premiums and reimbursements have increased steadily from 1999 to 2004.

TABLE 18.30   PhilHealth Benefits in 2009 (Unit: ₱)

Benefits	Hospital Tier		
	Primary	Secondary	Tertiary
Meals and accommodation (Not more than 45 days per patient per year)			
Case A	300	400	500
Case B	300	400	500
Case C	–	600	800
Case D	–	–	1,100
Drugs (Inpatient)			
Case A	2,700	3,360	4,200
Case B	9,000	11,200	14,000
Case C	–	22,400	28,000
Case D	–	–	40,000
X-ray and laboratory services (Inpatient)			
Case A	1,600	2,240	3,200
Case B	5000	7,359	10,500
Case C	-	14,700	21,000
Case D	-	–	30,000
Specialist service fees (₱/day)			
Case A			
GPs	300–1,200	300–1,200	300–1,200
Specialist hospitals	500–2,000	500–2,000	500–2,000
Case B			
GPs	400–2,400	400–2,400	400–2,400
Specialist hospitals	600–3,600	600–3,600	600–3,600
Case C			
GPs	–	500–4,000	500–4,000
Specialist hospitals	–	700–5,600	700–5,600
Case D			
GPs	–	–	600–6,000
Specialist hospitals	–	–	800–8,000
Surgical theater		RVU30 and below = 750;	30 and below = 1, 200;
Surgical relative value	500	RVU30–80 = 1,200;	RVU31–80 = 1,500;
Unit (RVU)		RVU81–600 = [2,200, 7 500]	RVU81–600 ≥ 3,500

Note: The statistical data reflects all NHIP members and their dependents.
Source: Retrieved from the official website of PhilHealth (http://www.philhealth.gov.ph).

It is reasonable for PhilHealth to reserve up to four years' worth of premium reimbursements as it is now facing increasing risk due to the introduction of a series of free programs. It is estimated that 25% of premiums are reimbursed to elderly adults aged over 60 and 25% to individuals aged under 20. However, PhilHealth has not published a detailed financial analysis regarding its revenues and expenditures. Nevertheless, the free services paid

TABLE 18.31 PhilHealth Special Benefit Packages

Benefit Packages	Unit	Benefits (₱)
OCDP	Each impoverished member for each LGU	300
MCP	Each case/childbirth	4,500
TB-DOTS	Each case	4,000
SARS package	Each case	50,000

Source: Retrieved from the official website of PhilHealth (http://www.philhealth.gov.ph).

to healthcare providers constitute a large proportion of PhilHealth reimbursements, and therefore might give rise to supplier-induced demand.

Table 18.32 shows the asset status of PhilHealth on March 31, 2005. Most of these assets were derived from long-term government bond investments.

4. Impact of Social Insurance Although the changes in the health status of the overall population or those of the impoverished individuals cannot be solely attributed to this universal health insurance program, we can still discuss the following effects of the NHIP.

1. *The NHIP made healthcare a top political priority.* Through the sponsored program, PhilHealth has put the accessibility of healthcare services to the top of the political agenda, at both the central and local levels. This in turn has facilitated the increase in funding for the health insurance of impoverished groups.
2. *It provides stable funding for the health sector.* In recent years, there have been severe cutbacks in the government budget due to high public debts. However, PhilHealth does not rely on the government budget, and secures much of its healthcare funds via premium

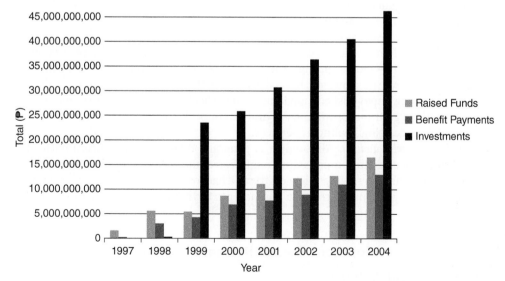

FIGURE 18.13 Analysis of PhilHealth's financial status from 1997 to 2004. *Source:* Retrieved from the official website of PhilHealth (http://www.philhealth.gov.ph).

TABLE 18.32   Financial Statements of PhilHealth from 2004 to 2005 (Unit: ₱)

Item	2004	2005
Short-term investments	11.8 billion	11.7 billion
Short-term government bonds	6.6 billion	10.2 billion
Special savings	5.3 billion	1.5 billion
Ownerships, factories, and facilities	600 million	1.1 billion
Land	500 million	900 million
Long-term investments	30.9 billion	36.9 billion
Long-term government bonds	30.3 billion	36.8 billion

Source: Retrieved from the official website of PhilHealth (http://www.philhealth.gov.ph).

contributions. Although the annual premiums vary with the economic performance of the Philippines, compared to relying only on the government budget, the NHIP has provided a more sustainable, stable and reliable funding source for the provision of healthcare services.

3. *It provides better health information.* PhilHealth has collected information on various disease types and other health-related information from NHIP-insured persons through its claims information system. However, this information is only limited to individuals enrolled in the NHIP. Its database also enables real-time updates, thereby outperforming the conventional database, which was only updated once every several years via periodic data collection, sampling, and surveys.

4. *It has given rise to vibrant public-sector organizations.* As a separate and independent self-regulatory organization, PhilHealth has created vibrant public-sector organizations that are open to new ideas and are testing those ideas. Among the many policy areas that require improvement, PhilHealth has positioned itself effectively within financial and legal frameworks in order to promote healthcare reforms through proper leadership and management.

5. *It has improved healthcare accessibility and financial protection for impoverished individuals.* PhilHealth has improved healthcare accessibility and financial protection for impoverished individuals through the Sponsored Program and the IPP. Its improvements in this area are, however, limited because of the low utilization rate of healthcare services among impoverished individuals. This reflects that indirect costs among these individuals (e.g., transportation costs and out-of-pocket expenses) remain prominent obstacles to accessing healthcare services.

6. *Healthcare service quality.* Although it is generally difficult to measure, PhilHealth's independent accreditation procedure might have improved the quality of healthcare services compared to relying solely on the DOH accreditation procedure. In the future, PhilHealth may also use its role as a purchaser to further promote the quality of healthcare services.

4. Issues and Development Trends in Health System Reforms

(1) Issues in Health Reforms

A World Bank report (World Bank, 2011) revealed several structural problems with the Philippine healthcare system: (1) excessively high drug prices have led to the unreasonable and irrational use of drugs. (2) There is an insufficient financial allocation for the prevention of new diseases, especially chronic noncommunicable diseases. (3) There is an overdependence on tertiary hospital services and underutilization of primary healthcare and specialist outpatient services. (4) The organization of the public hospital system is inefficient. (5) The quality of the health security system is insufficient to prevent low-quality and wastage of healthcare resources.

1. Strategic Issue 1 – Coverage of Informal Sector Workers   It has been predicted that voluntary household enrollment will lead to adverse selection. PhilHealth has strived to prevent such adverse selection, for instance, by limiting irregular annual premiums. The core of its strategy is to incentivize insurance companies (e.g., microfinance and cooperative organizations), to provide IPP to at least 70% of eligible members. It hopes to achieve the following "triple-win" situation.

1. *PhilHealth.* The replacement of individual insurance with group insurance will help prevent adverse selection and reduce the dropout rate, thereby further expanding coverage of the NHIP. PhilHealth also attempted to further reduce the dropout rate by encouraging health insurance agencies to cover those who are eligible to join the IPP. The specific regulations of this approach are as follows. First, insurance agencies will not receive payments if the minimum threshold is met, and the minimum premium will not be implemented. Second, there will be no discount and insurance agencies will not receive any reimbursement if the rate of participation falls below the 70% threshold due to dropout. Under this approach, PhilHealth will benefit from greater administrative efficiency if the eligible insurance agencies have more than 1,000 insured persons.

2. *Insurance agencies.* Insurance agencies are allowed to provide new products to insured persons in order to effectively meet their healthcare demands. In most cases, health insurance agencies hope to charge their insured persons the full premium rate while submitting the discounted amount to PhilHealth. The resulting profit margin can be used to cover the agencies' administrative costs and other flexible expenses. PhilHealth does not set exact specifications for these agencies regarding the use of these funds, but does provide ideas, suggestions, and technical support. Some studies have shown that the bad debt among certain microfinance organizations is mainly due to the expensive inpatient and pharmaceutical expenses incurred by insured patients, which often take priority over repayments. In the future, it is expected that future strategies will be developed to better secure the financial stability of these organizations.

3. *Insured persons.* Previous studies have shown that having a flexible payment system in place is more important than the ₱1,200 premium for workers. The success of the flexible payment system also depends on the extent to which the organization can innovatively design a flexible payment method for insured persons (e.g., weekly payments) and help resolve their difficulties when making payments (e.g., savings plans). PhilHealth targets well-managed insurance agencies with extensive and effective loan repayment systems. Managers of insurance agencies are required to provide PhilHealth with cheaper and more economical services if they introduce discounted premiums.

2. Strategic Issue 2 – Financial Protection   The law stipulates that "all Filipinos shall have access to affordable healthcare services." However, the goal of covering 70% of inpatient expenses has not yet been achieved, and the actual coverage rate is only around 30–45%. In practice, this coverage is highly variable and uncertain. A review of the HSRA in 2002 revealed that with the periodic increase in the reimbursement caps, PhilHealth has been unable to provide estimated support values for its reimbursements (Solon et al., 2002). The problem of determining PhilHealth's actual support value arises from the design of the NHIP, particularly in relation to the following: (1) PhilHealth benefits are designed to cover the "first peso," and (2) providers are allowed to impose additional charges if necessary (or if this can be endured by the market).

In summary, patient expenses, PhilHealth reimbursement caps, and out-of-pocket expenses are highly uncertain, making it difficult to generalize the support value given by PhilHealth. In many cases (e.g., in rural public hospitals), PhilHealth covers all medical expenses, whereas in some cases (e.g., private hospitals in major cities), only a small proportion of the medical expenses are covered and the remaining expenses are borne by the patients. Previous surveys have shown that the support value of PhilHealth was around 62% across the country, of which, the support values of public hospitals and private hospitals were 88% and 53%, respectively. However, this has not been confirmed via further studies.

Poor welfare and financial protection have reduced the value of insurance enrollment, thereby exacerbating the risk of adverse selection and the refusal of low-risk individuals to enroll. Understandably, these factors have increased the pressure on PhilHealth to improve its benefits. However, if the design of the benefit packages and PhilHealth's payment method for providers remain unchanged, these measures will only benefit providers, rather than insured persons.

3. Strategic Issue 3 – The Design of Benefit Packages and Payment Method for Providers A survey carried out in 1991, which studied randomly sampled inpatients from 132 hospitals in the Philippines, demonstrated that private hospitals increased their service prices to obtain greater benefits from PhilHealth (Gertler and Solon, 2000). The study estimated that private hospitals have imposed a 23.4% price markup for insured patients and a 60% price markup for private patients. Furthermore, the study estimated that while hospitals received about 86% of the benefit payments from PhilHealth via price discrimination, only about 14% of the received payment was used to support healthcare services for patients.

The study shows that when PhilHealth increases the reimbursement cap, private hospitals will simply raise their service prices in response. Thus, without prior determination of the final price, the increase in PhilHealth benefits will not improve the financial protection of insured persons.

Although PhilHealth has limited its own financial risks under the "first peso" plan, this risk transferred onto the patients instead, as they still have to pay for the remaining medical expenses after exceeding the reimbursement caps. Therefore, this plan has largely failed to constrain providers, and exposes patients to catastrophic medical fees that can potentially impoverish them. It has been suggested that PhilHealth could begin limiting the maximum amount payable by insured persons (i.e., the "second peso"), but the same problem may persist if the final price has not been negotiated, and patients will still be exposed to the issue of the "third peso."

(2) Future Development Trends

The international trend in health insurance reforms has been to expand health insurance coverage to informal sector workers and impoverished individuals, and to improve the delivery and quality of healthcare services. Under this general trend, many countries, including the Philippines, have also been promoting health reforms and development. Countries have accelerated the marketization and privatization of the healthcare industry in terms of facilities and funding to improve the efficiency of health security. For example, half of the hospitals in Indonesia have been privatized. Singapore is similarly advancing toward privatization: One of the most prominent features of Singapore's healthcare policies is that the government has been allowing the private sector to play a greater role in the name of reform. The various health insurance programs in Singapore, such as MediShield and Medisave, as well as the government policies concerning the management model used by private enterprises to administer hospitals, are considered clear steps toward healthcare privatization. These reforms have transformed the government into an administrator and not merely an investor. In Malaysia, the number of hospital beds and physicians in private hospitals has increased rapidly. In fact, these numbers are expected to exceed those of public hospitals in the near future. The Philippine healthcare system is similar to that of the US, specifically with regard to the large share of the private sector in the healthcare industry. However, the healthcare privatization of the Philippines has been impeded because of the country's slow economic development and the large impoverished population. In Thailand, public healthcare institutions still account for a large proportion of the total number of healthcare institutions, but their number has been gradually declining in recent years.

Various countries, including the Philippines, have been actively promoting the marketization of healthcare management because of the increasing healthcare expenditure in recent years. There are many causes for the growth in expenditure on both the demand side (e.g., population aging, higher living standards, changes in diseases) and the supply side (e.g., advancement in medical technology and pharmaceutical products). In countries such as the Philippines, government expenditure on healthcare security has always been limited. Hence, in order to ensure the continued development of healthcare security while also reducing healthcare costs, one of the options is to expand the management role of the private sector in healthcare (e.g., fundraising and hospital construction) and to impose medical fees on consumers who utilize public healthcare institutions. One of the latest development trends in the Philippine healthcare system is the collection of user fees for public facilities. Most hospitals in the Philippines have begun to charge patients a certain amount of medical fees in order to support their own daily expenses and operations. Similarly, Indonesia encourages private companies to invest in public hospitals and requires patients to pay 50% of all medical charges. Public hospitals in Thailand also charges patients 40% of all medical fees to support the stretched funds of these hospitals. In Malaysia, the operation and management of pharmacies and medical facilities in public hospitals have been entrusted to the private sector.

Policymakers in the Philippines generally believe that privatization and marketization will increase patients' cost awareness when selecting healthcare services. Furthermore, hospitals may improve their service quality and reduce their prices due to competition. In particular, the decentralization of the health security management system will enable healthcare institutions to take on greater responsibility for their patients. However, the marketization and privatization of the healthcare sector have also given rise to a number of public concerns. Although private healthcare institutions may improve healthcare services and encourage more effective use of healthcare resources, there are clear issues related to healthcare equality in the private sector. Private healthcare institutions are often established in cities, and only provide services to residents who can afford the medical expenses. Therefore, if wealthy residents prefer seeking medical attention in private healthcare institutions, the healthcare system will become divided into a public sector that primarily serves the poor and a private sector that primarily serves the rich. This scenario would, however, have a greater negative impact on the public sector, as it would lead to a lack of financial and political support for public hospitals. Moreover, although the privatization and marketization of the healthcare industry might help reduce the financial burden on the government, it will increase the cost of consumption, which will ultimately be unacceptable to impoverished individuals. Public concerns in this regard have also been exacerbated by the recent economic crisis. Similarly, the Malaysian government is aware that Malays who live in rural areas will be most affected by the overly rapid privatization and marketization of the healthcare industry. This is politically unfavorable to the ruling party, as they are its most determined supporters.

SECTION VI. THE HEALTH SYSTEM IN ARMENIA

1. Overview of Socioeconomics and National Health

(1) Overall Status

Armenia, officially the Republic of Armenia, is a small mountainous country located on the Eurasian border and the South Caucasus region. It covers a land area of 29,800 km^2, more than 90% of which is at least 1,000 meters above sea level. It is bordered by Turkey to the west, Iran to the south, Georgia to the north, and Azerbaijan to the east. The country is dominated by mountainous terrains, and its climate varies from dry subtropical to boreal climate depending on the topography.

Armenia is one of the republics that gained independence following the dissolution of the Soviet Union. Its capital is Yerevan. In 1992, the Republic of Armenia established ambassadorial-level diplomatic relations with China. In 2013, the total population of Armenia was 3.0221 million, 93.3% of which were Armenian, while the remaining ethnic groups included Russians, Kurds, Ukrainians, Assyrians, and Greeks.

Armenia is a small landlocked country with a majority Christian population. However, it has become a volatile and turbulent zone in the Caucasus because of its proximity to unstable Islamic countries and border disputes with neighboring countries.

(2) Economic Development

Agriculture is Armenia's main source of income, and its agricultural production is mainly concentrated in the lowland areas near the capital. Since its independence in September 1991, Armenia's economy has declined continuously due to various factors, such as a weak economic foundation, the Nagorno-Karabakh War, and economic blockades from Azerbaijan and Turkey. Armenia joined the World Trade Organization (WTO) in December 2002, after which its economy began to recover – until 2007, the country showed double-digit growth in GDP. Furthermore, Armenia's per capita income has increased rapidly and the living standards of Armenians have improved over the years. However, since the fourth quarter of 2008, its economic growth rate began to decline as a result of the inter-national financial crisis and fell drastically in 2009. In order to reduce the impact of the financial crisis, the Armenian government actively took a number of measures from 2010 to 2011, such as industrial restructuring, expansion of domestic demand, acceleration of infrastructure construction, and pro-agriculture policies, which have yielded positive out-comes. By 2013, the GDP and per capita GDP of Armenia were US$ 10.417 billion and US$ 3,447, respectively. However, Armenia is still classified by the World Bank as a lower-middle income country.

(3) Population Health Status

In 2013, the average life expectancy of Armenians was 70 years (males: 71 years; females: 78 years), which was lower than the average of Central Asia (76 years), but higher than the global average (70 years). Elderly adults aged over 65 years accounted for 10% of the total population. The under-five mortality rate in Armenia was 16 deaths per 1,000 live births, which was higher than the regional average (13 deaths per 1,000 live births), but lower than the global average (51%). Similarly, the maternal mortality rate in Armenia was 29 deaths per 100,000 live births, which was higher than the regional average (20 deaths per 100,000 live births) but lower than the global average (210 deaths per 100,000 live births). The male and female mortality rates in Armenia were 228 and 94 per 1,000 male/female adults, respectively. The incidence of tuberculosis has declined continuously over the years, reaching 52 cases per 100,000 people in 2012. The HIV-infected population accounted for 0.2% of the total population aged 15–49 years.

2. Healthcare System

(1) Overview of Healthcare System

The Armenian government implements a vertically managed and highly centralized healthcare system. In short, the postindependence Armenian healthcare system provides universal access to medical assistance and a comprehensive range of primary, secondary, and tertiary healthcare services. This healthcare system aims to provide universal health coverage and contribute to the protection and improvement of the population health status.

Armenia is divided into 11 provincial administrative units, each of which has its own hospitals and associated general hospitals that provide outpatient and primary healthcare services. In rural areas, there are health centers (which provide inpatient services), outpatient practices, and feldsher health posts. Residents are assigned to specific healthcare institutions and physicians according to their place of residence. The government bears the economic burden for both preventive and therapeutic services and ensures that these services meet specific quality standards. The law guarantees that all citizens have the right to access free healthcare, while also limiting their scope of choice; that is, the quality of healthcare services can only be included as a factor for assessing the performance of healthcare institutions or healthcare providers in the event of major incidents (e.g., fatal infectious diseases).

This system ensures free medical assistance and universal access to primary, secondary, and tertiary healthcare services. However, the allocation of healthcare funding and other resources are based solely on state regulations, and do not consider the public demand for healthcare services. Regional governments are directly responsible for the funding of their respective healthcare institutions, but their funds and funding mechanisms are determined by the state. This system has led to increased organizational capacity, redundancy of healthcare workers, excessive hospital beds, and uneven distribution of healthcare resources. In other words, there are ample highly skilled physicians in large-sized hospitals, but the number of primary care physicians is relatively inadequate and there is a shortage of healthcare workers in rural areas. Moreover, primary healthcare in Armenia is technologically underdeveloped and has low standards. The majority of healthcare resources are allocated to secondary healthcare and specialist care services, with an emphasis on the development of individual departments in hospitals. From the perspective of leaders and providers in the healthcare sector, the roles of hospitals and other inpatient institutions are uncertain, as the current focus of the healthcare system has been shifted to primary healthcare. Hospitals have a high degree of autonomy and their resources are still primarily based on equipment, tangible facilities, and opaque administrative expenses. Improvements in the quality and efficiency of healthcare services have been slow because of the lack of external or internal pressure and motivation.

Primary healthcare is a typical healthcare delivery system provided by first-line outpatient networks, which are affiliated with urban general hospitals and healthcare centers and determined according to the population size of a given community. In practice, the essence of primary healthcare services is the triage and referral of patients to different specialists and hospitals.

(2) Service Providers

Healthcare providers in Armenia are mainly divided into three tiers: national, regional, and municipal or community. After its independence, Armenia decentralized and restructured its public healthcare services. Apart from national public health and preventive services as well as some tertiary hospitals, the management and ownership of healthcare services have been delegated to regional governments (for primary healthcare) and municipal governments (for hospitals). The Ministry of Health (MOH) is responsible for the planning, regulation, funding, and implementation of healthcare services. Despite its reduced functions, the MOH plays a wider role in coordination and has increased its role in the formulation of national healthcare policies.

1. State Health Agency (SHA)   The SHA was established in 1998 as a publicly funded purchaser of healthcare services and was considered a preparatory step toward establishing a national social health insurance system. The SHA has a central office, as well as a capital city department and 10 regional branches (one in every province). It was initially created as a semi-governmental organization that was independent of the MOH. However, in 2002, it was brought under the jurisdiction of the MOH and was authorized to monitor the effective utilization of the state budgetary allocations from the MOH. Furthermore, it is also responsible for financial resource allocation based on a contractual mechanism with healthcare providers.

2. Other ministries and agencies
1. The Ministry of Finance is responsible for the verification and utilization of healthcare budgets, as well as the collection and disbursement of tax revenues, serving both the MOH and SHA.
2. The Ministry of Education is responsible for the undergraduate and postgraduate medical education of physicians.
3. The Ministry of Labor and Social Affairs is responsible for protecting the most vulnerable groups in society. In addition, together with the MOH, it is also responsible for providing healthcare services for the elderly, veterans, disabled individuals, etc.

3. Regional Governments   Following its restructuring of the regional governments, Armenia now has 11 regional governments. Due to the establishment of the SHA, these governments are no longer directly responsible for the funding of health insurance, but they retain some planning and regulatory authority in the daily management of healthcare services; that is, regional healthcare agencies are still accountable to the local government and must report regularly on their use of funds (Figures 18.14 and 18.15).

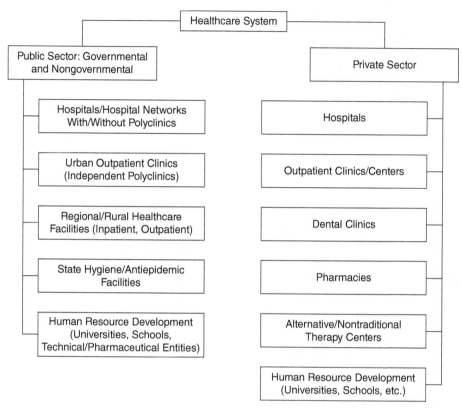

FIGURE 18.14 Overall design of the healthcare system in Armenia.

(3) Service Contents

The pre- and postindependence Armenian healthcare systems were both based on the Soviet model of healthcare services, which relied extensively on therapeutic services to reduce the burden of disease and mortality. Primary care physicians serve as "gatekeepers" of the system and account for only about 40% of all physicians.

1. Public Health In 2002, the Armenian sanitary and epidemiological services were consolidated to form the SHAEI under the MOH. The SHAEI consists of a headquarters office, 7 operations offices, 10 regional offices, and several other agencies. There are also 14 nonprofit testing centers, which were established to provide necessary laboratory controls, technical expertise, and public protection. The main functions of the SHAEI are: (1) ensuring the sanitary-epidemiological safety of the population; (2) investigating and monitoring certain entities in accordance with sanitary regulations; (3) protecting the public against communicable and noncommunicable diseases; (4) establishing sanitary-epidemiological safety standards and norms; (5) ensuring healthy living conditions; (6) disseminating knowledge and providing health education; and (7) identifying and preventing factors that adversely affect population health.

The core programs of public health include environmental and epidemiological surveillance, planned immunization, and health promotion.

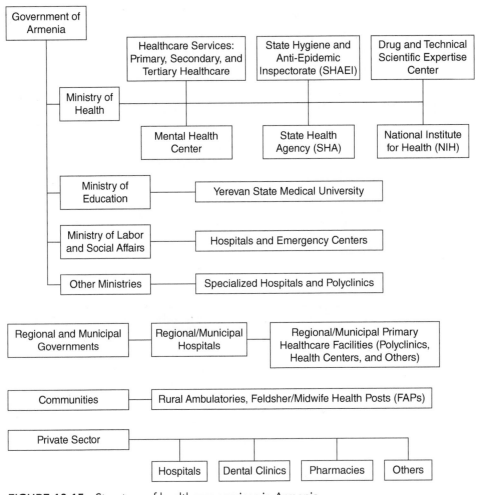

FIGURE 18.15 Structure of healthcare services in Armenia.

2. Primary Healthcare Primary healthcare is mainly provided by a network of first-contact outpatient facilities, including urban general hospitals, health centers, and rural outpatient clinics (the exact institution depends on the size of the population in a particular community). In general, a primary care physician serves a population of 1,200–2,000 adults, while a pediatrician is responsible for 700–800 children. The primary health-care facilities in Armenia include more than 400 outpatient clinics and general hospitals (among which 73 are located in the capital) and more than 600 emergency stations.

3. Inpatient services The main providers include general hospitals with hospital beds, maternity hospitals, clinics, and health centers. However, both the overall capacity and number of beds in Armenian hospitals are inadequate, and the hospitalization system remains poorly balanced due to the excess capacity and the number of healthcare workers.

4. Pharmaceutical care
An important indicator of the poor accessibility of healthcare services in Armenia is the poor accessibility of drugs, including essential medicines. There are virtually no

pharmacies or drugstores in community hospitals. Residents are thus required to travel to towns or major cities to purchase drugs.

5. Rehabilitation and Long-Term Care Rehabilitation and long-term care in Armenia generally consist of hospital-based clinical services for patients with chronic disease and temporary/permanent disabilities. Patients with severe physical and functional impairments in rural areas also often require long-term therapeutic or care services.

6. Palliative Care Despite being a signatory to the Council of Europe's recommendations on the organization of palliative care, palliative care services in Armenia have not been fully developed and still rely solely on oncological dispensaries and expert networks. A shortage of trained healthcare workers and financial protection are also some of the reasons for the slow progress in palliative services.

7. Mental Healthcare Mental healthcare services were poorly integrated into the previous Armenian healthcare system and lacked professionally trained social workers. After the founding of the Armenian Mental Health Foundation in 1996, mental health support plans were introduced as part of the community healthcare services, in order to integrate mental health services into routine healthcare.

8. Dental Healthcare Dental healthcare in Armenia is largely operated based on enterprises, with roughly 80% of the services provided in private for-profit clinics. Hence, dental healthcare services were the least affected by the social and economic transition.

9. Alternative/Complementary Medicine Alternative/complementary medicine mainly refers to traditional Armenian therapies, including acupuncture, herbal medicine, reflexology, physiotherapy, bio-resonance testing, and homeopathy, which require relatively short training courses. Alternative/complementary medicine can only be practiced by physicians with a university degree in clinical medicine and one year of professional work experience. Alternative/complementary medicine generally does not involve third-party payers and is entirely financed through out-of-pocket payments.

10. Maternal And Child Healthcare Maternal and child healthcare is mainly provided by outpatient general hospitals, but the services are limited in rural and remote areas. The government of Armenia has implemented a series of regional programs to help improve the quality of prenatal care and encourage breastfeeding, thereby reducing the under-five mortality rate.

3. Healthcare Funding

Public healthcare expenditures consist of recurrent expenses and capital expenditures in the government (central and regional) budgets, external loans and grants (including donations from international agencies and NGOs), and social (or compulsory) health insurance funds. The total healthcare expenditure is the sum of public and private healthcare expenditures and covers various healthcare services (preventive and therapeutic), family planning, nutrition programs, emergency care, etc. In 2012, the total healthcare expenditure in Armenia accounted for 4.5% of its GDP.

(1) Out-of-Pocket Payments

Reforms of the healthcare funding in Armenia have focused on diversifying the revenues for the healthcare sector and linking healthcare funding to the quality and volume of services provided. Given the limited availability of resources, economic reforms have also aimed to improve financial management and increase the financial sustainability and accountability of healthcare institutions. As the priority of current reforms is on improving the state budget and enhancing the effective use of resources, funding is still primarily derived from out-of-pocket payments, which account for about 65% of the total healthcare expenditure.

Out-of-pocket payments can be classified into three categories: formal copayments for services that are partially covered by the state budget; formal direct user fees for services not covered by state-funded healthcare packages; and informal payments for voluntarily received healthcare services that fall beyond the scope of the state reimbursement and user fee systems.

In 2009, the healthcare expenditure per capita of Armenia was US$132, which increased to US$150 in 2012. Personal out-of-pocket payments accounted for 93.8% of the total personal healthcare expenditure. In 2009–2012, the total healthcare expenditure of Armenia as a share of the GDP remained at around 4.5%.

(2) Voluntary Health Insurance (VHI)

In 2004, Armenia permitted the introduction and development of VHI. However, the development of VHI was severely restricted by the public's limited awareness and understanding of VHI, public skepticism of whether the quality and safety of healthcare services provided under the terms of this insurance scheme would be higher than those of the traditional system, and the relatively high amount of commercial insurance premiums.

(3) Basic Benefits Package (BBP)

Armenia introduced the BBP in 1997. This is a publicly funded service package specifying a list of services that are free and open for the entire population. It also specifies the population groups that are entitled to access any healthcare services for free. Other residents must fully cover their own expenses for healthcare services and drugs not listed in the BBP.

The BBP list has been periodically reviewed, and the scope of services has been expanded or reduced based on the level of funding available. However, this uncertainty has made both healthcare users and providers more cautious during the utilization/implementation of BBP. Furthermore, population groups that are entitled to free healthcare services are frequently required to pay for certain services because of the widespread presence of informal payments in healthcare facilities.

The Armenian government has made considerable effort to standardize the BBP and its assessment procedures to address the uncertainties arising from these annual adjustments. Currently, the coverage scope of the BBP includes inpatient services (e.g., emergency care, preventive care, obstetric and gynecological services, healthcare services for vulnerable populations, hemodialysis, and several important healthcare services, such as tuberculosis treatment); outpatient services (e.g., primary healthcare, medical care, prenatal and postnatal care, preenlistment examinations and treatment), sanitary-epidemiological services, and other healthcare measures.

(4) Other Funding Sources

In addition to humanitarian aid (donations of medical supplies and equipment), external healthcare funding in Armenia involves grants and loan projects provided in cooperation with the MOH. These projects, which are funded, recognized, and guaranteed by the UN, EU, and World Bank, are now the dominant form of external support in Armenia. In recent years, the US government-supported Armenia Social Transition Program (ASTP) has been serving as a complement to World Bank programs. The government of Japan has supported the upgrade and equipment purchase of many secondary and tertiary healthcare institutions in Armenia. In addition, the German government has enhanced and improved the infrastructure of general hospitals in Armenia by providing equipment and training funds as well as supporting a tuberculosis control center project, as part of an initiative for healthcare activities in the Caucasus.

4. Health System Reforms

(1) Reform Motivation

The greatest impetus for health reforms in Armenia is the structural imbalance of the existing healthcare system within the current economic environment, which has hampered the sustainability of this complicated and inefficient system. During the dissolution of the Soviet Union, the Armenian healthcare system suffered from a lack of materials and facilities, out-of-date medical equipment and supplies, oversupply and uneven distribution of healthcare workers, and healthcare workers with poor clinical skills. In addition, the healthcare system was characterized by an underutilization of primary healthcare and an overutilization of specialist and inpatient services, as well as considerable differences in healthcare infrastructure and resources between urban and rural areas. Since gaining independence in 1991, Armenia has experienced numerous hardships, such as economic crisis, political turmoil, and declining population health status.

Following the postindependence decentralization and reconfiguration of public services, the operation and ownership of healthcare services have been gradually delegated to regional governments (for primary healthcare services) and municipal governments (for most hospitals). The decentralization involved both the delegation of responsibility for service delivery and fundraising from the central government to regional healthcare agencies, as well as the privatization of hospitals and healthcare facilities. However, the privatization of healthcare facilities was too abrupt and lacked a systematic approach. Therefore, the Armenian government has suspended further privatization in recent years, pending a more comprehensive assessment and review of this strategy. In short, the process of decentralization has increased the level of autonomy and shared responsibility of healthcare providers. However, it has also brought considerable challenges due to the functional disintegration of the existing system.

(2) Reform Goals

The healthcare strategy in 2000 determined the general direction of healthcare development in Armenia. Based on a recognition of health and healthcare services as fundamental human rights, this strategy focused on implementing several major healthcare reforms: a repositioning of healthcare services toward a balanced partnership between primary healthcare and inpatient services; the promotion of disease prevention through controlling health determinants; and a shift from the narrow biomedical model toward a more socialized, diversified, and multisectoral approach to health and healthcare. Therefore, the development and strengthening of primary healthcare are major aspects of the Armenian health reform plan. Given the limited resources available, the reform aims to: (1) protect the constitutional right of the population to healthcare; (2) improve the utilization and volume of free public healthcare services; (3) establish and maintain a sustainable balance between social- and market-oriented values and the public healthcare system; (4) raise the public's awareness toward health; and (5) implement and standardize multisectoral cooperation and responsibility in healthcare services.

(3) Reform Contents

Armenia began reforming its healthcare sector at the early stages after its independence. The reform measures included changing not only the healthcare services of inpatient and outpatient institutions but also the financial and regulatory frameworks, with an overall aim of improving the efficiency and regulatory capabilities of the healthcare system. The Armenian government has promulgated a series of laws, such as the Program for Development and Reforms of the Health Care System of the Republic of Armenia 1996–2000 and the Law on Medical Aid and Services Provision to the Population. The Law on Medical Aid and Services Provision to the Population introduced various alternative funding approaches and effectively abolished the old healthcare system. Broadly, it stipulates: (1) the state shall ensure that everyone has the right to access free medical assistance and services within the scope of the state's health programs. (2) The state is responsible for developing and implementing health programs that enable it to fully fulfill its responsibilities for public health protection. (3) Each resident has the right to choose their healthcare providers. (4) Funding sources for health insurance include the state budget, insurance contributions, direct payments, and other legally recognized sources.

Subsequently, Armenia established the SHA as a purchaser of national health insurance services. The SHA later became the sole body responsible for reimbursing healthcare providers.

Although the central government retains considerable power, the reform of the healthcare sector led to a clear decentralization of the healthcare system. This was mainly achieved by the transfer of responsibility from the central to the local levels with regard to the delivery of primary and secondary healthcare services, as well as the transfer of financial responsibility from the central to local levels via the privatization of healthcare institutions (especially dispensaries and dental healthcare facilities).

1. Transfer of Responsibilities   The first phase of the transfer of responsibilities occurred between the mid-1990s and 1998, which involved the transfer of financial responsibility for the provision of statutory healthcare services from the central government to regional governments. Regional governments have a certain degree of autonomy with regard to negotiating contracts with regional healthcare providers, monitoring service quality, and amending regional budgets. However, the MOH retained its responsibility for pricing and defining the rights of the public to healthcare. At the beginning of the second stage, in 1998, the responsibility for the management of state financial resources for healthcare was completely transferred to the SHA. The SHA has since become the only governmental agency in Armenia with the authority to reimburse providers for their service packages. In addition, the responsibility for providing primary and secondary healthcare services has been transferred to regional governments, while the MOH is responsible for managing tertiary healthcare institutions.

2. Privatization   Privatization was achieved via the transfer or sale of public healthcare institutions to for-profit or nonprofit individuals or groups, and via changes in the legislative framework to allow entrepreneurs to establish private enterprises that included healthcare institutions. The MOH is responsible for the licensure and approval of such healthcare institutions. The government has established a series of policy objectives, including: (1) improving the transparency of financial flows in the healthcare sector; (2) mobilizing additional financial resources via private sector investments; (3) enhancing the effective and efficient use of healthcare resources; (4) improving the quality and diversity of healthcare services and providers; and (5) expanding the choices for healthcare users and facilitating a competitive environment.

At the same time, the government also stipulated that public health services, immunization, preventive services, control of infectious diseases, blood management services, and forensic medicine are not available for privatization.

However, during the process of privatization, the government has yet to adopt licensure and other approaches to ensure the quality of healthcare services, broad market access, or the capacity to regulate the market. The privatization efforts also lacked good regulatory and supervisory arrangements. These issues have raised concerns about potential financial mismanagement and the inability to fulfill social functions.

3. Healthcare Funding Reforms   Healthcare funding reforms in Armenia have focused on diversifying the revenues in the healthcare sector and linking healthcare funding with the quality and quantity of healthcare services provided. Reforms have also aimed at improving financial management and increasing the financial sustainability and accountability of the MOH.

To this end, in 1997, the government decided to use budgetary resources to target socially vulnerable groups and all socially important diseases. In 1998, the government introduced the BBP, a publicly funded service package, which specifies the population groups that are entitled to receive any type of healthcare services for free. Since then, the government has periodically reviewed the coverage scope of the BBP, expanding or reducing the breadth of services and population groups covered depending on the level of funding available.

Improving the financing mechanisms is crucial to the reforms and continuous transition of the Armenian healthcare system. The MOH is currently experimenting on different models to improve the efficiency, financial management, accountability, and financial sustainability of healthcare institutions. The core aim of this healthcare funding reform is to determine the scope and content of publicly funded services and benefits, thereby achieving the consolidation of healthcare resources. Currently, efforts to develop a system of National Health Accounts (NHAs) are moving forward, which may help improve the transparency of financial and decision-making information in the healthcare sector. The National Statistical Service has also conducted numerous public opinion polls to assess the outcomes of healthcare reform, in order to explore more effective mechanisms (e.g., PPS, user charges, risk pooling) as well as encourage fundamental discussion of social values and social mobilization.

Since Armenia gained independence, its healthcare system has undergone tremendous changes, culminating in the delegation of authority from the central to the regional level, and the transition toward substantial out-of-pocket payments from its citizens. Despite higher government investment in primary healthcare, the absence of relevant healthcare standards and quality assessment systems has limited the availability of basic and specialist healthcare services for many of those in need (e.g., the elderly, unemployed persons, women and children). These groups are unable to receive treatment from the nearest healthcare providers in a timely and convenient manner. Even when healthcare services are accessible, the quality is often in doubt because of the lack of healthcare standards and quality assessment systems. Many healthcare institutions still prefer or rely on informal payments, which render essential medicines, medical facilities, and medical technologies inaccessible to many vulnerable groups.

Despite the many challenges, Armenia is still actively reforming its healthcare system, shifting from an emphasis on therapeutic and epidemiological services to preventive services, family medicine, and community participation. The active and appropriate transition of Armenia towards primary and community healthcare is compelling and anticipated.

SECTION VII. THE HEALTH SYSTEM IN KYRGYZSTAN

1. Overview of Socioeconomics and National Health

(1) Overall Status

The Kyrgyz Republic (also known as Kyrgyzstan) is a Turkic-speaking landlocked country in Central Asia. It joined the Soviet Union on December 5, 1936, and declared its independence on August 31, 1991. The total land area of Kyrgyzstan is 199,900 km², and it is bordered by Kazakhstan to the north, Uzbekistan to the west, Tajikistan to the south, and China to the east. The capital, Bishkek, is near its northern border. At the end of 2013, the total population of Kyrgyzstan was 5.72 million, most of whom lived in rural areas. There are more than 80 ethnic groups in Kyrgyzstan, among which the Kyrgyz account for 71% of the total population; the other major ethnic groups include Uzbeks (14.3%) and Russians (7.8%). The official languages are Kyrgyz and Russian. The dominant religion in Kyrgyzstan is Sunni Islam, followed by Russian Orthodoxy. Kyrgyzstan is divided into seven regions (Chuy Region, Talas Region, Osh Region, Jalal-Abad Region, Naryn Region, Issyk-Kul Region, and Batken Region) and two independent cities (the capital, Bishkek, and the southern capital, Osh).

(2) Economic Development

The economy of Kyrgyzstan is based on multiple types of ownership. Agriculture is the dominant sector in Kyrgyzstan, and it has a weak industrial foundation. Its economy relies heavily on the production of raw materials. Kyrgyzstan suffered an economic recession in the early stage of its independence because of its discontinuation of economic relations with most post-Soviet states and radical reforms. In the early twenty-first century, the government of Kyrgyzstan adjusted its economic reform policies, gradually shifting toward the adoption of a market economy and implementing economic reforms centered on privatization and denationalization. As a result, the country has maintained a relatively low economic growth rate, restorative increases in industrial production, and relatively stable commodity prices. Furthermore, inflation has fallen to its lowest level since Kyrgyzstan's independence.

In 2013, the GDP and per capita GDP of Kyrgyzstan were US$7.226 billion and US$1,263, respectively, which were higher than were those in 2012. The World Bank Annual Report 2012 classified Kyrgyzstan as a low-income country.

(3) Population Health Status

In 2012, the average life expectancy of Kyrgyzstanis was 70 years (males: 66 years; females: 74 years), which was lower than the average of Central Asia (72 years) and the global average (71 years). The under-five mortality rate of Kyrgyzstan (27%) was higher than the regional average (13 per 1,000 live births), but lower than the global average (51 per 1,000 live births). Similarly, the maternal mortality rate (75 deaths per 100,000 live births) was higher than was the regional average (20 deaths per 100,000 live births), but lower than the global average (210 deaths per 100,000 live births). Both the male (279 per 1,000 adult males/females) and female adult mortality rates (135 per 1,000 adult males/females) were higher than the regional and global averages.

The incidence rate of tuberculosis increased from 138.2 cases per 100,000 people in 2003 to 175 cases per 100,000 people in 2011, which was higher than the regional average (56 cases per 100,000 people) and the global average (170 cases per 100,000 people). In 2001, the number of AIDS patients showed exponential growth due to various factors, such as widespread intravenous drug abuse, immigration, promiscuity, marginalization of vulnerable groups, and low public awareness of AIDS. In 2011, the incidence of AIDS in Kyrgyzstan (225 cases per 100,000 people) was lower than the regional average (263 cases per 100,000 people) and the global average (499 cases per 100,000 people). Although malaria was originally a rare disease in Kyrgyzstan, its incidence began to increase in 2002, eventually reaching 0.1 cases per 100,000 people in 2011.

As a landlocked country with mountainous terrain, Kyrgyzstan is highly susceptible to iodine deficiency. Previous studies have shown that up to 52% of adolescents in the northern region of Kyrgyzstan show signs of iodine deficiency, whereas the figure for the southern region is a staggering 87%. Similar to other regions of Central Asia, iron deficiency is common among women in Kyrgyzstan, mainly due to the male-oriented food choices of households.

2. Healthcare System

Prior to Kyrgyzstan's independence, its healthcare system was highly centralized and controlled by the Soviet Union. The Ministry of Health (MOH) of the Union of Soviet Socialist Republics (USSR) was the main healthcare planning and management agency of the Soviet Union. The healthcare services in the 15 Soviet Socialist Republics (SSRs) were supervised by their respective health ministries, but the authorities of these ministries were limited to implementing the supreme directives of the MOH of the USSR. This inherited convention remained the main problem facing healthcare management in Kyrgyzstan in the late 1990s.

Currently, the MOH of Kyrgyzstan is responsible for formulating national healthcare policies and clinical standards, which are implemented by local health authorities and healthcare providers. The healthcare system is divided into four government administrative levels: national, state (*oblast*), municipal, and district (*rayon*) levels. Local healthcare agencies at the oblast, municipal, and rayon levels are responsible for implementing orders from the MOH. In addition, the privatization of healthcare services has been subject to numerous restrictions. Private healthcare institutions mainly include outpatient clinics and pharmacies, but remain on a relatively small scale. In summary, the healthcare system in Kyrgyzstan is centralized under the MOH, which is responsible for healthcare affairs at each administrative level (Figure 18.16).

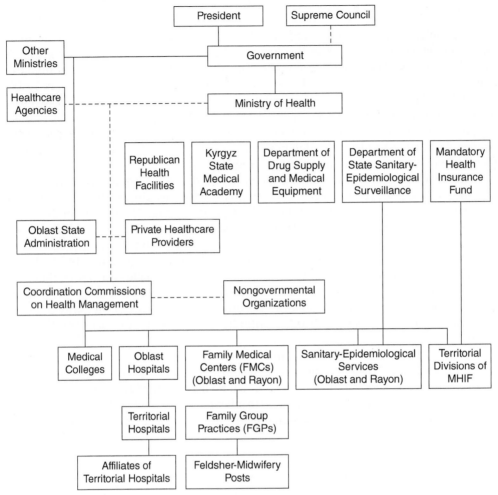

FIGURE 18.16 Organizational structure of the healthcare system in Kyrgyzstan.

(1) The Cabinet

The Cabinet of Kyrgyzstan is currently responsible for adopting healthcare policies, implementation plans, and healthcare development strategies that have been approved by the Supreme Council. The Cabinet also obtains funds and controls some of the national, oblast, and special programs related to health protection and national healthcare development. It is also responsible for reporting annually to the Supreme Council on the population health status and the implementation of the overall healthcare budget in Kyrgyzstan.

(2) MOH

The MOH is responsible for implementing healthcare policies and collaborating with other agencies to develop and implement national welfare programs and various other targeted healthcare programs. The MOH is responsible for the quality and quality control of healthcare services, as well as the safety and effectiveness of pharmaceutical products, medical products, and equipment. The MOH serves as a regulator for all healthcare-related organizations (including medical education), regardless of their affiliations and administrative level. The MOH is also responsible for the approval of policy and program documents for all organizations, but it is only directly responsible for the operation of a handful of national specialized healthcare agencies and tertiary healthcare institutions in Bishkek. In addition, the MOH coordinates and controls regional healthcare agencies via coordination commissions on health management. The MOH reports annually to the Cabinet on the population health status of Kyrgyzstan.

(3) Department of State Sanitary-Epidemiological Surveillance (SSES)

The SSES is primarily responsible for sanitary-epidemiological services, which form the foundation of public health services, and is directly accountable to the MOH. The director of the SSES is a medical epidemiologist and also the Deputy Minister of Health. The department was established in 1997 from the former Republican Sanitary-Epidemiological Station and the Sanitary-Epidemiological Department of the Ministry of Health.

(4) Department of Drug Supply and Medical Equipment (DDSME)

The DDSME is directly affiliated with the MOH. Its functions include formulating drug policies, and the surveillance and evaluation of drug quality. The department is responsible for the registration of pharmaceutical products and the licensure of pharmaceutical manufacturers and retailers. The DDPME was established in 1997 by merging the former Republican Centre on Standardization and Quality Control of Drugs and Medical Equipment, the Ministry of Health Department on Drugs and Medical Equipment, and the Ministry of Health Pharmacological Committee.

(5) Local Health Authorities

Local health authorities oversee healthcare institutions that provide primary and secondary healthcare services, including polyclinics, and oblast and rayon hospitals (except those owned by the central government and private enterprises). They are responsible for the delivery of healthcare services within their jurisdiction. Local health authorities implement national healthcare policies and local healthcare programs via coordination commissions on health management. In addition, they are also responsible for controlling the implementation of national and oblast healthcare programs, as well as targeted healthcare programs. They formulate and ensure the implementation of healthcare budgets. In addition, they are charged with improving the capacity and working environment of healthcare workers. These local health authorities are required to report annually to local councils on the overall health status of their jurisdiction.

(6) Other Agencies

Ministries and agencies other than the MOH also provide parallel healthcare services. The parallel system comprises seven ministries, five large state-owned joint stock companies, and various companies and organizations partially funded by the government. In 1998, parallel healthcare services accounted for approximately 6% of the total government healthcare expenditure. These healthcare institutions are directly accountable to their respective agencies and are funded by the government budget.

Since the 1990s, private healthcare institutions gradually expanded from pharmacies to healthcare providers. In 2003, the MOH issued 254 licenses for private practices, of which

49 were issued to legal entities and 205 to individuals. Private healthcare institutions may bid for public contracts and participate in national welfare programs. To date, these institutions have mostly been associated with pharmaceutical supply, mainly occurring under the Additional Drug Package provided by the Mandatory Health Insurance Fund (MHIF) on an outpatient basis. The public procurement of private healthcare services has also emerged.

The healthcare sector in Kyrgyzstan has witnessed the emergence of non-governmental professional associations, including associations of physicians, pharmacists, nurses, cardiologists, patients with diabetes, and blood donors. The Association of Family Group Practices and Hospital Association established in 1997 have cooperated closely with the MOH in health reforms.

Even after the dissolution of the Soviet Union, the national healthcare system in Kyrgyzstan has essentially followed the Soviet model. World Health Organization (WHO) statistics have shown that, in 2009, the total healthcare expenditure of Kyrgyzstan accounted for 6.8% of its GDP, with a per capita healthcare expenditure of US$152. In 2000–2010, there were 23 physicians, 57 nurses and midwives, 2 dentists, and 51 hospital beds per 10,000 people in Kyrgyzstan. As of May 2013, there were 24.7 physicians and 58.2 healthcare workers per 10,000 people. In 2007, there were 160 hospitals across Kyrgyzstan, among which most specialist hospitals (offering cardiology, surgery, pediatrics, obstetrics and gynecology, psychiatry, oncology, and otorhinolaryngology services) had been established in Bishkek. By contrast, most burn centers and orthopedics specialist hospitals had been established in Osh. Other types of hospitals, such as general hospitals, are distributed throughout the country. In addition, there were approximately 90 nursing homes and medical rehabilitation centers across the country. There are no pharmacy departments in any hospitals in Kyrgyzstan, and patients are required to purchase drugs from pharmacies using prescriptions issued by physicians.

In recent years, Kyrgyzstan has placed considerable emphasis on its relationship with the international community, in an effort to obtain foreign financial aid for its healthcare sector. According to news reports in Kyrgyzstan, countries such as the US, Denmark, Germany, Japan, and Switzerland, along with organizations such as the World Bank, Islamic Development Bank, Asian Development Bank, German Development Bank, and WHO (i.e., the UN), have provided substantial financial aid to the healthcare sector in Kyrgyzstan. Foreign financial aid accounts for 60% of the healthcare budget of Kyrgyzstan. In October 2005 alone, the World Bank and the German Development Bank provided US$15 million and €16 million, respectively, to assist Kyrgyzstan in comprehensive healthcare management, personalized healthcare, personnel training, etc. The government of Japan sponsored Kyrgyzstan with medical equipment worth US$21.5 million between 1995 and 2005. To date, the humanitarian aid offered by the US to Kyrgyzstan (primarily for the healthcare system) has reached US$290 million.

3. Healthcare Funding and Expenditure

(1) Current Status

Currently, the main funding sources of the healthcare system in Kyrgyzstan are (1) global budget revenues (national and local); (2) the MHIF; (3) public investment programs; and (4) out-of-pocket payments.

The World Bank's Public Expenditure Review 2004 reported that out-of-pocket payments represented the main source of healthcare funding, accounting for nearly half of the total healthcare funding in Kyrgyzstan. Furthermore, the global budget revenues (the central and local governments) accounted for 44% of the total healthcare funding in Kyrgyzstan, while the remaining healthcare funding was made up of public investment programs supported by the World Bank and Asian Development Bank (0.9%) and social insurance (4%). Around 32% of the global budget revenue was from the national budget and 68% from the local governments.

(2) Mandatory Health Insurance Fund (MHIF)

The MHIF is the "single payer" in the healthcare sector. It is responsible for pooling funds, purchasing healthcare services, and establishing healthcare budgets. In addition, the MHIF is charged with the quality assurance and the development of health information systems. The director of the MHIF is also the Deputy Minister of Health. The MHIF was established in 1997 as a foundation under the Cabinet but was subsequently transferred to the MOH in 1998. The MHIF is also accountable to the Ministry of Finance and local state administrations with regard to the utilization of budgetary resources and healthcare funds.

The MHIF is a compulsory health insurance scheme that prohibits members from withdrawing. Table 18.33 shows that the funding source for the MHIF varies across different populations. The MHIF does not serve as a funding source; rather, it accepts financial transfers from social funds and the national budget on behalf of certain insured groups. The MHIF pools funds from employees' income, which are also used to cover farmers. The funding for children, social security beneficiaries, pensioners, and military personnel is derived from the national budget. The insurance status of participants of this scheme is determined based on social security identification, pensioner's identification, or mandatory health insurance policies.

The deputy chairman of the MHIF, Almaz Imanbaev, stated that the MHIF covers 4.137 million Kyrgyzstan residents, which is 76.3% of the total population. He has further claimed

TABLE 18.33   Funding and Coverage of the MHIF in Kyrgyzstan

Population Group	Funding Source
Employees, including Formal Sector Employees	2% payroll contribution by employers
Civil servants and public enterprises	2% payroll contribution by employer (i.e., the government) to the Social Fund
Self-employed	Voluntary purchase of mandatory health insurance policies
Private Farmers	6% of the base rate of land tax
Employees of the Ministry of Defense, National Guard, and the Ministry of Interior	Contributions based on 1.5 times the minimum salary allocated from the national budget
Children under 16; school children under 18; and students of primary, secondary, and higher professional education institutions (except part-time and evening students) under 21	Contributions based on 1.5 times the minimum salary allocated from the national budget
Individuals with disabilities since childhood and individuals receiving social and state benefits	
Pensioners	
Registered unemployed persons	

that the MHIF covers 1.136 million workers, 389,000 farmers, 521,000 retirees, 1.7 million children under 16 years and other population groups, as well as more than 2,000 military personnel. Imanbaev reported that a plan to maximize the MHIF coverage for all citizens is currently being drafted. Socially disadvantaged groups are the main population lacking coverage.

The MHIF has implemented the State-Guaranteed Benefits Package (SGBP), which provides medical assistance to Kyrgyz citizens, and the Additional Drug Package, which provides outpatient and surgical services to MHIF-insured persons. The role of the MHIF in healthcare funding has increased substantially since 2001, whereby the MHIF has created a single pool of funds at the oblast level by pooling healthcare budgets from all areas (regions, cities, and districts). The MHIF purchased services from these funds for the entire oblast population using the same method employed nationally for insured persons, thereby becoming the sole purchaser of healthcare services at the oblast level. In mid-2002, this "single-payer" system was extended to two other oblasts (Naryn and Talas), with territorial and population coverages of 50% and 33%, respectively. By 2004, the entire country had come under the "single-payer" system.

Under the framework of a "single-payer" system, the MHIF administers the local healthcare budgets. A new financial planning system was established based on new standards, whereby purchases are decided on the basis of final outcomes or population needs (number of inpatient cases, total number of patients receiving primary healthcare, and regional population size for outpatient and sanitary-epidemiological providers) rather than the capacity (beds and personnel) of healthcare institutions. Furthermore, it aims to overcome regional disparities via fund distribution coefficients reflecting the remoteness and economic characteristics of the regional populations. This new planning system has the following major features and goals: (1) provide healthcare services to 100% of the population under the SGBP; (2) achieve purchaser–provider split with the MHIF serving as the sole purchaser of healthcare services; (3) integrate the sources of healthcare funding (budgetary funds, MHIF funds, and out-of-pocket payments); (4) pool budgetary funds at the oblast level; (5) substitute informal case payments with more transparent formal copayments; (6) allocate resources without restrictions from chapters and line-item budgets; and (7) improve the referral system from primary healthcare to higher levels of care by integrating it into the healthcare system.

Despite the clear separation of funding and pooling responsibilities between the Social Fund and the MHIF, the actual amount allocated to the MHIF has always been less than the expected amount. In 2002, only 54.8% of premiums paid by employers to the Social Fund were allocated to the MHIF. The allocation rate for pensioners was even lower, and none of the predetermined fund allocations were achieved in 2002. The lack of funding allocation from the Social Fund revenues has been attributed to the financial problems of the Social Fund itself. Therefore, funds that should have been allocated to the MHIF were used to cross-subsidize other sectors, particularly pensions. Since January 2003, Social Fund transfers to the MHIF have improved considerably – that is, the Social Fund was no longer permitted to be indebted to the MHIF. This new regulation was imposed by the agreement with the new IMF Poverty Reduction and Growth Facility (an IMF lending facility for low-income countries that focuses on national poverty reduction strategies).

(3) Out-of-Pocket Payments

In addition to the MHIF, there are four types of out-of-pocket payments in Kyrgyzstan's healthcare system: (1) informal under-the-counter cash payments or payments-in-kind for services and goods in public healthcare institutions that should have been provided free-of-charge; (2) purchase of goods and services from private providers, primarily outpatient drugs and private healthcare services purchased from private pharmacies and markets; (3) formal user fees; and (4) formal copayments made by patients to healthcare institutions that have been included in the single-payer system.

Informal out-of-pocket payments include under-the-counter payments made to healthcare workers, the purchase of drugs and medical supplies needed for the services offered by public healthcare institutions, and inpatient expenses for food and other nonmedical supplies. Informal out-of-pocket payments are common in Kyrgyzstan. By contrast, formal user fees are regulated by the Law on Extra-Budgetary Activities of Public Health Facilities. The prices of healthcare services must be approved by the State Commission on Anti-Monopoly Policy. Formal user fees are typically captured in healthcare budgets as "special income." Currently, special income includes nonmedical services (e.g., rent, transportation, nonhealth-related chemical and laboratory tests), healthcare services provided to foreigners, dental services (except those included in the SGBP), and healthcare services requested by individuals (e.g., plastic surgery, abortions, anonymous treatment).

Formal copayments for drugs, meals, and certain healthcare services under the SGBP constitute a major part of the single-payer system. The copayment system has been introduced into outpatient institutions and hospitals. Although the level of copayment is fixed, it can vary for patients exempt from copayments, between insured and uninsured patients, as well as among different types of medical interventions (e.g., treatments or surgeries in hospitals, high-priced or routine examinations in outpatient institutions). It is expected that this copayment system would replace informal cash payments.

As part of a comprehensive set of reforms to funding and purchasing in the single-payer system, the SGBP is considered the first major attempt to clearly define the responsibilities of the state in the delivery of healthcare services and to replace informal out-of-pocket payments with a transparent, formal copayment system. Although it has achieved initial outcomes, its sustainable, long-term success in replacing informal payments with formal payments relies heavily on the continuous maintenance and growth in government healthcare expenditures, which would enable cost savings in restructuring major components of the healthcare delivery system (Figure 18.17). In 2012, the government healthcare expenditure accounted for 7.1% of Kyrgyzstan's GDP.

(4) External Funding Sources

External funding sources include humanitarian aid, technical support, grants, and loans. The amount of foreign aid provided to Kyrgyzstan in the 1990s was enormous. According to the National Health Accounts (NHA) database, which accumulates data at the institutional level, the amount of foreign aid from 1998 to 2000 was 10% of the total healthcare expenditure in Kyrgyzstan.

However, the amount of foreign aid varies considerably each year because of the closure and initiation of relevant programs. The major donors supporting health reform in Kyrgyzstan include the World Bank, the WHO, the US Agency for International Development (USAID), the UK Department for International Development (DFID), and the Swiss Agency for Development and Cooperation (SDC). In early 2003, the Global Fund to Fight AIDS, Tuberculosis, and Malaria approved grants worth US$17 million and US$1.1 million to fund AIDS and tuberculosis programs, respectively.

The healthcare reform programs (*Manas* and *Manas Taalimi*) in Kyrgyzstan are administered by the Department of Health Care Reform (DHCR), which is accountable to the MOH.

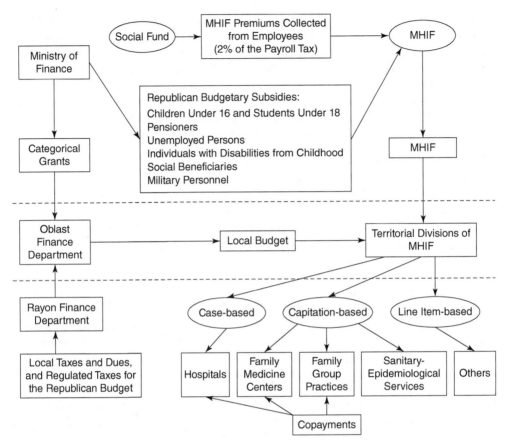

FIGURE 18.17   Financial flow in the single-payer system of Kyrgyzstan.

The DHCR coordinates donation activities in the healthcare sector. Many donors have supported the implementation of vertical healthcare programs targeting areas such as tuberculosis, AIDS, sexually transmitted diseases, and acute respiratory infections; family planning and reproductive health; immunization; and drug procurement. The WHO has supported the healthcare reform programs and a series of other activities, including upgrading and equipping healthcare institutions, as well as strengthening healthcare information systems and health funding reforms. The Asian Development Bank has supported similar activities in the southern region of Kyrgyzstan. The Swiss Agency for Development and Cooperation supported the restructuring of healthcare services and the development of primary healthcare in the Naryn oblast via the Swiss Red Cross, which included a new emphasis on community-based health promotion activities.

4. Health System Reforms

(1) Reform Background

1. Reform Motivation   Since gaining independence in 1991, Kyrgyzstan has undergone considerable economic and political changes. The severe economic recession and significant growth in poverty have led to reforms in all sectors of society. Furthermore, the drastic reduction in healthcare funds has had a negative impact on the quality of healthcare services, which may be one of the reasons for the deterioration in the overall health status of the population. This macroeconomic environment has contributed to the healthcare reforms in Kyrgyzstan.

2. Reform Goals (1) To improve the health status of the population. (2) To improve the accessibility and equality of healthcare services by eliminating differences in health indicators across regions and between urban and rural areas, as well as by protecting patients' right to healthcare services. (3) To improve the effectiveness and efficiency of the utilization of healthcare resources. (4) To improve the quality of healthcare services.

3. Reform Approaches In 1994, the MOH requested the WHO European Regional Office to assist in the establishment and implementation of a comprehensive healthcare reform program (MANAS). That same year, the USAID also began supporting the initial Issyk-Kul health reform pilot program via the Zdrav reform program. This program was synchronized with MANAS, and many of the specific measures implemented in the Issyk-Kul health reform were ultimately incorporated into MANAS in 1996.

The health reforms were implemented with the aforementioned objectives in mind, which have both improved primary healthcare services and achieved purchaser–provider split ahead of schedule. However, the SGBP, which was scheduled to be completed in 1997, only began being piloted in 2001.

(2) Reform Characteristics

1. Healthcare Funding – Single-Payer System The reform of healthcare funding is embodied in the "single-payer system," which integrates all previous positive developments. The single-payer system is characterized by: the purchaser–provider split in healthcare; coordination of the main healthcare funding sources; pooling of budgetary funds at the oblast level to overcome the previously fragmented funding arrangements; replacement of informal out-of-pocket payments with transparent, formal copayments; and resource allocation to providers according to their outputs rather than capacities. By contrast, the risks and challenges facing this single-payer system are reflected in the delayed payments made to healthcare providers due to insufficient, disrupted, or otherwise problematic Social Funds received by the local or central budgets. These delays can lead to a greater demand by healthcare providers for informal out-of-pocket payments in conjunction with copayments, thereby undermining public trust in the healthcare system. In addition, the regional economic disparities might also lead to varying levels of copayments across different oblasts. Another risk is that the rationalization of healthcare delivery will lag behind the increase in public utility taxes. Finally, legislative initiatives in healthcare delivery must be supported by a corresponding increase in financial allocations. Otherwise, the single-payer system will not be able to sustain itself, and will eventually fail.

2. Healthcare Delivery System The rationalization of public healthcare institutions is perhaps the most difficult reform to implement. Initiation of this reform was in fact delayed by immense political resistance until 2003. However, new economic instruments were adopted by these institutions that now operate under the single-payer system, which should be able to facilitate the rationalized construction of such institutions. The fragmented healthcare budget is the main challenge to reforming healthcare funding and the healthcare delivery system. A crucial part of healthcare funding reform is the pooling of funds at the oblast level, which would guarantee better risk sharing. Furthermore, healthcare institutions should be given greater budgetary autonomy as part of the complementary reforms. The flexibility of healthcare institutions in the allocation of internal resources has been greatly enhanced by the introduction of new provider payment methods, especially the copayment system.

(3) Reform Implementation

1. Reform Implementation Has Primarily Been the Responsibility of the MOH Since Kyrgyzstan's Independence   During the Soviet period, the planning, regulation, and management of the healthcare system in Kyrgyzstan were centrally controlled by the Soviet Union. Following the country's independence, the MOH of Kyrgyzstan assumed primary responsibility in planning, regulation, and management; however, it is gradually delegating its functions.

The overall management of the healthcare system mainly follows a top-down hierarchical model. The laws, decrees, and regulations adopted by the Supreme Council are subsequently issued by the MOH as orders that are compulsory for all publicly owned healthcare institutions. Then, the administrative department of each healthcare institution issues internal orders with timetables and divisions of responsibilities. Each institution must monitor the implementation of these orders and report the outcomes to the MOH.

The MOH directly administers all public healthcare institutions and the Kyrgyz State Medical Academy. The MOH appoints the heads of state healthcare organizations, and its approval is needed for the appointments of the heads of municipal healthcare organizations by local state authorities. The main administrative functions of the MOH include the development of guidelines that are compulsory for all healthcare providers, the licensure and accreditation of healthcare providers, and the establishment of quality assurance measures. The MOH also coordinates donation activities and provides humanitarian aid, as well as performing the central procurement of drugs and medical equipment for public healthcare institutions.

Furthermore, the MOH is responsible for financial planning and budgetary management. It establishes healthcare budgets based on national healthcare policies and healthcare revenue estimates; in particular, it investigates the scopes and types of healthcare services required for the population and the financial resources needed to provide these services. The role of the Ministry of Finance and local finance departments is crucial in the budgeting process, as both have financial authority over budgetary funds. However, following the introduction of the single-payer system, their roles in the healthcare sector have been limited to revenue collection. The single-payer system, including the responsibilities of the Ministry of Finance and other finance departments, has been described in detail in the sections on healthcare funding and expenditure, and financial resource allocation.

The local state administrations are responsible for healthcare planning and regulation below the national level. Prior to the major reform of local governments in 2000, these functions were fulfilled by oblast health departments. Following the abolition of these departments, these functions were delegated to oblast hospitals, which were then further delegated to supervisory councils for healthcare management. These councils later became the Coordination Commissions on Health Management in 2003.

The Coordination Commissions on Health Management are collegiate bodies consisting of local representatives of the central government, as well as representatives of the corresponding councils, local healthcare organizations, social security agencies, oblast finance departments, educational institutions, veterinary institutions, trade unions, and NGOs. A coordination commission is chaired by the head of the oblast government (or the mayor in Bishkek and Osh), who establishes and appoints all members of the commission. Each commission has two deputies, one of which is the head of an oblast healthcare institution, while the other is the head of the local MHIF department. The commission meets whenever necessary, but no less than once per quarter. The decisions of the coordination commissions are mandatory for all local healthcare institutions. Each coordination commission is accountable to its corresponding oblast state administration and the MOH.

At the level of healthcare institutions, leaders in healthcare planning, regulation, and management are appointed by the administration, which has financial and managerial autonomy. The head of an oblast or municipal healthcare institution is required to have a university degree and a professional education in medicine, economics, or administration, as well as a certificate of registration for healthcare management. The management of private healthcare providers, including healers (traditional medical practitioners), is based on licensure. Private healthcare providers must maintain and submit all the necessary documents and reports. The interaction and collaboration between private and public healthcare providers, including participation in the implementation of the SGBP, are based on contracts.

The participation of the public in healthcare planning remains limited. However, in some designated pilot areas, public feedback has been used in future planning. Presently, various studies have been conducted via interviews, focus groups, and participatory rural appraisal studies, with the aim of understanding people's experiences of the reforms and their overall expectations of the healthcare systems.

2. Decentralization (Localization) of the Healthcare System   As mentioned previously, the MOH is responsible for formulating national healthcare policies and clinical standards, but these functions are, in fact, implemented by local healthcare authorities and providers.

Recent reforms have divided the healthcare system into four government administrative levels: national, state (oblast), municipal and district (rayon). In addition, there are numerous national programs, such as immunization plans, that are operated by a separate vertical system. The fragmented healthcare budget is the main obstacle to reforming healthcare funding and the healthcare delivery system in Kyrgyzstan. One key aspect of the reform of healthcare funding is the pooling of funds at the oblast level (this reform was initiated in 2001 with pilots in Chui and Issyk-Kul, and has since been extended nationwide), which guarantees better risk sharing and breaks the integration of financing and provision, thereby preventing surplus material capacity. Healthcare institutions have also been given greater budgetary autonomy as part of the complementary reforms. The flexibility of healthcare institutions in the allocation of internal resources has been greatly enhanced by the introduction of the new provider payment methods, especially the copayment system.

Local governments are involved in oblast-level healthcare management through: (1) participation in the Coordination Commissions on Health Management; (2) budget transfers by oblast finance departments to the local department of the MHIF; (3) rationalization of healthcare institutions; (4) healthcare workforce policies; and (5) social protection of vulnerable groups by issuing "social passports" and funding the delivery of healthcare services for patients who are exempt from copayments.

3. Progressive Participation of NGOs   In recent years, some of the functions of the MOH have been delegated to NGOs. For instance, the accreditation of healthcare institutions has been entrusted to the Medical Accreditation Commission. Furthermore, the Association of Family Group Practices and the Hospital Association are responsible for overseeing the quality of healthcare services and the development of clinical protocols.

The private sector is still comparatively small and primarily consists of outpatient services and pharmacies. The privatization of the healthcare sector began with the pharmaceutical sector. Under the communist system, drugs were purchased centrally, and then sold at fixed, state-regulated prices. In 1992, numerous local pharmaceutical companies were merged into a conglomerate known as the Galenical Drugs Business Project, which was controlled by the state and led by Kyrgyzpharmindustria. Following the second wave of privatization in 1994–1995, these companies were further transformed into joint-stock companies or limited liability companies. The monopoly state-owned company, Kyrgyz Pharmacia, which was responsible for the procurement and distribution of drugs, was privatized in 1994. In 1996, the majority of pharmacies were fully privatized, with the exception of a handful of municipal pharmacies.

On the other hand, the privatization of other healthcare sectors is subject to more constraints. For instance, the privatization programs from 2001 to 2003 prohibited the privatization of healthcare institutions and other social infrastructure, with the exception of abandoned buildings and dental clinics. However, private healthcare providers are allowed to establish new private healthcare institutions.

The health reform in Kyrgyzstan has taken place within the context of a political and economic transformation, and severe economic pressure. In 1996, Kyrgyzstan initiated a comprehensive 10-year healthcare sector reform program with the support of foreign donors. Currently, the country has established a number of healthcare-related laws and regulations; introduced a mandatory health insurance system; implemented a new provider payment method (i.e., the introduction of the single-payer system has integrated all previous health reform outcomes and played a catalytic role in the reform); and restructured and enhanced primary healthcare services.

However, the health reform needs to be deepened even further. The structural adjustment of healthcare service delivery needs to be continued with an emphasis on the hospital and sanitary-epidemiological sectors. Furthermore, activities to prevent the spread of communicable diseases (especially tuberculosis, malaria, and AIDS) also need to be continued. In recent years, the average life expectancy of Kyrgyzstan has improved continuously but has remained relatively low. In addition, its maternal and infant mortality rates remain high. Citizens should be encouraged to take greater responsibility for their own health.

The health reform in Kyrgyzstan has provided important lessons for other transitional healthcare systems, mainly with regard to:

1. The development of the healthcare sector relies to a great extent on the economic and democratic development of the society as a whole.
2. It is difficult to reform the healthcare funding system if it is not integrated into the national financial system.
3. The success of health reforms should not lead to an immediate reduction in funding. The introduction of mechanisms to ensure more efficient resource utilization, while lowering the funding level, is likely to result in public distrust in the reform process.
4. The structural adjustment of the healthcare delivery system cannot be achieved solely by administrative measures, but must also consider the role of economic levers.
5. The coordination of donor activities is critical to the successful implementation of reforms.
6. There must be a professional and united reform team dedicated to understanding the essence of the reforms being made. One of the major obstacles to reforms could be

healthcare workers. Therefore, it is crucial to ensure that healthcare workers receive extensive education and are fully informed of the reform process. These measures should be integrated with financial and other incentives to improve the enthusiasm of healthcare workers and the overall quality of their healthcare services, as well as reduce the demand for informal fees. It is also crucial to enhance the awareness of the public and civic organizations about the contents of reform.

7. It is extremely difficult to develop a new legislative framework in the early stages of program development, as laws tend to lag behind the reform process. Therefore, the new reform programs should be piloted prior to being expanded nationwide.

8. It is crucial to monitor, assess, and obtain feedback on the reform outcomes in a timely and accurate manner, as well as to control and correct existing issues in a timely manner.

The equal access of all Kyrgyzstanis to healthcare services had been threatened by the dissolution of the Soviet Union's free universal healthcare system. Although the country has developed the SGBP and a list of essential medicines, about half of the healthcare funds still come from personal out-of-pocket payments, much of which are informal under-the-counter payments. Following the introduction of the "single-payer" system, these informal payments have been replaced with formal copayments to a certain extent, but low-income earners continue to face difficulties in accessing healthcare services and drugs. As the high patient expenses are associated with the low government reimbursement and the overall economic fragility of Kyrgyzstan, the government is unlikely to increase its expenditure in the near future. The MANAS Health Care Reform Program is scheduled to be terminated in 2006, and the MOH is currently developing a program to replace it. The new program will involve further reforms, vertical programs, and the integration of the general healthcare system, as well as the establishment of cross-sectoral health promotion strategies.

CHAPTER NINETEEN

Health Systems in Three African Countries

 SECTION I. THE HEALTH SYSTEM IN SOUTH AFRICA

1. Overview of Socioeconomics and National Health

South Africa, officially the Republic of South Africa, is the southernmost country in Africa. It is bordered to the east, west, and south by the Indian and Atlantic Oceans. South Africa mainly comprises of a vast plateau and is situated in semi-desert and desert regions at latitudes of 19°–33°S. More than two-thirds of the country has an arid climate and only a few rivers that serve as abundant water sources. South Africa is almost entirely located on the subtropical ridge and has a savanna climate. The country has a total land area of 1,219,090 km², with a population of 56.52 million by 2017, consisting of Black African (80.7%), white (8.0%), colored (8.8%), and Asian (2.5%) ethnic groups. Black South Africans can be further divided into nine major tribes: Zulu, Xhosa, Swazi, Tswana, North Sotho, South Sotho, Tsonga, Venda, and Ndebele, most of whom are Bantu-speaking. White South Africans mainly consist of Afrikaners of Dutch descent (formerly known as Boers; about 57%) and whites of British descent (about 39%), who mainly speak Afrikaans and English. Colored South Africans are the mixed-race descendants of whites, indigenous people, and slaves during the colonial era, who mainly speak Afrikaans. Most of the Asian South Africans are Indian (about 99%) and Chinese. There are 11 official languages in South Africa, among which English and Afrikaans have been adopted as the lingua francas. White South Africans, the majority of colored South Africans, and 60% of black South Africans are either Protestant or Catholic. About 60% of Asian South Africans practice Hinduism and 20% Islam. Some black South Africans practice a traditional African religion. Pretoria is the administrative capital, with a population of about 2 million; Cape Town is the legislative capital, with a population of about 2.9 million; and Bloemfontein is the judicial capital, with a population of about 650,000.

South Africa is considered a middle-income country, but there is a wide wealth gap: roughly two-thirds of the national income is concentrated among wealthy individuals, who account for only 20% of the total South African population. Since 1994, the government of South Africa has launched a series of socioeconomic development programs to improve the living environment of impoverished black South Africans through the establishment of housing, water, and electricity infrastructures, as well as the delivery of basic healthcare services. In 1997, the government issued the White Paper for Social Welfare, which listed poverty alleviation and social assistance for the elderly, disabled individuals, and minors as the priorities of social welfare. In 2010, the average life expectancies for men and women in South Africa were 53.3 and 55.2 years, respectively.

According to "OECD Economic Surveys: South Africa 2013," the GDP growth rate of sub-Saharan Africa increased from 3.5 percentage points in 2012 to 4.7 percentage points in 2013, which was due to the increase in domestic demands and investments. However, the GDP of South Africa only grew by 1.9 percentage points in 2013, as it is the largest economy in the region and its labor relations were affected by sluggish external demand. In 2011, the total healthcare expenditure in South Africa accounted for 8.5% of its GDP, which was slightly lower than the average of OECD countries (9.3%). Among the OECD countries, the US ranked first in healthcare expenditure as a share of the GDP (17.7%). The healthcare expenditure of a country is usually proportional to its national income; thus, countries with a higher GDP per capita tend to have greater healthcare expenditures. It is, therefore, unsurprising that the healthcare expenditure per capita of South Africa in 2011 (US$943) was lower than the average of OECD countries (US$3,339).

Public financial allocation is the main source of healthcare funding of OECD countries, with the exception of Chile, Mexico, and the US. In 2011, public funding in South Africa accounted for only 47.7% of the country's total healthcare expenditure, which was much lower than the average of OECD countries (72.2%) and very close to those of Chile (46.9%), Mexico (47.3%), and the US (47.8%).

In 2011, the number of physicians in South Africa accounted for only 0.7% of the total population, which was much lower than the average of OECD countries (3.2%). Similarly, the number of nurses in South Africa accounted for only 1.1% of the total population, which was also much lower than the OECD average (8.7%). Furthermore, in 2010, there were 2.4 hospital beds per 1,000 people in South Africa, which is about half the average of OECD countries (4.8 hospital beds per 1,000 people).

Over the past two decades, the life expectancies of OECD countries have somewhat improved, with the average value increasing from 74.7 years in 1990 to 80.1 years in 2011; in contrast, the average life expectancy of South Africa decreased significantly from 61.6 years to 52.6 years during that same period, mainly due to the HIV/AIDS epidemic. The infant mortality rate in OECD countries has also declined over the past two decades, from 10.9 deaths per 1,000 live births in 1990 to 4.1 deaths per 1,000 live births in 2011. However, South Africa maintained a very stable and high infant mortality rate (34.6 deaths per 1,000 live births in 2011) over the same period, which was also mainly due to the HIV/AIDS epidemic. UNICEF reported that 50% of HIV-positive infants in South Africa die from HIV-related illnesses before their second birthday (Table 19.1).

The proportion of adult smokers in many countries has declined over the past two decades. In 2009, the proportion of smokers in South Africa (13.8%) was much lower than was the average in OECD countries (20.9%). However, there was a significant difference in the proportion of smokers between males and females in South Africa: In 2009, the proportions of male and female smokers in South Africa were 24% and 8%, respectively.

TABLE 19.1 Comparison of Basic Health Conditions in South Africa in 2005–2012

Item	2005	2006	2007	2008	2009	2010	2011	2012
Total population	47,639,556	48,269,753	48,910,248	49,561,256	50,222,996	50,895,698	51,579,599	52,274,945
Population growth (%)	1.3	1.3	1.3	1.3	1.3	1.3	1.3	1.3
Average life expectancy (years)	51.6	51.6	52	52.6	53.5	54.4	55.3	56.1
Fertility rate (births per woman)	2.7	2.6	2.6	2.5	2.5	2.5	2.4	2.4
Adolescent fertility rate (births per 1,000 women aged 15–19 years)	63.8	61.5	59.2	57.5	55.8	54.2	52.5	50.9
Mortality rate for children under 5 (deaths per 1,000 live births)	79.1	76.5	72.5	69	63.1	52.9	47.2	44.6
Measles vaccination rate (% of infants aged 12–23 months)	63	64	62	64	78	74	78	79
Incidence rate of HIV/AIDS (population aged 15–49 years)	17.1	17.2	17.3	17.5	17.6	17.6	17.8	17.9
GDP growth (%)	5.3	5.6	5.5	3.6	-1.5	3.1	3.5	2.5

2. Healthcare System

(1) Organizational Structure and Management of the Healthcare System

South Africa has adopted a three-tier management model comprising the central, provincial, and municipal levels. The central level is responsible for unified policy formulation and overall planning, as well as supervising, managing, and assessing the distribution of social welfare funds to ensure that this distribution meets the requirements of the central government. The provincial (nine provinces nationwide) and municipal levels are responsible for the implementation of healthcare policies and plans. The central government has also established the Department of Social Development (DSD), and its main functions are: (1) to provide social security services for the general public; (2) to provide services for vulnerable groups, disabled individuals, low-income earners, and impoverished individuals. The DSD has a provincial office in each of the nine provinces, which cooperate with local governments in social security affairs.

Apart from the DSD, other governmental departments in South Africa are also involved in providing social security for its citizens: (1) the National Department of Health (NDoH) is responsible for health and maternity insurance, as well as for improving the residential and living environment of black South Africans; (2) the Department of Labor is responsible for unemployment benefits, whereby unemployed persons are eligible to receive four to six months of unemployment benefits. (3) The Department of Transport is responsible for determining the level of compensation for injuries from traffic accidents. Black South Africans live in predominately black areas, which typically have high rates of traffic accidents; the Department of Transport is responsible for establishing traffic accident insurance schemes for these areas.

Over the past decade, the government of South Africa has been studying the issue of including impoverished groups in the social welfare system. The total fiscal revenue of South Africa was ZAR1 trillion, of which ZAR46 billion was allocated to the DSD for assisting 8 million impoverished or disabled individuals. However, this government assistance is only available for the poorest South Africans due to the limited availability of funds. Specifically, only households with monthly incomes below ZAR800 are eligible for the assistance, which mainly includes: (1) unsupported elderly adults; (2) unemployed, disabled individuals; and (3) orphans. The age ranges for social grant eligibility are: elderly women aged over 60 years and elderly men aged over 65 years, and disabled women aged 18–59 years and disabled men aged 18–64 years. The government has also allocated some social welfare funds to support students and patients, build houses for low-income individuals, and provide assistance to veterans who participated in World War II. In addition, schools and hospitals are required to reduce school fees and medical charges, respectively, for impoverished individuals. Assessment and supervisory teams have been established at the central and provincial levels in order to inspect the implementation of social welfare policies in all regions. An Auditor-General has also been appointed to monitor the distribution of social grants. Furthermore, the central government has established the South African Human Rights Commission (SAHRC), which is responsible for reporting the formulation and implementation of social welfare policies to Parliament. Both the government and the President of South Africa attach great importance to SAHRC reports. The social welfare system is also monitored by non-governmental organizations (NGOs).

South Africa has implemented a completely open market economy, but there remains a wide wealth gap because of its long history of racial discrimination. Currently, there are very few job opportunities in South Africa, which has led to a remarkably high number of unemployed persons, accounting for nearly half of its total population. Over the past decade, the government of South Africa has been actively attempting to improve the employment rate and reduce the poverty rate. The Department of Labor also provides unemployment benefits to those who earn less than ZAR13,000 per year.

(2) Teaching Hospitals and Medical Schools

Approximately 900 medical students and 300 specialists graduate each year from seven medical schools in South Africa. Each medical school is affiliated with one or more large-sized teaching hospitals, which are equipped with 2,000–6,000 beds and are fully funded by the state through the respective provincial governments. Teaching hospitals are large-sized hospitals that provide tertiary and referral healthcare services and admit patients transferred from private hospitals. In addition, teaching hospitals are responsible for providing secondary healthcare services for impoverished individuals residing in the surrounding area. Due to fiscal austerity measures and an inadequate number of healthcare institutions, teaching hospitals also receive a large number of trauma, elderly, and other types of patients who are unrelated to medical education. This has resulted in a shortage of funds and talent in teaching hospitals, which have led to low enthusiasm and increased turnover among healthcare workers in these institutions. Recommendations to provide teaching hospitals with institutional autonomy and to collect service charges from private patients might enable the healthcare system to provide better research equipment and increase the salaries of full-time healthcare workers. Such changes are expected also to improve the quality of academic institutions. However, many scholars hold different views on this, believing instead that this may cause the government to reduce its financial allocations for the treatment of impoverished patients in teaching hospitals. As there are only seven medical schools in South Africa, with only a handful of senior academic positions across the country, it is foreseeable that many postgraduate students will seek employment in the private sector instead. Talent loss is another problem that has had a major impact on medical schools. Although some physicians have migrated abroad because of the apartheid system, many others do not return after studying abroad for the same reason. Furthermore, some physicians have stayed abroad in Western countries because of the excellent remuneration in those countries. However, it is still difficult to determine the impact of talent loss on the healthcare system in South Africa.

3. Health Security System

The healthcare system in South Africa consists of two parallel systems: the public healthcare system (a publicly funded healthcare system targeting individuals living in poverty or high-income individuals who refuse to purchase health insurance, accounting for roughly five-sixths of the total population) and the private healthcare system (targeting high-income individuals who have purchased health insurance, accounting for one-sixth of the total population).

(1) Formation of the Public Healthcare System

Before 1919, the healthcare system in South Africa underwent a continuous process of specialization, institutionalization, and organization, which were influenced by the UK, during which, various military hospitals and private hospitals were established, and a number of laws and norms were enacted to facilitate the coordination of the healthcare system. This coordination was further enhanced between 1919 and 1940 with the implementation of the Public Health Act. Then, in 1940–1950, healthcare policies were reformulated to eliminate structural deficiencies in the previous system. Thus, nearly every important aspect of the system was adjusted and reformed in some way, in order to establish a unified, comprehensive publicly funded healthcare system, whereby primary healthcare services were mainly delivered by healthcare centers. In 1950–1994, the healthcare system in South Africa was primarily characterized by racial discrimination and segregation, which affected not only the delivery of healthcare services but also the health status of South Africans. All healthcare policies during this period reflected the interests of the white minority. The government also aimed to establish a national healthcare service and made a gradual shift toward primary healthcare. After 1994, particularly April 27, 1994, a democratic government was elected, which established the new NDoH in an attempt to provide all South Africans with standardized, fair healthcare services. Following the abolition of apartheid, the healthcare system was gradually reformed into the current health security system. The government provides universal, low-cost public healthcare services to all citizens, while also allowing the establishment of private health insurance schemes to cover expensive healthcare services in private hospitals. Government expenditure accounts for about 42% of the total healthcare expenditure, out-of-pocket payments account for 10%, private health insurance schemes account for 45%, while the remaining 3% is covered by other funding sources. Public hospitals in South Africa provide universal, low-cost healthcare services to all citizens (free for low-income earners), and the resulting medical expenses are mainly covered by the government. The government of South Africa does not levy a special health insurance tax, and the National Treasury allocates funds from general tax revenues to each province, which in turn distributes the funds to public hospitals and public healthcare institutions for the reimbursement of medical expenses.

The public hospital system in South Africa has essentially achieved universal public healthcare coverage. Excluding the participants of private health insurance schemes, about five-sixths of the South African population utilizes public healthcare services. However, due to inefficient government management, the public hospitals in South Africa have relatively poor healthcare environments and service quality, which have also made it difficult for such hospitals to attract physicians and specialists. The numbers of general practitioners (GPs) and specialists per 1,000 patients in public hospitals are only 1/16 and 1/23 of those in private hospitals, respectively.

(2) Private Health Insurance

In 1998, South Africa adopted the Medical Schemes Act, which permits the establishment of private health insurance schemes. These are voluntary schemes for individuals, wherein premiums are shared between employees and employers. Furthermore, the government allows for pretax deductions on a proportion of the premiums. Private health insurance schemes in South Africa must operate on a non-profit basis, whereby surpluses must be retained within the scheme. Hence, they are in essence mutual-type commercial health insurance schemes. However, private health insurance schemes can hire market-oriented agencies to administer the schemes (scheme administrators or third-party administrators, TPAs), a managed care organization to control of the risks associated with medical expenses, or agents to promote the scheme. These market-oriented agencies are for-profit organizations that charge management fees. Private insurance schemes generally cover healthcare services provided at private hospitals, which tend to offer healthcare services of higher quality. As of the second quarter of 2008, there were about 112 private health insurance schemes in South Africa, which provided approximately 392 types of insurance plans. Currently, private health insurance schemes cover about one-sixth of the population in South Africa.

The government of South Africa has also established the Council for Medical Schemes (CMS) for the supervision of private health insurance schemes. The CMS is an NDoH-affiliated statutory body responsible for the supervision of the entry, service standards, and solvency of private health insurance schemes. Furthermore, it is responsible for overseeing scheme administrators and managed care organizations that cooperate with the scheme. The basic requirements of the CMS for health insurance schemes are: (1) the scheme must be open to the public for participation; (2) segregation of insured persons based on risk classification is prohibited – that is, the underwriting and differential pricing of insured persons according to age, medical history, and health status are prohibited; (3) the scheme must cover minimum health security services; (4) there must be excellent internal control and governance institutions. In summary, private health insurance schemes in South Africa are government-regulated, market-operated mutual health insurance schemes that purchase professional management services.

(3) Public–Private Partnership (PPP)

PPP is a unique feature of the healthcare sector in South Africa. It refers to any form of cooperation and interaction between the public and private sectors within the healthcare system. PPP aims to strengthen the role of hospitals in upholding universal health coverage, improve the infrastructure and services of hospitals, and enhance the institutionalization of hospitals. In addition, PPP aims to establish rules and regulations for improving the management and training of hospital professionals, as well as establishing a fair and reasonable insurance system. District healthcare systems in South Africa are jointly established by public and private hospitals. Furthermore, PPP was established to ensure the access of vulnerable groups to basic healthcare services through the development of clinics and basic healthcare programs. These efforts include: (1) providing free healthcare services for pregnant women and children under age six and free access to basic healthcare services; (2) establishing primary healthcare service packages and expanding tuberculosis control and immunization programs; (3) establishing hundreds of clinics to promote the delivery of integrated basic healthcare services, thereby improving the health status of South Africans.

Private health insurance schemes in South Africa are permitted to purchase external market-oriented management services, which can improve the professionalism of their management services and their risk management capabilities through the division of labor and market competition. For example, Discovery Health Pty. Ltd. has developed a client-oriented product structure and specialized risk management tools via the integration of medical, actuarial, operational, and technical expertise, and has created a set of highly refined customer services to meet varying customer needs. These efforts were intended to address the global challenge of controlling the risks associated with medical expenses, that is, scheme administrators must control medical expenses in order to ensure the sustainability of their schemes, which is in conflict with the desire of insured persons to spend more on their medical care. In terms of product structure, Discovery Health has introduced a three-tier product system that classifies healthcare services based on their frequency of use and cost. The company attracts most healthy insured persons to join the Vitality Club, which uses incentives to promote physical exercise, smoking, and drinking cessation, and a healthy lifestyle, in order to improve the overall health status and prevent diseases among customers. Furthermore, due to the relatively high moral hazard associated with common minor illnesses, the company uses customers' medical savings accounts to reimburse the medical expenses for these illnesses, which then leads customers to actively control their medical expenses. In contrast, the company provides the best possible healthcare services for costly, critical illnesses, as they have relatively low incidence rates and moral hazard.

Table 19.2 summarizes the challenges in sustainability and equality facing the healthcare system in South Africa. Most of these challenges are related to problems with the private health insurance schemes and the properties of PPPs. The inconsistency between public and private healthcare systems is widely considered the greatest barrier to the establishment of a fair healthcare system in South Africa. In its classification of healthcare systems, the WHO also considered this inconsistency as the main reason for the poor performance of South Africa's healthcare system.

(4) Medical Savings Account (MSA) Plans

MSA plans were established in 1994 in South Africa, and they form an important component of the country's medical schemes. These medical schemes are a type of conventional health insurance product provided by private health insurance companies based on the law of large numbers. MSA plans were initially established by the Medical Schemes Act, which came into effect in 2000.

The healthcare services covered by typical medical schemes can be divided into routine healthcare services and healthcare services for critical illnesses. The latter can be further divided into prescribed minimum benefits (PMBs) and above threshold benefits (ATBs). PMBs cover all emergency services, 270 defined medical conditions, and 28 defined chronic conditions without deductibles, out-of-pocket payments, and reimbursement caps. On the other hand, ATBs cover the medical expenses for critical illnesses with deductibles, out-of-pocket payments, and reimbursement caps. The reimbursement of routine healthcare services can be further divided into annual thresholds, MSAs, out-of-pocket payments and conventional medical schemes, among which the annual threshold and conventional medical schemes have deductibles, out-of-pocket payments, and reimbursement caps.

MSA plans are used to cover out-of-pocket expenses for various co-payment mechanisms. In South Africa, MSAs are more often considered as a means of tax avoidance because both the contributions and accrued interest of MSAs are tax exempt. Since 2000, the government of South Africa has enacted legislation stipulating that MSA annual contributions must not exceed 25% of the premiums of corresponding medical schemes, in order to prevent the excessive use of MSAs for tax avoidance. Moreover, the reimbursement scope of MSAs has been limited to out-of-pocket expenses and medical expenses beyond the coverage of medical schemes.

4. Status of Healthcare Funding

Most healthcare institutions in South Africa are funded by the National Treasury. In 2007, the total public hospital expenditure accounted for 3.05% of the GDP and 11.08% of the total government expenditure. Although the government covers about 40% of the healthcare expenditure, public hospitals still face immense pressure from serving roughly 80% of the South African population, whereas most of the country's healthcare resources are concentrated in private hospitals, which serve only 20% of the total population. In February 2007, the National Treasury allocated an additional ZAR 5.3 billion to the NDoH for human resources, control of the HIV/AIDS epidemic, hospital reconstruction, and tertiary healthcare services. In 2003, the government launched a hospital restructuring program with a budget of ZAR 1.9 billion to improve the performance of the public healthcare system through continuous improvement of the infrastructure, necessary equipment, and management skills of public hospitals. Under this program, local hospital management departments are given authority over various operational issues facing hospitals, such

TABLE 19.2 Challenges in Sustainability and Equality Facing the Healthcare System of South Africa

Challenges in Sustainability	Challenges in Equality
Category 1	Category 1
Stagnated growth of healthcare resources in the public sector	Tax-based funding:
Increase in the size of the population that is dependent on public healthcare services (especially high-risk individuals)	It is unclear whether the tax system is progressive, neutral, or regressive
—	Outcomes/utilization of healthcare services is not allocated based on patient needs
—	The government pays for the medical scheme premiums of each civil servant from the tax-based funds, and the premiums are 12 times those of individuals who rely on public healthcare services.
Category 2	Category 2
High annual growth rate of medical scheme premiums	PPP: The government provides substantial subsidies to the private healthcare sector
Reduced scope of service benefits	Tax exemption for medical scheme premiums
Increased co-payment rate	Funding for the training of healthcare workers, most of whom enter the private sector upon the completion of training
Decline in the number of insured persons	Medical scheme-insured persons are charged at a price lower than the cost recovery level in public hospitals
More healthcare resources are utilized to provide healthcare services for a minority of patients	—
Category 3	Category 3
One-quarter of persons insured by medical schemes are civil servants and their dependents	Cross-subsidization:
As the government covers two-thirds of the medical scheme premiums of civil servants, there is excessive growth in medical expenses, further decreasing the scarce government resources	Income (cross-subsidization of high-income earners for low-income earners): minimal, as the insurance premium rate is not determined according to income levels
Overreliance of medical schemes on the number of civil servants	Cross-subsidization related to health status (transfers from low-risk to high-risk insured persons): reduced levels due to the refinement of risk classification and risk pooling
Multiple scopes of service benefits	—
Refinement of risk pooling	—
Increased instability of individual insurance schemes	—

as financing and staffing, to ensure that the healthcare needs of local residents are met. In April 2006, there were 33,220 South African physicians registered under the Health Professions Council of South Africa (HPCSA), a supervisory agency for physicians. The HPCSA requires physicians who wish to renew their annual registration to comply with the Continuing Professional Development (CPD) program by attending periodic workshops, seminars, and refresher courses. PPPs were gradually formed to help resolve the shortage of resources and workforce in public hospitals. For instance, some private healthcare institutions began providing beds and healthcare services for patients in public hospitals. In addition, public hospitals have begun providing free screening and treatment regimens for AIDS and poverty-associated diseases, such as tuberculosis and cholera, which have a considerable impact (particularly HIV/AIDS) on the healthcare system of South Africa.

The healthcare funding system of South Africa is dominated by the public healthcare sector, that is, through total tax revenues. The public healthcare system in South Africa provides universal healthcare services to nearly the entire population through widely distributed service points. Furthermore, basic healthcare services are provided free of charge. However, public healthcare institutions have exceedingly long waiting times, and only a handful of physicians in these institutions provide basic healthcare services. These public healthcare institutions support the development of primary healthcare by providing free services for pregnant women and children.

In 2008, the healthcare system in South Africa began paying greater attention to the development of primary healthcare and the delivery of basic healthcare services. Currently, approximately 37% of GPs are employed by public hospitals, while the rest work in private hospitals. However, there is a shortage of GPs in public hospitals, with about one-third of positions being vacant, and a large number of healthcare workers have not renewed their registration with the HPCSA. Approximately 42% of nurses and 30% of physicians work in public hospitals. Nearly 62% of the total healthcare expenditure is spent on private hospitals, which only serve around 7 million patients; in contrast, about 38% of the total healthcare expenditure is spent on public hospitals, which serve nearly 35 million patients.

5. Health System Reforms

(1) Reform Background

Apartheid has had a lasting legacy of inequality in South Africa, and its impact is reflected on both the income level and access to social services. South Africa also faces an extreme degree of inequality in health status and access to healthcare services. The South Africa Demographic and Health Survey showed that most black South Africans are served in public hospitals, whereas most white and Indian South Africans are served in private hospitals. The racial conflicts and the HIV/AIDS epidemic in South Africa have resulted in a stagnated economic growth, which in turn has increased the medical expenses for treating these patients, thus further reducing the GDP and increasing poverty.

In 1983–1985, public healthcare expenditure increased alongside the GDP, but there was an extreme degree of inequality in the use of healthcare services. Only around 75% of South Africans had access to public healthcare services, the majority of whom were middle-income earners. In contrast, impoverished South Africans lacked access to public healthcare services, as hospitals were not easily accessible and despite the low charges, the medical expenses were too high for these individuals. Therefore, the delivery of basic healthcare services has become a top priority of healthcare system reform in South Africa. Twenty-five percent of impoverished South Africans could not receive healthcare in the event of illnesses. Furthermore, women and children living in impoverished areas faced more health issues. Public hospitals mainly provided healthcare services to the wealthy population. Hospitals accounted for 75% of the total public healthcare expenditure and were mainly academic institutions and tertiary hospitals, which primarily serve the wealthy.

There are two different systems for the delivery and funding of healthcare services in South Africa: the public healthcare system and the private healthcare system.

The government has adopted various policies and legal measures to promote the provision of more healthcare services in the public sector. However, there is a tendency to allocate more financial resources to private hospitals, which implies that they receive higher reimbursements and typically have better working environments and higher-end technologies. Hence, more healthcare workers are moving from public hospitals to private hospitals, resulting in a shortage of talent in public hospitals.

Following the establishment of a democratic government in 1994, the African National Congress (ANC) took power and began to eliminate racially discriminatory healthcare policies. Prior to this, most hospitals served only white South Africans, while 14 health departments were facing institutional separation and redundancy. Hence, the vast majority of South Africans did not have fair access to healthcare services, and rural residents often had to make long journeys to receive healthcare services in designated hospitals. Therefore, it became imperative to reform the healthcare system, including hospitals.

(2) Specific Reform Measures

1. Reform of the Management System   After taking power, the ANC accelerated the abolition of racially discriminatory healthcare policies and implemented a major health reform centered on basic healthcare services, in order to ensure sufficient control over local public healthcare services. Since 1994, hospital services and basic healthcare services have been provided by the nine provincial health departments. These provincial health departments allocate a portion of the healthcare budget to local authorities for the provision of basic healthcare services, which are free for children under the age of six years and pregnant or breastfeeding women.

The government has established district healthcare systems to ensure that local governments have control over the delivery, regulation, and coordination of public healthcare services. The government has also established more than 700 clinics and 125 mobile clinics, as well as refurbished further 2,298 clinics, in order to ensure the widespread availability and accessibility of healthcare services. The number of private hospitals and clinics has continued to increase alongside a growing preference for private hospitals among wealthy individuals.

The hospital system can be divided into the public healthcare system, which provides services to the majority of impoverished individuals, and the private healthcare system, which mainly serves a minority of employees. Private hospital services are provided to 23% of the total population, but the resulting medical expenses account for 60% of the total healthcare expenditure in South Africa. The majority of healthcare workers, with the exception of nurses, are employed in private hospitals. The government of South Africa has also explored innovative PPPs that involve contracting with the professional associations of relevant private hospitals for the delivery of healthcare services to patients in the public healthcare sector, in an effort to accelerate the development of district healthcare systems and increase the autonomy and efficiency of public healthcare providers.

In January 1995, the NHI Benefits Advisory Committee was established to help develop a healthcare system that ensures equal access to affordable, sustainable and efficient primary healthcare services for all South Africans. The total tax revenues, as well as the tax revenues and user fees levied by local authorities, cover 38.7% of the total healthcare expenditure in South Africa.

2. Reform of the Reimbursement Mechanism   The government of South Africa has significantly altered its funding arrangement via the introduction of fiscal federalism. This has affected the funding and budgetary affairs of the healthcare system, in order to enable local governments to allocate healthcare resources in a more equitable manner. The public healthcare sector mainly relies on tax revenues from the central government, as well as financial support from local governments. Funding sources for public hospitals also include user fees and social health insurance.

The distribution of public healthcare resources is primarily a redistribution at the national level. Its aim is to reduce the number of large-sized hospitals that provide tertiary healthcare services to poor and uninsured individuals, while also directing its main focus on basic and community healthcare services, which have long been neglected in South Africa. In addition, physicians were transferred to areas most in need of them by, for example, imposing more significant restrictions on areas in which primary care physicians can provide healthcare services.

In 2006–2007, the standard fee for each uninsured person for primary healthcare services in public hospitals was ZAR297. The total primary healthcare expenditure is funded by provincial health departments and district health bureaus and accounts for 20% of the total healthcare expenditure on public hospitals. The government has also established institutions, such as the South African Medical Research Council (SAMRC) (which provides therapeutic support and integrative therapies for tuberculosis, HIV, and AIDS), in order to improve the ability of public hospitals to screen for diseases. Furthermore, various means of support were also provided to uninsured HIV/AIDS and tuberculosis patients. There is an increasingly severe shortage of GPs, specialists, dentists, pharmacists, and psychiatrists in public hospitals, which can mainly be attributed to the poor remunerations for these personnel, leading to talent loss. Currently, social health insurance is the main source of healthcare funding and provides important opportunities for the establishment of PPPs. District healthcare systems in South Africa are jointly established by public and private hospitals. Moreover, the salary of physicians has also been raised to attract younger physicians. As of the end of 2007, comprehensive HIV/AIDS services were available in 362 public hospitals.

Although private practitioners or patients are allowed to access facilities in public hospitals, a corresponding user fee is levied on them to increase the incomes of these hospitals. Moreover, to ensure that vulnerable groups had sufficient access to healthcare services, the following individuals were eligible for free services prior to 1994: South Africans who request family planning and disinfection services, as well as vaccination and other measures to prevent infectious diseases; patients who participate in clinical trials; patients with infectious diseases and notifiable diseases (e.g., tuberculosis, leprosy, cholera, and sexually transmitted diseases); physical examinations for victims of assault and rape; organ, blood, milk, or tissue donors; and public healthcare workers with work-related injuries. There were also numerous free services for patients with chronic diseases, nutritional deficiencies, and mental illnesses. On May 24, 1994, the President announced that children aged under six years and pregnant women, as well as women at six weeks postpartum, are eligible for free healthcare services. The priority of basic healthcare was the development of clinics and basic healthcare programs, including: free healthcare services for pregnant women and children aged under six years; free access for all South Africans to basic healthcare services; establishing the district healthcare system; formulation of the Essential Medicines List (EML) and Medicines Act; development of mental healthcare services; expansion of human resources; provision of abortion services; establishment of rural clinics, etc. Primary healthcare packages were established, and tuberculosis control and immunization programs were expanded. Moreover, hundreds of clinics were established to improve the health status of South Africans by promoting the delivery of integrated, basic healthcare services.

3. Reform of the Operational Mechanism   South Africa is mainly aiming to promote the delivery of private healthcare services, while concurrently developing a more equitable public healthcare system. The public healthcare sector has faced considerable pressure as it needs to allocate resources to a universal basic healthcare system, which primarily provides Western medicine and traditional African medicine, in an attempt to establish a PPP-based healthcare system.

As noted earlier, PPP is a unique feature of the healthcare sector in South Africa. It refers to any form of cooperation and interaction between the public and private sectors within the healthcare system. The main purpose of PPP is to promote the development of private hospitals, while also establishing a more equitable and efficient healthcare system, thereby ensuring universal access to basic healthcare services. PPP was deemed necessary in the early days of the South African healthcare system, as public hospitals faced an increasingly severe shortage of specialists, dentists, pharmacists, and psychiatrists due to poor remunerations. The emergence of social health insurance as the main source of healthcare funding provided important opportunities for the establishment of PPP. On the one hand, South Africa began to promulgate policies that allowed healthcare technicians in public healthcare institutions to provide paid services in other healthcare institutions, such as working part-time in private healthcare institutions, in order to increase their incomes and motivate them to remain in public hospitals. On the other hand, the participation of private hospitals in South Africa was crucial for alleviating the shortage of healthcare resources, improving the accessibility of healthcare services, and meeting the diversified healthcare needs of the public. The operational mode of PPP serves as the final approach to the establishment of a healthcare system that is favorable to the sustainable development and equality of the entire health insurance industry, while also upholding the principle of equality in investments in the healthcare sector. PPP is aimed at strengthening the role of hospitals in universal health coverage, improving the infrastructure and services of hospitals, and enhancing the institutionalization of hospitals. In addition, PPP also aims to establish rules and regulations for improving the management and training of hospital professionals, as well as establishing a fair and reasonable insurance system for South Africans.

4. Reform of Resource Allocation   South Africa has faced extreme shortages in the healthcare workforce (particularly among physicians and nurses), as well as an uneven distribution in this workforce across different regions and between the public and private healthcare systems. In 2006, there were 0.77 physicians and 4.08 nurses per 1,000 people in South Africa; in 2007, there were 23.7 and 166.3 independent healthcare practitioners per 1,000 people in public and private hospitals, respectively. The government of South Africa has adopted a number of measures, including establishing various talent training programs, raising the salaries of physicians and nurses in public hospitals, encouraging private hospitals to establish medical schools, etc., in order to improve the rational allocation of healthcare resources. Public hospitals in South Africa have also been encouraged by the government to attract young physicians by raising physicians' salaries and improve the sharing of human resources by establishing regional human resource networks with private hospitals.

(3) Reform Development and Evolution

1. Commission on Old Age Pension and National Insurance (1928)   The Commission recommended that an NHI scheme be established to cover medical, maternity, and funeral benefits for low-income earners living in suburban areas.

2. Committee of Enquiry into NHI (1935)   The Committee recommended similar proposals to those made in 1928. Neither of those proposals was ever put into practice.

3. National Health Service Commission (1942–1944) The National Health Service Commission was a reform advocated by Dr. Henry Gluckman, which recommended the implementation of a National Health Tax to ensure the delivery of free healthcare services to all South Africans according to their specific needs, irrespective of race, color, wealth, or status. Health centers, which provide comprehensive primary healthcare services, would serve as core institutions of the healthcare system.

The Gluckman proposals were accepted by the government, but they were implemented successively as a series of measures rather than all at once. Ultimately, only the number of community health centers in South Africa increased to 44 within two years, whereas other aspects of the proposals were never implemented.

4. Health Care Finance Committee (1994) In the early 1990s, the spotlight was once again turned to the possibility of introducing partially mandatory health insurance, and several policy initiatives were formulated focusing on social or national health insurance. The Healthcare Finance Committee of 1994 recommended that formal employees and their immediate dependents form the preliminary core membership of social health insurance before it is expanded to other groups.

The Committee also suggested that there be a cooperative payment scheme, and that private funds, also known as private medical schemes, should act as financial intermediaries for funding healthcare providers. The Committee also proposed the establishment of a risk-equalization mechanism between individual insurance policies to help stabilize the health insurance industry. In other words, the segregation of insured persons based on risk classification, as well as differential pricing of insured persons according to their ages, medical history, and health status, were prohibited.

5. Committee of Inquiry on NHI (1995) The 1995 Committee of Enquiry on NHI fully supported the recommendations of the 1994 Health Care Finance Committee, with the exception of the benefits package. This NHI committee placed great emphasis on primary healthcare services.

6. The Social Health Insurance Working Group (1997) In 1997, the Social Health Insurance Working Group developed an administrative framework that resulted in the enactment of the Medical Schemes Act in 1998. This Act was intended to regulate private health insurance and reinforce the principles of open enrollment, community rating, PMBs, and better management mechanisms. Under this Act, private health insurance schemes become nonprofit and aim to cover medical expenses incurred by insured persons in private hospitals. Participation in private health insurance schemes is voluntary and the premium contributions can be shared between employees and employers. Nevertheless, the coverage for private healthcare services remained below 16%, as private insurance was only affordable to relatively wealthy individuals.

7. Committee of Inquiry into a Comprehensive Social Security for South Africa (2002) In 2002, the DSD appointed Prof. Vivienne Taylor to chair the Committee of Inquiry into a Comprehensive Social Security for South Africa. This Committee recommended that health coverage be made mandatory for formal sector employees who earn above a particular tax threshold. Furthermore, their premium contributions should be proportional to their incomes and collected as part of the health tax.

The Committee also recommended that the government establish a national healthcare fund for public facilities.

8. Ministerial Task Team on Social Health Insurance (2002)   In order to implement the recommendations of the Taylor Committee, the NDoH established the Ministerial Task Team on Social Health Insurance in 2002. The team drafted specific recommendations on social health insurance and how to achieve long-term outcomes via legislative and institutional mechanisms. However, the social health insurance model was not widely supported and the drafted recommendations were stalled.

9. Advisory Committee on NHI (2009)   In August 2009, the Advisory Committee on NHI was established to implement health reforms. A resolution initiating this reform was passed at the Polokwane conference in December 2007. In September 2010, the ruling party of South Africa, the ANC, formally proposed the establishment of NHI. The chairman of the ANC Subcommittee on Health, Dr. Zweli Mkhize, said that from 2012 onward, South Africa is expected to need another 14 years to progressively improve the NHI. In addition, the availability of funds has become a major bottleneck in the implementation of this enormous project: It is expected that the project will require upward of ZAR214 billion in 2020. Once fully established in 2025, the universal healthcare system is expected to require ZAR255 billion per year to sustain itself. The South African economic research institute, Econex, reported that the government could not afford such an immense investment in the implementation of the NHI. Moreover, implementation of NHI in South Africa would require an additional 10,000 GPs and 7,000–17,000 specialists.

(4) Reform Characteristics

1. Establishment of a Healthcare System Based on Basic Healthcare Services   The new government has established basic healthcare systems in each district to address the nation's healthcare issues. The establishment of a vigorous basic healthcare system with limited public resources is expected to play an important role in achieving healthcare equality.

2. Establishment of a PPP-based Operational Mechanism   In November 2001, during the National Health Summit, the concept of PPP was proposed and various measures were introduced to help promote cooperation and trust between the public and private sectors. The government encouraged PPP in order to expand the coverage of healthcare services while also improving the standards of such services. The key to healthcare services lies in the equal distribution of healthcare institutions, reduction of drug prices, expansion of healthcare expenditure, and engagement of the private sector in the delivery of healthcare services. Despite increasingly extensive public–private interactions, there remains an overall lack of cooperative mechanisms between these two sectors.

3. Establishment of a Healthcare System with a Legal Basis   The objectives of enacting laws are to reduce the degree of inequality among private healthcare institutions, control drug prices via the management of health insurance schemes that discriminate against chronic diseases, and enhance the control and management of private insurance schemes, thereby ensuring the access of uninsured persons to public healthcare services.

SECTION II. THE HEALTH SYSTEM IN EGYPT

1. Overview of Socioeconomics and National Health

Egypt, officially the Arab Republic of Egypt, was founded in 1952. It is located in northeastern Africa, and more than 96% of its landscape is desert. Egypt is the most populous country in the Middle East and the second most populous country in Africa. Furthermore, it is one of the four ancient civilizations and is one of the oldest countries in the world. Egypt has long been a leading country in the fields of economics and technology in Africa. Although Egypt is highly influential in both Africa and the Middle East, its economy is not optimistic, and the majority of Egyptians live below the poverty line. In particular, the turbulent political situation starting in early 2011 has had a serious impact on Egypt's economy. Furthermore, the country's extremely high birth rate has resulted in about 10 million unregistered citizens. European experts have estimated that the total population of Egypt may have reached 90 million, possibly even 100 million. Islam is the official religion of Egypt, and the majority of followers are Sunni, who account for 84% of the total population. The remaining 16% of the total population are Coptic Christians or followers of other religions. In 2013, the GDP of Egypt was US$262.7 billion. Overseas remittance, tourism, Suez Canal revenues, and the oil industry are the four largest sources of foreign exchange earnings in Egypt.

The Egyptian government follows a semi-presidential system. The capital city, Cairo, is the political and cultural center of Egypt, with an area of about 3,085 km^2 and a population of approximately 8 million. It is one of the most populous cities among Arabian and African countries. The famous pyramids of Giza and the Great Sphinx are located in the southwestern suburbs of Cairo.

2. Healthcare System and Structure

The social security system in Egypt was established in 1992 and has been reformed twice: in 1994 and 1995. The system mainly covers employees of government departments, agencies, and enterprises (including rural enterprises). Egyptian law has made participation in the government-run healthcare system compulsory, with the exception of individuals who choose to enroll in commercial health insurance. Approximately 17 million Egyptians are enrolled in government-run health insurance, whereby the employed population is administered by the Social Insurance Organization (SIO) under the Ministry of Manpower and Migration (MoMM), and the unemployed population is administered by the Health Insurance Organization (HIO) under the Ministry of Health and Population (MoHP). Civil servants are mainly enrolled in government-run insurance, but some are also enrolled in nongovernmental (mainly for-profit) insurance schemes.

The social security system of Egypt mainly consists of health insurance, work-related injury insurance, and pension insurance. Employers (i.e., enterprises) and employees pay 15% and 11% of the employee's salaries, respectively, as social insurance premiums; of which, 4% of the employers' contribution and 1% of the employees' contribution (a total of 5%) are set aside as health insurance premiums, with additional subsidies from the government. All health insurance premiums are transferred to the SIO of the MoMM, of which 1% is set aside as a premium for work-related injury insurance while the remaining 4% is administered by the HIO of the MoHP as health insurance premiums. The premiums for work-related injury insurance are used to cover the transportation and treatment of disabled workers, with a maximum reimbursement term of six months (180 days); any remaining medical expenses after exceeding the maximum reimbursement term are covered by disability benefits. The premium contributions of retirees aged 50–60 years account for a very small share (only about 5%) of the total premium contributions. Individuals who have retired after 60 years of age are entitled to receive a pension equivalent to 80% of their pre-retirement salaries (after tax deduction, the actual amount of pension is equivalent to 100% of their preretirement salaries). Retirees who wish to maintain their medical benefits generally have to pay premiums equivalent to 3% of their pensions at their own expense, without any contributions from their former employers.

Unemployed Egyptians can be eligible for the same medical benefits as employed persons by joining a health insurance scheme and paying their premiums to the relevant department. In addition, the government provides free basic health protection for uninsured, unemployed persons, who can seek medical treatment in hospitals established by the government and managed by the MoHP. All resulting medical expenses are covered using the 4% healthcare fund collected by the government. There is approximately one health center for every three or four villages in rural areas, providing free services to rural residents.

Following a period of economic liberalization in Egypt, there was a substantial increase in the revenues in certain industries, such as oil and banking. Commercial insurance began to emerge because the old social insurance system could no longer meet the demands of some high-income earners. Although all hospitals in Egypt used to be state-owned, private hospitals providing better services have since emerged. Following the implementation of numerous economic policies and increasing privatization, the number of private hospitals in Egypt has increased significantly, some of which have facilities comparable to those of public hospitals. Under these circumstances, some high-income earners began seeking medical attention in the higher-end private hospitals, leading to an increase in the consumer population and personal medical expenses. This prompted insurance companies to begin providing health insurance in order to compete with the National Health Insurance scheme.

Commercial health insurance primarily offers group coverage, with a lesser emphasis on individual coverage. Employers sign an agreement with insurance companies to participate in group health insurance. Employers with proof of participation in insurance policies that provide better benefits than do the government-run schemes are exempt from paying the 4% employer contribution but still need to pay the 1% employee contribution to the SIO. Commercial insurance typically offers better benefits and services, with a broader coverage area across Egypt (government-run schemes cover fewer hospitals). However, commercial insurance schemes impose an additional 10% administrative fee. The provision of commercial insurance schemes is supervised by the Insurance Review Organization and Misr Reinsurance. To reduce wastage, commercial insurance companies in Egypt have established a review committee comprising hospital healthcare workers and insurance companies to assess the necessity of hospitalization and expensive treatment regimens.

It should be noted that unemployed Egyptian women can only participate in commercial insurance. However, widowed Egyptian women who continue to pay a premium equivalent to 3% of their deceased husbands' salaries are entitled to receive the same health insurance benefits as their husbands.

3. Health System Reforms and Prospects

Egypt is a developing country where tourism is one of the main industries. The Egyptian government is aware of the importance of basic healthcare services for its residents and hence has been formulating relevant policies and reforming its healthcare sector. Egypt has a multi-tiered, segregated healthcare system. The government mainly provides preventive and therapeutic services. In 2005, Egypt had nearly 5,000 healthcare institutions with more than 80,000 beds. The HIO was established in 1964 to provide mandatory health insurance for employees, under the supervision of the MoHP. In 1992, the HIO's coverage expanded to widows and retirees. Furthermore, the Student Health Insurance Program (SHIP) was established for school children. The SHIP fund is derived from individual premiums paid by employees and the consumption tax on cigarettes. In 2004, there were roughly 30 million insured persons in Egypt. The private healthcare sector in Egypt comprises both for-profit and nonprofit organizations. It is difficult to determine the volume of private healthcare services in Egypt, as all medical expenses are covered by the patients themselves. Nevertheless, the MoHP estimated that in 2005, the number of beds in private healthcare institutions accounted for about 16% of the total number of hospital beds in Egypt. Although the healthcare services in the urban areas of Egypt are relatively accessible and modern, they are scarce and outmoded in low-income and rural areas. Most villages lack primary care institutions. Furthermore, most family planning institutions, public hospitals, and emergency centers are established in urban areas. The urban population accounts for only 44% of the total Egyptian population, but nearly 90% of large-sized hospitals are located in cities, and nearly 81% of the total working hours of physicians are taken up by the urban population.

A considerable amount of foreign aid and the relative political stability in the late 1990s provided a window of opportunity for reform of the Egyptian healthcare system. The Health Sector Reform Program (HSRP), jointly funded by the United States Agency for International Development (USAID), World Bank, European Union, African Development Bank, and Austrian Government, was officially launched in 1997 with the fundamental aim of improving the efficiency, funding, organization, and delivery of healthcare services in Egypt. This reform program sought to improve the overall health status of Egyptians by reducing the infant and under-five mortality rates and increasing the average life expectancy. Additionally, the reform program aimed to reduce the burden of infectious diseases by improving the country's primary healthcare services. The HSRP was launched on the basis of the social insurance model in an attempt to integrate the fragmented Egyptian healthcare funding structure into a single National Health Insurance Fund (NHIF). Furthermore, provincial branches of the NHIF known as Family Health Funds (FHFs) were established to help achieve the separation of funding and provision. These FHFs sign contracts with governmental, private, and nongovernmental providers for the delivery of basic healthcare services to registered beneficiaries.

In 1999, the HSRP launched pilot programs in three Egyptian provinces (Alexandria, Menoufia, and Sohag). The infrastructure of primary healthcare institutions in those pilot areas was improved through a newly implemented management system and well-trained family medical workers. This family medicine model is a holistic medical model designed to provide primary healthcare services to all members of a family. As part of this pilot program, Family Health Units (FHUs) were established, which employed family physicians, nurses, healthcare assistants, and administrative personnel to provide primary healthcare and general outpatient services to local residents. By November 2003, the pilot programs had established 66 FHUs, which increased to 643 FHUs in 2008. The aim was to reach 2,500 FHUs by the end of 2010.

The HSRP was initiated by Hosni Mubarak's government. However, Mubarak resigned after a 30-year rule in January 2011 as a result of mass protests, which severely affected one of Egypt's pillar industries, i.e., tourism, leading to numerous banks, shops, and factories being shut down. This Egyptian Revolution has had long-term adverse effects on the public healthcare system, particularly the implementation of the HSRP, which by that time had seen a number of achievements and was scheduled to be completed in 2015. The development of private healthcare institutions in Egypt has had a significant impact on the public healthcare system, as they tend to outperform public healthcare institutions in terms of service quality, clinical outcomes, and customer satisfaction. In contrast, public healthcare institutions, particularly those in rural areas, lack healthcare resources and a well-trained healthcare workforce. In addition, the salaries of workers in public healthcare institutions are much lower than of those employed in private healthcare institutions. As a result, the majority of physicians serving in public healthcare institutions also serve in private practices to compensate for their insufficient earnings. This public–private dichotomy in the healthcare system has had negative effects on the delivery of healthcare services. This is because it encourages inattentiveness among healthcare workers in public medical institutions, which drives patients into their private practices. Moreover, this system has led to a deterioration in the service quality of public healthcare institutions due to absenteeism and corruption.

Egypt has a relatively low healthcare expenditure, which accounts for only 3.7% of its GDP (World Bank, 2010). Despite such a low level of healthcare expenditure, private healthcare providers accounted for 57% of this expenditure in 2004, while the remaining 43% was accounted for by public healthcare institutions. Furthermore, almost half of the public healthcare institutions in Egypt face a shortage of medical equipment and healthcare workers. These factors might be major reasons for the relatively low average life expectancy (only 59 years) and the high prevalence of communicable diseases (e.g., schistosomiasis) in Egypt. The absence of health insurance schemes for vulnerable groups or informal workers is another major reason for these unfavorable health statistics.

Thus, we can see that the Egyptian health reform has progressed slowly for many years and achieved poor outcomes. Under the direct influence of the Jasmine Revolution in Tunisia, in February 2011, the Middle Eastern strongman Hosni Mubarak, who had been in power for 30 years, stepped down following the mass demonstrations and protests of the Egyptian Revolution. During the subsequent political transition, the conflict between the military and Egyptian Islamic authorities (represented by the Muslim Brotherhood) intensified, making the progress in health reform as unpredictable as the country's prospects for democratization.

During this political transition, the new round of health reforms must be implemented with great caution, and a set of pragmatic objectives must be established. To this end, it is necessary to reach a consensus on health reforms despite the value pluralism in Egypt. There are two important issues worthy of both the public's and healthcare workers' attention: (1) governance structure and anti-corruption issues; and (2) issues related to the healthcare workforce. However, health reforms must be further concretized to ensure its successful implementation, in order to resolve these two sets of issues. In addition, the officials of the MoHP should be held accountable for the reform outcomes in order to ensure that the healthcare services are well-received by the public.

The Egyptian Ambassador to the US, Sameh Shoukry, noted that the Egyptian health reform remains a priority on Egypt's social development agenda. At present, health reforms in Egypt have encountered numerous challenges resulting from the country's political situation. However, the most serious challenge is the allocation of financial resources to develop valuable human capital. In response to these challenges, promotion of population health is becoming an attractive reform option, and might become the basis for future health reforms. Apart from developing PPP, the most critical elements of the current Egyptian health reform are the establishment of financially sustainable health insurance programs to provide high-quality healthcare services, expand the coverage of basic healthcare services, improve the quality of family planning services, and establish and reinforce the consumer protection mechanism. Sameh Shoukry believed that postrevolutionary Egypt must continuously and comprehensively reform its healthcare sector to ensure that people have access to greater benefits and improved standards of welfare. In summary, the new

Egyptian government urgently requires strategic plans and investments for improving the health status of Egyptians. In particular, the government needs to establish public policies to overcome the enormous challenges posed by the public–private dichotomy in its healthcare system. It should strive to prevent the limited healthcare resources from being dominated by the private sector (which primarily serves the wealthy), in order to achieve an equal distribution of healthcare resources. Health reform is considered a key aspect of social reforms during this period of political transition; thus, the reforms in Egypt must be implemented in a prudent and pragmatic manner.

SECTION III. THE HEALTH SYSTEM IN MOROCCO

1. Overview of Socioeconomics and National Health

Morocco, officially the Kingdom of Morocco, is a country with a constitutional monarchy, located in the northwest of Africa. It is a bordered by Algeria to the east and the Atlantic Ocean to the west, and faces Portugal and Spain across the Straits of Gibraltar and the Mediterranean Sea to the north. In addition to Arabic, Morocco has numerous local languages, and French and Spanish are also spoken in the country. It has a lengthy coastline along the Atlantic Ocean (more than 1,700 km) that reaches past the Strait of Gibraltar to the Mediterranean Sea. Morocco has a complex terrain, including the Atlas Mountains in the center and the north; the Moroccan Plateau and the Sub-Saharan Plateau in the east and south; and long, narrow warm plains on the northwestern coast. Morocco has a pleasant climate throughout the year, with lush forests and blooming flowers, as heatwaves from the southern Sahara Desert are blocked by the Atlas Mountains. As a result, Morocco has been called "a cold country with a hot sun" and the "North African Garden." However, its climate is also that of a dry, tropical desert owing to the effect of the cold Canary Current. The Atlas Mountains run down the backbone of the country, with Toubkal having the highest peak (4,165 m) in the country.

According to Law 47-96 on Regions, which was adopted on September 10, 2003, Morocco (including Western Sahara) has been divided into 17 regions, 49 provinces, 12 prefectures, and 1,547 municipalities. More than 80% of Moroccans are Arab, while the remaining 20% are Berber. In 2006, the illiteracy rate of Moroccans was 38.4%. Sunni Muslims form the majority, and the remaining population is Jewish or Christian. In 2009, Morocco had a population of more than 32 million. In 2010, the GDP of Morocco was US$91.7 billion, and the GDP per capita was US$2,839. Furthermore, its economic growth rate was 3.2%, with an inflation rate of 1.4%.

2. Healthcare System

The Moroccan healthcare system is based on the healthcare system of France and comprises the public sector (including local health departments and military logistic health departments), the private nonprofit sector, and the private for-profit sector.

(1) Public Healthcare Sector

The public healthcare sector comprises Basic Healthcare Establishments (Etablissements de Soins de Santé de Base, ESSB) and Health Centers (Centros de Salud, CS). There are 1,653 ESSB in Morocco (416 ESSB in cities and 1,237 ESSB in rural areas). Twenty-seven percent of CS across the country is staffed with at least one physician. Nevertheless, 50% of rural residents still have problems seeking medical attention, and the rural healthcare system is still facing certain challenges. This is mainly due to the dispersed nature of rural populations, who live in 31,483 villages across the country. Villages with less than 500 residents account for 77% of all villages, while the remaining 23% of villages have 500–3,000 residents. Villages are far from each other, with poorly maintained road networks and transportation systems. The government has adopted the following strategies to improve the rural healthcare services in Morocco:

1. *Fixed healthcare.* This strategy is centered on CS, each of which is surrounded by several clinics that provide primary healthcare services in rural areas. Each clinic is headed by a nurse, who provides routine outpatient services, preventive services for infectious diseases, maternal and child healthcare services, and family planning services for approximately 15,000 residents. Each CS is equipped with 20–30 beds to serve approximately 45,000 residents and is responsible for the workforce allocation in clinics, epidemiological surveillance, primary healthcare, gynecological services, and health education. This fixed healthcare strategy is responsible for serving about 28% of rural residents in Morocco.

2. *Mobile healthcare.* This strategy involves the use of home visits, fixed-point healthcare, and mobile medical teams. Home visits are conducted by nurses who use motorcycles to visit their patients and provide preventive and family planning services. Fixed-point healthcare refers to the selection of a fixed venue for providing the same healthcare services as home visits. A mobile medical team is usually made up of at least two healthcare workers, and occasionally, a physician, who uses motorcycles to travel to villages and provide healthcare services that cannot be met by other means. These mobile medical teams also provide midwifery services for extremely underserved areas. The coverage rate of this mobile healthcare strategy is about 57% of rural residents in Morocco.

Taken together, these healthcare strategies cover up to 85% of rural residents, while the remaining 15%, especially those who live in remote and impoverished areas, are not covered because of the lack of facilities and healthcare workers. Traditional midwifery services are the main healthcare services provided to residents living in these areas. Urban areas of Morocco have better healthcare facilities, and the healthcare services are mainly provided via the fixed strategy. However, there are some underserved areas that require nurses to provide preventive and family planning services. Around 56.1% of urban residents seek medical attention in local ESSB. These healthcare services are free of cost, apart from the copayments required from patients. In 1991, 98 public hospitals provided a total of 26,000 beds, accounting for 86% of the total number of hospital beds in Morocco. The number of residents per hospital bed ranged from 64 to 1307, with an average of 984. Furthermore, 3,855 physicians were employed by the Ministry of Health, which accounted for 5% of the total number of physicians in Morocco, of whom, 59% were specialists. There were also 22,802 male and female nurses (healthcare assistants) in Morocco, as well as 4 military hospitals providing a total of 1,029 beds for local residents.

(2) Private Nonprofit Sector

In Morocco, some companies in the phosphate mining industry and the electric power industry, as well as the state-owned railways, invest in the healthcare system to provide healthcare services for their employees. One of the funding sources for the National Social Security Fund (Caisse Nationale de Sécurité Sociale, CNSS) is the collection of health insurance premiums jointly paid by employers and employees based on a certain percentage of employees' salaries. The CNSS is primarily responsible for providing health insurance funds for 800,000 salaried employees in private companies to compensate for their income losses due to sick leave and maternity leave and to provide family members of the deceased with death and disability benefits. The private nonprofit sector in Morocco has a total of 50,000–70,000 employees, 324 hospitals and clinics, and 1,800 hospital beds (accounting for about 6% of the total number of state-owned hospital beds).

(3) Private For-Profit Sector

There are 2,552 clinics and medical consulting centers, 110 outpatient clinics, 2,500 beds, 804 dental clinics, and 1,767 pharmacies across Morocco.

The total healthcare expenditure in Morocco accounted for 4% of its GDP, while the public healthcare expenditure accounted for 37% of the total healthcare expenditure. The public healthcare expenditure of Morocco is shared among the central government (30%), local governments (40%), and international healthcare cooperatives (30%). In 1993, the government of Morocco allocated a healthcare budget of 2.7 billion dirhams (the currency unit of Morocco), 74.5% of which was spent on hospitals. The remaining budget was spent on preventive services. Private sector expenditure accounted for 63% of the total healthcare expenditure.

3. Difficulties in Health Industry Development

Broadly speaking, the overall health status of Moroccans has greatly improved. Over the past 40 years, the infant mortality rate declined from 160 per 1,000 live births and 57.4 per 1,000 live births, while the average life expectancy increased from 47 to 66.8 years. The coverage of preventive vaccination has also increased from 5% to about 90%, and the incidence rate of infectious diseases among children has decreased considerably. Furthermore, there have been no reported cases of diphtheria and whooping cough since 1990. The incidence rate of measles also fell from 797.1 per 100,000 people in 1960 to 6.2 per 100,000 people in 1990. After 1990, there have been no reported cases of poliomyelitis, which has been the main cause of disability in Morocco in the past. In addition, malaria, schistosomiasis, and leprosy have basically been eradicated from the country. There have been only a few reported cases of trachoma in the southern region of Morocco. Although the number of beds has almost doubled, the average number of residents per hospital bed rose from 750 in 1960 to 864 in 1980 and later 943 in 1990 due to population growth. The promotion of social insurance in Morocco requires further development. Infectious disease control and maternal and child healthcare still represent major healthcare issues in Morocco. In 1992, there were 359 maternal deaths per 100,000 births, and only 17.5% of pregnant women living in rural areas had antenatal checkups. Furthermore, 87% of Moroccan women gave birth without assistance from healthcare workers. The infant and adolescent mortality rate in Morocco was 76.2 per 1,000 instead of percents in 1991, of which 26% was attributed to diarrhea. Diarrhea also caused nearly 18,650 deaths among children aged under 5 months in the same year. Moreover, there are about 25,403 new tuberculosis cases in Morocco each year, equivalent to about 10 per 100,000 people each year. The country's outdated medical equipment is far from capable of meeting its ever-growing healthcare needs. About 50% of the hospitals in Morocco were built many years ago and are in need of renovation, while about 60% of X-ray devices were purchased 15 years ago. In addition, there is also a wastage of human and material resources in hospital management that has led to inefficiency in their service delivery. There are also certain quantitative and qualitative issues with regard to the healthcare workforce in Morocco. On the one hand, there is an insufficient number of physicians. On the other hand, there is an overemphasis on the healthcare needs in urban areas, which has resulted in a bias for tertiary healthcare services that require a higher degree of specialization. This has further worsened the imbalance in the allocation of the healthcare workforce.

On top of the lack of financial resources, this crisis has been further intensified by the pressure of population growth. Despite closely engaging in family planning services, the total population of Morocco had reached 3.53 million in 2017, more than half of whom live in urban areas because of the tendency toward population concentration in such areas. In order to meet the healthcare needs of the country, it is expected that Morocco will require an additional 1,900 beds, 150 medical centers, and 1,100 physicians per year. Accordingly, Morocco must raise further 2 billion dirhams to establish another two medical colleges, as the existing two medical colleges are no longer sufficient.

CHAPTER TWENTY

Health Systems in Four Selected European Countries

 SECTION I. THE HEALTH SYSTEM IN RUSSIA

1. Overview of Socioeconomics and National Health

The Russian Federation is the largest country in the world, spanning two continents – Europe and Asia – covering a total area of 17 million km². It has land borders with 14 neighboring countries, and a coastline along the Arctic and Pacific Oceans. It is also connected to the Atlantic Ocean through the Baltic and Black Seas. Possessing the world's largest reserves of minerals and energy resources, Russia is the world's largest natural gas exporter, and the largest exporter of crude oil among non-Organization of Petroleum Exporting Countries (OPEC) members.

The overall health status of the Russian population has declined drastically since the dissolution of the Soviet Union in 1991. Furthermore, there has been a decreasing trend in the growth rate of the Russian population since the mid-1980s, which even showed negative growth in 1992. Presently, Russia has the lowest average life expectancy in Europe, particularly among men in Russia (nearly 13 years below the EU average).

The maternal mortality rate gradually declined from 68 deaths per 100,000 live births in 1998 to 39 deaths per 100,000 live births in 2000. However, this latter figure was still higher than that of other European countries. In addition, the neonatal mortality rate is a rather thorny issue in Russia, with some reports indicating that nearly 20% of newborns have birth defects and only 35% of newborns are "completely healthy."

Cardiovascular disease is the leading cause of death in Russia, which also has the highest mortality rate in Europe. Deaths from external causes, such as trauma and poisoning (e.g., homicide, suicide, alcohol intoxication) and deaths from cardiovascular diseases both peaked in 1994. Cancer is second only to external causes as the leading cause of death in Russia.

In 2012, the total population of the Russian Federation was 143.5 million. The country sported a GDP of US$2.015 trillion and a GNI per capita of US$127,000. The impoverished population, defined according to the national poverty line, accounted for 11.0% of the total population. These statistics reflect its status as a high-income, non-OECD country. The average life expectancy in Russia is 70 years (men: 65 years; women: 76 years), and the proportion of elderly individuals aged over 65 is 13% of the total population. In 2013, the mortality rate in Russia was 13%, with a maternal mortality rate of 24 deaths per 100,000 live births, an infant mortality rate of 9 deaths per 1,000 live births, and an under-five mortality rate of 10 deaths per 1,000 live births. The average life expectancy and GNI per capita are both lower than the average of all high-income, non-OECD countries. Its total healthcare expenditure accounted for 6.3% of its GDP, which is equivalent to a healthcare expenditure per capita of US$887.

2. Healthcare System

Following the dissolution of the Soviet Union, Russia's administrative systems, including its healthcare system, were decentralized. Specifically, the healthcare system was divided into the federal, regional (*oblast*), and municipal (*rayon*) levels.

According to the Constitution of the Russian Federation, the State is responsible for the legislation and protection of human rights, as well as protection of the rights and freedoms of its citizens, while the federal and regional governments are responsible for the coordination of healthcare-related issues.

In 1993, the "Fundamentals of the Legislation of the Russian Federation on Citizens' Health Protection" was promulgated. This law stipulated the following responsibilities for the federal government: protection of human rights and the rights and freedoms of citizens in relation to health protection; elaboration of federal health protection policies; elaboration and implementation of federal programs related to healthcare development, disease control, healthcare services, public health education, etc.; determination of the share of the healthcare expenditure in the federal budgets and elaboration of healthcare-related financial policies (i.e., tax exemptions, budget-related tariffs, and other expenses); management of federal assets related to healthcare; establishment of a unified federal statistics and financing system in healthcare; development of uniform standards and federal education programs for medical and pharmaceutical training, as well as the determination of healthcare specialties; organization and monitoring of compliance with quality standards in healthcare; development and approval of the basic mandatory health insurance (MHI) program and establishment of its annual premium rate; determination of the amount of subsidies for recipients of medicosocial care and pharmaceutical supplies; organization and implementation of the State Sanitary and Epidemiological Surveillance (SSES); development and approval of federal healthcare regulations, norms, and standards; organization of all healthcare systems in the Russian Federation; coordination of activities by the state, administrative and economic sectors, as well as activities among the regional, municipal, and private healthcare systems; formulation of technical specifications for medical expertise; and formulation of certification procedures for healthcare services and drugs (Figure 20.1).

The same law further stipulates the following responsibilities for regional governments: formulation and allocation of regional budgets; material and technical supply for regional healthcare institutions; approval of local MHI programs; establishment of additional subsidies for the recipients of medicosocial care and pharmaceutical supplies; coordination of healthcare-related activities among regional authorities and municipal and private

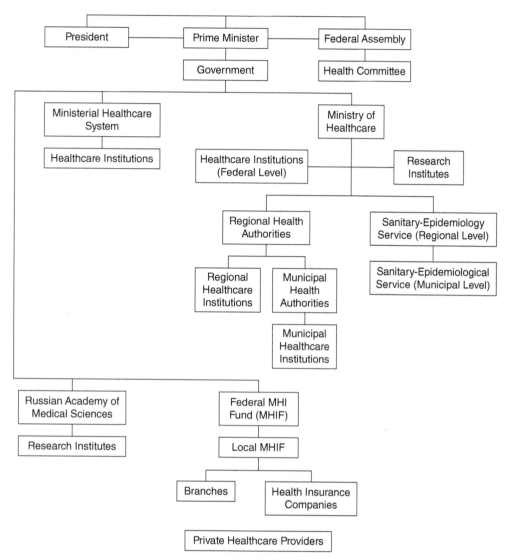

FIGURE 20.1 Organizational structure of the healthcare system in the Russian Federation.

healthcare systems; organization and coordination of training for healthcare workers; and licensure of medical and pharmaceutical activities within the respective regions.

Finally, the law stipulates the following responsibilities for the municipal (rayon) government: organization, maintenance, and development of municipal healthcare institutions; ensuring public health and welfare; and formulation of local healthcare budgets.

(1) Ministry of Healthcare

The federal Ministry of Healthcare is the highest administrative agency for healthcare, headed by a minister appointed by the prime minister and approved by the Federal Assembly. The Ministry of Healthcare is the central healthcare policymaking agency for the Russian Federation and possesses the nominal right to oversee the work and decisions delegated to each region. However, the Ministry of Healthcare cannot ensure the strict compliance of local governments to central directives because of the expanding authority of the oblasts, especially in terms of budgeting.

The primary responsibilities of the Ministry of Healthcare are: formulation and implementation of national healthcare policies; development and implementation of federal healthcare programs, including programs for diabetes, tuberculosis, health promotion, health education, disease prevention, forensic medicine, etc.; developing and presenting bills to the State Duma; governance of federal healthcare institutions; development of medical education and human resources; epidemiological and environmental health surveillance, along with health statistics; control of infectious diseases; development of healthcare regulations; development of national standards and recommendations for quality assurance in healthcare; drug control and certification; and disaster relief (disaster medicine).

Other federal healthcare agencies include highly specialized medical institutions that provide tertiary healthcare services.

The sanitary-epidemiological system is an independent agency within the Ministry of Healthcare. Unlike the other, decentralized healthcare administrative systems, it has a hierarchical structure. Municipal governments report to regional governments, which in turn report to the federal government. Each hospital is equipped with sanitary-epidemiological physicians and epidemiologists, who are charged with reporting epidemics to the sanitary-epidemiological system. This vertical system ensures the upward flow of epidemiological information and the downward dissemination of epidemic alerts.

The Ministry of Healthcare allocates a budget received from the Ministry of Finance to research institutions, the Russian Academy of Medical Sciences, Russian Academy of Sciences and medical colleges. Federal healthcare institutions account for about 4% of the total hospital bed capacity in Russia.

Currently, the federal government (i.e., the Ministry of Healthcare) controls only a small proportion (about 5%) of the total healthcare resources.

(2) Regional (Oblast) Level

The administrative agencies at this level are responsible for the management of regional healthcare. Before the establishment of the MHI system via the legislation in 1993, regional governments had full control over their respective regional healthcare funds. However, following the implementation of the MHI, they lost some of this control to the newly established MHIF. However, because the MHI system has only been partially implemented, the regional and local governments currently control only about two-thirds of the total public healthcare funds, so they retain a significant role in management. Each region must ensure its compliance with federal programs, particularly those focused on the control of the overall health conditions and infectious diseases. Although these federal programs are highly prioritized, individual regions do not actually have to report directly to the Ministry of Healthcare. Following the decentralization of the early- to mid-1990s, regional administrative agencies have wielded considerable autonomy. Indeed, some regional health authorities have actively participated in the formulation of reform schedules and the oversight of healthcare quality, while also employing programs similar to those of the federal government. However, some regional health authorities have not shown active engagement in such activities.

In terms of healthcare provision, regional healthcare institutions primarily consist of general hospitals with about 1,000 beds and children's hospitals with about 400 beds; both types of hospital have inpatient and outpatient departments to deliver healthcare services to the entire regional population.

There are also regional healthcare institutions specialized in infectious diseases, tuberculosis, psychiatric diseases, etc. In addition, about a quarter of pharmacies and more than 70% of diagnostic centers are regional institutions.

(3) Municipal (Rayon) Level

In many major cities, municipal governments are actively engaged in health reforms; however, in rural areas, the responsibilities of health authorities are more similar to those of hospital directors in central districts. Since the promulgation of the General Principles of Organization of Local Self-Government in the Russian Federation in 1995, municipal governments have not been required to report to the federal or oblast governments, although they must still comply with the orders issued by the Ministry of Healthcare. This has posed a problem for healthcare policy, since municipal governments need not comply with the health reforms or other policies being pushed by the oblast governments, and need only provide statutory healthcare services within their jurisdiction. In practice, many regional and municipal governments have developed a negotiating mechanism to ensure that regional health authorities retain their authority over local governments.

Urban regions generally have multidisciplinary municipal hospitals with about 250 beds, along with municipal children's hospitals with about 200 beds. In addition, there are emergency care hospitals, 700-bed hospitals specialized in infectious diseases and tuberculosis, maternity hospitals, psychiatric hospitals (some of which are considered regional hospitals), and disability hospitals. Most pharmacies, independent polyclinics, and some diagnostic centers are also administered at the municipal level.

Healthcare institutions in rural rayons typically include a central hospital with approximately 250 beds, which may also serve as polyclinics. Some rayons also have smaller-sized hospitals with about 100 beds. Additionally, there can be independent polyclinics (unaffiliated with hospitals), small-sized polyclinics or "outpatient hospitals," and health posts staffed by feldshers.

(4) Ministerial System

The ministerial system comprises ministries other than the Ministry of Healthcare and various state-owned enterprises, which traditionally have only provided healthcare services for their employees and dependents. For example, of the more than 20 ministries (e.g., Ministries of Defense, Railways, Marine and River Transport, Internal Affairs), most have their own polyclinic networks, some of which include inpatient institutions.

These healthcare institutions usually provide high-quality healthcare services, among which 18 parallel civil healthcare systems are funded by the federal (i.e., Ministry of Finance) budget. The military and security systems are funded by both the federal budget and extra-budgetary resources; the exact amount of the latter remains unknown, as they are not listed in any official statistics. Although the healthcare institutions affiliated with large-sized, state-owned enterprises are overwhelmed by the financial pressures related to maintaining their own healthcare services, the enterprises continue to establish healthcare institutions and fund their activities.

These parallel systems account for 15% of all outpatient institutions and 6% of inpatient institutions.

(5) Private Sector

There are signs indicating that private sector healthcare services are legally permissible and that the emerging private healthcare activities have potential for growth. However, the development of private sector healthcare remains limited. The healthcare sector has not yet seen rapid progression in privatization, which has overwhelmed a number of other sectors. At the international level, the privatization of the healthcare sector is widely rejected because of a belief that healthcare institutions and service providers should not be made profitable in order to ensure the equality and accessibility of healthcare services.

Hospitals can impose additional charges on top of the basic benefits package, but their profits must not exceed 5% of their officially reported revenues.

In addition, hospitals can provide beds to enterprises or voluntary health insurance (VHI) agencies that pay for employers and insured persons. However, the ownership of these hospitals remains almost exclusively in the public sector. Large-scale privatization is further hindered by legal uncertainties related to leaseholds purchased from the government. There are also certain issues regarding the establishment of nonprofit or "trust" hospitals, as it is difficult to determine the taxation of charitable organizations. Furthermore, public healthcare institutions have always held a certain degree of hostility towards the involvement of nongovernmental organizations (NGOs) in their conventional services.

On the other hand, the private sector has progressed considerably in developing drug supply, followed closely by dentistry and ophthalmology. Outpatient medications are excluded from the basic benefits package and have to be purchased directly from pharmacies, which were the first batch of enterprises to be approved for privatization by the Ministry of Healthcare. All essential dental care services are provided on a fee-for-service basis, but the majority of dentures and fillings are performed in the private sector. Other areas of development in the private sector include diagnostic centers, rehabilitation facilities, and certain specialist private clinics (or centers).

Currently, the State Duma is considering a bill that would regulate the private healthcare sector more. Indeed, the rapid and disorderly growth of the private healthcare sector has prompted an urgent need for effective regulation. The need is evidently related to the significant decline in government revenues.

3. Health Insurance System

(1) Mandatory Health Insurance (MHI)

1. Reform of the Funding System   Under the Soviet system, healthcare services were almost exclusively funded by government budgets at all levels. State-owned healthcare institutions were funded by their respective budgets, whereas rayons covered the expenses of healthcare institutions within their respective jurisdictions. In the late Soviet era, a small group of Russian academics attempted to implement generalized funding reform. Following the dissolution of the Soviet Union, the focus of their discussions of this reform shifted towards the specific situation in Russia.

Key considerations in establishing the new funding model of the Russian Federation were the severe shortage of healthcare funds at the time and the need for a steady flow of funds despite budget fluctuations. The system adopted in the UK and Nordic countries, where the governments served as single payers, was rejected as being too similar to the Soviet system. The out-of-pocket payment system, wherein patients would have to cover a large proportion of their medical expenses, was also rejected because it would have harmed equal access to healthcare services. As a result, the mandatory health insurance (MHI) system presented itself as the only solution. Due to the rapid introduction of market-oriented reforms in other economic sectors, the Russian Federation decided to introduce an MHI system that relies primarily on market forces to regulate the various issues facing the Russian healthcare system.

Therefore, in April 1993, the Russian Federation amended and reissued the Law on Health Insurance of the Citizens of the RSFSR (June 1991), which served as the basis for subsequent reforms of the health insurance system.

The key objectives of this law included introducing new nonbudgetary sources of funding to augment existing budgetary funds, establishing a fund coordination mechanism, and providing universal and comprehensive health coverage, while simultaneously giving patients the freedom to choose their preferred healthcare providers and insurance agencies. To achieve these objectives, it was necessary to improve the management level of the healthcare system and to introduce incentive mechanisms based on the principles of market competition among insurance agencies and healthcare providers.

The new funding system set forth in the Law on Health Insurance included the following elements: reforming the healthcare funding system by establishing nonbudgetary sources of revenues to increase the total amount of healthcare funds without displacing existing funding sources; establishment of a federal MHIF; establishment of regional MHIFs; the transfer of employers' payroll contributions to local and federal funds (equivalent to 3.4% and 0.2%, respectively) to maintain the balance between these two funds; local government payment for nonworking populations (although the specific amount is unclear); further clarification from the federal government regarding the previously undefined scope of insurance reimbursement, as well as permitting regional governments to define a minimum reimbursement level above the aforementioned requirements; permitting VHI to cover services beyond the basic MHI package; procurement of healthcare services on behalf of the public by private insurance companies and branches of local MHIFs (in regions where private insurance companies are unavailable, the local MHIFs are considered solely responsible for procurement until private insurance companies have been established); the pooling of all funds into local MHIFs, which pay insurance agencies based on risk-adjusted capitation; and insurance agencies pay providers on a pay-for-performance basis according to annually renegotiated fee standards agreed on by local MHIFs, regional health authorities, local governments, medical associations, and other relevant regional agencies.

1. *Composition of the new funding system.* Conceptually, the new system can be divided into four parts, as shown in Figure 20.2: Panel I comprises the funding sources; Panel II represents the agencies involved in financial management; Panel III lists the agencies involved in the organization and management of healthcare services provided to consumers; and Panel IV comprises the institutions engaged in the provision of healthcare services.

   The funding sources in Panel I include the federal and local budgets, employer contributions to the MHI and VHI schemes (if desired), and the contributions of citizens via VHI schemes and out-of-pocket payments. In 1990–1991, the federal and local budgets were estimated to have contributed to about 55% of the total healthcare funds; however, this share has subsequently declined to about 30% with the gradual increase in the MHI share over time.

   The federal budget is mainly allocated to the Ministry of Healthcare in Panel II (line 1) to support training, research, and public health activities, as well as large-scale investments and expensive healthcare services in Panel IV (line 6). The local budget is allocated to local health authorities (line 2) for supporting the same activities as

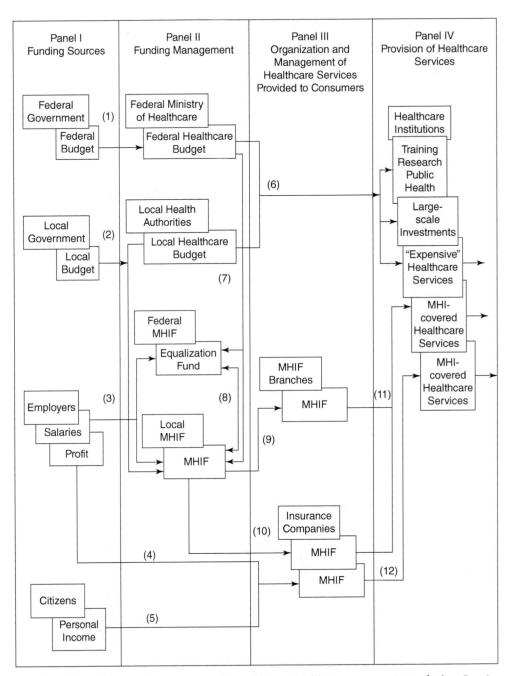

FIGURE 20.2 Schematic representation of the Health Insurance Act of the Russian Federation. *Source:* D. Chernochovsky, H. Barnum, and E. Potapchik, "Health System Reform in Russia: The Finance and Organization Perspectives." *Economics of Transition* 4, no. 1 (2010): 113–134.

the federal government but at the local level (line 6). Additionally, the local budget is allocated to partially subsidize the premium contributions of the nonworking and noncontributing populations (line 7). These payments are made on a capitation basis, as approved by the oblast government, but cannot be lower than the average of employers' premium contributions for each employee. The premium rates do not need to be established through legislation. Moreover, a portion of the local budgets is set aside to provide discretionary support for the delivery of healthcare services (line 7).

Another funding source involving employers (both private and government agencies) is the salary-based social insurance premium contributions paid by employers to MHIFs (line 3): to ensure equality, 0.2% of employees' salaries is paid to the federal fund and 3.4% to the local fund. Additionally, employers can, if they desire, purchase VHI for their employees to cover healthcare services that fall beyond the statutory coverage (line 4). The purchase of VHI can be subsidized by the government via tax relief. Individual citizens may also purchase VHI, if desired, and/or make out-of-pocket payments for their medical expenses.

Both the federal and local funds were established as independent, nonprofit agencies. They were initially responsible for the financial management of the health insurance system; eventually, however, they were also charged with the financial management of oblast healthcare systems (i.e., health insurance and budgets), thus becoming the coordinating body of oblast healthcare funds. A board has been established for each of these funds to serve as the governing body. In reality, however, the daily administration of the funds is carried out by the executive director only. Typically, the boards comprise representatives from government agencies, the Central Bank, health insurance companies, professional medical associations, trade unions, and insurance agencies. The objective of the federal fund is to ensure fair, accessible, and universal health coverage via the inter-regional redistribution of health insurance revenues. The federal fund (line 8) might be channeled to local funds in order to achieve this objective. The legislation does not stipulate the scale of these financial flows. Furthermore, additional federal budget revenues can be transferred into the federal or local funds in order to achieve inter-regional equality (line 7).

According to the legislation, two types of agencies are responsible for organizing and managing the healthcare services provided to consumers. As shown in Panel III, these agencies are all insurance agencies, including private for-profit insurance companies and local MHIF branches. These agencies sign a contract with providers (Panel IV) and funds are paid on a capitation basis by local MHIFs according to the contract (lines 9 and 10). The law allows insurance agencies to act as healthcare managers or providers via healthcare workers in their own institutions or by purchasing healthcare services from other providers. Therefore, despite not being explicitly stipulated in the legislation, the legislation has enabled the development of health maintenance organizations (HMOs) and preferred provider organizations (PPOs).

Panel III shows that health insurance can be divided into MHI and VHI, both of which can be provided by insurance agencies. According to the law, the establishment of local MHIF branches is a temporary measure in areas without insurance agencies or that are in the process of establishing such agencies. Some believe that this approach is suitable for rural and sparsely populated areas; it has been implemented since 1993.

Citizens are given two main rights: (1) the right to choose and periodically change their insurance agencies without their employers' influence, and (2) the right to choose their healthcare providers. It is clear that consumers' choice of healthcare providers is indirectly affected by their choice of insurance agencies, which sign contracts with healthcare providers. There are public and private healthcare providers (Panel IV) in Russia, both of which compete with each other for contracts with insurance agencies (i.e., local MHIF branches or insurance companies) (lines 11 and 12). The reimbursements given to providers are determined according to fee standards, which are predetermined through negotiations among insurance agencies, professional associations, and local health authorities.

2. *Characteristics of the new funding system.* The Health Care Reform Law promulgated in 1991 and amended in 1993 established the MHI system in order to address the issue of severe shortage of funds in the healthcare sector, while also conforming to the prevailing ideological trend toward a radical transition to a market-based economy. These goals were accomplished through purchaser–provider split, which improves the efficiency, quality, and equality of the healthcare system via market forces (Figure 20.3).

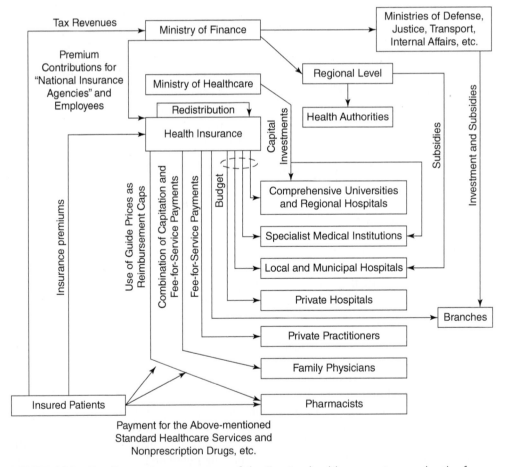

FIGURE 20.3 Funding and management of the Russian healthcare system under the framework of the Health Insurance Legislation. *Source:* D. Chernichovsky and E. Potapchik, "Health System Reform Under the Russian Health Insurance Legislation," *International Journal of Health Planning and Management* 12, no. 4 (1997): 279.

1. *MHIF*. A key feature of the new funding system is the establishment of the federal MHIF as well as various regional-level local MHIFs (one in each federal subject).

   The local MHIFs were established to collect and manage insurance revenues from a 3.6% payroll tax on employers on behalf of the working population and the premium contributions of regional governments on behalf of the nonworking population (children, retirees, unemployed persons, etc.), as well as to distribute these funds to insurance companies or MHIF branches. These agencies in turn subcontract healthcare services on behalf of their members.

   The insurance revenues from the 3.6% payroll tax are allocated to the oblast MHIFs (3.4%) and federal MHIF (0.2%). Each region is subsidized via transfer payments to ensure the inter-regional equalization of financial allocation. The federal and local MHIF committees were established as public nonprofit funding agencies. Although personnel from the Ministry of Healthcare serve as board members of the federal MHIF and are charged with its oversight, the federal MHIF is still an independent legal entity that does not need to report to the Ministry of Healthcare.

   The federal MHIF supervises and administers the operation of 89 local MHIFs, which correspond to the existing oblast administrative system. The key responsibilities of the federal MHIF include the implementation of the equalization mechanism and comprehensive regulation of the health insurance system.

   On the other hand, local MHIFs are responsible for collecting premium contributions and implementing state benefits programs.

2. *Independent third-party payment system*. The second key feature of the healthcare reform legislation is the establishment of an independent third-party payment system to purchase healthcare services on behalf of insured persons. These third-party payers include: (1) independent carriers (i.e., insurance companies) and (2) local MHIF branches, which are established in oblasts without insurance companies. Both the insurance companies and local MHIF branches receive funds from local MHIFs on a capitation basis according to their contracts. They are also expected to selectively sign contracts with healthcare providers to promote low-cost, high-quality healthcare services by encouraging competition among providers. The insurance companies and local MHIF branches are tasked with monitoring fund utilization and service quality, as well as encouraging a shift of focus towards primary healthcare and preventive medicine. They are also allowed to provide VHI.

   Legally recognized insurance agencies are permitted to operate as HMOs, PPOs, and general practitioners (GPs) that control the healthcare budgets of their patients. The legislation does not explicitly specify which of these forms the agencies must take, but it does stipulate that the form must be consistent with the direction of the agency's intended development.

3. *Expected outcomes of the new funding system*. The Law on Health Insurance is a flexible instrument established in an attempt to create a publicly controlled NGO-type institution within the healthcare system, while also allowing for the development of various organizational forms according to the particular preferences and capabilities of each region. Therefore, it is able to improve the utilization efficiency of healthcare resources while also maintaining equal, accessible, and universal health coverage, which were the major characteristics of the Soviet system.

   The implementation of the Law on Health Insurance was expected to have a number of benefits. First, the amount of total healthcare funds was expected to increase, as the Act stipulated that the health insurance fund was intended to supplement rather than replace budget funds. Statistics reported by the Ministry of Healthcare showed that the revenues from health insurance would increase the healthcare budget by 30% at the start of its implementation. Moreover, health insurance funding would constitute a stable and predictable funding source that would neither be affected by the budget fluctuation nor have to compete with other sectors for budget allocation, thereby resolving the financial shortages caused by the previous "residual principle."

The key feature of this approach is ensuring purchaser–provider split, which is known to improve the efficiency and quality of healthcare services. Accordingly, a healthcare service procurement system was established through contracts between the insurance agencies and providers in order to reinforce the regulation of existing incentive mechanisms, and eventually replace the previous "command-and-control" administrative system with a flexible competitive system driven by consumer demand. These changes were achieved through introduction of two levels of competition: (1) competition among insurance agencies for consumers to subscribe to their insurance policies, thus enabling consumers to select insurance agencies based on the quality of their contracted healthcare providers as well as the quality control of the insurance agencies. (2) Competition among hospitals, polyclinics, and other healthcare providers (both public and private institutions) for contracts with insurance agencies. These healthcare providers rely on payments specified by the contracts with insurance agencies rather than on budgets (for medical institutions) or salaries (for healthcare workers) for their revenues. For-profit insurance agencies (who lack a guaranteed income) tend to select healthcare providers that deliver high-quality and efficient healthcare services. On the other hand, providers that sign contracts with insurance agencies tend to be willing to deliver high-quality, low-cost healthcare services.

Not only would market mechanisms address the issue of inefficient and poor-quality healthcare services, but also it would also address the issue of excess capacity, as healthcare institutions that provide inefficient, expensive, or poor-quality services would be eliminated from the market because of the lack of contracts with insurance agencies. In summary, the freedom of consumer choice can drive the operation of market mechanisms, which in turn can help in meeting consumer demands.

(2) Positive Progress, Models, and Issues of the Reform

1. Positive Progress in Reform   The Health Care Reform Law was implemented in 1993, leading to the establishment of the federal and local MHIFs for the collection of insurance premiums. As of early 1994, a total of 78 regional funds, 587 branches, and 164 insurance companies were established. In the late 1990s, there were a total of 89 local MHIFs (one in each federal subject), 1,170 local MHIF branches, and 415 insurance companies. Since then, mergers and bankruptcies have whittled down the insurance companies to around 300. Furthermore, a large number of independent health insurance agencies emerged because of the continuous expansion of private insurance agencies in other areas (private insurance has been permitted since the late 1980s), which eventually led them to expand and diversify toward health insurance.

Despite facing numerous obstacles, the reform of healthcare funding has given rise to several positive developments. Particularly, the contractual approach has allowed for the clear delineation of responsibilities and a greater sense of accountability. The implementation of the new funding system also necessitated the development of new administrative and information management techniques. For instance, computerized information systems for healthcare services and standards for patients, providers, and insurance agencies were continuously developed. Although the pay-for-performance system has not been widely introduced, it still has significant potential for promoting efficiency while also increasing cost-consciousness and ensuring external quality control. Furthermore, there is now increased awareness of legal compliance and patients' rights, such that patients have begun seeking legal recourse with the support of insurance companies. The funds collected through health insurance have become more stable, and have even increased in some regions. In fact, existing public healthcare funds might have declined considerably in the absence of health insurance, as evidenced by the substantial funding reduction in other social sectors that rely solely on budgetary funds.

2. Models of Reform Implementation   More than a decade after the reform, the Russian healthcare funding system remains unstable and faces numerous challenges. For instance, the funding and service procurement mechanisms stipulated in the reform law have not yet been fully implemented in most regions, with the exception of Samara.

Samara is the largest industrial center in the Volga area, possessing a population of 33 million. It was one of the three regions that joined the New Economy Movement (NEM) in the late 1980s. Samara has displayed some positive reform outcomes because of its implementation of NEM: the average length of hospital stays fell by 7%, the number of "unnecessary" hospitalizations fell by 13%, emergency ambulance calls fell by 12%, and the number of hospital beds declined by 5,500.

In 1996, the Samara oblast passed "The Concept for Development of Health Care in Samara for 1996–2000," which includes the following objectives: modernization of the MHI system; prioritization of primary healthcare and GP training; rationalization of healthcare services by encouraging patients to seek secondary healthcare services only when necessary; development of multiple forms of ownership, including private practice; modernization of healthcare management, including quality control; and improvement of the rate of resource utilization.

In 1993, Samara adopted the federal MHI model, and has since achieved universal coverage. Furthermore, Samara collected 100% of insurance contributions in the first two quarters of 1999. This was the collective outcome of the following two measures: (1) the joint efforts of the local MHIFs in Samara to collect premium contributions from all enterprises, and (2) in 1998, the oblast Duma decided to reclaim responsibility for paying premium contributions on behalf of the nonworking population from the rayon governments; the resulting expenses were then included in the oblast budget. In fact, Samara is the only oblast that actually took responsibility for funding coordination in accordance with the 1993 legislation, and fully paid the premiums of the nonworking population. According to the relevant stipulations, these premiums are calculated as the total healthcare expenditure minus the premiums paid by the working population.

The success of Samara in collecting all premiums for the MHI implies that it is able to not only provide subsidized benefits programs to its citizens but also increase the number of items on the benefits list.

Its ability to provide an enhanced benefits package may also be attributed to its efforts to improve the cost-effectiveness of service delivery. In August 1995, the Samara oblast began reimbursing hospitals and polyclinics based on the principles of NEM. Polyclinics were reimbursed on a capitation basis according to the population size of their jurisdictions. Moreover, polyclinics were also charged with referring patients to inpatient care and covering all inpatient expenses – they became, in effect, budget-controllers. If the inpatient expenses were less than the capitation payments, the polyclinics could retain the balance; however, if the inpatient expenses exceeded the capitation payment, they had to cover the difference. This payment mechanism enabled cost-savings in inpatient services. The proportion of inpatient expenses in the total healthcare expenditure has substantially declined from 80% during the Soviet era to around 54%.

This mechanism has, however, evidently prevented patients from accessing necessary inpatient services purely due to financial reasons. In a survey on this issue, the majority of physicians interviewed firmly denied the existence of this phenomenon. However, under certain circumstances, they admitted that certain patients had to cover the medical expenses for diagnostic tests and inpatient care, even after being referred.

Most polyclinics in Samara have established day care facilities, which have significantly reduced the number of inpatients. Outpatient surgical facilities are also being developed.

In addition, the development of general practice services has gained increasing attention. In 1994, the regional medical university established a general practice department. That same year, it was estimated that among the 1,500 GPs in the Russian Federation, one-third were based in Samara. GPs were encouraged to work in teams of three (family physician, gynecologist or obstetrician, and pediatrician) in general clinics.

Samara is the only federal subject in the Russian Federation that has passed a law on private practice (1999), which allows psychiatrists and internists specialized in "social diseases," including drug and alcohol addictions, to engage in private practice.

Private practitioners can participate in the MHI system, whereas government-employed physicians typically serve in state-owned institutions; that is, they provide services in and receive salaries from hospitals and polyclinics. Although patients still lack the freedom to choose insurance companies or healthcare providers, certain privatization measures have facilitated a limited degree of competition. Furthermore, state-owned institutions may provide healthcare services on a private basis, but the number of private institutions remains limited because of the high service and operational costs.

Physicians serving in public institutions are paid salaries according to rigid scales that apply to all physicians in the Russian Federation. However, the opportunity to deliver paid services has given these physicians a legal mechanism to increase their incomes and compete with each other for patients who can afford their medical expenses. A proportion of the out-of-pocket payments for such services may be set aside as fixed capital investments. Hence, there are significant differences between healthcare institutions that offer and do not offer paid services, with the former being equipped with better instruments and facilities.

These innovative approaches adopted in Samara seemed to have resolved some of the issues that other regions of the Russian Federation are still trying to address. However, they have also given rise to other problems. Particularly, the approaches might have resulted in a two-tier healthcare system in Samara, where high-income earners are entitled to high-quality and convenient healthcare services, whereas low-income earners are provided with second-rate services and face problems with healthcare accessibility. The practice of allowing and encouraging paid services in a such large number of public healthcare institutions might have cultivated a certain degree of social risk by prompting physicians to exclusively serve patients that are able to pay in pursuit of profits, thereby damaging the interests of patients hoping to receive free healthcare services. Furthermore, it is worth noting that although Samara successfully collected all premium contributions for the MHI system, the funding remains inadequate to fully cover all promised healthcare benefits. Hence, there is still room for the development of paid services.

Nevertheless, Samara has progressed faster than most other regions in the Russian Federation in its promotion of reforms in accordance with the Health Insurance Act of 1993. In addition, it should be noted that the aforementioned risk factors are attributed to financial shortages rather than any inherent shortcomings in the new system.

3. Issues in the Implementation of the Reform

1. *Partial substitution of budgets by health insurance.* The implementation of health insurance payroll tax collection has provided ample funding for the healthcare sector. Indeed, the payroll tax seemed to continuously fund the healthcare system in the early stages of its implementation (1993–1994). Specifically, as expected, public healthcare funds increased by around 35% in 1993. However, in 1994–1995, some local governments began reducing their financial allocations to healthcare because healthcare institutions were being partially paid by the health insurance schemes. By 1997, public healthcare funds had declined by 27% compared to 1993. Other factors contributed to this decline, such as vague legislation regarding the level of capital investments by regional health authorities and the severe economic challenges facing many oblasts. As a result, health insurance funding has lost its supplementary role, and has partially replaced budget funding. However, it has also been argued that the economic difficulties of the 1990s would have greatly reduced the healthcare expenditure even if the healthcare system had remained completely dependent on budgetary funding. For example, the expenditures on education and cultural activities declined by 36% and 40%, respectively, when the GDP fell by 38% between 1991 and 1997; by contrast, the healthcare expenditure declined by only 21%. Therefore, the health insurance funds evidently have to some extent protected the healthcare system from being affected by large-scale budget cuts.

   The new insurance system's objective of increasing overall healthcare funding has not been achieved because of the severe funding shortage facing the entire healthcare system. Some experts have claimed that a sufficient amount of funding is needed to provide a universal, free benefits package; for that reason, they advised that the payroll tax for health insurance should be increased from 3.6% to 7%. However, this practice is not sustainable for many enterprises, which are now facing numerous financial difficulties, such that they are unable, or unwilling, to afford the current payroll tax of 3.6%.

2. *Regional fragmentation and incomplete implementation.* Of the 89 regions of the Russian Federation, approximately one-quarter have not yet established insurance companies. As a result, these regions are being served by local MHIF branches or local MHIFs. Although not stipulated in the Health Insurance Act of 1993, local MHIFs were eventually granted the right to act as insurance agencies that can purchase services directly from healthcare providers. Another quarter of these regions have adopted the third-party payment system (i.e., insurance companies and local MHIFs or their branches). Insurance agencies cannot foresee any potential profit in sparsely populated rural areas. Initially, local MHIF branches were intended to operate temporarily for about a year until the establishment of insurance agencies; however, their operation has continued past 1997. Currently, they have become a permanent feature of the rural

health insurance system. Furthermore, some regions have totally eliminated insurance agencies from the healthcare funding system, relying entirely on the direct payments made by local MHIFs. The expenses of the nonworking populations in many regions are covered completely by local budgetary funds rather than health insurance. However, even regions that make payments using health insurance have not achieved full compliance because of financial difficulties and their fear of power erosion. Therefore, these regional governments have preferred to fund healthcare institutions directly over paying the premium contributions. However, we foresee that the governments may stop reimbursing hospitals and polyclinics without penalty in the event of economic difficulties; instead, the institutions might face financial penalties for any delays in their premium contributions. Another reason for this is that some regional governments may want to undermine the operation of the health insurance system.

3. *Confusion caused by the dual funding source channels (budget and insurance).* In most regions, both budgetary and insurance funding co-exist, although there are considerable interregional variations in their arrangements. For example, in some areas, the budgetary funds are used to cover all outpatient expenses and the insurance funds to cover inpatient expenses. In other areas, the insurance funds are used to cover inpatient expenses only for adults. There are also areas where the insurance funds are used to cover the working population, whereas the budgetary funds are used to cover the nonworking population. The local MHIFs appear to be incapable of functioning as coordinating agencies for health insurance and budgetary funds. This has led to a serious problem – that is, healthcare providers receive conflicting information and incentives because of differences in the contractual agreement for service delivery and the payment methods adopted by service payers. As a result, planning and financial activities have become increasingly complex for healthcare providers.

   The presence of multiple payers who have varying priorities and motives is expected to lead to the dissemination of conflicting information to providers, which will inevitably result in confusion.

4. *Lack of competitive and selective contractual relationships.* The fundamental principle of health insurance reform is to introduce competition among insurance agencies and healthcare providers. As described earlier, competition was clearly absent in one-third of regional institutions, where local MHIFs or their branches had become monopolistic healthcare purchasers. Because potential insurance agencies cannot foresee profit in sparsely populated rural areas, real competition is only possible in urban areas, where insurance agencies have already been established. Indeed, it has been estimated that more than half of all insurance companies in Russia were established in the country's three largest cities: Moscow, St. Petersburg, and Ekaterinburg. However, competition remains absent in some regions even when those regions have more than one insurance company. In such regions, there is a division in the spheres of influence among insurance agencies. For example, the population of St. Petersburg has been divided into various sectors, each of which has its own healthcare fund. Under these circumstances, neither employers nor consumers have the right to choose, as the contracts signed between local MHIFs and insurance companies strictly limit their respective areas of service.

   Given the aforementioned circumstances, insurance agencies are rarely motivated to monitor their costs and quality, or to selectively sign contracts, due to the guaranteed participation of insured persons in their insurance policies. In fact, there is a general perception throughout the Russian Federation that insurance companies do not act as active service purchasers.

Competition among healthcare providers should comply with the selective contracting undertaken by healthcare purchasers. As mentioned previously, the competition among providers for contracts with insurance agencies has limited consumers' choice of providers (which is another approach for stimulating competition) due to their choice of insurance agencies. Thus, if consumers rely only on insurance agencies to indirectly choose their healthcare providers, competition among providers cannot be attained without selective contracting between insurance companies or local MHIF branches and providers.

However, in addition to the aforementioned, there are further constraints to the competition among healthcare providers in Russia in particular circumstances. One of the key barriers originated from the monopolistic practices inherited from hospitals and polyclinics of the Soviet era. In sparsely populated areas, the economies of scale have hindered the establishment of rival providers; that is, there is no room for new providers to form a competitive environment because of the high start-up costs, as well as various economic and regulatory barriers. Hence, the competition among providers can only be achieved in large urban areas with a relatively large number of insurance agencies. In reality, however, even urban areas have displayed a limited degree of competition.

Although selective contracting is regarded as crucial to the success of the new funding system, it has encountered various obstacles. There is particular resistance from health authorities, given that the domination of market mechanisms would diminish their authority to a certain extent. Hospital and polyclinic administrators often resist selective contracting as well, despite its potential for greater revenue, as it might influence their existing practices and give rise to uncertainties. Even the Russian public is uneasy with the notion of choosing between competing providers, and instead prefers to rely passively on the government to arrange everything. The head of the Moscow MHIF, a strong supporter of healthcare reforms, has also expressed his doubts about the driving force of competition when he noted that "basically all polyclinics in Moscow are the same – they have the same level of services, and the same qualification of physicians."

5. *Insurance companies are not always risk-bearing agencies.* Insurance companies are generally perceived as having "perverse" motives. On the one hand, they are private, for-profit organizations, which implies that they must bear all risks and losses in their pursuit of profit. However, they are generally unwilling to absorb these losses. On the surface, these losses are absorbed by the local MHIFs, although they can often avoid this by reducing their reimbursement rates to healthcare providers. As a result, patients are often the ultimate bearers of the losses through out-of-pocket payments to compensate for the shortage of public funds.

According to the 1993 legislation, insurance companies are entitled to receive prospective capitation payments from local MHIFs. As a result, they strive to minimize their reimbursements to providers by selecting highly efficient prospective payment methods, in order to maximize their profits.

However, local MHIFs eventually adopted a retrospective payment method for reimbursing insurance companies or local MHIF branches, thereby completely eliminating the enthusiasm of insurance companies to engage in selective contracting and to seek efficient, high-quality healthcare providers. The local MHIFs would cover the remaining expenses of insurance companies if the latter exceeded a predetermined amount. Insurance companies therefore began to earn their profits by collecting a fixed percentage of each activity billed to local MHIFs. Since insurance agencies now had guaranteed incomes, they were no longer motivated to promote cost savings among providers. Additionally, agencies were also willing to coordinate and collaborate with healthcare providers to increase the service volume in the pursuit of greater profits. In summary, so long as insurance companies do not act as actual risk-bearing agencies with guaranteed profits, they will not receive any of the potential profits from improved efficiency.

The earlier discussion mainly focused on insurance companies, but it is equally applicable to local MHIF branches, which are also unwilling to serve as risk-bearing agencies because they are a part of the MHI system.

6. *Decentralization of administrative and financial authority.* The Health Insurance Act was implemented on the basis of extensive decentralization of the administrative and financial authority held by the regional health insurance system.

The reimbursement of healthcare services provided to patients who actually reside in a different region has given rise to some serious issues. During the Soviet era, there was a network of specialized inter-regional clinical and diagnostic centers that served patients from neighboring rayons by reimbursing medical institutions for healthcare services that they provided to patients from nearby regions. This network permitted some rayons to provide a comprehensive range of healthcare services, whereas others could specialize in particular services. Permitting the public to utilize services in this manner was the outcome of comprehensive planning efforts at the central and regional levels. However, because of funding shortages in local MHIFs, it is no longer possible to provide a comprehensive range of healthcare services. Currently, patients who wish to receive treatments in neighboring oblasts must make out-of-pocket payments. The federal center is currently responsible only for federal programs. Inter-regional cooperation is a newly emerging trend in addressing this problem, but it still has not yielded any observable outcomes.

The breakdown of inter-regional collaboration has led to the disintegration of the healthcare system and regional "sovereignization." Currently, some regional governments wish to establish their own healthcare networks, thus leading to the duplication of services and unwise capital investment models. This trend has reduced the utilization efficiency of highly specialized services and facilities without creating a more competitive environment for healthcare providers.

Federal healthcare institutions are strongly influenced by reductions in the federal budget, as the MHI does not cover medical expenses in federal hospitals. This has led to the termination of numerous institutions. Thus, decentralization has had a clear adverse impact on federal clinical and research institutes. Other healthcare institutions have also been forced to rely on out-of-pocket payments for services that were previously free in order to remain viable. As a result, the majority of Russians do not have access to highly specialized therapeutic services, while many research institutes, due to a lack of federal funds, have been forced to close down.

7. *Inter-regional imbalances and shortcomings in the equalization mechanism.* According to the law, the federal MHIF requires premium contributions from employees equivalent to 0.2% of their wages in order to remove inter-regional differences. However, inter-regional economic disparities in Russia have progressed far beyond the ability of the federal MHIF to compensate because of various measures adopted to cope with the economic crisis in the 1990s. These inter-regional disparities have also increased continuously, with some regions having a strong industrial base, and others facing severe unemployment and budget deficits in their local governments. In 1992, the ratio of lowest-to-highest healthcare expenditure per capita in Russia was 1:4.3, which increased to 1:7.6 in 1998.

8. *Failure to change the structure of incentive practices in healthcare institutions.* According to the Health Insurance Act, healthcare providers can be reimbursed through various methods, including capitation, fee-for-service, and diagnosis-related group (DRG)-based payments, as well as any other method or combination of methods based on mutual agreements. This measure has provided flexibility for each region to decide its preferred reimbursement method. However, most regions have not made any significant changes in their reimbursement methods to healthcare workers since the Soviet era. The majority of physicians are salaried employees of healthcare institutions – that is, they are employees of regional governments. Despite innovations in hospital reimbursement methods, the primary reimbursement method remains retrospective. As a result, the incentive structure of polyclinics and hospitals has not only failed to improve service efficiency but also aggravated overutilization of the healthcare system. Although there are insurance companies in some regions, these companies passively pay healthcare providers, rather than making use of their potential to create the necessary incentives.

9. *Limited freedom of choice for consumers.* According to the law, consumers are free to choose their preferred insurance agencies; in other words, they are free to choose the providers contracted by their insurance agencies. This freedom of choice is crucial not only for ensuring consumer satisfaction, but also for promoting competition among insurance agencies and providers. However, the freedom of choice for consumers is generally limited because of the unavailability of insurance agencies in many regions. Even in regions with numerous insurance agencies, populations are often divided into individual sectors or spheres of influence for insurance companies, which has eroded consumers' freedom of choice. In such circumstances, patients have slightly more freedom to choose their preferred physicians in polyclinics. Such freedom of choice would help improve the service quality in an incentive system that rewards physicians for their service quality or workload. However, since the income of most physicians in the Russian Federation takes the form of fixed salaries, there is no corresponding increase in their incomes for the increased workload that comes with patients' greater preference for them. Therefore, the potential benefits of competition resulting from consumers' freedom of choice have been diminished.

10. *Inadequate regulation.* Overdecentralization of the healthcare administration has caused the federal government to lose much of its regulatory authority. Although the Ministry of Healthcare supports health insurance legislation, it has made no further effort to coordinate the various agencies within the healthcare system, which has effectively impeded the formation of the legal and regulatory foundation for the MHI. The government's negligence of the reform process has also led to a rapid and massive decentralization. Furthermore, the State has overemphasized the role of the market mechanism, regarding it as a panacea for all issues in the healthcare system without giving proper attention to the regulatory role of the government. For example, in the absence of regulatory measures, there has been a strong reliance on the mechanism of market competition to ensure that insurance companies fulfill their intended roles. Similarly, there is very weak regulatory control over the MHIF. Although the law permits insurance agencies to contract with public and private providers, it does not make a clear structural or regulatory distinction between public and private funding methods for MHI and VHI at either the insurer or the provider level. The ambiguity of these concepts has led to changes in the medical-seeking behaviors of poorly informed consumers, manipulation of publicly funded benefits packages, and collusion (rather than competition) between publicly funded insurance agencies and providers. The unclear division of responsibilities among different levels of governments and health insurance agencies,

as well as the poor policy coordination, have together exacerbated the inefficient utilization of healthcare resources.

11. *Roles of politics.* The introduction of new healthcare funding agencies has led to conflicts of interest and power struggles between the old and new systems. The Ministry of Healthcare and the Ministry of Finance, along with the regional health authorities, have been consistently opposing the establishment of insurance funds and insurance companies, as the latter have encroached upon their administrative and financial roles. In recent years, however, they seemed to have accepted this as part of the reality. The Ministry of Finance does not support the emergence of pooled funds that are completely beyond its control. Currently, some regional governments refuse to pay insurance contributions on behalf of the nonworking population, with the aim of undermining the insurance system in order to create an excuse for abolishing insurance agencies. Local authorities across the 12 regions of the Russian Federation have always hindered insurance funds and have used any collected funds to pay for non-healthcare-related programs, such as housing and construction.

In 1994, most regional health authorities began claiming control over the health insurance funds. However, at the same time, some regions held a positive attitude toward the new healthcare funding reform, particularly in regions with greater financial and administrative capacities. In 1995–1996, top health officials made attempts to revise the Health Insurance Act to limit the authority of the newly established insurance agencies. Their recommendations included abolishing the autonomy of the MHIFs, thus placing them under government jurisdiction, and eliminating publicly funded private insurance agencies. However, these efforts were blocked in the Federal Assembly because they represented the interests of a new insurance group comprising private insurance agencies and MHIFs. On the other hand, some regions (e.g., Kursk and the Mari El Republic) decided not to comply with the federal MHI system and stopped private insurance agencies from participating in funding activities. Notably, the Ministry of Healthcare once opposed the establishment of the health insurance system. However, its dissolution in 1996 marked the end of the campaign against insurance agencies and health insurance funds.

12. *Inadequacy of the reform legislation.* The architects of the health reform believed that the financial shortage was the fundamental issue facing the Soviet healthcare system. They hoped that the introduction of a new fundraising program would increase the total amount of funds available. Furthermore, some believed that other problems would be resolved by the new fundraising program. However, in emphasizing the financial shortage, the architects ignored the importance of cost-effectiveness, cost containment, and mechanisms for improving service efficiency. Additionally, the reform architects relied heavily on the belief that market-oriented reforms would improve system efficiency without recognizing that a strong economic, regulatory, and institutional environment, as well as strong political leadership, are prerequisites for successful reform.

(3) Future Development of Healthcare Funding

As mentioned previously, the implementation of the Health Insurance Act has encountered numerous unforeseen obstacles with unexpected outcomes. Over the years, these issues have prompted countless discussions and recommendations for introducing new reforms to healthcare funding in order to address them.

In 1997, two competing proposals were hotly debated in the Federal Assembly. One of the proposals was put forward by V. Starodubov (the Deputy Minister of Healthcare at that time, and later the Minister of Healthcare until 1999), who recommended the elimination of all insurance companies and placing health insurance funds under the control of regional and federal health authorities. This proposal essentially rejected the new system, returning to a centralized, tax-based healthcare funding model. The other proposal was put forward by Y. Goryunov (a member of the State Duma) with the aim of enhancing market relations by reinforcing the roles of insurance companies; NGOs related to licensing, accreditation, and inspection; and some private healthcare institutions. This proposal further urged the implementation of relevant regulations that required local budgets to pay the insurance contributions of the nonworking population. Although both proposals were debated by the Federal Assembly in 1998, they were eventually abandoned.

In 1999, representatives of the Ministry of Healthcare, the Federal MHIF, Ministry of Taxation, and other ministries and federal departments jointly established a working group to discuss recommendations made by the Governor of the Samara Oblast. He proposed increasing employers' contributions to health insurance premiums and reducing the amount of tax revenue allocated to regional healthcare budgets. This proposal aimed to increase the proportion of funds administered by MHIFs; however, it has not yielded any tangible outcomes.

Over the past two years, there have been discussions on the reorganization and merger of the social and health insurance sectors. In addition, the roles of insurance agencies in the newly reformed funding system have continued to stoke debate. In general, both health officials and employers view MHIFs, especially insurance companies, as unnecessary aspects of the healthcare funding system. Some have even accused MHIFs of passively mobilizing financial resources via increased management costs, which unnecessarily burden the healthcare system. On the other hand, the supporters of this new funding system have reported that it is impossible to conduct a fair assessment of a system that has yet to be fully implemented.

Most Russians are likely not aware of what the MHI is or who the accountable parties are, and hence have no opinions on it and would not object to its continued implementation.

In 1999, the State Duma passed the Law on Mandatory Health Insurance in its first hearing, but later faced considerable opposition and multiple failures in its enactment. This law aimed to diminish the importance of insurance agencies within the statutory funding system and offer regional governments the option to eliminate them whenever necessary. However, it has not been enacted because of continuous opposition by insurance agencies.

Discussions on the future development of this system are intensifying, and have given rise to a legislative draft that takes into account multiple factors. The new bill was contested in 2001 and early 2002 for the following important reasons:

1. Local MHIFs are currently accountable to their respective regional health authorities. The law recommends the establishment of a centralized social and health insurance system by reorganizing local MHIFs into regional branches of the federal fund.
2. The federal government covers the premium contributions of the nonworking population using the federal budget. Hence, the federal fund will have the following two funding sources: premium contributions paid by the working population and premium contributions paid using the federal budget on behalf of the nonworking population.
3. This system retains the role of insurance agencies and establishes additional conditions to facilitate competition among insurance agencies. These additional conditions include the freedom of all citizens to choose their preferred insurance agencies; stringent operating requirements for insurance agencies, such as the disclosure of operational plans and justification for selected services; and specification of service volume in contracts with healthcare providers.

The aforementioned third factor follows a different line of thought from the earlier two factors cited, as it favors a free-market-oriented perspective that enables insurance agencies to play important roles in the reformed system. The government seemed to favor this factor, meaning that it had a greater likelihood of being written into law. Still, there were still many problems that needed to be considered, several of which the new bill attempted to address, such as the fund pooling mechanisms; resolving excessive decentralization; creating new regulations for health insurance companies; selective contracting; the prospective payment system; issues related to severe financial shortage, such as cost-sharing; and reinforcement of planning in view of the overreliance on market mechanisms.

Recently, two additional issues have triggered discussion: (1) the possibility of using the federal budget to match the premium contributions paid out of regional budgets for the nonworking population; (2) the possibility of using pensions to cover the premium contributions of retirees.

However, it should be emphasized that this new bill has progressed slowly because of the various criticisms levied at it. As described earlier, it is widely believed that the present funding system operates in the interests of insurance companies rather than patients. This issue must be addressed in a future reform to the funding system. Some experts have also proposed that there is no clear legal basis for the management of public funds (i.e., the social insurance premiums collected by MHIFs) by private agencies, such as private insurance agencies. Furthermore, it has been suggested that there are many contradictions to regulations in the Civil Code regarding the operation of the MHI system. Some have also argued that it is inappropriate to use a single law to regulate both the MHI and VHI; a separate law is needed to address issues in the latter. There are numerous approaches to solving these issues, but it is likely to take some time to select the most desirable funding system in the future.

(4) Voluntary Health Insurance (VHI)

The VHI was officially approved in 1991 and the relevant regulatory laws were promulgated in 1992. VHI services can be provided to individuals or groups (e.g., corporate employees) and insured persons are entitled to receive additional services on top of those offered by the basic benefits package. VHI is provided only by private, for-profit insurance companies (nominally, these are joint ventures), but market entry is also permitted for nonprofit organizations. According to the Mandatory Health Insurance Act of 1993, VHI can be offered by private insurance agencies in the MHI system.

VHI plays a very limited role in the healthcare funding of the Russian Federation. In 1999, it was estimated that VHI accounted for only about 3.5% of the total healthcare funding. In general, VHI is only purchased by the rich as well as by a small number of employers for their employees (in addition to MHI premiums, foreign companies tend to provide private insurance for expatriate employees).

Private insurance companies tend to focus on the high-end market and provide additional services on top of the free healthcare services covered by the basic benefits package. Their focus has shifted toward providing better conditions and hotel-style services, as well as ensuring patients' access to prestigious medical institutions. Therefore, companies are willing to sign contracts with clinics and hospitals that previously belonged to the closed healthcare system and received more resources during the Soviet era. This makes them capable of ensuring their clients' access to treatment in better healthcare institutions with highly skilled healthcare workers, without having to fully cover the medical expenses (i.e., they are subsidized by public funds).

TABLE 20.1 Healthcare Funding Sources in Russia in 1995–2009 (Unit: %)

Funding Sources	Year														
	1995	1996	1997	1998	1999	2000	2001	2002	2003	2004	2005	2006	2007	2008	2009
Tax revenues (budget)	48.5	45.9	49.1	41.4	39.7	35.7	35.5	35.1	35.5	36.1	36.0	36.4	39.3	39.4	39.4
MHI	25.5	25.5	25.5	23.7	22.2	24.2	23.2	23.9	23.3	23.5	26.0	26.8	24.9	24.9	25.0
Out-of-pocket payments	16.9	18.1	18.1	23.0	27.5	30.0	30.5	30.9	32.8	33.2	31.3	30.0	29.7	29.1	28.8
Private insurance	1.6	2.0	2.0	2.2	2.6	3.2	4.7	4.1	4.2	3.5	3.1	3.7	3.4	3.8	3.9
NGO	2.8	2.9	3.0	2.4	1.8	1.7	1.8	2.0	2.0	1.9	1.8	1.5	1.4	1.4	1.4
Other out-of-pocket payments	4.8	5.6	6.6	7.3	6.2	5.2	4.3	4.0	2.2	1.8	1.8	1.6	1.3	1.4	1.5
Total	100.1	100.0	104.3	100.0	100.0	100.0	100.0	100.0	100.0	100.0	100.0	100.0	100.0	100.0	100.0

Source: WHO, 2011.

935

Hence, most benefits are offered by insurance companies exclusively to individuals who are already the most privileged in the healthcare system.

The government of the Russian Federation has amended VHI-related laws to improve the regulation of the system, expand its scope of coverage, and encourage more individuals to participate in VHI. The 1997 "Concept of Development of Healthcare and Medical Science in the Russian Federation" recommended the further development of VHI; nevertheless, there have been no initiatives since.

4. Healthcare Funding System and Financial Allocation

(1) Healthcare Funding System

1. Funding Sources and Structures According to official statistics, most healthcare services in the Russian Federation are co-funded via budgetary and insurance sources. Table 20.1 shows the share of each funding source over the last decade.

Table 20.2 shows the allocation of federal budgetary funds. The funds are allocated by the Ministry of Healthcare for training, medical research, public healthcare services, large-scale investments, and tertiary (i.e., highly specialized) healthcare services. The portion allocated to other agencies includes funding for the Russian Academy of Sciences and parallel healthcare systems. However, these funds do not completely cover all expenditures in the parallel systems, which are also funded by other ministries via extra-budgetary federal funds not included in the official statistics. Therefore, it is extremely difficult to determine the exact amount of expenditure of these parallel healthcare systems.

Regional healthcare budgets once constituted about 45% of the total healthcare fund; however, this proportion has declined significantly since 1992, bottoming out in 2002 at 35.1%; since then, it has risen again, stabilizing at 39.3–39.4% in recent years.

The budgetary funds of regional governments may be allocated according to the following two objectives: (1) to make direct payments for certain healthcare services (in the prereform system, many regions made payments in accordance with the specifications of the benefits package), and (2) to pay for the insurance contributions of the non-working populations. Regional governments have adopted a range of different allocation methods for their healthcare budgets.

The MHI system contributes a relatively large proportion of funds, and this proportion has been steadily maintained at about 25%. The financial shortage caused by the shrinking budgets has been compensated to some degree by the steadily increasing share of out-of-pocket payments. The proportion of funds allocated for services with charges has

TABLE 20.2 Healthcare Funding in the Russian Federal Budget (Unit: %)

Funding Sources	1999	2000
Ministry of Healthcare	81.5	79.4
Other agencies	18.5	20.6
Total	100	100

Source: Ministry of Finance of the Russian Federation, 2001.

increased more than fivefold (accounting for 8.4% of the total healthcare expenditure), especially for the purchase of drugs (pharmaceutical expenses have increased more than threefold, reaching one-quarter of the total healthcare expenditure in 1999).

Since patients purchase outpatient drugs at their own expense, the rise in these expenses has been attributed to the rapid increase in drug prices. The country has witnessed a rising trend in the adoption of VHI, although it still accounts for only a small proportion of the total healthcare funds.

It should also be noted that the premiums paid via budgetary funds for the nonworking population account for about one-fourth of the disposable MHIF. This, however, has been gradually falling since 1995, reaching about 5.2% in 1999. The health insurance premiums contributed by the working population accounted for approximately 16% of the total healthcare fund, while the premium contributions made on behalf of the nonworking population by regional healthcare budgets accounted for about 5% (which is far from sufficient to cover the health insurance premiums of this population). The nonworking population accounts for approximately 55.27% of the total Russian population, and members of this population incur healthcare expenditures that greatly exceeded those of the working population, who are mostly younger and healthier. In fact, there are numerous regions that partially cover or do not cover the premium contributions of their nonworking populations, which is the root cause of the financial shortage of the healthcare system.

Table 20.3 shows the funding sources of the MHI system and its development process. The share of budgetary funds dedicated to the premium contribution of the non-working population peaked in 1995 but subsequently fell steadily until 1998–1999, after which it began rising again.

The Institute for Social Research has conducted a series of surveys on the drug and healthcare expenses of Russian households. The results showed that the out-of-pocket payments for healthcare services in 1998 were significantly higher than were those officially reported by Goskomstat.

The shares of the different funding sources recalculated using new estimates for out-of-pocket payments are shown in Table 20.4.

The total out-of-pocket sources accounted for around 47.3% (nearly half) of the total healthcare fund, which was far higher than the general estimates and certainly far higher than the projected amount for a healthcare system providing free universal healthcare services. Table 20.4 also shows higher estimates for out-of-pocket payments, which may be attributed to the inclusion of under-the-table payments in the estimation.

TABLE 20.3 Funding Sources for the MHIF in Russia in 1994–2001 (Unit: %)

Funding Source	Year							
	1994	1995	1996	1997	1998	1999	2000	2001
Premium revenue	66.0	60.7	6.3	62.0	63.7	67.9	7.9	66.7
Budgetary funds for the nonworking population	19.3	27.4	25.2	22.1	22.4	22.4	25.2	26.6
Others (e.g., savings, penalties, fines)	14.7	11.9	13.5	15.9	13.9	9.7	2.9	6.7
Total	100	100	100	100	100	100	100	100

Source: Goskomstat of the Russian Federation, 2002.

Table 20.4 Shares of the Main Funding Sources Based on the Estimates for Out-of-Pocket Payments Calculated by the Institute for Social Research

Funding Sources	1998 (₽ billion)	1998 (%)
Federal budget	5.7	3.6
Regional healthcare budget	58.7	36.7
MHI premiums for the working population	20.0	12.5
Individual VHI premiums	3.8	2.4
Household healthcare expenses	32.3	20.2
Household drug expenses	37.0	23.1
Corporate healthcare expenses	2.6	1.6
Total	100.0	100.0

Source: Data of the Institute for Social Research, S. Shishkin, "Problems of Transition from Tax-Based System of Health Care Finance to Mandatory Health Insurance Model in Russia," *Croatian Medical Journal* 40, no. 2 (1999): 195–201.

2. Out-of-Pocket Payments   The majority of insurance schemes operating in the Russian Federation do not include cost-sharing provisions. Some of the major hospitals or outpatient services include only the following officially sanctioned charges: dental care; routine ophthalmological services (e.g., eye examinations); most medical aids and dental fillings; outpatient drugs; and other services that fall outside the coverage of the basic benefits package.

Dental care charges, prescription fees for patients in outpatient facilities, and service charges for dental fillings were imposed in accordance with standard practices inherited from the Soviet era. However, numerous categories of patients can be exempted from drug expenses. In line with official regulations, there has been no increase in the number of healthcare services that require out-of-pocket payments in major healthcare institutions. Despite these regulations, an increasing number of patients participated in healthcare funding during the 1990s. This, in part, can be attributed to an increase in drug costs due to the increasingly important role of the private sector in importing and distributing drugs.

Additionally, the growth of out-of-pocket payments can be attributed to medical charges that fall beyond the coverage of statutory funds, which have to be covered by patients at their own expense. Generally, if providers of free healthcare services are unable to cover their costs using public funds, they must charge for the delivery of healthcare services even if the services are legally required to be free of charge. The government is forced to accept these legally controversial practices as it is unable to provide the necessary funding, thus leading to a considerable degree of inequality: patients might either receive free services or have to make a full out-of-pocket payment, depending on the type of healthcare services or the place of delivery. The out-of-pocket expenses for inpatient care, especially surgical services, can exceed the monthly or even the annual salary of patients. Apart from these semi-legal service charges, there are also some under-the-table payments made to physicians and other healthcare workers, which will be discussed later in the section on "Under-the-table payments."

The Institute for Social Research has conducted a series of surveys on the drug and healthcare expenses of Russian households and found a considerable difference between the estimated out-of-pocket expenses and the widely cited official data. For instance, a survey carried out in January 1998 revealed that the total out-of-pocket payments, including under-the-table payments, accounted for 47%, or nearly half, of the total healthcare fund (Table 20.4). Furthermore, the survey showed that the expenses for drugs and medical devices accounted for 62% of the total out-of-pocket expenditure (from both official and unofficial statistics), followed by outpatient and inpatient services. Despite being much more expensive than primary healthcare services, inpatient services have a relatively lower utilization rate and thus account for a smaller proportion of the total healthcare expenditure.

Other household surveys have explored the total out-of-pocket expenditure in Russia. A survey reported in 2001 that about 10% of patients seeking medical attention made out-of-pocket payments, about half of whom paid officially at a cashier in amounts ranging from ₽2 to ₽3,000, whereas the remaining 56% gave cash or gifts to healthcare workers in amounts ranging from ₽10 to ₽3,000. Among inpatients, those who made out-of-pocket payments accounted for 15.4%, of whom 65.3% paid through official channels while 5.3% gave cash and gifts to healthcare workers.

These statistics reveal some of the inequalities in healthcare funding as a result of out-of-pocket drug and healthcare expenses. Particularly, the poorest group had less frequent outpatient visits and shorter hospital stays, and seldom purchased necessary drugs to save costs. However, their healthcare expenses as a percentage of their incomes were three times those of the richest group. One in 10 respondents claimed that in 1998, one of their family members did not receive the recommended inpatient services because of cost considerations. Half of the households believed that at least one of their members could not afford the recommended drugs at least once. Furthermore, more than 20% of households reported that one of their members did not receive the recommended cardiovascular drugs due to cost considerations. It must be noted that the rural population had higher out-of-pocket expenses as a percentage of their incomes compared to the urban population.

The share of payments made to private healthcare institutions was much higher than the share of households that received healthcare services in private healthcare institutions. For instance, the payments made for private dental services accounted for 60.7% of the total expenses for dental services, but only 19.8% of households sought medical attention in private dental clinics. However, a census carried out in 1999 revealed that the share of payments made for private dental services has decreased. Similarly, 15.3% of payments for inpatient services were made to private hospitals, but only 0.4% of households sought healthcare services in private hospitals. The survey clearly indicates that despite the widespread problem of under-the-table payments, private healthcare services are far more expensive than are those provided in public institutions. Evidently, it is difficult for impoverished individuals to access paid healthcare services because they are unable to afford the corresponding expenses. Thus, impoverished individuals are often deprived of their constitutional right to healthcare because of the shortage of free services and the widespread availability of paid services.

The growth of formal and informal private payments is attributed to an imbalance between the promise of free healthcare services and the reality of severe resource constraints. According to the WHO's index of fairness in financial contribution, the Russian Federation ranked 185th out of 191 countries. These increasingly prominent inequalities have made it imperative to revise the constitutional provisions for free healthcare services. In view of the severe financial shortage and the inability of the government to fulfill its commitments using the available public resources, some experts have proposed transferring a portion of the statutory healthcare expenditure to consumers in order to increase the available healthcare funds, raise cost awareness among consumers and, ironically, improve healthcare equality.

In most circumstances, the imposition of copayments would lead to increased inequality in healthcare funding because it would have a greater impact on low-income earners. However, the prevalence of legally controversial under-the-table payments in the Russian Federation has made the existing system susceptible to inequalities in healthcare access. Hence, the imposition of copayments might in fact reduce inequality in the current system.

One of the issues mentioned in the 1997 "Concept of Development of Healthcare and Medical Science in the Russian Federation" is the cost-sharing of healthcare services under the basic benefits package. However, this report does not specify a normative or legislative mechanism for the implementation of cost-sharing. According to official statements, the issue of cost-sharing has become a key topic in recent years; even so, no specific measures for the implementation of cost-sharing have yet been discussed. An economic program formulated in 2000 did give serious consideration to the use of copayments for healthcare services, but the government ultimately did not legalize this practice. Then, a presidential speech made in 2001 highlighted the problems arising from the prevalence of informal payments, but the possibility of legalizing copayments was not mentioned. Currently, it is believed that the cost-sharing approach will not be legalized in the near future for political reasons; nevertheless, the issue has been raised publicly and has received widespread attention. A sociological survey carried out by the European Community's Technical Assistance to the Commonwealth of Independent States and Georgia (TACIS) showed that some people in Moscow expressed a willingness to contribute their own financial resources to support healthcare funding.

Certain administrative agencies that oppose the federal law have taken steps to partially legalize the copayment approach. For example, the Health Authority of Perm Krai has established fixed charges for outpatient visits and daily hospital stays; Kaluga Oblast is considering the implementation of copayments for their promised healthcare services; and the Republic of Karelia withholds 80% of the pensions of inpatients to cover healthcare expenses.

3. Under-the-Table Payments   During the Soviet era, healthcare workers often received under-the-table payments as a form of supplementary income, although the actual situation of these payments is not publicly known. The collection of relevant data has been hindered by the reluctance of officials to admit to the existence of the phenomenon and the difficulty in valuing these payments, which are made in either cash or goods. However, a study conducted by the Soviet Sociological Institute in the 1980s revealed that the "black" portion of the healthcare economy accounted for about 17% of the total healthcare budget. More conservative estimates put the out-of-pocket payments for healthcare services at 7–10% of the total healthcare expenditure. Regardless of which dataset is more accurate, it is apparent that out-of-pocket payments are a significant funding source, especially payments made to physicians and nurses.

Under-the-table payments should be understood within the wider context of corruption in the Russian Federation. According to a two-year study on corruption funded by the Danish government and the World Bank, and carried out by the Russian Information Science for Democracy (INDEM), Russians collectively spent US$36 billion per year in bribery (equivalent to more than half of the government expenditure in 2002). Of this, US$2.5 billion was spent on "casual corruption," including the payments for normally free healthcare services. In fact, healthcare had the largest proportion of bribes of any other sector, at more than US$600 million. This survey also found that about 12 million Russians did not seek necessary medical attention because they could not afford to make these under-the-table payments. Undoubtedly, under-the-table payments will continue to serve as a major channel of healthcare funding. There is a wide gap between comprehensive healthcare services and the limited formal financial resources, and the absence of adequate informal funding sources has hindered the sustainability of the healthcare system.

A series of surveys conducted by the Institute for Social Research (in collaboration with the Legal and Regulatory Reform Project, Boston University) included under-the-table payments within their calculation of the out-of-pocket drug and healthcare expenses. In December 1997, the total amount of informal payments made by households for their drug and healthcare expenses accounted for 15.5% of the total out-of-pocket healthcare expenditure. In December 1998, there was a slight increase in the absolute amount spent by consumers on informal payments (from ₽4.6 in 1997 to ₽35.9 in 1998). However, the share of informal payments out of the total out-of-pocket expenditure declined to 11.5% in 1998 because of the increase in the total out-of-pocket healthcare expenditure. The amount of informal payments was twice the amount of officially reported legitimate payments.

Informal payments are made much less frequently in the private sector than in the public sector, and nearly all pertain to inpatient services. More specifically, under-the-table payments account for about one-third of inpatient expenses, most of which are made to physicians; the remaining payments for inpatient expenses are made to healthcare officials who arrange for hospital stays, nurses, and other hospital staff.

Informal payments are also frequently made for dental services. In December 1998, under-the-table payments for dental services accounted for an estimated 29.3% of the total out-of-pocket expenditure; most of these payments were made to dentists in private practice. The prevalence of under-the-table payments can be attributed to a desire for tax avoidance among healthcare providers. Moreover, by lowering the recorded medical expenses, the "surplus" of tax avoidance can be shared between patients and providers, thereby benefitting both parties.

Drugs and public outpatient services have the lowest amount of informal payments. It is also interesting to note that under-the-table payments made for inpatient services tend to be greater in rural areas than in urban areas. This might be because of the poor quality of healthcare services in rural healthcare institutions, which is consistent with the overall developmental trend of Russia. As mentioned previously, rural healthcare institutions usually impose higher out-of-pocket charges.

(2) Formulation of Third-Party Budgets and Resource Allocation

Figure 20.4 shows the operational flow of healthcare funds. The Ministry of Healthcare and the Ministry of Finance have adopted the annual budget cycle approach for reviewing the centrally funded portions of the healthcare system (i.e., direct ministerial costs, federal healthcare institutions, and support for core programs such as planned immunization), in order to facilitate nationwide funding via general taxation.

Additionally, the Ministry of Healthcare and the federal MHIF calculate the annual cost of the Program of State Guarantees for Medical Care Provision Free of Charge (PGG), which has been implemented nationwide. Adjustments are then made with the agreement of the Ministry of Finance based on the mortality and morbidity spectrum of each region. A target amount is established based on an annual cost estimation of each region using a nonrecommendatory and nonlegally-binding method. About two-thirds of the target amount are used for the PGG, under which the delivery of primary and secondary healthcare services is funded by the MHI system. The remaining one-third of the target amount is allocated to tertiary and specialized healthcare services, as well as regional programs funded by regional budgets.

The standard rate of employers' premium contributions is established by the federal government. By contrast, the premium contributions made by local governments on behalf of the nonworking population (i.e., the elderly, children, disabled individuals, and unemployed persons) have not been standardized by the federal government, and thus vary considerably across different regions. According to the Health Insurance Act of 1993, the total pool consisting of premium contributions and the budgetary and insurance funds should be integrated with the direct financial support for local governments, which is derived from various sources (e.g., taxes and rental incomes), in order to establish an overall fund for each region. However, in most situations, regional governments can only partially cover the premium contributions needed for the medical expenses of those incapable of self-care. Therefore, the actual amount of funds available to the MHI system is far lower than the target amount, averaging less than two-ninths of the target. The regional budgets, which are intended to cover the premium contributions of the nonworking population, are often preferable for directly channeling funds to healthcare institutions to enhance their control over fund utilization. The remaining one-third of the target amount (including those for tertiary healthcare services) is derived from the regional budgets. Most of these funds are channeled to regional healthcare institutions, while a small amount is channeled to federal healthcare institutions.

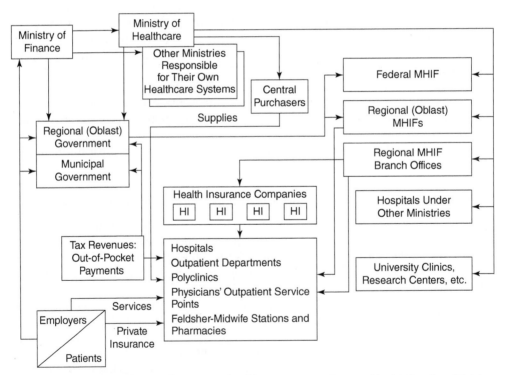

FIGURE 20.4 Capital flow in the Russian healthcare system. *Source*: Health Services Division, WHO Regional Office for Europe, 2010.

The total amount of regional funds is based more on the historical budgets of the healthcare institutions concerned than on the target amount established by the Ministry of Healthcare. The specific basis of its determination includes: the composition of healthcare workers, number of beds, and fixed costs; the earning ability of the local government; local customs and practices; and the operational status of local insurance systems (given that employers do not always fulfill their obligations).

In some situations, the flow of these two major funds is supplemented by direct contracts between enterprises and healthcare providers, as well as between insurance agencies and healthcare providers in the parallel system (the funding sources of which are completely independent of the system of the Ministry of Healthcare). In other circumstances, VHI schemes have increased the income of the healthcare sector by covering the medical expenses of insured persons in mainstream healthcare institutions. Both out-of-pocket and under-the-table payments have significantly increased the total healthcare budget in Russia. While these funding sources have neither been defined in detail during the formulation of third-party budgets nor truly publicly investigated, their contributions are crucial to the development of the healthcare sector.

Many regions also receive funds from the Ministry of Finance under the budgetary transfer payments of the social sector, which do not have separate allocations for healthcare, education, and other social expenditures. While the demand for regional healthcare must be assessed to determine the amount of transfer payments, regional governments nevertheless reserve the right to decide the amount allocated to healthcare and other social services on their own. As the decisions made by regional governments are not monitored, the financial information of each regional healthcare system is not included in the overall national budget. Regional governments also make transfer payments to rayon governments, which are free to determine the amount allocated to each activity. Furthermore, rayon governments can also raise their own funds via taxation. The healthcare funds transferred by the federal government to regional governments, and by regional governments to rayon governments, are not derived from those particular government levels, but are still listed in the official statistics as regional and municipal budgetary sources, respectively.

Some funds flow from regional governments to the federal government. In principle, the federal healthcare system should provide free services to each region in accordance with their respective quotas. However, this practice has not been successfully implemented because of a lack of federal resources. Thus, the use of healthcare services provided in federal institutions often requires payments from regional governments or patients. This quota system is implemented in 67 of the 273 federal inpatient institutions affiliated with the Ministry of Healthcare that are capable of providing high-tech services. The quotas are intended to cover about one-quarter of the service activities of these healthcare institutions, but the actual utilization rate of these institutions is much lower because of the required payments.

The premiums collected by the MHIF are transferred to insurance companies based on a weighted capitation formula. The insurance companies (or MHIF branches and local MHIFs in regions without insurance companies) sign contracts with healthcare providers based on DRG-based payments with the aim of improving service efficiency. The MHIF signs contracts directly with healthcare providers in the absence of insurance agencies in the region. The payment methods used reflect the priorities of third-party payers and the service volume of healthcare providers. In reality, however, healthcare funds are still allocated according to historical budgets, and little concern is given to the adoption of payment methods that can promote the efficiency of insurance agencies.

The federal MHIF aims to regulate capital flow and to fill the gaps in resources caused by varying wage bases across different regions by reallocating 0.2% of its total funds. However, this amount is insufficient to address the existing healthcare inequalities; hence, numerous areas in the healthcare sector continue to face a shortage of healthcare resources.

(3) Hospital Payments and Their Impact

1. Hospital Payments Historically, hospitals received budgetary funds based on the number of beds. Polyclinics received funds according to a similar method, albeit based on the number of outpatient visits (rather than hospital beds). The amount approved by the central government (which involves the consideration of various factors, such as inflation and economic growth) clearly reflected how hospital budgets increased each year. However, this had a negative impact on hospitals by prompting them to increase the number of beds in order to request more resources.

In order to address these issues, the healthcare funding system has shifted toward partial insurance-based payment models and made payments for inpatient services according to fixed prices based on DRGs. Moreover, hospitals have been forced to shorten the length of hospital stays through insurance-based pricing and to conduct more reasonable diagnostic tests. Polyclinics received payments through various methods, with the aim of encouraging them to treat patients in their outpatient settings rather than refer patients to hospitals. In addition, hospitals and polyclinics were entitled to receive about 30% of their funds from their respective oblast or rayon governments based on their actual costs. In reality, however, the new method of financial allocation is even more complicated than the older method, and the payment methods for hospitals have deviated from those conceived in the original model.

In areas with full implementation of insurance schemes, the local MHIFs sign contracts with insurance companies for the delivery of healthcare services to their insured persons. First, the local NHIFs make a prospective capitation payment to insurance companies on behalf of each insured person. Insurance companies then sign contracts with local healthcare providers (hospitals, polyclinics, and small clinics) for the delivery of healthcare services covered by the basic benefits package, which was jointly established by the Ministry of Healthcare and the federal MHIF. Previously, prices were established via local fee agreements, and while this basic model has been retained, local MHIFs now allocate the capitated funds to insurance companies retrospectively. Recently, a fundamental change in the payment method was introduced after reviewing the expenditures and reserves to prevent the misuse of funds. It has become clear that a large amount of funds (about US$100 million) have not been utilized rationally, with there being some cases of serious mismanagement in the past. The root cause of these issues lies in the transfer of large sums of money to insurance companies, which then use their capital reserves for speculative investments that often end in failure.

In the absence of insurance companies or local MHIFs (or federal MHIF branches), healthcare providers are paid retrospectively for their services. Retrospective payments can completely eliminate the possibility of cost savings in hospitals. Accordingly, the problems arising from this payment method are associated with two separate yet closely related factors: the role of insurance companies and the impact of this payment method on healthcare providers (i.e., hospitals).

2. Impact on hospitals In the 1990s, a number of new payment methods were introduced for healthcare providers, although the precise methods varied greatly by region. In 1997, most hospitals (58%) that had contracted with insurance funds had adopted a DRG-based payment system, whereas only 5.5% of hospitals had adopted the line-item budgeting method. Hence, we might make a conservative assumption that insurance companies have generally switched to the adoption of the new payment methods alongside the reform of insurance funds. Overall, approximately 80% of Russian hospitals have signed contracts with either an insurance fund or an insurance company, but it is difficult to determine the respective percentages.

Areas that have already implemented the new payment methods for hospitals are accustomed to only paying for services stipulated in their contracts with insurance funds or companies. On average, these methods are estimated to account for only about one-third of hospital revenue, while the remaining two-thirds come from regional budgetary funds, which still employ the line-item payment method based on their historical approach.

The implementation of the new payment methods for hospitals has undoubtedly brought a number of positive outcomes. These include the development of new clinical and financial information systems; increased collection and utilization of data on hospital utilization, patient DRGs, and costs; an overall increase in the awareness of cost-effectiveness; and increased concerns about quality.

However, improvement in hospital utilization through the introduction of these new payment methods has not materialized for two reasons: the first is related directly to the payment methods. Evidence has shown that the new payment methods have not been able to improve the efficiency of hospital providers. Despite showing a decreasing trend in many countries, the average length of hospital stay has remained largely unchanged in the Russian Federation. There have been signs indicating that, regardless of whether input- or output-based payment methods are adopted, hospital stays remain uniformly lengthy among the different regions. This is possibly because in most regions long hospital stays are used as a DRG reference value for determining reimbursement rates, thereby leading to reduced efficiency. Retrospective payments have also failed to inhibit the use of expensive hospital services. Furthermore, Moscow hospitals paid on a line-item basis have been found to have higher output values than do those paid on a DRG basis. Presently, the prevailing perception is that high bed occupancy rates imply more effective utilization of healthcare resources. On the other hand, prospective payment methods are only applied in certain circumstances. Effective penalties should be imposed for noncompliance with the relevant regulations concerning payments. In the absence of such penalties, some healthcare institutions might not provide the relevant services in accordance with their contracts after receiving payments.

The second reason for the lack of improvement in hospital behaviors is that the new payment methods account for only about one-third of the total hospital revenue, which has the following consequences: (1) the full implementation of the new payment methods has been hindered; (2) the coexistence of multiple payment methods has led to confusion and prevented the use of a rational approach for the financial management and planning of hospitals; and (3) the coexistence of old and new payment methods has resulted in conflicting and contradictory guidelines and motives.

Recently, emerging evidence has hinted at the increasing reluctance of patients to access healthcare services, which has led to an increase in the disease burden, especially for chronic illnesses. This increasing reluctance can be attributed to the general perception that the healthcare system is experiencing numerous problems and improper operation.

Moreover, an increasing number of inpatients might have to pay for "hotel-style services" at their own expense, and even bring their own food and bed sheets with them to the hospital. Under-the-table payments have also increased inpatient expenses, causing patients to be even more reluctant to seek medical attention in conventional healthcare institutions. Although this phenomenon should in theory reduce pressure on the insurance system, the actual outcome was not expected.

Neither the large-scale detachment of patients from the existing healthcare system nor the dependence of hospitals on debt for filling the financial gaps are sustainable strategies. Planners and policymakers are currently formulating the next set of reforms, which aim to improve the efficiency and control the cost of insurance. During this transition period, hospitals have continued to provide healthcare services based on physicians' medical judgments, without restricting the service volume. These hospitals continue to receive funds from local governments and/or insurance companies, as well as through other funding mechanisms, but their incomes remain insufficient to cover their actual costs in providing healthcare services. Although some of the financial gaps can be filled via semi-formal and informal out-of-pocket payments, the sustainability of these payment methods is unclear.

(4) Payment of Physicians

In 1991, the average income of healthcare sector personnel was equivalent to about 75.4% of the national average income. In Russia, the remuneration of physicians is currently similar to that of primary school teachers, and only slightly higher than that of nurses or feldshers. A general surgeon in a public hospital might earn only ₽1,500 (equivalent to US$50) per month, while a surgeon serving in a palatial private hospital in Moscow might earn up to US$1,500 per month. There is no distinction in terms of physician remuneration between primary and secondary healthcare institutions. However, specialists and physicians serving in hospitals might have slightly higher remuneration because they have more opportunities to upgrade their qualifications and undertake additional tasks.

All healthcare workers serving in the public sector are salaried, and most are employed indirectly by the levels of government responsible for their healthcare institutions. Their employment contracts determine the rate of remuneration and may specify the required number of working hours or shifts, workload (generally based on the number of patients within their areas of jurisdiction), or the scope of responsibilities. Recent adjustments have set requirements for postgraduate qualifications, work experience, and the scope of responsibilities for particular positions; however, the required workload or quality have not been specified.

The central government stipulates the basic salary level for healthcare workers because they are all employed by a particular level of government. Their salaries increase annually based on an estimated range of adjustments determined by the Ministry of Healthcare and the Ministry of Finance within the global constraints of the healthcare budget. Official decision-making bodies face little pressure because there are no independent trade unions representing the medical professions, and striking is illegal in Russia. However, there is widespread dissatisfaction regarding the rate of remuneration. Senior policymakers have realized that the current practice has largely dampened the enthusiasm of healthcare workers, which in turn could have a negative impact on healthcare outcomes. Currently, it is common to see physicians who put little or no effort into their work, receiving very few patients and frequently referring patients to other institutions, but who still receive the same monthly salaries as their more diligent and committed colleagues. This has undermined the enthusiasm of many hardworking healthcare personnel.

In response to these challenges, the Russian Federation initiated an expansion of the basic bonus pilot scheme during its healthcare reform. In the 1980s, the administrators of hospitals and polyclinics were given autonomy to award bonuses to personnel with good performance. Currently, the right of healthcare institutions to generate income and retain profits has been further expanded, making hospital administrators expect greater resources to establish performance-related incentive mechanisms.

Presently, bonuses are common practice in Russia. Supplementary income accounts for about 20% or more of physicians' monthly income, but in the absence of a formal performance appraisal mechanism, bonuses are distributed by board members regardless of physicians' performance. This practice lacks the support of any formal mechanisms. Furthermore, it allows for the worst case scenario: that is, senior healthcare workers, who are generally difficult to constrain, may abuse their power and influence the rational distribution of bonuses. However, we are optimistic that the administrators of hospitals and polyclinics will introduce different salary standards. Moreover, there is still hope that a more comprehensive salary formula will be established for healthcare workers to help link service outcomes (rather than workloads) with incentives.

Measures meant to improve performance via salaries have also been undermined by the prevalence of under-the-table payments. Both nurses and doctors receive under-the-table payments, but it is easier for the latter to earn additional income because of their greater power over resources, medications, diagnostic tests, and hospital admissions. These under-the-table payments are a source of informal income that contribute to the income gap between physicians, nurses, and feldshers. Additionally, physicians and specialists serving in hospitals have higher incomes than do GPs and primary care physicians.

Although the private sector is still underdeveloped in the Russian Federation, it offers more diverse remuneration methods for physicians. Healthcare workers serving in quasi-private, fee-for-service polyclinics that offer dental or ophthalmological services are paid salaries plus additional income from profit sharing. Physicians offering private consultations charge patients on a fee-for-service basis; they may retain 40–70% of their service charges if they work outside a clinic, while the remaining balance is used to cover operational costs.

The government has clearly recognized that an overall increase in salary is required to improve the motivation and performance of healthcare workers.

(5) Role of Insurance Companies

In regions with insurance companies, a case-based system (which is related to a DRG-based system), has been established through negotiation on the appropriate length of hospital stay, the appropriate packages of interventions and tests, and appropriate clinical standards expected for each case of a given condition. However, these insurance companies are not risk-bearing because they pay providers on a case-by-case or visit-by-visit basis and are reimbursed for each service item by local MHIFs. Furthermore, they do not limit the number of admitted cases or allow hospitals to determine healthcare demands via negotiation. Hence, there is a tendency toward "underwriting" healthcare services for the entire local population because of the lack of a formal mechanism that limits the service volume of hospitals. These contracts are established based on the contents of the basic benefits package, but do not specify the service volume to be purchased.

The role of health insurance companies has become increasingly limited to billing and bill processing. Presently, they earn their profits by charging a percentage of each paid intervention, rather than via the savings on their per capita expenditures for the covered population. Therefore, these companies are reluctant to reduce the service volume or encourage healthcare providers to reduce costs or unnecessary interventions. Health insurance companies have become agencies that merely receive commissions for processing hospitals' invoices. They rarely monitor the standards of hospital activities and are only concerned with the creation of added-value profits.

In 1996, a review of the insurance status in Moscow and St. Petersburg highlighted the inherent problems in the aforementioned situations. Generally, it is believed that insurance companies should not cover medical expenses that have exceeded the per capita limits. However, previous surveys revealed that local funds often made payments based on demand regardless of the medical expenses, while insurance companies imposed service charges at a flat rate of 8% on all processed invoices. This has evidently created new perverse motivations, causing insurance agencies to be unwilling to control their costs. It has, in fact, emboldened them to collude with healthcare providers to pursue the highest possible charges. The fact that most contracts were signed with hospitals has further promoted the advantages of secondary healthcare services over primary healthcare services. Although measures have been taken to prevent such improper practices, the practices have begun to affect the development of the insurance model itself.

5. Health System Reforms

(1) Healthcare Service Reforms

In the mid-1980s, the shortcomings of the Soviet healthcare system became increasingly apparent, and healthcare planners became aware of the need to address the oversupply and inefficiency of healthcare institutions, as well as the low enthusiasm of their employees. A series of reforms were introduced: particularly, pilot programs were launched in Kemorovo, Leningrad, and Samara to resolve the imbalance between secondary and primary healthcare services. These pilot programs were launched with the aim of examining the role of market mechanisms and the allocation of healthcare budgets in the primary healthcare sector. However, they have almost all been abandoned because of certain incidents.

The dissolution of the Soviet Union exposed and exacerbated the issues facing traditional healthcare management in Russia, which is in urgent need of reform. The overall health status of the population experienced a rapid decline, with considerable decreases being seen in the life expectancies of both men and women. There was a significant increase in the mortality rate of males in their teens to their forties. Russia also saw outbreaks of infectious diseases that had not been reported in decades. Moreover, there was an increasing trend in the morbidity and mortality rates of chronic diseases. This developmental trend in population health was further aggravated by the strains placed on the population by the economic chaos of the 1990s. Politicians, planners, and policymakers were all well aware of the need to reform the healthcare services to meet the increasing healthcare demands resulting from the wastage of healthcare resources and the duplication of healthcare institutions. However, because of the collapse of the tax base and other economic events, the healthcare expenditure of the Russian Federation decreased; in fact, the country was no longer able to maintain the funding level required to meet the healthcare demands of the Soviet era. Furthermore, there was a drastic decline in the efficiency of the healthcare system and the quality of healthcare services. The dissolution of the Soviet Union due to political unrest is an even more important factor underlying the current health system reforms. The Perestroika and Glasnost policies raised public expectations and triggered a demand for reforms, while the establishment of the new government brought hope for reform to policymakers and the general public alike. One of the key areas requiring urgent reform was the high degree of centralization. Decentralization was considered a critical component in all reform policies because it granted local governments greater decision-making autonomy, as well as served as a representative feature of a new political era.

Since the driving force of the reform process lay within issues related to capital investment, efficiency, and decentralization, reform measures had to focus directly on addressing these issues. The key reform measures subsequently carried out therefore focused on implementing the MHI nationwide to supplement tax-based capital investment, aiming to integrate all three funding approaches. In view of the critical financial shortage facing the Russian Federation, payroll-based insurance premium contributions came to be regarded as the only source of additional healthcare funds. The advantage of such funds is that they are earmarked specifically for healthcare services.

In addition, the Ministry of Healthcare supported reforms related to the training of GPs, the autonomy of hospital and polyclinic administrators, the income of employees, and planning and regulation. The aim of these reforms was to combine various measures and to gradually overturn the rigid, highly bureaucratic model of control through the decentralization of management and financial responsibilities, thereby improving the economic rationale and efficiency of decision-making in healthcare, as well as meeting the healthcare demands of patients and citizens.

Before 1991, under the Soviet healthcare system, there was a high degree of centralization, with the Supreme Soviet wielding ultimate authority. Regional administrative agencies were charged with the management of regional healthcare. The parallel system (also known as the ministerial system) comprised ministries other than the Ministry of Healthcare and state-owned enterprises. Traditionally, these enterprises only provided healthcare services for their employees and their families.

Under the Soviet system, the healthcare system was almost exclusively funded by government budgets at all levels. Healthcare institutions were funded by the respective republican budgets, while rayons covered the expenses of healthcare institutions within their jurisdiction. Similar to the parallel healthcare systems under other ministries, large enterprises (i.e., industrial and agricultural enterprises) also provided healthcare services to local populations and shared the resulting medical expenses. The main reason for the higher estimated out-of-pocket payments is the inclusion of under-the-table payments in the estimation. VHI plays a very limited role in the healthcare funding of the Russian Federation. External funding sources, including loans and grants provided by bilateral and multilateral agencies, also have limited roles in funding the healthcare system.

Due to the collapse of the tax base and other economic events, the healthcare expenditure of the Russian Federation has decreased and cannot even maintain the funding level necessary to meet the healthcare demands of the Soviet era. Furthermore, there has been a drastic decline in the efficiency of the healthcare system and the quality of healthcare services. The dissolution of the Soviet Union due to political unrest is an even more important factor underlying health system reforms. Decentralization was considered a critical component in all reform policies because it not only allowed local governments to have greater decision-making autonomy, but also served as a representative feature of a new political era. Since the driving force of the reform process lies with issues related to capital investment, efficiency, and decentralization, reform measures had to focus directly on addressing these issues. A series of key reform measures were in fact carried out, involving the implementation of MHI nationwide to supplement tax-based capital investment, which aimed to integrate all three funding approaches. In view of the critical financial shortage facing the Russian Federation, payroll-based insurance premium contribution came to be regarded as the only source of additional healthcare funds, with the advantage of being earmarked specifically for healthcare services. The Ministry of Healthcare has also supported reforms to the training of GPs, the autonomy of hospital and polyclinic administrators, the income of employees, and planning and regulation.

On October 8, 2013, the Minister of Health of Russia, Veronika I. Skvortsova, announced at the All-Russian Health Care Media Forum the "guarantee of free access to healthcare services for all Russian citizens in all government and municipal medical institutions in the Russian Federation." She stated that this provision will not be changed now and will not change in the future. All healthcare services covered by the national health protection schemes were made accessible to all Russian citizens throughout their lives. The minister also promised that the number of covered healthcare service items would increase annually.

However, this announcement does not imply that the Russian federal government will launch a new free healthcare policy. The principle of universal free healthcare has long been stipulated in the Constitution of the Russian Federation (1993). Therefore, this announcement was only a reaffirmation of the federal constitution. More specifically, Article 41 of the Constitution of the Russian Federation (1993) stipulates that all citizens have the right to healthcare and medical care, and that the government will provide free healthcare services to citizens using relevant government budgets, insurance premium contributions, and other funding sources. In practice, the healthcare funds of the Russian Federation are mainly derived from MHI premiums contributed by enterprises and institutions in accordance with the Law on Health Insurance of the Citizens of the RSFSR (passed in June 1991), and the allocation of federal budgets to the MHI. Of these methods, the premium contributions accounted for more than 90% of the total MHI revenue.

In other words, Russia has implemented a free healthcare policy. Note that the Minister of Health had to make these solemn announcements because of frequent rumors that the policy would be replaced with paid healthcare. President Vladimir Putin and Prime Minister Dmitry Medvedev have also both reiterated recently on different occasions that the right of citizens to access free healthcare services will not be abolished.

(2) Characteristics of Health System Reforms

1. Healthcare funding   In 1987–2001, a new economic system for funding was promoted in three pilot regions: St. Petersburg, Kemorovo, and Samara. These pilots were conducted with the aim of giving the healthcare system administrator greater flexibility and control over healthcare resources, in order to better meet the healthcare demand of patients. This would ultimately enhance the development of primary healthcare and avoid the risk of reduced service quality. The key objectives of the "Law on Mandatory Health Insurance" include introducing new, nonbudgetary funding sources to augment existing budgetary funds; establishing a fund pooling mechanism; and providing universal and comprehensive health coverage while giving patients the freedom to choose their preferred healthcare providers and insurance agencies.

2. Management of Healthcare Providers   The Kemorovo pilot, conducted in the late 1980s, was the first attempt to increase the authority of hospital administrators. Under the pilot system, administrators could decide the hiring and dismissing of hospital staff, negotiate salaries and bonuses, and make demands about employee performance. They were also given a certain degree of financial autonomy to generate income and retain profits within their respective hospitals or polyclinics, and they could make purchasing decisions independently without having to consider the opinions of service providers. Although this model has been widely adopted, in many cases, the managerial roles have shifted, and hospital administrators are expected to have greater autonomy in the new healthcare system.

3. Human Resources and Training　The training of GPs has received increasing attention in the Russian Federation. A two-year training program introduced in 1992 has ensured that general medicine is a specialty in its own right, thereby increasing the social status of family physicians while also improving their skills. The training of management skills and other relevant skills has also been initiated. For instance, the Moscow Medical Academy established the Faculty of Health Care Management to provide postgraduate training for hospital administrators.

4. Healthcare Legislation　Since 1991, the Russian Federation has promulgated a series of laws and regulations leading to the large-scale expansion of legislation on health and healthcare. Article 72 of the Constitution of the Russian Federation stipulates that the legislative basis of public healthcare services is jointly determined by the Russian Federation and its subjects. Each subject is mainly responsible for the health status of the populations residing in areas under its jurisdiction, as well as the organization, management, and funding of public healthcare services. Furthermore, these subjects have the right to implement laws that are applicable within its jurisdiction. These measures have improved the healthcare legislation system, provided a legal basis for reforming the healthcare system, and ensured the orderly implementation of health reforms.

5. Incomplete Reform of Healthcare Legislation　The health system reforms in the Russian Federation were carried out during a period of serious social turmoil and under enormous pressure from healthcare demands. The reforms successfully made various achievements and outcomes in the early stages, which can be attributed to various factors. However, because of the short duration of implementation, many of the important aspects of the reforms could not be achieved and the health index system remains imperfect.

SECTION II. THE HEALTH SYSTEM IN HUNGARY

1. Overview of Socioeconomics and National Health

(1) Overview of Socioeconomic Development

Hungary is located in central Europe, bordered to the north by Slovakia, to the east by Ukraine and Romania, to the south by Serbia and Croatia, and to the west by Slovenia and Austria. It covers an area of around 93,000 km², or roughly 1% of Europe's total geographical area. Hungary was a German ally in World War II, becoming occupied by Germany in 1944 and later being liberated by the Soviet Union. Since 1989, Hungary has established a stable, multiparty coalition system. The National Assembly (*Országgyűlés*) has

386 seats and a four-year election cycle. Since 1996, the country has been divided into seven regions, each consisting of three counties, with the exception of central Hungary (Budapest and Pest County). The country has a population of about 10.2 million, 99% of whom are Hungarian citizens. The largest minority group in Hungary is the Romani people. The official language of Hungary is Hungarian.

The Hungarian socioeconomic system began transitioning in the 1990s, and its economy has been gradually recovering from its lowest point since 1994. In recent years, the country has shown relatively good momentum in economic growth, making it one of the most rapidly developing transition countries in Eastern Europe. In 2001, Hungary spent 6.8% of its GDP on healthcare, and 75% of its healthcare expenditure came from public funds. In 2002, Hungary's GDP growth rate was 3.3%, while its GDP per capita was US$6,000. The average monthly salary of Hungarians was Ft122,500 (approximately RMB5,100). Hungary joined the European Union (EU) in May 2004. Hungarian health reform was carried out in response to its overall socioeconomic transition, and involved taking into consideration factors such as history (e.g., a healthcare system similar to the German model was implemented in the late nineteenth century to the twentieth century) and the current situation (e.g., the need to link up with the management systems of the UK, France, Germany, etc. after joining the EU). The Hungarian healthcare system is essentially established based on the German model of the social health insurance system. In 2012, the GDP per capita of Hungary was US$12.4601 billion. The macroeconomic indicators of Hungary in selected years from 1990 to 2012 are shown in Table 20.5.

(2) National Health Status

Hungary has a large elderly population – people aged over 60 years account for 20.6% of the total population. Since the 1980s, Hungary has been experiencing negative population growth; for instance, in 2002, the natural population growth was −3.5%. In 2012, the total population of Hungary was 52.50 million, with an average annual growth rate of −0.5%. The demographic indicators of Hungary in select years from 1990 to 2012 are shown in Table 20.6. In 2012, the total healthcare expenditure in Hungary accounted for 7.8% of its GDP, and the average life expectancy was 74.3 years (men: 70.9 years; women: 77.9 years). Hungary's mortality-based indicators in selected years from 1990 to 2012 are shown in Table 20.7. The leading causes of death in Hungary, in descending order, are: cardiovascular diseases, malignant neoplasms, digestive diseases (including liver disease), accidental injuries, poisoning, and violence. This trend in the health status of Hungarians continued until 2000, at which point the all-cause mortality rate was higher than the 27 other EU countries, while its mortality rates for malignant neoplasms and digestive diseases were higher than the 12 countries in the WHO European region.

2. Healthcare System

(1) Healthcare Resources

Hungary currently has 180 hospitals, 3.7 physicians per 1,000 population, and 3,000 dentists. There is a total of 5,125 family physicians, each of whom provides healthcare services to about 2,000 families. There are approximately 8 hospital beds per 1,000 people (a quarter of hospital beds are intended for long-term treatment and rehabilitation), and the average length of hospital stay is 8.5 days. Public healthcare institutions account for 90% of

TABLE 20.5 Macroeconomic Indicators of Hungary in 1990–2012 (Selected Years)

Indicators	Year					
	1990	1995	2000	2005	2010	2012
GDP (current US$, million)	33,056.1	45,561.4	46,385.6	110,321.7	127,503.3	124,600.5
GDP, PPP (current international US$, million)	92,662.1	92,738.3	121,466.6	171,223.5	211,348.9	224,549.2
GDP per capita (current US$, US$)	3,186.4	4,411.0	4,542.7	10,936.9	12,750.3	12,560.1
GDP, PPP (current international US$, US$)	8,932.2	8,978.5	11,895.7	16,974.6	21,134.8	22,635.2
Annual growth rate of GDP (%)	−3.5	1.5	4.2	4.0	1.3	−1.7
Total expenditure as a share of GDP (%)	−	52.1	42.0	42.7	44.8	44.3
Cash surplus/deficit as a share of GDP (%)	−	−8.9	−2.8	−7.4	−3.5	−2.6
Healthcare expenditure per capita (current US$, US$)	−	323.0	325.7	922.7	1,026.0	986.8
Healthcare expenditure per capita, PPP (constant price international $ in 2005, US$)	−	656.7	851.9	1,432.1	1,653.9	1,729.3
Total healthcare expenditure as a share of GDP (%)	−	7.3	7.2	8.4	8.0	7.8
Total labor force (million)	4.5	4.2	4.2	4.3	4.3	4.4
Total unemployment rate (%)	−	10.2	6.4	7.2	11.2	10.9
Real interest rate (%)	2.5	4.6	2.6	5.9	5.3	5.6
Official exchange rate (local currency unit per US$, period average)	63.2	125.7	282.2	199.6	207.9	225.1

Source: World Bank, 2012.

healthcare institutions in Hungary, while the remaining are private healthcare institutions. These public healthcare institutions are either affiliated with the Ministry of Health or the governments of autonomous regions.

(2) Healthcare System and Management Agencies

Hungary had once implemented a social insurance system from the late nineteenth century to 1950, after which it began to implement the Soviet healthcare system in the second half of 1950. After the transition, Hungary resumed its socialized healthcare system, which

TABLE 20.6 Demographic Indicators of Hungary in 1990–2012 (Selected Years)

Indicators	Year					
	1990	1995	2000	2005	2010	2012
Total population (million)	10.4	10.3	10.2	10.1	10.0	9.9
Female population (% of total population)	52.0	52.2	52.4	52.5	52.5	52.5
Population aged 0–14 years (% of total population)	20.4	18.1	16.8	15.5	14.6	14.6
Population aged over 65 years (% of total population)	13.5	14.3	15.1	15.7	16.7	17.0
Annual average population growth rate (%)	–1.0	–0.1	–0.3	–0.2	–0.2	–0.5
Population density (number of people per km²)	115.4	114.9	113.9	112.6	110.5	109.6
Total fertility rate (number of births per woman)	1.9	1.6	1.3	1.3	1.3	1.3
Crude birth rate (%)	12.1		9.6	9.7	9.0	9.1
Crude death rate (%)	14.0	14.1	13.3	13.5	13.0	13.0
Age dependency ratio (%)	51.3		47.0	45.4	45.7	46.3
Urban population (% of total population)	65.8	65.2	64.6	66.4	69.0	69.9

Source: World Bank, 2012.

TABLE 20.7 Mortality-Based Indicators of Hungary in 1990–2012 (Selected Years)

Indicators	Year					
	1990	1995	2000	2005	2010	2012
Total life expectancy at birth (years)	71.6	71.1	71.7	72.6	73.5	74.3
Male life expectancy at birth (years)	68.3		68.2	69.0	70.0	70.9
Female life expectancy at birth (years)	75.2	74.9	75.3	76.3	77.2	77.9
Mortality rate per 1,000 adult females (%)	132.7		114.5	107.4	—	—
Mortality rate per 1,000 adult males (%)	305.1	318.0	271.5	256.5	—	—

Source: World Bank, 2012.

is similar to that in Germany. In 1993, Hungary began reforming its healthcare system. Healthcare funds came to be raised through mandatory social health insurance, and the National Health Insurance Fund was established, which was used to cover healthcare expenditures. At present, the Hungarian healthcare system provides universal health coverage to the entire population.

There are three funding sources for the Hungarian health insurance fund: (1) mandatory social health insurance, where both employers and employees make premium contributions equivalent to 11% and 5%, respectively, of employees' total wages. These premium contributions in total account for 60% of the total health insurance fund. (2) Health insurance tax, whereby employers also have to pay €15 per month for each employee. This accounts for 20% of the total health insurance fund. (3) The government budget, where the government allocates a certain amount of its budget each year to the health insurance fund. This accounts for 20% of the total health insurance fund.

Currently, the total health insurance fund amounts to about €6 billion (approximately RMB60 billion), of which 50% is allocated to healthcare expenses, 30% to drug expenses, and the remaining 20% to cash expenditures (e.g., medical aids for disabled individuals and low-income earners). Additionally, about 150,000 Hungarians have joined supplementary insurance schemes and are entitled to receive better healthcare services. The scope of reimbursement for the health insurance fund includes family physician services, home-based care, inpatient services, and therapeutic services for critical illnesses and chronic diseases.

The organizational structure of the Hungarian healthcare system mainly comprises the following components, as shown in Figure 20.5.

1. Ministry of Health, Social and Family Affairs (MoHSFA) Aside from unemployment benefits (i.e., benefits for unemployment and early retirement), the Hungarian social and welfare system is administered and supervised by the MoHSFA, which is mainly responsible for implementing governmental healthcare, social, and family policies. The Minister is charged with the management, coordination, and organization of the health and social security systems, scientific research, healthcare and pension policies related to social insurance (in cooperation with the Ministry of Finance), and the administration of the National Health Insurance Fund (NHIF), the National Pension Insurance Fund (NPIF), and other legal obligations. The Minister is responsible for the planning of public hygiene and healthcare tasks, disease prevention, all public healthcare programs related to health promotion, and the administration of healthcare services provided by the National Public Health and Medical Officer Service (NPHMOS), national-level healthcare institutions, national research institutes and higher education institutions, and the Health Promotion Research Institute and the Office of Health Authorization and Administrative Procedures (OHAAP). Additionally, the Minister administrates the Social Policy Council, the National Health Council, and the National Disability Council, as well as supervises the Hungarian Medical Chamber and the Hungarian Chamber of Pharmacists via regulations. (Note: In May 2002, the government merged relevant departments to establish the MoHSFA, but government restructuring in October 2004 led to the MOHSFA being split into the Ministry of Youth, Family, Social Affairs and Equal Opportunities, which is charged with pensions, family, and social affairs, and the Ministry of Health, which is responsible for healthcare-related affairs.)

2. National Public Health and Medical Officer Service (NPHMOS) The NPHMOS is a public administrative agency that performs national tasks and implements a unified health management system. Its duties include public health and epidemiology; administrative licensing; sector-neutral occupational supervision; organization, monitoring, control, and prevention of diseases; and health improvement (i.e., health protection, health education, and health promotion). The NPHMOS supervises all natural and legal entities in Hungary, and companies that do not qualify as legal entities (except for Army, Navy, Air Force, and enforcement agencies, although the NPHMOS still has the right to conduct hygiene inspections in these agencies).

3. National Health Council The National Health Council is responsible for ensuring the long-term sustainability of healthcare policies and promoting user rights of healthcare and social services. The council participates in the drafting and decision-making processes of the government's healthcare policies by proposing projects and recommendations, commentary documents and opinions, and analyzing and evaluating the procedures for policy implementation. It plays an important role in identifying key areas for health improvement (which must be unanimously agreed by experts).

4. Medical Research Council   The Medical Research Council is an agency that provides recommendations, comments, consultation, and decision-making support to the Minister of Health. This council is primarily concerned with healthcare policies and healthcare-related (i.e., medical, pharmaceutical, and scientific) issues. Specifically, it coordinates with government-controlled research activities, provides recommendations for Hungarian and international research priorities, and assists in translating scientific findings into healthcare practices in Hungary. The council also advises on the design, implementation, documentation, and control of human clinical trials and biomedical studies to ensure that they meet international ethical, scientific, and therapeutic requirements. Furthermore, it also oversees the implementation of these activities. The council gives opinions on scientific research activities, reviews and assesses the establishment of new regional research ethics committees, and coordinates and promotes their standardized operations.

5. Professional Associations (Health Profession Associations)   Since 1994, there have been two major professional associations (for physicians/dentists and pharmacists) in the healthcare system that operate on a self-regulatory basis with compulsory membership. The responsibilities of these associations – called the Hungarian Medical Chamber and the Hungarian Chamber of Pharmacists – include personal management of professional affairs through directly selected agencies or officials within the legal framework; defining and representing professional ethics as well as economic and social interests; contributing to the formulation of healthcare policies; and promoting healthcare and pharmaceutical services. These associations are public institutions with public responsibilities and are entitled to government subsidies according to regulatory budgets. Membership of these associations is compulsory – only qualified members can practice medicine and pharmacy in Hungary. On March 4, 2004, the representative assembly officially established the Chamber of Health Professionals for nurses and related healthcare workers. Only members of this association can practice nursing and other related healthcare professions.

6. Medical Academies   Medical academies are the highest level of medical institution that provides recommendations and reviews. They are jointly administered by the Hungarian Medical Chamber and the Hungarian Chamber of Pharmacists, but their operating expenses are funded by the MoHSFA. Presently, there are 37 medical academies and 3 pharmaceutical academies under the MoHSFA. In addition to academies for medicine and pharmacy, there are also academies for nursing and other healthcare specialties. These academies produce, periodically review, and publish professional recommendations and guidelines within their respective specialties, as well as define the technical requirements and qualification certificates required for each position.

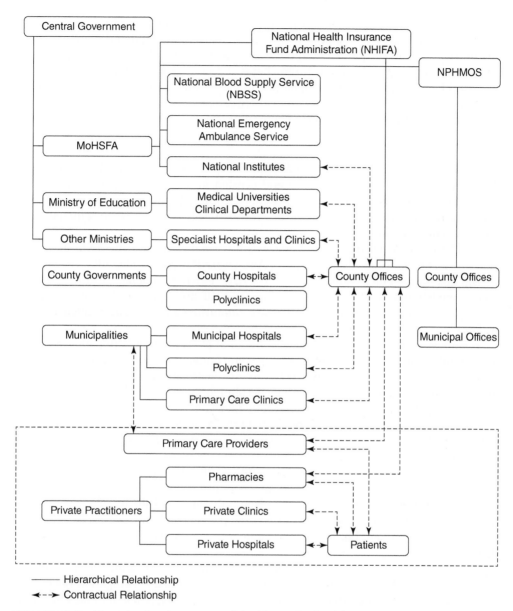

FIGURE 20.5 Organizational structure of the Hungarian healthcare system.

(3) Healthcare System and Hospital Management

1. Primary Healthcare In 1992, Hungary's regional GP system was replaced by the family physician system in order to accomplish two major goals. The first goal was to tie the remuneration of family physicians with the number of patients served by giving patients the freedom to choose their physicians. This clearly altered the physician–patient relationship. Since 1992, residents from other regions may apply to register with a preferred family physician, and patients within the jurisdiction of a specific family physician may choose family physicians in other regions. This change indicated that family physicians now had to compete with each other to keep their patients, which highlighted the importance of patient trust and satisfaction. Although the free choice of physicians had no practical significance in sparsely populated rural areas, it has had a very positive and significant impact on most other citizens. The second goal was to allow family physicians to serve as gatekeepers, as they are the first line of contact between patients and the healthcare system. However, under the current system, family physicians remain incapable of effectively performing their role as gatekeepers.

2. Social Insurance Fund and its Administrators Before 1988, the Hungarian social insurance (including health insurance and pension insurance) was part of the central budget. The Social Insurance Fund was established on January 1, 1989. The fund and its administrators were separated from the central budget to establish the National Social Insurance Fund Administration.

In 1993, the Social Insurance Fund was further divided into the NPIF and NHIF, while the National Social Insurance Fund Administration was divided into the National Pension Insurance Fund Administration (NPIFA) and the National Health Insurance Fund Administration (NHIFA). Both the NPIF and NHIF are supervised by the government of Hungary, while the NPIFA and NHIFA are administered by the government through the MoHSFA.

Healthcare services mainly include professional medical services (inpatient services) and general medical services for all citizens (general outpatient services), which are mainly provided by hospitals and family physicians, respectively. Healthcare institutions in Hungary are dominated by public institutions, which account for more than 90% of the total, while the remaining 10% are private hospitals that emerged following the economic transition. The latter are primarily specialist hospitals that provide advanced healthcare services (e.g., gynecological and surgical services) for high-income earners in order to meet the multi-level healthcare demands of patients.

Medical expenses are mainly covered by the NHIF, which enables patients to access free inpatient services and requires them to pay only a small fee for drugs when seeking outpatient services. The NHIF reimburses hospitals through DRG-based payments and allocates lump sums to family physicians based on the number of contracted residents. However, the government has capped the number of contracted residents for each family physician.

Public hospital directors are selected and appointed by the Ministry of Health or regional health authorities, mostly via competitive appointments. Hungarian public hospitals have similar internal management structures to that of public hospitals in China. Physicians in public hospitals are considered government employees, but public hospitals can also contract with private practitioners, who undertake relevant healthcare work in public hospitals according to the contract.

The NHIF is the main funding source of hospitals. For instance, more than 90% of the operating income for the two hospitals in Budapest is derived from the NHIF, while the remaining 10% is derived from out-of-pocket payments (5%) and other income sources (5%). Currently, the NHIF utilizes a DRG-based payment system for reimbursing hospitals, but it has also capped the income of hospitals to control blind expansion.

(4) Healthcare Funding Policies

Based on the purchaser–provider split introduced through the Hungarian health reform of 1990, the government must purchase healthcare services from hospitals on behalf of residents, rather than directly running the hospitals. Learning from other EU countries, Hungary has implemented a mandatory social health insurance scheme and the third-party payment system.

The NHIFA [abbreviated as OEP (*Országos Egészségbiztosítási Pénztár*) in Hungarian], was established in 1993 and is specialized in the administration of the NHIF. It has 41 regional offices with more than 4,000 employees and contracts with 154 hospitals nationwide each year to purchase healthcare services on behalf of residents. Together, the contracted hospitals have a total of 60,500 beds and 33,000 physicians. Similar to in Germany, a dual financial system has been adopted for the funding of Hungarian hospitals, whereby the government is responsible for investment projects, while the NHIFA is responsible for covering the operating expenses of hospitals. However, the government can only provide a very small amount of maintenance funds because of financial constraints.

In the early 1990s, a pay-for-performance system was introduced for reimbursing healthcare services. Other payment systems have also been employed for different healthcare services in Hungary. For instance, the NHIFA has adopted the capitation system for reimbursing family physicians and the fee-for-service system for outpatient services. The NHIFA has also introduced the DRG-based payment system for reimbursing inpatient services for acute diseases, which is based on the German point system. In addition, the NHIFA has also adopted a per-diem payment system, which is based on the DRG-based payment system in the US, to reimburse inpatient services for chronic diseases.

Hungary has a high personal income tax rate, with Hungarians having to set aside nearly 70% of their salaries for various taxes. Of this, 23.5% is used to cover health insurance premiums, with about 19.5% coming from employers and 4.0% coming from employees.

The Hungarian health insurance system is currently facing the following challenges: limited funds, with about 40% of the population (including the elderly, children, unemployed persons, and many individuals participating in the untaxed "black economy") being exempt from paying their insurance premiums while still being entitled to free healthcare services; the increasing application of new, expensive medical technologies; the continued increase in healthcare demand as patients receive more information; the increase in healthcare expenditure alongside population aging; and the continuous increase in a market orientation. Because of the limited funding of the NHIFA, hospitals have almost no autonomy and their development has been seriously restricted. Notably, the medical expenses of patients are not 100% covered by the NHIFA, whose share is adjusted based on the government budget. The amount of funds provided by the NHIFA is often inversely proportional to the number of healthcare services provided. Almost all hospitals in Hungary regularly experience financial losses. To compensate, a few hospitals collect rent from private companies for the lease of real estate. In general, however, hospital profits are usually very low, being just enough to repair equipment and instruments, but not sufficient for purchases and replacements.

Numerous new measures are being considered to address the financial shortage facing hospitals in Hungary, including designing basic service packages based on cost effectiveness; capping service-volume-based needs assessment; enhancing the purchasing role of the NHIFA; and attaching greater importance to quality assessment in the procurement process for healthcare services.

3. Reform Changes and Characteristics of the Healthcare System

(1) Historical Development of the Healthcare System

Health reforms in Hungary began in the mid-1980s when the liberals of the Communist Party took office and formulated a reform plan for restructuring the socialist healthcare system. The reform and its implementation were initiated before the first free election in 1990. Prior to 1991, the reform of the healthcare sector concentrated on decentralization, before shifting to cost containment after 1994.

1. Reforms in the Late 1980s   The Ministry of Social Affairs and Health established a Reform Secretariat, which provided policy advice based on international models and experiences. The Ministry also initiated numerous pilot experiments, including the restructuring of the DRG-based payment system. In 1987, the Information Center for Health Care was established. This body was responsible for the DRG system and served as a key agency in designing and administering the provider payment system. The legalization of private healthcare began in 1989. In 1990, the healthcare budget was transferred to the Social Insurance Fund.

2. Reforms from 1990 to 1994   In 1990, local governments in Hungary began regulating healthcare providers under the new contract model. The ownership of primary care surgeries, polyclinics, and hospitals, as well as regional obligations, was transferred from the central government to local governments. Furthermore, the central government established the "designated allowances" system to subsidize local governments on a conditional and proportional basis. In 1991, the NPHMOS was established to coordinate infectious disease surveillance, immunization, and public healthcare services in Hungary. In 1992, the Social Insurance Fund was divided into the NHIF and NPIF, each of which began to operate on a self-regulatory basis in 1993 after the election of trade union representatives. In 1992, "district physician services" were renamed "family physician services" and postgraduate training became required for medical practitioners. In addition, the capitation payment system and contractual model were introduced for family physician services. The sub-budgets of the NHIF were determined based on DRGs and per diem rates.

3. Reforms from 1994 to 1998   The first comprehensive economic stabilization measure was launched in 1995 for the provision of social welfare, which included healthcare services. Dental services were excluded from the scope of NHIF coverage, and subsidies for medical spa treatment were removed. Furthermore, the responsibility for occupational healthcare services was shifted to employers. In 1996 and 1997, the government also addressed the excessive scale of the hospital sector by removing more than 9,000 beds from the healthcare system. There were three aspects of the taxation strategy that reduced avoidance of social insurance premiums and increased the income of the NHIF: the rising premium rate of social health insurance, the reduction of employer-sponsored health insurance premium rate, and the collection of lump-sum tax. In 1997, the government restructured and weakened the autonomy of the NPIF, and proposed a fixed payment system that involved subsidizing 20% of the hospital budget without considering their actual performance. From 1994 to 1998, the government of Hungary successfully implemented cost containment measures, which led to a significant decline in the healthcare budget.

4. Reforms From 1998 to 2002 The government abolished the self-regulation of the Social Insurance Fund and took full control over the NHIF and NHIFA. The management of the NHIFA was transferred to the Prime Minister's Office. The upper limit on employees' health insurance premiums was abolished. A new Ministry of Health was established on January 1, 2001, which successfully regained control over the NHIFA from the Ministry of Finance (October 2000). A 10-year public health action program was launched to improve the life expectancy of males and females to 70 and 78 years, respectively (August 2001).

5. Reforms From 2002 to the Present Since 2002, reforms have placed more emphasis on healthcare planning and preventative measures. The National Assembly accepted the Johan Béla National Program for the Decade of Health, with the aim of improving the health status of Hungarians through various public health activities. Particularly, national screening programs for breast cancer, cervical cancer, and rectal cancer (2006) were introduced.

(2) Characteristics of Health System Reforms

1. Decentralization of the Healthcare System The central government still has decision-making and regulatory power over the healthcare system, but some of its responsibilities have been transferred to quasi-public agencies, while the remaining functions have been decentralized. While the government has retained decision-making and budgetary power over the NHIFA at the national level, its responsibilities for contract management and payment have been decentralized to the county level. In 1990, specific public health responsibilities and the relevant taxation power were decentralized to local governments, at which point the ownership of most healthcare institutions was transferred to local governments. As a result, local governments became the main healthcare providers in the Hungarian healthcare system.

2. Healthcare Funding The public healthcare fund receives finances from both central and local taxation, but is mainly derived from the premium contributions of the social health insurance scheme (i.e., the NHIF). The social health insurance scheme is a comprehensive welfare scheme with wide coverage (barring a few exceptions). Aside from for drugs, medical emergencies, prostheses, and medical spa treatment, patients make little or no copayment. Central and local taxation and private sources are the main complementary funding sources of social health insurance. While external sources currently have little effect on healthcare funding, the amount of private donations is expected to increase in the future alongside the increasing number of charitable organizations in the healthcare sector.

3. Healthcare Expenditures Of the total healthcare expenditure in 2000, Hungary allocated 36% to medical products, 30% to inpatient treatments, 16% to outpatient treatments, 6% to therapeutic services, and 5% to preventive and public healthcare services. The social health insurance system enables the central government to implement cost containment measures for most healthcare services through various methods. Particularly, the government controls the NHIF and drug expenditures.

4. Healthcare Delivery   The healthcare system is established based on the responsibility for healthcare delivery, which involves the principle of "providing healthcare services within respective jurisdictions." The Healthcare Act of 1997 (Government Decree No. 154/1997/16) stipulated that local governments are responsible for providing primary, secondary, and tertiary healthcare services, while the central government is responsible for providing (i.e., funding) public health, emergency ambulance services, blood supplies, and other healthcare services.

5. Management Structure of Hospitals   The government has introduced a DRG-based hospital reimbursement method for acute inpatient services, a hospital per diem payment method for chronic inpatient services, and a tripartite structure for top hospital management involving a financial director, a medical director, and a nursing director. In 1994–1998, the government implemented other reform measures in the hospital sector, abolishing the tripartite management structure and determining the minimum requirements for service delivery. Hospitals were obliged to establish a supervisory council and maintain a quality-control system. In 1998–2002, the government granted hospital administrators more autonomy by allowing and encouraging them to use their discretion in medical cooperation.

6. Human Resources and Training   The salaries of healthcare workers and other public employees are 50% greater than the average salary in Hungary. This is because of the government's introduction of a mandatory minimum wage system for highly educated employees (which is twice the minimum wage). Physicians and other nonmedical health-care workers are also given a "loyalty bonus" (equivalent to one year's salary) to enhance their enthusiasm if they have served in the healthcare sector for four years. Education for healthcare professionals is divided into secondary, post-secondary, and higher education levels, and is monitored by the Ministry of Education. The Ministry of Health is responsible for the supervision of vocational training.

4. Existing Issues and Development Trends in the Healthcare System

(1) Core Objectives of Optimization

In Hungary, the objectives of the healthcare system have been explicitly defined in various laws, regulations, and policy documents, or are implied in actions taken by the government. In the latter case, the objectives are not written or declared, but are inferred from actual policy measures. Generally, there is an unspoken consensus among the main political parties regarding the core objectives of the healthcare system, at least on a political level. As far as the codified policy objectives are concerned, the starting point has always been the Constitution of the Republic of Hungary, which defines health as a right of Hungarian citizens. Specifically, the Constitution declares that:

Hungarians living within the territory of the Republic of Hungary have the right to the highest level of physical and mental health.

The Republic of Hungary shall implement this objective through institutions of labor safety and healthcare, through the organization of medical care and the opportunities for regular physical activity, as well as through the protection of the urban and natural environment.

Throughout various legislative periods, government reform measures have often been challenged by opposition parties on the basis of these regulations. For example, welfare cuts have been challenged in the Constitutional Court as a violation of the "right to the highest level of physical and mental health." In Ruling No. 56/1995, the Constitutional Court stated that the right to health must be interpreted within the confines of economic performance, but also that welfare cannot be curtailed infinitely without violating numerous constitutional rights and principles. This ruling required the government to establish new laws on social insurance, which were eventually enacted in 1997 and have since become the most important legal basis for the objectives of the Hungarian healthcare system.

(2) Main Existing Problems

First, the Hungarian healthcare system has excessive healthcare resources. Various health management departments and insurance fund management agencies have noted that the existing numbers of hospitals and hospital beds are excessive and should be gradually reduced. Second, the overly rapid growth of healthcare expenditure has made it difficult to raise healthcare funds. Hungary implements a universal social insurance system with a relatively high degree of equality, but most patients lack a sense of responsibility for their own health. The overly rapid growth of healthcare expenditures, which has in turn overburdened the NHIF, can be attributed to factors such as the deeply-rooted concept of free access to healthcare services, the lack of cost control awareness, and population aging. Although the social insurance system provides universal health coverage, the insurance fund is mainly derived from existing labor income – that is, "the minority covers the majority." Currently, the labor force participation rate in Hungary is 30%–40%. There is also a relatively serious issue related to illicit workers, many of whom are highly paid but have a low tax return, which has made the fundraising process more difficult. Third, there is a lack of awareness of the importance of preventive healthcare. The preventive healthcare system has always been based on the Soviet epidemic prevention system, which has outdated disease prevention and control measures and places an inadequate emphasis on the prevention and treatment of chronic non-communicable diseases. Furthermore, Hungary is also facing serious problems stemming from unhealthy lifestyles, such as high rates of alcoholism and smoking, widespread obesity, and an irrational diet structure.

(3) Direction of Future Reforms

Health reforms in Hungary have become increasingly extensive, and the next step involves the following. (1) Reforms of the healthcare system: these reforms aim to further introduce market mechanisms, attract greater social capital investment to the healthcare sector, and establish more private hospitals in order to meet patients' multilevel healthcare demands and improve the service efficiency of public hospitals. (2) Controlling the growth of healthcare expenditure: currently, healthcare administrators are striving to encourage patients to visit family physicians, in order to conserve healthcare resources and reduce healthcare expenditure. (3) Reforms of disease prevention system: in response to changes in the population spectrum, disease spectrum, and causes of death, as well as the challenges presented by unhealthy lifestyles, Hungary has been considering reforms of the existing disease prevention system, which will enhance its intervention in the unhealthy lifestyles of its population and enable better control of chronic non-communicable diseases.

Since the mid-1990s, there have been substantial increases in the life expectancies of men and women in Hungary. However, numerous health outcomes remain poor, including the mortality rates of cancer, cardiovascular diseases, liver disease, and suicide, which place Hungary among the European countries with the worst health status. The mortality rate is especially high among middle-aged men, mainly due to their unhealthy lifestyles (i.e., the high prevalence of smoking and alcoholism and unhealthy diets). The activities of the National Public Health Plan (NPHP) have been significantly reduced in recent years because of inadequate funding in prevention and health promotion coupled with underdeveloped organization. Cross-sectoral activities are poorly coordinated and the issue of increasing healthcare inequality has not been addressed properly.

However, avoidable mortality indicators, such as infant and maternal mortality rates, and mortality rates from appendicitis and hernia, have displayed a more optimistic trend, as has the excellent immunization record in Hungary, which has achieved almost 100% coverage for children.

Hungary has a well-functioning single-payer health insurance system with nearly universal coverage. It has made a transition from an overcentralized system to a purchaser–provider split model with new payment methods, which have created incentives for increased technical efficiency. For example, Hungary launched a DRG-based payment system for hospitals in 1993, and has since accumulated a wealth of operational experience. Hungary also has a unique patient identification system that can provide information on the drug consumption and use of specialist inpatient and outpatient services for each patient. This is a rich, integrated dataset whose potential has yet to be fully realized in academic research and healthcare policymaking.

In Hungary, the management of the single-payer health insurance system has become increasingly blurred. The initial self-regulatory arrangement was quickly eliminated, and the governance structure of the NHIF went through a series of modifications that resulted in increased direct central control and reduced stakeholder participation, and has exposed the system to political pressure. These effects in turn led to reduced transparency and increasingly unpredictable funding arrangements. Although the large-scale and strategic reform measures intended to address the service management function of the system have not been achieved in most cases, there have been several useful technical improvements, particularly in the area of healthcare funding. These improvements include the successful introduction of health technology assessments (HTAs) and the establishment of incentives to intensify competition for generic drugs.

Nevertheless, the health reforms have been unable to improve the efficiency of resource allocation, despite the increased technical efficiency over time. Formal payments have survived health reforms over 20 years. Furthermore, a human resource crisis is emerging because of the aging of healthcare workers (especially physicians), staff shortages, and increasing migration.

Ensuring appropriate incentives to improve the efficiency in patient pathways has been adopted by successive governments. The Care Coordination System (CCS) was introduced as a pilot program in 1999. It has many innovative features and provided a country-specific response to the problem of allocation efficiency. However, it was eliminated in 2008 because it lacked a complete scientific evaluation.

Since 2004, cost containment has been the dominant objective of healthcare policies. Public healthcare expenditure has declined considerably to 5.1% of Hungary's GDP in 2009. This has had a direct impact on the growing human resource crisis. In addition, the efficiency gains resulting from cost containment have been used to reduce the national debt, rather than being reinvested in the healthcare sector. A key issue is the lack of an overarching, evidence-based strategy for the mobilization of healthcare resources. In the absence of such a strategy, the healthcare system remains vulnerable to the broader objectives of economic policies. The diversification of funding sources in the healthcare system seems to be expanding continually along with the latest strategic policy on taxation. However, it remains to be seen whether the integration of insurance premiums and budget transfers from general taxation are capable of providing a stable funding arrangement.

The government faces two major challenges in achieving a more efficient and fair service delivery system: restructuring the existing capacities based on an assessment of healthcare demands and addressing issues related to informal payments. There is some evidence suggesting that the introduction of user charges has reduced the magnitude of informal payments, albeit not substantially. However, other evidence suggests that user charges influence economic protection and funding equality, especially the protection of user charges. In addition, several existing programs could lead to substantial improvement if they could be further implemented. The new information system has made the healthcare system more transparent and accountable. Nevertheless, good governance requires more evidence-based and transparent policymaking, performance monitoring, and accountability at the healthcare policy level. Attempts have been made to measure the quality of healthcare services using various quality indicators, but further, more systematic attempts are necessary.

Finally, Hungary is a target country for cross-border healthcare, mainly for dental care and rehabilitative services. Therefore, the healthcare industry has been regarded by the government as a potential strategic area for economic growth and development.

 ## SECTION III. THE HEALTH SYSTEM IN THE CZECH REPUBLIC

1. Overview of Socioeconomics and National Health

The Czech Republic (often shortened to Czechia or *Česko* in Czech) was listed as a developed country by the World Bank in 2006. The Czech Republic officially joined the European Union on May 1, 2004. It covers a land area of 78,867 km², and is bordered by Germany to the west, Poland to the north, Slovakia to the east, and Austria to the south. The western part of the Czech Republic is known as Bohemia, whereas the eastern part comprises Moravia and Czech Silesia.

In 2012, the total population of the Czech Republic was 10.5 million, its GDP was US$196 billion, and its GNI per capita was US$18,130. It is classified as a high-income, non-OECD country. The life expectancy of its population is 78 years (men: 75 years; women: 81 years), which is lower than the average among other high-income, non-OECD countries. Approximately 16% of the population is over 65 years of age. The population mortality rate is 10%, with a maternal mortality rate of 5 deaths per 100,000 live births (2013), an infant mortality rate of 3 per 1,000 live births, and an under-five mortality rate of 4 per 1,000 live births. Its total healthcare expenditure as a share of GDP is 7.7%, and the healthcare expenditure per capita is US$1,432. Among the leading causes of death, circulatory system diseases were ranked first, followed by malignant neoplasms and then trauma and poisoning (2002). Other population health indicators are shown in Table 20.8.

The Czech health security system has three major characteristics: (1) universal social health insurance funded by individuals, employers, and the state; (2) diversified services that are mainly purchased by insurance funds via contracts with private outpatient service providers and public hospitals; and (3) the determination of coverage and compensation schemes based on negotiations between the major stakeholders.

TABLE 20.8 Health Indicators of the Czech Population in 1970–2012

Indicator	Year							
	1970	1980	1990	2000	2005	2006	2007	2012
Total population (million)	9.78	10.23	10.36	10.27	10.23	10.27	10.33	10.51
Population growth (%)	-0.65	0.00	0.01	-0.09	0.27	0.34	0.63	0.10
Fertility rate (no. of children)	1.93	2.10	1.89	1.16	1.28	1.33	1.44	1.50
Crude death rate (%)	12.60	13.10	12.50	10.60	10.60	10.20	10.10	10.30
Male crude death rate (%)	13.70	13.73	13.20	10.98	10.83	10.51	10.44	–
Female crude death rate (%)	11.50	12.56	11.77	10.26	10.27	9.85	9.84	–
Life expectancy (years)	69.67	70.30	71.53	75.21	76.19	79.82	77.10	78.10
Male life expectancy (years)	66.18	66.84	67.63	71.75	72.97	73.55	73.82	75.10
Female life expectancy (years)	73.33	73.92	75.51	78.61	79.32	80.00	80.30	81.20
Infant mortality rate (per 1,000 live births)	20.20	16.90	10.80	4.10	3.39	3.33	3.14	3.10
Under-five mortality rate (per 1,000 live births)	–	12.42	5.19	4.13	4.12	3.98	4.70	3.80

Source: World Bank, 2012.

2. Healthcare Organizations and the Regulatory System

(1) Healthcare Providers and Health Provision Institutions

The organizational structure of the healthcare service system in the Czech Republic is shown in Figure 20.6.

Healthcare services in the Czech Republic are mainly provided by private practitioners. The major types of healthcare provider include general practitioners (GPs) for adults, GPs for children and adolescents, primary care gynecologists, primary care dentists/stomatologists, outpatient specialists, hospitals, other inpatient institutions, emergency service and family health service centers, pharmacies, public health stations, and public health associations.

Inpatient services are provided by various specialist healthcare institutions in addition to hospitals, such as long-term care institutions, psychiatric institutions, rehabilitation institutions, day and night care institutions, tuberculosis and respiratory diseases institutions, and spa facilities. This network of healthcare institutions also includes pharmacies and other institutions that provide healthcare technologies.

On the other hand, outpatient and pharmacy services are almost completely privatized, and the owners of such institutions include physicians, pharmacists, and various other operators. According to the Act on Healthcare in Non-Governmental Healthcare Facilities (Act No. 160/1992 Coll.), all institutions providing outpatient services must be registered. Registration is predicated on these institutions meeting specific conditions for the provision of healthcare services; accordingly, institutions that do not meet these conditions are not permitted to register.

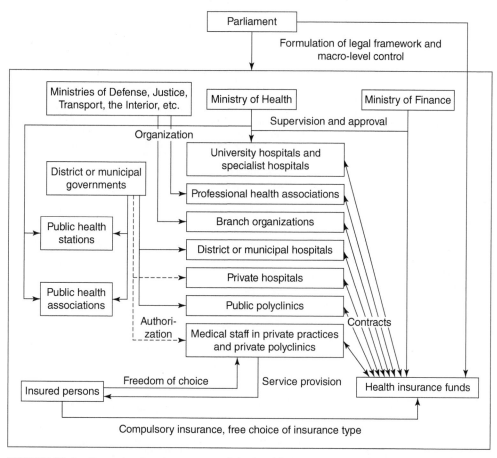

FIGURE 20.6 Organizational structure of the healthcare system in the Czech Republic.

(2) Administrative Agencies of Healthcare Services

The Ministry of Health has been designated the core administrative agency for health services by law. Its primary responsibilities include the administration of healthcare services; conducting public health research; direct administration of subordinate healthcare institutions; finding, protecting, and using natural therapeutic resources, natural medicinal springs, and natural mineral springs; conducting research and development of drugs and healthcare technologies for disease prevention, diagnosis, and treatment; administration of health insurance; and healthcare information systems. The organizational structure of the Ministry of Health is shown in Figure 20.7. In addition to the Ministry of Health, there are also a number of regional offices that administer at the regional level.

The Ministry of Health directly administers and controls healthcare institutions and organizations engaged in the provision of public health, as well as regional and interregional large hospitals. It is also responsible for teaching hospitals and specialist tertiary institutions. However, community-level administration by the Ministry of Health was abolished in 2002. Since then, private organizations have been permitted to operate small hospitals under specific conditions. Currently, a few dozen small hospitals have been privatized

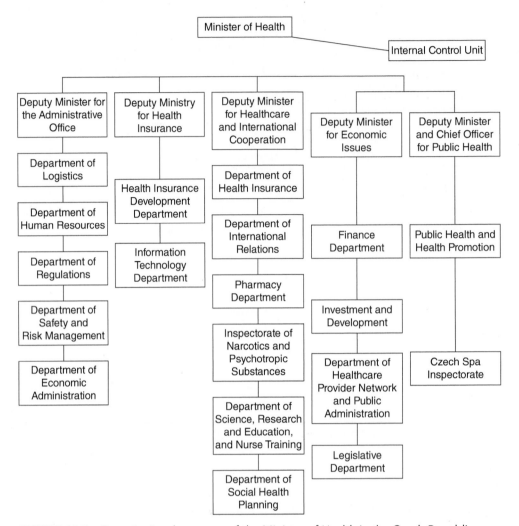

FIGURE 20.7 Organizational structure of the Ministry of Health in the Czech Republic.

and operate as trading companies. Note that these private hospitals are still required to raise funds through statutory health insurance.

Before 2002, the majority of hospitals in the Czech Republic were managed by the regional offices of the Ministry of Health. However, since January 2003, administrative authority was shifted to the districts, by the end of that same year, nearly all administrative work had been decentralized at the local level. Accordingly, past debts incurred by hospitals were transferred from the central government to the local governments.

Furthermore, all healthcare affairs originally handled by the regional departments were transferred to district governments, thus implying an increase in district authority. Nevertheless, this decentralization has also created a problem: that is, certain powers were not clearly defined, especially with regard to the construction of service monitoring networks and the evaluation of healthcare service quality. Because of these ambiguities in legislation, certain districts have converted their hospitals into private for-profit hospitals; other districts are still observing the situation. Moreover, the Ministry of Health has yet to achieve consensus on the nature of hospital services. Presently, a few dozen hospitals in the Czech Republic operate as limited liability companies.

3. Healthcare Funding and Universal Social Health Insurance

(1) Sources of Healthcare Funding

The Czech Republic has five sources of funding for healthcare services: health insurance, state budget, municipal budgets, cash payments, and donations. The implementation of voluntary insurance remains at the pilot stage. Currently, statutory health insurance is the main source of funding, accounting for 80% of the total funds.

Direct taxation of investment and noninvestment expenditures by the central and local governments is the second largest source of funding, accounting for 10% of the total funds (Table 20.9). Cash payments account for a relatively low share of the healthcare funding in the Czech Republic, at only 8.3% in 2002; this percentage was among the lowest in all OECD member countries. Voluntary health insurance accounts for a nonsignificant market share in the Czech Republic, at less than 0.1%.

(2) Health Insurance

On January 1, 1993, the Czech health security system shifted from tax-based financing to insurance-based financing. This new health insurance system introduced a method of fundraising through statutory health insurance, which requires all residents of the Czech Republic to enroll in health insurance.

The Czech health insurance system has extremely broad coverage: all permanent residents of the Czech Republic are eligible for health insurance, as are nonpermanent residents employed by a company registered in the Czech Republic. Every health insurance fund must accept any individual who meets the criteria for enrollment. Individuals who do not meet the criteria of statutory insurance can purchase contract-based health insurance. Individuals enrolled in statutory health insurance reserve the right to switch health insurance funds once every 12 months. Depending on the terms of the voluntary insurance and the range of health services covered, customers can choose either short-term or long-term insurance plans. Short-term plans (which last for less than 365 days) are suitable for short-term visitors, such as tourists or civil servants. Foreigners who have been granted visas for more than 90 days (except those who are granted work visas, given that they can participate in statutory health insurance if they are employed by companies registered in the Czech Republic) are able to enroll in long-term health insurance plans (duration of more than 365 days).

Currently, the entire health insurance system is dominated by nine major health insurance funds. The largest of these is the General Health Insurance Fund (GHIF), which covers approximately 68% of the total population.

The GHIF has 77 branches, one in each district (the traditional administrative unit of the country) of the Czech Republic. Each district branch is headed by a director, who is responsible for supervising their respective district and is accountable to a supervisory board (comprising three insured person representatives and two employer representatives) and a board of directors (comprising five insured persons representatives and four employer representatives). The insured person representatives are elected by their respective district assemblies, while the employer representatives are appointed by the district Chamber of Trade and Industry. The highest authority at the national level is the Assembly of Representatives,

TABLE 20.9 Major Funding Sources of the Czech Republic in 1991–2002 (Unit: %)

Funding Source	Year											
	1991	1992	1993	1994	1995	1996	1997	1998	1999	2000	2001	2002
Public taxation	96.8	95.4	94.8	94	92.7	92.6	91.9	91.9	91.9	91.6	91.4	91.7
(Direct taxation)	96.8	95.4	19.1	16.5	16.5	12.5	11.8	10.9	11.1	10.5	9.5	10.2
Statutory insurance (total)	–	–	75.7	77.5	76.2	80.1	80.1	80.1	80.1	81.1	81.9	81.5
Private	3.2	4.5	5.2	6.0	7.2	7.4	8.1	8.1	8.2	8.41	8.6	8.3
Cash payment	3.2	4.5	5.2	6.0	7.2	7.4	8.1	8.1	8.2	8.4	8.6	8.3

Source: 2003 National Budget, Ministry of Health (includes expenditures of other ministries, e.g., Ministry of Defense).

which is responsible for reviewing the annual report, annual accounts, and annual budget before these are approved by the Parliament. In addition, a board of directors is responsible for overall planning and decision-making, and consists of 30 members, including 10 government representatives (from the Ministry of Finance, Ministry of Health, and Ministry of Social Affairs), 10 insured person representatives (elected by Parliament), and 10 employer representatives (appointed by the Chamber of Trade and Industry). There is also a supervisory board comprising nine members (three each from the aforementioned groups of representatives).

For all other insurance funds, there are no laws specifying the number of members for the management board, board of directors, or supervisory board. However, the number of members must be equally distributed across the three representative groups (i.e., state representatives appointed by the Ministry of Health, insured person representatives elected by Parliament, and employer representatives appointed by the Chamber of Trade and Industry). Unlike the GHIF, the boards of directors of these funds have the power to appoint a director.

To start a new health insurance fund, applications must be submitted to both the Ministry of Health and the Ministry of Finance. The newly proposed fund must insure at least 50,000 people and have the required financial reserves stipulated in the law.

Individuals who do not meet the criteria for statutory health insurance can be covered by voluntary health insurance provided by the GHIF. However, voluntary health insurance is only supplementary and must be purchased from the GHIF. In other words, the Czech Republic does not permit the free choice of insurance funds. The criteria for insurance participation, scope of insurance coverage, rights and obligations of the insured persons and the insurance fund, payment method for insurance premiums, and other issues are clearly outlined in the "General Insurance Terms and Conditions" issued by the GHIF. A list of healthcare institutions that provide services under the voluntary health insurance can be obtained from all GHIF district branches. Voluntary health insurance is regulated by the Insurance Act (Act No. 363/1999 Coll.).

1. Health Insurance Funding Level   Health insurance is jointly funded by individuals, employers, and the state.

Premium contributions are defined by law as a specific percentage of pretax wages, whereby employees contribute 4.5% and employers 9% (for a total of 13.5%). The ceiling for contributions is six times the average wage in the Czech Republic. The percentage of contributions by self-employed individuals is about 13.5%; however, this should not exceed 35% of their profits. The law also specifies the minimum contributions for self-employed individuals, which are adjusted according to the inflation rate. In 2004, this minimum was Kč905 (approximately €28) per person per month. Because nearly 80% of self-employed individuals do not make or declare any annual profits, they are only required to pay the minimum contribution. This has led to discussions as to whether this part of the Health Insurance Act should be amended.

The Ministry of Finance contributes the same percentage of "wages" for those covered by state insurance. For example, in 2003, the monthly wage was Kč3,458 (approximately €108); hence, the Ministry of Finance contributed Kč467 (approximately €15) per person per month as a premium.

About 56% of the population is insured by the state under the GHIF. By law, the GHIF is responsible for providing insurance to the entire population, including those without an income, such as the unemployed, pensioners, children and dependents under the age of 26 years, students, women on maternity leave, military personnel, prisoners, and individuals receiving social welfare. Although children and pensioners can participate in any health insurance fund, most of them participate in the GHIF. The Ministry of the Interior (i.e., the police) and the Ministry of Defense (i.e., the military) have their own independent insurance systems, which originated from the healthcare system that existed before 1989. Large enterprises or specific categories of employment (e.g., mining industry, banking industry) usually organize their own insurance as well.

2. Mutual Competition Among Insurance Companies   Individuals are free to choose their insurance companies and are eligible to switch companies once per year. If a specific insurance company goes bankrupt, their customers are transferred to the GHIF. Health insurance companies are not permitted to make a profit, so any surplus funds must be deposited into a special account known as a reserve fund. The Ministry of Labor and Social Affairs, Ministry of Finance, and Ministry of Health all have members participating in the management boards of insurance funds throughout the country. Among these bodies, the Ministry of Health is responsible for the supervision of these management boards.

Recently, 18 health insurance companies have disappeared from the market. Some of these went bankrupt, whereas others were ordered by the government to suspend business because they did not meet the legal requirements for operation. A number of reasons have been cited for these issues, such as the limited risk diversification ability of small companies, excessive operating costs, and excessive number of special programs (e.g., special insurance for the chronically ill, asthmatics). Some funds were ultimately merged, whereas others were shut down.

The bankruptcy of insurance funds is regarded a major cause of the high amount of debt accrued by the healthcare system. This debt began to accumulate when healthcare providers could not be paid, who in turn could not pay their staff or suppliers. These financial difficulties are most prominent among hospitals, the majority of which are operating at some level of deficit. By the end of 2003, the deficit had increased to Kč6 billion (approximately €220 million), or nearly 4% of the total annual healthcare expenditure.

Thus, it seems that it was a mistake to assume that the different health insurance funds would compete with each other by providing different services. In the beginning, the health insurance funds offered a variety of services on top of those covered by the basic benefits package, in order to compete for insured persons. However, it later became evident that many health insurance companies did not have sufficient funds to pay even for the basic healthcare services. In 1994, the reimbursement of services not covered by the basic benefits package was restricted by law. Then, in 1997, the practice of competing through the offering of additional services was completely prohibited by law. In the end, these earlier bankruptcies led to a total ban on the provision of additional services by health insurance funds.

3. Redistribution of Premium Contributions   To reduce the potential for risk selection and alleviate the financial difficulties caused by adverse selection that many health insurance funds were facing, contributions to health insurance premiums were redistributed. More specifically, nearly 60% of the total premium contributions were redistributed according to a capitation formula by the GHIF. The capitation rate of insured persons over the age of 60 years was three times that of individuals below the age of 60 years.

In 2003–2004, a political consensus was reached on reforming the risk structure compensation scheme among the nine health insurance funds. After a two-year transition period, all premiums were reallocated according to the following two principles: (1) age and (2) factors reflecting the degree of resource utilization (e.g., treatment of chronic diseases or complications). Nevertheless, apart from age, it remains unclear as to which criteria are applicable to the new risk structure compensation scheme.

4. Existing Issues and Future Reforms for Health Insurance Funds   In recent years, the financial difficulties of health insurance funds have become increasingly prominent, especially those of the GHIF. These financial problems have been attributed to numerous factors, such as insufficient supervision and control of staff workloads, inadequate premium contributions, and difficulties in cost containment under the fee-for-service system. However, the primary reason might be the extremely high costs of the service provider network. Both health insurance funds and public administration are making relatively slow progress in restructuring the healthcare service network and actively purchasing services through selective contracts.

The problems stemming from loopholes in the administrative mechanisms can only be resolved through improvements in legislation. For example, the vast majority of premiums in this system are contributed by salaried employees and employers, whereas self-employed persons, who must also contribute premiums, might be entirely exempted or contribute at a reduced rate.

Since the beginning of 2003, a number of new recommendations have been proposed, in particular that the Ministry of Health should consider the introduction of deductibles. The Ministry of Health is also attempting to increase the cash flow into healthcare services through various measures, such as reducing the required reserve funds for health insurance funds.

(3) Financial Allocation and Capital Flow

1. Purchase of Healthcare Services   As funding for healthcare services is based on a set percentage of the population's income, the size of the overall budget for healthcare services is determined by the income levels of the insured persons. Expenses that cannot be covered by this budget are borne by the state and district budgets.

The rapid growth of healthcare expenditure has become the most pressing issue in the health reforms of the Czech Republic. Since 1990, healthcare expenditures have been increasing annually, peaking in 1992–1993 (when the health insurance system was introduced), while the expenditure per capita has increased by about 60%. Since then, the increase in expenditure per capita has declined somewhat, but it still remains high. For instance, for the GHIF, the expenditure per capita grew by 36% in 1994, 21% in 1995, 14% in 1996, and 9% in 1997; thus, it increased by a total of 105% between 1993 and 1997. Nearly 90% of the public financial resources of the healthcare system are raised and spent by health insurance funds, which makes these funds the most important resource allocators of the healthcare system (Figure 20.8).

Health insurance funds reimburse the expenses for healthcare services through contracts with hospitals and physicians. Initially, a fee-for-service payment method was adopted, whereby each service item on the fee schedule was assigned a corresponding number of reimbursement points. These points were then multiplied by the monetary value of each point (i.e., the point value) to obtain the reimbursement amount for each item, which

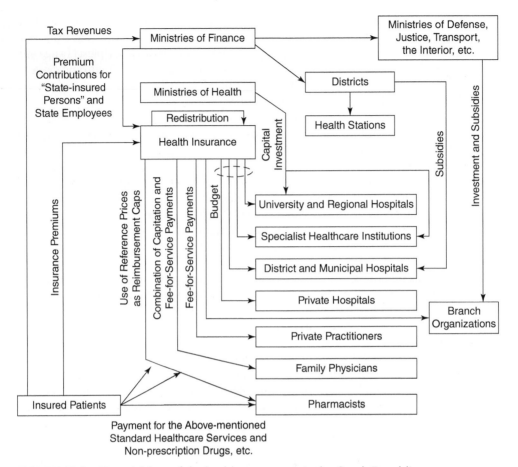

FIGURE 20.8 Financial flow of the healthcare system in the Czech Republic.

formed the basis of the payment. The point value was determined through multiple factors, including the maximum allowable value, the agreed value, and the overall reimbursement level of a given health insurance fund. The maximum point value was determined by the Ministry of Finance.

As insurance companies contracted separately, those that collected more premiums were able to offer higher payments for each point. This, in turn, gave service providers the incentive to encourage patients to switch from one insurance company to another in order to obtain greater reimbursements. However, in reality, the differences between healthcare insurance funds were insignificant because most funds would reference the GHIF when setting their reimbursement values. Furthermore, for all health insurance funds, increasing the reimbursement level of a specific item would reduce the point value because the upper limit of the overall reimbursement level had been predetermined.

Before 1994, health insurance funds did not have the power to restrict services covered under the insurance contract – that is, they were required to sign contracts with service providers with an unlimited scope on the services covered. This made insurance agencies serve as passive payers rather than as active service purchasers. However, legislation enacted in 1994 permitted certain restrictions to be implemented, with reduced reimbursements being provided for services that exceeded the restricted scope.

In 1997, the Parliament promulgated Act No. 48/1997 Coll. and several additional provisions that clearly specified which services could be restricted in the insurance contracts, and that permitted the use of payment methods other than the fee-for-service system. This reform also led to the formulation of a uniform point value, which is determined through negotiations between the insurance funds and service providers and requires the final approval of the Ministry of Finance. This 1997 act can be regarded as the most important reform made to healthcare financing since the health insurance system was established in 1992–1993.

In July 1997, the Ministry of Health issued a new list of procedures (service items) and assigned new point values. However, this list was met with opposition from both service providers and insurers. The former believed that the new point values would not cover the real costs incurred during the provision of healthcare services, whereas the latter believed that the premiums collected were insufficient to cover the predetermined scope of services. In 2003, about 3,800 items were specified as reimbursable services.

2. Fee Payments

1. *Payment of hospital fees.* Between 1993 and 1997, points were used to evaluate whether hospitals were carrying out activities according to their specific budget requirements. Under this system, hospitals were required to submit invoices to their affiliated insurance companies for the charges incurred by patients, which included the patient's identification code and a list of healthcare procedures provided. The total list included approximately 4,500 procedures, which were reimbursed based on the points assigned to these procedures and the number of times the procedures were performed. Hospitals were also required to invoice the number of reimbursable points for each day, which was in turn multiplied by the point value. Additionally, they received lump-sum payments for drug expenses. The point value was calculated as follows: any funds remaining after subtracting the material charges (which are reimbursed directly) were divided by the total number of points to obtain the point value. The value of each point was uniform throughout the country. However, as calculations were performed separately for each health insurance fund, there could be disparities among the different insurance companies.

   However, there were certain shortcomings in this point-based, fee-for-service system of hospital payment: that is, it caused hospitals (including outpatient institutions) to provide excessive services and overvalued the services of certain specialties (e.g., plastic surgery and ophthalmology). Furthermore, it did not offer subsidies for service providers with higher labor costs (especially in the capital city, Prague). Moreover, because the system did not reduce the length of hospital stay, the per diem rate of hospital beds has been adjusted proportionally since the end of 1994.

   Since mid-1997, hospital inpatient services have been reimbursed by health insurance based on a budget, which in turn is determined according to the expenses incurred during the same period in the previous year (while also taking into account the inflation rate).

   Since 2001, in addition to the budget, the payment of hospitals has included a flat fee calculated based on the number of cases treated. Due to frequent changes in regulations (twice a year), only the main principles of this payment are described: if the number of treated cases for a given year is lower than 101% compared to the previous year, then the full amount of the flat fee is paid per insured patient. If the number of treated cases for a given year is higher than 101% but lower than 105%

compared to the previous year, then half the amount of the flat fee is paid for each insured patient exceeding the threshold (the full amount is paid up to 101%). If the number of treated cases exceeds 105%, then 1/5 the amount of the flat fee is paid for each insured patient exceeding the threshold (the previous calculation methods are applicable up to 105%).

Currently, relevant government departments are preparing to introduce "diagnosis-related groups" (DRGs) to address certain existing problems. This will represent a major reform for hospitals.

2. *Payment of physician fees.* There are significant differences in income between physicians working in private institutions and physicians employed by the state. The majority of the latter work in state-owned hospitals and receive a fixed salary that is above the national average. In contrast, the income of physicians in private institutions is determined according to the service volume delivered. As mentioned earlier, the income of physicians was initially based on a pure fee-for-service system. However, because of the limited amount of overall funding, the provision of more services implied that the reimbursement for each service item would be reduced. Hence, to compensate for the decreased reimbursement rate, physicians would increase the number of services provided, which in turn further reduced the reimbursements received. Between 1993 and 1997, the GHIF's expenditure on each family physician increased by 31%, while that on each outpatient specialist increased by 258%. These increases could not be explained by the reduction in outpatient services provided by hospitals, given that the outpatient expenditure per capita had increased by 67%.

To break this vicious cycle, in 1997, the Ministry of Health and the GHIF introduced targeted reform measures for the payment of family physicians and specialists. First, a capitation system was introduced for family physicians. This involved dividing the target population into 18 groups based on age; for example, individuals aged 0–4 years were assigned a value parameter of 3.8; individuals aged 20–24 years were assigned a value of 0.9; individuals aged 60–64 years were assigned a value of 1.5; and individuals aged 85 years or above were assigned a value of 3.4. The number of patients served by each physician was uniformly limited, and exceeding this limit led to a smaller payment per capita. In addition, some family physician services (e.g., preventive examinations, home visits) were still based on the fee-for-service system; these services accounted for 30% of the total income of family physicians.

As for outpatient specialists, a lump-sum payment system was introduced in the second half of 1997. These payments were settled once per quarter, and the amounts were determined with reference to the levels in the same quarter in 1996 (while also taking into account the inflation rate). This same payment system was also adopted for hospitals. Full reimbursement of the lump-sum payment was only provided if the performance level of inpatient services in the hospital was at least 70% of that delivered in the same quarter of the previous year. This condition was proposed by the insurance companies based on information from the Ministry of Health, which indicated that 20–30% of the healthcare services provided were unnecessary (i.e., they were only intended to increase profits through earning more points). Statistics from the second half of 1997 showed that the service volume decreased by approximately 20%. In January 1998, further reforms were made to the reimbursement system for specialist outpatient services and a fee-for-service mechanism was once again implemented. However, because of the limits imposed by the state on service volumes, the reimbursement of specialists was no longer unlimited.

Furthermore, the point values used to calculate the amount of reimbursement began to be determined by the number of hours worked. For example, working up to nine hours per day awarded Kč1 per point, whereas working up to 12 hours per day awarded only Kč0.8 per point. Unlike office-based outpatient specialists, the reimbursement of outpatient services provided by hospitals and other healthcare institutions were still based on a lump-sum payment system. In July 1997, a special price list was established for the reimbursement of dental/stomatological services. On this list, the price of each service item is stated directly in Czech koruna instead of points, and some procedures are reimbursed using bundled payments. Services using aforementioned standard materials are covered entirely by the patients (as such, the insurance does not pay the standard price or the cost of standard materials). In summary, the previously mentioned reforms to the reimbursement systems for family physicians, outpatient specialists, and hospitals effectively changed the incentives of healthcare providers. These reforms also altered the prevailing tendency to provide patients with excessive or unnecessary services. In fact, the reimbursement mechanism caused certain physicians to minimize the services they provided due to the fact that these physicians still believed they were treating some patients "without reimbursement" (i.e., services provided after the physician's "limited working hours"). Nevertheless, it is important to note that the overall budget did not change and even increased for many physicians.

4. Trends in Health System Reforms

(1) Reform History of the Healthcare System

In the early 1990s, the Czech healthcare system underwent numerous reforms at an extremely rapid pace but with a relatively stable implementation process. However, since the late 1990s, healthcare reforms in the Czech Republic have slowed considerably.

More specifically, in the early 1990s, the Czech healthcare system underwent considerable reform. Most of these reforms were successfully implemented, and the overall progress of the reforms was relatively smooth. The reforms centered primarily on comprehensive reconstruction of healthcare institutions, the redistribution of power, and the establishment of a health insurance system.

However, from 1998 to 2004, only a handful of amendments were made to policies on healthcare provision and health insurance regulations. The fundamental statute for statutory health insurance – Act No. 48/1997 Coll. – was originally a temporary document for short-term application. Currently, it seems that its period of enforcement will continue even until the next election in 2021. Furthermore, during this period, partial reforms were made to address the most prominent issue in the healthcare system – healthcare financing. However, these reforms did not involve any major changes to the financial status of the statutory health insurance system.

(2) Overall Characteristics of Health System Reforms

1. Healthcare Funding   The Czech Republic has established nine health insurance funds responsible for financing the healthcare sector. The GHIF is the most important among them, accounting for the vast majority of the market. Health insurance financing is independent of state budget financing and emphasizes the humanization and democratization of healthcare. Subsequently, the introduction of statutory health insurance led to the establishment of a healthcare system with single-source financing. Still, there was a continued need to accrue more resources and to identify better methods of allocating these resources (e.g., a fee-for-service payment system). It was initially expected that more resources and better allocation methods would enhance the efficiency of the system; however, they may have led to the overutilization of healthcare services.

2. Healthcare Legal and Management Systems   A series of laws, regulations, and policy documents were successively issued during the healthcare reform process in the Czech Republic. After the 1998 election, the Czech Social Democratic Party formed a minority government. According to the party's electoral manifesto, entitled "Together for a Better Tomorrow," health was regarded as "a public property, society's source of wealth and better living, and not just a private property and good." Accordingly, all factors limiting social solidarity, including low income, disease, and population aging, were unacceptable. Subsequently, several proposed amendments to relevant legislations were introduced. For example, in 2000, the Ministry of Health submitted proposed amendments to the government for the Statutory Health Insurance Act, the Department, Professional, Company and Other Health Insurance Funds Act, the General Health Insurance Fund Act, and the General Health Insurance Fund Premiums Act. For a variety of reasons, these proposed amendments were never actually passed; still, at the very least, the proposals indicated that the government was aware of the necessity of promoting reforms through the introduction of relevant laws, regulations, and policy documents.

3. Role of International Exchange and International Organizations   The Czech Republic's entry into the European Union prompted adjustment to some of its laws. For example, the Parliament passed Act No. 123/2000 Coll. relating to medical devices, and Act No. 407/2001 Coll., which amended the "Addictive Substance Act" and "Protection of Public Health Act." Furthermore, the "Transplantation Act" was passed in 2004. Various international organizations have also been involved in the Czech reform process. For example, in 2004, the World Bank participated in the reform discussions in the Czech Republic. Such legislative adjustments and the assistance of international organizations have both played positive roles in promoting reform of the healthcare system in the Czech Republic.

(3) Experiences in Health System Reforms

The Czech healthcare system underwent extensive and rapid transformation in the early 1990s. The objectives of these reforms gradually became clearer as their impacts permeated the healthcare system. In 1989, the establishment of a humanized and democratized healthcare system that was independent of the financing of the state budget was considered a key issue. By the end of the reforms, a healthcare system with single-source financing was established through the introduction of statutory health insurance. However, it was still necessary to continue uncovering more resources and identifying more effective methods of resource allocation. It was initially expected that these methods (e.g., the fee-for-service reimbursement system) would enhance the efficiency of the system, but they may have actually resulted in the overutilization of healthcare services.

As noted earlier, the Czech healthcare system underwent major and rapid reform during the early 1990s, with the objectives of these reforms taking shape as they changed the healthcare system. In terms of healthcare provision, the population of the Czech Republic has essentially attained full coverage. To date, the successes of the system have outweighed the failures. However, the Czech healthcare system still has numerous problems. These problems could be resolved through the proposal of creative solutions that are free from bias and the formulation of policies that emphasize a balance of interests.

Currently, healthcare policymakers are most concerned about the system's financial instability as well as the deficits related to the statutory health insurance and hospitals. The Czech Republic has been actively attempting to address the increasing deficit in public finances. So far, however, the Ministry of Finance and central leadership have only attempted to address these deficits through limiting expenditures; no attempts have been made to increase management efficiency or to implement activities that enhance the capacity of the public sector (e.g., scientific research and education). Furthermore, the situation has been deteriorating due to political pressure to reduce the tax burden, which in turn would run the risk of increasing the socioeconomic burden on low- and middle-income groups. In addition, healthcare resources are still being wasted due to their ineffective use and the overutilization of or regional imbalances in certain services. Thus, it is necessary for political representatives and other relevant parties to discuss whether it is possible to fundamentally alter the principles of formulating healthcare policies. These principles primarily concern the feasibility of the reforms, and their alteration could resemble those reforms implemented in Slovakia under the influence of the World Bank: that is, private for-profit health insurance companies (joint-stock companies) would be able to administer the financial resources of statutory health insurance.

Indeed, in 2004, the World Bank played a role in the reform discussions of the Czech Republic. This suggests that the Czech Republic is considering enhancing the competition of statutory health insurance and increasing the autonomy of hospitals. Within this context, there is an ongoing effort to develop corresponding payment mechanisms for hospital services (i.e., DRGs).

It is now necessary to consider the direction in which the Czech healthcare system will develop. This is an extremely crucial issue that society is naturally highly sensitive to. Therefore, consistency must be maintained in the adoption and implementation of major political decisions in order to ensure optimal rationalization and effectiveness in all aspects of healthcare, including the quality of healthcare services, the financing of the healthcare system, and implementation of national health policies.

The development of health policies is determined by the positions of policymakers towards healthcare provision, specifically, whether to apply or limit market mechanisms. One of the options is to further "commercialize" the statutory health insurance system, thereby liberalizing the contractual relationships and encouraging competition among service providers. This involves combining the privatization of hospitals with higher cost-sharing with patients, a method of regulation known as the "invisible hand." Another option is to continue implementing the existing approach, that is, to continue relying on the "visible hand" to enforce regulation.

The systematic resolution of healthcare problems is likely to be an important issue for some time in the future; it is no longer possible to resolve each problem as it arises. Over the past decade, the lack of communication among the various stakeholders (i.e., policymakers; healthcare providers; representatives of health insurance funds, professional associations, and patient associations; and the public) has further complicated the healthcare problems.

The statutory health insurance has been clearly separated from the national budget, and the task of the latter involves merely providing investment subsidies to healthcare institutions. Nevertheless, there are a few economic incentives in this system that remain questionable. As mentioned earlier, during the decentralization process, the irregular subsidies allocated to indebted hospitals were not allocated in a standardized manner, which encouraged hospitals to engage in lobbying rather than perform the necessary structural adjustments and procedural reforms. Another problem was that hospitals were reimbursed retrospectively – that is, on the basis of past financial flows – which only partially reflected their actual output. This led to insufficient pressure on hospitals to improve their management, increase productivity, and maintain financial health.

Regardless of whether the government intends to increase the competition among health insurance companies or maintain the existing structure, there is still a pressing need to introduce a more advanced and equalized risk structure compensation scheme. Specifically, the government must consider adding more risk adjustment factors than just age in order to ensure more effective and fairer reallocation of resources. For example, losing the capacity to work could be an additional risk adjustment factor, as it could significantly improve the formula for reallocation.

Provisions concerning the benefits covered by statutory health insurance have been reviewed in detail. Arguably, these benefits include too many luxury and unnecessary services, such as nonprescription drugs and spas, which are mostly paid by patients themselves or supplementary health insurance in other European countries.

In addition, the failure to integrate accident insurance into the statutory healthcare system has been consistently criticized. Thus far, there is still no public accident insurance. Employers are required to purchase accident insurance for their workers from a private insurance company called "Kooperativa." Although accident insurance and health insurance are usually separate in other countries, the integration of the two is still regarded as an important measure.

As with other countries, a deeper problem in the overall healthcare system concerns the common lack of necessary qualifications among health insurance staff (knowledge on health economics, law, health insurance theory, epidemiological methods and actuarial calculations). In other countries, healthcare workers generally undergo a long training and qualification process before being hired, whereas the health insurance companies in the Czech Republic do not impose such requirements and their workers are essentially trained on the job. Furthermore, it will be a long and slow process to formulate and implement policies related to the required knowledge and qualifications of healthcare staff, as well as the requirements for attaining these qualifications. This is because the necessary knowledge has not been adequately integrated into the relevant educational programs at the undergraduate or graduate level (in healthcare, economics, and law).

A key problem with the current Czech healthcare system is the lack of sufficient evaluations of or attention to the development of the overall statutory health insurance system. Its current annual general reports are not satisfactory in this regard. Therefore, the Czech healthcare system should strive to learn more from other European countries and attempt to improve the overall transparency of its system.

SECTION IV. THE HEALTH SYSTEM IN BULGARIA

1. Overview of Socioeconomics and National Health

(1) Basic National Conditions

Bulgaria, officially the Republic of Bulgaria, is a country located in the Balkan Peninsula in southeastern Europe. It covers a land area of 110,993 km² and has a population of 7.6 million (as of 2009). The country is divided into 28 provinces. The ethnic composition of its population (which is a controversial estimate) is as follows: 85.8% Bulgarian, 9.7% Turkish, 3.4% Roma, and 1.1% other ethnic minorities.

Before the end of World War II, Bulgaria was a major agricultural country comprising numerous rural landowners. By the end of the 1980s, its economy had begun to decline; eventually, it became one of the poorest countries in Central Europe. In response, Bulgaria gradually began to transition from a planned economy to a market economy. However, in the wake of this transition, it faced serious difficulties and a sharp decline in its economy, only managing to resume sustainable growth in 1998. Government expenditure as a share of GDP decreased from 65.9% in 1990 to 34.9% in 1997, and increased to only 44.5% in 2000. After the economic transition, there was a sharp rise in the unemployment rate and widespread poverty, with as estimated 35% of the population living below the poverty line. By 2009, Bulgaria's GDP remained the lowest among the EU member states and was only 41% of the average level among the EU14 countries. In 2012, Bulgaria's GDP per capita was US$50.9752 billion. Table 20.10 shows the macroeconomic indicators of Bulgaria in 1990–2012.

All EU countries have shown an increase in the average life expectancy. Similarly, aside from a slight decline between 1989 and 1997, the life expectancy in Bulgaria has grown consistently since 1970, increasing from 71.2 years in 1980 to 74.3 years in 2012. In general, most of the mortality and morbidity indicators in Bulgaria are lower than the EU average. Table 20.11 shows the population indicators of Bulgaria between 1990 and 2012, and Table 20.12 shows the basic mortality indicators of Bulgaria for selected years between 1990 and 2012.

In 2009, the three major causes of death were circulatory system diseases (66.0% of all diseases), malignant neoplasms (15.9%), and respiratory system diseases (3.8%). Although infant and under-five mortality rates have been decreasing by 5–6% per year over the past decade, these indicators are still lagging far behind the averages of the EU12 and EU27 countries. Table 20.13 shows the composition of the causes of death in Bulgaria for selected years in 1980–2008.

The mortality rates of chronic diseases (e.g., cardiovascular and cerebrovascular diseases) and trauma have been increasing continuously in Bulgaria. This pattern is closely related to factors such as increasingly unhealthy lifestyles, unbalanced diets, deteriorating environmental conditions, and increasing poverty. The neonatal, under-five, and maternal mortality rates also deteriorated in the 1990s. The number of abortions has exceeded the number of births since 1980, and Bulgaria has the highest abortion rate in Europe. In 2003, the total healthcare expenditure of Bulgaria was about €850 million (approximately RMB8.5 billion), accounting for 4.8% of the GDP, and the annual healthcare expenditure per capita was about €100 (approximately RMB1000).

TABLE 20.10   Macroeconomic Indicators of Bulgaria in 1990–2012 (Selected Years)

Indicator	Year					
	1990	1995	2000	2005	2010	2012
GDP (current US$, million)	20,726	13,107	12,599	27,188	47,727	50,972
PPP (current international $, million)	47,066	46,508	50,919	75,924	106,553	117,192
GDP per capita (current US$)	2,377	1,555	1,579	3,733	6,453	6,977
GDP, PPP (current international $, US$)	5,399	5,533	6,232	9,809	14,408	16,041
Annual growth rate of GDP (%)	–9.1	2.9	5.7	6.4	0.4	0.8
Total expenditure as a share of GDP (%)	53.5	39.5	31.6	31.7	30.9	32.3
Cash surplus/deficit as a share of GDP (%)	–5.0	–5.1	–0.4	3.2	-3.5	-0.8
Healthcare expenditure per capita (current US$, US$)		81.6	97.7	273.5	480.2	515.5
Healthcare expenditure per capita, PPP (constant price International $ in 2005, US$)		290.2	385.0	718.7	1,053.1	1,177.1
Total healthcare expenditure as a share of GDP (%)		5.2	6.2	7.3	7.6	7.4
Total labor force (million)	4.1	3.8	3.4	3.4	3.4	3.4
Total unemployment rate (%)		15.7	16.2	10.1	10.2	12.3
Real interest rate (%)		10.5	4.4	1.2	8.1	7.4
Official exchange rate (local currency unit per US$, period average)	0.002	0.07	2.12	1.57	1.48	1.52

Source: World Bank, 2012.

TABLE 20.11   Population Indicators of Bulgaria in 1990–2012 (Selected Years)

Indicators	Year					
	1990	1995	2000	2005	2010	2012
Total population (million)	8.7	8.4	8.2	7.7	7.4	7.3
Female population (% of total population)	50.7	51.0	51.3	51.3	51.3	51.4
Population aged 0–14 years (% of total population)	20.3	17.9	15.7	13.7	13.3	13.5
Population aged over 65 years (% of total population)	13.2	15.1	16.6	17.4	18.3	18.9
Annual average population growth rate (%)	–1.8	–0.4	–0.5	–0.5	–0.7	–0.6
Population density (number of people per km²)	78.8	76.0	73.9	71.2	68.1	67.3
Total fertility rate (number of births per woman)	1.8	1.2	1.3	1.3	1.6	1.5
Crude birth rate (%)	12.1	8.6	9.0	9.2	10.2	9.5
Crude death rate (%)	12.4	13.6	14.1	14.6	14.9	15.0
Age dependency ratio (%)	50.3	49.3	47.6	45.1	46.3	48.0
Urban population (% of total population)	66.4	67.8	68.9	70.2	72.5	73.6

Source: World Bank, 2012.

TABLE 20.12   Basic Mortality Indicators of Bulgaria in 1990–2012 (Selected Years)

Indicators	Year					
	1990	**1995**	**2000**	**2005**	**2010**	**2012**
Total life expectancy at birth (years)	71.6	71.1	71.7	72.6	73.5	74.3
Male life expectancy at birth (years)	68.3	67.4	68.2	69.0	70.0	70.9
Female life expectancy at birth (years)	75.2	74.9	75.3	76.3	77.2	77.9
Mortality rate per 1,000 adult females (%)	98.0	99.9	98.8	92.4	88.3	—
Mortality rate per 1,000 adult males (%)	219.3	245.3	224.9	219.7	197.0	—

Source: World Bank, 2012.

TABLE 20.13   Composition of the Causes of Death for Bulgaria in 1980–2012 (Selected Years)

Cause of Death	Year					
	1980	**1990**	**1995**	**2000**	**2005**	**2008**
All causes	1,162.1	1,138.3	1,170.3	1,145.8	1,065.3	995.4
Infectious diseases	7.2	5.9	7.1	8.6	7.3	6.9
Tuberculosis	3.9	2.1	3.4	3.4	2.9	2.4
Circulatory system diseases	638.0	691.3	725.6	737.1	677.4	611.3
Ischemic heart disease	185.3	230.1	234.8	193.6	163.1	126.0
Malignant neoplasm	136.9	152.4	161.6	150.1	171.0	171.6
Cervical cancer	3.9	5.2	6.6	6.9	6.9	7.0
Breast cancer (female)	16.6	21.1	22.6	21.8	23.6	23.3
Tracheal, bronchial, and lung cancer	27.0	30.7	33.2	29.0	34.6	34.5
Diabetes	11.2	17.7	21.1	19.1	16.5	18. 1
Mental disorders, diseases of the nervous system and sensory organs	7.2	8.3	11.2	11.0	9.6	11.0
Respiratory system diseases	107.8	68.4	56.1	46.8	43.6	41.6
Digestive system diseases	27.6	33.6	37.2	30.0	33.1	34.8
Other causes (injury and poison)	61.1	60.9	62.7	52.4	45.0	44.9
Traffic accidents	16.0	18. 4	14.8	11.7	10.8	13.4
Suicide and self-harm	13.7	14.1	15.5	15.0	10.7	10.1

Note: The statistical data are expressed as the age-standardized mortality rate per 1,000 people for all ages.
Source: World Health Organization Regional Office for Europe, 2010.

2. Healthcare System

The Bulgarian Ministry of Health is responsible for the formulation of national health policies, as well as the organization and operation of the healthcare system. It is also in regular contact with all ministries related to public health, such as the Ministry of Finance; the Ministry of Transport; the Ministry of the Environment and Waters; the Ministry of Agriculture; the Ministry of Labor and Social Policy; and the Ministry of Education, Youth and Science.

In 1998, the passage of the Health Insurance Act (HIA) prompted reform of the Bulgarian healthcare system into a health-insurance-based system consisting of both compulsory and voluntary forms of health insurance. The key players in this system are insured persons, healthcare providers, third-party payers that represent the National Health Insurance Fund (NHIF) (the single payer of social health insurance [SHI]), and voluntary health insurance companies (VHICs).

The health insurance system (including the SHI and voluntary health insurance [VHI]) covers the diagnosis, treatment, rehabilitation, and drug expenses incurred by insured persons. In contrast, the Ministry of Health is responsible for providing and funding public health services, emergency care, transplantation, blood transfusion, tuberculosis treatment, and inpatient care for patients with mental health problems. In addition, the Ministry of Health is also responsible for planning and protecting the human resources of the health system, the development of medical science, and the collection and storage of data on population health and healthcare expenditure accounts. However, the Ministry of Health acknowledged in its National Health Strategy 2008–2013 that the quality and reliability of the information being collected has deteriorated since 1989, especially after establishment of the health insurance system.

All healthcare providers in Bulgaria are autonomous self-governing organizations. Private enterprises provide primary healthcare, dental care, and drug services, as well as most specialist outpatient services; there are also some private hospitals. By contrast, the state owns all university hospitals and national medical centers, national-level specialist hospitals, emergency centers, psychiatric hospitals, and transfusion and hemodialysis centers, as well as 51% of regional hospitals.

According to the stipulations of the HIA, it is compulsory for all Bulgarians to enroll in health insurance. Their rights as patients and insured persons are listed in the Constitution of Bulgaria, the Health Act, the HIA, as well as numerous other national and international acts and regulations. However, some studies have shown that Bulgarians do not have sufficient access to their rights as patients (as outlined in these legislations). Thus, although there are many patient organizations in Bulgaria, they do not play a substantive role in determining health priorities.

(1) Historical Development

The Balkan Wars (1912–1913) and World War I (1914–1918) caused the health and social status of Bulgarians to deteriorate, which necessitated social and health reforms by the government at that time. In 1918, the Act on Worker Insurance for Illness and Injury was introduced. Then, in 1924, the Social Insurance Act was adopted, which was followed one year later by the promulgation of the Employment Insurance Act. The Social Insurance Act mandated the participation of the employees of all enterprises and organizations, along with civil servants, in social insurance, as protection against accident, illness, childbirth, disability, and old age. It also established a social insurance fund that funded hospitals, nursing homes, clinics, community facilities, and worker housing. The Public Health Act of 1929 (which replaced the Public Health Act of 1903) defined hygiene and anti-epidemic standards, thereby enhancing prevention of social diseases and improving health education activities.

The first Ministry of Public Health was established in 1944. In 1946, the Act on Maternal and Child Health was adopted to establish a stable security system for maternal and child healthcare.

In 1949, the Bulgarian healthcare system was adjusted to form a centralized government-run system. In 1951, the National Assembly proposed the implementation of free universal healthcare services and organized the healthcare provision system on a regional basis. During this period, private hospitals and pharmacies were nationalized, thus prohibiting physicians and pharmacists from cooperating with private practices. In addition, a specialized system for the regulation of healthcare workers and a monitoring system for certain major diseases were established. Outpatient services were provided by physicians and specialists in regional general hospitals, while the government established a system for monitoring healthcare for pregnant women and children.

In 1973, a new Public Health Act was adopted, which emphasized environmental protection, behavioral factors, demographic issues, and the importance of community-based interventions in addressing health-related issues.

This period leading up to 1989 is referred to as a period of health system development within the context of centralized financing and management. During this period, a series of health and demographic issues became increasingly prominent, as did the clear lack of effective measures for reducing inefficiency in various healthcare sectors, wastage, and poor management of health system resources. Since 1989, however, major changes have occurred in the political sphere of Bulgarian society. The New Constitution of the Republic of Bulgaria was officially ratified in 1991. At this point, numerous systems underwent development and economic reforms were initiated. The public sector reforms followed a particularly unstable trajectory with frequent amendments to the reform objectives. Discussions on the need to reform the health system into a social healthcare system began during Bulgaria's transition from a centrally planned economy to a market economy.

The Health Insurance Act (1998), the Health Care Establishments Act (1999), the Professional Organizations Act (1998), and the Act on Drug and Pharmacy Administration in Human Medicine (1995) provided a legal basis for the health system reforms. The Public Health Act of 1973 remained in force until 2004, after which it was terminated and replaced by the Health Act of 2005. Changes to these laws have produced, in certain circumstances, discontinuities and disparities among new and existing laws, thereby leading to confusion in the roles and responsibilities of the different parties making up the healthcare system.

The establishment of the health insurance system began in 2000. Implementation of the system lagged behind the development of the economic sector. From July 1999, employers were required to share the social security contributions of their employees. This provided a funding source for the initiation of these reforms. Thus, Bulgaria transformed from a state-financed healthcare system into a social health insurance system. The reforms introduced market principles, decentralization, and diversity in the ownership of healthcare institutions and the provision of healthcare services.

The reforms produced three key players in the system: patients as purchasers, outpatient and inpatient institutions as providers, and public and private health insurance organizations as third-party payers. However, the incoherent reforms led to tensions and conflicting relationships among different healthcare sectors. Furthermore, the patient–physician relationship has become strained due to organizational changes and an unclear division of rights and responsibilities.

(2) System Overview

The Bulgarian Ministry of Health has absolute authority over the formulation of health policies through the National Health Strategy (NHS). At the district level, Regional Health Inspections (RHIs) are responsible for formulating and implementing the health policies in their respective provinces. The Bulgarian health system is a health-insurance-based system that combines compulsory SHI and VHI. The SHI is uniformly administered by a single payer – the NHIF – whereas the VHI is solely provided by for-profit joint-stock companies. This health insurance system (SHI and VHI) covers the diagnosis, treatment, rehabilitation, and medication of insured persons. Public health services, inpatient care for psychiatric patients, emergency care, transplantation, and transfusion are managed and funded by the Ministry of Health.

The SHI system was established with the introduction of the Health Insurance Act of 1998. The NHIF is the sole agency in charge of the SHI and hence occupies a monopolistic position by law. It is an autonomous public institution that is independent from national health administrative agencies (i.e., the government). This institution includes one central office located in Sofia, 28 regional offices (one in each district, known as Regional Health Insurance Funds [RHIFs]), and 108 municipal offices. The NHIF is the highest authority for the SHI and comprises representatives of the government, insured persons, and employers. Its mission is to guarantee insured persons' equal access to the healthcare system. The NHIF provides funding for healthcare and dental services, as well as drugs included in the basic benefits package. The benefits package and service prices are determined through negotiations between the NHIF and the Bulgarian professional associations of physicians and dentists. The results of these annual negotiations are signed into the National Framework Contract (NFC), which defines the rights and responsibilities of the NHIF, healthcare providers, insured persons, organizational procedures, and control mechanisms. Based on the NFC, the providers sign individual agreements with the RHIFs, which in turn sign agreements with all public and private healthcare institutions within their respective regions according to the standards of the NFC.

According to the Health Care Establishments Act of 1999, healthcare providers are independent market competitors. Healthcare providers are divided into three categories by law: (1) outpatient healthcare institutions (individual or group primary and specialist healthcare and dental care, medical and dental centers, diagnostic laboratories); (2) inpatient healthcare institutions (specialist and general hospitals for long-term treatment and rehabilitation); and (3) a cluster of institutions that includes emergency centers, mental health centers, comprehensive cancer centers, dermatology and venereal disease centers, medical-social care centers, hospices, hemodialysis centers, cell banks, etc. Regardless of the category, all healthcare providers must be registered in accordance with the Trade Law, Company Law, or other relevant legislations. Since 2011, primary healthcare institutions, most outpatient specialist medical and dental care institutions, pharmacies, and some hospitals have been included in the private sector. Furthermore, aside from emergency centers, all healthcare providers can contract with the NHIF and VHIC. Providers can also receive out-of-pocket payments for services not included in the insurance or when the provider is considered a third-party payer in the contract. In addition to the NHIF and out-of-pocket payments, district or municipal healthcare providers can receive payments from the Ministry of Health or municipalities.

Emergency care and public health services are organized and funded by the Ministry of Health. Bulgaria has 28 regional emergency centers (one in each district) as well as branch facilities in towns within each district. In 1999, the public health system was restructured to form 28 Regional Centers for Protection and Control of Public Health (RCPCPHs). In early 2011, these RCPCPHs merged with the district-level representative health agencies – the Regional Health Centers (RHCs) – to form RHIs, which combined the functions of the two institutions. The public health network also includes the National Center of Radiobiology and Radiation Protection, the National Center for Infectious Diseases, the National Center of Drug Addictions, the National Center of Health Informatics, and the National Center of Public Health Protection.

(3) Organizations

The organizations of the Bulgarian healthcare system are shown in Figure 20.9.

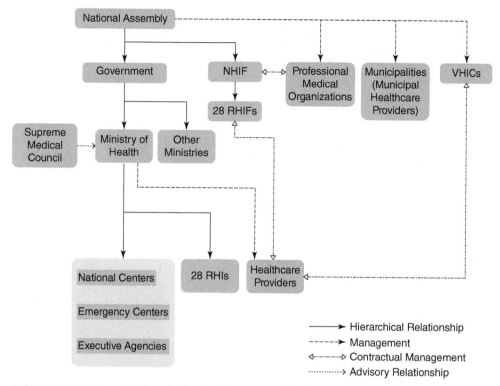

FIGURE 20.9 Organizations in the health system of Bulgaria.

1. National Assembly   Bulgaria is a parliamentary republic. The National Assembly – the country's parliamentary body – occupies an important position in the development of national health policies. Not only does it have the authority to approve the national budget, but it also holds the authority to approve the NHIF activities. Furthermore, in the early twenty-first century, a Parliamentary Commission on Health was established as part of the health reforms under the Constitution and the Rules for the Organization and Work of the National Assembly.

This Commission holds legislative power and reviews the health-related issues proposed by its members as well as other key issues raised by the National Assembly, Ministry of Health, or Director of the NHIF. Members of the Commission can also receive suggestions from professionals, professional associations, and non-governmental organizations. Furthermore, the Commission organizes and initiates public discussions and debates.

2. Ministry of Health   The Ministry of Health is responsible for the entire national health system. It administers the national healthcare budget and has executive power over the management of the national health system. The Minister of Health can introduce national health policies and implement national healthcare strategies. Additionally, the Minister presents the annual National Health Report and reports on the implementation progress of the National Health Strategy to the National Assembly.

The Ministry of Health is in charge of public health, health management, emergency care, blood transfusion, inpatient psychiatric care, medical and social care for children under the age of three, transplantations, and health information. It is also responsible for guaranteeing and maintaining the development of health interventions by healthcare institutions, medical technology, medical professional training, and medical science. The Ministry of Health supervises and is responsible for the health-related activities of the Council of Ministers, the Ministry of Defense, the Ministry of the Interior, the Ministry of Justice, and the Ministry of Transport.

It is also in charge of coordinating the roles of the various parts of the healthcare system, and funding the executive agencies responsible for pharmaceuticals and transplantation, as well as the national centers for public health, infectious diseases, health information, and so on. Furthermore, the Ministry of Health can also establish permanent or temporary advisory committees and expert work groups to support discussion and policymaking for specific issues, such as hospital restructuring, HIV/AIDS and sexually transmitted diseases, and treatments abroad.

3. Other Ministries   The Ministry of Health cooperates with the Ministry of Finance on the payment and allocation of healthcare system funds. This cooperation was deepened in 2010, when the Minister of Finance became the Deputy Prime Minister in charge of health financing. However, this also implies that without the approval of the Minister of Finance, the Ministry of Health is unable to make independent decisions related to financial issues.

Issues related to the training of healthcare workers require cooperation with the Ministry of Education, Youth and Science. In addition, cooperation with the Ministry of the Environment and Waters, as well as the Ministry of Agriculture and Food, is necessary to address issues related to public health, the environment, and food safety. Furthermore, the Ministry of Health acts in close cooperation with the NHIF, the Social Assistance Agency, and several committees established by the Council of Ministers, including the National Council on Narcotic Substances, the National Council on Medical Expertise, and the Central Ethics Commission.

4. Supreme Medical Council   The Supreme Medical Council is an advisory agency for the Ministry of Health. It includes five representatives from the Ministry of Health; five representatives from the Bulgarian Medical Association; three representatives from the Bulgarian Pharmaceutical Association; three representatives from the NHIF; one representative each from the Bulgarian Association of Health Professionals, the National Association of Municipalities, and the Bulgarian Red Cross Organization; and one representative from each medical school.

The Supreme Medical Council offers advice on national health strategies, drafts of healthcare-related bills, draft budgets, the annual reports of the Ministry of Health, the planning of admission quotas for undergraduates and graduates in healthcare professions, and issues related to medical ethics.

5. Supreme Council of Pharmacy   The Supreme Council of Pharmacy was established by the Ministry of Health. It consists of five representatives from the Ministry of Health, five representatives from the Bulgarian Pharmaceutical Association, two representatives from the NHIF, and one representative of the pharmaceutical faculty of each medical university. The Council provides advice on the main directions and priorities of pharmacy and pharmaceutical policies.

6. National Health Insurance Fund (NHIF)   The NHIF was established in 1999 in accordance with the Health Insurance Act of 1998. It consists of a central office and 28 regional offices and is administered by a Supervisory Board and a Governor of the Fund elected by the National Assembly. The NHIF budget is the main source of public funding for the healthcare system. The relationship between the NHIF and healthcare providers is based on the NFC as well as individual contracts signed with the providers. The NHIF reimburses insured persons for the basic healthcare services defined in the basic benefits package, as well as ensures their equal access to these services. The reimbursement levels for the healthcare services and products included in the basic benefits package are stipulated in the NFC. In addition, the NHIF supervises and monitors the behaviors of healthcare providers and imposes penalties on providers who appear to violate patient rights.

7. Professional Medical Organizations   Bulgaria has four professional medical associations that have been established by law: the Bulgarian Medical Association, Bulgarian Dental Association, Bulgarian Pharmaceutical Association, and Bulgarian Association of Health Professionals. These associations represent the rights and interests of their respective professionals, for whom membership is compulsory. Their activities include providing comments on draft bills, participating in the drafting of clinical guidelines, exploring ethical issues, and so on.

8. Regional Health Inspections (RHIs)   The public health administration at the district level is organized and executed by 28 RHIs. The RHIs are the local agencies of the Ministry of Health, and their functions include collecting, recording, handling, storing, analyzing, and providing health information; reviewing the quality of registered healthcare providers; implementing health information technology; organizing action plans for diseases and natural disasters; coordinating activities related to the implementation of national and regional health programs; guiding research on the demands for human resources in healthcare, and so on.

9. Municipalities   During the decentralization process, municipalities became owners of a major share of healthcare providers. Since 2011, the majority of specialist care institutions, nearly 70% of general hospitals providing active treatment, and some specialist hospitals providing active treatment have become municipal property. Municipalities participate in the ownership of district general hospitals as well. Local governments intervene in healthcare in the form of the Permanent Committees at the Municipal Councils and municipal healthcare offices. These Permanent Committees study the healthcare needs of residents and the problems in healthcare provision, and draft proposals for improvement. The municipal healthcare offices organize the healthcare services for the municipalities within the jurisdiction of the RHIs. In certain municipalities, Public Health Councils serve as advisory agencies to the Mayor's office.

10. Private Enterprises   Private healthcare enterprises were revived in the legislative reform plan of 1991. Since 2011, primary healthcare institutions, most outpatient specialist medical and dental care institutions, pharmacies, and some hospitals have been included in the private sector. In 2009, private hospitals accounted for more than 30% of all hospitals in the country. Private inpatient beds accounted for 11.4% of all hospital beds, which is much lower than the EU27 average of 36.2%. Furthermore, in 2009, private hospitals managed 14.3% of all inpatients. According to the National Center of Health Informatics, the utilization of private hospital beds is 1.5 times the national average, whereas bed turnover is comparable to the average of acute hospitals. Furthermore, there are significant differences in case mixes between private and public hospitals. The majority of private hospitals are specialist hospitals for surgery, gynecology, and ophthalmology. In accordance with the Health Care Establishments Act, private healthcare institutions can sign contracts with the NHIF in the same manner as public institutions. In addition, private healthcare institutions can also offer healthcare services beyond the scope of the SHI system and public health institutions.

11. Private Health Insurance Companies VHICs have largely failed to develop a sound market in Bulgaria; there are only 20 such companies registered. The Financial Supervision Commission (FSC) of the National Assembly is responsible for supervising VHICs. VHICs provide healthcare packages for preventive, outpatient, inpatient, and rehabilitation services that exceed the scope of the compulsory SHI.

The largest VHIC accounts for 15.4% of the VHI market share, while another six companies together account for 70.4%.

12. Nongovernmental Organizations (NGOs) There are more than 100 NGOs operating in the Bulgarian healthcare system. They are involved in treatment and prevention, environmental issues, patient rights, and the development and implementation of national health policies. Furthermore, NGO representatives and national experts are increasingly being included in discussions on effective supervision and other issues.

13. Medical Schools In 1917, the establishment of the Medical Faculty in Sofia hailed the beginning of medical education in Bulgaria. In 1972, the centralization of education prompted the revival of the Medical Academy, which included all medical faculties and universities in the country. At that time, immense academic potential was concentrated within the Medical Academy – it had more than 4,100 lecturers and 10,000 students. In 1990, medical schools were given greater autonomy. As of 2011, Bulgaria has four medical universities, on each in Sofia, Plovdiv, Varna, and Pleven. In addition, medical faculties have also been established at Sofia University and Trakia University of Stara Zagora. These universities offer master's degree programs in clinical medicine, dentistry, pharmacy, public health, and health management, as well as bachelor's programs in nursing, midwifery, and health management.

(4) Health Planning

Health policy priorities are defined in the National Health Strategy (NHS). Recently, the Ministry of Health formulated the NHS for 2008–2013, which aims to guide the establishment of an efficient and financially stable healthcare system that provides accessible and high-quality services to citizens, with the ultimate goal of achieving a healthy nation. The priorities for the development of the Bulgarian healthcare system outlined in the NHS are:

1. Implementing a "Health in All Policies" (HiAP) approach.
2. Improving population health by implementing active and effective health promotion, prevention, and rehabilitation programs that target major diseases in society.

3. Training and developing human resources in healthcare and enhancing their socioeconomic status.
4. Ensuring the financial stability of the healthcare system.
5. Improving the accessibility, quality, and efficiency of emergency medical care.
6. Adjusting and optimizing the management of inpatient healthcare.
7. Developing and establishing an integrated system of electronic data exchange in the healthcare system.

At the end of 2009, the Ministry of Health created a working group that began the reform of public hospitals. The aim was to ensure the quality of inpatient and outpatient services through an integrated approach that satisfied the varying levels of healthcare needs in the population. As part of the reform, the assets of public hospitals were divided between the government (51%) and the hospitals themselves (49%). As a result, health administrative agencies now participate in hospital management as representatives of government investors. Furthermore, hospitals have shifted from being fully funded by the government budget to joint funding from the government budget and health insurance funds. During the corporate reforms, public hospitals established councils (boards) consisting of investor representatives, as well as the leaders, experts, and senior management of public hospitals. For example, in a university hospital owned by the Ministry of Health, the council would comprise five members, including the Deputy Minister of Health, two professors from the affiliated university, the hospital director, and the deputy director. These councils meet on an average of once per month and decide on the major affairs of the hospital. The council also appoints a hospital director to engage in daily management of the hospital. Currently, the Bulgarian National Assembly is in the process of passing a law to privatize small urban hospitals, in order to reduce the number of hospitals and attract greater social capital.

3. Healthcare Resource Allocation

The framework for the planning and distribution of outpatient healthcare facilities is based on the territorial principle of the National Health Map and the district health maps. However, because of the lack of limits on the number of healthcare facilities in each district and the lack of clear stipulations for inpatient care, these healthcare facilities proliferated rapidly over the late 2000s. Investment in national or municipal healthcare facilities comes from the national or municipal share of the facilities' capital. However, there has been a decreasing trend in municipal funding for new investments and maintenance costs for local hospitals. The Ministry of Health has launched several investment projects to further build the healthcare infrastructure, to which healthcare institutions can apply.

The inadequate organization of primary healthcare, uneven geographical distribution of GPs, and the lack of incentives to provide primary and specialist healthcare have all resulted in increases in the utilization of specialist healthcare services and hospitalization rates. The number of acute beds per capita in Bulgaria is higher than the EU27 average, whereas the average length of hospital stay is slightly lower than both the EU27 and EU15 averages. Both of these indicators have shown a decreasing trend.

(1) Capital Stock and Investments

In 2009, there were 306 hospitals in Bulgaria. The Health Care Establishments Act of 1999 defined the types of hospitals according to different criteria and regulated the restructuring of existing public healthcare institutions. In 1999, most hospitals were publicly owned.

In 2008, the Regional Development Law divided the country into six regions: Northwestern, North-central, Northeastern, Southwestern, South-central, and Southwestern (Regional Development Law of 2008; Article 4 Paragraph 3). The Ministry of Health then conducted an analysis to provide support for the development of a concept of hospital system restructuring, which revealed significant regional inequalities in the hospital sector. The main aim of this concept was to ensure equal access to hospital care throughout the country.

More specifically, the analysis revealed that the Southwestern region had the highest number of hospitals (about 109), which were mainly concentrated in the district of Sofia and its capital city. According to the modern standards of medical specialties, the North-central, Northwestern, and Southeastern regions did not have any hospitals meeting the requirements of high technology and high specialization. The situation was even worse in the South-central and Northeastern regions, with the former being the only region without a university hospital.

Hospitals were also reported to show uneven distribution, oversupply of specific healthcare services, underutilization of medical equipment, and duplication of activities. This resulted in the gradual disqualification of staff members, who were unable to provide high-quality services, thereby forcing patients to seek treatment elsewhere. This was particularly evident when local hospitals focused on providing outpatient services to local residents, while also providing services available at district hospitals but at a lower volume and quality.

Before the introduction of the health insurance system, the daily expenses and investments of public healthcare institutions were fully funded by the state budget. At present, the state and municipalities provide subsidies that have been approved by the State Budget Act and the municipal budgets. These subsidies are set aside for the acquisition of long-term tangible assets, maintenance and restructuring costs, information technology and systems, and so on.

With municipal participation, the budget of the Ministry of Health covers the capital costs for state-owned hospitals, which increased from BGN6.1 million (€3.1 million) in 2000 to BGN17.7 million (€9.0 million) in 2009, for a total of BGN115.1 million over 10 years. The bulk of these costs concerned the renovation of hospital buildings and procurement of medical equipment. Since the restructuring of district hospitals in 2000, funds for capital/life cycle/maintenance have mainly been provided by the state. As a rule, the allocation of municipal funding for hospital maintenance is largely symbolic. In the rare instances where municipalities have provided funds for new investment or maintenance, these funds did not have a significant impact on the status of district hospitals. There has also been a persistent downward trend in funding for the investment and maintenance of municipal hospitals. Therefore, it is evident that capital investment has become a problem, and it may need to be prioritized in the health policy agenda.

In 2004, a revolving investment fund was established under the Ministry of Health investment program (i.e., the "Reforming the Health Sector" program), which was funded by a loan agreement between the World Bank and Bulgaria. This fund provides hospitals with interest-free loans to invest in healthcare infrastructure, such as equipment and furnishings. Its main aim is to provide sustainable investments in the healthcare system based on objective needs assessments and adequate planning. To this end, the fund has a transparent selection process with clear criteria, and beneficiaries are closely observed to ensure their compliance and quality. In the first phase of this fund (which ended in October 2007), contracts were signed with 30 healthcare institutions that were allocated about €5 million in funds. Since then, 23 further contracts have been signed (€3.5 million). These funds were integrated into the reimbursement process of each hospital. The Ministry of Health stores detailed information on the equipment purchased by each institution as well as the amounts due.

In addition, state-owned healthcare institutions can apply for funding under the 2007–2013 "Regional Development" operational program, which was approved by the European Commission in 2007. Bulgaria was allocated BGN148 million (€75.7 million), and the funds were received by the Ministry of Health through a program called "Support for reconstruction, renovation and equipping of public health establishments in urban agglomerations." The plan is to spend BGN79.9 million (€40.9 million) on hospitals, and about 20 hospitals from six regions are eligible to apply. Depending on the project, a maximum of BGN5–BGN10 million (€2.5–€5 million) can be spent on repairs, reconstruction, and renovations. The goal is to transform these hospitals into high-tech institutions that can provide highly specialized healthcare services across the country, thereby improving the quality and equality of hospital services as a whole. An additional BGN58 million (€30 million) is to be spent on the modernization of radiological equipment. Indeed, the aforementioned concept of hospital system restructuring (Ministry of Health, 2009) envisions the construction of three radiotherapy centers, which will be funded by this program. If this program is successful, Bulgaria will be eligible to participate in the EU healthcare fund, which amounts to €3 billion as of 2014.

(2) Development Trends in the Healthcare Workforce

Healthcare workers, with the exception of nurses, are abundant in Bulgaria. There is also an upward trend in the number of university-educated healthcare workers. The number of workers in each profession within the healthcare system has varied with the dynamic changes in overall workforce (WHO Regional Office for Europe, Ministry of Health, Adamov et al., 2010).

Compared to the number of specialists, the number of GPs is very low. In Bulgaria, general medicine was only introduced as a specialty in 2001. Before this – in 2000 – internists and pediatricians were given the opportunity to retrain as GPs in order to satisfy the demands of the new health insurance system. Of course, these physicians were originally not trained as GPs, and the implementation of official requirements for training physicians as gatekeepers has been delayed repeatedly. Surveys of beneficiaries indicate a lack of trust in GPs, low uptake of preventive examinations, and a preference for direct contact with specialized services over primary care. Inequalities are important in this context: the total number of GPs is relatively low (0.63 GPs per 1,000 people in 2008, which is lower than the EU average of 0.85) and nearly 17.8% of vacancies in impoverished areas were unfilled (World Bank, 2009). Furthermore, the number of GPs decreased by 8% in 2000–2008. As the average age of GPs is more than 50 years, it is expected that more GPs will retire over the next few years. The decreasing trend in GPs may be partially explained by number of students admitted to medical schools in the 1990s.

Between 1990 and 2000, the ratio of physicians in Bulgaria increased steadily. During this period, this figure was consistently higher than the averages of the EU12, EU15, and EU27 countries, and far higher than those of Romania and Poland, which had the lowest ratios of physicians in the region. In 2009, internists had the highest ratio (2 per 10,000 people), followed by gynecologists and pediatricians (1.8 per 10,000 people) and surgeons (1.6 per 10,000 people). This distribution has remained relatively stable over the past few years.

By contrast, the number of nurses per 1,000 people reduced by half between 1990 and 2002 (from a peak of 6.2 in 1990 to a trough of 3.6 in 2002). Bulgaria has a relatively low ratio of nurses compared to the EU average as well as other countries in the region. Since 2005, there has been a slight increase in the number of nurses. However, the majority of trained nurses seek employment abroad because of their low recognition and remuneration in Bulgaria. This has led to a considerable loss in the nursing workforce. In contrast, the ratio of midwives is higher than the EU27 average; however, this ratio is similarly showing a decreasing trend. In summary, in 2008, the number of physicians in Bulgaria was higher than the EU average, but the number of nurses was among the lowest in the European region.

Bulgaria has always been – and continues to be – the country with the highest ratio of dentists in Europe. Since 1990, this figure has been increasing steadily, peaking at 0.84 per 1,000 people in 2006 and decreasing slightly thereafter. This figure is about 40% higher than the EU12 average and 25% higher than the EU average. This phenomenon can be attributed to the increased admissions of dental students in the 1970s and 1980s, as well as the lack of pricing regulations for dental services in the 1990s (Georgieva et al., 2012). The drastic increase in the number of dentists in 1999 and 2000 is due to a law adopted at the end of 1999, which required dentists to formally register before they begin practicing. Due to the establishment of the Faculty of Dentistry at the Medical University of Varna, it is expected that the number of dentists will continue to increase. On the other hand, there has been a constant decline in the number of dental technicians, leading to a considerably uneven distribution between them and dentists.

The number of pharmacists increased steadily until 1990, and it exceeded the EU12 average for this period (Georgieva et al., 2012). However, this trend inverted in 1990 – between 1990 and 2000, the ratio of pharmacists per 1,000 people decreased from 0.48 to 0.12, respectively, causing Bulgaria to rank among countries with the lowest ratio of pharmacists in the EU. Unfortunately, newer data are not available. The significant decrease in the number of pharmacists and assistant pharmacists may be attributed to the fact that, at this point, only pharmacists who were affiliated with the pharmacist network of healthcare institutions were included in the data. This change in statistical methods renders the figures unreliable and explains why more up-to-date data are not available in the WHO Health for All (HFA) database. The general decrease in numbers may also be partially due to the fact that a large proportion of pharmacists are employed by foreign private pharmaceutical companies, which offer better remuneration and more flexible working hours. It is expected that the establishment of two new Faculties of Pharmacy in Plovdiv and Varna will help to increase the number of pharmacists in the future.

The use of complementary and alternative medicine (CAM) for the improvement of individual health is becoming more widespread in Bulgaria. The Health Act of 2005 legalized alternative treatments, such as homeopathy, acupuncture, acupressure, and other nontraditional methods, along with the use of nonmedicinal products with organic and mineral origins. All CAM providers must register their practice with their respective district centers and disclose their methods of practice. Only graduates with a master's in medicine or dentistry can practice homeopathy. All other CAM providers are allowed to practice after obtaining a bachelor's degree in medicine or after completing four semesters of medical studies and practice. Currently, there are 1,666 individuals with a master's degree in medicine or dentistry who have completed a homeopathy course.

4. Healthcare Funding Mechanism

The healthcare funding mechanism in Bulgaria is currently a mixed public–private healthcare financing system. Healthcare funds are jointly provided by the independent SHI, taxes, out-of-pocket payments, VHI premiums, corporate payments, donations, and external funds. The total healthcare expenditure as a share of the GDP increased from 5.3% in 1995 to 7.3% in 2008. Of the total healthcare expenditure in 2008, 36.5% was from out-of-pocket payments, 34.8% from SHI expenditures, 13.6% from Ministry of Health expenditures, 9.4% from municipal expenditures, and 0.3% from VHI expenditures.

In 2008, the public and private expenditures as shares of the total healthcare expenditure were 57.8% and 42.2%, respectively.

The main purchaser of healthcare services is the NHIF, which was established in 1998. This is the sole agency responsible for social insurance in Bulgaria. SHI contributions are fixed at 8% of the insured person's monthly income, which can also be paid by the employers or the state. The relationship between the NHIF and healthcare providers is based on contracts. The NHIF regularly revises the NFC in cooperation with the professional associations of physicians (and dentists); then, on the basis of this NFC, healthcare providers sign individual contracts with the district branches of the NHIF (i.e., the RHIFs), and are paid on a fee-for-service or capitation basis according to the services provided to the population. Public health services and services provided by national emergency centers, psychiatric hospitals, and children's homes for health and social care are funded by the Ministry of Health.

In 2008, out-of-pocket payments accounted for 86% of personal healthcare expenditures and 36.5% of the total healthcare expenditure. User fees apply to all patients, which include physician (dentist) consultations, laboratory tests, and hospitalization; however, a small minority of patients are exempt, including children, pregnant women, chronically ill patients, unemployed persons, and low-income groups.

VHI is funded by VHICs that are solely intended for voluntary health insurance. In addition to the benefits covered by the NHIF, all citizens are free to purchase different health insurance packages. Additionally, VHICs can also offer basic benefits packages covered by the NHIF. In VHI, the organizational relationships between purchasers and providers are based on integrated and reimbursement models. In 2010, less than 3% of the population had purchased some form of VHI.

(1) Healthcare Expenditure

The total healthcare expenditure as a share of the GDP in Bulgaria is comparable to the average of the European region. This total healthcare expenditure increased significantly between 1996 and 2003, eventually exceeding the EU12 average. It has declined slightly since 2006 and has remained relatively unchanged since. The average annual real growth rate of the total healthcare expenditure is positively correlated with the average annual GDP growth.

The healthcare expenditure per capita (in international purchasing power parity, $PPP) increased rapidly, from US$285 in 1995 to US$910 in 2008. This was due to the strong GDP growth. Furthermore, although the average annual growth rate was 1.1, this was still far lower than the EU average. The EU average for healthcare expenditure per capita in 2000 (US$1,220, $PPP) was three times that of Bulgaria, and two times that of Bulgaria in 2008 (US$1,968, $PPP).

Official statistics indicate that public expenditure as a share of the total healthcare expenditure decreased gradually from 100% during the transition period in 1989–1990 to 57.8% in 2008 (WHO Regional Office for Europe, 2011). This decreasing trend was stable (with occasional fluctuations), thereby reflecting the relative increase in person healthcare expenditure and the growing shortage of public healthcare resources. From an international perspective, Bulgaria's public healthcare expenditure (57.8%) is far lower than the averages of the EU12 (73.0%), EU15 (77.5%), and EU27 (76.6%).

In 2008, therapeutic and rehabilitation services accounted for the largest share of healthcare expenditure (53.6%). This was followed closely by expenditure on medical goods dispensed to outpatients (36.8%). Data from the National Statistical Institute for the same year indicate that 66.9% of public healthcare expenditure is spent on therapeutic and rehabilitation services. Although public health services, preventive care, and health promotion are the primary tasks of all health authorities, these services only account for 4.3% of the total healthcare expenditure. In 2008, the Ministry of Health spent only 1.4% of the total healthcare expenditure on preventive and public health services. In 2008, hospitals absorbed 41.0% of the total healthcare expenditure, followed by retailers (mainly pharmacies) (36.9%) and outpatient service providers (16.7%).

(2) Income Sources and Financial Flows

The main sources of income in the healthcare system include direct payments in the form of out-of-pocket payments, cost-sharing, and VHI premiums. The share of these income sources in the total healthcare expenditure increased from 26.7% in 1995 to 36.5% in 2008. By 2007, they accounted for 96% of all private healthcare expenditures, and was more than 86% in 2008.

Before the implementation of the SHI system, out-of-pocket payments in the healthcare system took the form of direct payments to private healthcare providers. After 2000, these direct payments were expanded to include cost-sharing and payments for services not covered by the NHIF. However, due to the establishment of the private healthcare system, the decentralization of power in public healthcare institutions, and the immaturity of the new SHI system, there was a sharp rise in out-of-pocket payments, which became the main source of income in 2000 (accounting for 40.4% of the total healthcare expenditure). The actual amount of private payments might be understated, as the data on out-of-pocket payments did not include informal payments. We assume that these make up a significant share of out-of-pocket payments.

The SHI represented the second largest source of income for the healthcare system (accounting for 34.8% of the total healthcare expenditure in 2008). The SHI is paid jointly by employees and employers, or individually by self-employed or unemployed individuals. The amount is linked to the income of the insured person. According to the HIA, insured persons must pay premiums based on a percentage of their total income. Self-employed persons must pay the full amount, whereas the contributions of employees are shared between the employer and employee. The dependents of employees and self-employed persons must pay additional premiums to obtain coverage. The premiums of pensioners and civil servants are paid by the state.

The third major source of income is from general taxation, which is nonearmarked revenue allocated to the Ministry of Health budget from the central budget and RHI income. Municipalities can also use local tax revenues to pay for healthcare services. About a quarter of the total tax revenues allocated to healthcare consist of transfers from the central budget to municipalities that are earmarked for healthcare.

(3) Funding Potential of Health Insurance

National tax revenues are no longer used to cover healthcare expenditures, apart from the premiums of pensioners and civil servants (which are covered by the state using social funds). In theory, there are advantages to relying on health insurance premiums rather than taxation: the funds are earmarked, the government does not have the right to use these funds for other purposes, and there is no need to compete with other sectors for financial resources.

Whether the changes in the financing methods of the Bulgarian healthcare system can successfully achieve a balance of income and expenditure will depend on the amount of premium contributions and the proportion of beneficiaries. In accordance with the HIA, Bulgaria's SHI provides universal coverage and its social insurance fund frequently requires government subsidies. The HIA also stipulates that the premiums of pensioners, civil servants, and unemployed persons are paid by the state and municipalities. However, this is an immense sum because of the high unemployment rate and population aging, making it a burden on the state and municipalities. Insufficient or delayed funding carries the risk of undermining the SHI.

Furthermore, the failure to collect premiums from the expected number of insured persons will lead to insufficient funds. In fact, collecting half the expected premiums under the Bulgarian SHI scheme is considered relatively good, which casts doubts on the possibility of achieving future balance of income and expenditure. This risk of imbalanced income and expenditure is further caused by the overly low income per capita of Bulgarians, which in turn results in insufficient premium contributions.

Nonsalaried workers in small private firms or small business owners can also affect premium contributions, as their incomes can be difficult to clarify. A similar issue has been reported in other transitioning countries. During the course of privatization, this category of workers has continued to increase, which has led to decrements in the financial resources of insurance funds, as it is very easy for these workers to avoid paying premiums.

In addition, the Bulgarian SHI stipulates that insurance premiums should be shared between employers and employees, whereby employers are required to contribute a fixed percentage of the employee's income. This has increased the expenditure of employers, who are then reluctant to employ more workers, thus keeping the unemployment rate high.

Employers may also hire informal workers to avoid paying their share of the health insurance premiums. According to a survey by the WHO Regional Office for Europe, the collection of premium contributions reported by the Bulgarian social insurance agency has been deteriorating. Furthermore, while the unemployment rate increased from 11% in 1993 to 16% in 1998, the number of employees remained relatively stable at around 3–3.3 million. This figure is clearly inaccurate, and can be attributed to the underreporting of the number of unemployed persons by private firms or the reporting of informal workers as formal workers. Furthermore, the overall number of informal workers has been increasing.

Therefore, the healthcare system cannot rely on funding from health insurance to guarantee an adequate and stable healthcare budget. The size of the budget must continue to depend on policy preferences and economic enforcement. In addition, economic development and the improvement of the financial system are indispensable conditions for the financial stability of the healthcare system.

5. Characteristics and Direction of Health System Reforms

(1) Reform Experiences and Characteristics

1. Until the end of the 1990s, the Bulgarian healthcare system remained on the periphery of reforms in the public sector. A few reforms were implemented in the early 1990s: (1) laws permitting the existence of private service providers were passed. (2) Medical associations were reestablished. (3) The responsibility for the provision of many healthcare services was transferred to local governments. Further, more radical reforms were

implemented in the late 1990s, including the introduction of an SHI system, in order to develop primary healthcare based on the GP model. This helped to rationalize the healthcare provision network.

2. During periods of economic crisis, reforms were implemented in a stepwise fashion. The reform strategy adopted by the Ministry of Health was based on the following principles: equality, cost-effectiveness, and service quality. In addition, education and training were provided for all healthcare, administrative, and paramedical personnel in the healthcare system. Previously unfamiliar concepts, such as general medicine, health insurance, and health promotion, became more widely accepted.

3. The first step in Bulgarian health reforms was the implementation of the Health Insurance Act of 1998, and the enactment of laws establishing professional organizations for physicians and dentists. Another pillar of these reforms was the Health Care Establishments Act of 1999, which outlined the various structural changes in the healthcare system. These laws laid the foundation for future reforms in the funding and service scope of the healthcare system.

4. These reforms have undoubtedly achieved some success. For instance, they have succeeded in substantially reducing the number of hospital beds, thereby reducing costs. This trend will most likely continue in the foreseeable future. In addition, the new insurance-based financial system is expected to increase efficiency, while also helping the fundraising efforts of the healthcare sector.

5. Patients are allowed to choose their GPs (family doctors). This feature of the reform was met with approval from patients. However, the strict enforcement of referrals for higher-level services has encountered some resistance, as it limits patients' choices. While consumers' right to choose their services has been extended through the expansion of private service providers, the introduction of formal copayments for medical expenses has affected the equality of services, especially for vulnerable groups. This is because these groups might not be covered by insurance and therefore might be excluded.

In the early 1990s, the Bulgarian health reforms had two main goals. The first was to improve population health, and the second was to establish a democratic and market-oriented healthcare system that could successfully meet the needs of Bulgarians. After 20 years, these goals have not yet been achieved. Hence, the need for healthcare system reform has become even more urgent. Improvements in the population health status are not satisfactory, and the main population health indicators are still far below the EU averages. Moreover, the general public and healthcare professionals are both dissatisfied with the healthcare system. In addition, the principles established by the new healthcare system have not been recognized. Although healthcare expenditure has increased threefold since the introduction of the SHI, there is still a shortage of financial resources, poor population health, and severe inequalities at all levels of the system.

The Bulgarian people are currently experiencing financial insecurity and the uneven distribution of financial burden. Maintaining equality within the Bulgarian health security system is a challenge, as it not only involves meeting wildly different healthcare needs, but also addressing socioeconomic gaps and geographical imbalances in the system. Currently, there are significant disparities in the quality and accessibility of healthcare services among different regions. Poverty is a serious barrier to the accessibility of health security, especially in a system so heavily dependent on formal and informal payments.

As with the healthcare systems of other EU countries, the Bulgarian system is characterized by limited centralization. This system gradually took shape under market conditions along with significant intervention by national health authorities. Material and financial resources coexist in the form of public and private ownership in Bulgaria.

At the district level, regional, subregional, and municipal authorities influence the administration of healthcare resources and organizations. Healthcare providers and professional associations are autonomous. There are multiple funding sources for the healthcare system, namely, health insurance funds, national and local budgets, and out-of-pocket payments. Market mechanisms are applied regardless of the ownership form. The healthcare needs of the population are covered through mandatory health insurance.

Although the Bulgarian healthcare system has the characteristics of a democratic, liberalized, and market-oriented system, it continues to show many weaknesses, which have led to an unsatisfactory population health status. Furthermore, there are health status inequalities between the urban and rural populations, and inequalities in the accessibility of the healthcare system have continued to grow throughout the reform process. The improvement rate of the population health status, as reflected by certain health indicators, does not yet meet reform goals.

In addition, the Bulgarian healthcare system is economically unstable. Healthcare institutions, especially hospitals, are faced with insufficient funding, and there is currently a lack of a transparent regulatory system for pricing. Hence, prices are determined not based on actual costs but on the available funds in the NHIF budget. Due to the NHIF's monopoly, market mechanisms do not play a role in public insurance, even though this is one of the major goals of the overall healthcare system. As of today, a large number of people are still not covered by statutory health insurance, and the VHI market requires further development.

(2) Problems with the Reforms

1. Decline in Population Health Status   Since its economic transition, Bulgaria has experienced economic recession and rising unemployment, which have led to a deterioration in population health. In particular, there have been increases in the incidence of infectious diseases; serious cases of neonatal diseases that have led to a mortality rate of 16%; and severe issues with tuberculosis, AIDS, and sexually transmitted diseases. Moreover, chronic noncommunicable diseases also have a major impact on the lives of the population.

2. Relative Surplus of Healthcare Resources and Funding Difficulties   Bulgaria has a surplus of healthcare resources, including healthcare institutions, hospital beds, and physicians. The government is currently adopting laws to adjust and suppress some of these resources. At the same time, because of the constraints of economic development, it is unlikely that the government will substantially increase its healthcare investment in the short term. This will likely have a significant impact on increasing health insurance funding and lead to the gradual expansion of the share of health insurance funds in healthcare expenditure.

3. Slow Pace of Reforms in the Public Hospital System   Bulgaria began reforming the healthcare system after its economic transition. One major reform was that the provision of general outpatient services was essentially transferred to private GPs. Although the corporate reforms of public hospitals began in 2000, based on our current understanding of the situation, there has been no substantial change in the daily operations and management of public hospitals.

(3) Future Reform Directions

According to the NHCS Action Plan, the 9 major goals of the Bulgarian development strategy for health reforms in 2008–2013 are:

1. In terms of public health, implement a set of national targeted programs focusing on the treatment and prevention of socially important diseases; increase public awareness of healthy lifestyles; improve the public health protection network; and guarantee the conditions for health promotion and prevention.
2. Guarantee the provision of higher-quality and accessible healthcare services.
3. Improve outpatient healthcare services.
4. Restructure hospital management and improve efficiency.
5. Comprehensively establish strict controls over drug quality, safety, and efficacy, and ensure the balanced supply of pharmaceutical and medical goods.
6. Comprehensively improve the educational quality of administrative personnel, improve the curriculum, and develop human resources.
7. Create an integrated system for the electronic exchange of healthcare data.
8. Increase public funding in healthcare, improve the public's awareness of VHI, and ensure the financial stability of the national healthcare system.
9. Participate in the activities of EU institutions and effectively absorb the EU Structural Funds, in order to achieve EU accession.

Although most of the goals related to quality improvement and hospital restructuring in the NHCS Action Plan had to be implemented by 2011, many of them were not achieved (e.g., establishing a patient safety system in compliance with European practice, linking accreditation assessment with payments, and expanding the network of long-term care and rehabilitation institutions).

A few amendments to the HIA are currently being prepared, which are intended to allow general insurance companies to offer VHI. This would abolish the requirement that VHI can only be provided by companies solely intended to offer this form of insurance (i.e., VHICs). Furthermore, insurance that can only cover specific risks might replace VHI (thereby enabling coverage of preventive activities along with other benefit packages). These proposed amendments were based on EU requirements. However, the Association of VHICs does not support these amendments, mainly because they do not allow VHICs to provide benefit packages, especially those for therapeutic and preventive care. Therefore, substantial changes to the current VHI system are still required.

At the end of 2010, the Minister of Health announced in an interview that from 2012, the clinical pathways will be replaced by DRGs as tools for hospital payments. Other announcements in early 2011 revealed that the application of electronic health records has been delayed, and that an integrated system for electronic data exchange will only be built in 2020.

Although there remain some uncertainties as to which specific changes to the healthcare system will actually be made, the ultimate goals of this system's future development are clear. The Biennial Collaborative Agreement between the Bulgarian Ministry of Health and the WHO Regional Office for Europe 2010/2011 lists the main priorities of future development. The medium-term priorities for collaboration in 2008–2013 are: (1) improve the organization, leadership, and management of the healthcare system and service provision (including crisis preparedness). (2) Reduce the health-related, social, and economic burden of infection diseases. (3) Enhance the health promotion and prevention of noncommunicable diseases. (4) Improve the surveillance and monitoring systems for environmental and food safety. (5) Reduce the health consequences of emergencies, disasters, crises, and conflicts, while also minimizing their social and economic impacts.

CHAPTER TWENTY ONE

Health Systems in Four American Countries

 SECTION I. THE HEALTH SYSTEM IN BRAZIL

1. Overview of Socioeconomics and National Health

(1) Basic National Conditions

Brazil, officially the Federative Republic of Brazil, declared its independence on September 7, 1822. It is the largest country in Latin America and the fifth most populous country in the world. Brazil is located along the eastern coast of Central and South America and is bounded by the Atlantic Ocean. It is the fifth-largest country in terms of land area, after Russia, Canada, China, and the US. It shares a border with Uruguay, Argentina, Paraguay, Bolivia, Peru, Colombia, Venezuela, Guyana, Suriname, and French Guiana. Brazil has vast areas of farmlands and rain forests. Because of its abundant natural resources and ample labor force, Brazil's GDP is ranked first in South America and tenth worldwide. It is a member of the Union of South American Nations. Historically, Brazil was a colony of Portugal, and its official language remains Portuguese. Brazil abolished slavery on May 13, 1888. On December 26, 2011, a think tank called the UK Center for Economics and Business Research announced the latest annual ranking of global economies, which revealed that Brazil had overtaken the UK, becoming the world's sixth largest economy.

In 2012, Brazil's total population was 198 million. Brazil has two main types of terrain: (1) highlands, which are more than 500 m above sea level and primarily distributed in the south; and (2) plains, which are less than 200 m above sea level and are distributed in the Amazon Basin in the north and west. The southeast region is the most populous region in Brazil; according to 2004 data from the Instituto Brasileiro de Geografia e Estatística (IBGE), this region has a population of more than 78 million, which is equivalent to 42% of the total population of Brazil.

Brazil is divided into 26 states and 1 federal district (the federal capital of Brasilia), which are further divided into 5,562 municipalities. Brasilia is located in the central Brazilian highlands. It was constructed in the late 1950s on a plateau at approximately 1000 m above sea level in the Goiás state of the Brazilian mainland, making it a capital city with one of the highest altitudes in the world. Brazil's industry is ranked first in Latin America. Its agricultural industry is particularly well-developed, and has given it the name the "World's 21st Century Breadbasket." It has a free market and an export-oriented economy. It is currently the world's seventh-largest economy and the second largest economy in the Americas. According to recent statistics by the World Bank, Brazil's GDP in 2012 was US$2.253 trillion. Brazil, together with China, India, Russia, and South Africa, form the BRICS countries. Brazil's socioeconomic development and population structure are very similar those of China. Hence, Brazil's reform measures and experiences in healthcare are valuable lessons for China's own health reforms.

(2) Healthcare System

Brazil's healthcare system is similar to the Nordic universal health system. The system was first established in the 1950s and has gradually developed since. Major changes occurred in Brazil's health security system around 1988 – specifically, the 1988 constitution enshrined health as a citizens' right and required the state to provide broad and equal access to healthcare services. In 1990, the Unified Health System (*Sistema Único de Saúde* [SUS]) was formally established to implement free universal healthcare. The SUS comprises all public health stations, hospitals, university hospitals, laboratories, pharmaceutical factories, blood banks, medical research institutions, and private healthcare institutions employed by Brazil's public health administration, and it comes under the unified leadership of the Federal Ministry of Health, State Health Secretariats, and municipal health departments. In this system, the responsibility for protecting citizens' health is shared among the federal, state, and municipal governments, with a particular emphasis on the role of municipal governments in healthcare management. The SUS covers 70% of the population, giving them access to free primary healthcare services. Besides surgical costs, all medical expenses are almost completely free. Hospitals even cover meal expenses for inpatients and the parents of hospitalized children. The procedures involved in seeking medical attention are uncomplicated. In general, patients initially visit the outpatient clinics of community hospitals, and may be referred to general or specialist hospitals by the community physician if they are found to have more serious conditions.

In addition to the SUS, Brazil has a subsystem known as the Supplementary Health System, which includes certain self-funded private healthcare institutions and private health insurance companies. Collectively, this system covers 25–30% of the population in Brazil. Compared to public hospitals, private healthcare institutions provide better medical equipment, healthcare workers, and health services. The full development of private healthcare institutions has enabled the diversification of Brazil's overall healthcare system, thereby presenting the population with greater choice.

According to data from the World Bank's official website in 2014 and the WHO's World Health Statistics 2013, Brazil has a higher birth rate (15.2% in 2011) and total fertility rate (1.8 births per woman) than does China; however, its mortality rate (6.2%) is slightly lower. Although the mortality rate of the overall population is relatively low, Brazil's infant and under-five mortality rates are still fairly high. Nevertheless, there has been a significant decrease in infant mortality rates compared to 1990. Specifically, in 1990, the infant mortality rate was 49 per 1,000 live births, which decreased to 14 per 1,000 live births in 2011 and then to 13.5 per 1,000 live births in 2013 (based on World Bank data); similarly, the under-five mortality rate decreased from 58% in 1990 to 16 in 2011%, and later to 12.3% in 2014.

In 2011, the average life expectancy of Brazilians was 74 years, which was seven years higher than that in 1990 and roughly similar to that in China. Brazil's overall population health status is approaching the level of moderately developed countries. Furthermore, in 2011, the incidence of elevated fasting blood glucose among adults aged over 25 years was 0.4% in males and 10% in females. Furthermore, the incidence of elevated blood pressure in males and females was 39.4% and 26.6%, respectively, and these rates were lower than were those in countries with similar income levels (Table 21.1).

Brazil places a great emphasis on disease prevention and maternal and child health, with the aim of reducing disease incidence and improving population health. The Ministry of Health has formulated a schedule for the types and doses of vaccinations required for children aged 1–10 years, adolescents aged 11–19 years, adults aged over 20 years, and elderly persons aged over 60 years. In fact, reporters of China's Xinhua News Agency found through interviews that every health station in Brazil had full-time staff in charge of vaccinations. According to the World Health Statistics 2013, in 2005–2012, Brazil's immunization coverage among one-year-olds was consistently above 95%.

As for Brazil's health infrastructure and resources, 89% of the population has access to the water supply system in Brazil (urban areas: 96%, rural areas: 58%) and 75% have access to sanitary toilets (urban areas: 83%, rural areas: 35%). As is evident, there are vast differences in health infrastructure between urban and rural areas in Brazil, implying that infectious diseases remain a major health risk among the Brazilian population. In addition, the percentage of the population that utilizes improved sanitation facilities increased from 67% in 1990 to 81% in 2010. Moreover, the number of physicians per 10,000 people was 17.6 and the number of hospital beds was 23. In 2010, government healthcare expenditure as a share of the total government expenditure was 10.7%, while the total healthcare expenditure as a share of the GDP was 9.0% (representing an increase of 2% compared to 2000). Government expenditure accounted for 47.0% of the total healthcare expenditure (an increase of 7% compared to 2000). Despite the government's substantial financial investments in the healthcare sector, government investment in public hospitals remains insufficient because of rising healthcare demand among the public. Thus, public hospitals have relatively poor environmental conditions, as well as long waiting times. In response,

TABLE 21.1 Comparison of Population Health Indicators Between Brazil and China

Indicator	1990	2011	
		Brazil	China
Birth rate (%)	—	15.2	11.93
Total fertility rate (%)	—	1.8	1.18 (2010)
Mortality rate (%)	—	6.2	7.14
Infant mortality rate (per 1,000 live births)	49	14	12.1
Under-five mortality rate (per 1,000 live births)	58	16	15.6
Life expectancy (years)	67	74	75

Sources: WHO World Health Statistics 2013; China 2012 Health Statistics Yearbook; data from the Sixth National Population Census of China; and World Bank database (http://data.worldbank.org.cn/country/brazil).

the government has been encouraging the private sector to establish healthcare institutions. This, coupled with the inability of public hospitals to satisfy the healthcare demands of the public, has caused private healthcare institutions to emerge rapidly in large numbers. The medical environment, medical equipment, service efficiency, technological level, and service quality of most private healthcare institutions are significantly superior to those of public hospitals. Therefore, high-income individuals tend to purchase commercial health insurance on top of their basic healthcare coverage, in order to seek medical attention from private healthcare institutions with better conditions in all respects.

2. Healthcare System

The healthcare delivery system in Brazil is composed of two major systems: the SUS and the Supplementary Health System. The SUS mainly includes government-run healthcare institutions, whereas the Supplementary Health System mainly includes private hospitals, clinics, private insurance, etc. The latter system is considered a necessary supplement to the public system.

(1) Evolution of the Healthcare System

Before the twentieth century, Brazil primarily concentrated on the control of infectious diseases, with a focus on solving the issues of potable water and sewage treatment, while also promoting trade development in coastal areas such as Rio de Janeiro. During this period, healthcare work was subservient to the goal of economic development. After the 1930s, Brazil began placing greater emphasis on public health, entering a phase of healthcare development centered on prevention. During this period, the worker's labor movement led to the promulgation and adoption of the Labor Code, which laid the foundation for protecting labor rights and gradually led to the establishment of health, pension, and maternity insurance.

From the 1920s to the 1960s, each industry began establishing its own hospitals, clinics, and other healthcare institutions to serve workers within the specific industry. Additionally, the government established public hospitals that provided services to farmers and impoverished individuals without insurance. The result was that employees of the formal sector, such as civil servants, workers, and bank employees, had both health and pension insurance. However, farmers and unemployed persons were excluded from the social security system, and thus could only rely on extremely limited, low-level services provided by the public health system. This led to a dual health security system, which remained in place until the end of the military dictatorship in 1988. A major consequence of this divided healthcare system is that although all Brazilians have, by law, the right to access free healthcare services provided by public healthcare institutions, severe shortages in government healthcare funds has impaired the accessibility of rural areas and impoverished groups to healthcare services. There are also serious inequalities in the healthcare services provided. In general, the fragmented healthcare system has led to considerable inefficiency in the system and poor health outcomes. An assessment by the WHO in 2000 revealed that although Brazil was ranked 54th in total healthcare expenditure per capita (estimated based on purchasing power) (China: 139th), it was ranked only 125th in terms of the overall performance of its healthcare system was ranked 125th (China: 144th), 112th in terms of health outcomes (China: 82nd), and 130th in terms of responsiveness (China: 88th). Furthermore, the equality of healthcare financing was the third lowest in the world.

Since the end of the 1980s, the strong democratic movement and promotion of the national health conferences in Brazil has led to the proposal of major reform concepts such as universal coverage, equality, continuity, and unification. Accordingly, health system reforms were implemented based on a strategy of decentralization – such that services have come to be mainly provided by state and municipal governments – leading to the creation of the SUS. With respect to these reforms, a WHO official based in Brazil, Prof. Julio Suarez, stated that after the military government stepped down, Brazil has made significant progress in the construction of its health system. The country's uniqueness lies in the fact that it did not follow the World Bank's recommendation for establishing a system based on social health insurance. Instead, Brazil formed a public service system funded by general taxation and centered on primary healthcare. This is the main feature that distinguishes Brazil from most other Latin American countries.

(2) Unified Health System (Sistema Único de Saúde, SUS)

Although it has a relatively unique financing system, the SUS is primarily funded via general taxation. The public service system mainly revolves around primary healthcare. Based on the concept of health equality, the ideological basis of the SUS is that all citizens have the equal right to health, meaning that every Brazilian has the right to access free healthcare services. These services are provided by all healthcare institutions in the health system. The implementation of the SUS has drastically reduced Brazil's infant mortality rate, controlled the spread of various infectious diseases and epidemics, and improved the overall health status of Brazilians.

1. Basic Concepts and Principles of the SUS In 1986, to address inequalities in the healthcare sector, the Brazilian government incorporated the SUS into its new Constitution, ensuring that it is the responsibility of all government levels to protect the health rights of citizens. The Constitution clearly stipulates the basic concepts and principles of the SUS: (1) healthcare for all. Every Brazilian citizen, regardless of race, region, religious beliefs, or socioeconomic status, is entitled to free healthcare from all levels of government-run healthcare institutions. (2) Everyone is equal before the SUS and shall be treated as needed, while acknowledging that different regions and groups (e.g., women, indigenous peoples, elderly individuals) have special healthcare needs; healthcare services shall thus be adapted according to local conditions and individual needs. (3) The SUS emphasizes comprehensive and systematic healthcare services, as well as the integration of prevention and treatment, thus unifying medical care, prevention, and health education. (4) The SUS emphasizes the organizational principles of "hierarchical management," "decentralization," and "social participation"; the functions and responsibilities of the federal, state, and municipal governments shall thus be clearly defined, and residents shall participate in the administration of the SUS management councils in their respective regions.

2. Organization and Management of the SUS In accordance with the provisions of the new Constitution, Brazil conducted extensive consultations with various parties and subsequently formulated two federal laws (which are equivalent to detailed implementation rules): Lei 8080/90 and Lei 8142/90. Lei 8080/90 sets forth strict stipulations on the specific contents for the organization and management of the SUS, as well as delegates authority over hospital management and clinical diagnosis and treatment to the primary level. Lei 8142/90 outlines strict stipulations on the funding sources and funding use of the SUS, as well as regulations for the fees charged by private healthcare institutions.

(3) Healthcare Network

Brazil's health administration system utilizes a vertical management approach and consists of three levels: community, municipal, and state. According to the statistics, Brazil currently has nearly 6,000 public hospitals and approximately 800,000 healthcare workers, while the number of patients discharged each year is about 12 million. Among the hospitals in Brazil, 73% are public and 27% are private. Of the latter, 22.7% are charitable hospitals run by public welfare organizations (e.g., churches), while the remaining are for-profit hospitals, a small proportion (about 200) of which are run by trade unions and foundations. The SUS collectively has 376,000 hospital beds, which account for 75.5% of all hospital beds in the country.

1. Composition of the Healthcare Network   The Brazilian healthcare network is composed of two major subsystems: (1) government-run healthcare institutions under the SUS; and (2) private hospitals and clinics under the Supplementary Health System. The government-run institutions are divided into three levels: community healthcare institutions, small hospitals, and large hospitals and institutions involved in public health (e.g., laboratories, pharmaceutical factories, blood banks, medical research institutions). These institutions are administered by the municipal health departments, State Health Secretariats, and Ministry of Health, respectively.

Community healthcare institutions form the foundation of the SUS. When residents fall ill, they must first seek medical attention from community health stations and will only be referred to higher-tier hospitals with better equipment and medical care if they cannot be treated by the physicians at the health station. The main responsibilities and functions of community health stations include (1) outpatient, emergency, and first consultation services; treatment of common and frequently occurring illnesses; and follow-up treatment and drug dispensation for chronic diseases in the elderly; (2) referral services and clinical observation. Patients with more serious conditions are reported in a timely manner to the municipal referral centers, which then arrange for the patients to receive medical attention from higher-tier hospitals. Patients who are temporarily unable to be transferred will remain at the community health station for clinical observation and treatment. (3) Public health and preventive services. Community health stations are staffed by full-time workers who administer vaccinations to children aged 0–10 years, adolescents aged 11–19 years, adults aged over 20 years, and elderly individuals aged over 60 years according to the regulations of the Brazilian Ministry of Health. Health stations are also engaged in the prevention and control of infectious diseases and perform follow-up treatment for certain major infectious diseases (e.g., AIDS, tuberculosis). (4) Maternal and child health services. These services include registration and prenatal checkups for pregnant women, childbirth and neonatal care, postnatal visits, etc. (5) Health education, disease rehabilitation, etc. The population served by Brazil's community healthcare institutions is generally on the scale of tens of thousands, with hundreds of patients being seen each day. Hence, these institutions undertake a considerable number of healthcare tasks.

Public hospitals are the pillars of the SUS. Their main responsibilities and functions are to: (1) admit patients referred from the community health stations or lower-tier hospitals who require hospitalization or surgical treatment, and provide emergency and rescue services (including major surgeries for organ transplantation, cancer, heart disease, and congenital defects). (2) Undertake national medical research. Public hospitals are equipped with large medical equipment (e.g., CT and MRI scanners), intensive care units, coronary care units, and central laboratories. Hence, much of Brazil's medical research and clinical experiments are conducted in public hospitals. (3) Undertake teaching and continuing education. The Brazilian government has stipulated that all medical students must complete their internships at public hospitals as medical residents upon graduation.

Care services are also provided by a large number of private hospitals and private healthcare institutions. These institutions have excellent medical environments and equipment, more meticulous technical services and consultations, and practitioners of greater skill. However, they also cost a considerable amount more to visit. Healthcare institutions run by various charitable organizations and churches also continue to play a key role in the SUS. The government has designated many of these hospitals as SUS healthcare institutions (based on a government evaluation). This entitles them to receive equipment and a certain amount of financial subsidies from the government, while also approving them to provide free healthcare services to a portion of the population. Private hospitals and clinics are an effective supplement to the public healthcare system. The government has conducted evaluations on many of these hospitals and designated them as SUS healthcare institutions. This entitles them to receive equipment, devices, and a certain number of financial subsidies from the government, while also approving them to provide free healthcare services to part of the Brazilian population.

2. Referral System of Public Healthcare Institutions In Brazil, patients must follow a strict procedure when seeking medical attention, which is characterized by two-way referrals based on the patients' conditions. Every city in Brazil has a dedicated referral office, which is primarily responsible for monitoring the daily use of resources (e.g., hospital beds) of each hospital and utilizing this information to direct the treatment process of patients in each healthcare institution in the city.

Patients must visit community healthcare institutions for their first consultation by booking an appointment. The community healthcare institutions then determine whether patients will remain at that institution or be transferred based on patients' conditions. If a patient must be transferred to a hospital for treatment, the community healthcare institution will contact the referral office directly, which in turn will contact and arrange for the transfer to a suitable hospital. After the patient has been transferred, if the large hospital believes that the patient does not meet the criteria for a critical illness and can be treated in a small hospital or community healthcare institution, then it will refer the patient back to the appropriate level of healthcare institution. In Hospital São Paulo and among surgical patients nationwide, the average length of hospital stay is eight days. After their stay, patients tend to be referred back to small hospitals and community healthcare institutions, and eventually to their homes (where they remain until they are fully recovered). The Brazilian government has provided excellent conditions for the functioning of this referral system. Communities are equipped with ambulances, which can be used to transfer patients to higher-tier hospitals specified by the referral office. As for critically ill patients, higher-tier hospitals will send physicians, nurses, and ambulances to pick up patients from the community. This significantly reduces the pressure on large hospitals because patients are kept within the community. Many hospitals also arrange for physicians to manage patients within the community, in order to decrease the length of hospital stay. For example, many diabetic patients visit the hospital to determine their treatment plans and are then allowed to return to their respective communities, where physicians regularly monitor their treatment. The strict procedures and referral system have enabled the full and rational utilization of Brazil's healthcare resources.

(4) Essential Medicines System

Brazil defines essential medicines as drugs that are vital and indispensable. The acquisition of essential medicines in Brazil is guaranteed by strong legislative protection, which aims to satisfy most of the population's health needs and to ensure the sustainable access of essential medicines for everyone.

1. Essential Medicines Policies   Although Brazil's SUS does not have explicit essential medicines policies, the measures that have been adopted in practice essentially adhere to the principles of essential medicine policies: purchasing generic drugs instead of patented drugs where possible, and limiting the number of drug types in secondary hospitals to fewer than 300. The procurement of drugs is mainly determined by the self-governing municipal health departments, although the procurement of expensive drugs must be approved by the state government. Brazil has a long-term essential medicines program. In 1970, the federal government established the Brazilian Drug Office (*Central de Medicamentos* [CEME]) to supply these drugs. Seventeen public pharmaceutical factories were opened to supply drugs for strategic public health programs. In 1986, after the establishment of the SUS, supplementary legislations were designed to assign the responsibility of drug provision to this system.

The National Drug Policy of 1998 enabled the free provision of essential medicines through the public health system.

2. Drug Administration Model   The National Health Surveillance Agency (Agência Nacional de Vigilância Sanitária, ANVISA) is responsible for supervising the production and circulation of drugs. The health administrations subordinate to the Ministry of Health, the health councils at all administrative levels, and private insurance agencies are responsible for supervising and managing the corresponding medical activities within their jurisdictions. No healthcare institution is permitted to provide discriminatory services or to refuse medical treatment without reason; otherwise, they are penalized by the health councils and other regulatory authorities.

3. Status of Rural and Primary Healthcare

(1) Basic Status

The proportion of population who live in rural areas in Brazil is less than 20%. This figure is even lower in developed areas in the south and southeast regions; the rural population accounts for only 6% of the total population in the Greater São Paulo area. Given the relatively small rural population, the government has not established healthcare networks in rural areas due to cost considerations. However, the issue of healthcare among the Brazilian rural population is not very serious. Investigations of economic affordability have revealed that due to the long-term implementation of private land ownership, the market economy, and the farm management system, farm owners are wealthier than are most urban residents, and hence have stronger economic affordability. Moreover, a considerable proportion of farm owners also have residences and businesses in cities, which enable them to access more convenient healthcare services. The healthcare conditions of farm workers are slightly poorer; however, each family owns at least one car and the nearest city is usually within one- to two–hours' drive, and thus should not pose any serious problems. Therefore, theoretically, Brazilian farmers should not face any problems in affording healthcare or in general face issues related to disease-induced poverty. Nevertheless, because of the inability of public healthcare services to meet demands, coupled with farmers' poorer awareness of disease prevention, a significant proportion of farmers do not receive good preventive healthcare services or timely treatment. This is especially the case for farmers living in remote areas, where the shortage of medical care and drugs is a prominent issue.

(2) Family Health Program and Regionalization Program

To better satisfy the medical and healthcare needs of farmers and the urban poor, as well as protect the health rights of these groups, federal and state governments have established a series of programs. Among them, the Family Health Program and Regionalization Program are two of the most important programs established by the federal government, the former of which has also received loan support from the World Bank.

1. Family Health Program (FHP) This program was established in 1994 by the federal government, and mainly targets the weaker areas of primary healthcare, maternal and child health, and disease control. The FHP represents a shift from the previous individualistic, passive, fragmented, treatment-based, and hospital-centered healthcare delivery model, replacing it with a family- and community-centered, continuous, and integrated primary healthcare system. In practice, the FHP involves forming family health teams that target different population areas. These teams are responsible for creating primary healthcare files for each family within their respective areas, analyzing the health risk factors in those areas, and identifying potentially vulnerable families and individuals. They also collaborate with community workers to conduct educational and preventive activities. Each team consists of at least 1 physician (a GP or family health physician), one nurse, one nurse aide, and four- to six community health advocates (CHAs). CHAs are community-dwelling, primary-level workers who are responsible for conducting family registration and home visits at least once a month within their areas; performing physical checkups for children under the age of two; ensuring the immunization and enrollment of school-age children; performing health education, advocacy, and guidance; maintaining environmental health, and so on. Each family health team generally serves 600–1,000 families, although they can serve up to 4,500 families. The FHP has developed rapidly since its inception. By 2000, nearly 3,059 municipalities (the tertiary-level administrative division; villages also fall within the jurisdiction of municipalities) from all states were participating in the program. At that time, there were 10,025 family health teams, each of which served about 3,450 individuals, thus covering approximately 37.9 million people in Brazil (i.e., 23% of the population). Currently, about 50% of the population is covered by the FHP. This rapid development is inextricably linked with the support of earmarked funds by the federal and state governments.

In addition to CHAs, each team received financial support from the federal government worth R$28,000. After 1999, the entire team (including CHAs) received an average of R$54,000 per year; teams that served larger populations could receive more funding. Newly established teams can receive an additional R$10,000 as starting funds. Physicians and nurses in these teams have higher salaries than do workers of the same categories in other public healthcare institutions. Since the implementation of the FHP, Brazilians have experienced significant improvements in their accessibility to healthcare services, such as prenatal and child healthcare, prevention of hypertension and cancer, etc.; currently, nearly all services are accessible by over 90% of the population.

2. Regional Management Program (RMP) The RMP is another major program initiated by the federal government, the purpose of which is to encourage physicians to serve in remote areas, such as the north, northeast, and central regions. Physicians who set up private practices in these areas will receive more registration fee subsidies from the government. More specifically, the standard registration fee subsidy for private practices in developed areas is US$4 per visit, whereas that in inland areas is US$5 per visit. Furthermore, the government guarantees that every RMP physician will receive a monthly salary of R$4,000–R%5,000, which is double the salaries of physicians in public healthcare institutions in developed urban areas. All RMP physicians are required to be GPs and must be selected by the government. As there is currently a shortage of GPs, the selection process is relatively challenging in practice.

3. Health Insurance System in Rural Brazil The Brazilian health insurance system was established in the 1920s; since, it has gradually evolved into a universal health insurance system covering all urban and rural residents nationwide. A key feature of the Brazilian health insurance system is that all citizens, both rich and poor, have the right to health security. Besides its broad coverage, the system has shown rapid development and high levels of benefits, placing it at the forefront of developing countries.

1. *Management of insurance system and provision of healthcare services.* The Brazilian health insurance industry is administered by the Ministry of Social Security, which has a National Health Insurance Council that operates its own healthcare insurance institutions. Insurance hospitals are divided into three tiers: tertiary, secondary, and primary. In addition to self-operated insurance healthcare institutions, the Council contracts with private hospitals and physicians. Patients who fall ill must first seek medical attention from primary healthcare institutions and can only be referred to secondary or tertiary institutions with the consent of physicians at the primary healthcare institutions. Patients who seek medical attention from hospitals or physicians without referrals must bear all costs at their own expense.
2. *Financing and payment of health insurance funds.* The rural health insurance funds in Brazil are financed via insurance premiums collected in the form of tax surcharges, together with appropriate subsidies from the National Treasury. As for the premiums of enterprise employees, the employees themselves contribute 8.5%–10% of their salary, while the employer contributes 17.5%. National taxes and government subsidies account for about 22% of the total insurance funds. Centralized collection and decentralized lump-sum utilization are implemented for health insurance funds; that is, the central Ministry of Social Security raises funds through banks and the National Treasury. After a review and a comprehensive balancing process by the Ministry, the funds are allocated to the states according to the actual medical needs of each state and region (based on the number of patient visits). The funds are then allocated by the states based on their respective budgets, with the approval of the state governor.

4. Health Insurance System and Financing

(1) SUS and Private Health Insurance System

Presently, Brazil's SUS covers 75.0% of all residents. Public healthcare institutions provide free treatments to patients and do not charge any medical fees. Furthermore, inpatients are entitled to three meals a day for free. All hospital expenses are paid by the government, and are determined using a DRG-like management method based on the hospital's workload and the cost of each DRG.

The private health insurance system covers 25%–30% of the Brazilian population. According to statistics by the Association of Private Health Insurance Companies, approximately 45–50 million people have purchased some form of private health insurance. Most are employees in the industrial and service sectors, for whom the companies collectively manage their health insurance. Some households or individuals contract directly with insurance companies to receive private health services or to ensure dual insurance coverage. Insurance companies determine the prices of services according to the insured amount and the contract with the private hospitals. The factors considered are: (1) the larger the number of insured persons included in the contracts with the hospitals, the cheaper the unit price of services. (2) Varying prices are charged for insured persons of different ages and genders; specifically, the contract prices of elderly individuals and women are higher. (3) Different prices are charged for different treatment measures and methods, and for different service contents. For example, the costs of specific surgeries and disease types must be negotiated with the insurance company.

(2) Financing

1. Financing Methods   The SUS is financed via public funds that are jointly raised by the three levels of government (national, state, and municipal). Brazil is the only South American country that uses a healthcare financing system based on general taxation. General taxation includes corporate income tax, business tax, consumption tax, social insurance tax, etc. The Constitution of Brazil requires the federal government to allocate 1%–2% of the GDP to healthcare expenses; in addition, healthcare expenses should account for no less than 15%, 12%, and 15% of the federal, state, and municipal budgets, respectively. The government healthcare expenditure in Brazil accounts for more than half of its total healthcare expenditure. However, due to imbalances in economic development among the states, the governments of 17 states (i.e., more than half of all states) are unable to afford the prescribed percentage of healthcare expenditure.

In 1967, Brazil created the National Institute of Social Security (Instituto Nacional de Previdência Social [INPS]), which was charged with administering employee health insurance. After 1988, this function was separated from the Ministry of Social Security and incorporated into the SUS. Brazil's private health insurance operates in a market-oriented manner, whereby premiums are collected based on disease risk and coverage is focused on services that are not included in the SUS. Thus, it is a useful supplement to the free public healthcare system. Brazil has 1,325 private health insurance companies, which cover more than 35 million individuals and receive a total annual premium income of about US$19 billion. Presently, the coverage rate of private health insurance is 19.7%; more specifically, the coverage rate in economically developed areas is 31%, whereas that of less developed areas is only 7%. However, since the service capacities of private hospitals are insufficient to meet demand, 46% of individuals enrolled in private health insurance still visit public hospitals for medical attention.

2. Historical Evolution   As with the UK and Sweden, Brazil's health insurance financing has progressed from occupation-based taxation to a national taxation mechanism based on general taxes. In the 1830s, the government introduced employer-based (i.e., occupation-based) health insurance for formal sector employees, civil servants, and semi-governmental employees. To fund this insurance, a social security fund based on general taxation was created, namely, the National Institute of Medical Assistance of Social Security (Instituto Nacional de Assistência Médica da Previdência Social [INAMPS]). However, since the INAMPS only targeted the formal economy, less than one-third of the population was covered, the majority of whom were concentrated in wealthier regions and cities. During the 1880s, the government consolidated various public programs in order to rationalize and restructure the complicated health insurance arrangements at that time into a unified national tax-based system.

Currently, the premiums of enterprise employees consist of the employee's contribution (8.5%–10% of their salary) and the employer's contributions (amounting to 17.5% of the employee's salary). Rural health insurance funds are financed through insurance premiums collected in the form of tax surcharges, together with appropriate subsidies from the National Treasury. National taxes and government subsidies account for about 22% of the total insurance funds. Centralized collection and decentralized lump-sum utilization are implemented for health insurance funds, with the central Ministry of Social Security raising funds through banks and the National Treasury. Following a review and a comprehensive balancing process by the Ministry, the funds are allocated to the states according to the actual medical needs of each state and region (based on the number of patient visits). The funds are then allocated by the states based on their respective budgets, after obtaining approval from the state governor.

5. Challenges and Reforms

(1) Main Existing Problems

Brazil's current healthcare system is based on reforms conducted in 1988. Although the system has been continuously refined for more than 20 years since then, it is still facing a number of problems:

1. Financial Pressure   The ratio of public healthcare spending is solidifying, which has led to a weakening of the macroeconomic regulation and control. As noted earlier, Brazil's "Budget Guidance Law" stipulates that healthcare expenditure should account for no less than 15%, 12%, and 15% of the federal, state, and municipal budgets, respectively. Although solidifying the ratio of public expenditure can guarantee healthcare investment to a certain extent, it has seriously weakened the government's capacity for macroeconomic regulation and control, thereby reducing its space for policy operations to cope with changes in socioeconomic development. Thus, the government is often powerless in the face of slow economic growth or sudden socioeconomic problems and is constantly under the dual pressure of legal conflicts and actual needs. The establishment of Brazil's universal health security system began in the 1950s. During the 1960s and 1970s, the Brazilian economy grew at an average rate of 10.1%, a phenomenon called the "Brazilian miracle"; this extensive growth ensured the smooth operation of the universal health security system. In the mid-1980s, the Brazilian economy fell into a severe recession and its GDP dropped noticeably. This led to a number of serious challenges for the free universal healthcare system, including insufficient funding and high levels of dissatisfaction among healthcare workers. Since the early 1990s, the Brazilian government has adopted a series of measures and its economic situation has improved somewhat. Nevertheless, the problems of universal health security have yet to be fundamentally resolved and the pressure on funding remains quite substantial.

2. Unsustainability of Free Comprehensive Healthcare Because of the low reimbursement levels for healthcare providers, the survival of hospitals has become unsustainable. The SUS reimburses hospitals through retrospective payments, which are based on inpatient diagnoses and per capita inpatient care. Furthermore, the low level of reimbursement for healthcare providers has led to a massive outflow of healthcare workers in public healthcare institutions toward the private healthcare system. The primary reason for this outflow is the low salaries of healthcare workers (mainly physicians) in public institutions. In order to increase their income, many healthcare workers have turned to private practice on top of working in public healthcare institutions or have left public hospitals completely to work in private hospitals. The flow of healthcare workers from public institutions to the private sector has further exacerbated the shrinking of public healthcare services; it has also led to provider-induced consumption and irregular medical practices. For example, individuals with a clearly coded diagnosis often opt for a more profitable diagnosis that is beyond their actual needs. Another example is that hospitals have attempted to increase their profits and induce demand by expanding the range of fee-charging services, as well as attracting and accepting the hospitalization of more insured patients. Nearly all public hospitals have begun providing fee-charging services, and in some hospitals, the volume of these services has actually exceeded that of free services. Indeed, in some public hospitals, the wards for insured patients provide much better amenities than do the free wards, almost to the point where they are on par with high-end hotels (being equipped with television, telephone, a sitting room, washrooms, etc.)

3. Uneven Distribution of Healthcare Resources Healthcare resources are unevenly distributed, and there is an absence of healthcare networks in rural areas. The Brazilian population is mainly concentrated in the developed southern region of the country. The varying levels of regional economic development and the consequent disparities in regional wealth are direct contributors to regional differences in healthcare standards. The substantial gap in income distribution among different groups is also another direct cause for the vast disparities in healthcare standards among these groups. Although the institutional design of the SUS was intended to provide universal coverage and various measures (e.g., the FHP) have been adopted to equalize healthcare services, the impact of inadequate funding has led to the concentration of healthcare institutions in urban areas, thereby giving rise to a number of issues in the SUS (e.g., limited coverage, inequalities, and poor quality). Some rural and remote areas have very poor accessibility to healthcare services because of the absence of healthcare institutions and physicians. It is also difficult for residents in remote areas to have normal access to the free healthcare system.

4. Inadequate Supply and Low Efficiency of Public Healthcare Services Although the Constitution stipulates that the protection of citizens' health is the responsibility of the government, and all levels of government have been annually increasing their investment in the healthcare industry, public health services, including primary healthcare, disease prevention, and basic treatments, are still insufficiently developed. Lack of access to healthcare is particularly prominent in Brazil's free healthcare system. Public hospitals commonly have long queues for outpatient services and drug dispensation, as well as long waiting times for hospitalization. Patients may have to wait several weeks for B-mode ultrasound, CT scans, or elective surgery; for major surgeries, some people may wait for more than one year. Therefore, people who are economically better off often choose to purchase private health insurance at their own expense in order to seek medical attention from private or union hospitals.

(2) Healthcare System Reforms

In recent years, the Brazilian federal government has focused its healthcare system reforms on primary healthcare services. The primary goal of these reforms is to enhance the capacity of primary healthcare services and improve healthcare quality, thereby enabling more people to receive medical attention at primary healthcare institutions and alleviating the pressure on higher-tier hospitals. The specific approaches adopted are as follows.

1. Establishing Family Health Teams Nationwide Family Health Teams (FHTs) are staffed depending on the needs of the population served, but generally consist of two to three GPs, several nurses and nurse aides, and social workers who have graduated from high school and received short-term training. The primary function of FHTs is to conduct surveys of family health. Each team generally serves 600–1,000 families. Their main tasks include planned immunization, maternal healthcare, health education, etc. Approximately 80% of the funding for FHTs comes from the federal government, 15% from the municipal government, and less than 5% from the state government. In terms of supervision, besides their internal management and regulation, FHTs receive external oversight by supervisory committees and complaint committees composed of representatives from the local community. The FHT program has enabled Brazil to achieve almost complete coverage for disease prevention, treatment, and health promotion services among its citizens.

2. Enhancing Government Financial Investments Public hospitals in Brazil are fully funded by the government. While the federal government is responsible for infrastructure (e.g., buildings) funding and equipment purchase, municipal governments are responsible for daily operating expenses. Around 30% of these expenses are allocated to the salaries of healthcare workers, while the remaining two-thirds are allocated to daily operations and drug expenses. Due to the implementation of a global budget system, hospitals do not tend toward profit-seeking to increase their healthcare revenues. In terms of obstetrics, the rate of Cesarean sections is lower than 15% in most public hospitals, which complies with WHO standards. However, in private hospitals, there are shockingly high rates – nearly 100% in some cases – despite the fact that the fees for Cesarean sections are relatively high (about US$833). Full-time hospital physicians work 40 hours per week, whereas specialists work 20 hours per week and spend their remaining time in private clinics or hospitals. Therefore, the income of specialists is higher than that of full-time hospital physicians. This has also resulted in a severe shortage of GPs in primary healthcare institutions.

3. Reforming the Public Health Administration System and Improving the Flexibility of Public Healthcare Institutions The former public health system in Brazil was directly administered by the federal government, which subsequently delegated its power to the state governments. In 1992, the Federal Ministry of Health further decentralized administrative power by delegating management of healthcare institutions previously administered by the State Health Secretariats to the municipal governments. These decentralized healthcare institutions remain a core component of the provision of healthcare services. The decentralization gave healthcare providers greater independence, particularly complete autonomy over high-level management as well as greater flexibility in the management of budgets, contracts, and expenditures.

4. Active Development of Private Healthcare Institutions and Health Insurance Agencies To address the inadequate supply of healthcare providers, the government has permitted private healthcare institutions and healthcare institutions run by charitable organizations to participate in the universal health security system and to undertake a certain volume of free healthcare services. First, the government has subsidized the free healthcare services provided by private healthcare institutions to a certain degree, and offers them certain tax exemptions, such as for business tax and the import tax on medical devices. Second, the government supports the healthcare institutions run by charitable organizations or churches by assisting them in building maintenance and equipment purchase, thereby giving them the capacity to provide free healthcare services.

Additionally, the government has supported the development of private healthcare institutions to encourage individuals who are economically capable to purchase private health insurance. Brazil and Argentina have both supported private healthcare institutions by allowing employers and employees to list the premiums for private health insurance as tax-deductible business expenses. This has encouraged the development of private health insurance as a supplement of the public health insurance system to better meet the multi-level healthcare needs of citizens.

SECTION II. THE HEALTH SYSTEM IN CUBA

1. Overview of Socioeconomics and National Health

(1) Basic National Conditions

Cuba, officially the Republic of Cuba, is an archipelago country located in the northern Caribbean Sea of North America. It has a land area of 110,860 km². The country's name is derived from a word in the Taino language, "coabana," which means "a great place" or "fertile land." In 2012, the total population of Cuba was 11.2479 million, 66% of which were white, 11% were black, 22% were mixed, and 1% were Chinese. The country is divided into 14 provinces and one special municipality. The majority of the population (75.3%) live in urban areas, while the remaining 24.7% live in rural areas. Its capital, Havana, is also the largest city in Cuba, sporting a population of approximately 2.19 million. Havana is the political, economic, cultural, and tourism center of Cuba, and is known as the "Pearl of the Caribbean."

Cuba is the only socialist country in the Americas. As a result of decades of embargo imposed by the US, the people of Cuba have faced manifold difficulties in maintaining their livelihood. Nevertheless, Cuba has achieved an average life expectancy of 78.3 years and a literacy rate of 99%, which has kept the country in a stably high position the ranking of countries by Human Development Index (HDI) for many years. In 2006, Cuba became the only country in the world to meet the World Wildlife Fund's (WWF) definition for sustainable development. In 2010, Cuba initiated market-oriented economic reforms.

(2) Population and Health Status

The Cuban government's healthcare philosophy is that "healthcare is the most fundamental human right of the highest priority." Cuba began health system reforms in the second year after the successful Cuban socialist revolution, recognizing that the duty of the socialist government to provide free healthcare services to all citizens. This principle was written into the Cuban Socialist Constitution. The specific measures included: (1) proposing an emergency training program to produce a large number of physicians to alleviate the urgent shortage; (2) focusing on the prevention and treatment of acute infectious diseases, with a special emphasis on the healthcare of vulnerable groups (e.g., women, children, and the elderly); (3) orienting the focus of healthcare work toward rural and primary healthcare.

According to statistical data from 2012, Cuba's neonatal mortality rate was 3 per 1,000 live births and its under-five mortality rate was 6 per 1,000 live births, which were the lowest in the Americas. Furthermore, Cubans have an average life expectancy of 79 years, putting Cuba high in the global rankings of life expectancy. Cuba has also become an aging country – approximately 16.2% of its population is aged above 60 years. In 2012, the number of hospital beds per 10,000 people was 58 and the number of psychiatric beds was 63. As of 2013, there were 67.2 physicians, 90.5 nurses (including midwives), 10.7 dentists, and 1.1 psychiatrists per 10,000 people. Cuba's prenatal care coverage and the ratio of births attended by skilled healthcare workers have both reached 100%. It is the first Latin American country to meet the primary healthcare standards set by the WHO.

2. Establishment and Development of the Health System

The development of the Cuban healthcare industry can be roughly divided into four stages.

(1) Reforms During Crisis (1959–1974)

Before the successful Cuban Revolution in 1959, Cuba's healthcare resources were extremely unevenly distributed, with rural areas in particular showing extensive shortages in healthcare services and drugs. The capital of Havana, which contained only 22% of the country's total population, still had nearly 60% of all physicians and 80% of all hospital beds in the country. By contrast, the majority of rural areas only had one hospital, and the government-funded healthcare system only covered 8% of the rural population. In the early stages after the success of the revolution, healthcare reforms were urgently needed. However, it was at this point that large numbers of physicians began fleeing the country, which further aggravated the shortage of healthcare workers. On the eve of the victory of the revolution, there were more than 6,300 physicians in Cuba; by 1963, this figure had been halved. Since 1960, the US has imposed an embargo on Cuba, thereby cutting off its traditional supply of drugs and medical equipment. As a result, Cuba's healthcare and health indicators began to decline, and certain infectious diseases re-emerged. The rapid population growth occurring during this time also further exacerbated the severity of the problem, plunging Cuba's healthcare industry into crisis.

In the face of these serious challenges, the Cuban government decided to initiate the implementation of a free universal healthcare system, declaring that all citizens had the equal right to access healthcare services and that all expenses should be borne by the State. Specific measures included: (1) proposing an emergency training program to produce a large number of physicians to alleviate the urgent shortage; (2) focusing on the prevention and treatment of acute infectious diseases, with a special emphasis on the healthcare of vulnerable groups (e.g., women, children, and the elderly); and (3) orienting the focus of healthcare work toward rural and primary healthcare. At the same time, the Cuban government merged the healthcare institutions left over from before the revolution, thereby forming a healthcare system unified under the leadership of the Ministry of Public Health (Ministerio de Salud Pública [MINSAP]).

Through tremendous effort, Cuba emerged from its healthcare crisis in 1974 and began the preliminary establishment of a new healthcare system centered on rural and primary healthcare. The number of physicians in the country increased to more than 10,000, which was essentially sufficient to meet its healthcare needs. The morbidity and mortality rates had finally fallen. Three major infectious diseases (polio, malaria, and diphtheria) were eradicated by 1971. Furthermore, the life expectancy increased by 10 years. From 1958 to 1968, Cuba's public health expenditure increased tenfold.

(2) Establishment of a Community-Centered Three-Tier System (1975–1983)

After the first stage, the healthcare industry in Cuba was on the right track, but its healthcare reforms were far from complete: The overall system was still hospital-centered, while preventive and therapeutic services could not be properly integrated; moreover, there were regional imbalances in the development and further expansion of coverage was needed. To address these issues, the MINSAP proposed the implementation of a "community-based healthcare model" in the mid-1970s, which marked a new phase in the country's health reforms.

By the mid-1970s, a three-tier healthcare system had been preliminarily established. In general, the primary healthcare network comprised small hospitals and polyclinics below the municipal (county) level; the secondary healthcare network consisted of central hospitals in provincial capitals and major cities; and the tertiary healthcare network consisted of national hospitals in the capital city. The main organizational form of this community-based healthcare model is the polyclinic. The government divided the jurisdiction of each municipality (county) into several health districts and required each district to establish polyclinics that undertake the main functions of the primary healthcare network. The construction of these polyclinics began in 1964; by 1974, there were 326 polyclinics in the country. The working principles of the primary healthcare network and the main tasks of the polyclinics are: (1) polyclinics are responsible for the healthcare-related affairs of all residents in the community, as well as coordinating with the secondary and tertiary networks, and collaborating with various groups and organizations within the community; they are accountable to the local governments. (2) The healthcare workers in polyclinics are organized into several health teams, which consist of specialists in internal medicine, pediatrics, obstetrics and gynecology, and dentistry; nurses; and psychologists and other personnel. These teams are responsible for the health of all citizens. (3) Prevention must be integrated with treatment, although the focus should be on prevention.

During this stage, Cuba's main health indicators were continually optimized. The life expectancy of Cubans increased by three years; the infant mortality rate decreased by 1 percentage point; immunization coverage reached all children nationwide; and infectious encephalitis was eradicated by 1981.

(3) Improvement of the Healthcare System and Establishment of the Family Doctor System (1984–1989)

The establishment of the three-tier system and the promotion of the community-based healthcare model were major advancements in Cuba's exploration of a healthcare system suited to its national conditions. Nevertheless, both the role and performance of the healthcare system still fell short of the original vision. This mainly manifested as inadequate prevention efforts, as well as a lack of breadth and depth of coverage. Therefore, continuing to explore better organizational forms for the primary healthcare network became the priority of Cuban health reforms in the early 1980s. Under the active recommendations of the public, the Cuban government began implementing the family doctor system in 1984.

The goal of the family doctor system is to provide residents with basic and universal healthcare services at the earliest possible point. Family doctors should have a comprehensive understanding of the patient's condition, including their family and surrounding environment. The family doctor system is a key component of the national healthcare system and the main carrier of the primary healthcare network. Family doctors are not only responsible for the patients, but also the health of all residents within their catchment area. After the implementation of the family doctor system, Cuban residents were given access to direct, comprehensive, convenient, and rapid healthcare services provided by the State. Each community was allocated a number of family doctors. In the 1980s, each family doctor was responsible for the healthcare of an average of 120 households or 600–700 residents. In general, each family doctor has a clinic staffed by one nurse. Family doctors tend to live above or near their clinics, which are open 24 hours. They usually receive patients in the morning and go on rounds in the afternoon; many are also required to work shifts in community-based polyclinics. Patients who cannot be treated in family doctor clinics and polyclinics are transferred to provincial or even central hospitals by the family doctors, who must also follow-up with patients' disease progression to coordinate their treatment. In addition, family doctors must perform regular physical checkups for residents to ensure that they fully understand the health status of each resident for whom they are responsible. Anyone considered unqualified in terms of technical skill and political ideology cannot become a family doctor. The government pays close attention to the lives of family doctors, providing them with high salaries and free housing and furniture, in order to allow them to focus on their work. Even while making substantial improvements to the primary healthcare network, the Cuban government did not neglect the construction of the tertiary healthcare network. Cardiovascular disease, cerebrovascular disease, and malignant neoplasms became the leading causes of death during this stage, leading to a greater demand for more advanced medical technology. To address this issue, the government adopted several measures, including providing sufficient funding, training high-level medical personnel, purchasing advanced medical equipment, and constructing more first-class hospitals and research institutions.

The continuous improvement in Cuba's healthcare standards was also inextricably linked with the rapid progress in pharmaceutical development and the medical device manufacturing industry. By the mid-1970s, Cuba's pharmaceutical production was sufficient to meet 80% of its domestic demand. By the end of the 1980s, Cuba was able to produce a number of drugs and medical devices that met advanced international standards.

In summary, during the third stage of development, the Cuban tertiary healthcare system was gradually refined and shaped to the point where all citizens could have access to physicians. These efforts have led Cuba to have some of the most advanced healthcare standards in the world.

(4) Challenges to the Existing System and New Developments (1990 to the Present)

Between 1989 and 1991, drastic political changes in Eastern Europe had a serious impact on Cuba, plunging the Cuban economy into crisis and once again causing a number of severe difficulties to arise in the healthcare industry. Despite the dire circumstances, the Cuban government and people both strove to ensure normal operation and continual improvement in the national healthcare network. In fact, a number of novel strategies and pathways were conceived to continue developing the healthcare sector under these new trends. For example, the shortage of drugs was resolved using a two-pronged policy: first, the use of traditional therapies, such as herbal medicine and acupuncture, was strongly advocated to reduce the dependence on chemical drugs; second, the pharmaceutical industry was actively grown, especially biotechnology and medical device manufacturing. Medical tourism was also developed during this period.

In summary, the development of the Cuban healthcare industry in the 1990s can be characterized by two major features: (1) the continued development of the healthcare industry and the further optimization of basic health indicators; (2) sudden growth in the pharmaceutical industry, especially the biopharmaceutical industry, which provided strong support for the development of the healthcare industry.

By the advent of the twenty-first century, the number of family doctors had exceeded 30,000. Thus, Cuba had essentially achieved full healthcare coverage for all members of society. Nevertheless, the government remained dissatisfied with its achievements, and thus it shifted its focus to addressing existing problems and deficiencies. These mainly involved the failure to transfer treatment of numerous diseases to the secondary network due to limitations in the conditions and level of the primary network. In response to this situation, the government began implementing a massive, multiyear, "extraordinary healthcare program" in 2002. The primary goal of this program was to further improve the quality of life of all age groups, and its basic idea was to ensure that primary healthcare services were more accessible to the public. Its main measures included: (1) enhancing the role of polyclinics. The first step was to upgrade all polyclinics; the second was to increase and procure medical equipment; and the third was to increase the functions of polyclinics by setting up rehabilitation and emergency services. In brief, polyclinics were given the capacity to diagnose and treat the majority of illnesses, such that most patients can be treated within the primary network; (2) enhancing the healthcare standards of healthcare workers in polyclinics. This involved large-scale training, as well as inviting well-known experts and professors to conduct advanced classes in polyclinics; furthermore, students became eligible able to pursue master's and doctoral degrees; (3) improving the quality of pharmaceutical services. Reforms were carried out to address the issues of drug shortages and inefficiency and irregularities in drug distribution, as well as to rationalize the structure of the pharmaceutical manufacturing industry.

Following the implementation of this program, polyclinics acquired the healthcare capacity of many large hospitals, and patients could obtain treatment from such clinics within 6 km of their location, on average; this distance has continually decreased with each improvement made to polyclinics. The ultimate goal of this reform is to ensure that Cuba is a global leader in healthcare. President Castro once said that, "Cubans will have the world's best health system and they will continue to enjoy all services for free."

3. Healthcare Delivery and Regulatory Systems

The most prominent features of the Cuban healthcare system are its complete and comprehensive national "three-tier healthcare delivery system" and "family doctor model," both of which have effectively alleviated the pressure on large hospitals. The Cuban government has merged all healthcare institutions in the country to form a healthcare system under the unified leadership of the MINSAP.

(1) Healthcare Delivery System in Cuba

1. Three-Tier Healthcare System By the 1970s, the MINSAP had begun creating a three-tier system. Since then, Cuba has established and refined a healthcare network with unique characteristics based on the functions and levels of its existing health service system. This network is divided into three tiers: community-based primary healthcare institutions, secondary healthcare institutions providing specialist medical services, and tertiary healthcare institutions. The primary, secondary, and tertiary networks together constitute the three-tier healthcare delivery system. The three tiers of healthcare network are described in more detail:

- The primary healthcare network (or basic healthcare network) consists of polyclinics and family doctors (primary healthcare).
- The secondary healthcare network (or intermediate healthcare network) consists of provincial and municipal hospitals and health laboratories.
- The tertiary healthcare network (or advanced healthcare network) consists of specialist hospitals and research institutes (e.g., the Institute of Cardiovascular and Lymphatic Diseases; the Institute of Tropical Medicine; the National Institute of Hygiene, Epidemiology and Microbiology).

Different healthcare institutions show a clear division of labor as well as close cooperation. The division of labor is mainly manifested in the high degree of hierarchy and high level of standards. For example, there are 12 specialist hospitals and research institutes throughout Cuba that are responsible for researching and resolving the challenges encountered in therapeutic and preventive care. Cooperation is mainly exhibited among the primary healthcare units, such as polyclinics. These units are staffed by clinicians, who treat diseases, and epidemiologists, who engage in disease prevention. There are also health inspectors who are responsible for the management of food, environmental, and other health inspections and supervision.

The primary healthcare network was the foundation and primary focus of the construction of the three-tier healthcare delivery system. It is responsible for the comprehensive treatment and prevention of diseases, as well as community advocacy for healthcare knowledge. Its main organizational form is the polyclinic; specifically, the government has divided each municipality (county) into several health districts, each of which must establish polyclinics to undertake the main functions of the primary healthcare network. The primary healthcare network is charged with the preliminary diagnosis and treatment of common and frequently occurring diseases. More serious cases are referred to the secondary network for treatment. Cases that cannot be treated in the secondary network are in turn referred to the tertiary network. Once the patient's condition has been treated, they may be transferred back to the community polyclinic for rehabilitative treatment. The ability of the Cuban three-tier healthcare network to implement community-based first consultation and two-way referrals relies heavily on the effective operation of its family doctor system.

2. Family Doctor Model   To fulfill its promises regarding population health in the revolutionary manifesto, the Cuban government began to revolutionize the healthcare system in the wake of the Cuban Revolution, with the primary goal of achieving "healthcare for all." In the mid-1970s to the early 1980s, Cuba established the three-tier healthcare system, which significantly improved its overall healthcare status. During this period, the main primary healthcare units were the polyclinics established in each health district within a municipality (county). These polyclinics were responsible for the healthcare-related affairs of all residents within their jurisdiction, as well as coordinating with the secondary and tertiary healthcare networks. However, because of their overly large service areas and excessive workload, the polyclinics were unable to achieve the required breadth and depth in their preventive work among residents. Thus, with the active support of the public, the

Cuban government began implementing the family doctor system in urban and rural areas in 1984, and later gradually expanded it throughout the country in the 1990s. The gradual expansion enabled the family doctor system to achieve a better organizational form for the primary healthcare network, which had its own unique appeal.

The urban population in Cuba accounts for more than 75% of the total population. Nevertheless, community healthcare work is both conducted in both urban and rural areas via polyclinics. These polyclinics are the basic healthcare units directly under the leadership of the municipal health department. Each city has a number of polyclinics based on its population size; in general, there is one polyclinic per 10,000 people. Within the jurisdiction of each polyclinic, there are also several healthcare points (i.e., family physicians), with each healthcare point serving about 600–800 residents.

(1) Family Doctor Clinics   In 1984, Cuba began establishing the Family Doctor Program (FDP), which was subsequently expanded to rural areas in 1990. The Cuban government set up family doctors in the communities and villages within the jurisdiction of each polyclinic based on the size and distribution of the population served. In general, each family doctor is responsible for providing healthcare to 120 households, or 600–800 residents. Their duties include providing primary therapeutic and preventive services to the households they serve, maintaining the health records of these households, and ensuring that everyone in their charge receives vaccinations and health checkups.

Each family doctor typically has a clinic located within a residential area, and these clinics are typically staffed by a single nurse who assists the family doctor. The FDP has achieved full coverage in Cuba, and the government allocates personnel based on the healthcare demands and development status of specific urban and rural areas, in order to reduce regional differences. This ensures a balanced distribution of healthcare resources throughout the country.

A family doctor clinic usually consists of a consultation room, a waiting room, a monitoring room, a kitchenette, and a bathroom. It is also equipped with the necessary medical equipment, such as adjustable beds, a refrigerator, an autoclave, a medicine cabinet, small medical devices, and drugs. Clinic facilities are generally provided for free by the government. Family doctors usually live above or near their clinics. Apart from returning home for the weekend and holidays, they tend to spend most of their time working and living at the clinic and are often highly integrated within the community; many form close friendships with the residents of their community. With the promotion of the family doctor system in urban streets and rural villages, family doctors have also gradually been introduced into schools, factories, ships, cooperatives, and other workplaces to ensure that all citizens have access to a physician. By the late 1990s, Cuba had 30,000 family doctors, which far exceeded the number in developed countries such as the US, UK, and Canada. Furthermore, healthcare coverage had extended to nearly every corner of the country, with a coverage rate of about 98%.

(2) Polyclinics   In Cuba's primary healthcare system, family doctors' work is complemented and managed by community-based polyclinics. Currently, there are 498 community-based polyclinics throughout Cuba, with one polyclinic handling the management of every 15–40 family doctors.

Polyclinics are primary healthcare institutions with the capacity to provide therapeutic services, disease prevention, and health inspection, while also undertaking certain health administration duties (management of subordinate healthcare points). Specifically, their constituent departments and functions are:

1. *Medical department.* Polyclinics only have emergency rooms and specialist clinics. The specialist clinics are run by one- to two specialists sent by higher-tier hospitals to provide consultation and treatment to residents one day a week. As such, polyclinics do not normally provide therapeutic services (except for emergency services).
2. *Disease prevention and health inspection department.* This department is responsible for immunization, epidemiological surveys, and environmental health protection within their jurisdiction, as well as collecting water and food samples for inspection by upper-tier regulatory bodies.
3. *Maternal and child health department.* This department is responsible for the census of gynecological diseases; and providing guidance and regular checkups for pregnancy, breastfeeding, and child nutrition.
4. *Medical education department.* This department comprises highly qualified experts with rich medical knowledge and substantial clinical experience. They are mainly responsible for enhancing the clinical skills and theoretical knowledge of family doctors within their jurisdiction. The methods adopted include concentrated learning and practical guidance at individual clinics.
5. *Psychological and behavioral medicine department.* Following changes in population disease patterns, the Cuban healthcare sector has, in recent years, begun to attach greater importance to the prevention of noncommunicable diseases. To this end, polyclinics have all been staffed by psychologists, and are equipped with psychological and behavioral counseling clinics.
6. *Logistics department.* Each polyclinic has its own canteen where employees can have their meals.

Polyclinics are open 24 hours, providing outpatient services from 8 a.m. to midnight, and emergency services from 8 a.m. to 4 a.m. Outside these hours, there are usually two family doctors on night shifts, effectively ensuring that patients can seek medical attention at any time. The normal operation of polyclinics at night is highly convenient for a large number of daytime workers, and it also appears to significantly improve the treatment efficacy and clinical outcomes of many diseases with high nighttime incidences. Polyclinics receive about 800–1,000 patients each day. Each polyclinic provides health management services to about 30,000–60,000 residents, implemented through 20–40 family doctor clinics.

Polyclinics provide 22 types of healthcare services to residents, and are equipped with pediatrics, gynecology, diagnostics, dermatology, psychiatry, statistics departments as well as clinical laboratories. The vast majority of polyclinics are also equipped with testing laboratories, X-ray machines, endoscopes, ultrasound machines, optometry machines, and emergency rooms. Hence, they can be considered as small outpatient hospitals.

Polyclinics are also responsible for family planning, emergency dental treatments, maternal and child healthcare and prevention, services for diabetic patients, management of pregnant women, and nursing care for the elderly. In addition, they are also responsible for investigating the causes of diseases occurring within their areas; studying the impacts of environmental factors and the lifestyles of community members on diseases; communicating, reporting, and researching solutions with community administrative leaders in a targeted manner; and conducting health education programs. Furthermore, polyclinics are also responsible for collecting patient records submitted by family doctors, which might need to be reported to the government at any time to ensure that Cuba's healthcare information is complete and easily accessed for statistical analysis. Polyclinics work closely with their subordinate family doctors. All patient information collected by the family doctors is entered into the polyclinic electronic database, such that the polyclinic doctors can immediately retrieve the relevant information from the database when patients visit the polyclinic.

(3) Family Doctor Service Model

1. *Comprehensive medical services.* Family doctors are the main carriers of the Cuba primary healthcare network, providing residents with early, basic, and universal healthcare services.

   First, they are responsible for treating common illnesses among patients. When residents fall ill, they first seek treatment from family doctors, who only refer cases that they cannot treat to higher-tier hospitals. Family doctors can diagnose and treat common diseases in internal medicine, surgery, pediatrics, and gynecology. For patients who require consultation, the responsibility can be shared among several neighboring family doctors. If a patient cannot be treated because of limitations in medical equipment or a unconfirmable diagnosis, the family doctor will accompany them to a higher-tier hospital for treatment, and is responsible for conveying the patient's medical history and past treatments to that hospital.

   Second, family doctors are responsible for carrying out healthcare work among residents, such as immunization, home visits, maternal healthcare and postnatal follow-ups, disease screening, and regular health checkups. Cuban family doctors must perform at least one health checkup per year for each resident, and women aged 25–65 years must receive at least one breast examination every three years.

   Third, family doctors are responsible for organizing various lectures to educate residents on healthcare or publicize important healthcare knowledge. This will help residents solve environmental health and dietary issues, improve their knowledge and ability to prevent diseases and maintain health, and induce all family members to consciously participate in healthcare, thereby reducing their disease incidence and improving their physical health. Family doctors are also required to maintain close links with various administrative agencies and groups, as well as communicate residents' health status and problems with their living and sanitation conditions, in order to strengthen the leadership of these departments in protecting the health of residents.

   Fourth, family doctors are required to establish household health records for each family under their charge. The contents of these records include household economic conditions, basic housing conditions, the presence of any pets, the presence of sources of infectious diseases, environmental-health-related factors of the surrounding area, and so forth. Additionally, the family doctor must also create a personal health card for every resident, including children. In summary, all affairs related to residents' health fall within the duties of family doctors. In his speech at the Third Congress of the Communist Party of Cuba, President Castro described family doctors as experts of comprehensive medicine, which is indeed a well-deserved title.

2. *24/7 service model.* Family doctor clinics in Cuba are open 24 hours a day. The typical work schedule for a family doctor is: upon waking up, the family doctor performs morning exercises with the local elderly residents. Subsequently, the family doctor may measure the blood pressure and pulse of these elderly residents, give suggestions on a healthy lifestyle, and answer any questions they may have. Then, the family doctor will begin their day of diagnosis and treatment. If there are no special circumstances, the family doctor will receive patients in their clinic in the morning, and make rounds in the afternoon. Home visits will be performed for patients unable to visit the clinic. Family doctors are also required to work regular shifts at their local polyclinic.

In addition, family doctors and nurses typically spend half a day each week at the polyclinic focused on their own learning or training in order to update their theoretical knowledge and master new techniques. They may be occasionally sent to upper-tier healthcare units for further study.

3. *Characteristics of family doctor services.* The effectiveness of the Cuban healthcare system is rooted in the primary healthcare system, particularly the family doctor system. The Cuban family doctor system has the following four major characteristics:

Prioritizing prevention. Family doctors tend to be readily available nearby when patients contract minor illnesses, which can help to prevent the occurrence of major illnesses. Common ailments such as colds, diarrhea, and cavities receive first-line treatment at family doctors, often on their first occurrence, which ultimately costs less and prevents major illnesses. Family doctors also take strict precautionary measures for at-risk populations. For example, they have a systematic set of preventive methods for pregnant women and neonates. During pregnancy and breastfeeding, family doctors or nurses may perform home visits with women daily to measure blood pressure, perform physical examinations, and enquire about the patient's condition. Family doctors and polyclinics occupy a key position in mother and child health programs, which have been heavily funded by the Cuban government. They play a major role in maternal health checkups and investigating the causes of maternal and fetal death, which have led to significant reductions in the maternal and neonatal mortality rates.

Focus on rehabilitation. Rehabilitative services are mainly provided to patients with chronic diseases and critical illnesses, or to post-trauma patients. Rehabilitative treatments are provided in a timely and persistent manner, which helps to improve their physiological function and enable them to lead a more normal life. This in turn reduces their likelihood of accruing higher medical expenses due to diseases caused by functional problems.

Timely intervention. This involves planning for the future and promoting future health. An emphasis is placed on community participation, whereby communities are guided by family doctors and relevant community organizations in discussions on the overall healthcare status of the community. Problems within the community are identified through these discussions, and suggestions for solutions are proposed.

Familiarity and convenience. Prevention and rehabilitation require a feasible and operable system, at the core of which is convenience. Family doctor clinics are situated within their community, and family doctors often live above or near the clinics. This implies that seeking medical attention is extremely convenient, as clinics are only a few minutes' walk away. Family doctors are tightly integrated into the community and are generally familiar to patients. Many are even able to recite the health statuses of everyone in their community from memory. Family doctors generally receive patients in their clinic in the morning and conduct home visits in the afternoon. Thus, patients need not even leave their homes to receive medical attention.

3. Analysis of the Operating Mechanism of the Service System

1. *Demand satisfaction.* In terms of satisfying healthcare demands, first, the broad coverage of Cuba's service networks and the national scope of the family doctor system have

guaranteed healthcare accessibility to all citizens. Second, community-based prevention, publicity, health checkups, and other services have generally satisfied residents' public health demands. Finally, the provision of fixed and familiar family doctors has improved patient–physician relationships, reduced oversight costs, and helped meet patients' demand for healthcare quality and service attitude.

2. *Cost containment.* This system has numerous advantages with regard to cost containment and the effective utilization of limited resources: (1) hierarchical services and two-way referrals can maximize the efficiency of the division of labor. (2) Family doctors act as gatekeepers for the tertiary healthcare network, thereby ensuring the rational distribution of resources in the tertiary network through control of referrals. (3) The healthcare resources in this system are distributed based on a rational pyramidal structure, whereby the primary healthcare network is the largest and receives the most investment and greatest emphasis. The service system fulfils its public health and disease prevention functions through the community healthcare services provided by family doctors, and prevents minor illnesses from developing into major diseases through timely and convenient first consultations, thus conserving healthcare resources.

3. *Prerequisites for effective operation.* The effective operation of the service system is based on two prerequisites: first, the hierarchy of healthcare services must have substantive functions along with horizontal and vertical differences. Otherwise, the three-tier network would not be able to achieve sufficient division of labor, diversion of resources, and resource conservation. Therefore, polyclinics must employ an adequate number of qualified GPs, while specialist or national hospitals must have sufficiently high healthcare standards that are complemented by advanced medical devices and other hardware. These qualities require the establishment of personnel training and education programs and medical research institutes. Second, family doctors must effectively fulfill their roles in health monitoring and disease prevention, and as gatekeepers of healthcare services. This naturally imposes relatively high requirements for the standards and professionalism of family doctors. Having physicians who are unable to make fair and reasonable judgments, while depriving patients of effective oversight and complaint channels, implies that the equality and efficiency of the system cannot be guaranteed. In practice, the network of relationships among family doctors and community residents can be both a regulator to improve patient–physician relationships, and a catalyst for rent-seeking behaviors. In cases of serious shortages in healthcare resources, physicians inevitably make decisions based on their personal preferences and closeness in relationships, or they may seek profits through under-the-table transactions. Thus, the lack of complaint channels and third-party supervision implies that the equality of the system cannot be guaranteed.

(2) Cuban Healthcare Workforce Training System

1. Development of the Workforce Training System   Before the successful 1959 revolution, the Cuban healthcare system was dominated by private physicians and private healthcare institutions. Following reforms, private physicians had no room to survive, and most of them opted to move abroad. By 1964, approximately half the physicians in the country had emigrated, mostly to the US. The extensive loss of professors that resulted from this emigration made it almost impossible for the only comprehensive medical school in Havana to resume normal classes.

To address the urgent shortage of healthcare workers, the government had to adopt active countermeasures. Medical students were given free medical education, and in return were required to serve in remote rural areas for one year upon graduation. This caused a substantial influx of youths from poor backgrounds into the medical profession. Since then, Cuba has trained a large number of physicians and provided them with job opportunities. By 1980, the number of physicians per 1,000 people in Cuba had exceeded that of the US.

In addition to the increase in the number of physicians brought about by the above recruitment policies, the Cuban government also controlled the structure and distribution of healthcare workers through the planning and organization of admission standards, specialty allocation, curriculum and training design, postgraduation assignments, and so on. Although the focus of Cuba's medical education program was on public health and primary healthcare, the actual enrollment of medical students was adjusted according to actual needs – that is, preferential policies were enacted for less favorable professions to attract more students. Furthermore, due to the importance of public health, only students in the top 10% of the graduation results were selected for employment in the public health sector. At the beginning of the reform, graduates were given mandatory assignments according to the needs of the country, in order to guarantee the balanced distribution of resources among different regions. Under the support of this policy, as of 1970, Cuba had established one regional hospital and one polyclinic in each province.

However, the mandatory assignments and fixed work were rather unfair to healthcare workers, so in the 1970s the system was adjusted to function as a remote-area rotation system. More specifically, in exchange for free higher education provided by the government, medical students had to serve for two years in remote rural areas that lacked healthcare. The gradual development of the healthcare education system produced enough healthcare workers to not only meet domestic demands, but also to have some sent abroad to provide international aid.

2. Medical Student Training Program   Cuba currently has about 60,000 physicians who have undergone formal training. The ratio of physicians to the population is 1:195, which is the highest in the world. By 1995, the number of physicians in Cuba had increased 20-fold compared to 1959. In addition, the Cuban government paid particular attention to recruiting medical students from different regions, social classes, and ethnicities. The result of this recruitment policy is that Cuban physicians have extremely diverse backgrounds (in terms of gender, economic background, social class, and ethnicity), and thus are able to serve diverse ethnic groups.

1. *Free education and training.* Since 1961, the Cuban government has trained its own physicians. A large convent was converted into a medical school without tuition fees and significantly expanded student enrollment. Due to shortages in material and human resources for healthcare, Cuba prioritized medical education and used free education to rapidly replenish the human capital reserves in the healthcare sector. This was undoubtedly the right choice to resolve the most difficult problem in reforming the healthcare system. First, the high rate of return on human capital investment partially explains the myth of the low-cost healthcare system in Cuba. Due to the extreme limitations in healthcare resources, investing in medical education was the most effective approach with the longest-lasting effect. Second, healthcare education was under the unified management of the State and was implemented through various education and recruitment programs. This made the professional structure and horizontal distribution

of healthcare workers nationwide more controllable, which facilitated the management of the overall healthcare system. This emphasis of the medical education system on public health and prevention also supported the fundamental position of community and primary healthcare services in the healthcare delivery system. Otherwise, the lack of sufficient GPs would have made the establishment of a primary healthcare and prevention network an empty promise.

2. *Specification of training curriculum.* Cuba has imposed very high requirements on the political ideology and professional quality of physicians, such that those who are not qualified in either regard cannot practice as physicians. Che Guevara, who was a physician, believed that physicians should serve patients meticulously, as well as dedicate themselves to the happiness of the people. The Cuban government requires every physician to embrace the highest humanistic sentiments toward their patients. Since 1960, all medical graduates have been obliged to abide by State assignments to rural or urban primary units for two to three years before they are permitted to move freely in the system. Upon graduation, about 97% of medical students are assigned to community-based health stations for a one-year internship, followed by two years of residency training. Physicians must have a firm grasp on biology, psychology, and sociology, as well as an understanding of how individuals integrate with their families and communities.

To become a family doctor, medical graduates must receive another two years of training. In 1983, a special family doctor training program was established in Cuba to cultivate qualified family doctors. From the first year onward, medical students are required to study basic medical knowledge while also undergoing practical training at polyclinics. The basic teaching content can be covered in six years, followed by another two years of training to become a family doctor; becoming a specialist requires a total of 10 years. Currently, Cuba has more than 33,000 family doctors nationwide, 97% of whom have an undergraduate degree.

Medical schools have formulated syllabuses specifically for training family doctors, which cover internal medicine, surgery, pediatrics, gynecology, mental and psychological health, sanitation and epidemic prevention, and so forth. The aim of the syllabus is to cultivate family doctors with a comprehensive base of knowledge and skills in various medical disciplines. In 1984, the outpatient department of a district hospital in Havana created a new model of healthcare delivery based on the principle of training family doctors. Its purpose was to provide students with the opportunity to practice consultations in family medicine under the guidance and assistance of teachers and experts, in order to gradually familiarize them with and help them master the knowledge and skills in clinical and social medicine required by family doctors. After completing the practical training for family doctors according to the syllabus, the students must pass an examination organized by a special committee in order to become family doctors. Full-fledge family doctors and nurses also spend half a day each week learning or training at the polyclinic, in order to update their own theoretical knowledge and master new techniques. Furthermore, family doctors or nurses are occasionally sent to upper-tier healthcare units for further study.

As students receive practical training at a very early stage, they are generally able to quickly master their jobs and easily integrate into the culture of the polyclinics. As a result, despite many years of healthcare shortages and poor infrastructure due to the political upheaval of the Soviet Union and the US embargo, the Cuban government has been able to rationally and flexibly implement effective utilization of its limited resources to gradually improve the health security of its population. Even during the economic crisis of 1990, Cuba ensured the smooth operation of its healthcare system and continuously enhanced its healthcare standards.

3. *Job assignment system.* Medical students receive free education but must serve for two years in remote areas upon graduating. This is the most unique aspect of the human resource distribution system in Cuban healthcare. This supporting policy has had the dual effect of expanding the healthcare workforce and regulating the regional balance of healthcare resources. For students, the losses incurred by serving for two years after graduation in remote areas is roughly equivalent to making deferred payments for their tuition fees. Since they are able to receive free education during their studies, using their labor after graduation in exchange for tuition fees is regarded as fair and reasonable. This can therefore be considered a type of transaction, carrying the corresponding rights and obligations thereof. It does not harm the overall rights of students to choose their education and employment. Furthermore, the system helps to promote the regional equality of the healthcare system and improves its efficiency by matching supply and demand.

The job assignment system is the organic combination of the healthcare education system with the healthcare delivery system. Education must serve the needs of employment. Hence, only by formulating education programs that fully comply with healthcare needs can a rational structure for healthcare professions and the optimal use of educational resources be achieved. On the other hand, adequate government investment and the construction of healthcare institutions have provided good prospects for medical education, such as a large number of suitable jobs and reasonable salaries. After all, only by ensuring the simultaneous growth of investments in tangible assets and medical education can the value of healthcare human resources be fully realized. The reason behind the successful implementation of the Cuban medical education policy is that it conformed to the trends and requirements of the overall health system reforms. The success of these overall reforms in turn is due to the close cooperation with the various supporting measures, such as the education system.

In addition, the lives of family doctors receive much attention from the government and are heavily supported by the public. The government provides these doctors with free housing and facilities, as well as relatively high salaries. Moreover, the public is extremely supportive of the work performed by family doctors. In some areas, the residents have even spontaneously organized the voluntary construction of clinics and housing for family doctors and nurses; some of these volunteer construction teams even consist of retirees. Due to this government attention and public support, the family doctor system in Cuba has developed rapidly. Nowadays, it plays a major role in the country's healthcare industry and has made important contributions to Cuba's status as a country with strong healthcare.

3. Cuban Medical Internationalism   In the Cuban healthcare system, resources are mainly invested in healthcare workers at the primary care level rather than in purchasing expensive drugs and equipment. As a result, the healthcare industry has become a high-tech, labor-intensive industry. Medical schools in Cuba have trained a large number of physicians to maintain an adequate supply of healthcare workers. Due to the ample healthcare workforce, Cuba is able to export healthcare services in exchange for much-needed oil. This process is known as Cuban medical internationalism. Cuba not only sends physicians to 60–70 countries, but also uses its vast medical school resources to train foreign physicians. The medical internationalism is helping Cuba reshape its global image, from the radical red of exporting revolution to the pure white of exporting healthcare.

This Cuban innovation began in 1998, when a large number of physicians and pharmacists were trained in Cuba to work in many other countries. The Latin American School of Medicine (la Escuela Latinoamericana de Medicina [ELAM]), located in Havana, has awarded 10,000 scholarships to foreign students. As of 2007, it has provided medical training to approximately 22,000 students from the Caribbean, Asia, Africa, and even the US. About 51% of these students were female. Currently, the education system has expanded its scope to cooperate with 64 countries. In 2005, Cuba sent 25,000 physicians and pharmacists abroad, which represents a sharp increase from the 5,000 in 2003. This indicates that an increasing number of countries have come to recognize the high level of medical education in Cuba. Venezuela and other countries have also begun to learn from the Cuban model. Cuba has utilized the "medical internationalism" to rapidly expand its influence and cooperation with other countries, which in turn have aided in Cuba's rapid development. At present, the Cuban economy is still growing rapidly – in 2006, it had a growth rate of 12.5%, and exhibited two-digit growth rates for two consecutive years.

Cuba has also adopted a unique training method for foreign medical students. Specifically, it does not expel students from this system. If a student fails their examination more than twice, they are transferred to other disciplines, such as laboratory testing or nursing. This system therefore assumes no distinction in the value of jobs, only the division of labor. Hence, everyone has their own strengths, and like the five fingers of a hand, everyone has a different function but is equally indispensable. Therefore, the teachers and students have an amiable relationship; while students are still under pressure, they remain happy. In addition, foreign students who complete their medical training in Cuba must leave after living in Cuba for eight years. Hence, the majority of these physicians will return to serve in their home countries.

(3) Healthcare Management and Supervisory Systems in Cuba

1. Management System   Before the Cuban Revolution in 1959, physicians were permitted to work simultaneously in public and private healthcare institutions. All physicians were members of national or regional physician associations, and were obliged to follow the rules of these associations as well as accept their management and supervision. The associations operated in a democratic manner, where members were able to participate in the decision-making. This self-governing form of management was dismantled when the healthcare system was taken under the centralized management of the State. In 1961, all healthcare resources and institutions were nationalized and centrally allocated by the MINSAP. Cuba gradually constructed a large number of public hospitals, all healthcare workers became government employees, and private practices were banned. The MINSAP is the central administrative agency of the overall system, and is responsible for the formulation of rules, allocation of institutions, and distribution of healthcare workers. In accordance with the country's administrative system, it divides healthcare institutions into three corresponding levels: national, provincial, and municipal, with local healthcare work being undertaken by local administrative agencies. This forms the administrative basis of the three-tier healthcare network.

Cuban health administration follows a dual leadership model. The supreme administrative body is the MINSAP, below which are the provincial health directorates. The selection and appointment of the provincial health director involves proposing three candidates by the MINSAP for each province (all of whom must be physicians), which is followed by discussions in the provincial assemblies to select one candidate from among the three as the health director. There are also municipal health directorates, and the appointment of the municipal health director similarly involves the proposal of three candidates by the provincial health director, followed by discussions in the municipal assemblies to select one candidate as the municipal health director. Furthermore, in order to strengthen the emphasis of local governments on healthcare, the Cuban government stipulates that the provincial (or municipal) health director must concurrently serve as the vice president of the provincial (or municipal) assembly.

2. Supervisory System The Cuban National Assembly of People's Power is the elected State authority tasked with overall supervision and decision-making. It is divided into the central and local assemblies. Municipal hospitals and polyclinics are directly accountable to the municipal assemblies. The provincial assemblies are elected by the municipal assemblies, and are responsible for formulating the policies of provincial hospitals as well as education and training centers. At the central level, the MINSAP and national healthcare institutions are subject to the leadership and supervision of the National Assembly. The National Assembly has the power to formulate and amend health plans, and to implement personnel adjustments in national healthcare institutions.

In order to ensure the responsiveness and accountability of the supervisory system, a number of public organizations and health councils assist with the supervision and decision-making of healthcare affairs. Following the 1959 revolution, public political organizations emerged in large numbers. The most influential among these were the Committees for the Defense of the Revolution (CDRs), whose original goal was to take charge of internal security and management of counter-revolutionary activities. By 1963, they had become the leading representatives of political decision-making and execution, and eventually came to play an active role in the healthcare sector. Other important organizations include the Federation of Cuban Women, National Association of Small Farmers, people's health councils, trade unions, and Municipal/Provincial/National Assemblies of People's Power. People's health councils are specifically responsible for assisting with the implementation of immunization, infectious disease control, maternal and child care, occupational health supervision, etc. They also provide suggestions and recommendations on the management of healthcare institutions, as well as the priorities and shortcomings of healthcare workers. The other public organizations mentioned earlier participate in the supervision and management of healthcare by sending elected representatives to the local people's health councils.

3. Analysis of the Operating Mechanisms of the Administrative and Regulatory Systems
1. *Unified management of healthcare resources.* The advantage of unified management is that it ensures the equal distribution of resources and optimal structural allocation. The mandatory assignment of personnel has enabled the availability of hospitals and physicians in both urban and rural areas, thus significantly enhancing the equality and accessibility of healthcare services. The centralized management of medical device procurement and healthcare project approval has also reduced wastage due to duplication, as well as diverted resources where they are most needed and most effective.
2. *Decentralized supervision of healthcare.* The local assemblies and public organizations are easily able to access information on the healthcare work being done within their communities, allowing them to successfully fulfill a supervisory role in order to promote

the implementation of healthcare programs and the improvement of service quality. However, it should be noted that the Cuban public organizations mentioned earlier differ from the social work or social service organizations in other western countries. Furthermore, they cannot be considered interest groups. These public organizations do not have much autonomy and are essentially political organizations. Their function is to protect the outcomes of the revolution through the supervision of healthcare work and participation in decision-making. Some studies have even suggested that hospitals in Cuba are not merely service venues – they are also public political venues where physicians are revolutionaries whose mission is to heal. This revolutionary fervor grants many healthcare workers a stronger sense of purpose, enabling them to devote much more effort into their work. However, pan-politicization is not the culture of a healthy society; the passion accompanying the victory of the revolution will no doubt fade over time. As it does, the balance of resources in healthcare institutions will gradually shift from the people to the political elite, leading to rent-seeking behaviors among physicians and other malpractices, and eventual deviation from the fair and rational system envisioned in the original design. The Cuban healthcare system is currently facing these issues.

3. *Prerequisites for effective mechanism operation.* Whether unified management can achieve the optimal allocation of resources is determined by the administrators' motivation, level of professionalism, information control, and capacity for resource allocation. The first prerequisite is motivation – there must be a set of incentive mechanisms to motivate the administrators to serve the people. Therefore, it is crucial to have a rational evaluation system and an effective supervisory system. This will ensure that there is objective feedback on the effectiveness of the mechanism, and provide the corresponding rewards and punishments, thereby constraining and regulating the behaviors of administrators. Second, the administrators must have sufficient professionalism and information channels to make correct judgments. Third, the ability to freely allocate resources according to the outcomes of scientific decision-making is necessary for the effective operation of the mechanism. The establishment and development of the healthcare system not only requires internal coordination, but also the close cooperation of and coordination with other systems.

The decentralized supervisory mechanism of the Cuban healthcare system partially satisfies the prerequisites for a unified management mechanism. The reliance on grassroots public organizations ensures that such supervisory work has a broad public base and excellent information channels. This not only provides direct incentives and constraints on daily healthcare services, but also provides appropriate information feedback for central decision-making and management. However, the nature of these supervisory organizations must be positioned more accurately and rationally. Autonomous community service-type public organizations, professional self-governing organizations, or nonprofit organizations representing the interests of the public are all positioning approaches worthy of reference. Cuba's complete reliance on national public opinion and the shaping of the political atmosphere to control healthcare behaviors is unsustainable.

4. Healthcare Funding System

Cuba's reform of its healthcare system was a crucial component of its socialist revolution. The socialist regime established after the Cuban Revolution had to seek affirmation internally while proving its superiority to the outside world. Cuba's core leader, Fidel Castro, regarded excellence in health indicators as a manifestation of national happiness and the superiority of socialism. Hence, he considered achievements and high international status in healthcare as a symbol of victory against imperialism. This overwhelming ideological control made it possible to achieve profound and radical reforms in the healthcare system.

The provision of universal health security, rapid improvement in health indicators, and elevation of national health status were important goals of the Cuban revolutionary government. As a result, the Cuban healthcare sector received sufficient attention and substantial investment, and the government dared to implement drastic reforms. The high centralization and planned economy of the Cuban government have enabled it to fully mobilize its social resources in support of the implementation of health system reforms.

(1) State Security Model of Free Universal Healthcare

In general, a country's healthcare financing system can take three forms: state security, social insurance, and free market. Among the aforementioned three models, the smaller the financing responsibility of the State, the greater the burden of personal expenses. The state security model uses the government budget as its basic financing channel, which largely guarantees that it has a source of funding. This model has been adopted in Cuba.

The Cuban healthcare system is known as the National Healthcare System (NHS) and is a type of state health security. Healthcare institutions are public and are funded by allocations in the government budget. The Cuban constitution stipulates that "protecting the right of all citizens to healthcare is the responsibility of the State"; hence, all citizens should have access to free healthcare services. Cuba's healthcare work is entirely under the unified responsibility of the State, and all private and market-based interventions are prohibited. All treatment, prevention, healthcare, and rehabilitation activities, as well as the salaries of healthcare workers, are borne by the state treasury. This ensures a strong material guarantee for the healthy development of the healthcare system. Overall, the government is responsible for the establishment of healthcare infrastructure; the construction of hospitals, clinics, medical schools, and medical research centers; the procurement of drugs and instruments; and the salaries of healthcare workers, teachers, and researchers.

In Cuba, the national health status is considered a barometer of government efficiency, and priority is given to government healthcare investment. Indeed, healthcare expenditure as a share of GDP and government healthcare expenditure as a share of the total government expenditure increased steadily from 6.7% and 11.9%, respectively, in 2000 to 10.4% and 14.5% in 2007. In order to highlight the importance of healthcare, the health director of each province (or municipality) concurrently serves as the vice president of the provincial (or municipal) assembly. All healthcare institutions have a single goal: to protect and promote national health, without consideration of profitability or subsistence.

In the late 1980s and early 1990s, Cuba fell into a crisis of survival due to the dual impact of drastic changes in the political environment of Eastern Europe and the US embargo. In the wake of the drastic changes in Eastern Europe, Cuba's healthcare investment plummeted from US$227 million in 1989 to US$56 million in 1993. Even so, not one hospital was closed down. Cuba even cut back spending on national defense in order to prioritize the development of healthcare. Since 1990, individuals were required to bear a small amount of medical expenses. However, apart from covering expenses for hearing aids, dentistry, plastic surgery, prosthetics, wheelchairs, crutches, and other medical devices, citizens still received free healthcare services. In recent years, Cuba has undergone substantial economic reforms, but its healthcare sector has remained virtually unchanged. After 1994, Cuba's healthcare investment resumed its growth, and the national health status continued to increase.

(2) Analysis of the Operating Mechanism of the Financing System

1. Protection of Social Equality Cuba implements a public healthcare system, where healthcare financing is completely dependent on national taxation, and the private sector is prohibited from participating in healthcare provision. All healthcare workers are government employees, and all citizens have the right to access free preventive, therapeutic, and rehabilitative services. In Cuba, the State bears sole responsibility for healthcare services. The principles of equality and universality are generally recognized in this system.

Universal healthcare security is a manifestation of social equality and social progress. Free healthcare services ensure that the people are not deprived of their right to healthcare due to poverty, thus guaranteeing the equal distribution of healthcare resources between the rich and poor, while also contributing to the protection and improvement of national health.

2. Containment of Rising Costs The costs of all healthcare expenses are borne by the State, including the salaries of healthcare workers. This income mechanism weakens the profit-seeking motivation of healthcare workers, thereby inhibiting the disorderly rise in healthcare expenses to a certain extent.

3. Right to Determine Allocation The prerequisites for the equality and efficiency of the Cuban healthcare financing system are adequate resources and a rational allocation mechanism. When there is a lack of healthcare resources, the demand for healthcare far exceeds the supply; however, since services are provided for free in this system, price cannot be a mediator to regulate supply and demand. Therefore, other factors must become the basis of allocation. Theoretically speaking, free healthcare should be allocated according to need, or at the very least, according to basic need. However, when the supply cannot even satisfy these basic needs, who should determine the allocation of resources? Which standards should be used? A more reasonable approach is to prioritize allocation based on chronology and urgency. However, because of the imperfections in the allocation and supervisory mechanisms, the system will gradually deviate from the ideal, eventually leading to the emergence of nonmonetized "exchanges" (e.g., greatness of political power and closeness of social relationships) to replace the functions of monetized prices. Although Cuba has an abundance of healthcare workers, it is currently lacking in medical devices, drugs, and other necessary resources. Hence, the concentration of healthcare resources among the political elite and individuals close to healthcare workers is common.

5. Healthcare Development and Reform Experiences

After the successful revolution in 1959, the Cuban government placed significant emphasis on healthcare, and gradually established a universal, government-funded healthcare system centered on prevention and primary healthcare and that encourages community participation, thus providing its citizens with timely, effective, convenient, and equal healthcare services (Table 21.2).

The Cuban healthcare system is considered one of the best in the world and has repeatedly been praised by the WHO. Based on a summary of our analysis, the experiences of the Cuban healthcare industry are as follows.

TABLE 21.2 Changes in the Main Indicators of the Cuban Healthcare System in 1959 and 2012

Main Indicators	1959	2012
Number of physicians	6,286 physicians, the vast majority of whom were in large cities and were engaged in private practice. In the early stages of the Cuban Revolution, around half these physicians decided to leave Cuba	75,600 physicians, half of whom are family doctors, with 100% healthcare coverage of rural areas
Infant mortality rate	Up to 60 per 1,000 live births	4.7 per 1,000 live births (2008 data)
Average life expectancy	Below 60 years	79 years
Healthcare status	Mainly infectious diseases, most can be prevented through immunization	Mainly noninfectious diseases, immunization program targeting 13 diseases
Medical education institution	Only one medical school	21 medical schools

(1) A Fundamental National Right That Is Free for Everyone

In Cuba, healthcare services are not products; instead, they are the most fundamental and important right of all citizens, and a manifestation of the superiority of the socialist system. The Constitution of Cuba clearly stipulates that every citizen has the right to access health protection and care. The State provides free medical and inpatient care through healthcare networks, polyclinics, hospitals, and prevention and professional treatment centers, in order to safeguard the health of the nation. Furthermore, the State also prevents disease outbreaks by promoting health education, regular health checkups, national immunization, and other public health campaigns. This is the cornerstone of the Cuban healthcare system. With this constitutional guarantee, Cuba has been able to prioritize national health, despite facing economic embargo, armed intervention, and even a crisis of survival. Through the emergency training of physicians, prevention and treatment of infectious diseases, strengthening healthcare for certain vulnerable groups (i.e., women, children, and the elderly), focusing on rural and community healthcare, and other measures, Cuba has rapidly improved its national health status, and successfully achieved universal healthcare coverage, thereby attaining its goal of providing accessible healthcare to all its citizens.

(2) Persistent Spirit of Exploration and Conformance to National Conditions

Cuba has a complicated healthcare system. It comprises three mutually complementary subsystems and is itself a subsystem of the overall social system in the planned economy. The reforms of the Cuban healthcare system are characterized by a sudden ideological and political breakthrough in the manifold resistance from vested interests; use of the State's capacity for centralized mobilization of resources to ensure the rapid construction of a new system following the destruction of the old system; and radical reforms, which prevent the various sequelae resulting from the incompleteness of gradual reforms, and thereby avoids the need to overcome the influence of path dependence when continuously attempting to patch up the system. The ideology of the Cuban socialist revolution has had a direct impact on healthcare workers, while the political supervision by public organizations have cultivated immense work pressure and considerable motivation in healthcare workers.

Cuba has established a relatively complete healthcare system but is still constantly trying to renew itself. After experiencing a period of difficulty in the 1960s, the Cuban healthcare industry gradually began to construct a three-tier healthcare system. The government's strategy of boosting the primary and tertiary networks, which would indirectly promote the secondary network, was able to solve a number of practical problems faced by the public while also improving healthcare standards. During the construction of the primary network, Cuba gained several decades of experience in exploration, such as its implementation of polyclinics and training of family doctors, and the subsequent equal development of both. Its persistent adherence to the principle of exploration has helped improve Cuba's healthcare standards continuously. Using the family doctor system as an example, Cuba has the highest number of family doctors per capita in the world, and its progress in this regard has yet to halt. In order to fully develop the role of family doctors, the Cuban government proposed to strengthen the work of polyclinics in the early twenty-first century. This would enable more diseases to be treated in the primary network and ensure that the healthcare services for citizens will reach new levels. This spirit of continuous improvement is a fundamental reason for the success of the Cuban healthcare industry.

(3) Implementation of "Three-Tier Healthcare" with a Focus on Grassroots Communities

In ascending order of hierarchy, the Cuban healthcare units are divided into family doctor clinics, polyclinics, and general or specialist hospitals. Each provides services at a different stage, thus forming a three-tier healthcare system. At the primary level are the family doctor clinics, which are the foundation of the Cuban healthcare system. Family doctors and nurses often live at or near their clinics and provide 24-hour service. They generally perform consultations in the morning and home visits in the afternoon, and aim to provide all residents in the community or village within their jurisdiction with diagnosis, treatment, care, immunization, and psychological counselling services. They are also responsible for health knowledge advocacy and helping to solve issues related to residents' health. At the secondary level are the polyclinics, each of which organizes and manages several family doctor clinics. These are equipped with X-ray and ultrasound machines, as well as other professional medical equipment, and provide residents within their jurisdiction with various specialty and auxiliary services (e.g., imaging, laboratory testing, rehabilitation). They are also responsible for local disease prevention. The practitioners in these two institutions are GPs who have received a six-year medical education. Altogether, polyclinics safeguard the physical health of 99% of residents nationwide. At the tertiary level are the general and specialist hospitals, which are responsible for the treatment of intractable diseases.

The focus of healthcare work in Cuba is on grassroots communities. About 80% of minor ailments in residents can be resolved quickly and safely within their community, thus effectively reducing the chances of minor illnesses developing into more serious conditions. Residents are generally able to obtain the services of a family doctor within 20 minutes; this fact left a deep impression on a group of health officials and physicians from the UK when they visited Cuba. As for patients with intractable or critical illnesses, the family doctors will transfer them in a timely manner to higher-tier polyclinics or general or specialty hospitals, but continue to participate in those patients' treatment and rehabilitation. In this way, Cuba not only achieves the unification of health education, disease prevention, diagnosis and treatment, and rehabilitation services within the community, but also ensures the organic linkage among different tiers of healthcare units, thereby forming a national disease surveillance and control system. This system guarantees the physical health of citizens, while also effectively controlling unnecessary hospital services, thus leading to both increased utilization of healthcare resources and equal allocation. Between 1985 and 1990 alone, the number of inpatients in Cuba was reduced by 15%.

(4) Rational Focus in Healthcare Work and Prominent Preventive Care

Healthcare in Cuba strives to treat both the symptoms and root cause of diseases, with a greater focus on the root causes. Similarly, while it pursues both disease prevention and treatment, it places a greater emphasis on prevention. More specifically, it attends to the long-term benefits and the balanced development of the overall system. Overall, it is centered on human health, endeavoring to strengthen disease prevention, health protection, and health promotion, rather than focus on disease treatment and control. This preventative focus is key to Cuba's outstanding health achievements.

Cuba has strengthened its health protection and health promotion activities through the departments of sanitary and epidemiological services, maternal and child healthcare, local disease control, and health inspection and quarantine, as well as good collaboration among healthcare institutions. The country has successively promoted and completed various programs and projects in diverse areas, such as disease prevention, drinking water and food safety, maternal and child healthcare, AIDS prevention, and promotion of healthy exercise. These have helped to rectify the poor lifestyles of residents, eliminate and control health risks, improve residents' awareness and sense of responsibility toward self-care, and reduce disease prevalence. Cuba currently has one of the lowest AIDS transmission rates in the world. It has the highest rate of births attended by skilled healthcare workers, as well as the best treatment and control of hypertension. Furthermore, since 1962, Cuba has strengthened its prevention and care services in order to reduce the physical and mental suffering of its people, while also reducing the country's economic burden and increasing the utilization rate of healthcare resources.

The combination of high-level primary public healthcare and community participation has made Cuba especially successful in controlling outbreaks of infectious diseases. In 1962, Cuba declared a "national immunization day" in the hopes of achieving universal immunization. By implementing universal immunization, Cuba successively eradicated polio and neonatal tetanus, as well as infectious diseases such as diphtheria, measles, and rubella. Infectious diseases are no longer the main causes of death among Cuba's population. In 1981, Cuba mobilized its communities to focus on eliminating mosquito breeding sites, which led to the rapid control of dengue fever. The control of HIV/AIDS was also achieved through national screening and centralized treatment. Table 21.3 shows the years in which infectious diseases were eradicated in the past 50 years.

The Cuban maternal and child healthcare system is also relatively complete. It mainly consists of 12 service items completed during health checkups for pregnant women, such as ultrasound diagnosis, assessment of alpha-fetoprotein levels, and various tests for hemoglobin, urine, serum, and HIV. Older pregnant women are also given cytogenetic tests. This system has led to significant changes in data related to maternal and child healthcare, as shown in Table 21.4.

TABLE 21.3 Eradication of Several Infectious Diseases in Cuba

Disease	Year Eradicated
Polio	1962
Malaria	1967
Neonatal tetanus	1972
Diphtheria	1979
Post-mumps meningoencephalitis	1989
Congenital rubella syndrome	1989
Measles	1993
Rubella	1995
Pertussis	1997

(5) Mobilization of Public Participation and Multilateral Cooperation

Widespread public mobilization and multilateral cooperation on healthcare issues have been considered important strategies in Cuba by the Pan American Health Organization. Whether conducting routine healthcare activities, such as hypertension control and environmental health, or emergency actions, such as eradicating malaria or controlling dengue fever, the Cuban government has always been able to garner the support and participation of community residents and related organizations.

Moreover, the Cuban Communist Party and national leaders have also led by example through their active participation. Fidel Castro and others took the lead in antismoking and AIDS prevention campaigns, which increased residents' awareness of the dangers of smoking and reduced their fear of AIDS. The Cuban government is always actively seeking the participation and support of public organizations and the public for both routine community healthcare work and emergency actions, including the eradication of epidemic diseases. The Federation of Cuban Women, for instance, assists in the screening of cervical cancer; the participation rate in such screening among women is 100% in many areas.

The public is also concerned about the healthcare industry, frequently offering advice and suggestions, which the government tends to fully respect. The Cuban government regards public participation as important for formulating appropriate healthcare policies. As such, the public, media, psychologists, and public organizations (e.g., the Federation

TABLE 21.4 Maternal and Child Healthcare in Cuba from Select Years Between 1970 and 2007

Indicator	Year									
	1970	1980	1990	1995	2000	2002	2003	2004	2006	2007
Infant mortality rate (per 1,000 live births)	38.7	19.6	10.7	9.4	7.2	6.5	6.3	5.8	5.3	5.3
Under-five mortality rate (%)	43.7	24.2	13.2	12.6	9.1	8.1	8	7.7	7.1	7.1
Proportion of infants with low birth weight (%)	10.3	9.7	7.6	7.9	6.1	5.9	5.5	5.5	5.4	5.3
Maternal mortality rate (per 100,000 live births)	—	—	—	4.8	4	4.1	4	3.9	4.9	2.13

of Cuban Women, trade unions) are actively involved in the management of healthcare work, particularly by offering suggestions and advice for its development. The extensive discussion and ample interaction among government departments, public organizations, and community residents not only enable the formulation of appropriate healthcare policies or measures, but also facilitate their smooth implementation and the formation of an effective supervisory and accountability system. In recent years, Cuba has also decentralized the decision-making power for healthcare policies to the newly established People's Councils, and promoted resident participation in efforts to affirm healthcare as a priority; these actions have further enhanced the effectiveness of healthcare policies.

By adhering to the principle of understanding the fundamentals and source, the Cuban healthcare industry has formed positive interactions within and outside the industry, which has promoted the overall economic and social development of the country. Within the industry, the healthcare sector has formed mutually beneficial ties with the pharmaceutical, environmental health, and maternal, child, and elderly care sectors, with the ultimate goal of improving the overall national health status. Outside the industry, the development of the healthcare sector has (1) promoted the employment of women; (2) improved national physical health, which in turn has promoted the development of the sports industry; (3) initiated medical tourism and enriched tourism projects; and (4) enabled a large number of healthcare workers to be sent abroad to support international cooperation. These developments have, in turn, further improved the quality of primary healthcare services and the development of the overall public health system.

(6) Effective Cost Containment and Improvement of Healthcare Performance

The performance of the Cuban healthcare system can be better reflected through international comparisons. WHO statistics indicate that among Cuba, the US, and China, Cuba has the lowest absolute amount of healthcare spending per capita and the best health indicators. Specifically, Cuba's healthcare expenditure per capita is less than 1/26 that of the US, but its average life expectancy is higher, under-five mortality rate is lower, and its healthy life expectancy is similar. China's healthcare expenditure per capita is slightly higher than that of Cuba, but its health indicators are far lower.

The reasons for the good performance of the Cuban healthcare system can be summarized as follows. First, the Cuban healthcare system has a rational hierarchical structure. The emphasis on public health and primary healthcare in Cuba has ensured that many diseases are effectively nipped in the bud, which saves a considerable amount of healthcare expenses. Second, the healthcare system has unified its financing, service delivery, personnel training, and supervisory systems, which has significantly enhanced its operational efficiency. The State-funded financing system and highly centralized management system form the material and institutional foundations of its universal health security system. They have also supported the establishment of the three-tier healthcare system and led the reform of the medical education system. The coordination between the medical education and healthcare delivery systems, the matching of personnel demand and supply, and the unification of specialty and training content with service direction have all improved the efficiency of the overall healthcare system and helped to conserve healthcare resources. Third, Cuba has low human resource costs. This is due to the ample supply of healthcare workers produced by the free education system in Cuba, and due to the inability of salaries to fully reflect the value of labor under a planned economy. Fourth, there is no cost inflation induced by third-party payments. As all healthcare workers in Cuba are government employees, their income is unrelated to the fees of the healthcare services they provide. Hence, there is no motivation for the overprovision of healthcare or the deliberate induction of demand, which in turn prevents excessive growth in healthcare expenditure.

 SECTION III. THE HEALTH SYSTEM IN CHILE

1. Overview of Socioeconomics and National Health

(1) Basic National Conditions

Chile, officially the Republic of Chile, covers a land area of 756,626 km². It is located in the southwest of South America, west of the Andes. It is bordered by Argentina to the east, Peru and Bolivia to the north, the Pacific Ocean to the west, and faces Antarctica across the ocean. Geographically, it is the narrowest country worldwide. The eastern part of Chile is occupied by the western slopes of the Andes Mountains, which cover one-third of its width from east to west. To the west is the Coastal Range, which has altitudes ranging from 300 to 2,000 m. Most of its terrain is coastal, extending all the way to the ocean in the south, where there are numerous coastal islands. The central region of Chile is a valley filled with alluvial soil, sporting an altitude of around 1,200 m. There are many volcanoes within its territory and earthquakes are frequent. The Chilean climate can be divided into three distinct regions: northern, central, and southern. The northern region is predominated by a desert climate; the central region has a subtropical Mediterranean climate with rainy winters and dry summers; and the southern region has a temperate, broad-leaved forest climate with frequent rain.

Chile is divided into 13 regions, 50 provinces, and 341 municipalities. According to the latest data by the World Bank, Chile's total population in 2012 reached 17.46 million. In terms of its demographic composition, mestizos (mixed European and Native American descent) account for around 75%, whites 20%, indigenous peoples 4.6%, and others 2%. The official language is Spanish, although Mapuche is used in many of the indigenous settlements. Nearly all (85%) of Chileans practice Catholicism and 2.4% practice Evangelism. Statistics indicate that in 2010 the total labor force was 7.58 million, while the total population in 2011 was 17.27 million.

Chile is a relatively wealthy country in Latin America and is listed in the World Health Statistics 2013 as a middle-income country. Chile is exceedingly rich in mineral, forestry, and aquatic resources. It has world's largest copper reserves and the largest known copper mine; hence, it is known as the "Kingdom of Copper." It is also the only producer of Chile saltpeter (sodium nitrate). Moreover, Chile's agricultural, fishery, and service industries are very well developed. In the 1980s, Chile achieved an average annual GDP growth rate of 7.7%. Despite its slower economic development in recent years, it is still one of the most developed countries in South America. According to World Bank data, Chile's GDP in 2012 was US$269.9 billion. The Chilean economy is recognized internationally as one of the strongest in the continent, and it is characterized by mining and raw material exports. At the same time, Chile also has a vast wealth gap, whereby the income of the richest 20% is 18.7 times that of the poorest 20%.

(2) Overview of Healthcare

As a middle-income country, Chile has outperformed other Latin American countries and countries with similar income levels in terms of its main health indicators, such as life expectancy, infant mortality rate, maternal mortality rate, and control of major infectious diseases. It has also eradicated or essentially eradicated smallpox, measles, polio, and malaria. More than 99.5% of pregnant women receive professional healthcare, and the malnutrition rate among infants and children is within 1%.

Regarding health outcomes, Chile is one of the highest performing countries in the world. According to the latest World Bank data and the WHO's World Health Statistics 2013, Chile's basic health indicators were: in 2011, its birth rate was 14.2%, while its total fertility rate was 1.8. This birth rate was slightly higher than that of China in 2011 (11.93%). In 2011, its mortality rate was 5.6%, which was slightly lower than that of China (7.14%). The infant mortality rate was 8 per 1,000 live births in both 2011 and 2012, representing a decrease of 0.8 percentage points from 1990. In 2011, the under-five mortality rate was 9 per 1,000 live births, representing a decrease of 1 percentage point from 1990, while in 2012, this indicator further decreased to 8.3 per 1,000 live births (Table 21.5).

In terms of healthcare resources, Chile has more than 990 hospitals, 600 medical centers, 1,850 primary healthcare posts, and nearly 40,000 hospital beds. Hospitals and medical centers are divided into public and private. The majority of these institutions are public, including public hospitals affiliated with the national healthcare system, all levels of primary healthcare center, and preventive care centers. Private institutions include for-profit or nonprofit polyclinics, specialist clinics, and hospitals. In 2011, the number of physicians per 10,000 people was 10.3, the number of hospitals per 10,000 people was 1.1, and the number of beds per 10,000 people was 20. The percentage of the population with access to good sanitation increased from 85% in 1990 to 99% in 2011. According to the World Health Statistics 2013, the coverage of public health in Chile has reached almost the entire population. For example, the immunization coverage of one-year-olds from 2005 to 2012 was 98–99%.

In 2010, Chile's healthcare expenditure as a share of its GDP was 7.4%, which was 3 percentage points lower than that in 2000. This ratio is slightly lower than the average relative to Chile's income level. Government expenditure accounted for nearly half (47.2%) of the total healthcare expenditure, which was an increase of about 4 percentage points compared to 2000. In contrast, the World Health Statistics 2013 indicate that personal out-of-pocket expenses as a share of the total healthcare expenditure was 52.8%, which was 4 percentage points lower than that of 2000.

A major feature of the Chilean healthcare system is the broad coverage of its social security system. Only 10% of the population is not enrolled in any insurance agencies, with the coverage rate being consistent across different income levels; that is, only 2% of the population of each income level are not covered. As a middle-income country, Chile has achieved a healthcare system with broad coverage primarily through its sustained economic growth, necessary institutional arrangements, effective healthcare financing mechanisms, and other economic and political factors.

An official of the Chilean Ministry of Health once proudly stated that Chile's health outcomes have benefited from the government's emphasis on public health and primary healthcare; the consistency and continuity of the government's social and public health policies over the past 100 years; and the gradual progress of public healthcare reforms. However, the official also stated frankly that the inefficiencies in certain healthcare institutions were caused by regional differences, inefficient utilization of healthcare resources, and outdated healthcare delivery models, all of which have affected the reform of public healthcare policies to a certain extent.

2. Healthcare System

The reform process of the Chilean healthcare system can be divided into three time periods: the centralized planning system under the National Health Service (Servicio Nacional de Salud [SNS]) (1952–1973), reforms in the 1980s under the military government (1973–1990), and the policy adjustments in the current democratic era (1990–2006).

TABLE 21.5 Basic Health Indicators of Chile in 1990 and 2011

Indicators	1990	2011
Birth rate (%)	—	14.2
Total fertility rate (%)	—	1.8
Mortality rate (%)	—	5.6
Infant mortality rate (per 1,000 live births)	16	8
Under-five mortality rate (%)	19	9
Life expectancy (years)	73	79

Source: China 2012 Health Statistics Yearbook, WHO World Health Statistics 2013, and World Bank official website (http://data.worldbank.org.cn/country/chile).

(1) Historical Evolution

1. First Stage – Beginning of Primary Healthcare and Health Insurance   In 1952, Chile created the SNS and concentrated nearly 90% of its healthcare resources in a single institution. Chile became the second country after the UK to establish free universal healthcare. The SNS operated for 27 years and established five important national programs (the Program for Maternal Health, Program for Child and Adolescent Health, Program for Elderly Adults, Program for Social Health, and Program for Environmental Health), which covered the majority of regions and populations. During this period (1952–1973), primary healthcare was carried out extensively, which enabled full coverage of childhood planned immunization and family planning. The extensive primary healthcare in turn helped to forge a culture of valuing health and played a major role in improving the health of Chileans. The comprehensive health insurance system established in 1952 stipulated that not only would the State formulate all policies related to health insurance, but also would administer specific healthcare affairs. Furthermore, the State would provide most healthcare services for free, such that the public sector would bear 90% of hospital expenses and more than 85% of patients' treatment expenses.

In 1968, Chile drafted the Curative Medicine for Employees Law, which included around 2.5 million employees in the public and private sector in the socialized system. Under the SNS system, Chile's global health indicators continued to improve, eventually becoming higher than were those of other Latin American countries.

This system carried on for nearly 30 years. However, as in other countries with government-run health insurance, by the late 1970s, Chile's health insurance system began to experience a profound crisis of efficiency. This crisis was characterized by the persistent increase in health insurance expenditure and the excessive financial burden on the State, which not only caused the health insurance system to become a bottleneck of economic development, but also a potential factor for social instability. The reform of the health insurance system was imminent by this stage.

2. Second Stage – Fundamental Transformation of Health Insurance   In the early 1980s, a change in Chile's political regime provided the ideal opportunity for a fundamental transformation of the health insurance system. Under the dominant influence of global economic liberalism at that time, the goal of these reforms to Chilean health insurance mainly involved saving costs, eliminating waste, fully developing potential, improving healthcare conditions, and reducing inequality. Thus, the healthcare system transitioned from a government-run system toward privatization and marketization.

In 1980, after Pinochet and his supporters overthrew the democratically elected president, thus establishing a military dictatorship, he adopted the tenets of neoliberalism to boost the economy. In accordance with the prescriptions of the Washington Consensus, large-scale privatization was carried out in the education and healthcare systems:: (1) introduction of private health insurance. In 1981, Chile redefined the role of the State in the healthcare system, established private health insurance agencies (Instituciones de Salud Previsional [ISAPREs]), reduced government funding allocation for healthcare institutions, and transformed the free education and healthcare services into fee-charging industries; (2) decentralization of responsibilities for primary healthcare to municipalities with poor financial capacity. This reform greatly weakened the provision of primary healthcare; (3) vigorous development of private hospitals. The healthcare policies adopted under the military government were based on three major principles: small government, free market, and support of private businesses. These principles were also considered key to economic development. The outcomes of Chile's global health indicators during this stage also demonstrated the effectiveness of such a system.

Although certain achievements were made in this stage, market competition did not improve national health or enhance the overall effectiveness of the healthcare system. For example, in 1960–1970, maternal and infant mortality rates both decreased at an annual rate of 2.5%, but these indicators remained virtually unchanged between 1970 and 1990, during the implementation of marketization.

3. Third stage – Clarification of Government Health Responsibilities   After a democratically elected government took office again, it began adjusting the healthcare development policies, emphasizing that the goal of healthcare reforms is not only to increase efficiency, but must also to uphold equality, meet the population's health needs, provide risk protection, and ensure service quality. Thus, it reinstated the role of the government in managing population health – that is, the government once again had a leading role in the financing, provision, and supervision of healthcare services. In this stage, the last major reform undertaken by the Chilean government was the promulgation of the Explicit Health Guarantees (Garantías Explícitas de Salud [GES]) in 2005. The GES obligated public and private compulsory health insurance agencies to provide coverage for 56 types of legally recognized health problems. Through the basic benefits package defined in this Act, the State was able to guarantee the accessibility, financing, and healthcare quality of various health problems for all citizens, thus ensuring that they are not discriminated on the basis of differences in insurance plans, gender, or income. This act marked a major reform of the Chilean healthcare system, bestowing beneficiaries with specific mandatory rights.

In general, the reforms of the healthcare system carried out by the Chilean government in the 1990s included (1) the reconstruction of the national healthcare system, and the implementation of decentralized management. The country was divided 27 regional healthcare centers, each of which contained different levels of hospitals, medical centers, and primary healthcare posts. The allocation of healthcare resources was determined through the coordination and negotiation among the Ministry of Health (Ministerio de Salud [MINSAL]), the National Health Fund (Fondo Nacional de Salud [FONASA]), and provincial governments. Furthermore, greater autonomy was granted to these regional healthcare centers. (2) The establishment of FONASA. FONASA is a public institution tasked with the collection, distribution, and management of healthcare resources, which also performs government healthcare functions. (3) Establishment of a dual health insurance system comprising private and public tracks. This dual-track system was developed by permitting private health insurance to enter the health insurance system. Workers can choose to enroll either in public or private health insurance. (4) Further improvement in the equality and efficiency of healthcare services. In terms of equality, workers were classified according to income levels to determine whether they would be fully covered by the government or partially covered by FONASA. In terms of efficiency, the different sectors of the healthcare system were clarified, while the responsibilities and management authority of the central and provincial health departments were defined. Finally, for the protection of patient interests, the standards of healthcare quality were reinforced and standards for patient waiting times were formulated.

(2) Healthcare System

1. Basic Healthcare System　A basic characteristic of the Chilean healthcare system is its compulsory social security system, which has recently reached a coverage of 90%. Although the marketization of health insurance operations has been encouraged and private insurance companies have been permitted to provide health insurance, enrollment in health insurance remains compulsory for eligible persons. That is, all individuals within the scope of this policy are required to enroll in health insurance. However, they are free to choose whether to enroll in public or private insurance. The targets of compulsory health insurance are limited to employees and retirees. Both the insured person and their dependents are considered insurance beneficiaries.

Chile's high level of healthcare coverage is closely related to the following factors. The first is Chile's sustained economic growth. The smooth implementation of a social security system requires immense economic support, particularly during the early stages (which are rife with moral hazards). Therefore, when there are sufficient public finances to cover these expenses, the implementation of this system will be easier. As a result, the implementation of health systems often occurs during periods of strong economic expansion. Additionally, Chile has a large group of people receiving free healthcare allowances (about one-fourth of the total population). Hence, the country requires sufficient resources to support this group. Stronger economic growth implies that the country is able to raise more taxes to support these expenses. Furthermore, economic growth also plays a crucial role in improving health outcomes. By comparing the infant mortality rates and life expectancies of certain Latin American countries, we can see that these two indicators are closely related to the level of economic development. Specifically, as the economic development improved, infant mortality decreased and life expectancy increased. Chile has the highest life expectancy in Latin America and a relatively low infant mortality rate. Likely, its performance on these two indicators is inseparable from its strong economic growth.

The second factor is high urbanization and income levels. Due to reduced management costs, the higher the population density in urban areas, the broader the coverage of the social security system. The rural population in Chile only accounts for slightly more than 10% of the total population. Hence, high urbanization is a driving factor for broad reforms. Moreover, the higher the internal income levels of an economy, the more likely it is able to bear the high management and operational costs needed for social security coverage. Chile is considered a middle-income country; the latest report of the International Monetary Fund (IMF) revealed that in 2010, Chile's income per capita was over US$11,500, and this is expected to reach US$16,192 by 2015. The purchasing power parity will also show a significant increase during those four years to US$19,379. These factors, to a certain extent, also explain the successful expansion of Chile's social security system.

The third factor is the existence of a competent and independent regulatory agency. Information asymmetry and adverse selection are the two most important and complex problems facing any health insurance market. Chile similarly faced these two problems in the early stages, when there were no regulatory agencies in place. For example, due to information asymmetry, insured persons faced difficulties in understanding and comparing the insurance products provided by FONASA and ISAPREs. In addition, due to adverse selection, certain high-risk groups were excluded from coverage by the ISAPREs, but were unable to seek assistance. Therefore, it was necessary for the government to set up regulatory agencies to ensure that the insurance market operated according to the rules of a perfectly competitive market, which would reduce these risks. Although the Chilean Superintendency of Health only began to regulate private insurers ten years after the implementation of the health insurance system, and public insurers after 20 years, the establishment of such regulatory agencies at the start of system implementation is a major learning point for other countries.

The final factor is that the formal labor market occupies a dominant position. Chile's experience demonstrates that joining the social security system and other formal labor market mechanisms are the most important factors for expanding the coverage of the healthcare system. If a country's institutions and laws strongly promote formality, especially the construction and development of a formal labor market, then the implementation of a health security system becomes easier. This is because under these circumstances, the administrative procedures for premium collections and other affairs are simplified, thus significantly enhancing the efficiency of the health security system while also providing sufficient convenience for expansion. Compared to other Latin American countries, Chile's overall economic performance and labor market are relatively formal (formal employment accounts for a relatively high proportion), which has provided crucial institutional support for the expansion of health security coverage.

2. Essential Medicines System   Currently, Chile's essential medicines system can be divided into two parts. The first includes primary and community healthcare institutions (including the vast majority of community polyclinics and family health teams, which are currently being rebuilt), where dozens of essential medicines are provided for free. These essential medicines are useful for managing common and frequently occurring diseases. However, essential medicines are not fixed and unchanging. Therefore, if patients require specific drugs for their clinical needs, these can be obtained for free through a fixed application procedure, pending the approval of the health and social security departments. The second part includes hospitals above the secondary tier, which do not have outpatient departments or pharmacies, only emergency departments and inpatient pharmacies, to meet their clinical needs. For patients covered by FONASA, 495 essential medicines are provided for free by inpatient pharmacies; other medicines must be applied for. As there are no mechanisms that involve "covering medical expenses with drug sales," the procurement and use of drugs are strictly determined according to clinical needs.

3. Health Administrative System   In terms of health administrative management, Chile also follows a unified management model for healthcare, health insurance, and drugs. Although the Institute of Public Health (ISP) and health financing authority (FONASA) are independent legal entities, they are both accountable to the MINSAL. They must perform drug regulation, along with the financing and allocation of healthcare funds, according to nationally standardized healthcare policies, thus forming a unified management system for healthcare, health insurance, and drugs.

Chile's administrative system is divided into 13 regions, 52 provinces, and 342 munici-palities. However, the functions of the provincial administrative units have blurred in recent years, and currently they lack substantive management tasks. Health management is not implemented via local health departments among the 13 regions. Instead, the country is divided according to the natural geography and demographic characteristics into 28 regional Health Services (Servicios de Salud [SS]), which are directly under the leadership of the MINSAL. Municipal health offices have a horizontal collaborative relationship with their corresponding municipal governments. Furthermore, the municipalities and health offices are directly responsible for organizing and managing hospitals and primary health-care institutions. Thus, within this environment of legislative, administrative, and judicial independence for municipalities, there remains a form of vertical management in local healthcare work. However, community participation plays a relatively significant role in the supervision of healthcare services.

4. Medical Aid System   Before the reform, Chilean social insurance utilized a pay-as-you-go system. The government was responsible for premium collection and fund management, while deficits in the social insurance sector were completely covered by state finances. Under this system, the government developed social assistance programs especially targeting the poor or groups with special needs. These programs were generally mixed with social insurance plans, making it difficult to form a self-contained system in terms of the funding sources and management system. Following the healthcare reforms, a mandatory savings system and a fully funded pensions system were established, while a proportion of Chile's health insurance came to be administered by private insurance com-panies. In addition, the fragmented social assistance programs were gradually separated from the social insurance system. Relevant institutions were established to implement the unified management of government social programs, and to coordinate their relationship with other social organizations and institutions. Thus, a more complete and organized social assistance system was formed.

Medical aid for impoverished groups is achieved through joint cross-subsidization of the government and other social groups, thereby embodying the spirit of mutual aid. In addition to the public health insurance system, Chile has several private health insurers. The government divides the population into five groups according to income level: A, B, C, D, and E. Group E represents high-income earners, who generally enroll in private insurance, while the other four groups generally participate in public insurance. Members of Group A do not have to pay insurance premiums, and all their medical expenses are covered by public funds. Members of Group B have to pay a certain percentage of premiums, while the rest is subsidized by the surplus of premiums in the public healthcare system paid by individuals in Groups C and D.

Chile's approach to healthcare funding ensures stable funding and the provision of comprehensive services that meet the healthcare needs of those living in poverty. Thus, the cross-subsidization of impoverished groups by the government and other social groups has embodied the spirit of mutual aid. However, this system has the following shortcomings: it requires a better definition of "impoverished groups" for healthcare services; it still has high management costs; the level of social equality is insufficient, as the contributors to the cross-subsidization are mostly middle- or upper-middle income earners, rather than high-income earners; and impoverished groups have low cost awareness, resulting in the waste of resources. In contrast to the universal healthcare system, this approach facilitates the flow of public resources toward groups that are most in need of services, and the total costs are relatively low. Hence, it is more commonly seen among developing and middle-income countries.

3. Analysis of the Health Insurance System

(1) Institutional Framework of the Health Insurance System

Chile has two major types of health insurance agency: public and private. In 2010, public and private health insurance agencies in Chile covered 68% and 32% of the population, respectively. More specifically, more than two-thirds of the population was covered by FONASA, while between one sixth and one fifth was covered by the state; the remainder of the population was covered by private insurance through universities or the military.

According to law, all non-self-employed workers in the formal sector, retirees receiving annuities, and self-employed persons enrolled in pension funds must participate in the compulsory health insurance system and contribute 7% of their income or annuity each month, with a monthly cap of US$2,000. Other individuals are also able to join this system, including independent workers, legally recognized impoverished individuals, and unemployed persons. With regard to the purchase of healthcare services, Chilean law requires FONASA to purchase the majority of its healthcare services from public hospitals and medical centers. Moreover, these institutions must also provide the majority of their services to FONASA, while the types and volume of services provided to private patients and the ISAPREs are subjected to strict limitations. As the main insurance agencies of the Chilean healthcare system, FONASA and ISAPREs have a competitive relationship, which forms one of the pillars supporting the efficient operation of Chile's health security system.

(2) Funding – Mixed Healthcare Funding System

Chile implements a mixed healthcare funding system that includes general taxation and social insurance taxes. Presently, universal coverage has essentially been achieved in Chile. However, since residents are free to choose between government-run social health insurance and private health insurance, this institutional design has effectively divided the population. Specifically, the majority of residents with good health status and high incomes have opted to enroll in private health insurance in order to access more timely and comfortable services; conversely, those with poor health status and low income are forced to remain in the public funding system (FONASA) in order to receive services from public hospitals and community clinics. This institutional arrangement does not allow for the social mutual aid function of insurance, where the rich subsidize the poor and the healthy subsidize the sick. Thus, it has received a relatively poor evaluation from the WHO.

Chilean law stipulates that all individuals with income must enroll in health insurance plans. Those enrolled in social health insurance contribute 7% of their wages as insurance premiums, and account for 73% of the population; the rest are enrolled in private health insurance, whose premiums exceed the statutory 7% and are at least 10% of their wages. Of Chile's total healthcare expenditure, compulsory premiums account for 17%, funds from general taxation for 28%, copayments for 27%, and other sources for 28%.

As Chile's administrative department for healthcare funds, FONASA is responsible for investment prioritization as well as the specific approaches used for investment of healthcare funds. Currently, the Chilean government has determined that primary healthcare should be prioritized for healthcare investment. Such prioritization has two components: (1) capitation fees, where the amount of transfer payments is calculated based on the population covered by each primary healthcare institution. These capitation fees are also adjusted according to the local level of economic development, demographic characteristics (e.g., ratio of impoverished groups, indigenous groups, women, and children), and incidence or prevalence of major diseases. Capitation fees generally account for 70% of the expenses or primary healthcare institutions. (2) Earmarked funds, which are allocated based on priority health intervention projects developed by the MINSAL and the workload involved in completing each project. These funds generally account for 30% of project funds. As for smaller-scale primary healthcare posts located in remote areas, the State allocates a fixed amount of funds based on their operational costs. Thus, we can see that Chile's healthcare investment has not stagnated through debate between supply-side or demand-side reimbursements, and instead has focused on ensuring greater equality and efficiency in the distribution of healthcare funds. The funding allocation for hospitals is 50% as determined by the volume of services provided, and the other 50% as determined by the hospital's operational costs. This approach avoids unnecessary debate over whether to purchase services or to directly subsidize hospitals using public funds.

(3) Policy Differences Between Public and Private Health Insurance Agencies

1. Public Health Insurance Agencies   As noted earlier, public health insurance agencies classify insured persons into five groups based on monthly income: A, B, C, D, and E. Group A includes legally recognized impoverished groups; Group B earns a monthly income of less than US$144; Group C earns a monthly income of US$144–225; Group D earns a monthly income of more than US$225; and Group E includes the minority of individuals with an exceptionally high income. The first four groups account for 41.2%, 31.5%, 12.8%, and 13.9% of the population, respectively. Individuals in Group E are not covered under public health insurance.

Public health insurance agencies provide insured persons with primary, secondary, and tertiary healthcare. Insured persons are also given subsidies for sick leave. Moreover, older women are entitled to five months of pre- and postnatal allowances. The key implication of this income-based classification is reflected in the copayment system. In general, Groups A and B have very low copayment rates, while Groups C and D have copayments of about 10% and 20%, respectively.

2. Private Health Insurance Agencies   Private health insurance agencies are the products of reforms in the healthcare and health insurance systems. Since their successful development in Chile, they have become the most profitable economic sector in the country, as evidenced by the increasing health insurance coverage of the population. Specifically, the population covered by private health insurance agencies has increased from 2.1 million (19% of the population) at their initial establishment to 3.8 million (32% of the population) currently.

3. Differences Between the Two Agencies   In Chile, the main differences between public and private health insurance agencies are:

1. *Difference in the premium rates of insured persons.* Public health insurance agencies essentially levy a uniform 7% health insurance tax, whereas private health insurance agencies charge different premiums based on the insured person's age, gender, household size,

health status, and other factors, at an average rate of 8.5%. Furthermore, the level of health security provided by private health insurance agencies is proportional to the amount of premiums paid.

2. *Difference in health insurance content.* The services covered by public health insurance include primary, secondary, and tertiary healthcare (in public hospitals), as well as healthcare services for major and critical illnesses. In contrast, private health insurance often does not cover healthcare services for major illnesses; hence, some insured persons in Chile are enrolled in both public and private health insurance.

3. *Significantly higher copayment ratios in private health insurance than in public health insurance.* This is the main method by which private health insurance controls "moral hazards." The level of health security provided by private health insurance plans are very low, but these plans are still popular because of the high service quality and efficiency. The copayment rates of public health insurance are determined based on income levels and are generally between 0% and 20%.

(4) Development of Private Health Insurance

In the early 1980s, the change in political regime provided an ideal opportunity for fundamentally transforming the health insurance system. Under the dominant influence of global economic liberalism at that time, the goals of these reforms to the Chilean health insurance system mainly were saving costs, eliminating waste, fully developing potential, improving healthcare conditions, and reducing inequality. Thus, the health insurance system transitioned from a government-run system toward privatization and marketization. At the same time, Chile also adjusted the health insurance management system and specific policy measures. In 1981, the National Health Service and the National Medical Service for Employees were restructured into the National Health Fund (FONASA) and National System of Health Services (Sistema Nacional de Servicios de Salud, SNSS), which fulfilled the government's responsibilities in the health insurance industry. At the same time, the central government began decentralizing some of its management authority over healthcare affairs; in particular, it delegated the management of primary health insurance to municipalities. However, the marketization of Chilean health insurance was incomplete and only partially privatized. Therefore, a dual health insurance system was formed comprising both public and private health insurance.

At the beginning of these health insurance reforms in Chile, despite the public's yearning for social healthcare and rejection of private health insurance, the government continued to adhere to the ideas of economic liberalism in its policies, resulting in the widespread persistent decline of public health insurance with social policy characteristics. The partial privatization of health insurance also led to the sustained expansion of private health insurance agencies, which gradually developed into the most profitable economic sector in Chile. From November 1990 to 1996, while there were no changes in the number of private health insurance agencies, the number of beneficiaries increased from 2.1 million in 1990 to 3.8 million in 1996, while the percentage of the population covered by private health insurance agencies under the compulsory health insurance system increased from 19% in 1990 to 32% in 1996. In 1990–1996, the healthcare expenditure per beneficiary covered by private health insurance agencies increased by 18%. However, in the late 1990s, the economic recession combined with the lack of innovative capacity of private health insurance agencies caused them to fail to provide new products to increase their market share. Hence, there was no major development in private health insurance, and the number of people enrolled in private health insurance barely increased after 1999.

The introduction of private health insurance agencies enhanced the cost awareness of the entire health insurance sector. Furthermore, the operations of public health insurance agencies have also achieved significant success. In 1981, reforms to the health insurance system led to a broad restructuring of the public health insurance system, which included stripping some of its functions and adhering more to consumer demands. Market mechanisms were also introduced, which significantly improved the efficiency of the system. In addition, the reforms led to a growth in demand for diagnoses and treatments, thereby increasing the total health insurance expenditure.

4. Evaluation and Summary of the Health System

(1) Characteristics of the Healthcare and Health Insurance Systems

1. Clear Reform Principles and Legal Guarantees The basic healthcare system of Chile has undergone three major reforms, each of which was based on clear reform principles. For instance, the basic principle of the first reform was to establish a health insurance system with universal coverage and guarantee the equality of healthcare services. The principle of the second reform was to improve the efficiency of healthcare services. The third reform embodied the principle of sustainability, which in turn was based on the guiding ideology of achieving balance between government intervention and market mechanisms, while enacting guarantees in the form of healthcare laws or even changes to the constitution.

2. Extensive Public Participation and High Reform Consensus Chile's reform principles and plans were all based on bottom-up public discussions in all sectors of society. The fundamental goal of such public participation was to avoid deviations in the reform direction. Chile has established health management committees to enhance the participation of community residents; these committees directly provide advice, supervision, and accountability for local healthcare work, thus improving the applicability of such work and the satisfaction of community residents. Furthermore, an emphasis on the equality of healthcare reforms and reforms targeting key health problems has become a basic concept adopted by health administrators of all levels. When introducing their local healthcare work, a director of a community health center in Chile covering only 30,000 people used a local population pyramid to describe the changes in disease patterns and ideas for coping strategies. This not only reflects the quality of the primary healthcare administrators, but also indicates the presence of a deep-rooted adherence to the equality of healthcare reforms.

3. A Health Administrative System that Integrates Healthcare, Health Insurance, and Drugs Chile adhered to the principles of comprehensiveness, uniformity, and efficiency in its establishment of a super-ministry based health administrative system that covers healthcare, health insurance, and drugs. Although the directors of FONASA and Superintendency of Health are appointed by the President, they are still accountable to the Minister of Health, which ensures the coordination of health security and health service policies. This system has also helped control the growth in total healthcare expenditure, which was only 7.4% of the GDP in 2010.

4. Compulsory Health Insurance with Broad Coverage A basic characteristic of the Chilean healthcare system is its compulsory social security system. The healthcare system has undergone three major stages of development, and the government's responsibilities for population health were clarified during the first stage. Recently, health insurance coverage reached upwards of 90%; in other words, only about 10% of the population are not enrolled in any insurance agencies.

5. Clear Government Responsibilities and Prominent Public Welfare Nature The public welfare nature of healthcare and health insurance in Chile is mainly reflected in two aspects of the system:

First, the premium rates of public insurance are linked to the income levels of beneficiaries, but not to their age, health status, or the total number of beneficiaries. All insured persons who have purchased public health insurance must contribute 7% of their income as premiums. As noted earlier, public health insurance agencies classify insured persons based on monthly income into Groups A, B, C, D, and E. Group A consists of legally recognized impoverished groups; Group B earns a monthly income of less than US$144, Group C earns a monthly income of US$144–225, Group D earns a monthly income of more than US$225, and Group E includes the minority of individuals with an exceptionally high income. The first four groups account for 41.2%, 31.5%, 12.8%, and 13.9% of the population, respectively. Individuals in Group E are not included in the coverage scope of public health insurance.

Second, the uninsured population is not limited to vulnerable groups, such as elderly, disabled, unemployed, and low-income individuals. In fact, the ratio of the uninsured population is consistent across all income levels (i.e., about 2% of each income level is uninsured). This system clearly stipulates that in addition to non-self-employed workers in the formal sector, retirees receiving annuities, or self-employed persons enrolled in pension funds, who must enroll in health insurance, other individuals (including independent workers, legally recognized impoverished individuals, and unemployed persons) are also able to join this system and receive the same healthcare services.

6. Integration of Social Insurance and Private Insurance to Ensure a Balance Between Equality and Efficiency Chile's healthcare reforms are exceedingly distinctive in that all three reforms were closely related to the government's views on achieving social and economic development. The first stage focused on public welfare and embodied the concept of big government. During this stage, the healthcare industry underwent rapid development, which led to substantial improvements in public health and population health status. However, the emphasis on equality and broad coverage also led to a sharp increase in demand and healthcare expenditure. This laid the foundation for the main theme of the second stage, which was the optimization of healthcare efficiency. This theme was similarly relevant to the government's focus on small government, big society. However, the consequences of focusing on efficiency were increased healthcare burden on the people and an increasing wealth gap, which threatened the equality and accessibility of healthcare services. These problems in turn gave rise to the themes of the third stage, which are currently advocated by the Chilean government: integrating social insurance and private insurance to ensure a greater balance between equality and efficiency. The coexistence of FONASA and ISAPREs has also given rise to a competitive relationship between the two, which has become a pillar supporting the efficient operation of the Chilean health security system. Nowadays, insured persons are free to choose whether to enroll in public or private health insurance.

(2) Existing Problems of the New Health Insurance System and Their Causes

Chile's new health insurance system is being increasingly criticized by the public, most of which are aimed at private health insurance companies. Two of the most prominent aspects are:

1. *"Cream skimming."* This is where private insurance companies skim off high-income and healthy individuals from the public insurance system to become their clients, while excluding those who are most in need of insurance (especially low-income earners) from the private insurance system.

   This mixed model of commercial and social insurance has been criticized because of its lack of equality, which is caused by the independent operation of these two forms of insurance. Social insurance, despite being a form of compulsory insurance, is not mandatory for everyone – it is only mandatory for employees and retirees. The service targets of commercial insurance are high-income groups. Because of the lack of government supervision, "cream skimming" has become evident in the Chilean commercial insurance market. Statistics have shown that in Chile, only 6.9% of elderly individuals aged over 65 years are covered by commercial health insurance, as opposed to approximately 26.7% of those aged 25–54 years. Due to the fragmentation of the commercial and social insurance markets, many individuals continue to be excluded from coverage under either form of insurance.

2. *Low protection provided by private health insurance.* This is mainly reflected in the very high levels of copayment rates (i.e., the proportion of healthcare expenses borne by the insured person). In addition, the "cream skimming" problem has given rise to a third problem that went largely unnoticed by the Chilean public: specifically, the massive outflow of high-income and healthy individuals from public health insurance agencies implied that the reform goal of the health insurance system – namely, to reduce public spending on healthcare – could not be achieved. Instead, public health insurance agencies attempted to improve their financial status by promoting new measures to attract high-income, healthy beneficiaries and to compete with private health insurance agencies, as well as by implementing a copayment system (which has existed since 1996). The implementation of the copayment system in public health insurance agencies led to a sharp increase in the personal burden of healthcare expenses, especially among those living in poverty.

   The causes of these problems mainly include:

1. *The dual-track system of health insurance and insurance pricing.* Public health insurance is administered by FONASA, and its premiums are unrelated to the number of insured persons or the demographic characteristics. All insured persons contribute 7% of their wages and receive the same level of insured services. In other words, the premiums of public health insurance increase with income, meaning that the price of insurance increases as a function of income. Because of differences in income level, high-income earners must pay a higher price to receive the same quality and quantity of healthcare services. Furthermore, public health insurance generally requires beneficiaries to receive healthcare services from public hospitals. Hence, those who opt for public health insurance inevitably face the many limitations of public healthcare providers, such as the low quality of healthcare services, inability to receive timely treatments, and long queues. On the other hand, the insured services under the private health insurance system are determined by the

individual's ability to pay. Premiums are based on the level of insurance required by the household and the risk status of each household member. There is thus an equivalent relationship between premiums and insurance level based on market principles, which is reflected in the equivalence and fairness of rights and obligations. Thus, higher premiums imply a higher quality and quantity of healthcare services, as well as greater convenience because patients can seek medical attention at any time without long queues. Therefore, high-income earners generally opt to enroll in private health insurance. High-income households also generally have better health status. By contrast, high-risk impoverished groups are only able to remain in public health insurance.

2. *Copayment system.* As the government has no clear policies on the copayment system, private health insurers have pursued their own interests and caused the copayment system to become a means to crowd out high-risk groups. Although the public health insurance sector has a copayment system, the same copayment ratio applies within the same group of people. In contrast, private insurers determine the copayment ratio of each beneficiary only after assessing their socio-economic conditions. Low-income groups tend to bear a higher proportion of healthcare expenses under private health insurance, as well as receive a lower level of economic protection. In effect, the copayment system sets up an additional barrier to the entry of lower-middle income groups into private health insurance. Generally, the level of economic protection provided by private health insurance agencies does not exceed one third of the healthcare expenses, with the lowest levels reaching below 10%. This implies that patients must bear 66% to 91% of the economic burden. Research has shown that individuals with healthcare expenses of less than 500,000 pesos per year pay 31.3% of the total expenses, whereas individuals with healthcare expenses exceeding 500,000 pesos per year pay 44.9% of the total expenses.

3. *The growth of private and public health insurance is not mutually reinforcing but mutually constraining.* The difference between the private and public health insurance systems is mainly in that they have two different types of contractual mechanisms. Insured persons are automatically sorted into two categories: low-income, high-risk individuals remain in the public health insurance system, whereas high-income, low-risk individuals must utilize the private health insurance system. This effectively destroys the subsidization mechanism of high-income to low-income earners in the public health insurance system. Not only does this fail to inhibit the growth in the investment of public health insurance agencies, but it in fact will increase that growth rate. In 1995, the Chilean government allocated US$932.8 million to public healthcare, equivalent to US$67.59 per capita, whereas public health insurance agencies cost US$8.7 million, equivalent to US$110.17 per capita. Chile's healthcare expenditure as a share of the GDP in 1985, 1990, and 1996 was 1.6%, 2%, and 2.3%, respectively. This trend was in conflict with the original intentions of Chile's health insurance reforms – namely, to reduce government burden. Thus, in order to improve their financial situation, public insurance agencies began to implement new plans to attract high-income insured persons to remain within the system. For example, medical allowances were provided to high-income earners, which enabled them to receive preferential treatment in public hospitals and required them to pay rather little healthcare expenses. This cultivated competition with private insurance agencies for attracting high-quality insured persons.

SECTION IV. THE HEALTH SYSTEM IN MEXICO

1. Overview of Socioeconomics and National Health

(1) Basic National Conditions

Mexico, officially the United Mexican States, has a land area of 1,972,550 km². It is the third largest country in Latin America and the 14th largest worldwide. Mexico is located in the southern portion of North America, and the northwestern tip of Latin America. It is the only passage between North and South America, and is commonly known as a "land bridge." Mexico is bordered to the north by the US; to the south by Guatemala and Belize; to the east by the Gulf of Mexico and the Caribbean Sea; and to the west by the Pacific Ocean and the Gulf of California. Mexico is divided into 31 states and 1 Federal District (Mexico City), which are further divided into municipalities (counties). The capital is Mexico City, which covers an area of approximately 1,485 km² and has a population of 20 million (including its satellite cities). It is the most populous city in Mexico.

Mexico is a major economic power in Latin America, and its GDP is second only to Brazil. However, there is also an extreme gap between the rich and poor. By 2017, 45% of the population lived in poverty, of which 18% lived in extreme poverty.

(2) Population and Health Status

As of 2012, the total population in Mexico was 116 million, making it second only to Brazil in Latin America and the 11th most populous worldwide. Mestizos (mixed European and Indigenous descent) accounted for 60% of the population, Indigenous peoples accounted for 30%, and European Mexicans accounted for 9%. According to a report published by the UN Human Settlements Program entitled "State of Latin American and Caribbean Cities 2012," Mexico had the largest number of emigrants of any country in 2010. The report found that in 2010, more than 30 million Latin Americans and Caribbean people lived in other countries. Among these, nearly 40% were Mexicans, implying that nearly 12 million Mexicans lived abroad (or about 10.7% of its total population). The official language in Mexico is Spanish, while 7.1% of the population speak indigenous languages. Most (89%) of the population are Roman Catholics, 6% are Protestants, and the remaining 5% belong to other religions or had no religion.

In 1983, through an amendment to the Mexican Constitution and the General Health Law, Mexico granted all individuals the basic right to health protection, and the "right to health protection for all Mexicans" was officially incorporated into the Constitution. In order to achieve the full coverage of healthcare services and health security, the Mexican government has implemented multiple reforms to the healthcare system. The aims of the reforms were to expand the accessibility of healthcare services, improve the service quality of the healthcare system, and establish a unified framework for the healthcare system. The most recent reform was the System for Social Protection in Health Act, which came into effect on January 1, 2004. The goal of this reform was to establish a universal health insurance system by 2010. This Act proposed a comprehensive reform approach, with the establishment of the Popular Health Insurance (PHI) being a major breakthrough that would ensure the gradual achievement of universal healthcare coverage.

Through promoting the coverage under the PHI, community healthcare funds were established for prevention and health improvement. Strengthening the prevention focus in particular reduced the dual burden of diseases. Indeed, one survey showed that early detection significantly improved for several noncommunicable diseases. By 2008, the incidence of malaria in Mexico had decreased by 60%, the number of people receiving treatment for rheumatism had increased sixfold, and the mortality rate of tuberculosis had decreased by 30%. Furthermore, the coverage of maternal immunization had reached 95%, making Mexico the country with the most comprehensive coverage for maternal immunization. According to WHO data, by 2012, Mexico's neonatal mortality rate had been reduced to 7 per 1,000 live births; its under-five mortality rate had decreased to 16 per 1,000 live births (from 25% in 2000); and its average life expectancy had increased from 71 to 76 years. Furthermore, with the broadening coverage of the PHI coverage, poorer households have received increasingly greater economic protection, and household impoverishment due to catastrophic healthcare expenditures has decreased by 20%.

2. Historical Evolution of the Health System

Over the past 180 years, the Mexican healthcare system has undergone four stages of development. The evolution and reform of the Mexican healthcare system have involved the continuous adjustment and refinement of the reform goals, policies, and strategies, and are a result of the country's complex social, economic, and political changes.

(1) Period of Preliminary Establishment

The modern healthcare system in Mexico was initially established in the early twentieth century. In this period, charitable hospitals for the poor, private hospitals for the middle class, and public hospitals for ordinary citizens emerged. The Mexican healthcare system can be precisely traced back the establishment of the Public Health Department (PHD) in 1917. In 1910, after the victory of the Mexican bourgeois revolution, the government incorporated the provision of healthcare and other social services into its range of functions. Hence, in 1917, the PHD was created to consolidate the scattered healthcare institutions, such as church hospitals and charitable organizations, and to preliminarily establish a few modernized healthcare institutions. However, because of the turbulent political situation at the time, the country's economic strength was limited, which meant that it was difficult for the government to play a major role in the formulation and implementation of social policies; instead, it could only provide limited funding and services for public health. Therefore, at that time, public healthcare services were mainly provided voluntarily by social welfare organizations, such as religious groups and charitable organizations. The PHD was only responsible for the management of public and private healthcare institutions, and its priorities were to improve the general sanitary conditions of farmers and prevent infectious diseases.

In the 1930s, the Mexican political regime completed its transition from "Caudilloism" to party politics, which objectively requires the government to be more actively involved in improving citizens' livelihood and other social affairs. In addition, the global economic crisis in 1929 was a heavy blow to Mexico, causing many of its people to fall on hard times. Dissatisfaction with the government manifested as workers' strikes, land grabbing by farmers, and a number of other events. Therefore, strengthening the construction of the public healthcare system became an important means for the government to express its concern for people's livelihood. However, due to the worsening economic crisis and the State's limited financial resources, the government was only able to enhance its management of existing public welfare organizations, including its ability to coordinate and integrate the healthcare services provided by these organizations. The government also sought to improve urban environmental health and the prevention of infectious diseases.

In 1937, Mexico formed the Ministry of Public Assistance (MPA). Together with the PHD, the MPA coordinated the healthcare policies of different healthcare providers and provided health protection for special groups, such as children, government employees, and military personnel. At the same time, certain rural cooperatives began providing healthcare services to their members, and health centers were established in urban areas and certain rural areas where conditions permitted. In 1943, the Mexican government merged the PHD with the MPA to form the Ministry of Health and Assistance (Secretaría de Salubridad y Asistencia [SSA]). The purpose of this merger was to provide healthcare services to impoverished individuals who were unable to enroll in basic social health insurance plans, further expand the scope of public healthcare coverage, and unify public health policies. However, the scope of services and level of benefits provided were extremely limited, such that some groups had no coverage at all.

(2) Period of Comprehensive Development

From 1943 to the 1970s, the Mexican healthcare system underwent a period of preliminary establishment and comprehensive development, gradually forming a complex and fragmented system comprising social health insurance agencies, the Ministry of Health, and numerous private insurance and healthcare institutions.

In 1943, the government integrated the functions of the PHD and MPA, thereby forming the SSA; expanded its healthcare functions for impoverished groups; and formulated comprehensive public health policies. Furthermore, it became jointly responsible with state governments for the provision of healthcare services and began implementing centralized management of healthcare institutions. The Ministry of Health also established the Children's Hospital of Mexico as the first "national health research institute." This institute was charged with providing complex tertiary healthcare services, specialty training, and scientific research. However, the majority of healthcare institutions were concentrated in cities during this period, and it was difficult for impoverished groups in rural areas to access public healthcare institutions. Furthermore, many households had to rely on their own financial abilities to receive low-quality and unregulated services from private practices.

Since the 1940s, basic social health insurance plans based on employment and economic statuses began to emerge among certain groups. Additionally, in 1943, the Mexican Institute of Social Security (Instituto Mexicano del Seguro Social [IMSS]) was established, which was responsible for the policies and management of social security schemes, including health and pension insurance. These insurance schemes were generally funded by employers, employees, and the Federal Government, each of whom contributed one third of the premiums. These insurance schemes were mainly established by different unions and industries. The IMSS health insurance covered both employees of the private sector and their dependents. However, the IMSS did not unify these scattered health insurance schemes; in fact, some of the schemes were not subjected to any form of IMSS control (even in terms of their funds and services). Subsequently, other mandatory social health insurance schemes were also established, including the health insurance for workers of Petroleos Mexicanos (PEMEX), the military, and their dependents. Later on, this fragmented health insurance system gradually occupied a dominant position in the Mexican healthcare system.

In 1959, the Institute of Social Security and Services for Government Workers (Instituto de Seguridad y Servicios Sociales de los Trabajadores del Estado [ISSSTE]) was established. This institute offered health insurance coverage for government employees and their dependents. The social insurance funds it used came from government funds (two thirds of the total) and employees' payroll taxes (one third).

The ISSSTE was specifically charged with providing healthcare services and other social welfare to government employees, thus further consolidating Mexico's fragmented healthcare system. Furthermore, in accordance with the Social Security Law, the Mexican government attempted to expand the beneficiaries of social health insurance in the hopes of incorporating temporary and rural workers into the health insurance system. However, these policies were not effectively or even fully implemented, leading to stagnated expansion of social health insurance.

The social security system only offered healthcare services to employees in the formal sector, and completely excluded workers in the informal sector and other low-income earners (in theory, the healthcare services of these groups should be provided by the SSA, but due to the shortage of government finances, the volume, and quality of healthcare services they received were extremely limited). Furthermore, this institutional arrangement, which was not based on need but on employment status and the ability to pay, caused social resources and government funding to begin tilting toward high-income earners with certain economic and political statuses. Finally, in terms of regional distribution, the majority of healthcare resources and services are concentrated in high-income areas, such as Mexico City, whereas the healthcare facilities and services provided in rural and less-developed areas were markedly insufficient. Over time, these two types of polarization became increasingly significant.

(3) Period of Regional Adjustment

The regional adjustment period for the Mexican healthcare system spanned the early 1970s to the late 1990s. The serious shortcomings in the Mexican government's financing equality of the healthcare system were gradually exposed, which prompted it to expand primary healthcare to rural areas and the urban poor who lacked healthcare, and to promote reform plans to address specific problems. However, the results were ineffective.

During the mid- and late 1960s, the government recognized that the uneven distribution of healthcare resources was threatening social solidarity and the effectiveness of its policies. Hence, special provisions were added to the Social Security Law requiring all temporary and agricultural workers to be covered under social insurance, which would be financed by the government. Its operation and management, on the other hand, would be undertaken by the IMSS. In the 1970s, all Mexican states used the IMSS and other social security systems to increase the accessibility of basic healthcare services and social protection for the poor. This granted some benefits of the social guarantees to rural residents and employees of the informal sector, thus enabling impoverished groups to utilize healthcare resources beyond the public health sector – that is, through the IMSS-COPLAMAR program (later renamed the IMSS-Solidaridad and IMSS-Oportunidades). This program was coordinated and administered by the IMSS Rural Affairs Department. Based on an agreement between the government and the IMSS, healthcare institutions under the IMSS were used to provide healthcare services to the urban and rural poor. Funds for this purpose were allocated by the federal government. Eventually, the program covered a population of 14 million. However, due to limited funding channels, the quality of healthcare services for these impoverished groups was far lower than was the quality of services for employees of the formal sector. Overall, the basic concept of this program was to provide low-level healthcare services to uninsured persons through government funding and social insurance (i.e., social health insurance), thereby achieving universal coverage of healthcare services. However, because of the economic downturn in the 1970s, these provisions were virtually unimplemented. Furthermore, this institutional separation impaired effective coordination between the IMSS and SSA, leading many policies and measures to be discounted or rendering them ineffective.

In the 1980s, the Mexican government began a new round of healthcare system reforms, the goal of which was still to achieve universal healthcare coverage and improve the quality of healthcare services. To expand the accessibility of healthcare services and improve the overall service quality of the healthcare system, the Mexican government established a more unified policy framework for national healthcare reforms; coordinated the activities of the service providers under the IMSS and Ministry of Health; and made its first attempt at transferring the responsibility of healthcare services to state governments. From 1984 to 1988, the first wave of decentralization reforms appeared, wherein the federal government began delegating its authority over healthcare services to local governments, thereby achieving comprehensive restructuring of authority and responsibility. The federal government's medical aid programs and healthcare services came to be directly provided by the state governments. Moreover, at the local level, the healthcare services provided by certain branch organizations of the IMSS and Ministry of Health and Assistance were integrated with those provided by local governments, in order to coordinate their policies. However, it should be noted that this first wave of decentralization involved only a partial delegation of the federal government's health administrative functions to local governments; full decentralization of health administrative authority was not achieved. Moreover, this reform was only implemented in 14 of the more economically developed states. To ensure the success of this reform, a Health Cabinet headed by the President was created via a presidential decree. This Cabinet provided political support and was responsible for coordinating the actions of relevant sectors. It was also charged with formulating the national healthcare system. By contrast, the SSA was responsible for formulating and coordinating national healthcare policies.

In 1983, by passing an amendment to the Mexican Constitution and the General Health Law, Mexico granted all individuals the basic right to health protection. Specifically, the amendment officially incorporated the "right to health protection for all Mexicans" into the Constitution. The subsequently enacted General Health Law was based on this particular provision. The SSA was renamed the Ministry of Health (MOH). In 1986, the National Health Council (NHC) was established. Its primary responsibility was to coordinate the health policies of the federal and state governments. Although this round of reforms came under the unified leadership of the president-headed Health Cabinet, and was supported by substantial preliminary preparation and planning, Mexico suffered yet another economic downturn during this period. This new financial crisis in Mexico led to a record low in federal finances, implying that the government did not have sufficient financial resources to cover the transitional costs of the reforms. On top of this, there was strong opposition from various interest groups, further hindering healthcare reforms and ultimately leading to their failure.

In the 1990s, the Mexican government proposed another round of healthcare system reforms. Thus, a second wave of decentralization reforms was initiated in Mexico. These reforms were essentially based on those attempted in the 1980s, but with more resolute and thorough delegation of responsibilities to local governments in order to provide citizens with more effective healthcare services. The remaining 18 states participated in the reforms, thus completing the decentralization reform plan. More functions and responsibilities in healthcare management were delegated to the state governments, which further enhanced the State Health Services (SHS). On the surface, these reforms appeared to weaken the central authority of the MOH. However, in essence, the reforms deepened the reach of the MOH at the grassroots level, helping it achieve a leading role in fulfilling its coordination, management, supervision, and evaluation functions. During this period, the MOH formulated the Reform Plan for the Health Service 1995–2000, which prioritized the expansion of several reforms in the basic health insurance, proposed the special "Coverage Extension Program" (CEP) to expand basic health insurance, and continued to provide healthcare services to low-income earners. Additionally, during the early 1990s, the Mexican government launched a poverty alleviation program for impoverished groups to counteract the impact of the financial crisis.

It should be noted that although the aforementioned measures had some impact on the expansion of healthcare coverage, they only partially satisfied the healthcare needs of low-income earners. Thus, further reforms were necessary. As of 2000, about 52% of the 100 million people in Mexico did not have health insurance. In addition, the different health insurance plans in Mexico each had independent legal, regulatory, and policy systems; independent management institutions and organizations; and independent healthcare institutions. Together, they formed a complex administrative system in which coordination of policies among the different sectors was extremely difficult, which in turn has influenced the overall performance of the Mexican healthcare reforms.

(4) Period of Overall Reform

Faced with the problems mentioned earlier, after 2000, Mexico implemented structural and institutional healthcare reforms, which were implemented comprehensively in the health security, service provision, and management system. The goal of these reforms was to achieve universal coverage of health insurance by 2010 in order to protect all citizens from the threat of disease. The reform strategy was to initially focus on uninsured populations and establish new insurance programs for vulnerable groups with the lowest income level, rather than rushing to reform the existing IMSS and ISSSTE; this strategy made the initiation and implementation of reforms easier. The MOH formulated the 2001–2006 National Health Program, which outlined the plans for comprehensive healthcare reforms. Specifically, the overall plan was to establish a social security system, using the formation of the PHI as its starting point, and thereby progressively attain universal health protection.

In April 2003, the System for Social Protection in Health (SSPH) Act was enacted, which came into effect on January 1, 2004. The goal of the SSPH Act was to achieve the universal coverage of the health insurance system by 2010. Specifically, it focused on strengthening the leadership role of the MOH, including its supervision, performance evaluation, and management of the overall healthcare system. In addition, it expanded the coverage of social health insurance to ultimately incorporate all uninsured individuals (who accounted for more than half the population at the time). The funding sources for these newly insured individuals included transfer payments from the federal and local governments, together with a small premium contribution from the individuals themselves. The share of these personal contributions was determined by their household income – specifically, the lower the household income, the lower the premium contribution, while the poorest 20% of households not being required to contribute any premiums. During the early stages, this program mainly targeted poor areas with limited social health insurance coverage. The SSPH sought to virtually eliminate the regional differences in public healthcare financing by 2010, and to achieve universal health insurance coverage by 2011. Mexico not only extended health insurance coverage to all citizens, but also reformed and integrated its vertically fragmented healthcare management, financing, and service functions.

In the midst of these healthcare system reforms, the new Mexican government began to integrate the supervisory agencies and supervisory work of public health and safety, including food and drug safety, environmental health, occupational health, import, and export inspection and quarantine, etc., in order to establish the MOH-led Department of Regulation and Health Protection. Comprehensive adjustments were then made to its organizational structure, goals, and functions, in order to alter the tradition of only strengthening supervisory functions in the healthcare process, and focus instead on the prevention of risk factors that threaten population health. Additionally, the supervisory functions that were originally scattered across different departments of the federal government were integrated, thus forming an "integrated health executive" in the truest sense, which reduced coordination costs and improved the efficiency of law enforcement.

The functions of the Department of Regulation and Health Protection were soon greatly expanded, forming nine major programs and covering the protection against and regulation of health risk factors in 248 industries. The functions specifically included the approval of conventional drug administrations, such as the supervision of medical devices, drugs, blood products, tissues, and organ transplants; toxicity and hazard testing of industrial products, such as pesticides, fertilizers, chemical products, and basic chemicals; supervision and testing of civilian products, such as food, tobacco, beverages, cosmetics, biological products, etc.; occupation health, such as the detection and prevention of occupation hazards; and environmental health, such as water, soil, air, and pollution testing.

Based on an overarching view of the reform process in Mexico's healthcare system, we can point to two principal ideas underlying the reforms: (1) coverage expansion, which involved incorporating uninsured individuals in the informal sector and unemployed households into the social health insurance system, thereby achieving universal coverage of social health insurance; and (2) integration of the existing "fragmented" institutional arrangements of the healthcare system. One specifically important measure in support of the latter was strengthening the leading role of the MOH in integrating healthcare resources, which ultimately helped achieve basic equality in the accessibility to healthcare services.

3. Healthcare Organizations and Service System

(1) Healthcare System

Since its establishment, Mexico's healthcare system has undergone multiple rounds of major reform, which eventually formed the basic framework of its current system. Broadly speaking, Mexico's health security and healthcare system comprises three components: the public healthcare system, social health insurance system, and private healthcare system (Table 21.6).

1. Public Healthcare System The public healthcare system mainly refers to the IMSS-Oportunidades program, which is led by the MOH and funded by the federal government. It is a social security program intended to provide social relief; it mainly provides healthcare services to rural remote areas and urban poor without social health insurance. The public healthcare system is financed by the government, and only provides uninsured persons with some basic healthcare services. However, the financing process is often restricted by the government budget; hence, its funding source is unstable. The future reform directions involve strengthening the management, supervision, and evaluation functions of the MOH, and integrating existing healthcare resources; focusing on promoting national health, sanitation, and epidemiological work, and transferring the responsibility for existing healthcare

TABLE 21.6 Healthcare Institutions and Composition of the Healthcare System in Mexico

Healthcare System	Healthcare Institutions	Year Established	Coverage Scope	Funding Source
Public healthcare system	Ministry of Health (MOH)	1979	Impoverished groups	Government
Social health insurance system — IMSS scheme	IMSS	1943	Formal sector employees	Employers, employees, and the government
ISSSTE scheme	ISSSTE	1960		Employees and the government
PEMEX scheme	PEMEX	1940	Government employees	Employees and companies
Popular Health Insurance (PHI)		2004	PEMEX employees	Government and some households
			Other uninsured populations	
Private health insurance system	Private institutions	—	High-income groups	Personal premium contributions

services to social health security agencies; and expanding the coverage of health insurance, in order to gradually incorporate uninsured groups into the PHI system.

2. Social Health Insurance System   Mexico has a diverse range of social health insurance schemes, several of which cover workers in the formal sector, have relatively stable funding sources, and provide higher-quality services. There are several different types of coverage under the social health insurance system.

The first is the social security program administered by the IMSS, which mainly covers all employees in the formal sector. The specific targets include enterprise workers, small business owners, and farmers. It provides coverage for about 50 million people, or roughly 50% of the total population. The funding for this comes from employers, employees, and the federal government. Employees contribute premiums based on a fixed percentage of their wages. This is the traditional social health insurance system in Mexico. Employees contribute an amount equivalent to about 2.25% of their monthly wages, employers contribute 6.3%, and the government subsidizes 0.45%.

The second is the social security program administered by the ISSSTE, which covers all government workers. It is funded by contributions from the insured individuals and the federal government and covers about 17 million people. There is also a health insurance program for military personnel.

The third is the PEMEX health insurance program, which mainly provides healthcare services to employees of the Mexican state oil company PEMEX and their dependents. This program is funded by contributions from the insured individuals and the federal government.

The fourth is the PHI, an insurance program established after the healthcare reforms in 2003 that seeks to address the inequalities in healthcare services and disease-induced poverty. This insurance scheme covers 40 million (40% of the population) impoverished

Mexicans without any insurance. It is funded by the federal government, state governments, and contributions from certain households, and purchases healthcare services from the MOH for its members.

3. Private Health Insurance System   The private health insurance system provides services to individuals who can afford them and who do not participate in the social health insurance system. Under this system, health service providers are more diversified. About 3 million rich Mexicans purchase private insurance and have access to higher quality healthcare services. However, some private institutions are not regulated, and some providers do not even have professional medical qualifications.

(2) Healthcare Institutions And The Healthcare System

Among Latin American countries, Mexico's social security system was established relatively early on and is fairly comprehensive. It provides coverage to the dependents of government workers, most households in the formal and informal sectors, and unemployed households. The different healthcare systems described earlier are administered by the ISSSTE, IMSS, and Federal MOH, and are operated by the branches of the ISSSTE, IMSS, and state health departments. In addition, the navy, Secretariat of National Defense, PEMEX, and other sectors (i.e., institutions) have their own social security systems and administrative agencies.

The IMSS is the largest social security institution in Latin America. Established in 1943, it provides healthcare services and nonmedical welfare across the lifespan to approximately 50 million formal-sector employees with a fixed income and their dependents. The system is funded by three parties: the federal government subsidizes each insured person based on 13.9% of the minimum wage standard of Mexico City in 1997 (adjusted annually based on the inflation rate); employers contribute the same amount of premiums; and insured persons contribute different amounts of premiums based on their wages. In 2009, the annual amount of personal contributions was about US$2,500 (about RMB17,000). Insured persons must seek medical attention from healthcare institutions that participate in the IMSS system. They can receive all healthcare services and drugs for free after contributing their premiums, although emergency services can be obtained from healthcare institutions outside the system. The IMSS has more than 3,000 primary, secondary, and tertiary healthcare institutions; emergency centers; family medicine centers; auxiliary medical services centers; and mobile hospitals. It also has 21 research institutes.

The ISSSTE, established in the 1960s, provides all healthcare services and nonmedical welfare to the employees of the federal government and a small proportion of state government employees. The nonmedical welfare services provided include pensions, mortgages, travel and hotel services, low-cost food, etc. Currently, about 2.8 million employees are enrolled; together with their dependents, the total number of insured persons is 10 million. The vast majority of these individuals are concentrated in cities, with upward of 30% being found in the capital of Mexico City. The ISSSTE system is funded by the federal government, state governments, and individuals. Compared to the IMSS system, the funding is higher but the operational mechanism of the health insurance is similar. Aside from emergency services, insured persons are also required to seek medical attention from healthcare institutions within this system. Moreover, a new reform act has permitted retired insured persons under the IMSS and ISSSTE to receive services provided by healthcare institutions participating in these systems.

The Federal MOH owns a small number of healthcare institutions that directly provide services to a small number of people. The Federal MOH also administers the PHI, a health security system that covers informal-sector and unemployed households. The PHI purchases services from healthcare institutions under the IMSS and ISSSTE. Note that the various social security systems in Mexico have each established their own healthcare institutions that directly provide services to insured persons; aside from emergency services, the systems are not interchangeable.

The three major healthcare systems and corresponding healthcare institutions in Mexico are summarized in Table 21.6. The Mexican health security system, particularly its achievement of universal coverage, has provided useful lessons to other countries. However, the fragmentation of the health security system remains the country's biggest problem (at least in the healthcare sector). The separate healthcare institutions owned by the different social security systems have led to the duplicate construction and multiparty planning of healthcare institutions. Moreover, the inability of insured persons under different systems to seek medical attention beyond their own systems has led to a wastage of healthcare resources and equality in utilizing healthcare services. To this end, the President of Mexico has made a commitment to integrate the scattered social security systems into a universal system by 2012, thereby ending the current state of fragmentation, establishing a more scientific and effective system, and providing citizens with better health security.

4. Health Security Financing and Allocation Mechanism

In 1983, an amendment to the Mexican Constitution and the General Health Law was passed in Mexico, thus granting all individuals the basic right to health protection. In April 2003, Mexico further amended the General Health Law and passed the SSPH Act. The most important change resulting from these legislative efforts was the provision of health security to individuals not covered under the traditional employment-based social security systems. Specifically, the Act stipulated that "all Mexicans have the right to join the health social security system," and required the establishment of a universal health insurance system by 2010. This has provided the healthcare financing in Mexico with a legal guarantee.

(1) Financing Structure of Health Insurance

As mentioned earlier, the Mexican health insurance program mainly comprises the IMSS, ISSSTE, and PHI (Table 21.7). There are also three major categories of insured persons: employees of private enterprises and their dependents (covered by the IMSS); employees of the public sector and their dependents (covered by the ISSSTE); and previously uninsured persons (covered by the PHI). The financing structure of the three health insurance schemes is based on a tripartite structure of power and responsibilities and is considered a mixed financing mechanism. The social insurance agencies of the IMSS, ISSSTE, and PHI systems have a similar structure. Furthermore, this structure includes the sharing of responsibilities and mutual aid among the federal government, state governments, and households.

The first major source of funding for these systems is government funding. This source of funding is a fixed healthcare investment made by the federal government for each household, which is also the social quota, thus ensuring equality among the three categories of people. More specifically, the government allocates a fixed amount of funds to each household, which is adjusted periodically based on inflation. The law clearly stipulates the amounts that the federal and state governments must bear. In 2004, the social quota of the federal government was 15% of the minimum wage, or about US$230 per year for each household.

TABLE 21.7 Funding Composition of Health Insurance in Mexico

Insurance Type	Insured Persons	Composition		
		Beneficiary	Co-contributor	Government
IMSS scheme	Employees of private institutions	Employees	Private employers	Federal and state governments
ISSSTE scheme	Employees of public institutions	Employees	Public employers	Federal and state governments
Popular Health Insurance (PHI)	Nonsalaried workers, independent workers, and other uninsured households	Dependents	Federal and state governments	-

The second funding source is the co-contribution. This funding involves matching the co-contribution funds for each category of insured persons and redistributing these funds among the different states. Within the IMSS system, these funds come from employers (i.e., for employees of private enterprises, the co-contributors are employers). Within the ISSSTE system, the government is the employer, so for employees of the public sector, the co-contributors are the public departments or units. As for the PHI, because of the lack of a clear employer, the co-contributors are the federal and state governments; the funds are negotiated and raised by the federal and state governments based on the development level of each state, thereby correcting the vast imbalances among the different states. Generally, the matching funds of the federal government are 1.5 times the social quota for medical expenses in each household, whereas the standard matching funds of the state governments are 0.5 times the social quota (these come from state taxes and other income).

The third source of funding is the contributions by the beneficiaries themselves or their dependents. These contributions are progressive in nature and help initiate income redistribution, given that the contributions are directly proportional to individual or household income. For employees of the private and public sectors, health insurance premiums are deducted directly from total wages based on their income level. As for previously uninsured populations, the amount of contribution is also progressive to ensure equality. The premiums contributed by each household are directly proportional to their income; in other words, households with higher income levels must contribute more premiums. The upper limit of the premiums contributed by this category of household is 5% of the household's disposable income. The poorest 20% of households, however, do not need to contribute premiums; instead, they must participate in relevant health programs.

(2) Funding Distribution of Health Insurance

The distribution of federal funds in the new healthcare system is mainly used to support four aspects: management and supervisory functions of the MOH, community healthcare services, services for noncritical illnesses, and expensive services for critical illnesses. Insurance funds are distributed at the federal and state levels. Based on actuarial calculations, the critical illness insurance funds receive 8% of the federal government's total social quota and the insurance matching funds of the federal and state governments. The remaining funds are used for primary healthcare services, while household contributions are collected and used at the state level. The fixed federal healthcare investment is distributed among the states according to a specific formula, the aim of which is to correct existing health problems as well as to account for regional differences, thereby achieving equal distribution. As the federal funds received by each state depend to a large extent on the number of households enrolled in the PHI, this breaks the old pattern of distribution based on historical habits and the number of healthcare workers.

More specifically, personal healthcare services are divided as: (1) primary and secondary healthcare services; and (2) expensive healthcare services provided by hospitals at the tertiary level and above. Primary healthcare services mainly target low-risk, common healthcare needs, and their expenses are borne by state governments. These specific services covered are all primary healthcare services provided by small-sized clinics and health centers, as well as basic specialist services provided by secondary hospitals. Critical illnesses have high risk and low probability, but the risk-sharing mechanism at the state level is relatively weak; hence, critical illness funds are raised at the federal level. The NHC is responsible for determining the reimbursement scope for critical illnesses, which includes cancer, cardiovascular disease, cerebrovascular disease, major trauma, long-term rehabilitation, AIDS, neonatal intensive care, organ transplantation, dialysis, etc. The reimbursement criteria include the burden of disease, cost-effectiveness indicators, and amount of resources.

(3) Popular Health Insurance (PHI)

1. Reform Process of the PHI   Since the 1990s, the Mexican healthcare system has faced three major problems: low public health expenditure, low health insurance coverage, and uneven distribution of healthcare expenditure per capita among different states. By the end of the twentieth century, half the population did not have health security, and the occurrence of impoverishment due to disease was serious. In view of the problems mentioned earlier, the new reforms of the Mexican healthcare system entered a pilot stage, which was centered on the gradual establishment of a social health security system for all citizens. The key to the effectiveness of this social health insurance system lay in the creation of the PHI, which targeted middle- and low-income groups as the main beneficiaries. By the end of 2006, 5 million households were covered by the PHI.

In 2001–2003, Mexico began piloting the PHI. Under the leadership of the MOH, the PHI was introduced in five states. In 2002, the National Commission of Social Protection was formed to supervise and manage the specific implementation of the program. The aim was to include all Mexicans under the program before 2010. This implied that Mexico was heading toward a universal health insurance system.

On May 15, 2003, the Mexican government promulgated the relevant laws. On January 1, 2004, the SSPH was enacted, and reforms were officially launched nationwide. The overall aim of these reforms was to create a universal health insurance system, and four specific reform goals were set: (1) to establish a progressive, predictable, and financially sustainable method to increase public health expenditure; (2) to increase allocation efficiency by ensuring that insurance funds are spent on cost-effective community intervention projects; (3) to prevent households from overspending on healthcare expenses by using collective mechanisms to manage risks effectively; and (4) to modify the incentives of the healthcare system by shifting the incentive mechanisms from the supply-side to the demand-side, in order to improve the quality, efficiency, and sensitivity to patient needs.

2. Funding and Payment Methods of the PHI

1. *Insurance funding.* The PHI provides financial protection for Mexicans who are not covered by other public insurance systems. As mentioned earlier, its funding structure is tripartite: (1) federal government subsidies, which are based on a fixed social quota made

by the federal government as the healthcare investment for each household; (2) state government subsidies, which are the matching co-contributions for different groups and the redistribution among different states; and (3) household insurance premiums, which are fixed amounts based on the level of household income. The upper limit is 5%, and households are required to participate in relevant health promotion activities at healthcare institutions. A proportion of the poorest households are exempt from paying premiums. The total sum of the three components amounts to US$680 per household on average. The main sources of funding are federal taxes and supplementary subsides by state governments. At the start of each year, the states formulate work plans and the state health departments report the list of insured persons to the Federal MOH. After the lists are reviewed by the Federal MOH, the Ministry of Finance directly allocates the subsidies to individual state health departments.

More specifically, the federal government first allocates health investments for each household; since 2004, this amount has been based on 15% of the minimum wage standard in Mexico City, and is known as the social quota. Subsequently, subsidies are allocated as government support for insured households. The amounts of these subsidies are 1.5 times the social quota (from the federal government) and 0.5 times the social quota (from the state governments). Finally, households prepay a small insurance premium based on their income levels. In order to improve financing equality, households that have participated voluntarily in this program are divided into 10 groups based on their income levels, such that those with higher income levels must pay higher premiums. The two groups with the lowest income levels are exempt from paying any premiums, but one of the perquisites for their enrollment is participation in health promotion activities. Households in Groups 3–7 with pregnant women and children under the age of five (born after 2006) are also exempt from paying premiums. As for households in the other groups, their premiums are based on a common fixed share of their disposable income, with an upper limit of 5%. However, for households in the top 10% in terms of income level, a two-stage payment has been established due to the vast disparity in income distribution within this population; hence, the amount of premiums ranges from US$55 to US$830 according to the different income groups. On average, the mean amount of household contributions in 2008 was US$360. The population eligible for this insurance includes all individuals who previously have not benefitted from social insurance, such as individual employers, unemployed persons, or individuals who have lost the ability to work. The majority of insured persons are impoverished groups or female-headed households.

2. *Insurance payments.* During the implementation of the PHI from 2004 to 2010, 14.3% of uninsured households (about 11 million households) were enrolled each year, and priority was given to low-income households. The PHI is designed to provide funds for personal healthcare services. It does not have its own healthcare institutions; instead, it purchases healthcare services from the IMSS and ISSTE systems, in order to provide protection for insured persons for specific services and drug lists.

The PHI has two personal healthcare service packages: the primary healthcare service package, which includes primary- and secondary-level interventions in general hospitals, and the high-complexity intervention package for critical illnesses. The costs are shared among the federal government, state governments, employers, and households. Household premium contributions increase with higher income levels. The funds for personal healthcare services under the basic health insurance are managed by state governments and are spent on basic services provided by health centers and general hospitals. The critical illness insurance funds are administered by the federal government and are spent on high-cost services in specialist hospitals.

Basic healthcare services include primary-level outpatient consultations and temporary care, as well as secondary-level basic inpatient services. Insured persons are able to access six major categories of healthcare service containing 266 items, as well as treatments for 116 pediatric diseases. The high-complexity interventions for critical illnesses are gradually being updated to form a prioritization mechanism based on clear, external criteria. The PHI Council is responsible for formulating the scope of critical illnesses, and the criteria are selected based on disease burden, cost-effectiveness, and available resources. Currently, the types of diseases eligible for critical illness interventions include cancer, cardiovascular disease, cerebrovascular disease, major trauma, long-term rehabilitation, AIDS, neonatal intensive care, organ transplantation, and dialysis. With the gradual increase in the amount of funds raise, the number of interventions has similarly increased, from 91 interventions and 168 drug treatments to 154 interventions and 173 drug treatments.

As primary healthcare services are mostly low risk and high frequency, the funds required for them can be pooled at the state level. However, the interventions for critical illnesses tend to have a low probability but high costs, making state-level pooling insufficient to counteract this type of risk; hence, a national-level risk pool was established. More specifically, from the supply-side perspective, it is more efficient to centralize the services for highly professional interventions.

In theory, the PHI can purchase healthcare services from the MOH system, IMSS system, and private healthcare institutions. However, currently, the service providers are still limited to healthcare institutions under the federal and state health departments. Different payment methods have been adopted by the PHI for healthcare institutions within the MOH system according to the services they provide: primary healthcare services are paid on a capitation basis, whereas critical illnesses are paid on a per-case basis. Nevertheless, both methods include the variable costs of the service items, while the fixed costs continue to be funded through traditional budget-based allocations. These two payment methods were merged after 2010.

3. Implementation Outcomes of the PHI To achieve the goal of universal coverage by 2010, nearly 1.5 million households were required to enroll in the PHI each year. In 2003, 614,000 households had enrolled, and by 2004, nearly 1,722,000 households had enrolled, which accounted for about 13% of all uninsured households. At the end of 2006, nearly 5.1 million households had enrolled in the PHI. In addition to the expansion of horizontal coverage, there has also been an increase in vertical coverage, which provides greater benefits. Based on cost-utility analyses, more comprehensive health security services have been provided to insured persons, from outpatient services to basic and advanced specialist services. Mexico's healthcare expenditure as a share of the GDP rose from 5.7% in 2000 to 6.8%. Among the poorest groups, the percentage of individuals with health insurance increased from 7% to 55%. Mexico has also constructed 1,700 new healthcare institutions nationwide, from rural health centers to large specialist hospitals. The vast gaps in the financial distribution and health expenditure per capita among the 32 states are also gradually narrowing. The new healthcare system is also not limited to disease treatment: community healthcare funds have been established for disease prevention and health improvement, while the strengthening of prevention has further reduced the dual burden caused by diseases. A survey showed that early detection had significantly improved for several non-communicable diseases.

Although 2005–2010 is a relatively short period of time, the changes have still been substantial. The incidence of malaria in Mexico had decreased by 60%, the number of people receiving treatment for rheumatism increased sixfold, and the mortality rate of tuberculosis decreased by 30%. Furthermore, the coverage of maternal immunization reached 95%, making Mexico the country with the most comprehensive coverage for maternal immunization. Moreover, the accelerated decline in maternal mortality reduced the maternal mortality rate by 20%, while the neonatal mortality rate fell by two-thirds by 2015. The number of male adolescent smokers has decreased by 17%, the number of people who receive a mammography has increased by 17%, and the number of people who received early cancer screening has increased by 32%. Finally, with broader coverage in public health insurance, poorer households have received greater economic protection, and the number of households impoverished by catastrophic healthcare expenditure has been reduced by 20%.

Afterword

SECTION I FEEDBACK AND THOUGHTS ON THE CHINESE VERSION OF *WORLD HEALTH SYSTEMS*

It has been three years since the publication of the Chinese version of *World Health Systems*. Before that, there were also two editions of *Medical Service and Insurance Systems in Developed Countries and Areas*. During these years, I have received a considerable amount of feedback and suggestions from my readers, much of which focused on the following proposal: since the book introduces and analyzes the health systems of numerous countries and areas, would it be possible to develop a formula that measures the degree of development of these systems?

This question has always troubled me. Given that the basic system, value orientation of development, and level of economic development are different for each country, is it truly feasible to measure and evaluate them using the same set of indicators? If not, then why do we use GDP as an indicator of the economic development of a country, area, or city?

This prompted me to begin thinking – if it is really possible to design a set of relatively reasonable measurement indicators for health systems, then what parameters should be included? What is a reasonable range for healthcare investment as a share of the GDP? What about investment indicators for other resources? Which of the many indicators of service process are easier to measure? What about the input–output efficiency? In addition to health outputs, how can we scientifically measure the degree of satisfaction?

There are countless such questions remaining. Nevertheless, I hope to take an exploratory step forward by attempting to create such an indicator. The basic route of design is as follows: (1) With reference to the ideas of Milton I. Roemer, the concepts of healthcare inputs, service process, and health outputs will first be explained using a diagram. (2) Then, these concepts will be illustrated using a set of measurable data, and weighted according to the different levels of importance. (3) Finally, these data and weights will be used to build a mathematical model, which will then be applied to measure and evaluate the different health systems. In applying the model, the indicators and weights will be further improved and modified depending on how they function during practical application. What shall we name this overall indicator? Let us call it the Medical System Index (MSI) for the time being.

SECTION II MAIN CONTENT OF THE MODEL

In his book *National Health Systems of the World*, Roemer described a basic model of health systems. We will draw on the basic ideas of this model to create several groups of categorical data, add the appropriate weights, and calculate the final MSI. The MSI can then be used to comprehensively evaluate the health systems of all countries and areas in the world, which will enable us to sort the countries and conduct specific indicator evaluations. These results will in turn allow us to identify the level of advancement and the deficiencies of each health system in order to achieve continuous improvement.

The MSI should evaluate the following five aspects of a health system:

1. *Healthcare resources.* This aspect includes healthcare inputs as a share of GDP, number of physicians per 1,000 people, number of nurses, number of hospital beds, number of medical equipment, drug supply, and so forth.
2. *Operation of healthcare institutions.* This aspect includes the diagnostic and treatment capacities of large hospitals, quantity and quality of surgeries, service volume and quality of community general practitioners and community nurses, residents' degree of satisfaction, community-based extension services, and so forth.
3. *Level of healthcare management.* This aspect concerns various strict management systems, laws and regulations, level of informatization, and equality and accessibility of healthcare services.
4. *Effective economic support.* This aspect relates to the coverage and equality of health insurance, input of social charity, and degree of government protection.
5. *Overall outcomes of healthcare services.* This aspect relates to the average life expectancy, infant mortality rate, maternal mortality rate, under-five mortality rate, disability-adjusted life years, and so forth.

Currently, the authoritative evaluation of health indicators is the Bloomberg Healthiest Country Index, which is calculated by the University of Washington Institute for Health Metrics and Evaluation.

 SECTION III CHALLENGES FOR FUTURE RESEARCH

We are still in the process of studying how to integrate practicality with feasibility of data quantification in the establishment of the MSI. For example, healthcare investment as a share of the GDP is around 10% among developed countries. It is 8% in the UK, where the equality of healthcare services is essentially guaranteed; however, the efficiency of its health system is low, and waiting times are long for common diseases. In contrast, healthcare investment as a share of the GDP is 17% in the US, where healthcare services are highly efficient but overly expensive and inequitable. So how should this indicator be integrated into the MSI model? Another example is that residents' degree of satisfaction with healthcare services can be measured using randomly sampled surveys, where professional interviewers conduct surveys using questionnaires face-to-face with service users. However, users' degree of satisfaction is subjective, and therefore is susceptible to errors during quantification and insufficiently objective. Unfortunately, I am not a mathematician and thus cannot implement the MSI as a mathematical model for now. Due to the time constraints of publishing this book, the ideas for establishing a comprehensive MSI model remain preliminary and would require further deliberation and research. I would like to use this as an opportunity to introduce my crude ideas, and invite all readers and experts to offer their valuable contributions in the hopes of completing and continuously refining this project, so that together we can jointly promote the continual improvement of health systems across the world.

Bibliography

Abel-Smith B. *An introduction to health: policy, planning and financing.* London and New York: Longman, 1994.

Abel-Smith B. The rise and decline of the early HMOs. *Milbank Memorial Fund Quarterly,* 1988, 66(4): 694–719.

Abel-Smith B, Creese A. Recurrent costs in the health sector – problems and policy options in three countries. Geneva: World Health Organization, 1989.

Abel-Smith B, Dua A. Community-financing in developing countries: the potential for the health sector. *Health Policy and Planning,* 1988, 3(2): 95–108.

Adamov V, Kolev K, Vrachovski D, Zahariev A, Marcheva A. Human resources of the health system in republic of bulgaria. *Cahiers de Sociologie et de Démographie Médicales,* 2010, 50(1): 6–120.

Aggarwal A. Impact evaluation of India's "Yeshasvini" community-based health insurance programme. *Health Economics,* 2010, 19(S1): 5–35.

Ai ZS. Development and analysis of Singapore's health insurance model. *Journal of Shanghai Tongji University: Natural Science Edition,* 1998, 19(9): 83–85.

Akerlof GA. The market for "lemons": quality uncertainty and the market mechanism. *Quarterly Journal of Economics,* 1970, 84(3): 488–500.

Armstrong A. A comparative analysis: new public management – the way ahead? *Australian Journal of Public Administration,* 1998, 57(2): 12–24.

Australian Government. National health reform: progress and delivery, 2011. http://www.yourhealth.gov.au/internet/yourhealth/publishing.nsf/Content/nhr-progress-delivery.

Australian Institute of Health and Welfare (AIHW). Australia's hospitals 2009–10: at a glance. Health services series no. 39. Cat. No. HSE 106. Canberra: Australian Institute of Health and Welfare, 2011.

Axel K. Health interview surveys in developing countries: a review of methods and results. *International Journal of Epidemiology,* 1983, 12(4): 465–481.

Baernighausen T, Sauerborn R, Zhang XP, et al. The mechanism of progressive development in Germany's health insurance. *Chinese Journal of Social Medicine,* 2000(1), 9–14.

Balarajan Y, Selvaraj S, Subramanian SV. India: Towards Universal Health Coverage 4 Health care and equity in India. *Lancet,* 2011, 377(9764): 505–515.

Bao JG. Australian health insurance and Queensland health system: investigation report. *Chinese Health Resources,* 2000, 3(3): 142–143.

Barr N, Whynes D. *Current issues in the economics of welfare.* Translated by He XB and Wang Y. Beijing: China Labor and Social Security Press, 2003.

Basch PF. *International health.* New York: Oxford University Press, 1978.

Bassetti M, Di Biagio A, Rebesco B, et al. Impact of an antimicrobial formulary and restriction policy in the largest hospital in Italy. *International Journal of Antimicrobial Agents,* 2000, 16(3): 295–298.

Beaver C, Zhao Y, McDermid S, et al. Casemix-based funding of Northern Territory public hospitals: adjusting for severity and socio-economic variations. *Health Economy,* 1998, 7(1): 53–61.

Berndt ER. Pharmaceuticals in US health care: determinants of quantity and price. *Journal of Economic Perspectives,* 2002, 16(4): 45–66.

Beveridge W. *Social Insurance and Allied Services* (Cmd. 6404) [The Beveridge Report], Alabaster Passmore & Sons Limited, November 1942.

Bhat R. Regulation of the private health sector in India. *International Journal of Health Planning and Management*, 1996, 11(3): 253–274.

Bhattacharjya AS, Sapra PK. Health insurance in China and India: segmented roles for public and private financing. *Health Affairs*, 2008, 27(4): 1005–1015.

Bi J. Research on the orientation of government science and technology management based on the theory of public goods. *Science & Technology Progress and Policy*, 2011, 11: 69.

Black D. Inequalities in health. *American Journal of Public Health*, 1991, 105(21): 23–27.

Blanpain J, Delesie L, Nys H. *National health insurance and health resources: The European experience.* Cambridge, MA: Harvard University Press, 1978.

Bloom G, Lucas H, Suhua C, et al. Financing health services in poor rural areas: adapting to economic and institutional reform in China. IDS Research Report 30. Sussex, UK: Institute of Development Studies, 1995.

Bloom G. Managing health sector development: markets and institutional reform. *Neoliberalism and the Development Policy Debate.* New York: Oxford University Press, 1991.

Boards of Trustees of the Federal Hospital Insurance and Federal Supplementary Medical Insurance Trust Funds. 2002 Annual Report. Germany, 2003.

Bradshaw J. The conceptualization and measurement of need: a social policy perspective. In Jennie Popay and Gareth Williams (eds.), *Researching the people's health.* London-New York: Routledge, 1994.

Brown LD. Exceptionalism as the rule? US health policy innovation and cross-national learning. *Journal of Health Politics, Policy and Law*, 1998, 23(1): 35–51.

Brown TM, Cueto M, Fee, E. The World Health Organization and the transition from "international" to "global" public health. *American Journal of Public Health*, 2006, 96(1): 62–72.

Bryndová L, Pavloková K, Roubal T, et al. Czech Republic: health system review. *Health Systems in Transition*, 2009, 11(1): 1–122.

Bunyavanich S, Walkup RB. US public health leaders shift toward a new paradigm of global health. *American Journal of Public Health*, 2001, 91(10): 1556–1558.

Bureau of Statistics. Canada Health Survey 2002. Ottawa: Department of Health Studies, 2003.

Cai RH. *Encyclopedia of China's health insurance system reforms.* Beijing: China Personnel Press, 1996.

Cai RH. *Health insurance practical training materials.* Beijing: Peking University Medical Press, 1999.

Canadian Association of Medical Clinics. *New horizons in health care: proceedings of first international congress on group medicine.* Winnipeg, MB: Wallingford Press, 1970.

Canadian Institute for Health Information. *Canada's health care providers, 2000 to 2009 – a reference guide.* Ottawa, ON: CIHI, 2011a.

Canadian Institute for Health Information. *National health expenditure trends, 1975 to 2011.* Ottawa, ON: CIHI, 2011b.

Cao Y. Implementation of free healthcare in Russia. *Contemporary Social Science Perspective*, 2013(11): 51–52.

Chan CK, Yang Y, Zhao MJ. 30-Baht for the treatment of all diseases – an experiment of the healthcare system in Thailand. *Medicine and Philosophy: Humanities and Social Science Edition*, 2007, 28(10): 7–8, 13.

Chang F, Zhang ZW. Structural analysis of policies for foreign drug compensation regulations. *China Pharmacy*, 2010(33): 3076–3078.

Chen AY. International comparison of healthcare cost containment and its insights for China. *International Medicine and Health Guidance News*, 2005, 23: 9–11.

Chen DJ, Luo YW. Japan's health insurance system and its insights for China. *Japanese Studies*, 2002, 3: 52–58.

Chen FZ. *Manual of reforms in the urban employee basic medical insurance.* Beijing: Seismological Press, 1999.

Chen PY. Introduction of Singapore's white paper on government healthcare policy. *Foreign Medicine (Hospital Management)*, 1995, 3: 94–103.

Chen SX. *A study on the poverty problem in the United States.* Wuhan: Wuhan University Press, 2000.

Chen TJ, Chou LF, Hwang SJ. Application of concentration ratios to analyze the phenomenon of "next-door" pharmacy in Taiwan. *Clinical Therapeutics*, 2006, (28)8: 1225–1230.

Chen X. Australian federal health insurance system. *Chinese Health Service Management*, 2002, 4: 245.

Chen Y, Wei X, Xie Y. Major practices and characteristics of public hospital reforms in South Africa. *Chinese Journal of Health Policy*, 2012, 5(8): 18–21.

Chen YF, Zhang L. Comparative analysis on the healthcare systems of the BRIC countries. *Chinese Health Economics*, ISTICPKU, 2013, 32(3): 5–7.

Chen YF. Comparative study on the healthcare systems of the BRIC countries. Doctoral Dissertation. Wuhan: Huazhong University of Science and Technology, 2011.

Chen ZX, Meng CX, Zhou ZT. *Hospital leadership.* Shanghai: Shanghai Scientific & Technical Publishers, 2002.

Cheng J, Zhao W. Healthcare expenditure in the process of population aging: analysis of experiences in WHO member states. *Chinese Journal of Health Policy*, 2010, 2(4): 57–62.

Cheng XM, Luo WJ. *Health economics.* Beijing: People's Medical Publishing House, 2003: 67–71.

Cheng XM. *Health insurance.* Shanghai: Fudan University Press, 2003.

China Labor Consultation Network. Investigation report on the health insurance in Germany and Hungary. 2009-05-06. http://www.51shebao.com.

Chou YJ, Yip WC, Lee CH, et al. Impact of separating drug prescribing and dispensing on provider behaviour: Taiwan's experience. *Health Policy and Planning*, 2003, 18(3): 316–329.

Chu TY. Constructing a service-oriented government: an investigation on the multidimensional theory. *Nanjing Journal of Social Sciences*, 2007, (9): 81–87.

Chu XY, Han PF, Huang LJ, et al. Overview of health system reforms in Hungary. *Chinese Journal of Social Medicine*, 2008, 25(5): 271–273.

Chu XY, Huang LJ, Han PF, et al. Overview of health system reforms in Russia. *Chinese Journal of Social Medicine*, 2009, 26(4): 220–222.

Chu ZH. Health system reforms and implementation in Singapore. *Foreign Medicine (Health Economics)*, 1994, 11(4): 145–148.

Chu ZH. Non-profit hospitals in the United States. *Health Economics Research*, 2001, (7): 41–42.

Cichon M. Health sector reforms in central and eastern Europe: paradigm reversed. *International Labour Review*, 1991, 130(3): 311–327.

Claudia J. Flawed but fair: Brazil's health system reaches out to the poor. Geneva: World Health Organization, 2008.

Cleary MI, Murray JM, Michael R, et al. Outpatient costing and classification: are we any closer to a national standard for ambulatory classification systems? *The Medical Journal of Australia*, 1998, 169(Suppl): 26–31.

Commons JR. *Institutional economics.* Beijing: The Commercial Press, 1997.

Cong SH. *Economic theory of social security.* Beijing: SDX Joint Publishing Company, 1996.

Constitution of the Republic of South Africa. (No. 108 of 1996). Statutes of the Republic of South Africa – Constitutional Law 38: 1241–1331. http://www.info.gov.za/documents/constituti.

Coopers, LD. *Costing and pricing contracts, pricing in hospitals: a case study.* London: NHS Management Executive, 1990.

Coovadia H, Jewkes R, Barron P, et al. The health and health system of South Africa: historical roots of current public health challenges. *Lancet*, 2009, 374(9692): 817–834.

Creese A. Global trends in health care reform. *World Health Forum*, 1994, 15(4): 317–322.

Creese A. User charge for health care: a review of recent experience. Current concerns. SHA paper number 1. Geneva: World Health Organization, Division of Health Service Strengthening, 1990.

Cui ZW, Jia GT, Fu XM, et al. Direction of Japan's health system reforms. *Foreign Medicine (Health Economics)*, 2000, 17(1): 13–15.

Dahlgren G, Whitehead M. *Policies and strategies to promote equity in health.* Geneva: World Health Organization, 1992.

Dai T, Wang XW, He P. Characteristics of the economic incentive mechanism for healthcare workers in Hong Kong and Taiwan. *Health Economics Research*, 2007, (8): 16–18.

Dai WD. Comparison and thoughts on the healthcare systems of BRIC countries. *Journal of Huazhong University of Science and Technology*, 2011, 25(2): 113–119.

Dang T, Antolin P, Oxley H. Fiscal implications of aging: projections of age-related spending. OECD Economics Department Working Papers, No. 305. Paris: OECD Publishing, 2001.

David BH, Kemp KB. *The management of health care technology in nine countries.* New York: Springer, 1982.

David H, Megan N. South African health review 1995. Durban: health system trust. (2004-05-05) [2011-10-21]. http://www.hst.org.za/sahr/chap4.htm.

Davies AM. Epidemiology and the challenge of aging. *International Journal of Epidemiology*, 1985, 14(1): 9–21.

DeNavas-Walt C, Proctor BD, Smith JC. *Income, poverty, and health insurance coverage in the United States: 2010.* Washington, DC: US Department of Commerce, 2011.

Deng DS. *A study on the social security system in the United States of America.* Wuhan: Wuhan University Press, 1999.

Deng F, Lü JH, Gao JM, et al. Comparative analysis of healthcare resources and health expenditures among BRICS countries. *Chinese Health Economics*, 2014, 2: 94–96.

Department of Health, Government of the Hong Kong Special Administrative Region. Preview of the public health service charges for the Department of Health, 2011. https://www.dh.gov.hk/chs/useful/useful_fee/useful_fee_css.html.

Department of Health. Health sector reform agenda: Philippines 1999–2004. Manila: Department of Health, 1999.

Department of Health. White paper for the transformation of the health system in South Africa. Pretoria: Department of Health, 1997.

Devadasan N, Criel B, Van Damme W, et al. Performance of community health insurance in India: findings from empirical studies. *BioMed Central*, 2012, 6(1): 9.

Diamond P. Privatization of social security: lessons from Chile. *Latin American Studies*, 2010, 32(6): 64–71.

Dimova A, Rohova M, Moutafova E, et al. Bulgaria: health system review. *Health Systems in Transition*, 2012, 14(3): 1–186.

Ding DX, Ma YN. Insights for China from the payment methods of medical assistance in foreign countries. *Health Economics Research*, 2009, 8: 22–24.

DOH. Department of Health, government of the Philippines, 2005. http://www.doh.gov.ph.

Dong QJ, Li GH. Reform of healthcare finances in Bulgaria. *Foreign Medicine (Health Economics)*, 2002, 19(4): 159–162.

Duan K. *Contemporary American insurance.* Shanghai: Fudan University Press, 2001.

Duan YF, Wang XW. Reform and development trends in Japan's healthcare system. *Foreign Medicine (Health Economics)*, 2002, 19(4): 166–170.

Duckett SJ. Casemix funding for acute hospital inpatient services in Australia. *Medical Journal of Australia*, 1998, 169(8): S17–S21.

Duckett SJ. Hospital payment arrangements to encourage efficiency: the case of Victoria, Australia. *Health Policy*, 1995, 34(2): 113–134.

Eberstadt N. World population prospects and the global economic outlook: the shape of things to come. *SSRN Electronic Journal*, 2011.

Eggleston K, Ling L, Qingyue M, et al. Health service delivery in China: a literature review. *Health Economics*, 2008, 17(2): 149–165.

Ellis RP, Alam M, Gupta I. Health insurance in India: prognosis and prospectus. *Economic and Political Weekly*, 2000, 35(4): 207–217.

Epstein AM. Medicaid managed care and high quality, can we have both? *Journal of the American Medical Association*, 1997, 278(19): 1617–1621.

Epstein AM. US teaching hospitals in the evolving health care system. *Journal of the American Medical Association*, 1995, 273(15): 1203–1207.

Eucken W. *The foundations of economics: History and theory in the analysis of economic reality.* Translated from the German by T. W. Hutchison. Chicago: University of Chicago Press, 1951.

Evans JR, Hall KL, Warford J. Shattuck lecture – health care in the developing world: problems of scarcity and choice. *New England Journal of Medicine*, 1981, 305(19): 1117–1127.

Fan GG, Nan F. A survey on the uneven distribution of healthcare resources in northeastern Mexico. *Foreign Medicine (Health Economics)*, 2006, 3: 140–144.

Fan VY, Mahal A. Learning and getting better: rigorous evaluations of health policy in India. *National Medical Journal of India*, 2011, 24(6): 235–237.

Fan WS. Principles of intergovernmental transfer and distribution of health resources. *Foreign Medicine (Health Economics)*, 2000, 17(1): 32–34.

Fan WS. Reforms of healthcare cost containment in Western countries. *Foreign Medicine (Health Economics)*, 1996, 3: 121–122.

Fang L. Business strategies adopted by Thai insurance companies for the adjustment of health insurance. *Insurance Studies*, 1999, 8: 48–49.

Feng L, Yang SM. Current status and insights from the "separation of prescribing and dispensing" in foreign countries, Taiwan and Hong Kong. *China Pharmacy*, 2005, 16(24): 1907–1909.

Feng XW, Wang H, Cheng G. Brazil's health system reforms and its insights for China. *Medicine and Society*, 2007, 20(12): 30–32.

Fleury S, Belmartino S, Baris E. Reshaping health care in Latin America: a comparative analysis of health care reform in Argentina, Brazil, and Mexico. *Revista Panamericana De Salud Pública*, 2000, 9(43): 130–131.

Fragonard B. Forecast of health insurance trends. French Department of Social Security website, 2006, http://www.security-sociale.fr/institutions/hcaam/rapport2007/hcaam_rappport2007.pdf.

François-Xavier S. Public sector reforms in France – Healthcare, social contract and markets. Translated by Zhang CY, Ma JP. *Journal of Chinese Academy of Governance*, 2010, 5: 139–140.

Friedman M. From "Created Equal," an episode of the PBS *Free to Choose* television series (1980, vol. 5 transcript).

Fries JF. Aging, natural death, and the compression of morbidity. *New England Journal of Medicine*, 1980, 303(3): 130–135.

Fu C. Introduction to the healthcare system in Hong Kong. *Progress in Health Policy Research* (internal publication), 2009, 7: 9–11.

Fu C, Zhang G. Insights and lessons from the healthcare management system in Taiwan. *Chinese Health Resources*, 2007, 10(1): 24–25.

Fu DY, Lan LJ. The health security systems of India, Brazil and Mexico and their insights for China. *Medicine and Philosophy: Humanities and Social Science Edition*, 2011, 32(19).

Fu HP, Su JT, Dan N, et al. Methods and experiences in centralized drug procurement by the Hospital Authority in Hong Kong. *Health Economics Research*, 2010, 9: 38–40.

Fu ZZ. Evaluation of Taiwan's health insurance system. The Second Cross-Straits High-Level Forum on Hospital Health Insurance Management, Nanjing, 2010.

Fuchs VR. Managed care and merger mania. *Journal of the American Medical Association*, 1997, 277(11): 920–921.

Fudan University. *The social security system in Japan – a joint discussion on China's social security system reforms*. Shanghai: Fudan University Press, 1996.

Furnas B. *American health care since 1994*. Washington, DC: Center for American Progress, 2009.

Furubotn EG, Richter R, *Institutions and economic theory, the contribution of the new institutional economics*. Ann Arbor: The University of Michigan Press, 1998.]

Gaál P, Szigeti S, Csere M, et al. Hungary health system review. *Health Systems in Transition*, 2011, 13(5): 1–266.

Gaál P. *Health systems in transition: Hungary* (2004). Translated by Shen J, Ren W. Beijing: Peking University Medical Press, 2008.

Gallai S, Dobos B, Yuan T, et al. An analysis of healthcare reforms in Hungary (1990–2010). *Journal of Public Administration*, 2010, 3(5): 25–64.

Gan JB. A historical materialist perspective – the fundamental causes of poverty and underdevelopment in developing countries. *Jianghai Academic Journal*, 1999, 5: 103–105.

Gao B. Innovations in the theory of economic development in the era of globalization. *Journal of Nanjing University: Philosophy, Humanities and Social Sciences*, 2013, 50(1): 13–26.

Gao DL. Drug administration and cost containment in Germany. *Foreign Medicine (Health Economics)*, 1999, 16(4): 147–151.

Gao DL. Healthcare reforms in Germany. *Foreign Medicine (Health Economics)*, 1999, 16(3): 97–102.

Gao DL. Medical equipment management and cost containment in Germany. *Foreign Medicine (Health Economics)*, 2000, 17(1): 410.

Gao M, Lin C, Sun W. The truth behind Russia's "free universal healthcare." *Times Figure*, 2013, 11: 64–65.

Gao XQ, Zhao MG. Overview and insights of the healthcare system in the Russian Federation. *Modern Hospital Management*, 2014, 12(2): 22–24.

Ge HY. India's healthcare system and its insights for China. *Decision-Making Reference for Hospital Leadership*, 2009, 11: 41–44.

General Statistics Office (GSO). *Niengiamthongke (Statistical Yearbook)*. Hanoi: Statistical Publishing House, 2008.

Georgieva M., Moutafova E. Hospital performance measurement in Bulgaria. *Health Reforms in South East Europe*. Palgrave Macmillan, 2012, 179–189.

German Federal Ministry of Health. Health reform 2000 (draft). Berlin: German Federal Ministry of Health, 1999.

Gertler P, Solon O. *Who benefits from social health insurance in developing countries?* Berkeley: University of California Press, 2000.

Giang TL. Social health insurance in Vietnam: current issues and policy recommendations. ERIA Research Project Report, 2009, 10: 292.

Gilson L, McIntyre D. Post-apartheid challenges: household access and use of health care in South Africa. *International Journal of Health Services*, 2007, 37(4): 673–691.

Gong YL, Yan F. *Social medicine*. Second edition. Shanghai: Fudan University Press, 2005.

Goudge J, Russell S, Gilson L, et al. Illness-related impoverishment in rural South Africa: why does social protection work for some households but not others? *Journal of International Development*, 2009, 21(2): 231–251.

Government of Canada. Healthy Canadians – a federal report on comparable health indicators. 2008. http://www.hc-sc.gc.ca/hcs-sss/pubs/system-regime/index-eng.php.

Government of United Kingdom. Department of Health – Spending Review 2010. London: The Stationery Office Limited, 2011.

Graser W. *Health insurance in practice: international variations in financing, benefits, and problems*. Oxford: Jossey-Bass, 1991.

Grossman M. *The demand for health: a theoretical and empirical investigation*. NBER Books, 1972, 137(2): 279.

Guan X. Insights for China from the recent reforms of the UK National Health Service. *Chinese Health Resources*, 2010, 13(1): 48–50.

Guo SZ. Characteristics of recent developments in health insurance and experiences in cost control in foreign countries. *Chinese Health Economics*, 1998, 5: 60–61.

Guo SZ. Social security – basic theories and international comparison. Shanghai: Shanghai University of Finance & Economic Press, 1996.

Guo WB, Zhang L, Zhang CY. A review of payment methods for health insurance expenses. *Health Economics Research*, 2011, 10: 23–26.

Guo Y, Liu PL, Xu J. Global health and national strategies. *Journal of Peking University: Health Sciences*, 2010, 3: 247–251.

Guo Y, Xie Z. Bridging the gap in one generation – theory on the social determinants of health and its international experience. *Journal of Peking University: Health Sciences*, 2009, 41(2): 125–128.

Haley DR, Beg SA. The road to recovery: Egypt's healthcare reform. *The International Journal of Health Planning and Management*, 2012, 27(1): 83–91.

Ham C. Learning from the tigers: stakeholder health care. *Lancet*, 1996, 347(9006): 951–953.

Hamed A. Egypt's transition towards a third wave of health sector reform. http://egyhealthcare.info/archives/306.

Han FQ. Comparison and insights of the community health services in China and Australia. *Chinese General Practice*, 2005, 8(18): 1506–1507.

Hao J. A study on the sustainable development of the New Rural Cooperative Medical System. Master's Thesis. Tianjin: Tianjin University of Finance and Economics, 2013.

Hao L. Challenges of Taiwan's "dual-track system" in the separation of prescribing and dispensing. *China Pharmacy*, 2008, 12: 40–42.

Hao ZM, Tian W, Cao Y. Current status and reforms in Japan's public hospitals. *Chinese Hospital Management*, 2009, 29(8): 66–67.

He ZW. Reform of public hospital management in Hong Kong and development ideas of the Hospital Authority. Bimonthly Forum of the Shanghai Health Development Research Center, 2011, 14–18.

The Health Care Study Group. Understanding the choices in the health care reform. *Journal of Health Politics, Policy and Law*, 1994, 19(3): 499–541.

Healthoo Information. Comparative analysis of policies for controlling drug expenditures in developed countries. 2002-6-12. http://www.healthoo.com/A9/200206/A9_20020612194900_96028.asp.

Heshmat S. *Managerial economics in health.* Translated by Ying XH. Beijing: Peking University Medical Press, 2004.

Hollingsworth JR, Hage J, Hanneman RA. *State intervention in medical care.* Ithaca, NY: Cornell University Press, 1991.

Hong Kong Department of Health. HealthyHK website. http://www.healthyhk.gov.hk.

Hong Kong Food and Health Bureau website. http://www.fhb.gov.hk.

Hong Kong Hospital Authority website. http://www.ha.org.hk.

Hu AP, Wang MY. *Managed healthcare: healthcare services and health insurance in the United States of America.* Beijing: Higher Education Press, 2010.

Hu DD, Sui D, Huang LJ, et al. Overview of health system reforms in Armenia. *Chinese Journal of Social Medicine*, 2008, 25(4): 219–221.

Hu L. Reforms and insights of the National Health Service in the United Kingdom. *Health Economics Research*, 2011, 3: 21–23.

Hu R. India: poorest accessibility to healthcare services. *Chinese Community Doctors*, 2012, 28(44): 23.

Hu S, Tang S, Liu Y, et al. Reform of how health care is paid for in China: challenges and opportunities. *Lancet*, 2008, 372(9652): 1846–1853.

Hu SL. Drug pricing policies in developed countries. *Medicine Economic News*, 2011. http://www.yyjjb.com.cn/html/2011-08/03/content_147675.htm.

Hu SL. Evaluating the new framework of health system performance – an introduction to the World Health Report 2000. *Health Economics Research*, 2000, 7: 5–7.

Hu SL. Introduction to Medicare in the United States of America. *Health Economics Research*, 2006, 12: 41–42.

Hu SY. *Health insurance and service system.* Chengdu: Sichuan People's Publishing House, 2001.

Huang ED, Li WP. Insights from world healthcare reforms (5). Reference value of healthcare reforms in France. *China Hospital CEO*, 2011, 14: 68–71.

Huang ED. Lessons from the French health service financing and payment mechanism for China. *Chinese Health Economics*, 2008, 27(5): 77–81.

Huang JQ, Yang J. Implications and principles of constructing a hospital formulary system. *Health Economics Research*, 2008, 9: 7–8.

Huang QM, Huang DX, Guo YY, et al. United medical group: positive exploration of a Chinese managed healthcare model. *Journal of Shanghai Jiaotong University: Medical Science*, 2010, 30(8): 919–924.

Huang SF. Insights from certain healthcare systems in developed countries. *Journal of Guangxi University: Philosophy and Social Science*, 1995, 2: 87–89.

Huang YX. A few theoretical questions about social equality. *Contemporary World and Socialism*, 2011, 3: 144–147.

Huby M, Dix G. Evaluating the social fund. UK: Social Policy Research Unit, University of York, 1992.

Hurst J. The reform of health care: a comparative analysis of seven OECD countries. Paris: OECD, 1992.

Intaranongpai S, Hughes D, Leethongdee S. The provincial health office as performance manager: change in the local healthcare system after Thailand's universal coverage reforms. *International Journal of Health Planning and Management*, 2012, 27(4): 308–326.

Intellectual Property Laboratory. Research and insights of drug patent protection in the USA. 2011-07-03. http://zhangchu.fyfz.cn/art/1018791.htm.

International Union of School and University Health and Medicine. School Health Symposium. Stockholm, Sweden, 1975.

Japan Ministry of Health and Welfare. Annual report on health and welfare 1999–2000. Seeking for new image of the elderly as social aging proceeds into the 21st century. Tokyo: Japan International Corporation of Welfare Services, 2001.

Jia YC, Li B. Understanding China's health insurance reforms from a Thai perspective. *Management Observer*, 2008, 11: 203–204.

Jiang A. Comment on the neoliberal health system reforms in Latin America. *Foreign Medicine*, 2007, 24(4): 178–183.

Jiang AH, Wang YT. Government responsibility in healthcare services – experiences and insights from Cuba. *Globalization*, 2013, 9: 50–58.

Jiang DS. A masterpiece on the theory of developmental economics – commentary on the *Dual Sector Model* by Lewis. *Management World*, 1990, 02: 220–222.

Jiang L. An analysis on the Australian health security system. Master's Thesis. Wuhan: Wuhan University of Science and Technology, 2009.

Jiang LG, Wang W. Insights from the healthcare systems of BRICS countries for China's healthcare reforms. *Contemporary Economic Research*, 2014, 3: 38–41.

Jiang SZ. Government responsibility and educational equality: an investigation based on public goods theory. *Modern University Education*, 2011, 6: 7–10.

Jiang XC, Xu J. Investigation and thoughts on Brazil's healthcare system. *Chinese Primary Health Care*, 2003, 17(7): 93–95.

Jiang Y. Remuneration in public hospitals in Hong Kong. Hong Kong: Hong Kong Research Team of the China Hospital Management Association, 1999.

Jiang ZQ, Xu WL. A brief discussion on the economic theory system of wealthy nations and people established in *The Wealth of Nations* by Adam Smith. *Shanghai Journal of Economics*, 1986, 05: 17–21.

Jin CL. Progress in Japan's health insurance reforms. *Chinese Health Resources*, 1999, 2(1): 39–40.

Jin WG. How Singapore achieved universal health insurance (I). *Chinese Health Insurance*, 2011, 4: 65–67.

Jin XR. Commentary on Lewis' classical dual-sector model of developmental economics. *World Economic Studies*, 1988, 04: 72–78.

Jin ZF. *The social security system in South Korea*. Shanghai: Shanghai People's Publishing House, 2011.

John TJ, Dandona L, Sharma VP, et al. India: towards universal health coverage 1 continuing challenge of infectious diseases in India. *Lancet*, 2011, 377(9761): 252–269.

Jongudomsuk P. Effect of capitation payment on resource allocation and financing of public hospital in Thailand. Conference paper. *Asia Healthcare & Insurance*, 2003, 06: 88–90.

Kaiser. KPMG survey of employer-sponsored health benefits, 1996 and 1998. Chicago, IL: Health Research and Educational Trust (HRET), 1999.

Kaiser. Survey of employer-sponsored health benefits, 1999 and 2000. Chicago, IL: Health Research and Educational Trust (HRET), 2001.

Kalimo E. Health service needs: measurement of levels of health. WHO Regional Publications, European Series No. 7, 1988: 64–71.

Kasper W, Streit ME. *Institutional economics: Social order and public policy*. UK: Edward Elgar Publishing, 1998.

Kassirer JP. Mergers and acquisitions – who benefits? Who loses? *New England Journal of Medicine*, 1996, 334(11): 722–723.

Kendig H, Duckett S. *Australian directions in aged care: the generation of policies for generations of older people*. Australian Health Policy Institute Commissioned Paper Series 2001/05, Australian Health Policy Institute, University of Sydney, 2001.

Keynes JM. *The general theory of employment, interest, and money*. Palgrave Macmillan, 1936.

Kickbush I. The need for a European strategy on global health. *Scandinavian Journal of Public Health*, 2006, 34(6): 561–565.

Kim HJ, Chung W, Lee SG. Lessons from Korea's pharmaceutical policy reform: the separation of medical institutions and pharmacies for outpatient care. *Health Policy*, 2004, 68(3): 267–275.

Knaul FM, Arreola-Ornelas H, Méndez-Carniado O, et al. Reform of universal health insurance in Mexico. *Comparative Economic & Social Systems*, 2009, 4: 61–68.

Kong DS, Li W, Yao SL. A report on the treatment of 100 cases of spondylosis by the medical team sent to Cuba. *The Journal of Cervicodynia and Lumbodynia*, 2001, 02: 142–143.

Korea National Health Insurance Corporation. Major indicators of the national health insurance by year. Seoul, Korea: Korea National Health Insurance Corporation, 2002, http://www.nhic.or.kr.

Kuang L. Managed healthcare – the mainstream of US health insurance operations. *Foreign Medicine (Hospital Management)*, 2000, 2: 49–52.

Kubiak A. *The voice of general public and business people on corruption*. Stefan Batory Foundation Warsaw, 2003.

Kumar M. Towards universal health coverage in India. *Lancet*, 2011, 377(9777): 1568–1569.

Kuszewski K, Gericke C, Busse R. *Health care systems in transition: Poland*. Copenhagen: WHO Regional Office for Europe, 2005.

Kuszewski K, Gericke C. *Health systems in transition: Poland* (2005). Translated by Luo Yi. Beijing: Peking University Medical Press, 2007.

Kuttner R. Columbia/HCA and the resurgence of the for-profit hospital business. *New England Journal of Medicine*, 1996, 335(6): 446–451.

Kwon S. Changing health policy process: policies of health care reform in Korea. *Journal of Health Politics, Policy and Law*, 2005, 30(6): 1003–1026.

Kwon S. Pharmaceutical reform and physician strikes in Korea: separation of drug prescribing and dispensing. *Social Science & Medicine*, 2003, 57(3): 529–538.

La Forgia G, Somil Nagpa S. *Government-sponsored health insurance in India: are you covered?* Washington, DC: World Bank Group, 2012.

Lalonde M. A conceptual framework for health. *RNAO News*, 1974, 30(1): 5.

Lee EK, Malone DC. Comparison of peptic-ulcer drug use and expenditures before and after the implementation of a government policy to separate prescribing and dispensing practices in South Korea. *Clinical Therapeutics*, 2003, 25(2): 578–592.

Lei HC. Methods and experiences in the allocation and management of large-scale medical equipment in foreign countries. *Foreign Medicine (Health Economics)*, 2000, 17(1): 14.

Lei M. Cuban healthcare and health system. *Global Science, Technology and Economic Outlook*, 1999, 11: 44–45.

Levin LS, Katz AH, Holst E. *Self-care: lay initiatives in health*. New York: Prodist, 1976.

Levitt R, Wall A. *The reorganized national health service*. London: Chapman & Hall, 1992.

Li AL. Health services in Australia. *Foreign Medicine (Hospital Management)*, 1994, 11(4): 156–159.

Li C. A study on the reform regulations of China's health security system. Master's Thesis. Xi'an: Xi'an University of Science and Technology, 2012.

Li C. *Social security systems in western Europe*. Beijing: China Social Sciences Press, 1989.

Li GH. A study on the health service system in Sweden. *Foreign Medicine (Health Economics)*, 2006, 23(2): 49–55.

Li GH. Comment on the health insurance model in Canada and its development. *Foreign Medicine (Health Economics)*, 2005, 22(1): 511.

Li GH. Comment on the reforms of the health insurance system in France. *Foreign Medicine (Health Economics)*, 2007, 24(3): 102–107.

Li GH. Overview of the reforms in the health insurance system of Sweden. *Foreign Medicine (Health Economics)*, 2001, 18(3): 100–105.

Li J. A management model with the participation of commercial insurance companies in social health insurance. Master's Thesis. Chengdu: Southwestern University of Finance and Economics, 2012.

Li J. *A study on the health security system in Sweden.* Shanghai: Fudan University School of Economics, 2010.

Li JC. Socialist equality: theory, history and reality. *Journal of the Party School of the Central Committee of the CPC*, 2011, 01: 5–9.

Li JH, Fan MS. Insights for China from the reforms of the French health insurance system. *Medicine and Philosophy*, 2010, 31(8): 44–46.

Li L, Chen QL. The impact of population changes on the healthcare system. In Zeng Y, Li L, Lin YF (Eds.), *China's population and economic development in the 21st century.* Beijing: Social Sciences Academic Press, 2006. 221–235.

Li L, Liu HL. Investigation report on Hungary and the Czech Republic. *Chinese Journal of Rehabilitation*, 2006, 05: 348.

Li L. The experiences of Singapore and Thailand in medical assistance and its implications. *Economic Research Guide*, 2012, 3: 213–214.

Li LB. Overview and trends in contemporary global health – World Health Summit and introduction to the Philadelphia Agreement. *Journal of Preventive Medicine of Chinese People's Liberation Army*, 2005, 23(4): 311.

Li MH. Comparison of rural health insurance systems in China and abroad. *World Agriculture*, 2013, 9: 79–84.

Li MJ, Zhou HS. Changes in Singapore's healthcare system – a review of the healthcare system in Singapore. *Foreign Medicine (Hospital Management)*, 2002, 1: 38–40.

Li QY. Resolving the conflicts of social harmony based on the theory of equality by Marx and Engels. *Contemporary Economic Research*, 2007, 10: 12–16.

Li WQ. Impact of the universal health insurance system on healthcare quality. The Second Cross-Straits High-Level Forum on Hospital Health Insurance Management, Nanjing, 2010.

Li X, Ye L. Insights for China from Germany's drug pricing and compensation mechanisms. *Chinese Health Resources*, 2010, 13(6): 307–309.

Li XH, Li QM, Cao S. Japan's reforms in the "separation of prescribing and dispensing" and its insights for China. *Modern Business*, 2009, 36: 206–208.

Li YF, Gao XC. New analysis on the evolution of the health system in China. *Chinese Health Economics*, 2007, 26(8): 20–23.

Li YH. Comparative study of the basic health security systems in China and Russia. *Foreign Medicine (Health Economics)*, 2012, 29(4): 145–148.

Li YN. *Ethical issues in economics.* Beijing: SDX Joint Publishing Company, 1995.

Li YQ. The role of governments in the healthcare market. *Foreign Medicine (Health Economics)*, 1996, 1: 5–8.

Li YW. Lessons and insights from the health insurance systems of Germany and the Czech Republic. *Labor Security World*, 2009, 11: 50–50.

Li Z (ed.). *Social security theory.* Beijing: China Labor and Social Security Press, 2007.

Li Z, Wang BZ, Zhou Y. Analysis on the current status and issues of healthcare supervision in China. 2007. http://www.doc88.com/p-138418808261.html.

Li Z. *Social security theory.* Beijing: China Labor and Social Security Press, 2001.

Li ZJ, Wang ZC, Zhu ML. *Research and lessons from the universal health insurance system in Taiwan.* Beijing: China Financial Publishing House, 2007.

Liang H, Sun XM, Lei HC, et al. New health reform policies and rational drug use. *Chinese Health Economics*, 2002, 21(1): 56–58.

Liang H, Sun XM, Zhu Y. Design of medical assistance policies for the poor in Shanghai. *Journal of Community Health Care*, 2002, 3(3): 153–157.

Liang H, Sun XM. Theoretical development of community health service and policy focus. *Journal of Community Health Care*, 2002, 10: 16.

Liang HC. *Health insurance systems in foreign countries.* Beijing: Joint Press of the Beijing Medical University and Peking Union Medical College, 1992.

Liang LL, Langenbrunner JC. The path of development to universal health coverage: an external perspective. *Chinese Journal of Health Policy*, 2013, 6(2): 1–3.

Liang XY. The vertical model allows us to provide a seamless service – the CEO of Providence Health Care, Carl Roy, discusses the comparison between Chinese and Canadian hospitals. *Contemporary Medicine*, 2003, 9(5): 28–29.

Liang Y, Shao R. Comparison of foreign health insurance models and its insights for China. *Shanghai Medical & Pharmaceutical Journal*, 2007, 28(6): 257–259.

Liang Z, Ke JP, Sun NS, et al. A study on the healthcare system in Australia. *Foreign Medicine (Health Economics)*, 2001, 18(2): 49–55.

Liao LL. An introduction to the casemix payment method in Japan's health insurance. *Foreign Medicine (Health Economics)*, 2006, 23(4): 167–170.

Lin MQ. An exploration on the separation of prescribing and dispensing (I). *Chinese Journal of Hospital Pharmacy*, 1998, 18(3): 132–135.

Lin V, Smith J, Fawkes S. Public health practice in Australia: the organized effort, 2nd edition. *Australia Journal of Primary Health*, 2015, 21(1): 115.

Ling Y. Public spending on treatments abroad by the British. *Decision & Information*, 2002, 4: 56–57.

Liu B, Li XF, Lu ZX. The transition of the Slovakian healthcare system. *Medicine and Society*, 2006, 19(7): 62–65.

Liu CJ, Li W, Yao L. Impact and implications of Australia's community health service and general practice on China. *Chinese General Practice*, 2004, 7(21): 1545–1550.

Liu DM, Long LR. New progress in foreign theories on social comparison and its implications – joint discussion of its impact on the theory of equality. *Journal of Huazhong University of Science and Technology: Social Science Edition*, 2008, 05: 103–108.

Liu H, Tang XL. Investigation report on Singapore's Central Provident Fund. Compilation of Foreign Investigation Reports in 1997 by the State Economic System Reform Commission, 1998.

Liu HY, Cui ZW. Japan's health system and its reforms. *Foreign Medicine (Health Economics)*, 2000, 17(2): 49–51.

Liu J, Li XR, Zhou SJ, et al. 16 years of experiences and insights from the operations of the national health insurance system in Taiwan. *Soft Science of Health*, 2012, 26(2): 104–107.

Liu J, Zhang G, Ai XJ, et al. A review of healthcare reforms in Hungary and Bulgaria (I). *Chinese Health Resources*, 2005, 8(4): 184–185.

Liu J, Zhang G, Ai XJ, et al. A review of healthcare reforms in Hungary and Bulgaria (II). *Chinese Health Resources*, 2005, 8(5): 234–235.

Liu JT, Guo Y, Chen NS, et al. What is a "good" health policy? *Chinese Hospital Management*, 2007, 27(4): 3–6.

Liu JX. Comparing the current status of universal health insurance and healthcare service systems in various countries. Cambridge, MA: Harvard University: 2002 Global Symposium on Health Care, 2002.

Liu L, Wan Y. Investigation report on the property rights reform of healthcare institutions by the Ministry of Health and World Health Organization Cooperation Projections (I). *China Health Industry*, 2005, 2: 90–92.

Liu L, Wan Y. Investigation report on the property rights reform of healthcare institutions by the Ministry of Health and World Health Organization Cooperation Projections (II). *China Health Industry*, 2005, 3: 80–82.

Liu LL. The social medical assistance systems of various countries and its insights for the establishment of social medical assistance for the urban poor in China. *Population & Economics*, 2006, 1: 65–70.

Liu QJ. *Developing countries and international institutions*. Beijing: China Renmin University Press, 2010.

Liu SJ. Why China's status as a "developing country" poses a problem. *Qiushi*, 2011(11): 33–36. http://www.qstheory.cn/zxdk/2011/201111/201105/t20110530_83225.htm.

Liu TG. Reflection on the public goods theory – joint discussion on the ideas for livelihood policies under the demand spillover theory. *Chinese Public Administration*, 2011, 9: 22–27.

Liu TG. The breakthrough and establishment of traditional public goods theory – joint discussion on positioning of government function in the post-public goods era. *Journal of Beijing Administration Institute*, 2011, 3: 12–17.

Liu WH. *Social security systems in developed countries*. Beijing: Current Affairs Press, 2002.

Liu X, Chou YL. A reexamination of Cuba's healthcare system: operating mechanisms and practical experiences. *Latin American Studies*, 2010, 32(6): 51–56.

Liu XY. Review of healthcare systems in developing countries. *Academic Journal of Shanxi Provincial Committee Party School of CPC*, 2006, 29(2): 74–76.

Liu XY. Thailand's universal health coverage and its insights for China. *Chinese Journal of Health Policy*, 2014, 7(2): 11–16.

Liu Y, Zhang L. Research progress in the performance evaluation of healthy systems. *Medicine and Society*, 2008, 06: 22–23.

Liu Y, Zhang L. Research progress on the theoretical framework for the performance evaluation of healthy systems. *Medicine and Society*, 2008, 21(8): 29–31.

Liu YJ. Insights from Thailand's "30-Baht Scheme" for health insurance in China. *Health Economics Research*, 2011, 04: 45–47.

Liu YZ, Zhang CY. Current status, problems and countermeasures of the economic and healthcare security for the elderly. *Population & Economics*, 2003, 1: 12–16.

Liu ZY. Status of rehabilitation care in Cuba. *Foreign Medicine (Hospital Management)*, 1999, 3: 50–51.

Lu J. Reform process and prospects of the healthcare system in China. *China Collective Economy*, 2012, 16: 74–75.

Lü XJ. *Social security system in Japan*. China: Economy & Management Publishing House, 2000.

Lu ZX, Jin SG. *Community health services in foreign countries*. Beijing: People's Medical Publishing House, 2001.

Luo YW. *Comparison of international social security systems*. Beijing: China Economic Publishing House, 2001.

Ma C, Yao X, Zhang XY. Comparison of the healthcare status in China and Russia. *Journal of Xinjiang Medical University*, 2011, 34(7): 770–773.

Ma D, Ren R. Health security system in Brazil. *Medicine and Philosophy*, 2007, 28(10): 1–3.

Ma J, Zhang CH, Fang XR, et al. Insights from the Philippine health system for the medical assistance of vulnerable groups in China. *Chinese Health Economics*, 2006, 25(1): 75–77.

Ma LH. Economic policies related to drug production, marketing and compensation in foreign countries (Europe and USA). *Proceedings of Health Economics Training and Research Network in China*. Shijiazhuang: Hebei Science and Technology Press, 1998.

Ma Q, Jiang LM. Comparison and lessons of the four major models of health security systems in the contemporary era. *Chinese Health Service Management*, 2008, 25(12): 815–816, 824.

Ma QY. Interpretation of "public service." *Chinese Public Administration*, 2005, 2: 78–82.

Ma S, Sood N. *A comparison of the health systems in China and India*. Santa Monica, CA: RAND Corporation, 2008.

Ma XJ, Wang XW. Comparative study on the performance evaluation framework and trends of international health service systems. *Chinese Journal of Health Policy*, 2009, 2(7): 52–56.

Magrini A. New approaches to analysing prescription data and to transfer pharmacoepidemiological and evidence-based reports to prescribers. *Pharmacoepidemiology and Drug Safety*, 2002, 11(8): 721–726.

Mahal A, Yazbeck AS, Peters DH, et al. The poor and health services use in India. Health, Nutrition and Population (HNP) Discussion Paper. Washington, DC: The World Bank, 2001.

Majerol M, Newkirk V, Garfield R. The uninsured: a primer. Suitland, MD: The Kaiser Commission on Medicaid and Uninsured, 2007.

Mao QA. *Analysis of the health insurance system in the United States of America*. Beijing: China Medical Science Press, 1994.

Mao SJ. Reform trends of the social health insurance in Germany. *Foreign Medicine (Health Economics)*, 2002, 19(3): 126–130.

Mao XL. How was the Cuban universal healthcare system established? *Study Monthly*, 2007, 7: 44–46.

Mao XL. The establishment and improvement of the universal healthcare system in Cuba. *China Party and Government Officials' Forum*, 2007, 223(6): 39–41.

Mao XL. Universal health security system in Cuba. *Scientific Decision-Making*, 2007, 8: 54–55.

Marmot MG, Adelstein AM, Bulusu L. Immigrant mortality in England and Wales 1970–1978. In *OPCS studies of medical and population subjects* (No. 47). London: HMSO, 1984.

Masami H. Health service in Japan. In Marshall W. Raffel (ed.), *Comparative health systems*, 335–370. University Park: Pennsylvania State University Press, 1984.

Maslow AH. *Maslow on self-transcendence*. Translated and edited by Shi L. Tianjin: Tianjin Academy of Social Sciences Press, 2011.

Matsuda S. Regulatory effects of health examination programs on medical expenditures for the elderly in Japan. *Social Science & Medicine*, 1996, 42(5): 661–670.

Maxwell RJ. *Health and wealth: An international study of health-care spending*. Published for Sandoz Institute for Health and Socio-Economic Studies by Lexington Books (Lanham, MD), 1981.

McGuire A, Henderson J, Mooney G. *The economics of health care: an introductory text*. London: Routledge & Kegan Paul, 1994.

Medicine Economic News. Lessons from the separation of prescribing and dispensing in Japan, September 15, 2006. http://www.hyey.com/MemberServices/ArtcleCharge/ShowArticle.aspx?ArticleID=75898.

Meimanaliev A-S, Ibraimova A, Elebesov B, et al. *Health systems in transition: Kyrgyzstan*. Translated by Situ SJ. Beijing: Peking University Medical Press, 2007.

Meng QY, Yao L. *Theory and practice of urban medical assistance in China*. Beijing: China Labor and Social Security Press, 2007.

Meng QY. Universal health coverage: From concept to action. *Chinese Journal of Health Policy*, 2014, 7(2): 1–4.

Mill JS. *Utilitarianism* (1863). Cambridge University Press, 1973.

Ministry of Civil Services, MCA [2005] No. 121, *Notice on accelerating the work of rural medical assistance*. China: Ministry of Civil Services, 2005.

Ministry of Civil Services, Ministry of Health, and Ministry of Finance, MCA [2003] No.158, *Opinions on the implementation of rural medical assistance*. China: Ministry of Civil Services, Ministry of Health, and Ministry of Finance, 2003.

Ministry of Finance and Ministry of Civil Services, MOF & MCA [2005] No. 39, *Opinions on strengthening the management of urban medical aid funds*. China: Ministry of Finance and Ministry of Civil Services, 2005.

Ministry of Health. *China Health Statistics Yearbook (2012)*. China: MOH, 2012.

Ministry of Health. MOH issued a briefing on China's NRCMS pilot situation. China: Official website of the Central People's Government of the People's Republic of China, September 28, 2006. Available at http://www.gov.cn/xwfb/2006-09/28/content_401003.htm.

Ministry of Health International Cooperation Unit. *Health systems in transition – Sweden (2005)*. Beijing: Peking University Medical Press, 2007.

Ministry of Health of Singapore. *Annual Report 2001*. Singapore: Ministry of Health, 2001.

Ministry of Health of Singapore. *State of health 1998 – the report of the director of medical services*. Singapore: Ministry of Health, 1998.

Ministry of Health of Singapore. *State of health 2000 – the report of the director of medical services*. Singapore: Ministry of Health, 2000.

Ministry of Health of Singapore. *State of health 2001 – the report of the director of medical services*. Singapore: Ministry of Health, 2001.

Ministry of Health Research Team for Maternal and Child Health. *Organizational form of healthcare in Mexico*. Maternal and Child Health Care of China, 1990, 5: 45.

Ministry of Health, Labour and Welfare of Japan. Annual reports on health and welfare 1998–1999. Social security and national life. Japan: Ministry of Health, Labour and Welfare, 2009.

Ministry of Health. Affordable health care: a white paper. Singapore: SNP Publishers, 1993.

Ministry of Health. Blue paper on the national health plan. Singapore: Ministry of Health, 1983.

Ministry of Health. *Pillars of health – a pictorial record of public health care facilities in Singapore*. Singapore: Ministry of Health, 1994.

Ministry of Labor, Invalids, and Social Affairs (MOLISA). Mot so van deve chinh sach bao dam xa hoi onuoc ta hien nay (the current situations of social protection in our country). Vietnam: MOLISA, 1993–2009.

Ministry of Public Health (MOPH). *Health survey in rural China (in Chinese)*. China: Ministry of Public Health, 1986.

Mossialos E, Oliver A. An overview of pharmaceutical policy in four countries: France, Germany, the Netherlands and the United Kingdom. *International Journal of Health Planning Management*, 2005, 20(4): 291–306.

Müller-Armack, Alfred. *The principles of the social market economy* (1965). The Social Market Economy, 1998.

Mu HZ (ed.). *International comparison of social security systems*. Beijing: China Labor and Social Security Press, 2007.

Mu HZ. *The establishment and improvement of the social security systems in developing countries*. Beijing: People's Publishing House, 2008.

National Bureau of Statistics of China. *National statistical yearbook*, 2011. http://www.stats.gov.cn/tjsj/ndsj/2011/indexch.htm.

National Center for Health Statistics. Health, United States, 2010: with special feature on death and dying. Hyattsville, MD: National Center for Health Statistics, 2011.

National Center for Health Statistics. National household survey 1999. Washington, DC: National Center for Health Statistics, 1990.

National Health Insurance. Department of Health of the Republic of South Africa website. 2011. http://www.doh.gov.za.

New Industrial Economy. Diverse paths to healthcare reform: experiences of developed countries. 2012-05-06. http://finance.jrj.com.cn/opinion/2012/05/06200313007391.shtml.

Nguyen TVH. *Voluntary social insurance in Vietnam*. Vietnam: Ministry of Labour, Invalids and Social Affairs, 2009. https://slideplayer.com/slide/5988196/.

Ni SM, Dong M. Investigation on the healthcare and health insurance system in Argentina and Chile. *Guide of China Medicine*, 2007, 2: 111–114.

Niu XQ. Comparative study of health security in China and Mexico. *China Business (Theoretical Research)*, 2012, 22: 43–44.

Noeikhiew N. Takeover of private hospitals. Democrat deputy leader says someone speculating on failure of Bt 30 health scheme. Bangkok, Thailand: The Nation, 2003.

Nordberg E. Invisible needs, past household health survey in third world countries: a review of method. MPH Thesis. Gothenburg: Nordic School of Public Health, 1986.

Normand C, Weber A, Carrin G, et al. Social health insurance: a guidebook for planning. *Journal of Public Health*, 2015, 12(4): 250–258.

Obama's call for an "assembly" of healthcare reforms. Ningbo Evening News. 2010-3-20. http://daily.cnnb.com.cn/nbwb/html/2010-03/20/content_175067.htm.

OECD. *The reform of health care – a comparative analysis of seven OECD countries*. Paris: Organisation for Economic Co-operation and Development, 1992, pp. 19–27.

Office for Population Census and Surveys (OPCS). General household survey. London: OPCS, 1993.

Office of Foreign Lending, Ministry of Health of China. Lessons and insights from the US health service management system for rural health development in China. *Chinese Health Economics*, 2008, 27(11): 75–80.

Opinions of the CPC Central Committee and the State Council on Deepening the Reform of the Medical and Health Care System. CPC Central Committee and State Council, 2009-03-17. http://www.lawinfochina.com/display.aspx?lib=law&id=7416&CGid=.

Pan J, Xu F, Liu GE, et al. Insights from the establishment of Taiwan's universal health insurance system for the healthcare reforms in mainland China. *Chinese Health Economics*, 2011, 7: 42–44.

Park S, Soumerai SB, Adams AS. *Antibiotic use following a Korean national policy*. Oxford, England: Oxford University Press, 2005.

Parker RL, Hinman AR. Use of health services. *American Journal of Public Health*, 1982, 72(9 Suppl): 71–77.

Patel V, Chatterji S, Chisholm D, et al. Chronic diseases and injuries in India. *Lancet*, 2011, 377(9763): 413–428.

Paul VK, Sachdev HS, Mavalankar D, et al. Social determinants of health. *Central European Journal of Public Health Supplement*, 2007, 15: S30–S32.

Pauly MV. The evolution of health insurance in India and China. *Health Affairs*, 2008, 27(4): 1016–1019.

Pei LK, Liu CJ, Legge D. *Challenges of universal healthcare system – insights from the Australian health system*. Beijing: People's Medical Publishing House, 2008.

Pei XG. The three foundations of China's theoretical economics. *Academic Journal of Zhongzhou*, 2005, 2: 21–26.

Pharmaceutical Price Regulation Scheme. Seventh report to Parliament, UK. 205. PMPRB Annual Report, 2001–2002, Canada, 2003.

PhilHealth. *The PhilHealth chronicles: the journey towards universal social health insurance*. Pasig City, Philippines: Corporate Planning Department, Philippine Health Insurance, 2004.

Philip M. The impact of the economic crisis on health and health care in Latin America and the Caribbean. *WHO Chronicle*, 1986, 40(4): 152–157.

Philippines National Health Accounts. 2003. http://www.nscb.gov.ph/stats/pnha/2003/default. asp. Data also accessed from World Health.

Phua KH. Privatization and restructuring of health services in Singapore. Occasional paper 5. Singapore: Times Academic Press, 1991.

Pigou AC. *The economics of welfare*. London: Macmillan and Co., 1920.

Popovich L, Potapchik E, Shishkin S, et al. Russian federation: health system review. *Health Systems in Transition*, 2011, 13(7): 1–190.

Prakongsai P, Limwattananon S, Tangchoroensathien V. The equity impact of the universal coverage policy: lessons from Thailand. *Advances in Health Economics and Health Services Resource*, 2009, 21: 57–81.

The Price Association of China, Fudan School of Public Health, and Shanghai Health Development Research Center. *The Policy of Pharmaceutical Pricing Management from a Global Perspective*, 2011: 207–217.

Price Division of the National Development Reform Commission of the People's Republic of China. Overview of drug price management in France, 2007. http://jgs.ndrc.gov.cn/jgqk/ t20071119_173105.htm.

Prinja S, Bahaguna P, Pinto AD, et al. The cost of universal health care in India: a model based estimate. *PLoS One*, 2012, 7(1): e30362.

Qi BC. The action principles and management of the Russian Medical Association. *Chinese Health Economics*, 1996, 15(6): 57.

Qi CJ. Changes and reforms of the healthcare system in Mexico. *Latin American Studies*, 2010, 32(4): 43–48.

Qi RG, Gao YQ, Xia B, et al. China should learn from the Thai model of rural health insurance. *Financial Times*, 2007-10-01.

Qin J, Qin ZH. Reward mechanisms for the remuneration of general practitioners in the UK. *Foreign Medicine (Health Economics)*, 1999, 16(2): 72–75.

Qing SM, Sun J. Understanding China's healthcare reforms from the perspective of Cuba public healthcare. *China Development*, 2013, 4: 43–47.

Qiu JX, Zhao LH. Insights for China from the rural healthcare systems of Japan, Thailand, South Korea and Brazil. *China Pharmaceuticals*, 2007, 16(14): 4–6.

Qu C, Zang XH. Experimental methods in the study of public goods theory. *Economic Perspectives*, 2003, 7: 27–31.

Raffel MW, Xia ZM. Health system reforms in Czechoslovakia. *Foreign Medicine (Health Economics)*, 1993, 10(3): 121–127.

Ramani KV, Mavalankar D. Health system in India: opportunities and challenges for improvements. *Journal of Health Organization and Management*, 2006, 20(6): 560–572.

Rao M, Rao KD, Kumar AKS, et al. India: towards universal health coverage 5. Human resources for health in India. *Lancet*, 2011, 377(9765): 587–598.

Ramsay G. *An essay on the distribution of wealth*. Edinburgh: Black, 1836.

Ratha D, Timmer H. *Resource book of community-based health care organization social health insurance schemes in the Philippines*. Global Economic Prospects 2006, Washington, DC: World Bank Group, 2003.

Rechel B, Duboi C-A, McKee M, et al. *The health care workforce in Europe: learning from experience*. Trowbridge, Wilts: The Cromwell Press, 2006.

Reddy KS, Patel V, Jha P, et al. India: towards universal health coverage 7. Towards achievement of universal health care in India by 2020: a call to action. *Lancet*, 377(9767): 760–768.

Ren LM, Liu JR. Analysis and suggestions on the model for combining urban medical assistance with the basic health insurance system of urban residents – a case study of Guangzhou. *Chinese Health Service Management*, 2010, 27(8): 525–528.

Ren R, Huang ZQ. *Development framework and strategies of the health security system in China*. Beijing: Economic Science Press, 2009.

Ren R. *Development framework and strategies of the health insurance system in China*. Beijing: Economic Science Press, 2009.

Ren R. Reform of the healthcare system in Australia (I). *Foreign Medicine (Health Economics)*, 2000, 17(1): 18-26.

Research team for the health insurance systems of three countries. An investigation on the health insurance systems of Brazil, Argentina and Mexico. *Chinese Health Economics*, 1989, 2: 59–64.

Research team of the National Development and Reform Commission and the Ministry of Health. Basic experiences and insights from Poland's health system reforms. *Macroeconomic Management*, 2005, 11: 58–60.

Research Unit in Health and Behavioural Change (RUHBC). *Changing the public health*. Chichester: Wiley, 1989.

Robertson AH. *Social security in the United States of America*. Translated by Jin YJ, et al. Beijing: China Renmin University Press, 1995.

Robertson P. *Rethinking need: the case of criminal justice*. Aldershot: Dartmouth, 1991.

Rodwin MA, Okamoto AE. Physicians' conflicts of interest in Japan and the United States: lessons for the United States. *Journal of Health Politics, Policy and Law*, 2000, 25(2): 343–375.

Roemer MI. *National health systems of the world*. New York: Oxford University Press, 1991.

Roemer MI, Roemer JE. The social consequences of free trade in health care: a public health response to orthodox economics. *International Journal of Health Services*, 1982, 12(1): 111–129.

Russian Government. *The concept of development of public health and medical science in the Russian Federation*, November 5,1997.

Sankar D, Kathuria V. Health system performance in rural India: efficiency estimates across states. *Economic and Political Weekly*, 2004, 39(13): 1427–1433.

Sapelli C, Torche A. The mandatory health insurance system in Chile: explaining the choice between public and private insurance. *International Journal of Health Care Finance and Economics*, 2001, 1(2): 97–110.

Savedoff W. Tax-based financing for health systems: options and experiences. Beijing, 2004, [2007-05-06]. WHO. http://www.WHO.EIP/FER/DP.

Scholkopf M. The hospital sector in Germany: an overview. *World Hospitals and Health Services*, 2000, 36(3): 13.

Shanxi Science Network. Use of computers and chromosomal information to broaden existing drug uses in the US. 2011-08-19.

Shao HY, Peng X. Comparison of international experiences in drug pricing and compensation policies. *Price: Theory & Practice*, 2011, 9: 69–70.

Shen HL. The health insurance systems in Germany and France and their insights for China. *Chinese Health Service Management*, 2000, 16(7): 441–442.

Sheng XB. Establishment of healthcare needs and framework of performance evaluation in the UK. *Foreign Medicine (Health Economics)*, 2001, 18(2): 65–70.

Sheng YT. Hospital and health insurance in the United States of America. *Chinese Journal of Hospital Administration*, 2002, 18(1): 61–62.

Shi G, Lei HC, Gao WZ. Investigation report on the health reforms of Brazil and Chile. *Health Economics Research*, 2008, 6: 13–18.

Shi G, Lei HC. Challenges and reforms of the healthcare system in India – an investigation report on India's healthcare system (II). *Chinese Health Economics*, 2008, 27(9): 95–96.

Shi G, Lei HC. Overview of the healthcare system in India – an investigation report on India's healthcare system (I). *Chinese Health Economics*, 2008, 27(8): 91–94.

Shi X, Zhou LL. Insights for China from the medical assistance system for vulnerable groups in foreign countries. *Chinese Health Economics*, 2007, 26(11): 78–80.

Shu Z, You CM, Nie JG. Overview of health system reforms in Kyrgyzstan. *Chinese Journal of Social Medicine*, 2009, 26(4): 222–223.

Singapore Ministry of Health. http://www.moh.gov.cn/publicfiles/business/htmlfiles/zwgkzt/ptjnj/year2010/index2010.html.

Singapore Ministry of Health. http://www.moh.gov.sg/content/moh_web/home/statistics/Health_Facts_Singapore/Population_And_Vital_Statistics.html.

Smith A. *The Wealth of Nations*. Bantam Classics, 2003.

Smith BM. Trends in health care coverage and financing and their implications for policy. *New England Journal of Medicine*, 1997, 337(14): 1000–1003.

Solon O, Panelo C, Gumafelix E. *A review of the progress of health sector reform agenda implementation*. Manila: Department of Health, 2002.

Song DP, Ren J, Zhao DH, et al. Overview of Mexico's health security system and its insights for China. *Chinese Journal of Health Policy*, 2010, 3(7): 49–51.

Song LZ, Zhao XY, Liu XF. *Comparative study of health insurance systems in foreign countries*. Beijing: Joint Press of the Beijing Medical University and Peking Union Medical College, 1994.

Song XD. Mexico provides health security to its rural residents. *Outlook Weekly*, 2001, 43: 18.

Song XJ, Liu G. The proportions of two types of industrial upgrading and the basics of economics – comparison and synthesis of Western economics and Marxist economics. *Qilu Journal*, 2013, 5: 107–111.

Spf in Vietnam. Working paper of Ministry of Labor, Invalids and Social Affairs. 2003. http://www.socialsecurityextension.org/gimi/gess/RessShowResource.do? resource.

Stevens A, Gabbay J. Needs assessment. Health Trends, 1991, 23(1): 20-23.

Stigler GJ. The economics of information. *Journal of Political Economy*, 1961, 69(3): 213–225.

Strindhall M, Henriks G. How improved access to health care successfully spread across Sweden. *Health Care Management Review*, 2007, 16(1): 16–24.

Su F, Wei L. Health insurance in Sweden: high welfare and broad covarage. *China Hospital CEO*, 2014(7): 80–83.

Su QY. Comparative study of the pension insurance systems in China and Vietnam. *Labor Security World: Theoretical Edition*, 2011, 8: 54–58.

Su S, Wu D. Current status of the drug pricing systems in developed countries. *Prices Monthly*, 2002, 3: 33–34.

Sun BY. *Contemporary British and Swedish social security systems*. Beijing: Law Press, 2000.

Sun BY. New political economics and contemporary public administration. *Journal of Beijing Administration Institute*, 2002, 3: 20–24.

Sun H, Song LL, Wei CY. Preliminary investigation on the development trends of urban and rural medical assistance systems. *Subnational Fiscal Research*, 2013, 9: 66–68.

Sun HB. Health diplomacy in Cuba. *Latin American Studies*, 2007, 5: 52–55.

Sun J. WHO concept of basic drugs and national practices. *Chinese Journal of Health Policy*, 2009, 2(1): 38–42.

Sun LH, Sun Q. Successful experiences of foreign countries in the selection of basic drugs and its insights for China. *China Pharmacy*, 2010, 21(4): 4513–4516.

Sun TD, Tong YQ, Ma ZH. Health equality – the cornerstone of public policies for establishing healthy cities. *Chinese Rural Health Service Administration*, 2007, 27(10): 723–725.

Sun XM, Cheng XX, Bao Y. Practice and research of community health services in Shanghai (I). *Chinese Journal of Health Policy*, 1999, 11: 18–22.

Sun XM, Cheng XX, Bao Y. Practice and research of community health services in Shanghai (II). *Chinese Journal of Health Policy*, 1999, 12: 13–16.

Sun XM, Hong L, Yuan C, et al. Survey of the medical financial assistance schemes of the urban poor in Shanghai. *International Journal of Health Planning and Management*, 2002, 17(2): 91–112.

Sun XM, Liang H, Tian WH. Reform and development of community health services. *Journal of Community Health Care*, 2002, 1(1): 17.

Sun XM, Liang H. Development of community health services from a four-dimensional perspective. *Chinese Journal of Health Policy*, 2002, 4: 24–26.

Sun XM, Zhang G, Zhao DD, et al. A study on the existing issues and countermeasures of health resources in Shanghai. *Chinese Journal of Health Policy*, 1998, 11: 10–12.

Sun XM. Background, opportunities and challenges of health development in Shanghai in the 21st century. *Health Economics Research*, 1984, 8: 15–16.

Sun XM. Comparative study of constrained models of healthcare services. *Chinese Health Service Management*, 2001, 3: 164–166.

Sun XM. Health access and health financing in rural China. PhD Thesis. UK: Keele Publishing House, 1996.

Sun XM. Impact of China's accession to the WTO on the healthcare market in Shanghai. *Chinese Journal of Health Policy*, 2000, 3: 20–22.

Sun XM. Major trends in the health development of Shanghai in the 21st century. *Chinese Journal of Health Policy*, 1999, 9: 21–23.

Sun XM. *Medical service and insurance system in developed countries and areas*, 2nd ed. Shanghai: Shanghai Scientific and Technical Publishers, 2012.

Sun XM. Meeting challenges head-on – implementation of the healthcare reform package decided by the State Council in Shanghai's health system. *Chinese Health Economics*, 2000, 1: 28–29.

Sun XM. Strategic thinking in the reform of the public hospital management system. *Journal of Community Health Care*, 2002, 2(5): 305–307.

Sun XY, Guo Y, Sun J. Validating the integration of the health belief model and planned behavior theory. *Journal of Peking University: Health Sciences*, 2009, 41(2): 129–134.

Sun Y. Reform of Russia's health security system and its prospects. *Theory Research*, 2011, 26: 79–80.

Sun ZG. Investigation report on healthcare system reforms in Canada, the United States and Mexico. China: National Development and Reform Commission, 2012. https://www.douban.com/group/topic/31780288/.

Supon L, Phusit P. Why has the universal coverage scheme in Thailand achieved a pro-poor public subsidy for health care? *BMC Public Health*, 2012, 12(Suppl1): S6.

Takegawa S, Sato H. *Corporate protection and social security*. Translated by Li LM, Zhang YC. Beijing: China Labor and Social Security Press, 2003.

Tan CT. Understanding the origin of economic development theory from the history of ideas in bourgeois economics. *Wuhan University Journal: Social Science Edition*, 1982, 3: 20–26.

Tang JC, Chen LY. A study on the development of the insurance market in Vietnam. *Around Southeast Asia*, 2012, 10: 48–54.

Tang JC. Implications of "free healthcare" in Russia. *Chinese Health Human Resources*, 2013, 11: 16.

Tang XL. The origin of the UK National Health Service and several major reforms. *Chinese Health Resources*, 2001, 4(6): 280–282.

Task Force of the State Council Development Research Center. Evaluation and recommendations for the healthcare system reforms in China. *China Development Review*, 2005, Supplement 1.

Tatara K. Prescribing and dispensing in Japan: conflict of interest? *Clinical Medicine*, 2003, 3(6): 555.

Temple W. *Citizen and churchman*. London: Eyre & Spottiswoode, 1941.

Thailand-country cooperation strategy: at a glance. 2010. http://www.who.int/countryfocus/cooperation_strategy/ccsbrief_tha_en.pdf.

Thailand-country health profile, global health observatory. 2011. http://www.who.int/gho/countries/tha.pdf.

Thailand-country statistics, global health observatory. 2011. http://apps.who.int/ghodata/?vid=19400&theme=country.

Thailand: 30-Baht coverage alone is sufficient for everyone to afford medical treatment. *Xinhua Daily Telegraph*, 2006-04-12.

Thailand: sustaining health protection for all. The World Bank Group, 2012. http://www.worldbank.org/en/news/video/2012/08/27/slideshow-thailand-sustaining-health-protection-for-all.

Tian CR. "One-package" management of health insurance hospitals in Mexico. *Labor Security Communications*, 2000, 9: 41.

Tian CR. Health insurance system in Mexico. *Labor Science of China*, 1989, 11: 35–37.

Tilley I. *Managing the internal market*. London: Paul Chapman Publishing Ltd., 1993.

Toh C. Impact of a free market system on medicine in Singapore. *Singapore Medical Journal*, 1997, 38(1): 7–10.

Tran TMO. An assessment of health care for the poor in Vietnam social insurance enrollments surge. 2011. http://www.dz-times.net/post/social/social insu.

Tu HB. An investigation on the health insurance system and drug price supervision in Canada and Mexico. *China Price Supervision and Inspection*, 2005, 11: 37–39.

United Nations Children's Fund. *The state of the world's children*. Washington DC: United Nations Children's Emergency Fund (UNICEF), 1999.

United Nations. *Opinion polls in 2000*. New York: United Nations, 2000.

United Nations. *Population aging 1999*. New York: United Nations, 2000.

US Census Bureau, Population Division. Annual estimates of the population for the United States, regions, states, and Puerto Rico: April 1, 2010 to July 1, 2011. *Washington, DC: US Census Bureau, Population Division*, 2011.

US Social Security Administration. *Global Social Security Systems – 1995*. Beijing: Huaxia Press, 1997.

Vickrey W. Counterspeculation, auctions, and competitive sealed tenders. *Journal of Finance*, 1961, 16(1): 8–37.

Wang CB, Ding JB. Effective path selection in public policies under the perspective of social equality – A theoretical interpretation of public policy effectiveness. *Jilin University Journal, Social Sciences Edition*, 2012, 2: 61–66.

Wang DS, Rao KQ. Reform and development of the healthcare system in Brazil and Argentina. *Chinese Health Economics*, 2006, 25(11): 7880.

Wang F. Universal health insurance – the most affordable Taiwanese miracle. Communist Party Members, 2009, 24.

Wang FC. Development of public goods theory and its implications for China's fiscal issues. *Finance & Trade Economics*, 2000, 9: 23–27.

Wang H, Li NN. Reform development of the health security systems in foreign countries and its implications. *Academics*, 2010, 4: 219–223.

Wang HY, Niu ZS. Development trends in the cost containment mechanisms for health insurance. *Foreign Medicine (Health Economics)*, 1998, 15(3): 97–100.

Wang HY. Comparative analysis of international health insurance models and reform development. *Foreign Medicine (Health Economics)*, 1999, 16(2): 49–63.

Wang HY. International development trends in the cost containment mechanisms for health insurance. *Chinese Health Economics*, 1998, 8: 13–15.

Wang J. The path to the separation of prescribing and dispensing in Taiwan and Japan. *China Pharmacy*, 2011, 7: 48–49.

Wang JX. Necessity and feasibility of the "separation of prescribing and dispensing." China Pharmaceutical Commerce. 2012-03-12. http://jiankang.cntv.cn/20120312/100535.shtml.

Wang LJ. Insights from the Cuba healthcare model for China's healthcare reforms. *Pharmaceutical Education*, 2009, 25(4): 1–3.

Wang M. The compulsory health insurance system in Japan. *China Insurance*, 2001, (6): 60–61.

Wang N, Wang J. The development history of Cuba's healthcare system and its implications. *Chinese Journal of Social Medicine*, 2009, 26(1): 19–22.

Wang N. Evaluation of Cuba's healthcare system and its insight for China. *Latin American Studies*, 2009, 2: 50–55.

Wang Q, Liu LH. Reform and development trend of the payment method for general practitioners in the UK. *Chinese Health Economics*, 2008, 27(12): 82–85.

Wang Q. Comparative study of health resources in China and the world. Master's Thesis. Beijing: Peking Union Medical College, 2013.

Wang Q. Comparative study of the economic development theory by Lewis and Schultz. *Economic Review*, 2011, 1: 20–24.

Wang RH. The four dimensions of healthy people and society: new concept of four-dimensional health. *Social Outlook*, 2007, 12: 5–9.

Wang RL, Nie C. Insights and explorations on the current status of home care in Japan. *Chinese Journal of Preventive Medicine*, 2010, 11(11): 1151–1152.

Wang W. A summary of China's health security research in 2009. *Chinese Journal of Health Policy*, 2010, 3(2): 34–39.

Wang W. Issues and reform of Japan's healthcare system. *Japanese Studies*, 2002, 3: 99–109.

Wang X. Thailand's 30-Baht healthcare scheme and its insights for the New Rural Cooperative Medical Scheme in China. Master's Thesis. Jinan: Shandong University, 2013.

Wang XJ. Comparative study on the health security systems in Taiwan and Mainland China. Master's Thesis. Wuhan: Wuhan University of Science and Technology, 2011.

Wang XJ. Hong Kong Hospital Authority: overview, organizational structure and operational mechanism. *Progress in Health Policy Research* (internal publication), 2009, 7: 16–37.

Wang XL. Comparison and thoughts of payment methods for health insurance in foreign countries. *Chinese Hospital Management*, 1999, 4: 10–12.

Wang XW, Liu LH. A review of the development trends and basic theoretical models of international healthcare systems. *Chinese Journal of Social Medicine*, 1995, 2: 53–56.

Wang XW, Liu LH. Comparative study on the management model of health systems in developed countries. *Health Economics Research*, 1995, 5: 18–20.

Wang YX, Li Q, Dong QL, et al. Overview of health system reforms in Poland. *Chinese Journal of Social Medicine*, 2008, 25(1): 18–19.

Wang ZM, Yang ZJ. Health insurance system in Mexico. *Medicine and Philosophy: Humanities and Social Science Edition*, 2007, 28(12): 45–47.

Ward R, Chen JY. Health care in Mexico. *Foreign Medicine (Health Economics)*, 1988, 5(3): 34–37.

Wei X, Guo Y, Shen J. The health systems in five countries of Central Asia and their reform policies. *Chinese Health Economics*, 2010, 29(8): 94–96.

Weng XY. *Are Americans unable to afford healthcare? The inside story of the war on Obamacare.* Beijing: China Machine Press, 2011.

Weng YH. Thailand's health insurance system and its insights for China. *Postgraduate Journal of Zhongnan University of Economics and Law*, 2012, 3: 120–124.

White A, Nicolaas G, Foster K, et al. *Health survey for England 1991.* London: HMSO, 1993.

Whitehead M. *The concepts and principles of equity and health.* Copenhagen: World Health Organization, 1990.

Whitehead M. *The health divide, inequalities in health.* Harmondsworth: Penguin, 1992.

WHO Centre for Health Development. The development of community health care in Shanghai: emerging patterns of primary health care for the ageing population of a megalopolis. *WHO Centre for Health Development*, 2004, 4(1): 61.

Wiggins D. *Needs, values and truth.* Oxford: Blackwell, 1987.

Wikipedia. Health insurance in the United States. https://en.wikipedia.org/wiki/Health_insurance_in_the_United_States. Last edited on January 15, 2019.

Wilkinson RG. Income and mortality. In Wilkinson RG (Ed.), *Class and health: research and longitudinal data.* London: Routledge, 1988. 88–114.

World Bank. A worldwide overview of facts and figures. *World Bank Other Operational Studies*, 2012.

World Bank. Bulgaria. *World Bank Other Operational Studies*, 2009.

World Bank. Czech Republic. [2014-5-1]. http://data.worldbank.org/country/czech-republic.

World Bank. Discussion briefs, World Bank Philippines country office. 2005.

World Bank. Egypt: Health sector reform and financing review. *World Bank Other Operational Studies*, 2010.

World Bank. Latest PPP data taken from world development indicators. 2002. http://siteresources.worldbank.org/ICPINT/Reesources/Table1_1.pdf.

World Bank. Philippines data at-a-glance information. 2005. http://devdata.worldbank.org/AAG/phl_aag.pdf.

World Bank. Philippine health sector review. *World Bank Other Operational Studies*, 2011.

World Bank. Russian Federation. [2014-5-1] http://data.worldbank.org/country/russian-federation.

World Bank. *World development report*. Washington, DC: World Bank, 1985.

World Bank. *World development report 1986*. New York: Oxford University Press, 1986.

World Bank Database. Poland. http://data.worldbank.org.cn/country/poland#cp_wdi.

World Data Bank. Development data. 2013. http://databank.worldbank.org/data/home.aspx.

World Health Organization. *A report of the health and health insurance (unpublished document WHO/SHS/NHP/ 94.3)*. Geneva: World Health Organization, 1994.

World Health Organization. *Assessment of health systems' crises preparedness – Poland*, 2009, http://www.euro.who.int/__data/assets/pdf_file/0007/112201/E93850.pdf?ua=1.

World Health Organization. Best practices for achieving universal health coverage. *Chinese Journal of Health Policy*, 2013, 3: 10.

World Health Organization. *Economic strategies in support of Health for All: financing health development, options, experiences and experiments, including selected case studies*. Geneva: World Health Organization, 1987, 95.

World Health Organization. Evaluation of recent changes in the financing of health services. Report of a WHO Study group. *WHO Technical Report Series*, 1993, 78(8): 1–74.

World Health Organization. *Global status report on noncommunicable diseases* 2014. Geneva: World Health Organization, 2014.

World Health Organization. *Governance for health in the 21st century: a study conducted for the WHO Regional Office for Europe*. Geneva: World Health Organization, 2011.

World Health Organization. *Intersectoral action for health*. Geneva: World Health Organization, 1986.

World Health Organization. *The public/private mix in national health systems and the role of ministers of health (unpublished document WHO/SHS/NHP/91.2)*. Geneva: World Health Organization.

World Health Organization. Prevention of perinatal morbidity and mortality. *Public Health Papers* No. 42. Geneva: World Health Organization, 1972.

World Health Organization. *Social health insurance, selected case studies from Asia and the Pacific*. Geneva: World Health Organization, 2005.

World Health Organization. *The world health report – health systems financing: the path to universal coverage*. Geneva: World Health Organization, 2010.

World Health Organization. *The world health report 1997: conquering suffering, enriching humanity*. Beijing: People's Medical Publishing House, 1998.

World Health Organization. *The world health report* 2000. Beijing: People's Medical Publishing House, 2001.

World Health Organization. World health statistics 2010. Geneva: World Health Organization, 2010. https://www.who.int/whosis/whostat/2010/en/.

World Health Organization. World health statistics 2011. Geneva: World Health Organization, 2011. https://www.who.int/gho/publications/world_health_statistics/2011/en/World Health Organization. World health statistics 2014. Geneva: World Health Organization, 2014. http://www.who.int/gho/publications/world_health_statistics/2014/en/.

World Health Organization. http://www.who.int/en.

World Health Statistics (2012–2014). Geneva: World Health Organization, 2012-2014.3.

World Health Statistics 2013. Geneva: World Health Organization, 2013. http://www.who.int/gho/publications/world_health_statistics/2013/en/.

Wu CJ, Lu ZN, Wang YF. Impact analysis of social health insurance on the equality of community healthcare institutions. *Chinese General Practice*, 2005, 8(17): 1426–1427.

Wu D. Overview of the health insurance system in France. *China Labor and Social Security*, 2009, 5: 61–62.

Wu HH. New progress in modern theories of economic development. *Economic Perspectives*, 1995, 4: 53–56.

Wu LX. Cuba – one of the poorest countries has the best public health system. *China Reform: Rural Edition*, 2003, 8: 42–46.

Wu M. An analysis on the economic development of the BRICS countries. Jilin University course paper, 2012. http://www.doc88.com/p-1416191645667.html.

Wu NN, Li Q, Ma LN, et al. Health system reforms in Sweden. *Chinese Journal of Social Medicine*, 2007, 24(4): 235–237.

Wu RT. *Information management of health insurance*. Beijing: China Labor and Social Security Press, 2002.

Wu RT. International comparison and policy selection of health security systems. Doctoral Dissertation. Beijing: Chinese Academy of Social Sciences, 2003.

Wu RT. *International comparison of health security systems*. Beijing: Chemical Industry Press, 2003.

Wu RX, Ye L. A review of price management policies for patented drugs in the UK. *China Pharmacy*, 2009, 7: 483–485.

Wu S. Experiences and insights from the health security systems of Brazil, Egypt and other developing countries. *Chinese Journal of Public Health Management*, 2014, 1: 26–28.

Wu W. Latest research progress on Western public goods theory. *Finance & Trade Economics*, 2004(4): 88–92.

Wu YB, He RX, Cai JN. Insights from world healthcare reforms (7). Russia: from government leadership to a missing role. *China Hospital CEO*, 2011, 16: 54–58.

Xi XR. The "failure" of free healthcare in Russia. 2013-10-10 (928) [2014-09-20]. http://view.163.com/special/reviews/medicalinsurance1010.html.

Xia WB. Establishing a socialist view of equality – learning from Deng Xiaoping's theory of social equality. *Journal of Peking University: Philosophy and Social Sciences*, 1999, 36(2): 17–23.

Xia ZM. Evaluation of the pilot health insurance scheme in Haiphong City, Vietnam. *Foreign Medicine (Health Economics)*, 1995, 3: 125–126.

Xiang G. Population status of Hungary. *International Forum*, 1990, 1: 45–49.

Xiao HH, Guo ZH, Rao XB. Insights from Australia for the selection of the Basic Drug List in China. *China Pharmaceutical Affairs*, 2008, 22(11): 961–968.

Xiao YM. Efficiency and equality: challenges to the humanist view of equality – joint discussion on the social equality theory of reform. *Theoretical Investigation*, 1996, 4: 86–88.

Xie HJ, Li YL. A study on the social insurance system in Vietnam. *Around Southeast Asia*, 2011, 8: 62–66.

Xie SY. An analysis on the reforms of the health insurance system in Chile. *Comparative Economic & Social Systems*, 2006, 5: 88–91.

Xie Z, Liu PL, Guo Y. Global actions, progress and insights in the formulation of the Millennium Development Goals in healthcare. *Journal of Peking University: Health Sciences*, 2013, 45, 3: 495–498.

Xiong BJ. *Population aging and sustainable development*. Beijing: Encyclopedia of China Publishing House, 2002.

Xiong CW. On educational and social equality – a reflection based on Parsons' theory. *Journal of the Chinese Society of Education*, 2007, 7: 5–10.

Xiong JP, Ma LN, Lu ZX, et al. Overview of health system reforms in Bulgaria. *Chinese Journal of Social Medicine*, 2008, 25(3): 150–151.

Xu HT. An investigation on the health insurance in Japan. *Health Economics Research*, 2002, 5: 36–37.

Xu JZ. A study on the public-private partnership model of health service provision in China. Master's Thesis. Shanghai: Shanghai Jiaotong University, 2009.

Xu M. The separation of prescribing and dispensing in major countries in the world. *China Pharmaceutical Commerce*, 2012. http://jiankang.cntv.cn/20120313/100574.shtml.

Xu MJ, Zhang XH, Liang WJ. Comparative study on the health security systems of China and ASEAN countries. *Medicine and Philosophy (A)*, 2013, 34(12): 67–69.

Xu Q. *A study on British cities*. Shanghai: Shanghai Jiaotong University Press, 1995.

Xu XS. Theoretical positioning of social equality issues. *Journal of Humanities*, 2000, 1: 10–15.

Xu YC. What China can learn from Russia in healthcare reforms. *Medicine Economic News*, 2013-10-30, A11.

Xu YY, Liu DH, Wang X, et al. Measurement of national health system performance and conceptual framework of statistical indicators. *Chinese Journal of Health Statistics*, 2006, 23(5): 386–389.

Xu ZJ. Economic characteristics of different health service models and an exploration on China's model of healthcare reform. *China Cancer*, 2007, 16(11): 872–875.

Xu ZR. *Theories and experiences of urban medical assistance during social transition*. Beijing: China Economic Publishing House, 2010.

Yan HP. A comparative study on the economic development theories of Adam Smith, Karl Marx and Joseph Alois Schumpeter. *Journal of Zhongnan University of Economics and Law*, 2003, 2: 37–43.

Yan Q, Wei M. *Social development theory: the perspective of developing countries*. Second edition. Nanjing: Nanjing University Press, 2005.

Yan ZX. Japan's health insurance system and its insights for China. *Contemporary Economy of Japan*, 1999, 5: 31–35.

Yang FS. Population status of Hungary. *Eastern Europe*, 1998, 3: 64.

Yang HF, Chen CG. The rural health insurance systems in Mexico and Brazil and its insights for the establishment of the New Rural Cooperative Medical Scheme in China. *Latin American Studies*, 2004, 5: 50–53, 58–64.

Yang HQ. *World Economic Outlook: Insights for China from the reforms of the social security systems among EU countries*. Washington, DC: International Monetary Fund (IMF), 1999.

Yang HS. *Healthcare in the United States of America*. Hefei: University of Science and Technology of China Press, 2002.

Yang HY. A brief discussion on the helath insurance system in France. *Études Françaises*, 2006(4): 80–82.

Yang JR, Zu ZY. An analysis on the underlying causes of the income gap among Chinese farmers in the 1990s. *Journal of Sichuan University: Philosophy and Social Science*, 2001(4): 5–13.

Yang SF. Healthcare reforms in Egypt and the difficulties of democratization. *Chinese Rural Health Service Administration*, 2013, 33(2): 151–153.

Yang SH. The healthcare miracle of Cuba. *Information China (e-Healthcare)*, 2013, 3: 24–25.

Yang SJ, Wang SL. The construction of Cuba's public healthcare system and its insights for China. *China Pharmaceuticals*, 2009, 18(14): 3–5.

Yang WP, Yang SG. A comparative study of social security reforms among the UK, USA and Japan. *Theory and Practice of Finance and Economics*, 2005, 26(5): 32–35.

Yao JH. The health insurance system in Australia. *Chinese Health Economics*, 2006, 6(25): 49–50.

Yao SM, Yao JR. The rise of the BRICS countries and their development prospects. *Macroeconomic Management*, 2012, 28(8): 84–86.

Ye P, Yang B, Wang KY, et al. Overview of the training and utilization of general practitioners in some developed countries. *Journal of Military Surgeons in Southwest China*, 2007, 9(2): 112–113.

Yi YN. A comparative study on the management systems of social health insurance in foreign countries. *Chinese Health Economics*, 1995, 14(2): 17–19.

Yi YN. A comparative study on the payment methods of health insurance in foreign countries. *Comparative Study of Foreign Health Insurance*, 1994, 9.

Yi YN. Adjustment and changes in the health economic policies of Western developed countries. *Chinese Health Economics*, 1996, 7: 8.

Yi YN. Characteristics of health economic policies in countries with market economies and its insights for China. *Health Economics Research*, 1996(7): 19–21.

Yiengprugsawan V, Kelly M, Seubsman SA, et al. The first 10 years of the Universal Coverage Scheme in Thailand: review of its impact on health inequalities and lessons learnt for middle-income countries. *Australasian Epidemiologist*, 2010, 17(3): 24–26.

Yin RX, Hu DY. Reflections on the achievements of the Cuban healthcare system – valuable lessons for China. *Chinese Journal of Medicinal Guide*, 2008, 6: 807–809.

Ying XH, Xu K, Hu SL, et al. A model for the medical assistance of the urban poor. *Chinese Health Resources*, 1999, 2(1): 26–28.

Yip W, Hsiao W. China's health care reform: a tentative assessment. *China Economic Review*, 2009, 20(4): 613–619.

Yoder RA. Are people willing and able to pay for health services? *Social Science & Medicine*, 1989, 29(1): 35–42.

Yong SH. An analysis on the performance of the universal health insurance system in Taiwan. *Economic Research Guide*, 2009, 2: 192–193.

You CM, Feng YM. Overview of health system reforms in the Czech Republic. *Chinese Journal of Social Medicine*, 2009, 26(2): 85–86.

You JF, Bian W. Reform issues of the health insurance system in Japan. *Foreign Medicine (Health Economics)*, 1998, 15(3).

Yu GJ, Ma Q. Health system in transition – Poland. *Chinese Health Resources*, 2007, 10(3): 153–156.

Yu GJ. Construction of regional medical associations. *Chinese Health Insurance*, 2009, 4: 33–35.

Yu J. Constructing a harmonious socialist society based on the orientation of social policies – a discussion from the perspective of the equity theory of organizational behavior. *Mao Zedong Thought Study*, 2007, 6: 109–111.

Yu JF, Zhang SY. The institutionalist paradigm of economic development theory and its comparison. *Economic Review*, 2012, 9: 14–18.

Yu LW, Xu WG. An analysis on the implementation path of the corporate governance structure in regional medical associations. *Chinese Hospitals*, 2010, 14(12): 35–37.

Yu QQ. International practice and insights in the cost containment of medical assistance. *Chinese Health Economics*, 2008, 27(12): 13–15.

Yu W. *Dynamics of international social security – construction of a universal health security system.* Shanghai: Shanghai People's Publishing House, 2013.

Yuan BB. Universal health coverage: a global movement requiring support by research evidence. *Chinese Journal of Health Policy*, 2014, 7(2): 5–10.

Yuan F, Mei Z. Dialectical thinking on the bottom-line theory of equality. *Theoretical Front in Higher Education*, 2010, 2: 44–48.

Yue GZ, Pan H. International comparison of operation models for managed healthcare and its policy insights. *China Economist*, 2005, 12: 11–12.

Yuen PP. The corporatization of public hospital services in Hong Kong: a possible public choice explanation. *Asian Journal of Public Administration*, 2014, 16(2): 165–181.

Zeng XY. A summary of studies on government failures in health security among foreign countries. *Development Studies*, 2009, 1: 54–57.

Zhan GB, Wang YH. Insights for China from the NHS reforms in the UK. *Nanjing Social Medicine*, 2010, 9: 36–42.

Zhang BR, Wang XG. An analysis on the recent changes and trends in the economic development theory and policies of North Korea. *Northeast Asia Forum*, 2004, 13(3): 49–54.

Zhang DC. Five development strategies of the Hong Kong Hospital Authority. *Chinese Hospital Management*, 1997, 17(7): 23–25.

Zhang DW. Basic experiences and insights from the healthcare work in Cuba. *Journal of the Party University of Shijiazhuang City Committee of CPC*, 2011, 9: 29–32.

Zhang GH, Tong FF. Analysis of contract economics in reforms of the health insurance system. *Journal of Jiangxi University of Finance and Economics*, 2006, 2: 23–26.

Zhang KL. Rural healthcare system in Thailand and its implications. *Socialism Studies*, 2010(3): 112–116.

Zhang KT. *Policy research on community services of population aging.* National Policy Research Report on Aging. China: The National Working Commission on Aging, 1999.

Zhang LF. The health insurance system in Japan and its reform measures. *Japanese Studies,* 2003, 1: 42–45.

Zhang Q. Reflections on the current status of the American health insurance system. *Chinese Health Economics,* 2007, 26(6): 79–80.

Zhang Q. *Theory, system and operation of health security in China.* Beijing: China Labor and Social Security Press, 2002.

Zhang QL. Healthcare costs and its containment in the United States of America. *Journal of World Economy,* 2002, 6: 53–59.

Zhang RR. The most important secret of health performance in France. *Outlook,* 2010, 35: 30–31.

Zhang W. Recent status of drug administration in Taiwan and progress in the separation of prescribing and dispensing. *Capital Medicine,* 2000, 7(3): 4–6.

Zhang WY. Different challenges faced by the hospitals of three BRICS countries. *China Hospital CEO,* 2010, 6(4): 26–27.

Zhang WZ. On Egypt's economic reform. *West Asia and Africa,* 1993, 3: 44.

Zhang X, Hattori S, Nghia BT. Technical assistance to the socialist republic of Vietnam for developing the social security system. Working paper of Asian Development Bank. https://www.adb.org/documents/tam/vie/tamvie34357.pdf.

Zhang XT, Fang HJ. On the development of China's non-profit private health insurance system. *Insurance Studies,* 2009, 8: 39–44.

Zhang XT. Current status and lessons of health insurance system in the United States of America. *Foreign Medicine (Health Economics),* 2002, 19(3): 98–101.

Zhang Y. The Marxist theory of equality and the principle of equality in the socialist market economy. *Teaching and Research,* 2006, 2: 19–25.

Zhang YF, Feng XS. Research and development on health system performance. *Medicine and Society,* 2013, 26(10): 35–38.

Zhang YH, Guo F, Wang Q, et al. Measurement results and analysis of China's total healthcare expenditure in 2010. *Chinese Health Economics,* 2012, 31(4): 5–11.

Zhang YJ. The past and present of the health insurance plan in Vietnam. *Chinese Health Insurance,* 2011, 2: 64–66.

Zhang YX. The Marxist theory of social equality and the issues of equality in contemporary Chinese society. *Social Sciences in Yunnan,* 2010, 6: 19–23.

Zhang YZ. Comment on the reforms of the social security system in Russia. *Central Asian and East European Market Research,* 2002, 6: 13–20.

Zhang ZY, Sun L. Definition and measurement framework for universal health coverage. *Chinese Journal of Health Policy,* 2014, 7(1): 19–22.

Zhang ZY. The relationship of market failure in the healthcare domain with government intervention. *Journal of Chifeng College (Natural Science Edition),* 2010, 26(8): 56–60.

Zhao B, Yan C. Health security system in Singapore. *Southeast Asian and South Asian Studies,* 2009, 4: 48–52.

Zhao FC, Li CW. Health insurance and medical assistance systems in foreign countries, its methods of convergence and insights for China. *Review of Economic Research,* 2011, 46: 52–60.

Zhao L. A legal study on drug patent protection under the TRIPS agreement. Master's Thesis. Dalian: Dalian Maritime University, 2008.

Zhao M. *An analysis on social security theory and institutional reform.* Beijing: China Financial and Economic Publishing House, 1999.

Zhao R. Social healthcare system in Cuba. *Global Science, Technology and Economic Outlook,* 2003, 6: 59.

Zhao XP. Lessons from the universal health insurance system in Taiwan. *Chinese Health Insurance,* 2011, 7: 68–70.

Zhao YJ, Wang LS. Comparative analysis on the health insurance systems of China, USA and Thailand. *Chinese Health Economics,* 2009, 11: 41–44.

Zhao YS, Yang J. Insurance for workers – development and reform of the Employees' Health Insurance in Japan. *Chinese Health Insurance*, 2009, 4: 65–68.

Zhao YS. Characteristics of health security in Japan and its lessons for China. *Chinese Health Insurance*, 2010(1): 60–63.

Zhao YS. Japan's health security system and a comparison between China and Japan, special column (1). Insurance for all citizens – an overview of the health security system in modern Japan. *Chinese Health Insurance*, 2009(2): 62–64.

Zhao YS. Japan's health security system and a comparison between China and Japan, special column (3). Coordinating urban and rural universal health insurance system – development and current status of Japan's national health insurance. *Chinese Health Insurance*, 2009, 4: 65–68.

Zhao YS. Japan's health security system and a comparison between China and Japan, special column (4). Coping with population aging – reforms in Japan's health security system for the elderly. *Chinese Health Insurance*, 2009(5): 65–68.

Zhao YS. Japan's health security system and a comparison between China and Japan, special column (5). The last line of defense in national health – development and current status of Japan's medical assistance system. *Chinese Health Insurance*, 2009(6): 64–67.

Zhao YS. Japan's health security system and a comparison between China and Japan, special column (6). Japan's development of community health services and creation of long-term care insurance. *Chinese Health Insurance*, 2009(7): 63–66.

Zhao YS. Japan's health security system and a comparison between China and Japan, special column (9). Development and current status of Japan's healthcare delivery system. *Chinese Health Insurance*, 2009(10): 60–63.

Zhao YS. Japan's health security system and a comparison between China and Japan, special column (10). Development and reform of Japan's health insurance laws. *Chinese Health Insurance*, 2009(11): 64–67.

Zheng BW. Information asymmetry and health insurance. *Comparative Economic & Social Systems*, 2002(6): 8–15.

Zheng Y, Yang ZH. Theoretical analysis on the correlation of social security and social equality. *Taxation and Economy*, 2011, 4: 51–55.

Zhou GS, Pan XL, Li KL. An exploration on the basis for the performance evaluation of physicians' workload. *Hospital Management Forum*, 2008, 25(12): 20.

Zhou HY. Insights from the US Medical School Rural Track for medical education in China. *China Higher Medical Education*, 2011, 2: 114–115.

Zhou JY. Improving the utilization efficiency of healthcare resources – exploring the construction of regional medical associations in Shanghai. *Hospital Directors' Forum*, 2009, 6(6): 12–15.

Zhou L, Ren R, Wang WJ. Reform of the health security system in Mexico and its lessons for China. *Medicine and Philosophy: Humanities and Social Science Edition*, 2007, 28(10): 4–6.

Zhou SD. A study on Marxist theory of economic development centered on labor and division of labor. *Socialism Studies*, 2013, 1: 8–14.

Zhou SQ. *Policies and ideas – a discussion on reform of urban health security system.* Guizhou: Guizhou People's Publishing House, 2002.

Zhou Y. Characteristics and reform practices of the payment system in Canadian health insurance. *Chinese Health Resources*, 2005, 8(4): 185–187.

Zhou YB. *Capitation and multi-tiered security – characteristics of health insurance in Thailand.* China Social Insurance, 1999, 12: 34.

Zhu J. Changes in the Chinese health security system: Path dependence and transcendence. Master's Thesis. Beijing: Capital University of Economics and Business, 2010.

Zhu K, Xie Y, Li CQ, et al. Experiences and insights from the management system of the community health service in the UK. *Chinese Primary Health Care*, 2010, 24(6): 19–21.

Zhu K, Xie Y, You CM, et al. Public-private partnerships of healthcare in South Africa and its implications. *Chinese Journal of Health Policy*, 2009, 2(6): 57–60.

Zhu XQ, Liu XQ. Overview of implementing the health insurance system in Vietnam. *Foreign Medicine (Health Economics)*, 1995, 04: 148–152.

Zhu Y, Sun XM, Liang H. Evaluation of practices in the medical assistance policies for the poor in Shanghai. *Journal of Community Health Care*, 2002, 3(3): 158–161.

Zhu YH. Introduction to the point-based global budget system in the universal health insurance of Taiwan. *Progress in Health Policy Research*, 2012, 2.

Zhu ZG. An economic analysis in the reforms of the rural health insurance system. *Health Economics Research*, 2010, 3: 13–16.

Zollner D, Kohler PA, Zacher KF (eds.). *The evolution of social insurance 1881–1981*. London: Francis Printer, 1982.

Zong XB. What are the procedures for the selection of the drug list in the UK? *Chinese Health Insurance*, 2010(8): 62.

Zou FL. Establishing health insurance fee standards based on disease classification and grading – insights from the health insurance accounting and payment methods in Australia. *Medicine and Society*, 2002, 15(6): 21–22.

Zou GB, Hao Q. Comparison of reforms in the social security systems of several developed countries. *World Economic Papers*, 2002, 2: 50–56.

Zou LZ, Jiang Q. The healthcare market and the operating mechanisms of the market economy. *Chinese Health Economics*, 1996, 5: 13–15.

Index